The Shoulder

£135   WE 810 ROC

£135   WE 810 ROC

The Shoulder

FOURTH EDITION
VOLUME ONE

EDITORS

Charles A. Rockwood, Jr, MD
Professor and Chairman Emeritus
Department of Orthopaedics
The University of Texas Health Science Center
at San Antonio
San Antonio, Texas

Michael A. Wirth, MD
Professor and Charles A. Rockwood Jr, MD Chair
Department of Orthopaedics
The University of Texas Health Science Center
at San Antonio
San Antonio, Texas

Fredrick A. Matsen, III, MD
Professor and Chairman
Department of Orthopaedics and Sports Medicine
University of Washington School of Medicine
Medical Director
University of Washington Sports Medicine
Seattle, Washington

Steven B. Lippitt, MD
Professor
Department of Orthopaedics
Northeastern Ohio Universities College of Medicine
Northeast Ohio Orthopaedic Associates
Akron General Medical Center
Akron, Ohio

Associate Editors

Edward V. Fehringer, MD
Associate Professor
Department of Orthopaedic Surgery and Rehabilitation
University of Nebraska College of Medicine
Omaha, Nebraska

John W. Sperling, MD, MBA
Professor
Department of Orthopedic Surgery
Mayo Clinic
Rochester, Minnesota

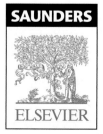

SAUNDERS

ELSEVIER

SAUNDERS
ELSEVIER

1600 John F. Kennedy Boulevard
Suite 1800
Philadelphia, PA 19103-2899

THE SHOULDER
ISBN: 978-1-4160-3427-8

Notice

Knowledge and best practice in this field are constantly changing. As new research and experience broaden our knowledge, changes in practice, treatment, and drug therapy may become necessary or appropriate. Readers are advised to check the most current information provided (i) on procedures featured or (ii) by the manufacturer of each product to be administered, to verify the recommended dose or formula, the method and duration of administration, and contraindications. It is the responsibility of the practitioner, relying on his or her own experience and knowledge of the patient, to make diagnoses, to determine dosages and the best treatment for each individual patient, and to take all appropriate safety precautions. To the fullest extent of the law, neither the Publisher nor the Editors assumes any liability for any injury and/or damage to persons or property arising out of or related to any use of the material contained in this book.

The Publisher

Library of Congress Cataloging-in-Publication Data
The shoulder / [edited by] Charles A. Rockwood Jr. . . . [et al.] ; associate editors, Edward V. Fehringer, John W. Sperling.—4th ed.
    p. ; cm.
    Includes bibliographical references and index.
    ISBN 978-1-4160-3427-8
 1. Shoulder—Diseases. 2. Shoulder—Surgery. I. Rockwood, Charles A.
    [DNLM: 1. Shoulder. 2. Shoulder Joint. WE 810 S55861 2009]
    RC939.S484 2009
    617.5′72—dc22   2008029883

Acquisitions Editor: Daniel Pepper
Developmental Editor: Agnes Hunt Byrne
Publishing Services Manager: Tina Rebane
Senior Project Manager: Amy L. Cannon
Multimedia Producer: Bruce Robison
Design Director: Gene Harris

Printed in China

Last digit is the print number: 9 8 7 6 5 4 3 2 1

Dedication

We dedicate these volumes first to our families, who have given us their fullest support and encouragement during our careers as shoulder surgeons. Without their constant love, we would have accomplished little. We next dedicate our work to the thousands of individuals who have consulted us regarding their shoulder problems with the hope that our efforts would enable them to regain comfort and function. Without their confidence in our efforts, we would have been unable to develop the knowledge of what works best and when.

Finally, we dedicate this book to all those who are captivated by the shoulder and who continue to pursue greater insights into its function, its malfunction, and the effective treatment of its clinical disorders. Without bright new minds applied to the many challenges presented by this complex and fascinating joint, our field would not be better tomorrow than it is today.

CAR
FAM
MAW
SBL
EVF
JWS

Foreword *to the Fourth Edition*

I am grateful for the opportunity to offer this Foreword for the fourth edition of this unique text on the shoulder—with an emphasis on the role of surgical treatment.

In the 1980s, when the first edition of *The Shoulder* was conceived, there was a tremendous need for the collection and organization of the information and wisdom that had been developed to date about the care of shoulder injuries and diseases. Ideas were changing rapidly, and technology was advancing at a fast pace.

There was an expanded understanding of the classification of fractures of the proximal humerus, and there were emerging improvements in fixation methods. The impingement syndrome was being embraced, and there was dramatically increased success with repair of torn rotator cuff tendons. Total joint arthroplasty had proven itself in the hip and the knee; there was a question about whether this would translate effectively to the shoulder. The biomechanics of shoulder instability were being developed, and the applications of these basic concepts to clinical treatment were emerging. The arthroscope was being applied effectively to the evaluation and care of rather simple knee problems, and there was a tremendous opportunity to develop and mature effective applications of this tool for the shoulder. As easily recognized, there was a steaming cauldron, if you will, of new knowledge demanding an organized expression, and that demand was answered by this text.

The basic idea to fully collect the information, to organize it, and to express it in a readable way was the genesis of *The Shoulder*. During the subsequent decades, the information available about the shoulder through courses, journals (particularly international journals), and other more focused textbooks has literally exploded.

It is a wish fulfilled that these editors, with the contributions of many insightful authors, have carried on with the initial concept, expanding and reorganizing materials in light of this new knowledge. We readers expect a careful display of surgical anatomy and biomechanics, new information about clinical evaluation and imaging, a rethinking of the directions for care of fractures about the shoulder, a large section on the application of arthroscopy to the evaluation and care of shoulder problems, the introduction of new ideas about the care of rotator cuff–related problems, carefully organized presentations on basic concepts that can be applied to the understanding of shoulder instability, and many, many other lesser, but not unimportant, subjects, that all of us encounter in the evaluation and treatment of patients. This text delivers on the materials just listed and contains supporting chapters extensively referenced so that the readers can easily access the information codified by the authors.

We must be very thankful to these gifted educators who have chaired innumerable continuing medical education courses, who have developed fellowships, who actively participate in clinical and basic research on the shoulder, and who have been involved with other texts for sticking with their original idea and actively pursuing the incorporation of new materials. Readers can count on this as a reliable source, a database if you will, against which other ideas can be compared. Readers not only will know where we stand on current issues after reading this text but also will be able to understand how we arrived at current thinking and treatment of a large variety of subjects in this anatomic region.

ROBERT H. COFIELD, MD
Caywood Professor of Orthopedics
Mayo Clinic College of Medicine
Mayo Clinic
Rochester, Minnesota
October 2008

Foreword *to the Third Edition*

Publishing companies do not re-issue books that are inaccurate, unused, or unpopular. So, there is a good reason to be excited about the third edition of *The Shoulder*, edited by Drs. Rockwood, Matsen, Wirth, and Lippitt. Not too long ago, as history is measured, we considered ourselves to be in the early stages of learning about the shoulder joint—its functional anatomy, its injury patterns, and, very importantly, its optimal treatment.

Since the first edition of this book, our technical capabilities in imaging, instrumentation, and pain control have improved tremendously. Chapters dealing with these aspects of shoulder care reflect this heightened scrutiny. Continuing interest in and understanding of both developmental and functional anatomy allow us to comprehend the biomechanics of not only the pathologic shoulder but also the normal shoulder. Without a clear picture of normal shoulder function, our devising and refinement of correctional procedures would lack a clear direction.

The editors have succeeded in assembling a panel of chapter authors with acknowledged skills in shoulder diagnosis and management. Perhaps more importantly, the contributing authors also demonstrate a commitment to the pursuit of better understanding and more effective treatments, rather than just relying on traditional methods. And, even more importantly, these authors are also discriminating about incorporating some of these newer techniques that may represent a triumph of technology over reason.

Finally, some of you know, and most of you can imagine, how much work it is to write and assemble a quality text such as this. It is our considerable good fortune to have these editors at the forefront of our profession, willing and able to undertake this arduous task, and producing a work of such outstanding breadth and quality.

FRANK W. JOBE, MD
Kerlan-Jobe Orthopaedic Clinic
Centinela Hospital Medical Center
Inglewood, California
January 2004

Foreword *to the First Edition*

It is a privilege to write the Foreword for *The Shoulder* by Drs. Charles A. Rockwood, Jr, and Frederick A. Matsen, III. Their objective when they began this work was an all-inclusive text on the shoulder that would also include all references on the subject in the English literature. Forty-six authors have contributed to this text.

The editors of *The Shoulder* are two of the leading shoulder surgeons in the United States. Dr. Rockwood was the fourth President of the American Shoulder and Elbow Surgeons, has organized the Instructional Course Lectures on the Shoulder for the Annual Meeting of the American Academy of Orthopaedic Surgeons for many years, and is a most experienced and dedicated teacher. Dr. Matsen is President-Elect of the American Shoulder and Elbow Surgeons and is an unusually talented teacher and leader. These two men, with their academic knowhow and the help of their contributing authors, have organized a monumental text for surgeons in training and in practice, as well as one that can serve as an extensive reference source. They are to be commended for this superior book.

CHARLES S. NEER, II, MD
Professor Emeritus, Orthopaedic Surgery
Columbia University
Chief, Shoulder Service
Columbia-Presbyterian Medical Center
New York, New York

Preface

Dear Readers,

Thank you for sharing our interest in the body's most fascinating joint: the shoulder. Where else could you be so challenged by complex anatomy, a vast spectrum of functional demands, and diverse clinical problems ranging from congenital disorders to fractures, arthritis, instability, stiffness, tendon disorders, and tumors?

The two of us (CAR and FAM) have been partners in the shoulder for more than 25 years. Although we have never practiced together, it became evident early on that the San Antonio and Seattle schools of thought were more often congruent than divergent—whether the topic was the rotator cuff, instability, or glenohumeral arthritis. We even agree that all rotator cuff tears cannot be and should not be attempted to be repaired!

But our story is not the only story. In these volumes we pay great respect to those with new, contrasting, or even divergent ideas, be they in other parts of the United States or abroad. We are most grateful to the chapter authors new to this fourth edition who have done much to enhance the value and completeness of *The Shoulder*.

As health care becomes one of the costliest expenses for the people of our country and others, we must now consider not only whether diagnostic tools are accurate and therapeutic methods are effective but also the appropriateness of their use and their value to individual patients (i.e., benefit of the method divided by the cost). We will be the best stewards of health care resources if we can learn to avoid ordering tests that do not change our treatment and avoid using therapies that are not cost-effective. This may be, in fact, our greatest challenge.

How can we learn what works best across the spectrum of orthopaedic practice when our knowledge is based on the relatively small and probably nonrepresentative sample of cases published in our journals? We are surely a long way away from fulfilling Codman's "common sense notion that every hospital should follow every patient it treats, long enough to determine whether or not the treatment has been successful, and then to inquire, 'If not, why not?' with a view to preventing similar failures in the future."

In preparing this the fourth edition of *The Shoulder*, we have been joined again by editors Michael A. Wirth and Steven B. Lippitt. New to this edition are associate editors Edward V. Fehringer and John W. Sperling. All are outstanding (and younger) shoulder surgeons who have helped us immeasurably in our attempts to expand the horizon of the book while still honing in on the methods preferred by the authors selected for each of the chapters.

We encourage you to be aggressive in your pursuit of new shoulder knowledge, critical of what you hear and read, and conservative in your adoption of the many new approaches being proposed for the evaluation and management of the shoulder. We hope this book gives you a basis for considering what might be in the best interest of your patients. We hope you enjoy reading this book as much as we enjoyed putting it together.

Best wishes to each of you—happy shouldering!

CHARLES A. ROCKWOOD, JR, MD
FREDERICK A. MATSEN, III, MD
MICHAEL A. WIRTH, MD
STEVEN B. LIPPITT, MD
October 2008

Contributors

Christopher S. Ahmad, MD
Associate Professor of Orthopaedic Surgery, Center for Shoulder, Elbow and Sports Medicine, Columbia University; Attending, Columbia University Medical Center, New York, New York
The Shoulder in Athletes

Answorth A. Allen, MD
Associate Attending Orthopaedic Surgeon, Hospital for Special Surgery; Associate Professor, Clinical Orthopaedic Surgery, Weill Medical College of Cornell University, New York, New York
Shoulder Arthroscopy: Arthroscopic Management of Rotator Cuff Disease

David W. Altchek, MD
Attending Orthopaedic Surgeon, Sports Medicine and Shoulder Service, Hospital for Special Surgery, New York, New York
Shoulder Arthroscopy: Thrower's Shoulder

Laurie B. Amundsen, MD
Assistant Professor, Department of Anesthesiology, University of Washington Medical Center, Seattle, Washington
Anesthesia for Shoulder Procedures

Kai-Nan An, PhD
Professor and Chair, Division of Orthopedic Research, Mayo Clinic, Rochester, Minnesota
Biomechanics of the Shoulder

Ludwig Anné, MD
Former Fellow, Alps Surgery Institute, Annecy, France
Advanced Shoulder Arthroscopy

Carl J. Basamania, MD
Orthopaedic Surgeon, Triangle Orthopaedic Associates, Durham, North Carolina
Fractures of the Clavicle

Alexander Bertlesen, PAC
Certified Physician Assistant, Department of Orthopaedics and Sports Medicine, University of Washington, Seattle, Washington
Glenohumeral Instability

Kamal I. Bohsali, MD
Attending Orthopedic Surgeon, Shoulder and Elbow Reconstruction, Memorial Hospital; Staff, Orthopedics, St. Luke's Hospital; Private Practice, Bahri Orthopedics and Sports Medicine, Jacksonville, Florida
Fractures of the Proximal Humerus

John J. Brems, MD
Shoulder Fellowship Director, Cleveland Clinic Foundation, Euclid Orthopaedics, Cleveland, Ohio
Clinical Evaluation of Shoulder Problems

Stephen F. Brockmeier, MD
Surgeon, Perry Orthopedics and Sports Medicine, Charlotte, North Carolina
Shoulder Arthroscopy: Arthroscopic Management of Rotator Cuff Disease; Shoulder Arthroscopy: Thrower's Shoulder

Robert H. Brophy, MD
Assistant Professor, Orthopaedic Surgery, Washington University School of Medicine, St. Louis, Missouri
Shoulder Arthroscopy: Acromioclavicular Joint Arthritis and Instability

Barrett S. Brown, MD
Surgeon, Fondren Orthopedic Group, Houston, Texas
Shoulder Arthroscopy: Biceps in Shoulder Arthroscopy; Shoulder Arthroscopy: Thrower's Shoulder

Ernest M. Burgess, MD†
Former Clinical Professor, Department of Orthopaedics, University of Washington; Endowed Chair of Orthopaedic Research, University of Washington School of Medicine; Senior Scientist, Prosthetics Research Study, Seattle, Washington
Amputations and Prosthetic Replacement

Wayne Z. Burkhead, Jr, MD
Clinical Professor, Department of Orthopaedic Surgery, University of Texas Southwestern Medical School; Attending Physician, W. B. Carrell Memorial Clinic; Attending Physician, Baylor University Medical Center; Attending Physician, Presbyterian Hospital of Dallas, Dallas, Texas
The Biceps Tendon

Gilbert Chan, MD
Visiting Research Fellow, Clinical Research, Joseph Stokes Jr Research Institute, Children's Hospital of Philadelphia, Philadelphia, Pennsylvania
Fractures, Dislocations, and Acquired Problems of the Shoulder in Children

Paul D. Choi, MD
Assistant Clinical Professor of Orthopaedic Surgery, Keck School of Medicine, University of Southern California, Los Angeles, California
Fractures, Dislocations, and Acquired Problems of the Shoulder in Children

Jeremiah Clinton, MD
Acting Clinical Instructor, Department of Orthopaedics and Sports Medicine, University of Washington, Seattle, Washington
Glenohumeral Arthritis and Its Management

Michael Codsi, MD
Staff Surgeon, Department of Orthopedic Surgery, Everett Clinic, Everett, Washington
Clinical Evaluation of Shoulder Problems

Michael J. Coen, MD
Assistant Professor, Department of Orthopaedic Surgery, Loma Linda University School of Medicine, Loma Linda University Medical Center, Loma Linda, California
Gross Anatomy of the Shoulder

†*Deceased*

Robert H. Cofield, MD
Professor, Department of Orthopedics,
Mayo Clinic College of Medicine;
Consultant, Department of Orthopedic
Surgery, Mayo Clinic, Rochester, Minnesota
*Management of the Infected Shoulder
Arthroplasty*

David N. Collins, MD
Surgeon, Adult Reconstruction and
Shoulder, Arkansas Specialty Orthopaedics,
Little Rock, Arkansas
Disorders of the Acromioclavicular Joint

Ernest U. Conrad, III, MD
Professor of Orthopaedics, University of
Washington School of Medicine; Director
of Sarcoma Service, Director of Division of
Orthopaedics, and Director of Bone Tumor
Clinic, Children's Hospital, University of
Washington, Children's Hospital and
Medical Center, Seattle, Washington
Tumors and Related Conditions

Frank A. Cordasco, MD, MS
Associate Attending Orthopaedic Surgeon,
Sports Medicine and Shoulder Service,
Hospital for Special Surgery; Associate
Professor of Orthopaedic Surgery, Weill
Medical College of Cornell University,
New York, New York
*Shoulder Arthroscopy: Acromioclavicular
Joint Arthritis and Instability*

Edward Craig, MD, MPH
Attending Orthopaedic Surgeon, Sports
Medicine and Shoulder Service, Hospital
for Special Surgery; Professor of Clinical
Surgery, Weill Medical College of Cornell
University, New York, New York
*Shoulder Arthroscopy: Arthroscopic
Management of Arthritic and Prearthritic
Conditions of the Shoulder*

Jeffrey Davila, MD
Former Fellow, Hospital for Special
Surgery, New York, New York
Shoulder Arthroscopy: SLAP Tears

Anthony F. DePalma, MD†
Former Chairman, Orthopaedic Surgery,
Thomas Jefferson University Hospital,
Philadelphia, Pennsylvania
*Congenital Anomalies and Variational
Anatomy of the Shoulder*

David M. Dines, MD
Professor of Orthopaedic Surgery, Weill
Medical College of Cornell University;
Assistant Attending, Orthopaedic Surgery,
Hospital for Special Surgery, New York;
Chairman and Professor of Orthopaedic
Surgery, Albert Einstein College of
Medicine at Long Island Jewish Medical
Center, New Hyde Park, New York
*Evaluation and Management of Failed
Rotator Cuff Surgery*

Joshua S. Dines, MD
Clinical Instructor of Orthopaedic Surgery,
Weill Medical College of Cornell
University; Assistant Attending, Sports
Medicine and Shoulder Service, Hospital
for Special Surgery, New York, New York
*Evaluation and Management of Failed
Rotator Cuff Surgery*

Mark C. Drakos, MD
Resident, Department of Orthopaedic
Surgery, Hospital for Special Surgery,
New York, New York
*Developmental Anatomy of the Shoulder
and Anatomy of the Glenohumeral Joint;
Shoulder Arthroscopy: Biceps in Shoulder
Arthroscopy*

Anders Ekelund, MD, PhD
Associate Professor, Department of
Orthopaedic Surgery, Capio St. Görans
Hospital, Stockholm, Sweden
*Advanced Evaluation and Management
of Glenohumeral Arthritis in the Cuff-
Deficient Shoulder*

Neal S. ElAttrache, MD
Associate Clinical Professor, Department
of Orthopaedic Surgery, University of
Southern California School of Medicine;
Associate, Kerlan-Jobe Orthopaedic Clinic,
Los Angeles, California
The Shoulder in Athletes

Bassem ElHassan, MD
Assistant Professor of Orthopedics,
Mayo Clinic, Rochester, Minnesota
The Stiff Shoulder

Nathan K. Endres, MD
Fellow, Harvard Shoulder Service,
Massachusetts General Hospital, Brigham
and Women's Hospital, Boston,
Massachusetts
The Stiff Shoulder

Stephen Fealy, MD
Assistant Attending Orthopaedic Surgeon,
Hospital for Special Surgery; Assistant
Professor of Orthopaedic Surgery, Weill
Medical College of Cornell University,
New York, New York
*Shoulder Arthroscopy: Acromioclavicular
Joint Arthritis and Instability*

Edward V. Fehringer, MD
Associate Professor, Department of
Orthopaedic Surgery and Rehabilitation,
University of Nebraska College of
Medicine, Omaha, Nebraska
Rotator Cuff

John M. Fenlin, Jr, MD
Director, Shoulder and Elbow Service,
Rothman Institute; Clinical Professor of
Orthopaedic Surgery, Thomas Jefferson
University, Philadelphia, Pennsylvania
*Congenital Anomalies and Variational
Anatomy of the Shoulder*

John M. (Jack) Flynn, MD
Associate Chief of Orthopaedic Surgery,
Children's Hospital of Philadelphia;
Associate Professor of Orthopaedic
Surgery, University of Pennsylvania School
of Medicine, Philadelphia, Pennsylvania
*Fractures, Dislocations, and Acquired
Problems of the Shoulder in Children*

Leesa M. Galatz, MD
Associate Professor, Orthopaedic Surgery,
Washington University School of Medicine,
St. Louis, Missouri
Complications of Shoulder Arthroscopy

Seth C. Gamradt, MD
Assistant Professor of Orthopaedic Surgery,
David Geffen School of Medicine at
University of California Los Angeles,
Los Angeles, California
*Shoulder Arthroscopy: Arthroscopic
Treatment of Shoulder Instability*

Charles L. Getz, MD
Clinical Instructor, Orthopaedic Surgery,
Rothman Institute, Philadelphia,
Pennsylvania
*Congenital Anomalies and Variational
Anatomy of the Shoulder*

Guillem Gonzalez-Lomas, MD
House Staff, Physician/Surgeon Residency,
Columbia University, New York,
New York
The Shoulder in Athletes

†*Deceased*

Thomas P. Goss, MD
Professor of Orthopaedic Surgery,
Department of Orthopaedics, University of
Massachusetts Medical School; Attending
Orthopaedic Surgeon and Chief of
Shoulder Surgery, University of
Massachusetts Memorial Health Care,
Worcester, Massachusetts
Fractures of the Scapula

Manuel Haag, MD
Former Fellow, Alps Surgery Institute,
Annecy, France
Advanced Shoulder Arthroscopy

Peter Habermayer, MD
Professor, ATOS Praxisklinik, Heidelberg,
Germany
The Biceps Tendon

Manny Halpern, PhD
Assistant Research Professor, New York
University School of Medicine; Certified
Professional Ergonomist, Occupational and
Industrial Orthopaedic Center, New York
University Hospital for Joint Diseases,
New York, New York
Occupational Shoulder Disorders

Jo A. Hannafin, MD, PhD
Attending Orthopaedic Surgeon and
Assistant Scientist, Hospital for Special
Surgery; Professor of Orthopaedic Surgery,
Weill Medical College of Cornell
University, New York, New York
*Shoulder Arthroscopy: Arthroscopic
Treatment of Shoulder Stiffness and
Calcific Tendinitis of the Rotator Cuff*

Laurence D. Higgins, MD
Chief, Sports Medicine, and Chief, Harvard
Shoulder Service, Department of
Orthopaedic Surgery, Brigham and
Women's Hospital, Boston, Massachusetts
The Stiff Shoulder

Jason L. Hurd, MD
Orthopedic Surgeon, Sanford Clinic
Vermillion, Vermillion, South Dakota
Occupational Shoulder Disorders

Joseph P. Iannotti, MD, PhD
Maynard Madden Professor and Chairman,
Orthopaedic and Rheumatologic Institute,
Cleveland Clinic, Cleveland, Ohio
*Emerging Technologies in Shoulder
Surgery: Trends and Future Directions*

Eiji Itoi, MD, PhD
Professor and Chair, Department of
Orthopaedic Surgery, Tohoku University
School of Medicine; Director, Department
of Orthopaedic Surgery, Tohoku University
Hospital, Sendai, Japan; Professor of
Bioengineering, Mayo Medical School and
Director, Biomechanics Laboratory,
Division of Orthopedic Research, Mayo
Clinic, Rochester, Minnesota
Biomechanics of the Shoulder

Kirk L. Jensen, MD
Director, East Bay Shoulder, Orinda,
California
*Radiographic Evaluation of Shoulder
Problems*

Christopher M. Jobe, MD
Professor and Chair, Department of
Orthopaedic Surgery, Loma Linda
University School of Medicine, Loma Linda
Medical Center; Consulting Staff, Jerry L.
Pettis Memorial Veterans Administration
Hospital, Loma Linda, California
Gross Anatomy of the Shoulder

Anne M. Kelly, MD
Assistant Attending Orthopaedic Surgeon,
Hospital for Special Surgery, New York;
Attending Orthopaedic Surgeon, North
Shore University Hospital at Glen Cove,
Glen Cove, New York
*Shoulder Arthroscopy: Biceps in Shoulder
Arthroscopy*

Christopher D. Kent, MD
Assistant Professor, Department of
Anesthesiology, University of Washington
Medical Center, Seattle, Washington
Anesthesia for Shoulder Procedures

Laurent Lafosse, MD
Surgeon, Orthopedic and Sport
Traumatology, Clinique Générale
d'Annecy, Annecy, France
Advanced Shoulder Arthroscopy

Clayton Lane, MD
Surgeon, Alabama Orthopaedic Clinic,
Mobile, Alabama
*Shoulder Arthroscopy: Arthroscopic
Management of Arthritic and Prearthritic
Conditions of the Shoulder*

Peter Lapner, MD
Assistant Professor, University of Ottawa;
Orthopaedic Surgeon, The Ottawa
Hospital, Ottawa, Ontario, Canada
Calcifying Tendinitis

Kenneth Lin, MD
Orthopaedic Surgeon, Proliance Surgeons,
Monroe, Washington
The Biceps Tendon

Steven B. Lippitt, MD
Professor, Department of Orthopaedics,
Northeastern Ohio Universities College of
Medicine, Northeast Ohio Orthopaedic
Associates, Akron General Medical Center,
Akron, Ohio
*Glenohumeral Instability; Rotator Cuff;
Glenohumeral Arthritis and Its
Management*

Joachim F. Loehr, MD
Professor and Consultant Orthopaedic
Surgeon, Clinic Director, ENDO-Klinik,
Hamburg, Germany
Calcifying Tendinitis

John D. MacGillivray, MD
Assistant Attending Orthopaedic Surgeon,
Sports Medicine and Shoulder Service,
Hospital for Special Surgery; Assistant
Professor of Orthopaedic Surgery, Weill
Medical College of Cornell University,
New York, New York
*Shoulder Arthroscopy: Arthroscopic
Management of Rotator Cuff Disease*

Frederick A. Matsen, III, MD
Professor and Chairman, Department of
Orthopaedics and Sports Medicine,
University of Washington School of
Medicine; Medical Director, University of
Washington Sports Medicine, Seattle,
Washington
*Glenohumeral Instability; Rotator Cuff;
Glenohumeral Arthritis and Its
Management*

Jesse McCarron, MD
Staff Surgeon, Shoulder Section,
Department of Orthopaedic Surgery,
Cleveland Clinic Foundation, Cleveland,
Ohio
Clinical Evaluation of Shoulder Problems

Bernard F. Morrey, MD
Professor of Orthopedic Surgery, Mayo
Clinic, Rochester, Minnesota
Biomechanics of the Shoulder

Andrew S. Neviaser, MD
Resident, Department of Orthopaedics,
Hospital for Special Surgery, New York,
New York
*Developmental Anatomy of the Shoulder
and Anatomy of the Glenohumeral Joint*

Stephen J. O'Brien, MD, MBA
Associate Attending Orthopaedic Surgeon, Shoulder and Sports Medicine Service, Hospital for Special Surgery; Associate Attending Professor of Surgery, Orthopaedics, Weill Medical College of Cornell University; Assistant Scientist, New York–Presbyterian Hospital, New York, New York
Developmental Anatomy of the Shoulder and Anatomy of the Glenohumeral Joint; Shoulder Arthroscopy: Biceps in Shoulder Arthroscopy

Brett D. Owens, MD
Adjunct Assistant Professor, Department of Surgery, Uniformed Services University of Health Sciences, Bethesda, Maryland; Assistant Professor, Texas Tech University Health Science Center; Director, Sports Medicine and Shoulder Service, William Beaumont Army Medical Center, El Paso, Texas
Fractures of the Scapula

Wesley P. Phipatanakul, MD
Assistant Professor, Department of Orthopaedic Surgery, Loma Linda University School of Medicine, Loma Linda Medical Center, Loma Linda, California
Gross Anatomy of the Shoulder

Robin R. Richards, MD, FRCSC
Professor of Surgery, University of Toronto; Director, Upper Extremity Reconstructive Service, Head, Division of Orthopaedic Surgery, and Medical Director, Neuromusculoskeletal Program, St. Michael's Hospital; Surgeon-in-Chief, Sunnybrook Health Sciences Centre, Toronto, Ontario, Canada
Effectiveness Evaluation of the Shoulder; Sepsis of the Shoulder: Molecular Mechanisms and Pathogenesis

Charles A. Rockwood, Jr, MD
Professor and Chairman Emeritus, Department of Orthopaedics, The University of Texas Health Science Center at San Antonio, San Antonio, Texas
Radiographic Evaluation of Shoulder Problems; Fractures of the Clavicle; Disorders of the Sternoclavicular Joint; Glenohumeral Instability; Rotator Cuff; Glenohumeral Arthritis and Its Management

Scott A. Rodeo, MD
Associate Attending Orthopaedic Surgeon, Hospital for Special Surgery, New York, New York
Shoulder Arthroscopy: Arthroscopic Management of Rotator Cuff Disease

Robert L. Romano, MD
Former Clinical Professor, Department of Orthopaedics, University of Washington School of Medicine; Staff Physician, Providence Medical Center, Seattle, Washington
Amputations and Prosthetic Replacement

Ludwig Seebauer, MD
Chairman, Center of Orthopaedics, Traumatology and Sportmedicine, Klinikum Bogenhausen, Academic Hospital of the Technical University of Munich, Munich, Germany
Advanced Evaluation and Management of Glenohumeral Arthritis in the Cuff-Deficient Shoulder

Peter T. Simonian, MD
Clinical Professor, Department of Orthopaedic Surgery, University of California, San Francisco, Fresno, California
Muscle Ruptures Affecting the Shoulder Girdle

David L. Skaggs, MD
Associate Professor, Orthopaedic Surgery, University of Southern California; Associate Director, Children's Orthopaedic Center, Children's Hospital of Los Angeles, Los Angeles, California
Fractures, Dislocations, and Acquired Problems of the Shoulder in Children

Douglas G. Smith, MD
Professor, Department of Orthopaedic Surgery, University of Washington School of Medicine, Harborview Medical Center, Seattle, Washington
Amputations and Prosthetic Replacement

John W. Sperling, MD, MBA
Professor, Department of Orthopedic Surgery, Mayo Clinic, Rochester, Minnesota
Management of the Infected Shoulder Arthroplasty

Robert J. Spinner, MD
Professor, Neurologic Surgery, Orthopedics and Anatomy, Mayo Clinic, Rochester, Minnesota
Nerve Problems About the Shoulder

Scott P. Steinmann, MD
Associate Professor, Department of Orthopedic Surgery, Mayo Clinic, Rochester, Minnesota
Nerve Problems About the Shoulder

Daniel P. Tomlinson, MD
Orthopedic Surgeon, Crystal Run Healthcare, Middletown, New York
Shoulder Arthroscopy: Arthroscopic Treatment of Shoulder Stiffness and Calcific Tendinitis of the Rotator Cuff

Hans K. Uhthoff, MD
Professor Emeritus, University of Ottawa; Attending Physician, Ottawa Hospital, General Campus, Ottawa, Ontario, Canada
Calcifying Tendinitis

Todd W. Ulmer, MD
Team Physician, Warner Pacific College; Orthopaedic Surgeon, Columbia Orthopaedic Associates, Portland, Oregon
Muscle Ruptures Affecting the Shoulder Girdle

Tom Van Isacker, MD
Former Fellow, Alps Surgery Institute, Annecy, France
Advanced Shoulder Arthroscopy

Jennifer L. Vanderbeck, MD
Orthopedic Surgeon, Cumberland Orthopedics, Vineland, New Jersey
Congenital Anomalies and Variational Anatomy of the Shoulder

James E. Voos, MD
Resident, Department of Orthopedics, Hospital for Special Surgery, New York, New York
Developmental Anatomy of the Shoulder and Anatomy of the Glenohumeral Joint

Christopher J. Wahl, MD
Assistant Professor, Department of Orthopaedics and Sports Medicine, University of Washington, Bellevue, Washington
Shoulder Arthroscopy: General Principles

Gilles Walch, MD
Surgeon, Clinique Sainte Anne Lumière, Lyon, France
The Biceps Tendon

Jon J. P. Warner, MD
Chief, Harvard Shoulder Service; Professor of Orthopaedic Surgery, Harvard Medical School, Massachusetts General Hospital, Boston, Massachusetts
The Stiff Shoulder

Russell F. Warren, MD
Surgeon-in-Chief, Hospital for Special Surgery; Professor of Orthopaedics, Weill Medical College of Cornell University, New York, New York
Shoulder Arthroscopy (Chapter Editor); Shoulder Arthroscopy: General Principles; Shoulder Arthroscopy: Arthroscopic Treatment of Shoulder Instability

Anthony S. Wei, MD
Former Research Fellow, Kerlan-Jobe Orthopaedic Clinic, Los Angeles, California
Complications of Shoulder Arthroscopy

Jason S. Weisstein, MD, MPH
Assistant Professor, Orthopaedics and
Sports Medicine Sarcoma Service,
University of Washington; Medical
Co-Director, Northwest Tissue Center;
Surgeon, Bone and Joint Center, University
of Washington Medical Center, Seattle,
Washington
Tumors and Related Conditions

Gerald R. Williams, Jr, MD
Director, Shoulder and Elbow Center,
Rothman Institute, Jefferson Medical
College, Philadelphia, Pennsylvania
*Emerging Technologies in Shoulder
Surgery: Trends and Future Directions*

Riley J. Williams, III, MD
Member, Sports Medicine and Shoulder
Service and Clinician-Scientist, Research
Division, Hospital for Special Surgery;
Associate Professor, Weill Medical College
of Cornell University, New York, New York
*Shoulder Arthroscopy: Arthroscopic
Treatment of Shoulder Instability*

Michael A. Wirth, MD
Professor of Orthopaedics and Charles A.
Rockwood Jr, MD Chair, Department of
Orthopaedics, The University of Texas
Health Science Center at San Antonio,
University Hospital, San Antonio, Texas
*Fractures of the Proximal Humerus;
Disorders of the Sternoclavicular Joint;
Glenohumeral Instability; Rotator Cuff;
Glenohumeral Arthritis and Its
Management*

Joseph D. Zuckerman, MD
Walter A. L. Thompson Professor of
Orthopaedic Surgery and Chairman,
Department of Orthopaedic Surgery, New
York University School of Medicine; Chair,
New York University Hospital for Joint
Diseases, New York, New York
Occupational Shoulder Disorders

Contents

VOLUME ONE

CHAPTER 1
Developmental Anatomy of the Shoulder and Anatomy of the Glenohumeral Joint 1
Stephen J. O'Brien, MD, MBA, James E. Voos, MD, Andrew S. Neviaser, MD, and Mark C. Drakos, MD
Comparative Anatomy 1
Embryology. 5
Postnatal Development 11
Adult Glenohumeral Joint 12

CHAPTER 2
Gross Anatomy of the Shoulder 33
Christopher M. Jobe, MD, Wesley P. Phipatanakul, MD, and Michael J. Coen, MD
History 33
Bones and Joints 38
Muscles 48
Nerves. 67
Blood Vessels 79
Bursae, Compartments, and Potential Spaces 87
Skin. 93

CHAPTER 3
Congenital Anomalies and Variational Anatomy of the Shoulder. 101
Jennifer L. Vanderbeck, MD, John M. Fenlin, Jr, MD, Charles L. Getz, MD, and Anthony F. DePalma, MD
Variational Anatomy of the Shoulder 101
Common Malformations of the Shoulder 117
Rare Anomalies 126

CHAPTER 4
Clinical Evaluation of Shoulder Problems. 145
Michael Codsi, MD, Jesse McCarron, MD, and John J. Brems, MD
Patient History. 145
Physical Examination 152
Special Tests 162

CHAPTER 5
Radiographic Evaluation of Shoulder Problems 177
Kirk L. Jensen, MD, and Charles A. Rockwood, Jr, MD
Fractures of the Glenohumeral Joint. 177
Anterior Instability 183
Posterior Humeral Head Compression Fractures Associated With Anterior Dislocation: The Hill–Sachs Defect 186
Posterior Instability 188
Glenohumeral Arthritis. 191
Glenohumeral Arthroplasty. 192
Clavicle 194
Acromioclavicular Joint and Distal Clavicle. 194
Sternoclavicular Joint and Medial Clavicle. 197
Rotator Cuff. 199
Scapula 206
Calcifying Tendinitis. 207
Biceps Tendon. 207

CHAPTER 6
Biomechanics of the Shoulder 213
Eiji Itoi, MD, PhD, Bernard F. Morrey, MD, and Kai-Nan An, PhD
Shoulder Complex 213
Glenohumeral and Scapulothoracic Joint Motion 217
Shoulder Motion 222
Shoulder Constraints 230
Muscle and Joint Forces. 250

CHAPTER 7
Effectiveness Evaluation of the Shoulder. 267
Robin R. Richards, MD, FRCSC
History 267
Development of Outcome Measures. 268
Types of Outcome Measures 268
Application of Outcome Measures 269
Assessing Outcome Measures. 270
Specific Outcome Instruments 271
Author's Current Practice 275
Future Developments. 275
Summary 275

CHAPTER 8
Anesthesia for Shoulder Procedures 279
Christopher D. Kent, MD, and Laurie B. Amundsen, MD
Anesthesia. 279

Neurologic Injury After Shoulder Procedures 285
Preoperative Considerations 287
Intraoperative Considerations 287
Postoperative Considerations 289
Summary 291

CHAPTER 9
Fractures of the Proximal Humerus 295
Kamal I. Bohsali, MD, and Michael A. Wirth, MD
Anatomy 295
Mechanism of Injury 297
Clinical Evaluation 297
Imaging 297
Classification 298
Methods of Treatment 300
Authors' Preferred Method of Treatment 307
Complications After Arthroplasty 325
Results After Arthroplasty 326
Reverse Shoulder Arthroplasty for Primary
and Secondary Management of Proximal
Humerus Fractures 326
Late Complications of Proximal Humerus Fractures . . . 327

CHAPTER 10
Fractures of the Scapula 333
Thomas P. Goss, MD, and Brett D. Owens, MD
Anatomy 333
Classification of Fractures of the Scapula 334
Clinical Features 335
Associated Injuries and Complications 335
Radiographic Evaluation 336
Types of Fractures and Methods of Treatment 336
Other Disorders 364
Authors' Preferred Method of Treatment 368

CHAPTER 11
Fractures of the Clavicle 381
Carl J. Basamania, MD, and
Charles A. Rockwood, Jr, MD
Historical Review 381
Anatomy 382
Morphology and Function 383
Function 385
Classification of Clavicle Fractures 389
Mechanism of Injury 394
Clinical Findings 396
Radiographic Evaluation 401
Differential Diagnosis 404
Complications 406
Treatment 413
Postoperative Care 419
Authors' Preferred Method of Treatment 419

CHAPTER 12
Disorders of the Acromioclavicular Joint 453
David N. Collins, MD
Developmental Anatomy 453
Anatomy and Function 453
Excision of the Distal Clavicle 457
Biomechanics of Acromioclavicular Motion 463
Spectrum of Disorders 466

Evaluation 467
Traumatic Disorders 474
Nontraumatic Disorders 514

CHAPTER 13
Disorders of the Sternoclavicular Joint 527
Michael A. Wirth, MD, and Charles A. Rockwood, Jr, MD
Surgical Anatomy 527
Mechanism of Injury 533
Classification of Problems of the
Sternoclavicular Joint 534
Incidence of Injury to the Sternoclavicular Joint 537
Signs and Symptoms of Injuries to the
Sternoclavicular Joint 539
Radiographic Findings of Injury to the
Sternoclavicular Joint 539
Treatment 542
Authors' Preferred Method of Treatment 551
Complications of Injuries to the
Sternoclavicular Joint 557
Complications of Operative Procedures 558

CHAPTER 14
Sepsis of the Shoulder: Molecular Mechanisms
and Pathogenesis 561
Robin R. Richards, MD, FRCSC
History 561
Septic Anatomy of the Shoulder 562
Microanatomy and Cell Biology 563
Classification 564
Pathogenic Mechanisms of Septic Arthritis
and Osteomyelitis 565
Microbial Adhesion and Intra-Articular Sepsis 568
Bacterial Pathogens 569
Clinical Presentation 570
Laboratory Evaluation 571
Complications 574
Treatment 575
Outcome 578
Prevention 579
Author's Preferred Method of Treatment 579
Summary 580

CHAPTER 15
Fractures, Dislocations, and Acquired Problems
of the Shoulder in Children 583
Paul D. Choi, MD, Gilbert Chan, MD, David L. Skaggs, MD,
and John M. Flynn, MD
Fractures of the Proximal Humerus 583
Fractures of the Clavicle 594
Fractures of the Scapula 604

CHAPTER 16
Glenohumeral Instability 617
Frederick A. Matsen, III, MD, Steven B. Lippitt, MD,
Alexander Bertlesen, PAC, Charles A. Rockwood, Jr, MD,
and Michael A. Wirth, MD
Historical Review 617
Relevant Anatomy 622
Mechanics of Glenohumeral Stability 629
Types of Glenohumeral Instability 651

DISLOCATION

Clinical Findings 661
Injuries Associated With Anterior Dislocations 666
Injuries Associated With Posterior Dislocations 678
Treatment 678

RECURRENT DISLOCATION

Evaluation 684
Treatment 700

VOLUME TWO

CHAPTER 17

Rotator Cuff **771**

*Frederick A. Matsen, III, MD, Edward V. Fehringer, MD,
Steven B. Lippitt, MD, Michael A. Wirth, MD, and
Charles A. Rockwood, Jr, MD*

Historical Review 771
Relevant Anatomy and Mechanics 775
Clinical Conditions Involving the Cuff 799
Incidence of Rotator Cuff Defects 800
Clinical Findings 802
Clinical Conditions Related to the Rotator Cuff 808
Shoulder Function and Health Status in Clinical
Conditions of the Rotator Cuff 809
Imaging Techniques 810
Differential Diagnosis 817
Treatment 819

CHAPTER 18

**Evaluation and Management of Failed Rotator
Cuff Surgery** **891**

Joshua S. Dines, MD, and David M. Dines, MD

Diagnosis 891
Failed Repairs 892
Persistent Subacromial Impingement 897
Stiffness 899
Heterotopic Ossification 902
Acromial Stress Fracture 903
Deltoid Insufficiency 903
Conclusion 906

CHAPTER 19

Complications of Shoulder Arthroscopy **909**

Anthony S. Wei, MD, and Leesa M. Galatz, MD

Early Reports and Reviews 909
Anesthesia-Related Complications 910
General Surgical Complications 911
Complications Specific to Shoulder Arthroscopy 914
Bupivacaine-Induced Chondrolysis 918
Summary 918

CHAPTER 20

Shoulder Arthroscopy **921**

Edited by Russell F. Warren, MD

20A. General Principles **921**

Christopher J. Wahl, MD, and Russell F. Warren, MD

History 921
Anatomy 922
Positioning, Portals, and Diagnostic Arthroscopy 929
Summary 939

**20B. Arthroscopic Treatment
of Shoulder Instability** **940**

*Seth C. Gamradt, MD, Riley J. Williams, III, MD,
and Russell F. Warren, MD*

Pathoanatomy 940
Diagnosis and Diagnostic Arthroscopy in
Shoulder Instability 941
Management of Post-Traumatic Anterior Instability 942
Arthroscopic Management of Posterior Instability 950
Arthroscopic Management of Multidirectional
Instability 952
Postoperative Management and Return to Play 956
Complications of Stabilization Surgery 957
Conclusions 957

**20C. Arthroscopic Management of Rotator
Cuff Disease** **961**

*Stephen F. Brockmeier, MD, Answorth A. Allen, MD,
John D. MacGillivray, MD, and Scott A. Rodeo, MD*

Arthroscopic Management of Impingement
Syndrome 961
Arthroscopic Rotator Cuff Repair 964
Arthroscopic Management of Subscapularis Tears 980

**20D. Acromioclavicular Joint Arthritis
and Instability** **984**

*Robert H. Brophy, MD, Stephen Fealy, MD, and
Frank A. Cordasco, MD, MS*

Anatomy of the Acromioclavicular Joint 984
Excision of the Distal Clavicle 984
Stabilization of the Acromioclavicular Joint 990

**20E. Arthroscopic Treatment of Shoulder
Stiffness and Calcific Tendinitis
of the Rotator Cuff** **993**

Daniel P. Tomlinson, MD, and Jo A. Hannafin, MD, PhD

Primary Adhesive Capsulitis 993
Secondary Adhesive Capsulitis 998
Secondary Shoulder Stiffness 998
Calcific Tendinitis 1000

**20F. Arthroscopic Management of Arthritic and
Prearthritic Conditions of the Shoulder** **1002**

Clayton Lane, MD, and Edward V. Craig, MD, MPH

Osteoarthritis 1002
Inflammatory Synovitis and Arthritis 1007
Renal Arthropathy 1008
Osteonecrosis 1008
Arthroscopy After Hemiarthroplasty and Total
Shoulder Arthroplasty 1008
Summary 1009

20G. Biceps in Shoulder Arthroscopy **1011**

*Barrett S. Brown, MD, Anne M. Kelly, MD,
Mark C. Drakos, MD, and Stephen J. O'Brien, MD, MBA*

Diagnosis of Biceps Pathology 1011
Treatment 1013
Coexisting Diagnoses 1018
Conclusion 1019

20H. SLAP Tears **1020**

Jeffrey Davila, MD

Anatomy 1020
Biomechanics 1021
Classification 1021
Diagnosis 1022
Surgical Management 1024

Surgical Technique. 1025
Paralabral Ganglion Cysts. 1026
Conclusions. 1028

20I. Thrower's Shoulder. **1029**
Barrett S. Brown, MD, Stephen F. Brockmeier, MD,
and David W. Altchek, MD
Internal Impingement. 1030
Diagnosis of Thrower's Injury 1031
Treatment 1033
Conclusion 1043

CHAPTER 21
Advanced Shoulder Arthroscopy **1045**
Laurent Lafosse, MD, Manuel Haag, MD,
Tom Van Isacker, MD, and Ludwig Anné, MD
Evolution of Shoulder Arthroscopy. 1045
The Shoulder as a House. 1045
The Arthroscopic Portals 1046
Shoulder Pathology by Area. 1047

CHAPTER 22
Glenohumeral Arthritis and Its Management **1089**
Frederick A. Matsen, III, MD, Jeremiah Clinton, MD,
Charles A. Rockwood, Jr, MD, Michael A. Wirth, MD, and
Steven B. Lippitt, MD
Mechanics of Arthritis and Arthroplasty 1089
Clinical Findings and Evaluation. 1107
Treatment 1131
Complications 1222
Revision. 1229

CHAPTER 23
Advanced Evaluation and Management of Glenohumeral
Arthritis in the Cuff-Deficient Shoulder. **1247**
Anders Ekelund, MD, PhD, and Ludwig Seebauer, MD
History and Biomechanics of Reverse Arthroplasty . . . 1247
Classification of Cuff Tear Arthropathy 1249
Differential Diagnosis. 1254
Evaluation 1255
Treatment 1255
Complications and Their Management 1274

CHAPTER 24
Management of the Infected Shoulder
Arthroplasty **1277**
John W. Sperling, MD, MBA, and Robert H. Cofield, MD
Patient Evaluation 1277
Treatment 1279
Summary. 1282

CHAPTER 25
Calcifying Tendinitis **1283**
Hans K. Uhthoff, MD, Peter Lapner, MD,
and Joachim F. Loehr, MD
Historical Review. 1283
Anatomy 1283
Incidence. 1284
Classification 1285
Pathology 1286
Pathogenesis 1288

Clinical Findings 1291
Radiology 1293
Laboratory Investigations 1295
Complications 1296
Differential Diagnosis. 1296
Treatment 1296
Conclusion 1304

CHAPTER 26
The Biceps Tendon. **1309**
Wayne Z. Burkhead, Jr, MD, Peter Habermeyer, MD,
Gilles Walch, MD, and Kenneth Lin, MD
Historical Review. 1309
Anatomy 1312
Function of the Biceps Tendon 1321
Classification of Bicipital Lesions 1326
Incidence. 1329
Etiology. 1330
Prevention 1331
Clinical Features of Bicipital Lesions. 1331
Diagnostic Tests. 1334
Complications 1339
Differential Diagnosis. 1339
Treatment 1341
Summary. 1355

CHAPTER 27
Nerve Problems About the Shoulder **1361**
Scott P. Steinmann, MD, and Robert J. Spinner, MD
Clinical Evaluation 1361
Musculocutaneous Nerve Injury 1362
Axillary Nerve 1363
Spinal Accessory Nerve 1366
Long Thoracic Nerve 1369
Suprascapular Nerve 1372
Thoracic Outlet Syndrome 1374
Parsonage–Turner Syndrome (Brachial Plexus
Neuropathy) 1376
Brachial Plexus Injuries 1377

CHAPTER 28
Muscle Ruptures Affecting the Shoulder Girdle **1389**
Todd W. Ulmer, MD, and Peter T. Simonian, MD
General Principles of Rupture
of the Musculotendinous Unit 1389
Rupture of the Pectoralis Major 1390
Rupture of the Deltoid. 1394
Rupture of the Triceps 1395
Rupture of the Biceps 1397
Rupture of the Serratus Anterior. 1399
Rupture of the Coracobrachialis 1400
Rupture of the Subscapularis 1400
Rupture of the Pectoralis Minor 1401
Rupture of the Supraspinatus 1401
Rupture of the Infraspinatus. 1401
Rupture of the Teres Major 1402
Conclusion 1402

CHAPTER 29
The Stiff Shoulder. **1405**
Nathan K. Endres, MD, Bassem ElHassan, MD,
Laurence D. Higgins, MD, and Jon J. P. Warner, MD
Definition 1405

Classification 1405
Normal Motion and Pathomechanics 1406
Pathophysiology 1408
Diagnostic Criteria 1409
Epidemiology. 1410
Predisposing Factors 1410
Evaluation 1412
Natural History 1414
Treatment 1414
Authors' Preferred Treatment 1423
Summary. 1428

CHAPTER 30

The Shoulder in Athletes. 1437
*Neal S. ElAttrache, MD, Guillem Gonzalez-Lomas, MD,
and Christopher S. Ahmad, MD*
Sports-Specific Biomechanics 1437
Asymptomatic Throwing Shoulder Adaptation 1446
Throwing Shoulder Conditions. 1449
Evaluation of the Overhead Athlete 1454
Treatment 1455
Traumatic Injuries 1472
Neurovascular Injuries 1479
Conclusion 1483

CHAPTER 31

Occupational Shoulder Disorders. 1489
*Manny Halpern, PhD, Jason L. Hurd, MD,
and Joseph D. Zuckerman, MD*
Occupational Shoulder Disorders 1490
Degenerative Joint Disease. 1495
Prevention. 1496
Outcomes of Treatment 1499
Evaluation of Upper Extremity Disability
and Impairment. 1501
Current Disability Compensation Systems 1503
Private Insurance Companies 1505
Conclusion 1506

CHAPTER 32

Tumors and Related Conditions 1509
Jason S. Weisstein, MD, MPH, and Ernest U. Conrad, III, MD
Historical Review. 1509
Anatomy 1510
Staging and Classification of Tumors 1512
Incidence of Neoplasms. 1530
Clinical Features 1532
Radiographic and Laboratory Evaluation. 1534
Complications of Tumors. 1536
Differential Diagnosis. 1536
Surgery 1538
Authors' Preferred Methods of Treatment 1550

CHAPTER 33

Amputations and Prosthetic Replacement. 1557
*Douglas G. Smith, MD, Robert L. Romano, MD,
and Ernest M. Burgess, MD*
Types of Amputations 1557
Precipitating Factors. 1558
Specific Procedures 1558
Prosthetic Rehabilitation. 1568

CHAPTER 34

**Emerging Technologies in Shoulder Surgery:
Trends and Future Directions. 1577**
Joseph P. Iannotti, MD, PhD, and Gerald R. Williams, Jr, MD
Biological Enhancement of Rotator Cuff Repair 1577
Computer Navigation and Minimally Invasive
Shoulder Replacement 1579
Management of Glenoid Bone Loss in Shoulder
Arthroplasty. 1580
Alternative Bearing Surfaces. 1581
Conclusions. 1583

Index i

DVD Video Contents

DISK ONE

CHAPTER 4
Clinical Evaluation of Shoulder Problems
4-1   Inspection
4-2   Palpation
4-3   Range of Motion
4-4   Differences Between Active and Passive Ranges
4-5   External Rotation at 90 Degrees of Abduction
4-6   Jobe Test
4-7   Stability Assessment
4-8   Rotator Cuff Testing
4-9   Slap Tests
4-10   Humeral Head Translation
4-11   Sulcus Sign
4-12   Anterior Translation
4-13   Apprehension Relocation
4-14   Posterior Instability (Jerk Test)
4-15   Posterior Instability (Supine Jerk)
4-16   Painful Arc
4-17   Kennedy Hawkins Impingement Test
4-18   Modified Neer Test
4-19   Internal Rotation Resistance Stress Test
4-20   Subcoracoid Impingement Test
4-21   O'Brien (Active Compression) Test
4-22   Crank Test
4-23   External Rotation Lag (Abduction)
4-24   External Rotation Lag (Adduction)
4-25   Bear Hug
4-26   Napoleon Test
4-27   Belly Press Test
4-28   Lift-Off Test

CHAPTER 11
Fractures of the Clavicle
Surgical Technique for Intramedullary Fixation
11-1   Patient Positioning
11-2   Incision
11-3   Drilling and Tapping Intermedullary Canal
11-4   Insertion of Clavicle Pin
11-5   Securing Pin
11-6   Soft Tissue Closure

CHAPTER 12
Disorders of the Acromioclavicular Joint
12-1   Surface Anatomy and Skin Incision
12-2   Exposure of the Acromioclavicular Joint
12-3   Reapproximation of the Coracoid Clavicular Ligaments
12-4   Drilling of the 3/16-Inch Hole Down Through the Clavicle in a Skeleton
12-5   Drilling of the 9/64-Inch Hole Down Through the Clavicle in a Skeleton
12-6   Insertion of the Coracoclavicular Screw During Surgery
12-7   Repair of the Deltotrapezius Fascia

CHAPTER 13
Disorders of the Sternoclavicular Joint
13-1   Sternoclavicular Reconstruction

CHAPTER 16
Glenohumeral Instability
16-1   Pathology
16-2   Incision
16-3   Exposing the Subscapularis
16-4   Incising Subscapularis
16-5   Visualizing Pathology
16-6   Roughening the Glenoid
16-7   Bone Tunnels
16-8   Suture Passing
16-9   Reattaching Capsule
16-10 Repairing Subscapularis
16-11 Skin Incision, Identification of the Musculocutaneous and Axillary Nerve, and Division of the Upper Two Thirds of the Subscapularis Tendon
16-12 Division of Anterior Capsule, Elevation of the Perthes/ Bankart Lesion, and Bankart Repair With Biodegradable Suture Anchors
16-13 Performing the Capsular Shift Procedure, and Repair of the Subscapularis Tendon

DISK TWO

CHAPTER 17
Rotator Cuff
Wirth's Technique of Open Rotator Cuff Repair
With Restore Orthobiological Implant
17-1   Introduction
17-2   Surgical Technique

CHAPTER 20
Shoulder Arthroscopy
20-1   Arthroscopic Treatment of the Stiff Shoulder
20-2   Impingement Syndrome
20-3   Repair of the Full-Thickness Rotator Cuff Tears:
Small to Medium
20-4   Biceps Tenodesis
20-5   Arthroscopic Rotator Cuff Repair
20-6   Biceps Tenotomy
20-7   Arthroscopic Anterior Stabilization/Bankart Repair
20-8   Arthroscopic Stabilization/Capsular Plication for MDI
20-9   Arthroscopic Posterior Stabilization l
20-10 Capsular Plication
20-11 Partial Thickness RTC Repair
20-12 SLAP Repair

CHAPTER 22
Glenohumeral Arthritis and Its Management
22-1   Surface Anatomy and Skin Incision
22-2   Elevation of the Deltoid off of the Scapula
22-3   Exposure of the Shaft of the Humorous and
Identification of the Axillary Nerve
22-4   Removal of the Remains of the Rotator Cuff Tissue
22-5   Removal of Cartilage and Decortication of the Glenoid
Fossa and Humeral Head

22-6   Arm Is Positioned in 10 to 20 Degrees of Flexion and
Abduction and in 40 to 50 Degrees of Internal Rotation
and Is Temporarily Stabilized With Steinmann Pin
22-7   Positioning the Malleable Template Across the Scapula
and Down the Humerus
22-8   Fixation of the Reconstruction Plate to the Scapula,
Pointing out the Importance of Getting Long Screws
Down Through the Plate of the Spine of the Scapula
and Down Into the Neck of the Scapula

Rockwood's Technique—Arthrodesis
22-9   Insertion of a Cortical Screw in the Humerus

Matsen's Technique—Total Shoulder Arthroscopy
22-10 Templating
22-11 Incision
22-12 Subscapularis Incision
22-13 Humeral Exposure
22-14 Humeral Reaming
22-15 Humeral Preparation
22-16 Subscapularis Capsule Repair
22-17 Glenoid Preparation and Insertion
22-18 Humeral Head Selection
22-19 Impaction Humeral Placement
22-20 Closure

Rockwood's Technique—Arthroplasty
22-21 Introduction
22-22 Skin Incision and Approach
22-23 Resection of the Humeral Head, Reaming
the Intermedullary Broach
22-24 Technique for Using Anchor Peg Glenoid Prosthesis
22-25 Selection of Proper Head Size and Soft Tissue
Balancing
22-26 Insertion of Final Prosthesis and Repair
of Subscapularis Tendon

Developmental Anatomy of the Shoulder and Anatomy of the Glenohumeral Joint

Stephen J. O'Brien, MD, MBA, James E. Voos, MD, Andrew S. Neviaser, MD, and Mark C. Drakos, MD

As humans evolved to assume an orthograde posture, the scapulohumeral complex underwent changes to facilitate prehension and comply with the demands of a non–weight-bearing joint. Over time, the inherent osseous articular congruity of the upper limbs was sacrificed for soft tissue stability to achieve a greater degree of mobility at the glenohumeral joint.

In this chapter we focus initially on the developmental anatomy of the shoulder girdle and then on the anatomy of the adult glenohumeral joint. Since the third edition, several studies and new technologic developments have advanced our anatomic and biomechanical understanding of the glenohumeral joint. We review these findings concerning the fetal aspect of shoulder development and then discuss in detail the gross anatomy of the remainder of the pectoral girdle.

COMPARATIVE ANATOMY

General Development

The forelimb in humans is a paired appendage whose evolutionary roots can be traced to the longitudinal lateral folds of epidermis in the fish species *Rhipidistian crossopterygian*.[1] These folds extend caudad from the region just behind the gills to the anus (Fig. 1-1). The pectoral and pelvic fins developed from the proximal and distal portions respectively and were the predecessors of the human upper and lower limbs (Fig. 1-2).[2]

Muscle buds, along with the ventral rami of spinal nerves, migrated into these pectoral fins to allow for coordinated movement. Peripheral fibers repeatedly divided to form a plexus of nerves, and different regions of muscle tissue often combined or segmented as function evolved.

Cartilage rays called *radials* (Fig. 1-3) arose between muscle buds to form a support structure, and the proximal portions of these radials coalesced to form basal cartilage, or *basilia*. The radials began to fuse at their base and eventually formed a concrescent central axis, or *pectoral girdle* (Fig. 1-4). These paired basilia eventually migrated ventrally toward the midline anteriorly to form a *ventral bar*, which corresponds to the paired clavicles in some mammals, as well as the *cleitrum*, a membranous bone that attached the pectoral girdle to the skull. The basilia also projected dorsally over the thorax to form the precursor of the scapula. Articulations within the basilia eventually developed at the junction of the ventral and dorsal segments (glenoid fossa) with the remainder of the pectoral fin, which corresponds to the glenohumeral joint in humans (Fig. 1-5).

As these prehistoric fish evolved into amphibians, their osseous morphology also changed to adapt to waterless gravity. The head was eventually freed from its attachments to the pectoral girdle, and in the reptile, the pectoral girdle migrated a considerable distance caudally.[3] The pelycosaurus of the late Paleozoic Era (235-255 million years ago) is among the oldest reptiles believed to have been solely land dwellers.[4] These early tetrapods ambulated with the proximal part of their forelimbs held in the horizontal plane and distal part flexed at a 90-degree angle in the sagittal plane. Locomotion was attained by rotation of the humerus in its longitudinal axis. The cleitrum disappeared entirely in this reptilian stage.

Whereas structural stability was primarily achieved via osseous congruity in these early reptiles, the shoulder evolved to dispense more flexibility and mobility in subsequent species. The basic mammalian pattern developed with articulations arising between a well-developed clavicle and sternum medially and a flat, fairly wide scapula laterally. The coracoid enlarged during this period, and

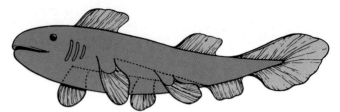

FIGURE 1-1 Paired lateral longitudinal folds of epidermis of the fish extending caudad from the region just posterior to the gills to the anus.

FIGURE 1-2 The pectoral and pelvic fins from the proximal and distal portions of the paired longitudinal lateral folds. These fins are the precursors of the upper and lower limbs.

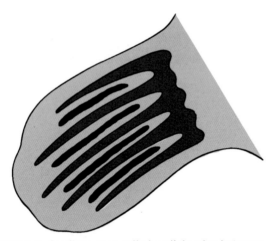

FIGURE 1-3 Cartilage rays called *radials* arise between muscle buds formed as a support structure for the limb. The proximal portions of these radials coalesce to form basal cartilage, or basilia.

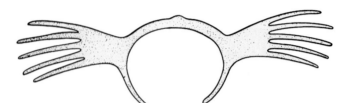

FIGURE 1-4 The paired basilia come together in the midline to form the primitive pectoral girdle. As these basilia migrate, they form a bar that is the precursor to the paired clavicles.

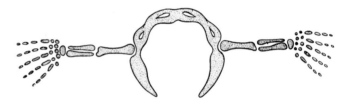

FIGURE 1-5 Articulations within the basilia develop at the junction of the ventral and dorsal segments, which form the primitive glenoid fossa.

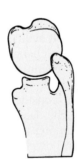 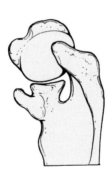 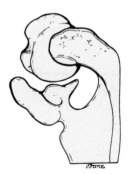

FIGURE 1-6 The coracoid and acromion have progressively enlarged in response to functional demands of the orthograde posture.

the scapular spine developed in response to new functional demands (Fig. 1-6). Four main variations on this scheme are seen.[5] Mammals adapted for running have lost their clavicle to further mobilize the scapula, and the scapula is relatively narrowed. Mammals adapted for swimming also have lost the clavicle, although the scapula is wider and permits more varied function. Shoulder girdles modified for flying have a large, long, well-developed clavicle with a small, narrow, curved scapula.

Finally, shoulders modified for brachiating (including those of humans) developed a strong clavicle, a large coracoid, and a widened, strong scapula.

Other adaptations in the erect posture were relative flattening of the thorax in the anteroposterior dimension, with the scapula left approximately 45 degrees to the midline (Fig. 1-7), and evolution of the pentadactyl limb with a strong, mobile thumb and four ulnar digits. This pentadactyl limb is very similar to the human arm as we know it.

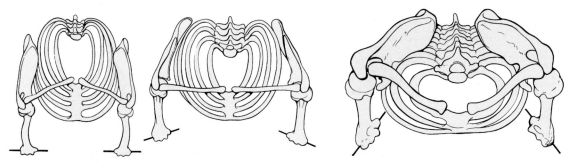

FIGURE 1-7 The anteroposterior dimension of the thoracic cage has decreased over time, with the scapula approximately 45 degrees to the midline. The scapula and glenoid fossa have also assumed a more dorsal position in the thoracic cage. This change in position led to the glenoid fossa's being directed laterally. Consequently, a relative external rotation of the humeral head and an internal rotation of the shaft occurred.

In approaching the more human form, we now discuss evolution of the different regions of the shoulder and pectoral girdle separately.

Development of Individual Regions

The Scapula

The scapula in humans is suspended by muscles alone and clearly reflects the adaptive development of the shoulder. It has shifted caudally from the cervical position in lower animals, and as a result, the shoulder is freed from the head and neck and can serve as a base or platform to facilitate arm movement. The most striking modification in the development of the bone of the scapula itself is in the relationship between the length (measured along the base of the spine) and the breadth (measured from the superior to the inferior angle) of the scapula, or the *scapular index* (Fig. 1-8).[6] This index is extremely high in the pronograde animal with a long, narrow scapula. In primates and humans, the scapula broadens, and the most pronounced changes are confined to the infraspinatus fossa. This modification has been referred to as an increase in the infraspinatus index.

Broadening of the infraspinatus fossa results in a change in the vector of muscle pull from the axillary border of the scapula to the glenoid fossa and consequently alters the action of the attached musculature. This adaptation allows the infraspinatus and teres minor to be more effective in their roles as depressors and external rotators of the humeral head. The supraspinatus fossa and muscle have changed little in size or shape over time; the acromion, which is an extension of the spine of the scapula (see Fig. 1-6), has enlarged over time. In pronograde animals, the acromion process is insignificant; in humans, however, it is a massive structure overlying the humeral head. This change reflects the increasing role of the deltoid muscle in shoulder function. By broadening its attachment on the acromion and shifting its insertion distally on the humerus, it increases its mechanical advantage in shoulder motion.

The coracoid process has also undergone an increase in size over time (see Fig. 1-6).[6] We have performed biomechanical studies in which it was shown that with the shoulder in 90 degrees of abduction, the coracoid extension over the glenohumeral joint can mechanically limit anterior translation of the humerus relative to the glenoid. In one shoulder that we tested after sectioning

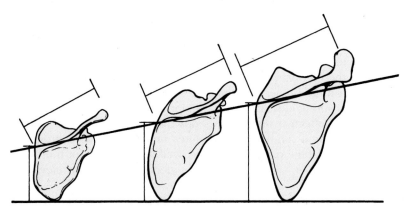

FIGURE 1-8 The size of the infraspinous fossa has gradually enlarged over time relative to the length of the scapular spine. This relative increase has led to a decrease in the scapular index.

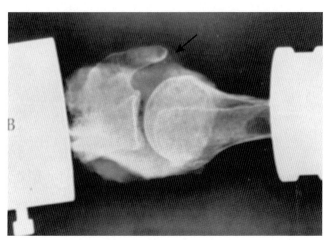

FIGURE 1-9 An x-ray view of an abducted shoulder shows a large overlap of the coracoid over the glenohumeral joint, which may restrict anterior translation.

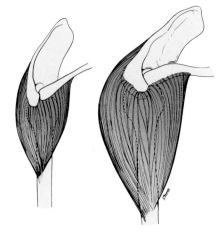

FIGURE 1-10 The deltoid muscle has migrated distally over time to improve the lever arm on the humerus.

of the capsule, the shoulder would not dislocate anteriorly in full abduction until after the coracoid process was removed (Fig. 1-9).[7]

Humerus

Like the scapula, the humerus has undergone several morphologic changes during its evolution. The head of the humerus has moved proximally, underneath the torso, as well as from the horizontal plane to a more vertical resting orientation. The insertion site of the deltoid has migrated distally to improve the lever arm of the deltoid muscle (Fig. 1-10).[6,8]

In addition, the distal humeral shaft underwent an episode of torsion relative to the proximal end of the humerus, thereby making the humeral head internally rotated relative to the epicondyles.[6] As the thoracic cage flattened in the anteroposterior plane, the scapula and glenoid fossa assumed a more dorsal position in the thoracic cage, which led to the glenoid fossa being directed more laterally (see Fig. 1-7). As a consequence, external rotation of the humeral head and internal rotation of the shaft relative to it occurred and led to medial displacement of the intertubercular groove and decreased size of the lesser tuberosity relative to the greater tuberosity. The resultant retroversion of the humeral head has been reported to be 33 degrees in the dominant shoulder and 29 degrees in the nondominant shoulder relative to the epicondyles of the elbow in the coronal plane.[9]

The other effect of this torsion on the humerus is that the biceps, which was previously a strong elevator of the arm, is rendered biomechanically ineffective unless the arm is externally rotated. In this fashion it can be used as an abductor, which is often seen in infantile paralysis.

Clavicle

The clavicle is not present in horses or other animals that use their forelimbs for standing. In animals that use their upper limbs for holding, grasping, and climbing, however, the clavicle allows the scapula and humerus to be held away from the body to help the limb move free of the axial skeleton. In humans, it also provides a means of transmitting the supporting force of the trapezius to the scapula through the coracoclavicular ligaments, a bony framework for muscle attachments, and a mechanism for increasing range of motion at the glenohumeral joint.

Scapulohumeral Muscles

The scapulohumeral muscles include the supraspinatus, infraspinatus, teres minor, subscapularis, deltoid, and teres major. The supraspinatus has remained relatively static morphologically but has progressively decreased in relative mass (Fig. 1-11).[8] The deltoid, on the other hand, has more than doubled in proportional representation and constitutes approximately 41% of the scapulohumeral muscle mass. This increase in size also increases the overall strength of the deltoid. In lower animals, a portion of the deltoid attaches to the inferior angle of the scapula. In humans, these fibers correspond to the teres minor muscle and explain the identical innervation in these two muscles by the axillary nerve.

The infraspinatus is absent in lower species; however, in humans, it makes up approximately 5% of the mass of the scapulohumeral muscles. The subscapularis has undergone no significant change, except for a slight increase in the number of fasciculi concomitant with elongation of the scapula, and it makes up approximately 20% of the mass of the scapulohumeral group. This adaptation allows the lower part of the muscle to pull in a downward direction and assists the infraspinatus and teres minor to act as a group to function as depressors as well as stabilizers of the head of the humerus against the glenoid during arm elevation.

Axioscapular Muscles

The axioscapular muscles include the serratus anterior, rhomboids, levator scapulae, and trapezius. All these

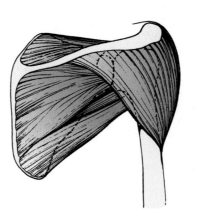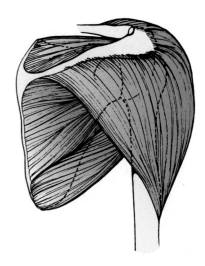

FIGURE 1-11 The supraspinatus muscle has remained relatively static morphologically but has progressively decreased in mass relative to the infraspinous muscles, although the enlarged deltoid muscle can be appreciated. The increased importance of the deltoid is evidenced by its increase in relative size.

muscles (except the trapezius) originated from one complex of muscle fibers arising from the first eight ribs and the transverse processes of the cervical vertebrae and inserting into the vertebral border of the scapula. As differentiation occurred, the fibers concerned with dorsal scapular motion became the rhomboid muscles. The fibers controlling ventral motion developed into the serratus anterior muscle. Finally, the levator scapulae differentiated to control cranial displacement of the scapula. The trapezius has undergone little morphologic change throughout primate development.

This group of muscles acts to anchor the scapula on the thoracic cage while allowing freedom of motion. Most authorities report the ratio between glenohumeral and scapulothoracic motion to be 2:1.[6,10] The serratus anterior provides horizontal stability and prevents winging of the scapula.

Axiohumeral Muscles

The axiohumeral muscles connect the humerus to the trunk and consist of the pectoralis major, pectoralis minor, and latissimus dorsi. The pectoral muscles originate from a single muscle mass that divides into a superficial layer and a deep layer. The superficial layer becomes the pectoralis major, and the deep layer gives rise to the pectoralis minor. The pectoralis minor is attached to the humerus in lower species, whereas in humans it is attached to the coracoid process.

Muscles of the Upper Part of the Arm

The biceps in more primitive animals has a single origin on the supraglenoid tubercle and often assists the supraspinatus in limb elevation. In humans, the biceps has two origins and, because of torsional changes in the humerus, is ineffective in shoulder elevation unless the arm is fully externally rotated.

The triceps has not undergone significant morphologic change, but the size of the long head of the triceps has been progressively decreasing.

EMBRYOLOGY

Prenatal Development

Three germ layers give rise to all the tissues and organs of the body. The cells of each germ layer divide, migrate, aggregate, and differentiate in rather precise patterns as they form various organ systems. The three germ layers are the ectoderm, the mesoderm, and the endoderm. The ectoderm gives rise to the central nervous system, peripheral nervous system, epidermis and its appendages, mammary glands, pituitary gland, and subcutaneous glands. The mesoderm gives rise to cartilage, bone, connective tissue, striated and smooth muscle, blood cells, kidneys, gonads, spleen, and the serous membrane lining of the body cavities. The endoderm gives rise to the epithelial lining of the gastrointestinal, respiratory, and urinary tracts; the lining of the auditory canal; and the parenchyma of the tonsils, thyroid gland, parathyroid glands, thymus, liver, and pancreas. Development of the embryo requires a coordinated interaction of these germ layers, orchestrated by genetic and environmental factors under the influence of basic induction and regulatory mechanisms.

Prenatal human embryologic development can be divided into three major periods: the first 2 weeks, the embryonic period, and the fetal period. The first 2 weeks of development is characterized by fertilization, blastocyst formation, implantation, and further development of the embryoblast and trophoblast. The embryonic period comprises weeks 3 through 8 of development, and the fetal period encompasses the remainder of the prenatal period until term.

The embryonic period is important because all the major external and internal organs develop during this time, and by the end of this period, differentiation is practically complete. All the bones and joints have the form and arrangement characteristic of adults. Exposure to teratogens during this period can cause major congeni-

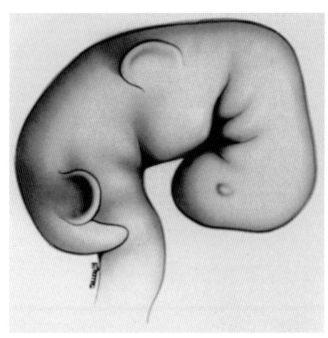

FIGURE 1-12 Because development of the head and neck occurs in advance of the rest of the embryo, the upper and lower limb buds are disproportionately low on the embryo's trunk.

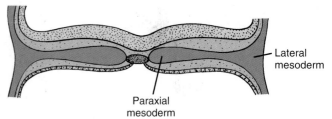

FIGURE 1-13 The mesoderm in the upper limb bud is developed from somatic mesoderm and consists of a mass of mesenchyme (loosely organized embryonic connective tissue). It eventually differentiates into fibroblastic, chondroblastic, and osteoblastic tissue.

tal malformations. During the fetal period, the limbs grow and mature as a result of a continual remodeling and reconstructive process that enables a bone to maintain its characteristic shape. In the skeleton in general, increments of growth in individual bones are in precise relationship to those of the skeleton as a whole. Ligaments show an increase in collagen content, bursae develop, tendinous attachments shift to accommodate growth, and epiphyseal cartilage becomes vascularized.

Few studies have focused on prenatal development of the glenohumeral joint. The contributions by DePalma and Gardner were essential but did not emphasize clinical correlations between the observed fetal anatomy and pathology seen in the postnatal shoulder.[11-13] Most studies of the developing shoulder have focused primarily on bone maturation. Analysis of soft tissue structures of the developing shoulder, such as the joint capsule and the labrum, is still incomplete. Studies have not thoroughly evaluated the inferior glenohumeral ligament complex, which has been shown to be an integral component for stability in the adult.[14] The seminal studies of the fetal glenohumeral joint were completed before the role of the soft tissue structures in shoulder stability was elucidated. We now have a greater appreciation of the anatomy and biomechanics of the static and dynamic stabilizers of the glenohumeral joint and their role in shoulder stability.

Embryonic Period

The limb buds are initially seen as small elevations on the ventrolateral body wall at the end of the fourth week

of gestation.[15] The upper limb buds appear during the first few days and maintain a growth advantage over the lower limbs throughout development. Because development of the head and neck occurs in advance of the rest of the embryo, the upper limb buds appear disproportionately low on the embryo's trunk (Fig. 1-12). During the early stages of limb development, the upper and lower extremities develop in similar fashion, with the upper limb bud developing opposite the lower six cervical and the first and second thoracic segments.

At 4 weeks, the upper limb is a sac of ectoderm filled with mesoderm and is approximately 3 mm long. Each limb bud is delineated dorsally by a sulcus and ventrally by a pit. The pit for the upper limb bud is called the *fossa axillaris.* The mesoderm in the upper limb bud develops from somatic mesoderm and consists of a mass of mesenchyme, which is loosely organized embryonic connective tissue. Mesenchymal cells can differentiate into many different cells, including fibroblasts, chondroblasts, and osteoblasts (Fig. 1-13). Most bones first appear as condensations of these mesenchymal cells, from which a core called the *blastema* is formed.[15,16] This development is orchestrated by the apical ectodermal ridge (Fig. 1-14), which exerts an inductive influence on the limb mesenchyme, promoting growth and development.

During the fifth week, a number of developments occur simultaneously. The peripheral nerves grow from the brachial plexus into the mesenchyme of the limb buds. Such growth stimulates development of the limb musculature, where in situ somatic limb mesoderm aggregates and differentiates into myoblasts and discrete muscle units. This process is different from development of the axial musculature, which arises from the myotomic regions of *somites,* or segments of two longitudinal columns of paraxial mesoderm (Fig. 1-15). Also at this time, the central core of the humerus begins to chondrify, although the shoulder joint is not yet formed. There is an area in the blastema called the *interzone* that does not undergo chondrification and is the precursor of the shoulder joint (Fig. 1-16). The scapula at this time lies at the level of C4 and C5 (Fig. 1-17),[17] and the clavicle is beginning to ossify (along with the mandible, the clavicle is the first bone to begin to ossify).

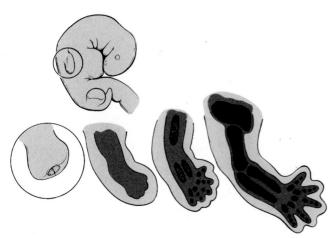

FIGURE 1-14 The apical ectodermal ridge exerts an inductive influence on the development of the upper limb.

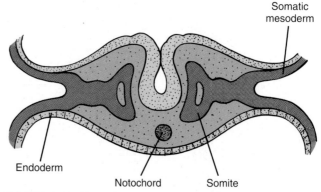

FIGURE 1-15 The axial musculature develops from myotomic regions of somites, which are segments of two longitudinal columns of paraxial mesoderm. This tissue differs from somatic mesoderm, from which the limb develops.

During the sixth week, the mesenchymal tissue in the periphery of the hand plates condenses to form digital rays. The mesodermal cells of the limb bud rearrange themselves to form a deep layer, an intermediate layer, and a superficial layer. This layering is brought on by differential growth rates.[18] Such differential growth in the limb also stimulates bending at the elbow because the cells on the ventral side grow faster than those on the dorsal side, which stretches to accommodate the ventral growth. The muscle groups divide into dorsal extensors and ventral flexors, and the individual muscles migrate caudally as the limb bud develops. In the shoulder joint, the interzone assumes a three-layered configuration, with a chondrogenic layer on either side of a loose layer of cells.[19] At this time, the glenoid lip is discernible (Fig. 1-18), although cavitation or joint formation has not occurred. Initial bone formation begins in the primary ossification center of the humerus. The scapula at this time undergoes marked enlargement and extends from C4 to approximately T7.

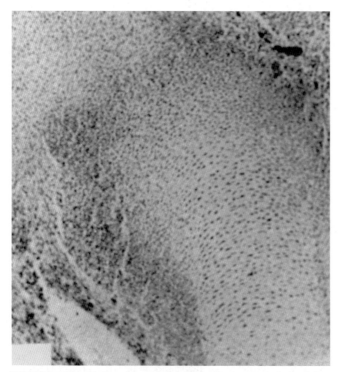

FIGURE 1-16 At 5 weeks of gestation the central core of the humerus begins to chondrify, but a homogeneous interzone remains between the scapula and the humerus. (From Gardner E, Gray DJ: Prenatal development of the human shoulder and acromioclavicular joint. Am J Anat 92:219-276, 1953.)

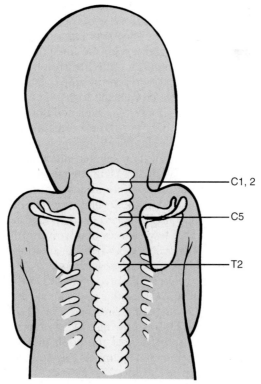

FIGURE 1-17 By the fifth week of gestation the scapula lies at the level of C4 and C5. It gradually descends as it develops. Failure of the scapula to descend is called *Sprengel's deformity.*

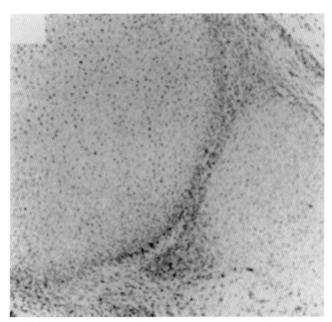

FIGURE 1-18 At 6 weeks' gestation (21 mm), a three-layered interzone is present, and the beginning of development of the glenoid labrum is evident. (From Gardner E, Gray DJ: Prenatal development of the human shoulder and acromioclavicular joint. Am J Anat 92:219, 1953.)

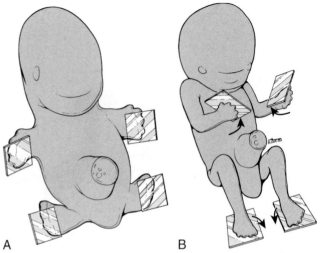

FIGURE 1-19 A, After the seventh week of gestation, the limbs extend ventrally, and the upper and lower limb buds rotate in opposite directions. **B,** As a result, the radius occupies a lateral position in the upper limb, whereas the tibia assumes a medial position in the lower limb, although they are homologous bones.

Early in the seventh week, the limbs extend ventrally and the upper and lower limb buds rotate in opposite directions (Fig. 1-19). The upper limbs rotate laterally through 90 degrees on their longitudinal axes, with the elbow facing posteriorly and the extensor muscles facing laterally and posteriorly.[15] The lower limbs rotate medially through almost 90 degrees, with the knee and extensor musculature facing anteriorly. The final result is that the radius is in a lateral position in the upper limb and the tibia is in a medial position in the lower limb, although they are homologous bones. The ulna and fibula are also homologous bones, and the thumb and great toe are homologous digits. The shoulder joint is now well formed, and the middle zone of the three-layered interzone becomes less and less dense with increasing cavitation (Fig. 1-20). The scapula has now descended and spans from just below the level of the first rib to the level of the fifth rib.[20] The brachial plexus has also migrated caudally and lies over the first rib. The final few degrees of downward displacement of the scapula occur later when the anterior portion of the rib cage drops obliquely downward.

By the eighth week the embryo is about 25 to 31 mm long, and through growth of the upper limb, the hands are stretched with the arms pronated (Fig. 1-21). The musculature of the limb is now also clearly defined. The shoulder joint has the form of the adult glenohumeral joint, and the glenohumeral ligaments can now be visualized as thickenings in the shoulder capsule.[15,21]

Although certain toxins and other environmental factors can still cause limb deformities (e.g., affecting the vascular supply), it is the embryonic period that is most vulnerable to congenital malformations, with the type of abnormality depending on the time at which the orderly sequence of differentiation was interrupted. One important factor in gross limb abnormalities, such as amelia, involves injury to the apical ectodermal ridge, which has a strong inductive influence on the limb mesoderm. Matsuoka and colleagues have mapped the destinations of embryonic neural crest and mesodermal stem cells in the neck and shoulder region using Cre recombinase–mediated transgenesis.[22] A precise code of connectivity that mesenchymal stem cells of both neural crest and mesodermal origin obey as they form muscle scaffolds was proposed. The conclusions suggested that knowledge of these relations could contribute further to identifying the etiology of diseases such as Klippel-Feil syndrome, Sprengel's deformity, and Arnold-Chiari I/II malformation.[22] Clearly, the timing of embryologic development is critical for understanding anomalies and malformations and is an area of further study.

Fetal Period

Fetal development is concerned mainly with expansion in size of the structures differentiated and developed during the embryonic period. By the end of the 12th week, the upper limbs have almost reached their final length. Ossification proceeds rapidly during this period, especially during the 13th to 16th weeks. The first indication of ossification in the cartilaginous model of a long bone is visible near the center of the shaft. Primary centers appear at different times in different bones, but usually between the 7th and 12th weeks. The part of the bone ossified from the primary center is called the *diaphysis*. Secondary centers of ossification form the epi-

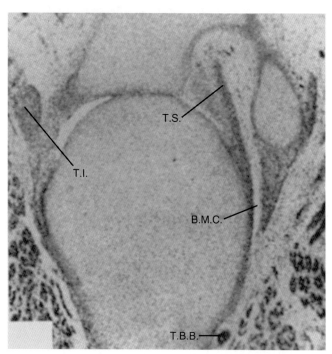

FIGURE 1-20 By the seventh week the glenohumeral joint is now well formed, and the middle zone of the three-layered interzone becomes less and less dense with increasing cavitation. The tendons of the infraspinatus (T.I.), subscapularis (T.S.), and biceps (T.B.B.) are clearly seen, as is the bursa of the coracobrachialis (B.M.C.). (From Gardner E, Gray DJ: Prenatal development of the human shoulder and acromioclavicular joint. Am J Anat 92:219-276, 1953.)

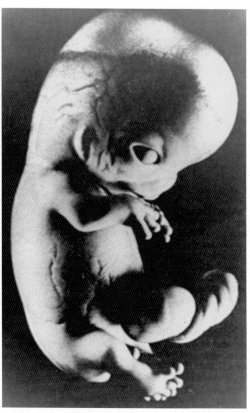

FIGURE 1-21 At the eighth week of gestation this embryo is about 23 mm long; through growth of the upper limb, the hands are stretched and the arms are pronated. The firm musculature is now clearly defined.

physis. The physeal plate separates these two centers of ossification until the bone grows to its adult length. From the 12th to the 16th week, the epiphyses are invaded by a vascular network, and in the shoulder joint, the epiphysis and part of the metaphysis are intracapsular. The tendons, ligaments, and joint capsule around the shoulder are also penetrated by a rich vascular network during the same time in the fetal period, that is, the third to fourth month of gestation.

A morphologic study of the prenatal developing shoulder joint concluded that the most important changes take place around the 12th week of prenatal life.[23] At about this time the glenoid labrum, the biceps tendon, and the glenohumeral ligaments formed a complete ring around the glenoid fossa and led the authors to believe that these structures play a role in stabilizing the joint as well as increasing the concavity of the glenoid fossa. The glenoid labrum consists of dense fibrous tissue and some elastic tissue but no fibrocartilage (as seen in the meniscus of the knee). The acromioclavicular joint develops in a manner different from that of the shoulder joint. Its development begins well into the fetal period (not the embryonic period), and a three-layered interzone is not seen as it is in the glenohumeral joint (Fig. 1-22). Most of the bursae of the shoulder, including the subdeltoid, subcoracoid, and subscapularis bursae, also develop during this time.

Fealy and colleagues studied 51 fetal glenohumeral joints from 37 specimens to evaluate shoulder morphology on a gross and histologic level and compare it with known postnatal anatomic and clinical findings in fetuses from 9 to 40 weeks of gestation.[24] Specimens were studied under a dissecting microscope, histologically, and with the aid of high-resolution radiographs to evaluate the presence of ossification centers. Fetal gross anatomy and morphology were similar to that of normal postnatal shoulders in all specimens. As noted previously, only the clavicle and spine of the scapula were ossified in the fetal shoulder. The humeral head and glenoid gradually and proportionally increased in size with gestational age. Comparative size ratios were consistent except for the fetal coracoid process, which was noted to be prominent in all specimens (Fig. 1-23).

In study by Tena-Arregui and colleagues,[25] frozen human fetuses (40 shoulders) were grossly evaluated arthroscopically with similar findings. They concluded that the anatomy observed was easier to discern than what is observed in adult shoulder arthroscopy[25] (Fig. 1-24).

Coracoacromial Arch Anatomy

By 13 weeks of gestation, the rotator cuff tendons, coracoacromial ligament (CAL), and coracohumeral ligament

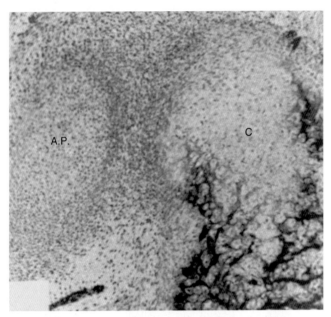

FIGURE 1-22 The acromioclavicular joint develops in a manner different from that of the shoulder joint. A three-layered interzone is not present as it is in the glenohumeral joint. A.P., acromion process; C, clavicle.

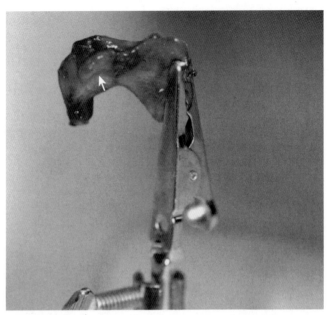

FIGURE 1-23 The fetal shoulder has a proportionally large coracoid process (*arrow*).

are present. The acromion is cartilaginous and consistently has a gentle curve that conforms to the superior aspect of the humeral head, similar to a type II acromion (Fig. 1-25).[26-28] These data suggest that variations in acromial morphology are acquired.

A macroscopic and histologic study performed by Shah and associates analyzed 22 cadaveric shoulders to establish what, if any, developmental changes occur in the differing patterns of acromia.[29] In all the curved and hooked acromia (types II and III), a common pattern of degeneration of collagen, fibrocartilage, and bone was observed, consistent with a traction phenomenon. None of these changes were exhibited by the flat acromion (type I). They therefore supported the conclusion that the different shapes of acromion are acquired in response to traction forces applied via the CAL and are not congenital.

The CAL consists of two distinct fiber bundles that lie in the anterolateral and posteromedial planes, as it does in the mature shoulder.[30] Histologic studies show that the CAL continues posteriorly along the inferior surface of the anterolateral aspect of the acromion. The CAL has well-organized collagen fiber bundles by 36 weeks of gestation.

In a study by Kopuz and colleagues, 110 shoulders from 60 neonatal cadavers were dissected and analyzed to look for CAL variations.[31] Three CAL types were identified: quadrangular, broad band, and V shaped. Histologic analysis showed that V-shaped ligaments had a thin central tissue close to the coracoid. The data suggest that the primordial CAL is broad shaped but assumes a quadrangular shape because of the different growth rates of the coracoid and acromial ends. In addition, broad and

V-shaped CALs account for the primordial and quadrangular types, and Y-shaped ligaments account for the adult types of the single- or double-banded anatomic variants, respectively. They concluded that various types of CALs are present during the neonatal period and that the final morphology is determined by developmental factors rather than degenerative changes.

Glenohumeral Capsule and Glenohumeral Ligaments

The anterior glenohumeral capsule was found to be thicker than the posterior capsule. The fetal shoulder capsule inserted onto the humeral neck in the same fashion as in the mature shoulder and was found to be confluent with the rotator cuff tendons at their humeral insertion. Superior and middle glenohumeral ligaments were identifiable as capsular thickenings, whereas the inferior glenohumeral ligament was a distinct structure identifiable by 14 weeks of gestation. Anterior and posterior bands were often noticeable in the ligament, consistent with the known inferior glenohumeral ligament complex (IGHLC) anatomy in the adult shoulder.[14] The anterior band of the IGHLC contributed more to formation of the axillary pouch than did the posterior band.

Histologically, the fetal IGHLC consists of several layers of collagen fibers that are highly cellular and have little fibrous tissue during early development. This tissue becomes more fibrous later in gestation. Polarized light microscopy demonstrates that these fibers are only loosely organized but are more organized than adjacent capsular tissues are. Arthroscopic images of the superior glenohumeral ligament have revealed a defined attachment to

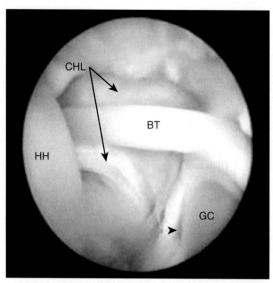

FIGURE 1-24 Arthroscopic view of the left shoulder of a 35-week-old fetus. CHL, coracohumeral ligament; BT, biceps tendon; HH, humeral head; GC, glenoid cavity.

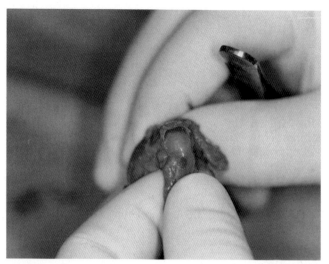

FIGURE 1-25 The fetal acromion process is cartilaginous and adherent to the superior aspect of the humeral head, thus giving the acromion a gentle curve, which is similar to an adult type II acromion.

the humeral head, forming an intersection of the biceps tendon as it enters the bicipital groove and the attachment of the upper edge of the subscapular muscle tendon.[25]

A rotator interval defect was noted in fetuses by 14 weeks of gestation. This capsular defect was seen consistently in the 1-o'clock position in a right shoulder or the 11-o'clock position in a left shoulder. The interval defect was often covered by a thin layer of capsule that extended from the middle glenohumeral ligament and passed superficially to the defect. Removal of this capsular layer revealed a clear defect between the superior and middle glenohumeral ligaments. Histologic examination of the interval defect in a 19-week-old specimen revealed a thin surrounding capsule with poorly organized collagen fibers. To our knowledge, this is the first suggestion that the capsular defect is not acquired. Specimens with larger rotator interval defects had greater amounts of inferior glenohumeral laxity. Closure of a large rotator interval defect in adults has been shown to be effective treatment of inferior glenohumeral instability.[32-34]

Glenoid

The fetal glenoid has a lateral tilt of the superior glenoid rim relative to the inferior rim in the coronal plane; in contrast, the adult shoulder is more vertically oriented. The labrum was noted at 13 weeks of gestation. The anterior and posterior aspects of the labrum became confluent with the anterior and posterior bands of the IGHLC, respectively. Detachment of the anterosuperior labrum at the waist of the comma-shaped glenoid was noted in specimens after 22 weeks of gestation, and such detachment corresponds to an area of variable labral detachment seen in mature shoulders. Gross discoloration of the glenoid hyaline cartilage in the inferior half of the glenoid is noted in specimens at 30 weeks in approximately the same area as the bare spot that is seen in the mature shoulder. No histologic evidence could be found of a bare area of glenoid hyaline cartilage as seen in the adult glenohumeral joint, and thus it may be acquired.

POSTNATAL DEVELOPMENT

Postnatal development of the shoulder is concerned mainly with appearance and development of the secondary centers of ossification, because the soft tissues change only in size after birth. Development of the individual bones is discussed separately.

Clavicle

The clavicle, along with the mandible, is the first bone in the body to ossify, during the fifth week of gestation. Most bones in the body develop by endochondral ossification, in which condensations of mesenchymal tissue become cartilage and then undergo ossification. The major portion of the clavicle forms by intramembranous ossification, in which mesenchymal cells are mineralized directly into bone. Two separate ossification centers form during the fifth week, the lateral and the medial. The lateral center is usually more prominent than the medial center, and the two masses form a long mass of bone. The cells at the acromial and sternal ends of the clavicle take on a cartilaginous pattern to form the sternoclavicular and acromioclavicular joints. Therefore, the clavicle increases in diameter by intramembranous ossification of the periosteum and grows in length through endochondral activity at the cartilaginous ends. The medial clavicular epiphysis is responsible for the majority of longitudinal growth (Fig. 1-26). It begins to ossify at 18 years of age and fuses with the clavicle between the ages of 22 and 25 years. The lateral epiphysis is less constant; it often appears as a

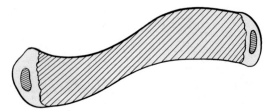

FIGURE 1-26 The medial clavicular epiphysis is responsible for most of the longitudinal growth of the clavicle. It fuses at 22 to 25 years of age. The lateral epiphysis is less constant; it often appears as a wafer-like edge of bone and may be confused with a fracture.

wafer-like edge of bone just proximal to the acromioclavicular joint and can be confused with a fracture.

Scapula

The majority of the scapula forms by intramembranous ossification. At birth, the body and the spine of the scapula have ossified, but not the coracoid process, glenoid, acromion, vertebral border, and inferior angle. The coracoid process has two and occasionally three centers of ossification (Fig. 1-27). The first center appears during the first year of life in the center of the coracoid process. The second center arises at approximately 10 years of age and appears at the base of the coracoid process. The second ossific nucleus also contributes to formation of the superior portion of the glenoid cavity. These two centers unite with the scapula at approximately 15 years of age. A third inconsistent ossific center can appear at the tip of the coracoid process during puberty and occasionally fails to fuse with the coracoid. It is often confused with a fracture, just like the distal clavicular epiphysis.

The acromion has two and occasionally three ossification centers as well. These centers arise during puberty and fuse together at approximately 22 years of age. This may be confused with a fracture when an unfused apophysis, most often a meso-acromion, is visualized on an axillary view. This finding is not uncommon and is often seen in patients with impingement syndrome.

The glenoid fossa has two ossification centers. The first center appears at the base of the coracoid process at approximately 10 years of age and fuses around 15 years of age; it contributes as well to the superior portion of the glenoid cavity and the base of the coracoid process. The second is a horseshoe-shaped center arising from the inferior portion of the glenoid during puberty, and it forms the lower three fourths of the glenoid.

The vertebral border and inferior angle of the scapula each have one ossification center, both of which appear at puberty and fuse at approximately 22 years of age.

Proximal Humerus

The proximal end of the humerus has three ossification centers (Fig. 1-28): one for the head of the humerus, one

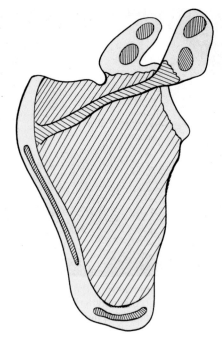

FIGURE 1-27 The coracoid process has two (sometimes three) centers of ossification. A third inconsistent ossific center can appear at the tip of the coracoid process during puberty, and occasionally this center fails to fuse with the coracoid. It may be confused with a fracture. The acromion has two (occasionally three) ossification centers as well; an unfused apophysis is not an uncommon finding and is often manifested as impingement syndrome.

for the greater tuberosity, and one for the lesser tuberosity. The ossification center in the humeral head usually appears between the fourth and sixth months, although it has been reported in *Gray's Anatomy*[35] to be present in 20% of newborns. Without this radiographic landmark, it is often quite difficult to diagnose birth injuries. The ossification center for the greater tuberosity arises during the third year, and the center for the lesser tuberosity appears during the fifth year. The epiphyses for the tuberosities fuse together during the fifth year as well, and they in turn fuse with the center for the humeral head during the seventh year. Union between the head and the shaft usually occurs at approximately 19 years of age.

ADULT GLENOHUMERAL JOINT

Bony Anatomy

The adult glenohumeral joint is formed by the humeral head and the glenoid surface of the scapula. Their geometric relationship allows a remarkable range of motion. However, this range of motion is achieved with a concurrent loss of biomechanical stability. The large spherical head of the humerus articulates against—and not within—a smaller glenoid fossa. This relationship is best com-

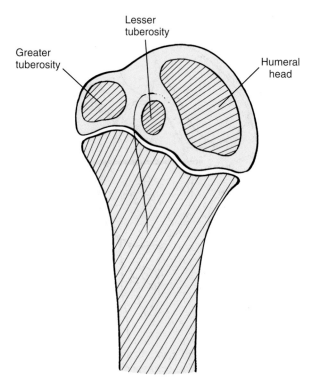

FIGURE 1-28 The proximal end of the humerus has three ossification centers: for the head of the humerus, for the greater tuberosity, and for the lesser tuberosity.

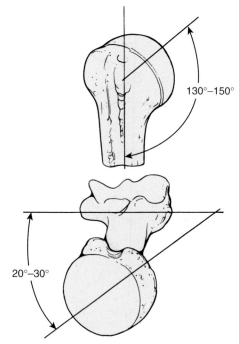

FIGURE 1-29 The neck and head of the humerus have an angle of inclination of 130 to 150 degrees in relation to the shaft (*top*) and a retrotorsion angle of 20 to 30 degrees (*bottom*).

pared with a golf ball sitting on a tee, with stability conferred by the static and dynamic soft tissue restraints acting across the joint.

The head of the humerus is a large, globular bony structure whose articular surface forms one third of a sphere and is directed medially, superiorly, and posteriorly. The head is inclined 130 to 150 degrees in relation to the shaft (Fig. 1-29).[1,36-38] Retroversion of the humeral head can be highly variable both among persons and between sides in the same person. Pearl and Volk found a mean of 29.8 degrees of retroversion in 21 shoulders they examined, with a range of 10 to 55 degrees.[39] The average vertical dimension of the head's articular portion is 48 mm, with a 25-mm radius of curvature. The average transverse dimension is 45 mm, with a 22-mm radius of curvature.[40] The bicipital groove is 30 degrees medial to a line passing from the shaft through the center of the head of the humerus (Fig. 1-30). The greater tuberosity forms the lateral wall, and the lesser tuberosity forms the medial wall of this groove.

The glenoid cavity is shaped like an inverted comma (Fig. 1-31). Its superior portion (tail) is narrow and the inferior portion is broad. The transverse line between these two regions roughly corresponds to the epiphyseal line of the glenoid cavity.[11] The glenoid has a concave articular surface covered by hyaline cartilage. In the center of the cavity, a distinct circular area of thinning is often noted. This area, according to DePalma and associ-

ates,[11] is related to the region's greater contact with the humeral head, as well as to age (Fig. 1-32). The average vertical dimension of the glenoid is 35 mm, and the average transverse diameter is 25 mm. Previous studies by Saha[41-43] noted that the glenoid may be either anteverted or retroverted with respect to the plane of the scapula. He found that 75% of the shoulders studied had retroverted glenoid surfaces averaging 7.4 degrees and that approximately 25% of the glenoid surfaces were anteverted 2 to 10 degrees. With regard to vertical tilt, the superior portion of the superior/inferior line of the glenoid is angled an average of 15 degrees medially with regard to the scapular plane, thus making the glenoid surface on which the humeral head lies relatively horizontal (Fig. 1-33).

Based on contact surface studies in 20 shoulders, Saha originally[41] classified glenohumeral articulations into three types: A, B, and C. In type A, the humeral surface has a radius of curvature smaller than that of the glenoid and has a small circular contact area. In type B, the humeral and glenoid surfaces have similar curvatures and a larger circular contact area. In type C, the humeral surface has a radius of curvature larger than that of the glenoid. The contact is limited to the periphery, and the contact surface is ring shaped. However, Soslowsky and colleagues examined 32 cadaveric shoulders using precise stereophotogrammetry and found that mating glenohumeral joint surfaces had remarkably high congruency, all falling

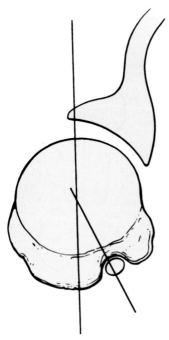

FIGURE 1-30 The bicipital groove is 30 degrees medial to a line that passes from the shaft through the center of the head of the humerus.

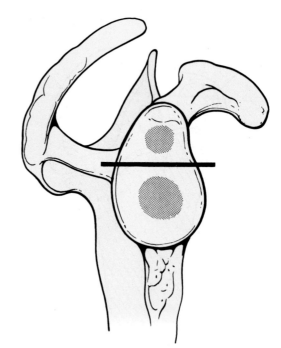

FIGURE 1-31 The glenoid cavity is shaped like an inverted comma. The transverse line corresponds to the epiphyseal line of the glenoid cavity.

into the type B category. Some 88% had radii of curvature within 2 mm of each other, and all cases were congruent to within 3 mm. Humeral head-to-glenoid ratios were 3.12:1 and 2.9:1 for male and female cadavers, respectively. These authors attributed the relative instability of the shoulder not to a shallow or incongruent glenoid but instead to the small surface area relative to the larger humeral head.[44]

The glenoid labrum is a rim of fibrous tissue that is triangular in cross section and overlies the edge of the glenoid cavity (Fig. 1-34). It varies in size and thickness, sometimes being a prominent intra-articular structure with a free inner edge and at other times being virtually absent. Previously, the labrum was likened to the fibrocartilaginous meniscus of the knee; however, Moseley

and Overgaard showed that it was essentially devoid of fibrocartilage, except in a small transition zone at its osseous attachment.[45] The majority of the labrum is dense fibrous tissue with a few elastic fibers. It is, however, important for maintaining glenohumeral stability.[10,46-51] The labrum is responsible for increasing the depth of the glenoid cavity by up to 50%, as well as for increasing the surface area contact with the humeral head.[47,50] It can also act as a fibrous anchor from which the biceps tendon and glenohumeral ligaments can take origin.

The long head of the biceps tendon passes intra-articularly and inserts into the supraglenoid tubercle. It is often continuous with the superior portion of the labrum. Previous studies by DePalma and associates[11] have shown that considerable variation may be present in this struc-

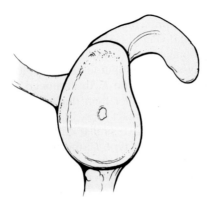

FIGURE 1-32 A bare area is often noted in the center of the glenoid cavity; this area may be related to greater contact pressure and also to age.

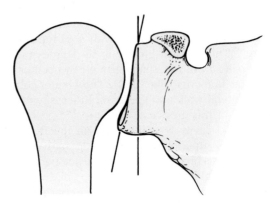

FIGURE 1-33 The superior portion of the superoinferior line of the glenoid is angled at an average of 15 degrees medially with regard to the scapular plane.

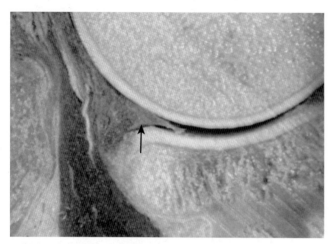

FIGURE 1-34 The glenoid labrum, a rim of fibrous tissue triangular in cross section, overlies the glenoid cavity at the rim or edge. It can have a striking resemblance to the meniscus in the knee.

ture. It can exist as a double structure, it can be located within the fibrous capsule, or, as in one case, it can be absent from within the joint. Electromyographic analysis of shoulder motion demonstrates that despite its presence within the joint, the long head of the biceps is not involved in glenohumeral motion.[52] It can contribute to shoulder pathology in may ways, however. In older patients, especially from the fifth decade onward, failure of the rotator cuff can lead to significant biceps degeneration through superior migration of the humeral head. Such degeneration is manifested as thickening, widening, and shredding. Andrews has also described similar changes in younger throwers.[53-56]

Shoulder Capsule

The shoulder capsule is large and has twice the surface area of the humeral head. It typically accepts approximately 28 to 35 mL of fluid; it accepts more fluid in women than in men. However, in pathologic conditions, this amount varies.[57] For example, in patients with adhesive capsulitis, the shoulder capsule accept only 5 mL or less of fluid, whereas in patients with considerable laxity or instability it can accept larger volumes of fluid.

The capsule is lined by synovium and extends from the glenoid neck (or occasionally the labrum) to the anatomic neck and the proximal shaft of the humerus to varying degrees. The capsule often extends and attaches to the coracoid process superiorly (via the coracohumeral ligament) and on either side of the scapular body (via the anterior and posterior recesses). It can extend down along the biceps tendon for variable lengths and across the intertubercular groove of the humerus. The joint capsule blends with ligamentous structures arising on nearby bony landmarks and contains within its substance the glenohumeral ligaments, including the inferior glenohumeral complex. All of these structures show great variation in size, shape, thickness, and attachment.

The coracohumeral ligament is a rather strong band that originates from the base and lateral border of the coracoid process just below the origin of the coracoacromial ligament (Fig. 1-35). It is directed transversely and inserts on the greater tuberosity. The anterior border is often distinct medially and merges with the capsule laterally. The posterior border is usually indistinct from the remaining capsule. Some authors believe that phylogenetically it represents the previous insertion of the pectoralis minor, and in 15% of the population, a part of the pectoralis minor crosses the coracoid process to insert on

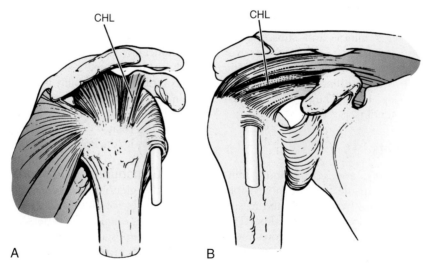

FIGURE 1-35 The coracohumeral ligament (CHL) is a strong band that originates from the base of the lateral border of the coracoid process, just below the coracoacromial ligament, and merges with the capsule laterally to insert on the greater tuberosity. This ligament may be important as a suspensory structure for the adducted arm. **A,** Lateral view. **B,** Anteroposterior view.

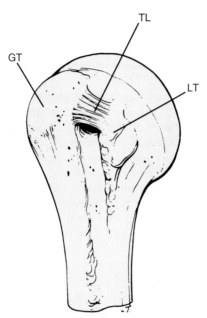

FIGURE 1-36 The transverse humeral ligament (TL) consists of transverse fibers of the capsule extending between the greater tuberosity (GT) and the lesser tuberosity (LT); it contains the tendon of the long head of the biceps in its groove.

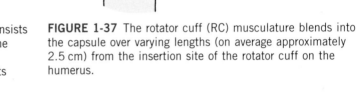

FIGURE 1-37 The rotator cuff (RC) musculature blends into the capsule over varying lengths (on average approximately 2.5 cm) from the insertion site of the rotator cuff on the humerus.

the humeral head.[35] Although the biomechanical contribution of this ligament is not yet fully known, it appears to have static suspensory function for the humeral head in the glenoid cavity when the arm is in the dependent position. With abduction, the ligament relaxes and loses its ability to support the humerus.

The transverse humeral ligament (Fig. 1-36) consists of a few transverse fibers of capsule that extend between the greater and lesser tuberosities; it helps contain the tendon of the long head of the biceps in its groove.

On all sides of the shoulder capsule except the inferior portion, the capsule is reinforced and strengthened by the tendons of the rotator cuff muscles, that is, the supraspinatus, infraspinatus, teres minor, and subscapularis (Fig. 1-37). The tendons blend into the capsule over varying lengths and average approximately 2.5 cm. The most prominent of these is the tendinous portion of the subscapularis anteriorly (Fig. 1-38). They form the musculotendinous, or capsulotendinous, cuff.

Glenohumeral Ligaments

The glenohumeral ligaments are collagenous reinforcements to the shoulder capsule that are not visible on its external surface. They are best appreciated in situ arthroscopically without distension by air or saline (Fig. 1-39). Their function depends on their collagenous integrity, their attachment sites, and the position of the arm.

Superior Glenohumeral Ligament

The superior glenohumeral ligament is a fairly constant structure present in 97% of shoulders examined in the

classic anatomic study by DePalma and in 26% to 90% of specimens in an anatomic study conducted at our institution.[11,51] Three common variations are seen in its glenoid attachment[11]: it arises from a common origin with the biceps tendon; it arises from the labrum, slightly anterior to the tendon; or it originates with the middle glenohumeral ligament (Fig. 1-40). It inserts into the fovea capitis and lies just superior to the lesser tuberosity (Fig. 1-41).[58] The size and integrity of this ligament are also quite variable. It can exist as a thin wisp of capsular tissue or as a thickening similar to the patellofemoral ligaments in the knee.

Biomechanical studies that we have performed show that it contributes very little to static stability of the glenohumeral joint.[59] Selective cutting of this ligament did not significantly affect translation either anteriorly or posteriorly in the abducted shoulder.

Its contribution to stability is best demonstrated with the arm in the dependent position, where it helps keep the humeral head suspended (along with the coracohumeral ligament and rotator cuff). Its relative contribution is contingent upon its thickness and collagenous integrity.

Middle Glenohumeral Ligament

The middle glenohumeral ligament shows the greatest variation in size of all the glenohumeral ligaments and is not present as often as the others. In 96 shoulders studied by DePalma and colleagues,[11] it was a well-formed, distinct structure in 68 cases, poorly defined in 16 cases, and absent in 12 cases. We found that it was absent in approximately 27% of the specimens that we studied.[51] In an individual specimen, it may be either quite thin or as thick as the biceps tendon (Fig. 1-42). When present,

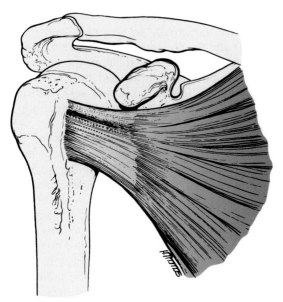

FIGURE 1-38 The subscapularis muscle inserts into the lesser tuberosity with the most superior portion and has a distinct thickening that can resemble a tendon.

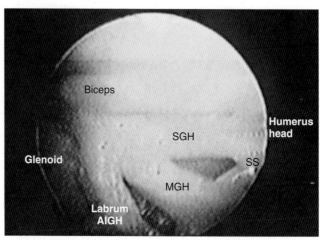

FIGURE 1-39 The glenohumeral ligaments are best appreciated by arthroscopic visualization without distention with air or saline. In this view, the various glenohumeral ligaments are seen as they appear from a posterior portal view. AIGH, anterior inferior glenohumeral ligament; MGH, middle glenohumeral ligament; SGH, superior glenohumeral ligament; SS, subscapularis.

it arises most commonly from the labrum immediately below the superior glenohumeral ligament or from the adjacent neck of the glenoid. It inserts into the humerus just medial to the lesser tuberosity, under the tendon of the subscapularis to which it adheres (see Fig. 1-41).[58] Other variations are seen in which the middle glenohumeral ligament has no attachment site other than the anterior portion of the capsule, or it can exist as two parallel thickenings in the anterior capsule. Its contribution to static stability is variable. However, when it is quite thick, it can act as an important secondary restraint to anterior translation if the anterior portion of the inferior glenohumeral ligament is damaged.[59]

Inferior Glenohumeral Ligament

The inferior glenohumeral ligament is a complex structure that is the main static stabilizer of the abducted shoulder. Although it was originally described as triangular, with its apex at the labrum and its base blending with the capsule between the subscapularis and the triceps area, Turkel and colleagues[58] expanded on the anatomic description by calling attention to the especially thickened anterior superior edge of this ligament, which they called the *superior band of the inferior glenohumeral ligament* (Fig. 1-43). In addition, they called the region between the superior band and the middle glenohumeral ligament the *anterior axillary pouch* and called the remainder of the capsule posterior to the superior band the *posterior axillary pouch*.

With the advent of arthroscopy, we have been able to study the joint in situ and appreciate capsular structures that were disrupted when examination was done by arthrotomy. By inserting the arthroscope from anterior and superior portals, in addition to the traditional poste-

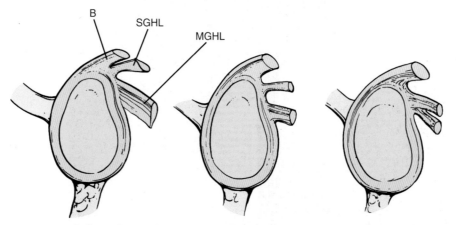

FIGURE 1-40 Three common variations of the origin of the superior glenohumeral ligament (SGHL). B, biceps tendon; MGHL, middle glenohumeral ligament.

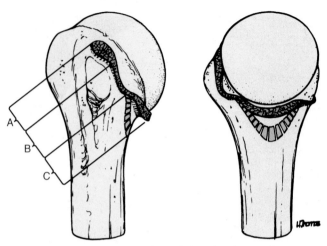

FIGURE 1-41 Attachment sites of the glenohumeral ligaments. *Left,* the superior glenohumeral ligament inserts into the fovea capitis line just superior to the lesser tuberosity (A). The middle glenohumeral ligament inserts into the humerus just medial to the lesser tuberosity (B). The inferior glenohumeral ligament complex has two common attachment mechanisms (C). It can attach in a collar-like fashion (*left*), or it can have a V-shaped attachment to the articular edge (*right*).

rior portals, and by observing the joint without distention by air or saline, we have found that the inferior glenohumeral ligament is more complex than originally thought. It is a hammock-like structure originating from the glenoid and inserting into the anatomic neck of the humerus (Fig. 1-44),[14] and it consists of an anterior band, a posterior band, and an axillary pouch lying in between. We have called this structural arrangement the *inferior glenohumeral ligament complex.* The anterior and posterior bands are most clearly defined with the arm abducted.

In some shoulders, the anterior and posterior bands can only be visualized grossly by internally and externally rotating the arm at 90 degrees of abduction (Fig. 1-45). With abduction and external rotation, the anterior band fans out to support the head, and the posterior band becomes cord-like (Fig. 1-46). Conversely, with internal rotation, the posterior band fans out to support the head, and the anterior band becomes cord-like.

The IGHLC takes its origin from either the glenoid labrum or the glenoid neck and inserts into the anatomic neck of the humerus. The origins of the anterior and posterior bands on the glenoid can be described in terms of the face of a clock. In our anatomic study (Fig. 1-47),[14] the anterior band of each specimen originated from between 2 o'clock and 4 o'clock and the posterior band between 7 o'clock and 9 o'clock. On the humeral head side, the IGHLC attaches in an approximately 90-degree arc just below the articular margin of the humeral head. Two methods of attachment were noted. In some specimens, a collar-like attachment of varying thickness was located just inferior to the articular edge, closer to the articular edge than the remainder of the capsule (Fig. 1-48). In other specimens, the IGHLC attached in a V-shaped fashion, with the anterior and posterior bands attaching close to the articular surface and the axillary pouch attaching to the humerus at the apex of the V, farther from the articular edge (Fig. 1-49).

The IGHLC is thicker than the capsule adjoining it anteriorly and posteriorly (Fig. 1-50), although considerable variation exists. The inferior glenohumeral ligament is thicker than the anterior capsule, which in turn is thicker than the posterior capsule.

The anterior and posterior bands of the IGHLC also show great variation in thickness, but we have been able to identify them in all specimens (Figs. 1-51 and 1-52).[14] Grossly, the anterior band is usually easier to distinguish than the posterior band because it attaches higher on the

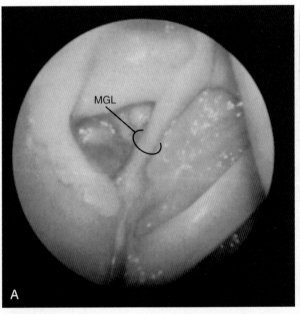

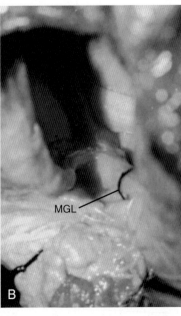

FIGURE 1-42 The middle glenohumeral ligament (MGL) has great variability. It can exist as a thin wisp of tissue (**A**), or it may be as thick as the biceps tendon (**B**).

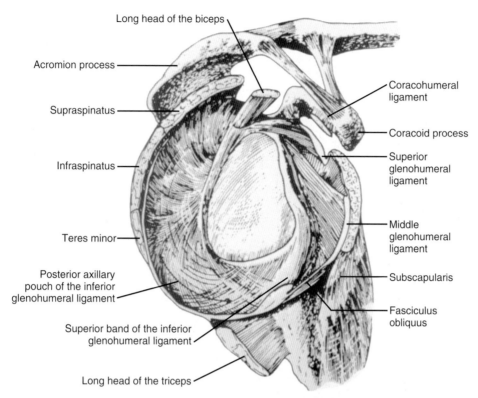

FIGURE 1-43 The anatomic description by Turkel and colleagues of the inferior glenohumeral ligament called attention to the anterior–superior edge of this ligament, which was especially thickened; they called this edge the *superior band of the inferior glenohumeral ligament*. However, no posterior structures are defined. (From Turkel SJ, Panio MW, Marshall JL, Girgis FG: Stabilizing mechanisms preventing anterior dislocation of the glenohumeral joint. J Bone Joint Surg Am 63:1208-1217, 1981.)

glenoid and is generally thicker. However, the anterior and posterior bands can be of equal thickness, and occasionally the posterior band is thicker than the anterior band.

Histologically, the IGHLC is distinguishable from the remainder of the shoulder capsule, and the anterior band,

axillary pouch, and posterior band are distinct structures.[14] Even in cases in which the bands were poorly defined macroscopically, they were easily distinguishable histologically; in fact, the posterior band is easier to distinguish histologically than the anterior band because of a more abrupt transition from the thin posterior capsule.

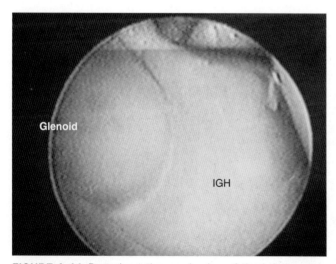

FIGURE 1-44 Posterior arthroscopic view of the inferior glenohumeral (IGH) ligament complex. It is a hammock-like structure originating from the glenoid and inserting onto the anatomic neck of the humerus.

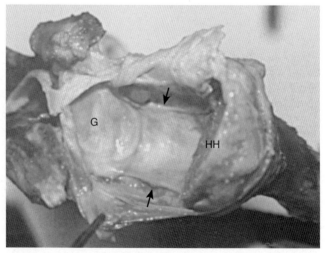

FIGURE 1-45 The anterior and posterior ends of the inferior glenohumeral ligament *(black arrows)* complex are clearly defined in this picture of an abducted shoulder specimen with the humeral head (HH) partially resected. G, glenoid.

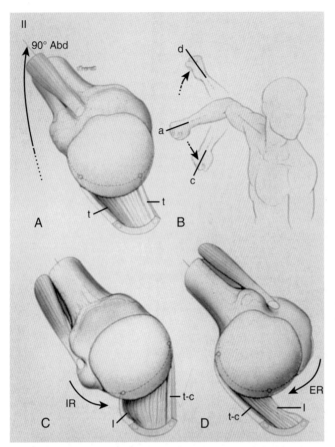

FIGURE 1-46 A, The inferior glenohumeral complex is tightened during abduction. **B,** During abduction and internal or external rotation, different parts of the band are tightened. **C,** With internal rotation (IR), the posterior band fans out to support the head, and the anterior band becomes cord-like or relaxed, depending on the degree of horizontal flexion or extension. **D,** On abduction and external rotation (ER), the anterior band fans out to support the head, and the posterior band becomes cord-like or relaxed, depending on the degree of horizontal flexion or extension. a, neutral; Abd, abduction; c, internal rotation; d, external rotation; l, loose; t, anterior and posterior band of glenohumeral ligament; t-c, tight, cord-like.

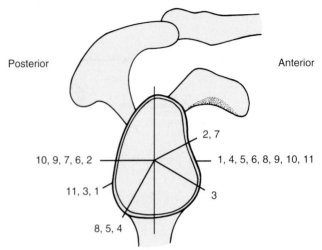

FIGURE 1-47 The glenoid attachment sites of the anterior and posterior bands. In 11 cadaver specimens (indicated by *number labels*), the anterior band originated from various areas between 2 o'clock and 4 o'clock and the posterior band from areas between 7 o'clock and 9 o'clock.

inner layer, oriented at 90 degrees to the middle layer. The inner layer is displaced outward at the expense of relative thinning of the outer layer. This finding can be appreciated quite well in coronal views of the posterior band (Fig. 1-56).

The transition from the posterior band to the axillary pouch is less distinct, and the axillary pouch exhibits a gradual intermingling of the coarse longitudinal inner fibers with the sagittal transverse fibers, which are continuous with the transverse fibers of the middle layer (Fig. 1-57). In the axillary pouch region, the outer layer is attenuated and virtually disappears.

The anterior band also exists as an abrupt thickening of the inner layer of the anterior capsule, although the distinction is not as marked histologically as the transition with the posterior band and the posterior capsule. The

The shoulder capsule consists of a synovial lining and three well-defined layers of collagen (Fig. 1-53). The fibers of the inner and outer layers extend in the coronal plane from the glenoid to the humerus. The middle layer of collagen extends in a sagittal direction and crosses the fibers of the other two layers. The relative thickness and degree of intermingling of collagen fibers of the three layers vary with the different portions of the capsule.

The posterior capsule is quite thin (Fig. 1-54). The three layers of the capsule are well seen, but the outer layer is least prominent and quickly blends into a layer of loose areolar tissue outside the capsule.

The posterior band of the IGHLC exists as an abrupt thickening in the capsule (Fig. 1-55). This thickening is due mostly to the presence of increased, well-organized, coarse collagen bundles in the coronal plane within the

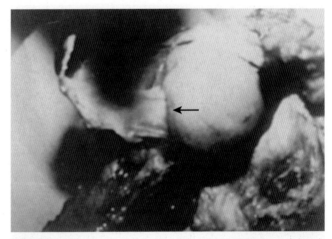

FIGURE 1-48 An example of a collar-like attachment *(arrow)* of the inferior glenohumeral ligament complex just inferior to the articular edge and closer to the articular edge than the remainder of the capsule.

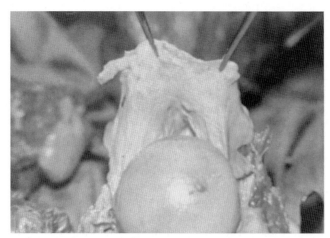

FIGURE 1-49 A V-shaped attachment of the inferior glenohumeral ligament complex of the humerus, with the axillary pouch attaching to the humerus at the apex of the V farther from the articular edge.

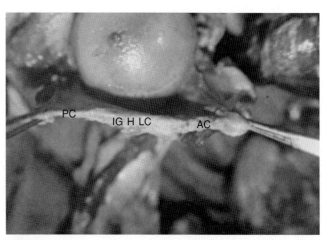

FIGURE 1-50 The inferior glenohumeral ligament complex (IGHLC) is thicker than the anterior capsule (AC) and the posterior capsule (PC).

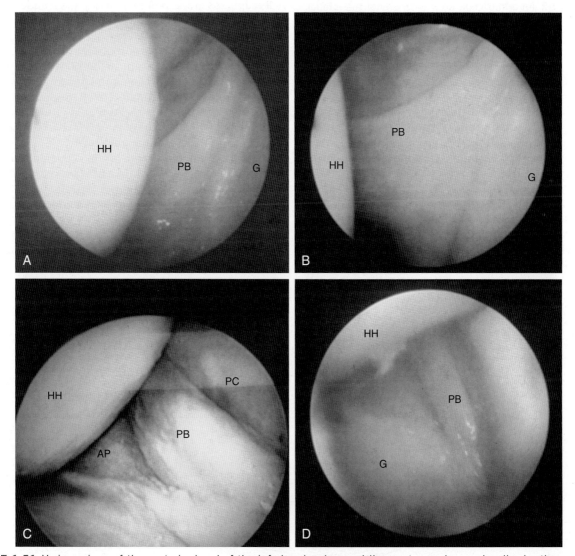

FIGURE 1-51 Various views of the posterior band of the inferior glenohumeral ligament complex as visualized arthroscopically from an anterior portal. **A** and **B** show the distinct configuration of the posterior band (PB) with internal and external rotation. During internal rotation, the posterior band fans out to support the humeral head (HH). **C** and **D** show two superior portal views of the posterior band, the posterior capsule (PC), the axillary pouch (AP), and the glenoid (G).

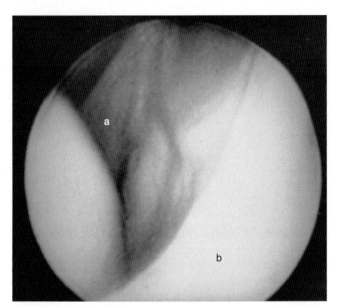

FIGURE 1-52 An arthroscopic view anteriorly of the inferior glenohumeral ligament complex showing the anterior and posterior bands (a and b) and the intervening axillary pouch.

more precise collagen orientation, similar to the posterior band, can be seen, and in the coronal view in Figure 1-58, we can see that the histologic picture is virtually identical to that of the posterior band seen in Figure 1-56. As we again approach the axillary pouch, these bundles lose their precise organization and intermingle with the fibers of the middle layer.

The capsule anterior to the IGHLC is qualitatively thicker than the capsule posterior to the IGHLC, mainly because of the relative increase in thickness of the middle layer. Extensive intermingling of the middle and outer layers of the capsule takes place in this region (see Figs. 1-50 and 1-53).

This view of the IGHLC functioning as a hammock-like sling to support the humeral head (Fig. 1-59) gives a unifying foundation to understand anterior and posterior instability in the human shoulder and explains how damage in one portion of the shoulder capsule can affect the opposite side. This concept has clinical significance for treating instability disorders of the shoulder.

Bursae

Several bursae are present in the shoulder region, and a number of recesses are found in the shoulder capsule between the glenohumeral ligaments. Two bursae in particular have clinical importance: the subacromial bursa, which is discussed later, and the subscapular bursa. The subscapular bursa lies between the subscapularis tendon and the neck of the scapula (Fig. 1-60), and it communicates with the joint cavity between the superior and middle glenohumeral ligaments. It protects the tendon of the subscapularis at the point where it passes under the base of the coracoid process and over the neck of the scapula. This bursa is linked to the coracoid process by a suspensory ligament, and in 28% of specimens dissected by Colas and associates, the subscapular bursae merged with the subcoracoid bursae, forming a unique wide bursa in this region.[60] The subscapular bursa often houses loose bodies in the shoulder, and it is also a region in which synovitis of the shoulder may be most intense, where small fringes, or villi, can project into the joint cavity.

Though uncommon (and not in communication with the joint cavity), another bursa may be present between the infraspinatus muscle and the capsule. Other synovial recesses are usually located in the anterior portion of the capsule. The number, size, and location of these recesses depend on topographic variations in the glenohumeral ligaments. DePalma and associates[11] described six common variations or types of recesses in the anterior

SAGITTAL SCHEMATIC OF HISTOLOGY

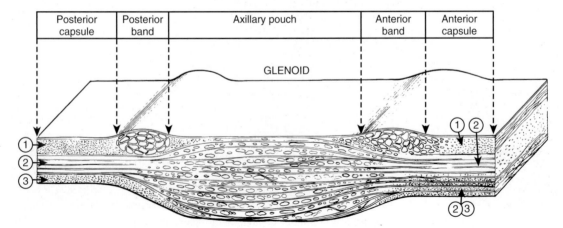

FIGURE 1-53 Schematic representation of the histologic layers of the shoulder capsule. The capsule consists of a thin synovial lining and three well-defined layers of collagen (see text).

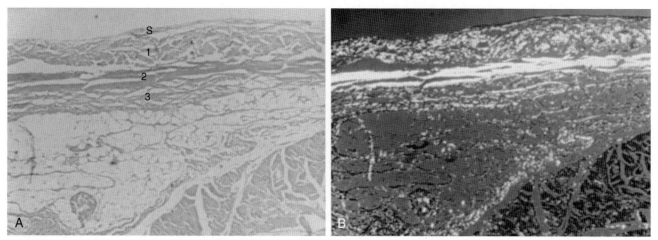

FIGURE 1-54 The posterior capsule is quite thin, and all three layers of the shoulder capsule along with the synovium (S) can be seen in these hematoxylin and eosin (**A**) and polarized (**B**) views. The posterior capsule quickly blends into a layer of loose areolar tissue outside the capsule.

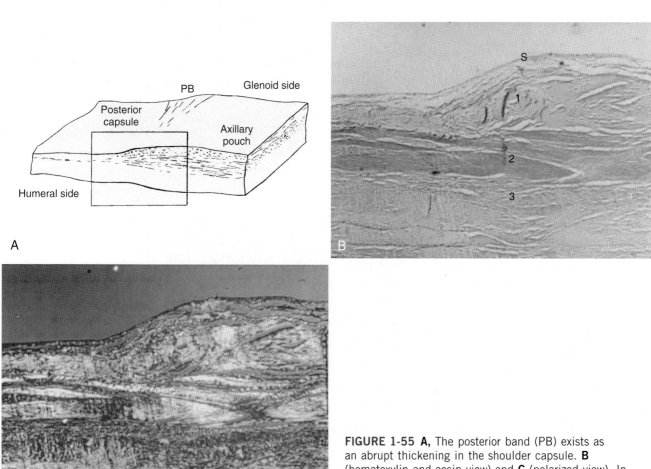

FIGURE 1-55 A, The posterior band (PB) exists as an abrupt thickening in the shoulder capsule. **B** (hematoxylin and eosin view) and **C** (polarized view), In these sagittal views, the thickening can be seen in the inner layer of the capsule.

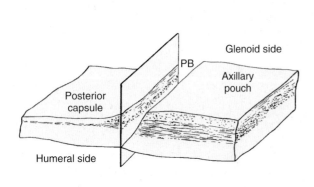

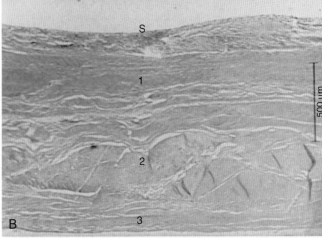

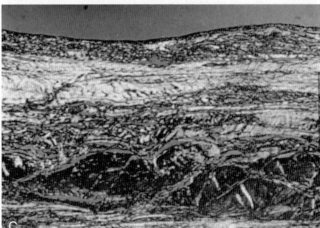

FIGURE 1-56 A, The precise organization of the posterior band (PB) is shown. In **B** (hematoxylin and eosin view) and **C** (polarized view), coronal views demonstrate three well-defined layers in this region.

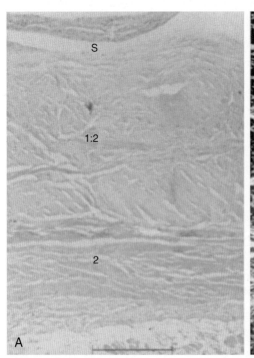

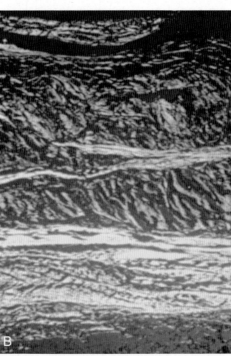

FIGURE 1-57 In **A** (hematoxylin and eosin view) and **B** (polarized view), sagittal views of the axillary pouch show blending of the inner and middle layers and a continuation of the outermost layer.

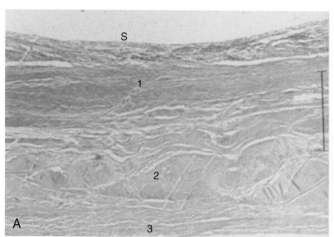 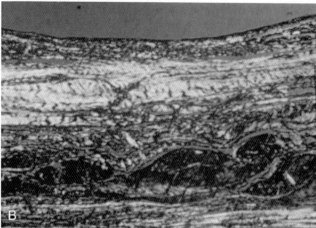

FIGURE 1-58 In **A** (hematoxylin and eosin view) and **B** (polarized view), the more precise collagen orientation returns in the region of the anterior band, as seen in these coronal views. These views are virtually identical with those of the posterior band in Figure 1-56.

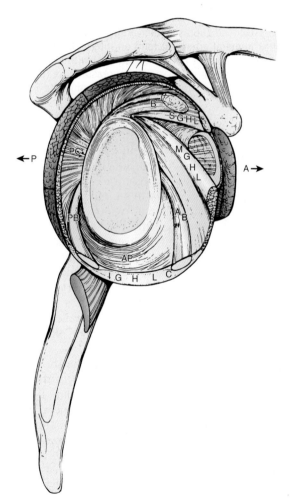

capsule (Fig. 1-61), which are really variations in the opening of the subscapularis bursa: type 1 (30.2%) has one synovial recess above the middle glenohumeral ligament; type 2 (2.04%) has one synovial recess below the middle glenohumeral ligament; type 3 (40.6%) has one recess above and one below the middle glenohumeral ligament; type 4 (9.03%) has one large recess above the inferior ligament, with the middle glenohumeral ligament being absent. In type 5 (5.1%), the middle glenohumeral ligament is manifested as two small synovial folds, and type 6 (11.4%) has no synovial recesses, but all the ligaments are well defined. Regardless of the type in which the recesses are found, the recesses show extreme variability. DePalma thought that if the capsule arises at the

FIGURE 1-59 Anatomic depiction of the glenohumeral ligaments and inferior glenohumeral ligament complex (IGHLC). A, anterior; AB, anterior band; AP, axillary pouch; B, biceps tendon; MGHL, middle glenohumeral ligament; P, posterior; PB, posterior band; PC, posterior capsule; SGHL, superior glenohumeral ligament.

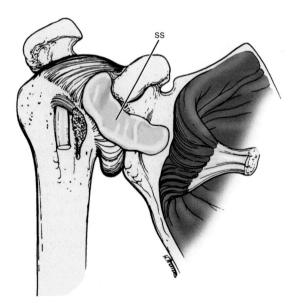

FIGURE 1-60 This subscapular (SS) bursa connects anteriorly and inferiorly under the coracoid process in the anterior portion of the capsule. Loose bodies are often found in this region.

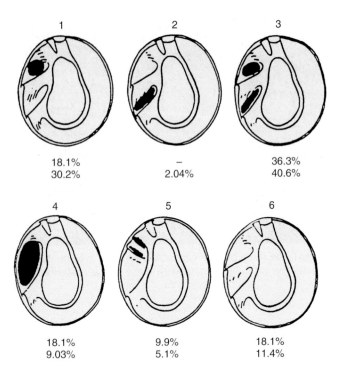

1	2	3
18.1%	–	36.3%
30.2%	2.04%	40.6%

4	5	6
18.1%	9.9%	18.1%
9.03%	5.1%	11.4%

FIGURE 1-61 Variations in the types of anterior recesses in the capsule. The original percentages of DePalma are listed (top lines), along with percentages from more recent anatomic studies (bottom lines).

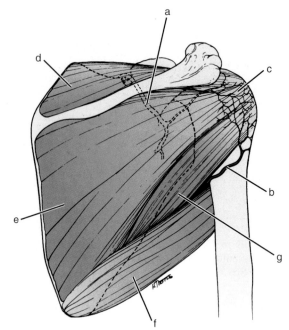

FIGURE 1-62 The suprascapular artery (a) and the posterior circumflex humeral artery (b) form an interlacing pattern on the posterior portion of the rotator cuff (c) with several large anastomoses. Also depicted are the supraspinatus (d), infraspinatus (e), teres major (f), and teres minor (g).

labrum or glenoid border of the scapula, few, if any recesses will be present. If the capsule begins farther medially on the scapula or glenoid neck, however, the synovial recesses are larger and more numerous. He believed that the end result of such recesses was a thin, weakened anterior capsule that can predispose the shoulder to instability.

Others refer to this general area of the anterior capsule as the *rotator interval*,[61] which they define as the space between the superior border of the subscapularis and the anterior border of the supraspinatus. This interval includes the region of the superior glenohumeral ligament and coracohumeral ligament, in addition to the middle glenohumeral ligament. Plancher and colleagues[62] found the average area of this region to be 20.96 mm². Some authors believe that enlargement of the interval can cause instability in certain shoulders and that it should be surgically obliterated during stabilization procedures.[61,63] Dynamic testing has shown that the subscapularis and supraspinatus dimensions as well as the total area of the rotator interval decrease significantly with internal rotation and open with external rotation. Imbrication procedures are performed with the arm in neutral to avoid loss of motion or insufficient tightening.[62]

Microvasculature

Rotator Cuff

Six arteries regularly contribute to the arterial supply of the rotator cuff tendons: suprascapular (100%), anterior circumflex humeral (100%), posterior circumflex humeral (100%), thoracoacromial (76%), suprahumeral (59%), and subscapular (38%).[64,65] The posterior circumflex humeral and suprascapular arteries form an interlacing pattern on the posterior portion of the cuff with several large anastomoses. These vessels are the predominant arteries to the teres minor and the infraspinatus tendons (Fig. 1-62). The anterior humeral circumflex artery supplies the subscapularis muscle and tendon and anastomoses with the posterior humeral circumflex over the tendon of the long head of the biceps (Fig. 1-63). In addition, a large branch of the anterior humeral circumflex artery enters the intertubercular groove and becomes the major blood supply to the humeral head.

Branches of the acromial portion of the thoracoacromial artery supply the anterosuperior part of the rotator cuff, particularly the supraspinatus tendon (Fig. 1-64), and often anastomose with both circumflex humeral arteries. The subscapular and suprahumeral arteries (named by Rothman and Parke to describe a small vessel from the third portion of the axillary artery to the anterior rotator cuff and lesser tuberosity) make only a minimal contribution.[65] Approximately two thirds of shoulders have a hypovascular zone in the tendinous portion of the supraspinatus just proximal to its insertion. Less commonly, the infraspinatus (37%) and the subscapularis (7%) also have a poorly perfused area. This area of hypovascularity corresponds to the common areas of degeneration. The hypovascular regions may be present at birth,[66] however,

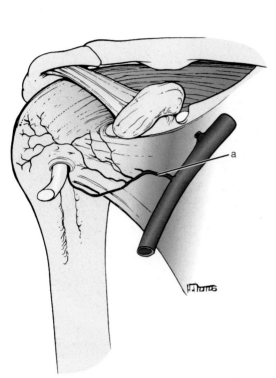

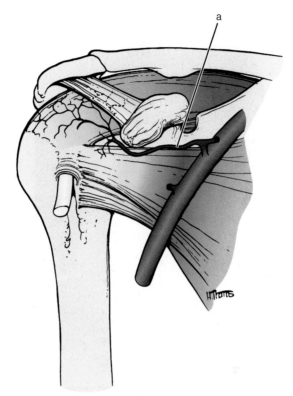

FIGURE 1-63 The anterior humeral circumflex artery (a) supplies the subscapularis muscle and tendon and anastomoses with the posterior humeral circumflex over the tendon of the long head of the biceps. In addition, a large branch of the anterior humeral circumflex enters the intertubercular groove and becomes the major blood supply to the head.

FIGURE 1-64 The acromial branch (a) of the thoracoacromial artery supplies the anterosuperior portion of the rotator cuff, particularly the supraspinatus tendon.

and a significant decrease in vascularity with aging and degeneration can be seen.

Rathbun and Macnab[66] demonstrated that in this hypovascular critical zone in the rotator cuff, vascular filling depends on the position of the arm, with less filling noted when the arm is in adduction (Fig. 1-65). Most likely, filling is also chronically impeded by advanced impingement, with the humeral head and rotator cuff impinging on the acromion, compressing the hypovascular zone, and limiting the potential for repair of small attritional

tears in these locations. This mechanism has never been proved, however.

Glenoid Labrum

The glenoid labrum is supplied by small branches of three major vessels supplying the shoulder joint: the suprascapular artery, the circumflex scapular artery, and the posterior humeral circumflex artery (Fig. 1-66). These vessels supply the peripheral attachment of the labrum through small periosteal and capsular vessels (Fig. 1-67).

FIGURE 1-65 The hypovascular critical zone in the rotator cuff in abduction (**A**) and adduction (**B**). Pure filling depends on the position of the arm, with less filling noted when the arm is in adduction. (From Rathbun JB, Macnab I: The microvascular pattern of the rotator cuff. J Bone Joint Surg Br 52:540-553, 1970.)

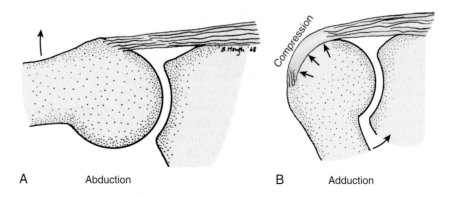

A   Abduction   B   Adduction

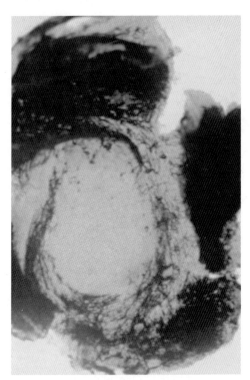

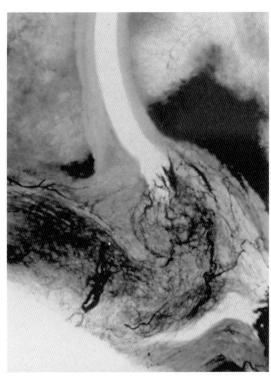

FIGURE 1-66 Microvasculature of the shoulder capsule and labrum. The inferior glenohumeral ligament complex has increased vascularity with regard to the remainder of the posterior capsule, which is relatively devoid of significant vasculature.

FIGURE 1-67 The vasculature of the labrum's edge is shown. Small periosteal and capsular vessels are visible.

Although the extent of these microvascular patterns is variable throughout the labrum, they are usually limited to the outermost aspect of the labrum, with the inner rim being devoid of vessels. This arrangement is similar to that observed in the menisci in the knee.[48]

Capsule and Glenohumeral Ligaments

The glenohumeral capsule and ligaments have a predictable blood supply, with contributions from the suprascapular, circumflex scapular, posterior circumflex scapular, and anterior circumflex arteries.

In a study by Andary and Petersen, adult cadaveric shoulders were analyzed to further characterize vascular patterns to the glenohumeral capsule and ligaments.[67] They found that the arterial supply to the capsule is centripetal, entering superficially and then penetrating deeper. There are four distinct regions of the capsule receiving consistent patterns of vascularity. The anterior and posterior circumflex scapular arteries enter the capsule laterally. The suprascapular and circumflex scapulars enter the capsule medially and arborize with the humeral circumflex vessels as they all converge on the middle of the capsule. The anterior humeral circumflex supplies the anterior part of the lateral aspect of the capsule. The posterior part of the lateral capsule is supplied by the posterior humeral circumflex. Medially, the periosteal network of the anterior aspect of the scapula supplies the anteromedial capsule, and branches of the circumflex

scapular and suprascapular arteries supply the capsule posteriorly. Perforating arteries from the rotator cuff tendons and muscle enter the capsule superficially in the midsubstance and at the humeral insertion, then penetrate to deeper layers.

The predominant arterial supply of the shoulder capsule is oriented in a horizontal fashion. This orientation is particularly evident in the region of the IGHLC.[14,67] The anterior and inferior aspects of the shoulder capsule demonstrate a denser vascular network than does the thin posterior capsule. However, a watershed region of hypovascularity was noted in the anterior aspect of the capsule near the humeral insertion in 5 of 12 specimens.[67] The authors correlated these findings with an associated hypovascular region in the critical zone of the supraspinatus tendon. Based on these results, they warn that surgical approaches to the shoulder that separate the rotator cuff from the underlying capsule can compromise the perforating vascularity to the capsule. Furthermore, laterally based incisions will probably cross the dominant horizontal vessels of the shoulder capsule.

Innervation

The superficial and deep structures of the shoulder are profusely innervated by a network of nerve fibers that are mainly derived from the C5, C6, and C7 nerve roots (the C4 root can make a minor contribution).[20,68] The

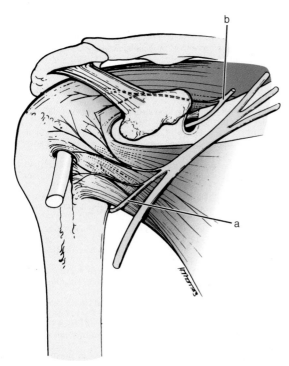

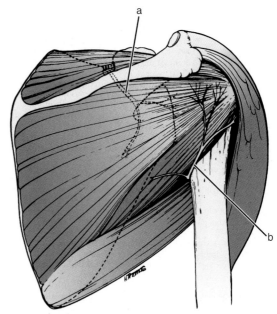

FIGURE 1-69 Posterior innervation of the shoulder joint. The primary nerves are the suprascapular (a) and the axillary (b).

FIGURE 1-68 Innervation of the anterior portion of the shoulder. The axillary (a) and suprascapular (b) nerves form most of the nerve supply to the capsule and glenohumeral joint. In some cases the musculocutaneous nerve sends some twigs to the anterosuperior portion of the joint.

innervation of the joint itself follows Hilton's law, which states that nerves crossing a joint give off branches to the joint, providing its innervation. Therefore, nerves supplying the ligaments, capsule, and synovial membrane of the shoulder are medullary and nonmedullary fibers from the axillary, suprascapular, subscapular, and musculocutaneous nerves. Occasional contributions are made from small branches of the posterior cord of the brachial plexus. The relative contributions made by any of these nerves are inconsistent, and the supply from the musculocutaneous nerve may be very small or completely absent.

After piercing the joint capsule, branches from these nerves form a network, or plexus, to supply the synovium. Anteriorly, the axillary nerve and suprascapular nerve provide most of the nerve supply to the capsule and glenohumeral joint. In some instances, the musculocutaneous nerve innervates the anterosuperior portion. In addition, the anterior capsule may be supplied by either the subscapular nerves or the posterior cord of the brachial plexus after they have pierced the subscapularis (Fig. 1-68).

Superiorly, the nerves making the primary contributions are two branches of the suprascapular nerve, with one branch proceeding anteriorly as far as the coracoid process and coracoacromial ligament, and the other branch reaching the posterior aspect of the joint. Other nerves contributing to this region of the joint are the axil-

lary nerve, musculocutaneous nerve, and branches from the lateral anterior thoracic nerve. Posteriorly, the chief nerves are the suprascapular nerve in the upper region and the axillary nerve in the lower region (Fig. 1-69). Inferiorly, the anterior portion is primarily supplied by the axillary nerve, and the posterior portion is supplied by a combination of the axillary nerve and lower ramifications of the suprascapular nerve.

Alpantaki and colleagues have performed an immunohistochemical staining study on cadavers to elucidate the innervation to the long head of the biceps tendon.[69] The authors found that thinly myelinated or unmyelinated sensory neurons provided innervation to this tendon. This supports the concept that the long head of the biceps tendon may be the pain generator in patients with shoulder pathology and is an area of ongoing study.

REFERENCES

1. Evans FG, Krahl VE: The torsion of the humerus: A phylogenetic survey from fish to man. Am J Anat 76:303-337, 1945.
2. Neal HV, Rand HW: Chordate Anatomy. Philadelphia: Blakiston, 1936.
3. McGonnell IM: The evolution of the pectoral girdle. J Anat 199:189-194, 2001.
4. Jenkins FA Jr: The functional anatomy and evolution of the mammalian humero-ulnar articulation. Am J Anat 137:281-297, 1973.
5. Bechtol CO: Biomechanics of the shoulder. Clin Orthop Relat Res (146):37-41, 1980.

6. Inman VT, Saunders M, Abbott LC: Observations on the function of the shoulder joint. J Bone Joint Surg Am 26:1-29, 1944.

7. O'Brien SJ, Schwartz RS, Warren RF, et al: Capsular restraints to anterior-posterior motion of the abducted shoulder: A biomechanical study. J Shoulder Elbow Surg 4:298-308, 1995.

8. Kent BE: Functional anatomy of the shoulder complex. A review. Phys Ther 51:947, 1971.

9. Kronberg M, Brostrom LA, Soderlund V: Retroversion of the humeral head in the normal shoulder and its relationship to the normal range of motion. Clin Orthop Relat Res (253):113-117, 1990.

10. Halder AM, Itoi E, An KN: Anatomy and biomechanics of the shoulder. Orthop Clin North Am 31:159-176, 2000.

11. DePalma AF, Callery G, Bennett GA: Shoulder joint: Variational anatomy and degenerative regions of the shoulder joint. Instr Course Lect 6:255-281, 1949.

12. Gardner E: The embryology of the clavicle. Clin Orthop Relat Res 58:9-16, 1968.

13. Gardner E, Gray DJ: Prenatal development of the human shoulder and acromioclavicular joints. Am J Anat 92:219-276, 1953.

14. O'Brien SJ, Neves MC, Arnoczky SP, et al: The anatomy and histology of the inferior glenohumeral ligament complex of the shoulder. Am J Sports Med 18:449-456, 1990.

15. Moore KL: The Developing Human. Philadelphia: WB Saunders, 1982.

16. Streeter W: Developmental horizons in human embryology. Carnegie Institute Series on Embryology 151. Washington, DC: Carnegie Institute, 1949.

17. Lewis WH: The development of the arm in man. Am J Anat 1:145-183, 1902.

18. Singleton MC: Functional anatomy of the shoulder. Phys Ther 46:1043-1051, 1966.

19. Haines RW: The development of joints. J Anat 81:33-55, 1947.

20. Gardner E: The innervation of the shoulder joint. Anat Rec 102:1-18, 1948.

21. Johnston TB: The movements of the shoulder joint: A plea for the use of the "plane of the scapula" as the plane of reference for movements occurring at the humero-scapular joint. Br J Surg 25:252-260, 1937.

22. Matsuoka T, Ahlberg PE, Kessaris N, et al: Neural crest origins of the neck and shoulder. Nature 436:347-355, 2005.

23. Aboul-Mahasen LM, Sadek SA: Developmental morphological and histological studies on structures of the human fetal shoulder joint. Cells Tissues Organs 170:1-20, 2002.

24. Fealy S, Rodeo SA, Dicarlo EF, et al: The developmental anatomy of the neonatal glenohumeral joint. J Shoulder Elbow Surg 9:217-222, 2000.

25. Tena-Arregui J, Barrio-Asensio C, Puerta-Fonolla J, et al: Arthroscopic study of the shoulder joint in fetuses. Arthroscopy 21:1114-1119, 2005.

26. Aoki M, Ishii M, Usui M: The slope of the acromion and rotator cuff impingement. Orthop Trans 10:228, 1986.

27. Bigliani LU, Morrison DS, April EW: The morphology of the acromion and its relationship to rotator cuff tears. Orthop Trans 10:228, 1986.

28. MacGillivray JD, Fealy S, Potter HG, et al: Multiplanar analysis of acromion morphology. Am J Sports Med 26:836-840, 1998.

29. Shah NN, Bayliss NC, Malcolm A: Shape of the acromion: Congenital or acquired—a macroscopic, radiographic, and microscopic study of acromion. J Shoulder Elbow Surg 10:309-316, 2001.

30. Fealy S, April EW, Khazzam M, et al: The coracoacromial ligament: Morphology and study of acromial enthesopathy. J Shoulder Elbow Surg 14:542-548, 2005.

31. Kopuz C, Baris S, Yildirim M, et al: Anatomic variations of the coracoacromial ligament in neonatal cadavers: A neonatal cadaver study. J Pediatr Orthop B 11:350-354, 2002.

32. Field LD, Warren RF, O'Brien SJ, et al: Isolated closure of rotator interval defects for shoulder instability. Am J Sports Med 23:557-563, 1995.

33. Harryman DT 2nd, Sidles JA, Harris SL, et al: The role of the rotator interval capsule in passive motion and stability of the shoulder. J Bone Joint Surg Am 74:53-66, 1992.

34. O'Brien SJ, Drakos MC, Allen AA: Arthroscopic assisted rotator interval closure. Tech Shoulder Elbow Surg 3:74-81, 2002.

35. Williams PL, Warwick R (eds): Gray's Anatomy. Philadelphia: WB Saunders, 1980.

36. Cyprien JM, Vasey HM, Burdet A, et al: Humeral retrotorsion and glenohumeral relationship in the normal shoulder and in recurrent anterior dislocation (scapulometry). Clin Orthop Relat Res (175):8-17, 1983.

37. Osbahr DC, Cannon DL, Speer KP: Retroversion of the humerus in the throwing shoulder of college baseball pitchers. Am J Sports Med 30:347-353, 2002.

38. Reagan KM, Meister K, Horodyski MB, et al: Humeral retroversion and its relationship to glenohumeral rotation in the shoulder of college baseball players. Am J Sports Med 30:354-360, 2002.

39. Pearl ML, Volk AG: Coronal plane geometry of the proximal humerus relevant to prosthetic arthroplasty. J Shoulder Elbow Surg 5:320-326, 1996.

40. Iannotti JP, Gabriel JP, Schneck SL, et al: The normal glenohumeral relationships. An anatomical study of one hundred and forty shoulders. J Bone Joint Surg Am 74:491-500, 1992.

41. Saha AK: Theory of Shoulder Mechanism: Descriptive and Applied. Springfield, Ill: Charles C Thomas, 1961.

42. Saha AK: Dynamic stability of the glenohumeral joint. Acta Orthop Scand 42:491-505, 1971.

43. Saha AK: The classic. Mechanism of shoulder movements and a plea for the recognition of "zero position" of glenohumeral joint. Clin Orthop Relat Res (173):3-10, 1983.

44. Soslowsky LJ, Flatow EL, Bigliani LU, et al: Articular geometry of the glenohumeral joint. Clin Orthop Relat Res (285):181-190, 1992.

45. Moseley HF: Recurrent dislocation of the shoulder. Postgrad Med 31:23-29, 1962.

46. Bankart ASB: The pathology and treatment of recurrent dislocation of the shoulder joint. Br J Surg 26:23-29, 1938.

47. Bigliani LU, Kelkar R, Flatow EL, et al: Glenohumeral stability. Biomechanical properties of passive and active stabilizers. Clin Orthop Relat Res (330):13-30, 1996.

48. Cooper DE, Arnoczky SP, O'Brien SJ, et al: Anatomy, histology, and vascularity of the glenoid labrum. An anatomical study. J Bone Joint Surg Am 74:46-52, 1992.

49. Kelkar R, Wang VM, Flatow EL, et al: Glenohumeral mechanics: A study of articular geometry, contact, and kinematics. J Shoulder Elbow Surg 10:73-84, 2001.

50. Lippitt S, Matsen F: Mechanisms of glenohumeral joint stability. Clin Orthop Relat Res (291):20-28, 1993.

51. O'Brien SJ, Warren RF, Schwartz E: Anterior shoulder instability. Orthop Clin North Am 18:395-408, 1987.

52. Yamaguchi K, Riew KD, Galatz LM, et al: Biceps activity during shoulder motion: An electromyographic analysis. Clin Orthop Relat Res (336):122-129, 1997.

53. Andrews JR, Carson WG Jr, McLeod WD: Glenoid labrum tears related to the long head of the biceps. Am J Sports Med 13:337-341, 1985.

54. Andrews JR, Dugas JR: Diagnosis and treatment of shoulder injuries in the throwing athlete: The role of thermal-assisted capsular shrinkage. Instr Course Lect 50:17-21, 2001.

55. Andrews JR, Gidumal RH: Shoulder arthroscopy in the throwing athlete: Perspectives and prognosis. Clin Sports Med 6:565-571, 1987.

56. Andrews JR, Kupferman SP, Dillman CJ: Labral tears in throwing and racquet sports. Clin Sports Med 10:901-911, 1991.

57. Neviaser JS: Adhesive capsulitis of the shoulder (the frozen shoulder). Med Times 90:783-807, 1962.

58. Turkel SJ, Panio MW, Marshall JL, et al: Stabilizing mechanisms preventing anterior dislocation of the glenohumeral joint. J Bone Joint Surg Am 63:1208-1217, 1981.

59. Schwartz E, Warren RF, O'Brien SJ, et al: Posterior shoulder instability. Orthop Clin North Am 18:409-419, 1987.

60. Colas F, Nevoux J, Gagey O: The subscapular and subcoracoid bursae: Descriptive and functional anatomy. J Shoulder Elbow Surg 13:454-458, 2004.

61. Nobuhara K, Ikeda H: Rotator interval lesion. Clin Orthop Relat Res (223):44-50, 1987.

62. Plancher KD, Johnston JC, Peterson RK, Hawkins RJ: The dimensions of the rotator interval. J Shoulder Elbow Surg 14:620-625, 2005.

63. Rowe CR: The Shoulder. New York: Churchill Livingstone, 1988.

64. Fealy S, Adler RS, Drakos MC, et al: Patterns of vascular and anatomical response after rotator cuff repair. Am J Sports Med 34:120-127, 2006.

65. Rothman RH, Parke WW: The vascular anatomy of the rotator cuff. Clin Orthop Relat Res 41:176-186, 1965.

66. Rathbun JB, Macnab I: The microvascular pattern of the rotator cuff. J Bone Joint Surg Br 52:540-553, 1970.

67. Andary JL, Petersen SA: The vascular anatomy of the glenohumeral capsule and ligaments: An anatomic study. J Bone Joint Surg Am 84:2258-2265, 2002.

68. DePalma AF: Surgery of the Shoulder. Philadelphia: JB Lippincott, 1983.

69. Alpantaki K, McLaughlin D, Karagogeos D, et al: Sympathetic and sensory neural elements in the tendon of the long head of the biceps. J Bone Joint Surg Am 87:1580-1583, 2005.

BIBLIOGRAPHY

Adler H, Lohmann B: The stability of the shoulder joint in stress radiography. Arch Orthop Trauma Surg 103:83-84, 1984.

Andersen H: Histochemistry and development of the human shoulder and acromioclavicular joints with particular reference to the early development of the clavicle. Acta Anat (Basel) 55:124-165, 1963.

Bardeen CR, Lewis WH: Development of the limbs, body wall and back in man. Am J Anat 1:1-26, 1901.

Basmajian JV, Bazant FJ: Factors preventing downward dislocation of the adducted shoulder joint. An electromyographic and morphological study. J Bone Joint Surg Am 41:1182-1186, 1959.

Bennett WF: Visualization of the anatomy of the rotator interval and bicipital sheath. Arthroscopy 17:107-111, 2001.

Bost F, Inman VT: The pathological changes in recurrent dislocation of the shoulder. J Bone Joint Surg Am 3:595-613, 1942.

Bretzke CA, Crass JR, Craig EV, et al: Ultrasonography of the rotator cuff. Normal and pathologic anatomy. Invest Radiol 20:311-315, 1985.

Brodie CG: Note on the transverse-humeral, coracoacromial, and coracohumeral liagments of the shoulder. J Anat Physiol 24:247-252, 1890.

Brooks CH, Revell WJ, Heatley FW: A quantitative histological study of the vascularity of the rotator cuff tendon. J Bone Joint Surg Br 74:151-153, 1992.

Brooks DB, Burstein AH, Frankel VH: The biomechanics of torsional fractures. The stress concentration effect of a drill hole. J Bone Joint Surg Am 52:507-514, 1970.

Buechel FF, Pappas MJ, DePalma AF: "Floating-socket" total shoulder replacement: Anatomical, biomechanical, and surgical rationale. J Biomed Mater Res 12:89-114, 1978.

Burkart AC, Debski RE: Anatomy and function of the glenohumeral ligaments in anterior shoulder instability. Clin Orthop Relat Res (400):32-39, 2002.

Camp J, Cilley EI: Diagrammatic chart showing time of appearance of the various centers of ossification and union. Amer J Roentgenol 26:905, 1931.

Ciochon RL, Corruccini RS: The coraco-acromial ligament and projection index in man and other anthropoid primates. J Anat 124:627-632, 1977.

Clark JM, Harryman DT 2nd: Tendons, ligaments, and capsule of the rotator cuff. Gross and microscopic anatomy. J Bone Joint Surg Am 74:713-725, 1992.

Codman EA: Rupture of the supraspinatus tendon and other lesions in or about the subacromial bursa. In Codman: The Shoulder. Brooklyn: G Miller, 1934, pp 262-312.

Cole BJ, Rodeo SA, O'Brien SJ, et al: The anatomy and histology of the rotator interval capsule of the shoulder. Clin Orthop Relat Res (390):129-137, 2001.

Corruccini RS, Ciochon RL: Morphometric affinities of the human shoulder. Am J Phys Anthropol 45:19-37, 1976.

Corruccini RS, Ciochon RL: Morphoclinal variation in the anthropoid shoulder. Am J Phys Anthropol 48:539-542, 1978.

Corruccini RS, Ciochon RL: Morphometric affinities of the human shoulder. Am J Anat 45:19-38, 1978.

Craig EV: The posterior mechanism of acute anterior shoulder dislocations. Clin Orthop Relat Res (190):212-216, 1984.

Crass JR, Craig EV, Feinberg SB: Sonography of the postoperative rotator cuff. AJR Am J Roentgenol 146:561-564, 1986.

De Smet AA: Arthrographic demonstration of the subcoracoid bursa. Skeletal Radiol 7:275-276, 1982.

DePalma AF: Surgical approaches to the region of the shoulder joint. Clin Orthop 20:163-184, 1961.

DePalma AF, Cooke AJ, Prabhakar M: The role of subscapularis in recurrent anterior dislocation of the shoulder. J Bone Joint Surg Am 3:595-613, 1942.

Deutsch AL, Resnick D, Mink JH: Computed tomography of the glenohumeral and sternoclavicular joints. Orthop Clin North Am 16:497-511, 1985.

Deutsch AL, Resnick D, Mink JH, et al: Computed and conventional arthrotomography of the glenohumeral joint: Normal anatomy and clinical experience. Radiology 153:603-609, 1984.

Dickson JA, Humphries AW, O'Dell HW: Recurrent Dislocation of the Shoulder. Baltimore: Williams & Wilkins, 1953.

Eberly VC, McMahon PJ, Lee TQ: Variation in the glenoid origin of the anteroinferior glenohumeral capsulolabrum. Clin Orthop Relat Res (400):26-31, 2002.

Edwards H: Congenital displacement of the shoulder joint. J Anat 62:177-182, 1928.

Eiserloh H, Drez D Jr, Guanche CA: The long head of the triceps: A detailed analysis of its capsular origin. J Shoulder Elbow Surg 9:332-335, 2000.

Engin AE: On the biomechanics of the shoulder complex. J Biomech 13:575-590, 1980.

Freedman L, Munro RR: Abduction of the arm in the scapular plane: Scapular and glenohumeral movements. A roentgenographic study. J Bone Joint Surg Am 48:1503-1510, 1966.

Garn SM, McCreery LD: Variability of postnatal ossification timing and evidence for a "dosage" effect. Am J Phys Anthropol 32:139-144, 1970.

Garn SM, Rohmann CG, Blumenthal T: Ossification sequence polymorphism and sexual dimorphism in skeletal development. Am J Phys Anthropol 24:101-115, 1966.

Garn SM, Rohmann CG, Blumenthal T, et al: Developmental communalities of homologous and non-homologous body joints. Am J Phys Anthropol 25:147-151, 1966.

Garn SM, Rohmann CG, Blumenthal T, et al: Ossification communalities of the hand and other body parts: Their implication to skeletal assessment. Am J Phys Anthropol 27:75-82, 1967.

Gay S, Gay RE, Miller EF: The collagens of the joint. Arthritis Rheum 23:937-941, 1980.

Gerber C, Ganz R: Clinical assessment of instability of the shoulder. With special reference to anterior and posterior drawer tests. J Bone Joint Surg Br 66:551-556, 1984.

Hollinshead WH: The Back and limbs. In Hollinshead WH: Anatomy for Surgeons. Philadelphia: Harper & Row, 1982, pp 617-631.

Hovelius L, Lind B, Thorling J: Primary dislocation of the shoulder. Factors affecting the two-year prognosis. Clin Orthop Relat Res (176):181-185, 1983.

Huber DJ, Sauter R, Mueller E, et al: MR imaging of the normal shoulder. Radiology 158:405-408, 1986.

Ilahi OA, Labbe MR, Cosculluela P: Variants of the anterosuperior glenoid labrum and associated pathology. Arthroscopy 18:882-886, 2002.

Jost B, Koch PP, Gerber C: Anatomy and functional aspects of the rotator interval. J Shoulder Elbow Surg 9:336-341, 2000.

Kaltsas DS: Comparative study of the properties of the shoulder joint capsule with those of other joint capsules. Clin Orthop Relat Res (173):20-26, 1983.

Keibel F, Mall FP: Manual of Human Embryology. Philadelphia: JB Lipponcott, 1912, pp 379-391.

Kieft GJ, Bloem JL, Obermann WR, et al: Normal shoulder: MR imaging. Radiology 159:741-745, 1986.

Kummel BM: Spectrum of lesions of the anterior capsular mechanism of the shoulder. Am J Sports Med 7:111-120, 1979.

Last RJ: Anatomy. New York: Churchill Livingstone, 1978.

Ljunggren AE: Clavicular function. Acta Orthop Scand 50:261-268, 1979.

Lucas DB: Biomechanics of the shoulder joint. Arch Surg 107:425-432, 1973.

McLaughlin HL, Cavallaro WU: Primary anterior dislocation of the shoulder. Am J Surg 80:615-621, 1950.

McLaughlin HL, MacLellan DI: Recurrent anterior dislocation of the shoulder. II. A comparative study. J Trauma 7:191-201, 1967.

Middleton WD, Reinus WR, Melson GL, et al: Pitfalls of rotator cuff sonography. AJR Am J Roentgenol 146:555-560, 1986.

Mink JH, Richardson A, Grant TT: Evaluation of glenoid labrum by double-contrast shoulder arthrography. AJR Am J Roentgenol 133:883-887, 1979.

Nelson CL, Razzano CD: Arthrography of the shoulder: A review. J Trauma 13:136-141, 1973.

Neviaser RJ: Anatomic considerations and examination of the shoulder. Orthop Clin North Am 11:187-195, 1980.

Odgers SL, Hark FW: Habitual dislocation of the shoulder joint. Surg Gynecol Obstet 75:229-234, 1942.

O'Rahilly R, Gardner E: The timing and sequence of events in the development of the limbs in the human embryo. Anat Embryol (Berl) 148:1-23, 1975.

Ovesen J, Nielsen S: Experimental distal subluxation in the glenohumeral joint. Arch Orthop Trauma Surg 104:78-81, 1985.

Ovesen J, Nielsen S: Anterior and posterior shoulder instability. A cadaver study. Acta Orthop Scand 57:324-327, 1986.

Ovesen J, Sojbjerg JO: Lesions in different types of anterior glenohumeral joint dislocation. An experimental study. Arch Orthop Trauma Surg 105:216-218, 1986.

Oxnard CE: Morphometric affinities of the human shoulder. Am J Phys Anthropol 46:367-374, 1977.

Palmer ML, Blakely RL: Documentation of medial rotation accompanying shoulder flexion. A case report. Phys Ther 66:55-58, 1986.

Pappas AM, Goss TP, Kleinman PK: Symptomatic shoulder instability due to lesions of the glenoid labrum. Am J Sports Med 11:279-288, 1983.

Peat M: Functional anatomy of the shoulder complex. Phys Ther 66:1855-1865, 1986.

Petersson CJ: Degeneration of the gleno-humeral joint. An anatomical study. Acta Orthop Scand 54:277-283, 1983.

Petersson CJ, Redlund-Johnell I: Joint space in normal gleno-humeral radiographs. Acta Orthop Scand 54:274-276, 1983.

Poppen NK, Walker PS: Normal and abnormal motion of the shoulder. J Bone Joint Surg Am 58:195-201, 1976.

Poppen NK, Walker PS: Forces at the glenohumeral joint in abduction. Clin Orthop Relat Res (135):165-170, 1978.

Post M: Surgical and Non-Surgical Management. Philadelphia: Lea & Febiger, 1988.

Prodromos CC, Ferry JA, Schiller AL, et al: Histological studies of the glenoid labrum from fetal life to old age. J Bone Joint Surg Am 72:1344-1348, 1990.

Reeves B: Experiments on the tensile strength of the anterior capsular structures of the shoulder in man. J Bone Joint Surg Br 50:858-865, 1968.

Resnick D: Shoulder arthrography. Radiol Clin North Am 19:243-253, 1981.

Rockwood CAJ, Green DP: Fractures in Adults. Philadelphia: JB Lippincott, 1983.

Rothman RH, Marvel JP Jr, Heppenstall RB: Anatomic considerations in glenohumeral joint. Orthop Clin North Am 6:341-352, 1975.

Rothman RH, Marvel JP Jr, Heppenstall RB: Recurrent anterior dislocation of the shoulder. Orthop Clin North Am 6:415-422, 1975.

Rowe CR, Sakellarides HT: Factors related to recurrences of anterior dislocations of the shoulder. Clin Orthop 20:40-48, 1961.

Rozing PM, Obermann WR: Osteometry of the glenohumeral joint. J Shoulder Elbow Surg 8:438-442, 1999.

Samilson RL: Congenital and developmental anomalies of the shoulder girdle. Orthop Clin North Am 11:219-231, 1980.

Sarrafian SK: Gross and functional anatomy of the shoulder. Clin Orthop Relat Res (173):11-19, 1983.

Steinbeck J, Liljenqvist U, Jerosch J: The anatomy of the glenohumeral ligamentous complex and its contribution to anterior shoulder stability. J Shoulder Elbow Surg 7:122-126, 1998.

Gross Anatomy of the Shoulder

Christopher M. Jobe, MD, Wesley P. Phipatanakul, MD, and Michael J. Coen, MD

HISTORY

During the Renaissance, a unique style of painting called *glazing* was developed. The artist applied to the canvas thin, transparent coats of different colors. The deep layers of paint, viewed through the more superficial layers, yielded a color variant and perception of depth that was not attainable with a single layer of paint. El Greco, Titian, and Rubens were among the artists who used glazing.

A study of the history of shoulder anatomy reveals that our current picture of the shoulder was constructed in a similarly layered fashion. Much of what we know about the shoulder was worked out in significant detail in the classical age. Even the earliest studies of the present era cited in this chapter refer to structures defined by previous workers. We have found that subsequent studies do not deflect from the earlier work but serve to explain or bring into sharper focus certain elements of those studies. Rarely does later work obliterate the significance of earlier work.

The stimulus for research and publication comes from three sources: the discovery of a new disease, the invention of a new treatment, and the arrival of a new method of studying anatomy. Perpetuation of the knowledge gained depends on the philosophic outlook and interest of the time and place in which it was discovered. Since publication of the first and second editions of *The Shoulder*, there has been a geometric expansion in the study of shoulder anatomy, much of it performed by authors of chapters in this text. So much study has in fact been carried out by these authors that we might suggest a fourth stimulus to anatomic study: the need to fill out a logical framework. When constructing chapters, writers often make a logical framework of what they themselves would like to know about their subject. The framework is then filled in as far as possible from the available sources. Remaining gaps in the framework provide a stimulus to anatomic study.

Before the Renaissance, the main barriers to anatomic study were religious and personal proscriptions against the dissection of human cadavers and different philosophic ideas regarding the laws of nature. As a result of these prejudices, early contributions were not advanced, and because they were not reconfirmed, they were lost to humanity. In a dialogue written in the warring states period (5th century BC), Huang Ti described the unidirectional flow of blood in arteries and veins. Huang Ti, the Yellow Emperor of China who lived around 2600 BC, is the mythologic father of Chinese medicine.[1-3]

This and other indications of anatomic study were buried in a heavily philosophic treatise about the yin and yang influences on the human body. (Recent work in traditional Chinese medicine correlates the yang acupuncture meridians with the course of postaxial nerve branches of the posterior cord and the yin meridians with the preaxial nerve branches of the medial and lateral cords.[4]) Over the centuries, this Daoist orientation led to a deemphasis on surgical anatomy and a resultant prejudice against surgery. Although Chinese anatomic observations were subsequently carried out by physicians who witnessed executions, the "death of a thousand cuts," and bodies disinterred by dogs after an epidemic, the philosophic climate was unfavorable for propagation and use of this information.[1] Therefore, a lasting description of circulation awaited rediscovery by John Harvey in the more receptive atmosphere of the 17th century, approximately 2000 years later.

The handling of dead bodies was prohibited in India, except when preparing them for cremation; however, Sustruta, in the 6th century BC, devised a frame through which flesh was dissected away from the deeper layers with stiff brooms.[5,6] He correctly described the two shoulder bones (clavicle and scapula) at a time when the West thought of the acromion as a separate bone. In the same era, Atroya fully described the bones of humans. Alcmaeon performed animal dissection around 500 BC in Greece.[6] The significance of these discoveries was lost because further study was not conducted.

Hippocrates was probably the first physician whose ideas regarding shoulder anatomy were perpetuated.[7] Writing in the 5th century BC, his discussion of articulations began with the shoulder, and much of his work focused on this joint. His writings applied to clinical rather than basic science. Although Hippocrates referred to "the unpleasant if not cruel task" of dissecting cadavers, we must assume that he witnessed dissections because he gave explicit instructions for obtaining exposure of portions of the shoulder anatomy to prove a clinical point.[6,8] He also described the position of nerves of the axilla when discussing his burning technique for treatment of anterior dislocation of the shoulder, and in his assessment of patients, he noted that some have a "predisposing constitution" to dislocation. He demonstrated knowledge of acromioclavicular separation, palsies of the shoulder, and growth plate fractures.[8]

Herophilus (circa 300 BC), the father of anatomy, dissected some 600 cadavers at the medical school in Alexandria and started an osteology collection. This collection is the first recorded evidence of what might be called a scientific approach in that he dissected more than just a few cadavers and performed his dissections for description rather than for pathologic analysis.[6] Early authors such as Celsus accused him of vivisection, but this allegation is unjustified.[6] His permanent anatomic collections, particularly of bones, contributed to the medical knowledge of the late Greek and early Roman eras. In the late Republic and early Empire, new proscriptions against dissection, some of which were written into law, stemmed the progress that had been made. Celsus (30 BC-41 AD), who was not a physician but an encyclopedist, collected the medical knowledge of the day and advocated the performance of human dissection, but the prohibition continued.[3,6]

Despite such barriers to the study of human anatomy, advances were made sporadically by gifted physicians in unique situations. Galen, a Greco-Roman physician who practiced in Pergamum and then in Rome during the 2nd century AD, contributed greatly to the early knowledge of anatomy. He is the father of the study of clinical anatomy and, because he was the surgeon for gladiators in Pergamum, might also be considered the father of sports medicine.[9] His writings on the "usefulness of the human body parts" contain the earliest effort at detailed anatomy of the shoulder. In discussing the bones and joints of the shoulder, he described the thin ligaments of the glenohumeral joint and observed that the rim of the glenoid was often broken with dislocation. Galen attributed the frequency of dislocation of the shoulder, in comparison to other joints, to an "antagonism between diversity of movement and safety of construction." He

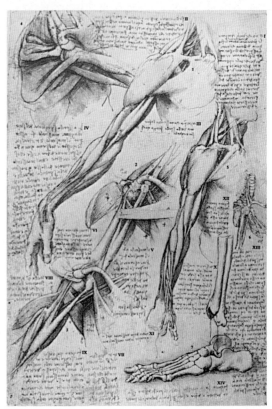

FIGURE 2-1 A page from Leonardo da Vinci's *Notebooks from Anatomical Study*. When compared with other illustrations of the time, the accuracy is striking. This particular dissection is interesting because the acromion is shown as a bone separate from the rest of the scapula. Other illustrations in the *Notebooks from Anatomical Study* show the acromion united. In Leonardo's accompanying notes, neither the fused nor the unfused state is considered normal. (From Windsor Castle, Royal Library. Copyright 1990, Her Majesty Queen Elizabeth II.)

described the anatomic principle of placing joints in a series to increase motion so that "the additional articulation might supply the deficiency of the first articulation." He also provided a complete description of all the muscles and their subdivisions, although he did not apply the Latin names used today.[9]

In describing the nerves, Galen referred to a sympathetic trunk and a plexus but did not apply names or recognize a standard construction of the brachial plexus. Instead, he considered the plexus to be a necessary method of strengthening support to the nerves. He described terminal branches of the brachial plexus, including the dorsal scapular, axillary, median, ulnar, and radial nerves. Galen also described the accessory spinal nerve. He noted the axillary artery, carotid artery, and lymph glands about the shoulder.[9] In short, he provided an impressive outline of shoulder anatomy, even by 21st-century standards.

Many differences between Galen's writings and modern descriptions relate to the fact that he performed only

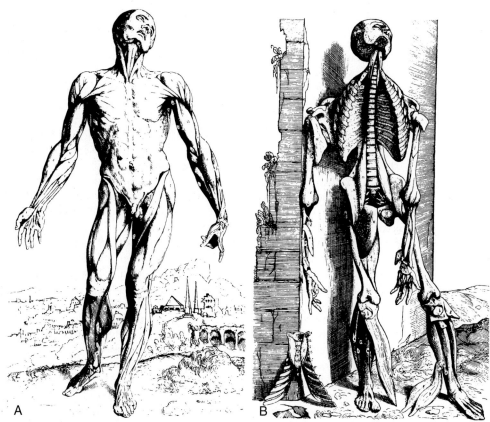

FIGURE 2-2 The first and last of Vesalius' series of illustrations demonstrating dissection of muscles of the human body. Note how his artists represent the body with dynamic strength when the muscles are intact (**A**) and show collapse and lack of support with removal of the muscles (**B**). Present-day artists who have visited the site of Vesalius' work say that many of the buildings in the background are still standing. (From Saunders JB, O'Malley CD: The Illustrations From the Works of Andreas Vesalius of Brussels. New York: World Publishing Company, 1950.)

animal dissection. He perpetuated the erroneous idea that the acromion is a separate bone, a concept that continued into the Renaissance. In addition, his writings on the acromion probably do not refer to the acromion as we know it but to the acromioclavicular joint.[9]

Shortly after Galen's time, Christianity became dominant in the Roman empire, which led to intensification of the preexisting laws against cadaveric dissection.[3] For centuries, no anatomic studies were performed on human material in Europe or in the Muslim empire. Although the Muslims were more successful in preserving the Galenic writings, their religion prohibited illustration. Perhaps the very completeness of Galen's studies contributed to the suppression of anatomic studies. Centuries passed with no new knowledge of human anatomy being acquired.[6]

When the Greek and Roman literature was reintroduced from the East, scholasticism was the dominant academic philosophy in the West. The scholastic philosophers Abelard and Thomas Aquinas depended heavily on deductive reasoning for any original contributions that they made and did not use observation or experimentation.[3,6] In view of the rich sources that reappeared from the East, one can understand how a scholar could absorb a much larger volume of information from ancient writings than from the slow and laborious process of experimentation.

Finally, during the Black Plague of 1348, the papacy allowed necropsy to be performed for the first time to elucidate the cause of death from the plague but not for anatomic study. Interestingly, when dissection for the purpose of teaching anatomy was reintroduced, it was not investigational but simply demonstrated the precepts of Galen.[6]

One of the greatest leaps in anatomic illustration occurred among Renaissance painters interested in accurate representation, some of whom dissected in secret and became serious students of anatomy (Fig. 2-1). Although their purpose was illustration and not new discovery, the increase in accuracy of illustrations in the notebooks of Leonardo da Vinci in comparison to older anatomic textbooks is quite remarkable.[6] Leonardo, in his early notebooks, was seeking to illustrate ideas from Mondino's dissection manual, which Mondino derived from Galen. The bulk of his drawing, however, is made up of his own observations, often independent of Galen.[10] Leonardo also recognized the value of dissecting multiple specimens:

And you who say that it is better to look at an anatomical demonstration than to see these drawings, you might be right, if it were possible to observe all the details shown in these drawings in a single figure, in which with all your ability you will not see . . . nor acquire a knowledge . . . while in order to obtain an exact and complete knowledge of these . . . I have dissected more than ten human bodies.[10]

In his shoulder illustrations, he shows fused and unfused acromia without notation regarding which was abnormal. His notations are largely instructions to himself, such as "draw the shoulder then the acromion," rather than observations of the incidence of variations.[10]

Anatomic study with clear illustration steadily increased over the next century. In 1537, Pope Clement VII endorsed the teaching of anatomy, and in 1543, Vesalius published his textbook *De Fabrica Corporis Humani* (Fig. 2-2).[11] Vesalius, although criticized for questioning the work of Galen during his early teaching career, was able to correct some of Galen's misconceptions. He described the geometry of muscles and contributed the concept of the dynamic force of the body, as illustrated in a vivid portrayal of progressive muscle dissection of the cadaver. In his artist's illustrations, the cadaver appears to lose more tone as each muscle layer is removed until, finally, in the last picture, the cadaver has collapsed against a wall. Vesalius demonstrated the vessels of the shoulder, and his drawings include an accurate illustration of the brachial plexus. The only element missing is the posterior division of the lower trunk (Fig. 2-3). He accurately portrayed rotation of the fibers of the costal portion of the pectoralis major.[11] His drawings also include material from comparative anatomy and indicate where these structures would lie if they were present in a human. This work was the starting point of scientific anatomy.[6]

The functions of muscles were deduced early from their shortening action and their geometry. While caring for patients during an anthrax epidemic, Galen asked them to perform certain arm motions. Because of his knowledge of anatomy, he was able to determine, without painful probing, exactly which muscle he was observing at the base of the anthrax ulcers typical of the disease and how close these ulcers were to vital nerves or vessels.[6] Modern biomechanics still benefits from study of the geometry of muscles.[12]

The dynamic study of muscles was made possible with the development of electrical equipment. DuBois-Reymond invented the first usable instrument for the electrical study of nerves and muscles in the early 19th century, and Von Helmholtz first measured the speed of nerve conduction.[6] Duchenne studied the action of muscles by electrically stimulating individual muscles through the skin, and like his predecessors, he began with the shoulder and emphasized that joint (Fig. 2-4). Duchenne also recognized that muscles rarely act individually and that this limited the accuracy of his method. He studied all the superficial muscles of the shoulder, including the trapezius, rhomboid, levator scapulae, serratus anterior, deltoid, supraspinatus, infraspinatus, teres minor, subscapularis, latissimus dorsi, pectoralis major, teres major, and triceps.[6,13,14] Subsequent developments in electromyography enabled researchers to measure muscle activity initiated by the patient.[14]

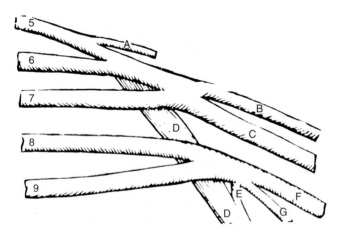

FIGURE 2-3 An illustration of the brachial plexus from Vesalius's textbook. There is reason to believe that Vesalius did this illustration himself. Note the absence of the posterior division of the lower trunk contributing to the posterior cord. (From Vesalius A: The Illustrations From the Works of Andreas Vesalius of Brussels, ed JB Saunders and CD O'Malley. New York: World Publishing Company, 1950.)

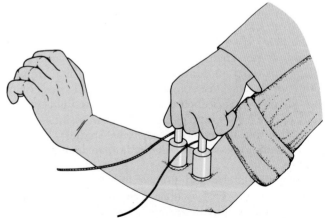

FIGURE 2-4 Duchenne's illustration of his technique for direct muscle stimulation. Like many of his great predecessors, he begins his text with a discussion of the shoulder. (From Duchenne GB: Physiology of Movement, ed and trans EB Kaplan. Philadelphia: WB Saunders, 1959.)

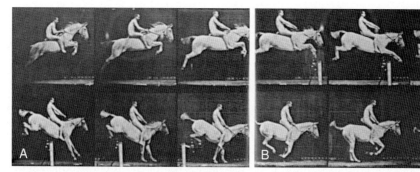

FIGURE 2-5 An example of the work of Eadweard Muybridge. This was the first time that high-speed photography was applied to the study of motion, both animal and human. This information, combined with the laws of Newtonian physics, brought about the birth of modern kinesiology. (From Muybridge E: Animals in Motion. New York: Dover, 1957.)

Functional anatomy was further elucidated by the science of physics. Aristotle studied levers and geometry and wrote about the motion of animals. Galen wrote about muscle antagonists. Leonardo da Vinci discussed the concept of centers of gravity in his notebooks. However, it was Sir Isaac Newton's physics that made possible the studies that we perform today. In the late 19th century, Eadweard Muybridge[15] published photographic studies of a horse in motion, and he later photographed human motion in rapid sequence to examine the action of the various levers of the body (Fig. 2-5). It was rapid-sequence photography that elucidated the synchrony of glenohumeral and scapulothoracic motion.[6,16] Braune and Fischer first applied Newtonian physics to functional anatomy.[17,18] In their classic studies, they used cadavers to establish the center of gravity for the entire body and for each segment of the body, the first detailed study of the physics of human motion based on such information.[7] Awareness of the great motion of the shoulder made it one of the first areas where overuse was described.[19]

The first thorough study of any joint combining all the techniques of the historical investigators was performed on the shoulder by Inman, Saunders, and Abbott.[20] This landmark work used comparative anatomy, human dissection, the laws of mechanics, photography, and the electromyogram.[20] All subsequent publications on the function of the shoulder might support or contradict findings in this study, but all cite it.[12]

Cadaveric dissection and other research continue to add to our knowledge of the shoulder and to our understanding of the findings of these early giants in the field. Exciting studies are presented at meetings and wherever the shoulder is a topic of discussion. These studies are stimulated by the same three sources that have inspired anatomists throughout history. The first stimulus is a new disease or a new understanding of an old disease. The premiere example here is the studies of impingement syndrome. The second stimulus is the invention of new technology for treatment, such as when the arthroscope activated renewed interest in variations in the labrum and ligaments of the shoulder.[21] The third is the invention of a new technique to study anatomy. In the past, this has occurred with Duchenne's electrical stimulus, the electromyogram, and the fluoroscope.[16] More recently, biochemistry, the electron microscope, magnetic resonance imaging (MRI), and laser Doppler vascular evaluation have stimulated new interest. All these techniques have deepened our understanding of previous findings in the shoulder rather than totally altered the picture (Fig. 2-6).

The final layer of paint in our portrait of shoulder anatomy has not been applied, and we are unlikely to see the day when further study is not required. Scholasticism appears to be creeping into medical school educa-

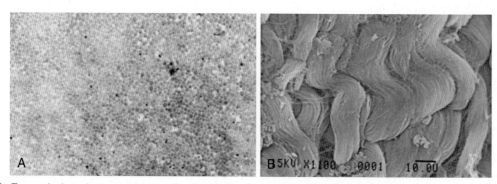

FIGURE 2-6 A, Transmission electron micrograph of collagen fibers of the subscapularis tendon. **B,** Scanning electron micrograph of the inferior glenohumeral ligament showing collagen fibers and fiber bundles.

tion. This trend is probably an unfortunate byproduct of the information surge of the late 20th and early 21st century, a phenomenon similar to the reappearance of Galen's writing in the era of scholasticism. More time is spent memorizing accumulated information at the cost of research experience. Although at present a revolution in surgical technique and technology has sent a generation of surgeons back to the anatomy laboratory,[21] one must not forget to encourage an interest in anatomy research in medical students.

In keeping with the concept of a layered portrait, the material in this chapter is arranged in a layered fashion. Discussion begins with the innermost layer, the bones and joints, the most palpable and least deformable structures of the shoulder. They are the easiest to visualize and are the best-understood anatomic landmarks. We then reveal the muscle layers that produce motion of the shoulder and the nerves that direct the muscles and provide sensation. We discuss the vessels that control the internal environment of the tissues of the shoulder and, finally, the skin that encloses the shoulder.

The central theme of the shoulder is motion. The amount of motion in the shoulder sets it apart from all other joints and accounts for the ways the shoulder differs from all other regions of the body.

BONES AND JOINTS

The orthopaedic surgeon thinks of bones primarily as rigid links that are moved, secondarily as points of attachment for ligaments, muscles, and tendons, and finally, as the base on which to maintain important relationships with surrounding soft tissue. Treatment of fractures has been called the treatment of soft tissues surrounding them.[22] In relation to pathology, bones are three-dimensional objects of anatomy that must be maintained or restored for joint alignment. Bones exist in a positive sense to protect soft tissue from trauma and provide a framework for muscle activity. In a negative sense, they can act as barriers to dissection for a surgeon trying to reach and repair a certain area of soft tissue. Loss of position of the bone can endanger soft tissue in the acute sense, and loss of alignment of the bone can endanger the longevity of the adjacent joints.

Joints have two opposing functions: to allow desired motion and to restrict undesirable motion. The stability of joints is the sum of their bony congruity and stability, the stability of the ligaments, and the dynamic stability obtained from adjacent muscles. The shoulder has the greatest mobility of any joint in the body and has the greatest predisposition to dislocation.

This great range of motion is distributed to three diarthrodial joints: the glenohumeral, the acromioclavicular, and the sternoclavicular. The last two joints, in combination with the fascial spaces between the scapula and the chest, are known collectively as the *scapulothoracic articulation*.[20] Because of the lack of congruence in two diarthrodial joints (the acromioclavicular and sternoclavicular joints), motion of the scapulothoracic articulation is determined mainly by the opposing surfaces of the thorax and scapula. About one third of the total elevation takes place in this part of the shoulder; the remainder occurs in the glenohumeral cavity. The three diarthrodial joints are constructed with little bony stability and rely mainly on their ligaments and, at the glenohumeral joint, on adjacent muscle. The large contribution of the scapulothoracic joint to shoulder function and to axial body mechanics has been emphasized since the 1990s.

The division of motion over these articulations has two advantages. First, it allows the muscles crossing each of these articulations to operate in the optimal portion of their length-tension curve. Second, the glenohumeral rhythm allows the glenoid to be brought underneath the humerus to bear some of the weight of the upper limb, which decreases demand on the shoulder muscles to suspend the arm. Such division of motion is especially important when the muscles are operating near maximal abduction and they are at that point in their length-tension curve where they produce less force.[23,24] Study of the ultrastructure of ligaments and tendons about the shoulder is in its infancy, but preliminary studies show little difference in terms of collagen biochemistry and fiber structure.[25,26]

Our discussion of the bones and joints proceeds from the proximal to the distal portion of the shoulder and includes the joint surfaces, ligaments, and special intra-articular structures. Joint stability and the relative importance of each of the ligaments to that stability are elaborated. We discuss the morphology of bones as well as their important muscle and ligament attachments. Finally, the relationship of bones and joints to other important structures in the shoulder is demonstrated.

Sternoclavicular Joint

The sternoclavicular joint, which is composed of the upper end of the sternum and the proximal end of the clavicle, is the only skeletal articulation between the upper limb and the axial skeleton.[27] In both the vertical and anteroposterior dimensions, this portion of the clavicle is larger than the opposing sternum and extends superiorly and posteriorly relative to the sternum.[27,28] The prominence of the clavicle superiorly helps create the suprasternal fossa. The sternoclavicular joint has relatively little bony stability, and the bony surfaces are somewhat flat. The ligamentous structures provide the stability of the joint. The proximal surface of the clavicle is convex in the coronal plane but somewhat concave in the transverse plane. The joint angles posteromedially in the axial plane. In the coronal plane, the joint surface is angled medially toward the superior end; the joint surfaces are covered with hyaline cartilage. In 97% of cadavers, a complete disk is found to separate the joint into two compartments (Fig. 2-7). The disk is rarely perforated.[29,30] The intra-articular disk is attached to the first rib below

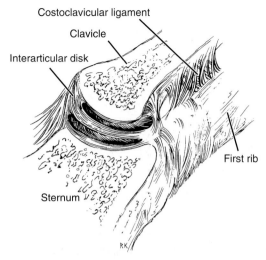

FIGURE 2-7 Cross section of the sternoclavicular joint. A complete disk separates the joint into two compartments. The disk has a firm attachment to the first rib inferiorly and to the ligaments and superior border of the clavicle superiorly.

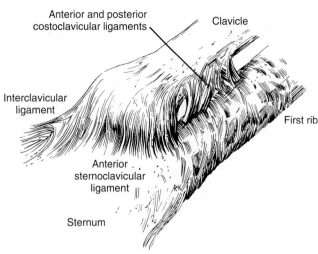

FIGURE 2-8 The exterior of the sternoclavicular joint. This illustration does not show the strongest of the ligaments: the posterior sternoclavicular ligament and the posterior partner of the anterior sternoclavicular ligament. The other important ligaments are shown in their appropriate anatomic relationships.

and to the superior surface of the clavicle through the interclavicular ligament superiorly. The disk rarely tears or dislocates by itself.[31]

The major ligaments in the joint are the anterior and posterior sternoclavicular or capsular ligaments (Fig. 2-8). The fibers run superiorly from their attachment to the sternum to their superior attachment on the clavicle. The most important ligament of this group, the posterior sternoclavicular ligament, is the strongest stabilizer to the inferior depression of the lateral end of the clavicle.[32] The paired sternoclavicular ligaments are primary restraints so that minimal rotation occurs during depression of the clavicle.

The interclavicular ligament runs from clavicle to clavicle with attachment to the sternum, and it may be absent or nonpalpable in up to 22% of the population.[25] The ligament tightens as the lateral end of the clavicle is depressed, thereby contributing to joint stability.

The anterior and posterior costoclavicular ligaments attach from the first rib to the inferior surface of the clavicle. The anterior costoclavicular ligament resists lateral displacement of the clavicle on the thoracic cage, and the posterior ligament prevents medial displacement of the clavicle relative to the thoracic cage.[33] Cave thought that these ligaments acted as a pivot around which much of the sternoclavicular motion takes place.[34] Bearn found that they were not the fulcrum in depression until after the sternoclavicular ligaments were cut. They are the principal limiting factor in passive elevation of the clavicle and are a limitation on protraction and retraction.[32] Perhaps the costoclavicular ligaments allow the good results reported for proximal clavicle resection.[33]

In the classic study on stability of the sternoclavicular joint, Bearn[32] found that the posterior sternoclavicular or capsular ligament contributed most to resisting depression of the lateral end of the clavicle. He performed serial ligament releases on cadaver specimens and made careful observations on the mode of failure and the shifting of fulcrums. This qualitative observation is a useful addition to computerized assessment of joint stability.

Although reliable electromyographic studies demonstrate that the contribution of the upward rotators of the scapula is minimal in standing posture, permanent trapezius paralysis often leads to eventual depression of the lateral end of the scapula relative to the other side, although this depression may be only a centimeter or two.[32] Bearn's experiment probably should be replicated with more sophisticated equipment to produce length-tension curves and to quantitatively test the response of the joint to rotational and translational loading in the transverse and vertical axes, as well as the anteroposterior axis that Bearn tested qualitatively.[32]

Motion occurs in both sections of the sternoclavicular joint: elevation and depression occur in the joint between the clavicle and the disk,[27] and anteroposterior motion and rotatory motion occur between the disk and the sternum. The range of motion in living specimens[20] is approximately 30 to 35 degrees of upward elevation. Movement in the anteroposterior direction is approximately 35 degrees, and rotation about the long axis is 44 to 50 degrees. Most sternoclavicular elevation occurs between 30 and 90 degrees of arm elevation.[20] Rotation occurs after 70 to 80 degrees of elevation. Estimation of the limitation of range of motion as a result of fusion is misleading because of secondary effects on the length-

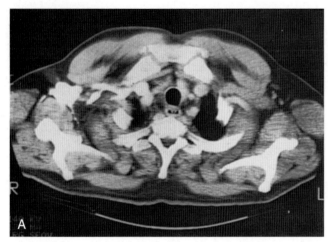
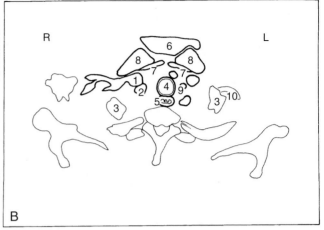

FIGURE 2-9 This contrast-enhanced CT scan (**A**) and line drawing (**B**) illustrate some of the more important anatomic relationships of the sternoclavicular joint, including the trachea and the great vessels. The structures are labeled as follows: *1,* junction of the subclavian and jugular veins; *2,* innominate artery; *3,* first rib; *4,* trachea; *5,* esophagus; *6,* sternum; *7,* sternohyoid muscle origin; *8,* clavicle; *9,* carotid artery; and *10,* axillary artery.

tension curve of the muscles of the glenohumeral joint and the ability of the glenoid to help support the weight of the arm. Fusion of the sternoclavicular joint limits abduction to 90 degrees.[12,16]

The blood supply to the sternoclavicular joint is derived from the clavicular branch of the thoracoacromial artery, with additional contributions from the internal mammary and the suprascapular arteries.[27] The nerve supply to the joint arises from the nerve to the subclavius, with some contribution from the medial supraclavicular nerve.

Immediate relationships of the joint are the origins of the sternocleidomastoid in front and the sternohyoid and sternothyroid muscles behind the joint. Of prime importance, however, are the great vessels and the trachea (Fig. 2-9), which are endangered during posterior dislocation of the clavicle from the sternum—a rare event that can precipitate a surgical emergency.[22,35,36]

An open epiphysis is a structure not commonly found in adults. The epiphysis of the clavicle, however, does not ossify until the late teens and might not fuse to the remainder of the bone in men until the age of 25 years.[32,36] Therefore, the clavicular epiphysis is a relatively normal structure within the age group at greatest risk for major trauma. The epiphysis is very thin and not prominent, which makes differentiation of physeal fractures from dislocations difficult. Instability of the sternoclavicular joint can result from trauma but, in some persons, develops secondary to constitutional laxity.[37]

Clavicle

The clavicle is a relatively straight bone when viewed anteriorly, whereas in the transverse plane, it resembles an italic S (Fig. 2-10).[38] The greater radius of curvature occurs at its medial curve, which is convex anteriorly; the smaller lateral curve is convex posteriorly. The bone is somewhat rounded in its midsection and medially and relatively flat laterally. DePalma[38] described an inverse relationship between the degree of downward facing of the lateral portion of the clavicle and the radius of curvature of the lateral curve of the clavicle.

The obvious processes of the bone include the lateral and medial articular surfaces. The medial end of the bone has a 30% incidence of a rhomboid fossa on its inferior surface where the costoclavicular ligaments insert and a 2.5% incidence of actual articular surface facing inferiorly toward the first rib. The middle portion of the clavicle contains the subclavian groove where the subclavius muscle has a fleshy insertion (Fig. 2-11). The lateral portion of the clavicle has the coracoclavicular process when present.

The clavicle has three bony impressions for attachment of ligaments. On the medial side is an impression for the costoclavicular ligaments, which at times is a rhomboid fossa. At the lateral end of the bone is the conoid tubercle, on the posterior portion of the lateral curve of the clavicle and the trapezoid line, which lies in an anteroposterior direction just lateral to the conoid tubercle. The conoid ligament attaches to the clavicle at the conoid tubercle and the trapezoid ligament attaches at the trapezoid line. The relative position of these ligament insertions is important in their function.[27,28,38]

Muscles that insert on the clavicle are the trapezius on the posterosuperior surface of the distal end and the subclavius muscle, which has a fleshy insertion on the inferior surface of the middle third of the clavicle. Four muscles originate from the clavicle: The deltoid originates on the anterior portion of the inner surface of the lateral curve; the pectoralis major originates from the anterior portion of the medial two thirds; the sternocleidomastoid has a large origin on the posterior portion of the middle third; and the sternohyoid, contrary to its name, does

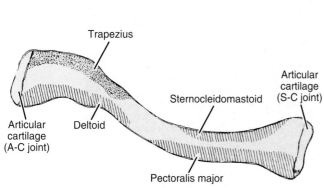

FIGURE 2-10 Anterior view of the right clavicle showing its italic S shape; the origins of the deltoid, pectoralis major, and sternocleidomastoid muscles; and the insertion of the trapezius muscle. Note the breadth of the sternocleidomastoid origin. A-C, acromioclavicular; S-C, sternoclavicular.

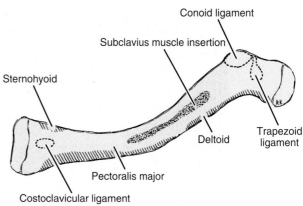

FIGURE 2-11 Posterior view of the right clavicle showing its major ligament insertions and the origins of the deltoid, pectoralis major, and sternohyoid muscles. Also shown is the subclavian groove where the subclavius muscle has its fleshy insertion.

have a small origin on the clavicle, just medial to the origin of the sternocleidomastoid.

Functionally, the clavicle acts mainly as a point of muscle attachment. Some of the literature suggests that with good repair of the muscle, the only functional consequences of surgical removal of the clavicle are limitations in heavy overhead activity[39,40] and that its function as a strut[41] is therefore less important. This concept seems to be supported by the relatively good function of persons with congenital absence of the clavicle.[42] However, others have found that sudden loss of the clavicle in adulthood has a devastating effect on shoulder function.

Important relationships to the clavicle are the subclavian vein and artery and the brachial plexus posteriorly. In fact, the medial anterior curve is often described as an accommodation for these structures and does not form in Sprengel's deformity, a condition in which the scapula does not descend. Therefore, the attached clavicle does not need to accommodate.[43-45] The curve is a landmark for finding the subclavian vein.[46] This relationship is more a factor in surgery than in trauma because the bone acts as an obstruction to surgeons in reaching the nerve or vessel tissue that they wish to treat. In trauma, clavicular injury usually does not affect these structures despite their close relationship, and nonunion is rare.[47] Most cases of neurovascular trauma fall into two groups: injury to the carotid artery from the displaced medial clavicle and compression of structures over the first rib.[48]

Acromioclavicular Joint

The acromioclavicular joint is the only articulation between the clavicle and the scapula, although a few persons, as many as 1%, have a coracoclavicular bar or joint.[49,50] Lewis[50] reported in his work that about 30% of cadavers had articular cartilage on their opposing coracoid and clavicular surfaces, without a bony process on the clavicle directed toward the coracoid.

The capsule of the acromioclavicular joint contains a diarthrodial joint incompletely divided by a disk, which, unlike that of the sternoclavicular joint, usually has a large perforation in its center.[29,30] The capsule tends to be thicker on its superior, anterior, and posterior surfaces than on the inferior surface. The upward and downward movement allows rotation of about 20 degrees between the acromion and the clavicle, which occurs in the first 20 and last 40 degrees of elevation.[20] It is estimated that many persons have even less range of motion because in some cases, fusion of the acromioclavicular joint does not decrease shoulder motion.[22] DePalma found degenerative changes of both the disk and articular cartilage to be the rule rather than the exception in specimens in the fourth decade or older.[29]

The blood supply to the acromioclavicular joint is derived mainly from the acromial artery, a branch of the deltoid artery of the thoracoacromial axis. There are rich anastomoses between this artery, the suprascapular artery, and the posterior humeral circumflex artery. The acromial artery comes off the thoracoacromial axis anterior to the clavipectoral fascia and perforates back through the clavipectoral fascia to supply the joint. It also sends branches anteriorly up onto the acromion. Innervation of the joint is supplied by the lateral pectoral, axillary, and suprascapular nerves.[27]

The ligaments about the acromioclavicular articulation and the trapezoid and conoid ligaments have been studied extensively (Fig. 2-12). Traditionally and more recently, it has been reported that anteroposterior stability of the acromioclavicular joint was controlled by the acromioclavicular ligaments and that vertical stability was controlled by the coracoclavicular ligaments.[22,51] A serial cutting experiment involving 12 force-displacement measurements was performed with more sophisticated equipment.[52] Three anatomic axes of the acromioclavicular joint were used, and translation and rotation on each axis in both directions were measured. The results of the

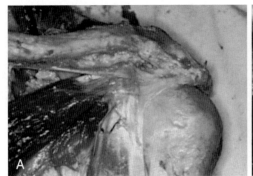
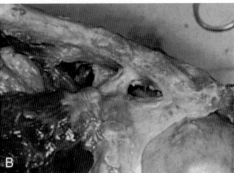

FIGURE 2-12 These photographs show the acromioclavicular joint complex before (**A**) and after (**B**) excision of the clavipectoral fascia, which was rather prominent in this specimen. Note the thickness of the coracoclavicular ligaments and their lines of orientation, which are consistent with their function. Note also the breadth and thickness of the coracoacromial ligament.

experiment confirmed previously held views, particularly when displacements were large.

The acromioclavicular ligaments were found to be responsible for controlling posterior translation of the clavicle on the acromion. (In anatomic terms, this motion is really anterior translation of the scapula on the clavicle.) The acromioclavicular ligaments were responsible for 90% of anteroposterior stability, and 77% of the stability for superior translation of the clavicle (or inferior translation of the scapula) was attributed to the conoid and trapezoid ligaments. Distraction of the acromioclavicular joint was limited by the acromioclavicular ligaments (91%), and compression of the joint was limited by the trapezoid ligament (75%), as discussed later.

The unique findings of the study were the contribution during small displacements. The acromioclavicular ligaments played a much larger role in many of these rotations and translations than in larger displacements, which

might reflect shorter lengths of the acromioclavicular ligaments. At shorter displacements, greater load is applied to the fibers of the acromioclavicular ligaments for the same displacement.

Interpretation of the stability attributed to the acromioclavicular ligaments needs to reflect the additional role that they play in maintaining integrity of the acromioclavicular joint. Although we would expect the linear arrangement of the collagen of the acromioclavicular ligaments to resist distraction, it makes little sense that the acromioclavicular ligaments would resist compression with these fibers, yet 12% to 16% of compression stability in the study was attributed to the acromioclavicular ligament. Maintenance of the integrity of the acromioclavicular joint, particularly the position of the interarticular disk, might be the explanation. We would not expect the acromioclavicular ligament to resist superior translation of the clavicle were it not for the presence of an intact joint

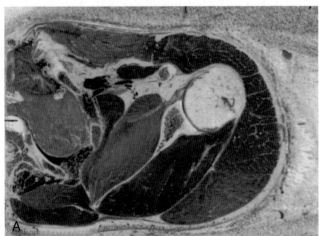
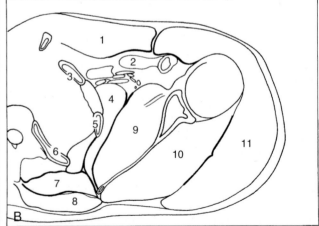

FIGURE 2-13 Photograph (**A**) and diagram (**B**) of a cross section of the scapula at the midportion of the glenoid. The thinness of most of the scapula and its most important bony process, the glenoid, can be seen, as well as the way the muscle and ligaments increase the stability of this inherently unstable joint by circumscribing the humeral head. Hypovascular fascial planes are emphasized. Note that the artist's line is wider than the plane depicted. The labeled structures include *1*, pectoralis major; *2*, pectoralis minor; *3*, first rib; *4*, serratus anterior; *5*, second rib; *6*, third rib; *7*, rhomboid; *8*, trapezius; *9*, subscapularis; *10*, infraspinatus; and *11*, deltoid.

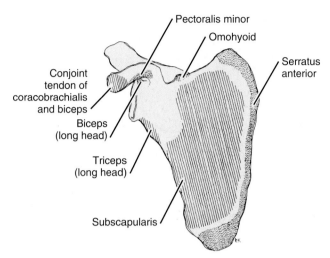

FIGURE 2-14 Anterior view of the scapula showing the muscle origins of the anterior surface *(striped pattern)* and the muscle insertions *(stippled pattern).* Ligaments and their origins and insertions are not illustrated.

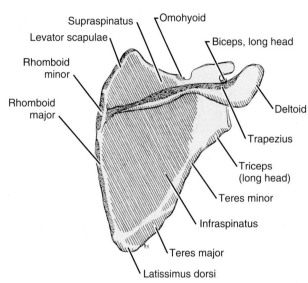

FIGURE 2-15 Posterior view of the scapula illustrating the muscle origins and muscle insertions.

below it creating a fulcrum against which these ligaments can produce a tension band effect.[52]

It is seldom that these ligaments are called on to resist trauma, and their usual function is to control joint motion. As noted earlier, this joint has relatively little motion, and muscles controlling scapulothoracic motion insert on the scapula. To a large extent, the ligaments function to guide motion of the clavicle.[53] For example, the conoid ligament produces much of the superior rotation of the clavicle as the shoulder is elevated in flexion.[12]

The distal end of the clavicle does not have a physeal plate. Todd and D'Errico,[54] using microscopic dissection, found a small fleck of bone in some persons that appeared to be an epiphysis, but it united within 1 year. We have not seen this structure at surgery or by roentgenogram. Probably the articular cartilage functions in longitudinal growth as it does in a physis.

Scapula

The scapula is a thin sheet of bone that functions mainly as a site of muscle attachment (Fig. 2-13). It is thicker at its superior and inferior angles and at its lateral border, where some of the more powerful muscles are attached (Figs. 2-14 and 2-15). It is also thick at sites of formation of its processes: the coracoid, spine, acromion, and glenoid. Because of the protection of overlying soft tissue, fractures usually occur in the processes via indirect trauma. The posterior surface of the scapula and the presence of the spine create the supraspinatus and the infraspinatus fossae. The three processes, the spine, the coracoid, and the glenoid, create two notches in the scapula. The suprascapular notch is at the base of the coracoid, and the spinoglenoid, or greater scapular

notch, is at the base of the spine. The coracoacromial and transverse scapular ligaments are two of several ligaments that attach to two parts of the same bone. Sometimes an inferior transverse scapular ligament is found in the spinoglenoid notch. This transverse ligament and ganglia of the labrum might all be factors in suprascapular nerve deficits. Seldom studied is the coracoglenoid ligament, which originates on the coracoid between the coracoacromial and coracohumeral ligaments and inserts on the glenoid near the origin of the long head of the biceps.[55] The major ligaments that originate from the scapula are the coracoclavicular, coracoacromial, acromioclavicular, glenohumeral, and coracohumeral.

The coracoid process comes off the scapula at the upper base of the neck of the glenoid and passes anteriorly before hooking to a more lateral position. It functions as the origin of the short head of the biceps and the coracobrachialis tendons. It also serves as the insertion of the pectoralis minor muscle and the coracoacromial, coracohumeral, and coracoclavicular ligaments. Several anomalies of the coracoid have been described. As much as 1% of the population has an abnormal connection between the coracoid and the clavicle: a bony bar or articulation.[49] Some surgeons have seen impingement in the interval between the head of the humerus and the deep surface of the coracoid.[56-58] The coracohumeral interval is smallest in internal rotation and forward flexion.

The spine of the scapula functions as part of the insertion of the trapezius on the scapula and as the origin of the posterior deltoid. It also suspends the acromion in the lateral and anterior directions and thus serves as a prominent lever arm for function of the deltoid. The dimensions of the spine of the scapula are regular, with less than 1.5-cm variation from the mean in any dimen-

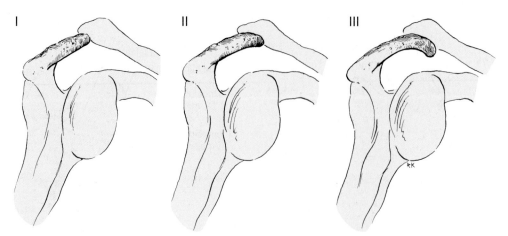

FIGURE 2-16 The three types of acromion morphology defined by Bigliani and colleagues. Type I, with its flat surface, provided the least compromise of the supraspinatus outlet, whereas type III's sudden discontinuity, or hook, was associated with the highest rate of rotator cuff pathology in a series of cadaver dissections.

sion. Recently, reconstruction of the mandible has been devised by using the spine of the scapula. Sacrifice of the entire spine, including the acromion, has a predictably devastating effect on shoulder function.[59,60]

Because of the amount of pathology involving the acromion and the head of the humerus, the acromion is the most-studied process of the scapula.[61] Tendinitis and bursitis have been related to impingement of the head of the humerus and the coracoacromial arch in an area called the *supraspinatus outlet*.[62] When viewed from the front, a 9- to 10-mm gap (6.6-13.8 mm in men, 7.1-11.9 mm in women) can be seen between the acromion and the humerus.[63] Recent advances in x-ray positioning allow better visualization of the outlet from the side or sagittal plane of the scapula.[64]

Several methods of describing the capaciousness of this space or its tendency for mechanical discontinuity have been devised. Aoki and colleagues[65] used the slope of the ends of the acromion relative to a line connecting the posterior acromion with the tip of the coracoid of the scapula to determine the propensity for impingement problems. Bigliani and associates[66] separated acromia into three types (or classes) based on their shape and correlated the occurrence of rotator cuff pathology in cadavers with the shape of the acromion on supraspinatus outlet radiographs (Fig. 2-16). Their classification is generally easy to use, but the transition between types is smooth, so some inter-interpreter variability will occur in those close to the transitions. Type I acromia are those with a flat undersurface and the lowest risk for impingement syndrome and its sequelae. Type II has a curved undersurface, and type III has a hooked undersurface. As one would expect, a type III acromion with its sudden discontinuity in shape had the highest correlation with subacromial pathology.

A more recent report by Banas and associates comments on the position of the acromion in the coronal plane (the lateral downward tilt). In their series of 100 MRI procedures, increasing downward tilt was associated with a greater prevalence of cuff disease.[67] The remainder of the roof of the supraspinatus outlet consists of the coracoacromial ligament, which connects two parts of the same bone. It is usually broader at its base on the coracoid, tapers as it approaches the acromion, and has a narrower but still broad insertion on the undersurface of the acromion; it covers a large portion of the anterior undersurface of the acromion and invests the tip and lateral undersurface of the acromion (Fig. 2-17). The ligament might not be wider at its base and often has one or more diaphanous areas at the base.[68] Because of the high incidence of impingement in elevation and internal rotation, acromia from persons older than the fifth decade often have secondary changes such as spurs or excrescences.

In addition to static deformation of the acromion, one would expect an unfused acromion epiphysis to lead to deformability of the acromion on an active basis and decrease the space of the supraspinatus outlet.[69] Neer, however, found no increased incidence of unfused epiphyses in his series of acromioplasties.[70] Liberson[71] classified the different types of unfused acromia as preacromion, meso-acromion, meta-acromion, and basiacromion centers (Fig. 2-18). In his series, an unfused center was noted on 1.4% of roentgenograms and bilaterally in 62% of cases. The meso-acromion–meta-acromion defect was found most often (Fig. 2-19).

The glenoid articular surface is within 10 degrees of being perpendicular to the blade of the scapula, with the mean being 6 degrees of retroversion.[72] The more caudad portions face more anteriorly than the cephalad portions.[73] This perpendicular relationship, combined with the complementary orientation of the scapula and relationships determined by the ligaments of the scapulohumeral orientation, makes the plane of the scapula the most suitable coronal plane for physical and radiologic examination of the shoulder. The plane of the glenoid defines the sagittal planes, whereas the transverse plane remains the same.[74]

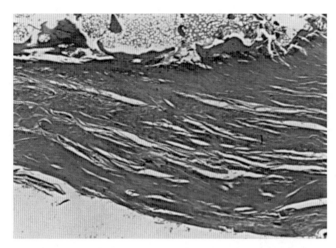

FIGURE 2-17 Photomicrographic view (×12) of the insertion of the coracoacromial ligament into the undersurface of the acromion. It can continue as far as 2 cm in the posterior direction. Note the thickness of the ligament in comparison to the bone.

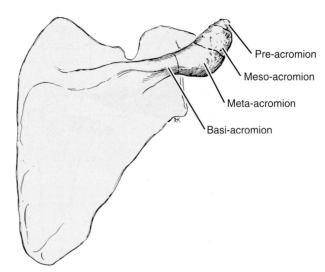

Pre-acromion

Meso-acromion

Meta-acromion

Basi-acromion

FIGURE 2-18 Different regions of the acromion between which union can fail to occur.

The blood supply to the scapula is derived from vessels in muscles that have fleshy origin from the scapula (see the section "Muscles"). Vessels cross these indirect insertions and communicate with bony vessels. The circulation of the scapula is metaphyseal; the periosteal vessels are larger than usual, and they communicate freely with the medullary vessels rather than being limited to the outer third of the cortex. Such anatomy might explain why subperiosteal dissection is bloodier here than over a diaphyseal bone.[75] The nutrient artery of the scapula enters into the lateral suprascapular fossa[60] or the infrascapular fossa.[76] The subscapular, suprascapular, circumflex scapular, and acromial arteries are contributing vessels.

Muscles not previously mentioned that originate from the scapula are the rotator cuff muscles: the supraspinatus, infraspinatus, teres minor, and subscapularis. At the superior and inferior poles of the glenoid are two tubercles for tendon origin, the superior for the long head of the biceps and the inferior for the long head of the triceps. At the superior angle of the scapula, immediately posterior to the medial side of the suprascapular notch, is the origin of the omohyoid, a muscle that has little significance for shoulder surgery but is an important landmark for brachial plexus and cervical dissection. The large and powerful teres major originates from the lateral border of the scapula. Inserting on the scapula are all the scapulothoracic muscles: the trapezius, serratus anterior, pectoralis minor, levator scapulae, and major and minor rhomboids.

Humerus

The articular surface of the humerus at the shoulder is spheroid, with a radius of curvature of about 2.25 cm.[12]

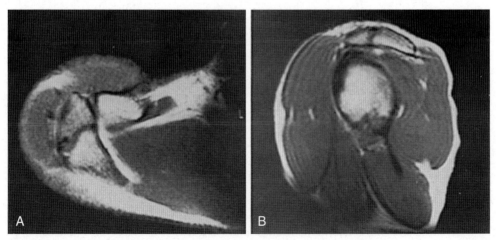

FIGURE 2-19 Transverse (**A**) and sagittal (**B**) MRI sections of an unfused meso-acromion.

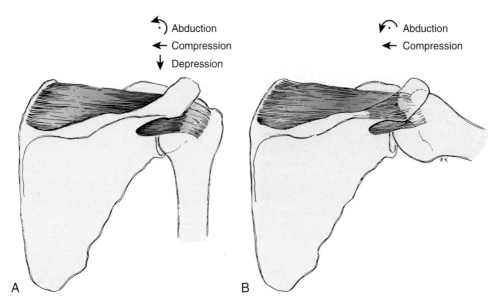

FIGURE 2-20 A, In neutral position, initiation of the use of the supraspinatus muscle produces a compressing force, and because the supraspinatus circumscribes the spheroid of the humeral head, a head depression force is generated. **B,** In the abducted position, when the force of the deltoid muscle does not produce as much vertical shear force, there is loss of the prominence of the spheroid and therefore loss of the head-depressing force of the supraspinatus. An abduction moment and joint compression force remain.

As one moves down the humerus in the axis of the spheroid, one encounters a ring of bony attachments for the ligaments and muscles that control joint stability. The ring of attachments is constructed of the two tuberosities, the intertubercular groove, and the medial surface of the neck of the humerus. Ligaments and muscles that maintain glenohumeral stability do so by contouring the humeral head so that tension in them produces a restraining force toward the center of the joint (Fig. 2-20). In this position, the spheroid is always more prominent than the ligamentous or muscle attachments. For example, when the shoulder is in neutral abduction and the supraspinatus comes into play, the greater tuberosity, which is the attachment of this tendon, is on average 8 mm less prominent than the articular surface, and thus the tendon contours the humeral head.[77] In the abduction and external rotation position, contouring of the supraspinatus is lost. The anterior inferior glenohumeral ligament now maintains joint stability, and its attachments are less prominent than the articulating surface.

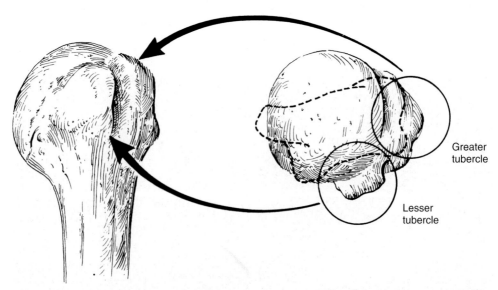

FIGURE 2-21 The head of the humerus is retroverted relative to the long axis of the humerus. The bicipital groove in the neutral position lies approximately 1 cm lateral to the midline of the humerus. Note the posterior offset of the head.

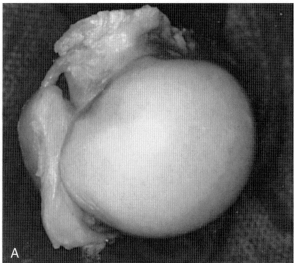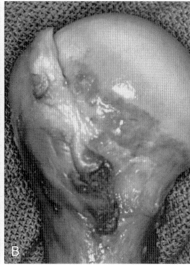

FIGURE 2-22 A, Superior surface of the humeral head, where the rotator cuff attaches immediately adjacent to the articular cartilage. The lesser tubercle is superior and the greater tubercle is to the left, with the bicipital groove and transverse humeral ligament between them. **B,** Posterior view of the humeral head and the gap between the articular surface and the attachment of the capsule and the tendon. This area is the anatomic neck of the humerus.

With the arm in the anatomic position (i.e., with the epicondyles of the humerus in the coronal plane), the head of the humerus is retroverted in relation to the transepicondylar axis. In addition, the average retrotorsion is less at birth than at maturity.[78] How much retroversion has been a topic of debate. Boileau and Walch[79] used three-dimensional computerized modeling of cadaveric specimens to analyze the geometry of the proximal humerus. They found a wide variation of retroversion ranging from −6.7 degrees to 47.5 degrees. These findings have helped revolutionize shoulder arthroplasty and brought about the development of the third-generation shoulder prosthesis, or the concept of the anatomic shoulder replacement. This concept centers around the great range in retroversion among different people. The surgical goal is restoring individual patient anatomy. Setting prosthetic replacements at an arbitrary 30 to 40 degrees of retroversion might not be optimal and does not account for individual anatomic variability.[79] The intertubercular groove lies approximately 1 cm lateral to the midline of the humerus.[72,80] The axis of the humeral head crosses the greater tuberosity about 9 mm posterior to the bicipital groove (Fig. 2-21).[81] The lesser tubercle (or tuberosity) lies directly anterior, and the greater tuberosity lines up on the lateral side. In the coronal plane the head-to-shaft angle is about 135 degrees.[77] This angle is less for smaller heads and greater for larger ones. The head size (radius of curvature) correlates most strongly with the patient's height.[77]

The space between the articular cartilage and the ligamentous and tendon attachments is referred to as the *anatomic neck of the humerus* (Fig. 2-22). It varies in breadth from about 1 cm on the medial, anterior, and posterior sides of the humerus to essentially undetectable over the superior surface, where no bone is exposed

between the edge of articular cartilage and the insertion of the rotator cuff. The lesser tubercle is the insertion for the subscapularis tendon, and the greater tubercle bears the insertion of the supraspinatus, infraspinatus, and teres minor in a superior-to-inferior order. Because of its distance from the center of rotation, the greater tubercle lengthens the lever arm of the supraspinatus as elevation increases above 30 degrees. It also acts as a pulley by increasing the lever arm of the deltoid below 60 degrees.[82] The prominence of the greater tubercle can even allow the deltoid to act as a head depressor when the arm is at the side.[83] Below the level of the tubercles, the humerus narrows in a region that is referred to as the *surgical neck of the humerus* because of the common occurrence of fractures at this level.

The greater and lesser tubercles make up the boundaries of the intertubercular groove through which the long head of the biceps passes from its origin on the superior lip of the glenoid. The intertubercular groove has a peripheral roof referred to as the *intertubercular ligament* or *transverse humeral ligament*, which has varying degrees of strength.[58,84] Research has shown that the coracohumeral ligament is the primary restraint to tendon dislocation.[85-87] The coracohumeral ligament arises from the coracoid as a V-shaped band, the opening of which is directed posteriorly toward the joint. In most cases, it histologically represents only a V-shaped fold of capsule and has no distinct ligamentous fibers.[88] Tightening of this area does affect shoulder function. The ring of tissue making up the pulley constraining the biceps tendon consists of the superficial glenohumeral ligament (floor) and the coracohumeral ligament (roof).

Because the biceps tendon is a common site of shoulder pathology, attempts have been made to correlate the anatomy of its intertubercular groove with a predilection for pathology (Fig. 2-23).[27] It was thought that biceps tendinitis resulted from dislocation of the tendon secondary to a shallow groove or a supratubercular ridge[84] and an incompetent transverse humeral ligament. Meyer[84] attributed the greater number of dislocations of the biceps tendon on the left to activities in which the left arm is in external rotation, a position that should have been protective. Current opinion is that dislocation of the tendon is a relatively rare etiology of bicipital tendinitis, that most cases of bicipital tendinitis can be attributed to impingement,[63] and that dislocation of the tendon is not seen except in the presence of rotator cuff or pulley damage.

Walch and colleagues[89] analyzed long head of biceps dislocations. They found that in 70% of cases, dislocation of the long head of the biceps was associated with massive rotator cuff tears. In particular, in only 2 of 46 cases was the subscapularis intact. It is possible that the theory of variable depth of the intertubercular groove also applies to the impingement syndrome as an etiology. A shallow intertubercular groove makes the tendon of the long head of the biceps and its overlying ligaments more prominent and therefore more vulnerable to impingement damage.[70]

The intertubercular groove has a more shallow structure as it continues distally, but its boundaries, referred to as the *lips of the intertubercular groove*, continue to function as sites for muscle insertion. Below the subscapularis muscles, the medial lip of the intertubercular groove is the site of insertion for the latissimus dorsi and teres major, with the latissimus dorsi insertion being anterior, often on the floor of the groove. The pectoralis major has its site of insertion at the same level but on the lateral lip of the bicipital groove. At its upper end, the intertubercular groove also functions as the site of

entry of the major blood supply of the humeral head, the ascending branch of the anterior humeral circumflex artery, which enters the bone at the top of the intertubercular groove or one of the adjacent tubercles.[90,91]

Two shoulder muscles insert on the humerus near its midpoint. On the lateral surface is the bony prominence of the deltoid tuberosity, over which is located a large tendinous insertion of the deltoid. On the medial surface, at about the same level, is the insertion of the coracobrachialis.

The humerus, as part of the peripheral skeleton, is rarely a barrier to dissection. The essential relationships to be maintained in surgical reconstruction are the retrograde direction of the articular surface and this surface's prominence relative to the muscle and ligamentous attachments. Longitudinal alignment needs to be maintained, as well as the distance from the head to the deltoid insertion. In fractures above the insertion of the deltoid that heal in humerus varus, or in cases of birth injury that cause humerus varus, the head-depressing effect of the supraspinatus is ineffective in the neutral position when the shear forces produced by the deltoid are maximal.[92] Interestingly, patients with congenital humerus varus rarely complain of pain but have limitation of motion.[93] The important relationships to the humerus in the region of the joint are the brachial plexus structures, particularly the axillary and radial nerves and the accompanying vessels.

MUSCLES

The orthopaedic surgeon views muscles in several ways. First, they produce force. Second, they are objects of dis-

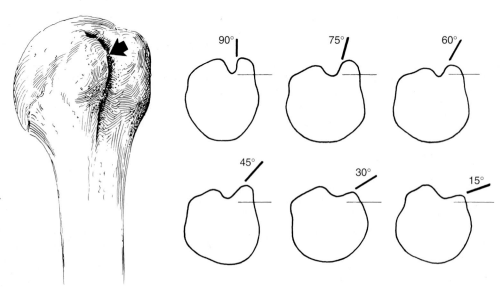

FIGURE 2-23 Variations in shape and depth of the intertubercular or bicipital groove *(arrow)*. Formerly it was believed that a shallow groove combined with the supratubercular ridge of Meyer, a ridge at the top of the groove, predisposed to tendon dislocation. Bicipital disease is now thought to result from the impingement syndrome. (Redrawn from Hollinshead WH: Anatomy for Surgeons, vol 3, 3rd ed. Philadelphia: Harper & Row, 1982.)

section in terms of repairing, transferring, or bypassing them on the way to a deeper and closely related structure. Finally, muscles are energy-consuming and controllable organs for which blood and nerve supply must be maintained.

A brief review of interior anatomy is in order. The force generators within the structure of muscle are the muscle fibers, which are encased in a supporting collagen framework that transmits the force generated to the bony attachments. Each fiber's excursion is proportional to the sum of the sarcomeres or, in other words, its length. Muscle strength is a product of its cross-sectional area or the number of fibers.

The internal arrangement of muscle fibers can affect strength (Fig. 2-24). If all the fibers of a muscle are arranged parallel to its long axis, the muscle is called *parallel* and has maximal speed and excursion for size. Other muscles sacrifice this excursion and speed for strength by stacking a large number of fibers in an arrangement oblique to the long axis of the muscle and attaching to a tendon running the length of the muscle. This type of arrangement is referred to as *pennate* or *multipennate*. Strength again is a product of the number of fibers; however, because of the oblique arrangement of the fibers, the strength in line with the tendon is obtained by multiplying this strength by the cosine of the angle of incidence with the desired axis of pull. Its excur-

sion is also a product of this cosine times the length of these shorter fibers. Some muscles, such as the subscapularis in its upper portion, have multipennate portions in which excursion is so short and the collagen framework so dense that the muscle acts as a passive restraint to external rotation of the glenohumeral joint (e.g., at 0 and 45 degrees of abduction).[94-96]

The complex arrangement of the shoulder into several articulations that contribute to an overall increase in mobility is also important in terms of the function of muscle. First, the multiple joint arrangement demands less excursion of the muscles that cross each articulation, thereby allowing each joint's muscles to operate within the more effective portions of their length-tension curves. Second, joint stability requires that joint reaction forces cross the joint through the bony portions. Muscles of the shoulder serve not only to bring joint reaction forces to the glenohumeral joint in the area of the glenoid but also to move the glenoid to meet the joint reaction forces.[97] This need for multiple muscles to function in each motion complicates the diagnosis and planning of tendon transfer.[98]

Actions of muscles have been measured in terms of standard movements such as abduction in the plane of the scapula, forward flexion of the shoulder, and internal and external rotation of the shoulder in neutral abduction. Studies have also been done on rehabilitation-associated activities such as scapular depression, an activity per-

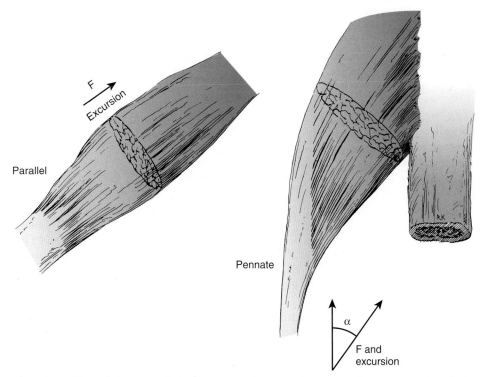

FIGURE 2-24 Muscles whose fibers have a parallel arrangement have maximal excursion and speed of contractility because both force and excursion are parallel to the long axis of the muscle. In a pennate arrangement, multiple fibers with shorter length can be stacked to obtain a greater cross-sectional area. Not all of this strength is in the desired direction, nor is the excursion. The effective force and excursion are projections of these vectors on the described directions, the magnitudes of which are products of the cosine of the angle times the excursion or force (F) magnitude.

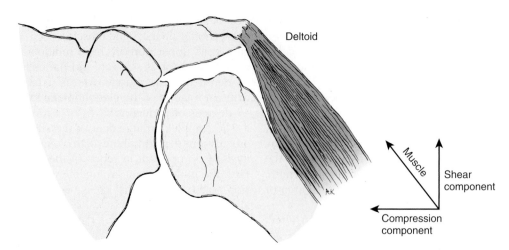

FIGURE 2-25 The action of muscles at the joint surface can be projected into two perpendicular vectors: a compression vector aimed directly at the articular surface and a shear vector producing motion tangential to the joint surface.

formed by patients using a wheelchair or walker. More complex motions of daily life and the actions of athletes are currently under research.[99] Because the upper extremity can be positioned many ways, an infinite number of studies can be performed.

A muscle performs its activity entirely by shortening its length. The action that results and the level of each muscle's activity depend on two conditions: the position at the beginning of an activity and the relationship of the muscle to the joint. The muscle vectors of the shoulder can be divided into two components with respect to the joint surface (Fig. 2-25). One component produces shear on the joint surface, and the other produces compression and increases the stability of the joint. Muscles of the shoulder can make an additional contribution to stability by circumscribing the protruding portions of the humeral spheroid, a continually directed shear force creating compression to increase stability.[12,100] Stability depends on the joint reaction force vector crossing the joint through cartilage and bone, the tissues designed for compression stress. A useful oversimplification of the contributions of shoulder muscles to stability is that the glenohumeral muscles strive to direct the joint reaction vector toward the glenoid and the muscles controlling the scapula move the glenoid toward the force.

Externally applied resistance, including the force of gravity on the action that is being performed, is an additional determinant of which muscles will be active in a particular motion. At high levels of performance, the level of training becomes important in determining how a muscle is used. People who are highly skilled may be more adept than the less trained at positioning their skeletons so that they use less muscle force in retaining joint stability. Such positioning allows more muscle force to be used in moving the limb.[101]

Two examples illustrate the variability of muscle action in performing the same activity. The first is elevation of the scapula (Fig. 2-26). When the subject is in the anatomic position and is performing an elevation in the scapular plane or in forward flexion, the main elevators of the scapula are the upper fibers of the trapezius, the serratus anterior, and the levator scapulae. In studies of overhead activity[102] it was found that the orientation of the throwing arm relative to the spine in different activities such as tennis, baseball, and so forth was similar, but that the arm in relation to the ground was more vertical for heavier objects. The relationship of the humerus to the scapula and the scapula to the main axial skeleton, however, was little changed. Such a finding ought to be anticipated because these muscles are already operating within the optimal portion of Blix's curve for their activity. Further arm elevation is obtained by using the contralateral trunk muscles, with the upper part of the trunk bending away from the throwing arm and creating a more vertical alignment of the throwing arm relative to the ground. Rotation of the scapula also begins earlier when elevating heavier objects.[103] By producing a more level glenoid platform, this maneuver allows the glenoid rather than the muscles to bear more of the weight of the thrown object. In a sense, one might consider the contralateral trunk muscles to be elevators of the scapula.

In another athletic maneuver, the iron cross performed by some gymnasts, the arm is again in 90 degrees of abduction, and the entire weight is placed on the hands. The upward force on the hands is counterbalanced by the adduction force generated by the latissimus dorsi and the lower portion of the pectoralis major. Because of the shorter lever arm of these muscles, balancing forces are much greater than the upward forces on the hands (see Chapter 6). Therefore, the joint reaction force on the humeral side tends to run in a cephalocaudad direction. The other muscle active in this enforced adduction is the teres major, which brings the lower portion of the scapula toward the humerus. In this maneuver, the hands are in a fixed position and the teres major acts as an upward rotator of the scapula. Because the teres major is active only against strong resistance,[104] it could be postulated

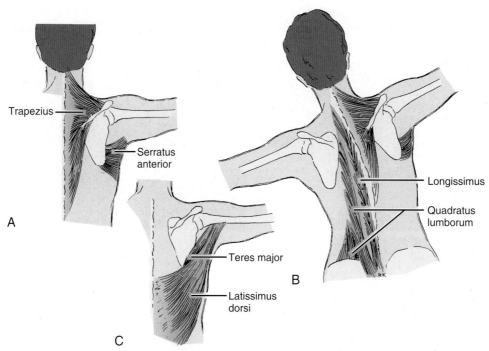

FIGURE 2-26 Three different ways muscles produce elevation of the scapula. **A,** Pure elevation of the scapula in the scapular plane, as might occur in a throwing motion. **B,** When throwing a heavier object, more elevation of the scapula is necessary to allow the glenoid to bear extra weight. Because the muscles of the shoulder are already operating at the optimal points of their length-tension curve, further elevation must be obtained by using the contralateral trunk muscles to produce contralateral flexion of the spine. **C,** An upward moment on the upper limb, such as in the iron cross maneuver, must be resisted by a greater force in the latissimus dorsi. The resultant caudad-directed joint reaction vector must meet the bone of the glenoid. This scapular elevation is produced by the teres major.

that elevation of the scapula may be the major action of the muscle.

As objects of surgical intervention, the important issues with muscles are tissue strength and resting positions that can be used to guard repairs. Muscles are also approached for the purpose of transfer. In such cases, attachment to bone, excursion of the muscle, phase activity innervation, and nutrition are important.

Tendons are attached to bone by interlocking of the collagen of the tendon with the surface of the bone (direct insertion) or by continuation of the majority of collagen fibers into the periosteum (indirect insertion) (Fig. 2-27).[105] Direct insertions have a transition zone from the strong but pliable collagen of the tendon to the hard and unyielding calcified collagen of the bone. The transition begins on the tendon side with nonmineralized fibrocartilage, then mineralized fibrocartilage, and finally bone. Thus, there is no sudden transition in material properties at bone attachments, and collagen is present in amounts necessary to bear the stresses generated.

When all the force generated by a muscle is borne by a single narrow tendon, this attachment tends to become a collagen-rich direct insertion and provides the surgeon with a firm structure to hold sutures. When the area of attachment to bone is broad, the same layered arrangement can exist, but most of the collagen goes into periosteum in what is called *indirect attachment*. As the

muscle force is spread over a broad area, these attachments tend to become collagen poor, or fleshy, with little collagen to hold sutures. When these areas of muscle are mobilized, a portion of contiguous periosteum is left attached to the muscle to increase the amount of collagen available to hold sutures during reattachment. Direct insertions are not traversed by blood vessels, but indirect insertions are (Fig. 2-28).[105]

Muscles are generally approached as barriers to dissection because they overlie an area that the surgeon wants to reach. When they cannot be retracted, it is more desirable to split tendons or muscles than it is to divide them. Often, however, there are limits to splitting. For example, in the deltoid, where the axillary nerve runs perpendicular to the fibers of the muscle, the amount of splitting that can be performed is limited (Fig. 2-29). The trapezius should not be split in its medial half because of the course of the spinal accessory nerve.[106]

As viable structures, muscles require functioning vessels and nerves. Knowledge of these structures is necessary to avoid damage, particularly when rather ambitious exposures or transfers are contemplated. The procedure is more complicated when the surgeon wants to split a muscle or when a muscle is supplied by two separate nerves or two separate vessels.

The internal nerve and vessel arrangements in some muscles of the shoulder have been carefully studied.

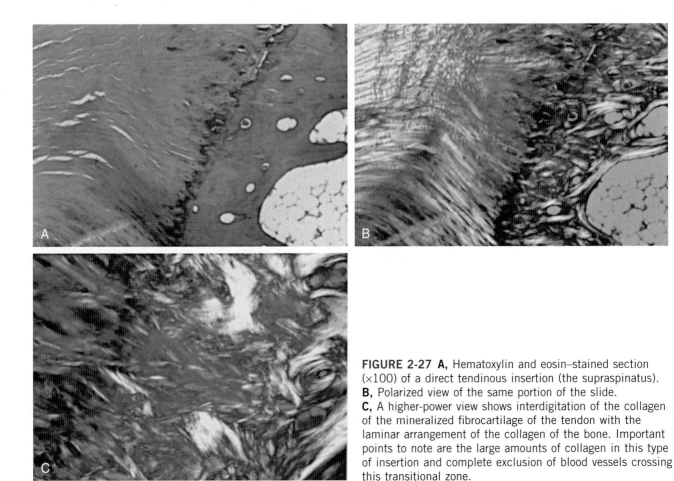

FIGURE 2-27 A, Hematoxylin and eosin–stained section (×100) of a direct tendinous insertion (the supraspinatus). **B,** Polarized view of the same portion of the slide. **C,** A higher-power view shows interdigitation of the collagen of the mineralized fibrocartilage of the tendon with the laminar arrangement of the collagen of the bone. Important points to note are the large amounts of collagen in this type of insertion and complete exclusion of blood vessels crossing this transitional zone.

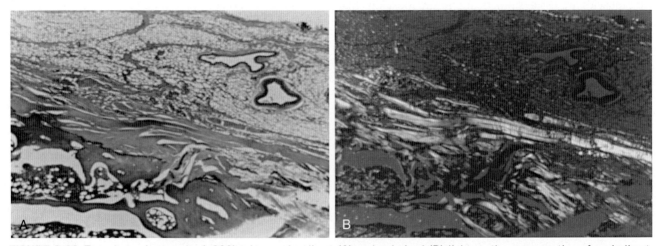

FIGURE 2-28 Two photomicrographs (×200) taken under direct (**A**) and polarized (**B**) light on the same section of an indirect muscle insertion (the deltoid). Note the thinner and looser arrangement of the collagen fibers. Only a few of the fibers interdigitate with the bone; most fibers continue into the collagen of the periosteum and from there into the indirect insertion of the trapezius. In an indirect attachment, blood vessels cross from bone to tendon.

Much of this work was done in the 1930s by Salmon but has not been available in the English literature until recently.[76] Research has been conducted by microvascular surgeons,[107] who suggest a classification system based on the vessels of the muscle (Fig. 2-30). Type I muscle circulation has one dominant pedicle. Type II has one dominant pedicle with an additional segmental supply. Type III has two dominant pedicles. Type IV, the most problematic type for transfer, has multiple segmental arterial supplies. It is this segmental arterial supply that limits the amount of muscle that can be transferred without endangering the viability of the muscle. Several segmental vessels must be maintained in these muscles. Type V has one dominant vessel with a number of secondary supplies. A similar type of classification could be developed for the internal nerve anatomy of these muscles inasmuch as the nerves often follow the same connective tissue support structures into the muscle.

Perhaps the most elegant conceptualization of circulation is the idea of the angiosome. As described by Taylor and Palmer, an angiosome is a block of tissue supplied by a dominant vessel.[108] The human body is then a three-dimensional jigsaw puzzle composed of these angiosomes. Each angiosome is dependent on its dominant vessel. Adjacent angiosomes have vascular connections that discourage interangiosome flow under normal circumstances but are capable of dilating under stress. An example of an applied stress is the delayed transfer of a flap, which allows the control vessels to dilate and capture adjacent tissue that might have become necrotic had the flap been moved at the first procedure.[76]

The arterial and venous angiosomes of a muscle correspond very closely, and the vessels travel together in the connective tissue framework of the muscle. The inter-

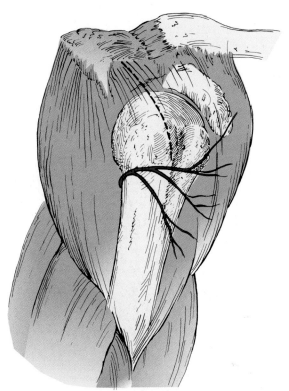

FIGURE 2-29 The position of the axillary nerve transverse to the fibers of the deltoid limits the extent of a deltoid-splitting incision in the anterior two thirds of the muscle. (From Jobe CM: Surgical approaches to the shoulder. Techniques in Orthopaedics 3[4]:3, 1989, with permission of Aspen Publishers, Inc. Copyright © January 1989.)

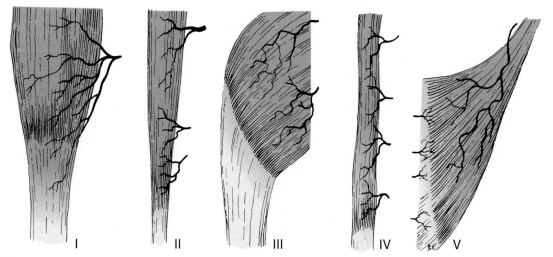

FIGURE 2-30 The five arrangements of blood vessels supplying muscle. Type I has one dominant vessel. Type II has a dominant vessel with one or more additional segmentally supplying vessels. Type III has two dominant pedicles. Type IV is the most difficult type to transfer because of multiple segmental supplies rather than one or two dominant supplies on which a muscle transfer may be based. Type V has a large dominant vessel with a number of small secondary supplies. (Redrawn from Mathes SJ, Nahai F: Classification of the vascular anatomy of muscles: Experimental and clinical correlation. Plast Reconstr Surg 67:177-187, 1981.)

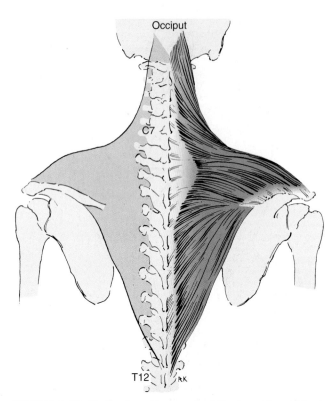

FIGURE 2-31 Textbook arrangement of the trapezius origins and insertions. The muscle originates from the occiput, the nuchal ligament, and the dorsal spines of vertebrae C7 through T12. It inserts on the acromion, the spine of the scapula, and some distal part of the clavicle. The trapezius is subdivided functionally into upper, middle, and lower fibers.

angiosome arterial control vessels are the choke arterioles, whose mode of function is obvious. The venous control is somewhat more complex because of the presence of valves in muscle veins that can be as small as 0.2 mm in diameter.[109] These valves create unidirectional flow toward the vascular pedicle. The control veins between adjacent angiosomes are free of valves except for each end. These valves are oriented to prevent entry of blood into the control vein. Venous congestion can then lead to dilatation and valve incompetence. Because the flow in these veins can be in either direction, they are called *oscillating veins.*[109]

The smaller vessels within muscles tend to run parallel to the muscle fibers.[76,109] Exceptions are the main branches to the muscle, which must cross perpendicularly to reach all of their smaller watersheds.[76] Knowledge of the anatomy of both the large and small vessels allows the placement of muscle-splitting incisions between and within angiosomes while avoiding division of the main branch vessel.

The discussion of muscles proceeds as follows. Individual muscles are discussed in terms of origin and insertion, with comments on the type of attachment to bone. We then move on to discuss the boundaries of muscles and their functions that have been described to date. Innervation of muscles are discussed in terms of the nerve

or nerves and the most common root representation. We then describe the vascular supply and its point or points of entry into the muscle, with brief mention of anomalies. The muscles are separated into four groups for purposes of discussion. First are the scapulothoracic muscles that control the motion of the scapula. The second group consists of the strictly glenohumeral muscles that work across that joint. Third, we discuss muscles that cross two or more joints. Finally, we discuss four muscles that are not directly involved with functioning of the shoulder but that are important anatomic landmarks.

Scapulothoracic Muscles

Trapezius

The largest and most superficial of the scapulothoracic muscles is the trapezius (Fig. 2-31). This muscle originates from the spinous processes of the C7 through T12 vertebrae.[110] The lower border can be as high as T8 or as low as L2. The upper portion of the trapezius above C7 takes its origin off the ligamentum nuchae, and two thirds of specimens have an upper limit of origin as high as the external occipital protuberance.[110] Insertion of the upper fibers is over the distal third of the clavicle. The lower cervical and upper thoracic fibers have their insertion over the acromion and the spine of the scapula. The lower portion of the muscle inserts at the base of the scapular spine. On the anterior or deep surface, the muscle is bounded by a relatively avascular space between it and other muscles, mostly the rhomboids. Posteriorly, the trapezius muscle is bounded by fat and skin.

As a whole, the muscle acts as a scapular retractor, with the upper fibers used mostly for elevation of the lateral angle.[111] Although some of the other fibers might come into play, only the upper fibers were found by Inman and colleagues to be consistently active in all upward scapular rotations.[20] The muscle follows a cephalocaudal activation as more flexion or abduction is obtained.[111] In forward flexion, the middle and lower trapezius segments are less active because scapular retraction is less desirable than in abduction.[20] Suspension of the scapula is supposed to be through the sternoclavicular ligaments at rest; electromyographic studies show no activity unless there is a downward tug on the shoulder.[32] The muscle must provide some intermittent relief to the ligaments of the sternoclavicular joint because paralysis of the trapezius produces a slight depression of the clavicle, although not as much as one might expect.[32] The major deformity is protraction and downward rotation of the scapula.[16]

The amount of depression might depend on the amount of downward loading of the limb with a paralyzed trapezius.[112] There appears to be a characteristic deficit seen in trapezius paralysis in which the shoulder can be brought up only to 90 degrees in coronal plane abduction but can be brought much higher in forward flexion.[112-114] In one case of congenital absence of the trapezius and the rhomboids, the patient compensated by using forward flexion to elevate the arm and lordosis of the lumbar spine to bring the arms up. When the arms had reached the vertical position, he would then release his lumbar lordosis and hold the elevation with the serratus anterior.[115] Acquired loss of trapezius function is less well tolerated.[16,116] A triple muscle transfer of levator scapulae, rhomboideus major, and minor can be performed to treat trapezius palsy.[117]

The accessory spinal nerve (cranial nerve XI) is the motor supply, with some sensory branches contributed from C2, C3, and C4. The nerve runs parallel and medial to the vertebral border of the scapula, always in the medial 50% of the muscle (Fig. 2-32).[106] The arterial supply is usually derived from the transverse cervical artery, although Salmon found the dorsal scapular artery to be dominant in 75% of his specimens.[76] The blood supply is described as type II,[107] a dominant vascular pedicle with some segmental blood supply at other levels. Huelke[118] reported that the lower third of the trapezius is supplied by a perforator of the dorsal scapular artery, and the upper fibers are supplied by arteries in the neck other than the transverse cervical artery. Other authors have attributed the blood supply of the lower pedicle to intercostal vessels.[109] Trapezius muscle transfers are based on supply by the transverse cervical artery.

Rhomboids

The rhomboids are similar in function to the midportion of the trapezius,[20] with an origin from the lower ligamentum nuchae at C7 and T1 for the rhomboid minor and T2 through T5 for the rhomboid major (Fig. 2-33). The rhomboid minor inserts on the posterior portion of the medial base of the spine of the scapula. The rhomboid major inserts into the posterior surface of the medial border from the point at which the rhomboid minor leaves off down to the inferior angle of the scapula. The muscle has, on its posterior surface, an avascular plane between it and the trapezius. The only crossing structure here is the transverse cervical artery superiorly or a perforator from the dorsal scapular artery. On the deep surface is another avascular fascial space that contains only the blood vessel and nerve to the rhomboids. On the muscle's deep surface inferiorly, the rhomboid major is bounded by the latissimus at its origin. Superiorly, the rhomboid minor is bounded by the levator scapulae.

The action of the rhomboids is retraction of the scapula, and because of their oblique course, they also participate in elevation of the scapula. Innervation to the rhomboid muscle is the dorsal scapular nerve (C5), which can arise off the brachial plexus in common with the nerve to the subclavius or with the C5 branch to the long thoracic nerve. The nerve can pass deep to or through the levator scapulae on its way to the rhomboids and can contain some innervation to the levator. The dorsal scapular artery provides arterial supply to the muscles through their deep surfaces.

Levator Scapulae and Serratus Anterior

Two muscles, the levator scapulae and serratus anterior, are often discussed together because of their close rela-

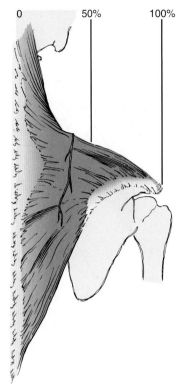

FIGURE 2-32 Course of the spinal accessory nerve relative to the trapezius muscle. If the spinal origins are taken as the 0 point of the muscle length and the acromion as the 100% length, the nerve and major branches are all in the medial 50% of the trapezius. The major course is parallel and medial to the vertebral border of the scapula. (From Jobe CM, Kropp WE, Wood VE: The spinal accessory nerve in a trapezius splitting approach. J Shoulder Elbow Surg 5:206-208, 1996.)

tionship in comparative anatomy studies (see Fig. 2-33). The levator scapulae originates from the posterior tubercles of the transverse processes from C1 through C3 and sometimes C4. It inserts into the superior angle of the scapula. The muscle is bounded in front by the scalenus medius and behind by the splenius cervicis. It is bounded laterally by the sternocleidomastoid in its upper portion and by the trapezius in its lower portion. The spinal accessory nerve crosses laterally in the middle section of the muscle.[27]

The dorsal scapular nerve may lie deep to or pass through the muscle. In specimens in which the dorsal scapular artery comes off the transverse cervical artery, the parent transverse cervical artery splits, the dorsal scapular artery passes medial to the muscle, and the transverse cervical artery passes laterally.

Ordinarily, the dorsal scapular artery has a small branch that passes laterally toward the supraspinatus fossa. In at least a third of dissections, these vessels supply the levator with circulation.[119]

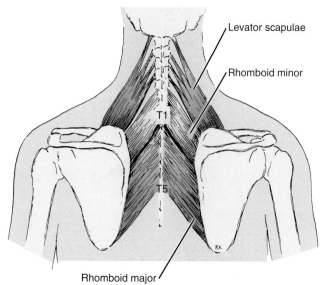

FIGURE 2-33 Rhomboids and the levator scapulae. The dominant orientation of the fibers of these muscles and their relative positions along the medial border of the scapula are shown.

The levator acts to elevate the superior angle of the scapula. In conjunction with the serratus anterior, it produces upward rotation of the scapula.[12] That the levator (Fig. 2-34) has a mass larger than the upper trapezius is illustrated properly only by comparing the two muscles in cross section; in most illustrations, it is obscured by overlying musculature.[12] Some authors speculate that this muscle also acts as a downward rotator of the scapula.[27] Innervation is from the deep branches of C3 and C4, and part of the C4 innervation is contributed by the dorsal scapular nerve.

The serratus anterior originates from the ribs on the anterior lateral wall of the thoracic cage. This muscle has three divisions (Fig. 2-35). The first division consists of one slip, which originates from ribs 1 and 2 and the intercostal space and then runs slightly upward and posteriorly to insert on the superior angle of the scapula. The second division consists of three slips from the second, third, and fourth ribs. This division inserts along the anterior surface of the medial border. The lower division consists of the inferior four or five slips, which originate from ribs 5 to 9. They run posteriorly to insert on the inferior angle of the scapula, thus giving this division the longest lever and most power for scapular rotation.

The serratus anterior is bounded medially by the ribs and intercostal muscles and laterally by the axillary space. Anteriorly, the muscle is bounded by the external oblique muscle with which it interdigitates, where this muscle originates from the same ribs.

The serratus anterior protracts the scapula and participates in upward rotation of the scapula. It is more active in flexion than in abduction because straight abduction requires some retraction of the scapula. Scheving and Pauly found that the muscle was activated by all movements of the humerus.[120] The serratus operates at a higher percentage of its maximal activity than does any other shoulder muscle in unresisted activities.[12,121] Absence of serratus activity, usually because of paralysis, produces a winging of the scapula, with forward flexion of the arm and loss of strength in that motion.[122,123] Muscle transfer to replace the inferior slips mainly restores only flexion.[124]

Innervation is supplied by the long thoracic nerve (C5, C6, and C7). The anatomy of this nerve has been studied intensely because of events in which injury has occurred. The nerve takes an angulated course across the second rib, where it can be stretched by lateral head tilt combined with depression of the shoulder.[125] The blood

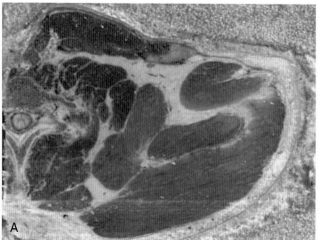

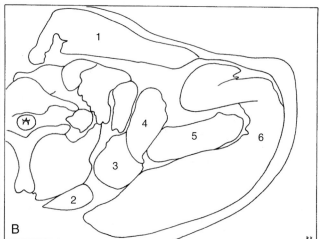

FIGURE 2-34 Photograph (**A**) and diagram (**B**) of a transverse section at a level slightly higher than the superior angle of the scapula showing the considerable girth of the levator scapulae, seen in cross section. Most of the other muscles noted are shown in their longitudinal section. The structures are as follows: *1*, sternocleidomastoid; *2*, rhomboid minor; *3*, levator scapulae; *4*, superior slip of the serratus anterior; *5*, supraspinatus; and *6*, trapezius.

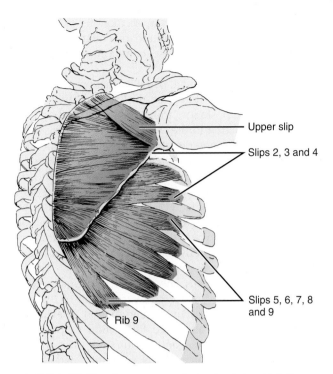

FIGURE 2-35 The three groups of muscles into which the slips of the serratus anterior are divided. The upper slip comes off the first two ribs and the first intercostal space and inserts at the upper edge of the medial border of the scapula. The slips coming off ribs 2, 3, and 4 insert on the broad major portion of the medial border; the slips from ribs 5, 6, 7, 8, and 9 converge on the inferior angle of the scapula.

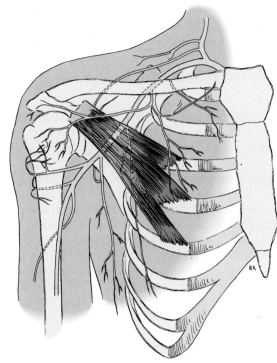

FIGURE 2-36 The pectoralis minor is an important landmark as an anterior border of the axillary space, as well as for dividing the axillary space into its proximal, middle, and distal portions. It acts in protraction and depression of the scapula.

supply to the serratus is classically stated to be through the lateral thoracic artery.[27] Often, however, the thoracodorsal artery makes a large contribution to the blood supply, especially when the lateral thoracic artery is small or absent. The lateral thoracic artery is the most commonly anomalous artery, originating from the axillary artery. The thoracodorsal artery can supply up to 50% of the muscle. The upper slips are supplied by the dorsal scapular artery.[76] There, additional contributions from the intercostal and internal mammary arteries are found.

Pectoralis Minor

The pectoralis minor has a fleshy origin anterior on the chest wall, from the second through the fifth ribs, and inserts onto the base of the medial side of the coracoid with frequent (15%) aberrant slips to the humerus, glenoid, clavicle, or scapula (Fig. 2-36).[123,126,127] The most common aberrant slip is the continuation across the coracoid to the humerus in the same path as the coracohumeral ligament. Its function is protraction of the scapula if the scapula is retracted and depression of the lateral angle or downward rotation of the scapula if the scapula is upwardly rotated. Innervation is from the medial pectoral nerve (C8, T1).

Blood supply is through the pectoral branch of the thoracoacromial artery.[27] Reid and Taylor reported in their

injection studies, however, that this vessel does not provide a constant supply to the pectoralis minor; another source is the lateral thoracic artery.[128] Salmon found multiple tiny arteries direct from the axillary that he called the *short thoracic arteries*.[76]

Absence of the muscle does not seem to cause any disability.[129] This muscle was thought to never be absent when the entire pectoralis major is present,[27] but Williams reported one case, verified at surgery, in which the pectoralis minor was missing from beneath a normal pectoralis major.[129] Bing reported three other cases in the German literature.[130]

Subclavius

The subclavius muscle is included with the scapulothoracic muscles because it crosses the sternoclavicular joint, where most of the scapulothoracic motion takes place (Fig. 2-37). It has a tendinous origin off the first rib and cartilage and a muscular insertion on the inferior surface of the medial third of the clavicle. The tendon has a muscle belly that is pennate in structure. The tendon, 1 to 1.5 inches long, lies mainly on the inferior surface of the muscle.[131] Its nerve supply is from the nerve to the subclavius. The blood supply is derived from the clavicular branch of the thoracoacromial artery or from the suprascapular artery.[76,128] The action of this muscle is to stabilize the sternoclavicular joint while in motion—particularly with adduction and extension against resistance, such as hanging from a bar (i.e., stabilization in intense activity).[132]

Glenohumeral Muscles

Deltoid

The largest and most important of the glenohumeral muscles is the deltoid, which consists of three major sections: the anterior deltoid, originating from the lateral third of the clavicle; the middle third of the deltoid, originating from the acromion; and the posterior deltoid, originating from the spine of the scapula.[133] Typical of broadly based muscles, the origin is collagen poor throughout its breadth. Insertion is on the deltoid tubercle of the humerus. It is a long and broad insertion. Klepps[134] found that the anterior, middle, and posterior deltoid muscle fibers merged into a broad V-shaped tendinous insertion with a broad posterior band and a narrow anterior band. They found that the deltoid insertion in the vast majority of specimens was separated from the pectoralis major insertion by less than 2 mm. The axillary and radial nerves were not very close to the deltoid insertion.[134]

The deltoid muscle's boundary on the external side is subcutaneous fat. Because of the amount of motion involved, the subacromial bursa and fascial spaces bound the deep side. The axillary nerve and posterior humeral circumflex artery, the only nerve and the major blood supply of the muscle, also lie on the deep side. The pectoralis major muscle lies anteromedially. The clavicular portion of this muscle shares many functions with the anterior third of the deltoid. Within the boundary of the two muscles is the deltopectoral groove, where the cephalic vein and branches of the deltoid artery of the thoracoacromial trunk lie.

The three sections of the deltoid differ in internal structure and function (Fig. 2-38). The anterior and posterior deltoid sections have parallel fibers and a longer excursion than the middle third, which is multipennate and stronger and has a shorter excursion (1 cm). The middle third of the deltoid takes part in all motions of elevation of the humerus.[12] With its abundant collagen, it is the portion of the muscle most commonly involved in contracture.[135]

Elevation in the scapular plane is the product of the anterior and middle thirds of the deltoid, with some action by the posterior third, especially above 90 degrees.[136] Abduction in the coronal plane decreases the contribution of the anterior third and increases the contribution of the posterior third. Flexion is a product of the anterior and middle thirds of the deltoid and the clavicular portion of the pectoralis major, with some contribution by the biceps (Fig. 2-39). The contribution of the latter two muscles is so small that it is insufficient to hold the arm against gravity without the deltoid.[137] In summary, the deltoid is active in any form of elevation, and loss of deltoid function is considered a disaster.[138]

The deltoid contributes only 12% of horizontal adduction. It was suggested that the lower portion of the posterior deltoid has some activity in adduction. Shevlin and coworkers, however, attributed this action to providing an external rotation force on the humerus to counteract the internal rotation force of the pectoralis major, teres major, and latissimus dorsi—the major adductors of the shoulder.[136] The deltoid accounts for 60% of strength in horizontal abduction.[139] The deltoid muscle's relationship to the joint is such that it has its shortest leverage for elevation in the first 30 degrees,[12] although in this position leverage is increased by the prominence of the greater tubercle.[82] Gagey and Hue have shown that the deltoid can contribute to head depression at the initiation of elevation.[83]

The anterior third of the deltoid is bounded on its deep surface by the coracoid, the conjoint tendon of the cora-

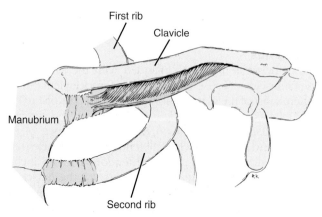

FIGURE 2-37 The subclavius muscle has a pennate structure and a long tendon on its inferior surface.

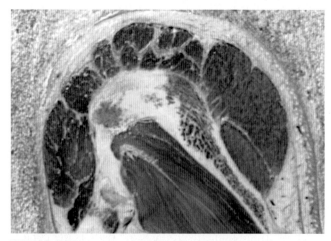

FIGURE 2-38 A cross section taken just below the origin of the right deltoid demonstrates the relative positions of the three divisions of the deltoid and the differences in their internal structure. The middle deltoid, being multipennate, has an abundance of internal collagen. The anterior third (on the *left*) and the posterior third (on the *right*) tend to be parallel in structure or partially unipennate adjacent to the septum that separates them from the middle third.

cobrachialis, and the short head of the biceps and the clavipectoral fascia. The posterior portion of the deltoid is bounded on its deep surface by the infraspinatus and teres minor and by the teres major muscle on the other side of the avascular fascial space. The deltoid has very dense fascia on its deep surface. The axillary nerve and the posterior humeral circumflex vessels run on the muscle side of this fascia.[140]

Innervation of the deltoid is supplied by the axillary nerve (C5 and C6), which enters the posterior portion of the shoulder through the quadrilateral space and innervates the teres minor in this position. The nerve splits in the quadrilateral space, and the nerve or nerves to the posterior third of the deltoid enter the muscle very close to their exit from the quadrilateral space and travel in the deltoid muscle along the medial and inferior borders of the posterior deltoid. Interestingly, the posterior branch extends 6 to 8 cm after it leaves the quadrilateral space.[98] The branch of the axillary nerve that supplies the anterior two thirds of the deltoid ascends superiorly and then travels anteriorly, approximately 2 inches inferior to the rim of the acromion. Paralysis of the axillary nerve produces a 50% loss of strength in elevation,[139] even though the full abduction range is sometimes maintained.[141] Its vascular supply is largely derived from the posterior humeral circumflex artery, which travels with the axillary nerve through the quadrilateral space to the deep surface of the muscle.[27,28,76,133] The deltoid is also supplied by the deltoid branch of the thoracoacromial artery, with rich anastomoses between the two vessels. The deltoid artery travels in the deltopectoral groove and sends branches to the muscle.[76] Numerous additional arteries are also present. The venous pedicles are identical to the arterial pedicles,[109] except that the cephalic vein is quite dominant, especially for the anterior third of the deltoid.

Rotator Cuff

Before discussing the rotator cuff muscles individually, some remarks about the cuff as a whole are in order. Although made up of four separate muscles, the rotator cuff is a complex arrangement. The muscles can appear separate superficially, but in their deeper regions they are associated with each other, with the capsule underneath, and with the tendon of the long head of the biceps.[139]

In their deeper regions, the tendons send fascicles into their neighbors. The most complex of this sharing occurs at the bicipital groove, where the fascicles of the supraspinatus destined for the insertion of the subscapularis cross over the groove and create a roof. Conversely, the fascicles of the subscapularis tendon that are headed for the supraspinatus insertion create a floor for the groove by undergoing some chondrometaplasia.[139]

Also in their deeper regions, muscles and tendons attach to the capsule. Again, the most complex of these arrangements occurs at the rotator interval. In this region the coracohumeral ligament contributes fibers that envelop the supraspinatus tendon. This relationship is most apparent on the deep surface, where it is visible to the arthroscopist as a curved cable running from the anterior edge to the back of the supraspinatus tendon and on into the infraspinatus to create a laterally based arch or suspension bridge.[142] This arrangement creates a thicker region of the cuff visible on ultrasound.

Supraspinatus

The supraspinatus muscle lies on the superior portion of the scapula. It has a fleshy origin from the supraspinatus fossa and overlying fascia and inserts into the greater tuberosity. Its tendinous insertion is in common with the infraspinatus posteriorly and the coracohumeral ligament anteriorly. This complex tendon formation is common to the rotator cuff. The superficial fibers are longitudinal and

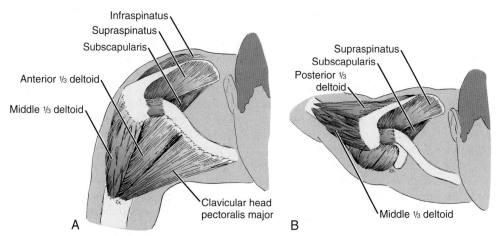

FIGURE 2-39 Function of the deltoid. **A,** The middle and anterior thirds of the deltoid function together with the clavicular head of the pectoralis major in forward flexion. **B,** In horizontal abduction, the posterior third of the deltoid is active and the anterior third is inactive. The middle third of the deltoid is active in all motions of the glenohumeral joint.

give the tendon the appearance of a more discrete structure. These more superficial fibers have larger blood vessels than the deeper fibers do. The deeper fibers run obliquely and create a nonlinear pattern that holds sutures more effectively. This tendon sends fibers anteriorly with the coracohumeral ligament over the bicipital groove to the lesser tuberosity. The anterior edge of the tendon is enveloped by the coracohumeral ligament. The anterior portion of the supraspinatus is more powerful than the posterior half, with the muscle fibers inserting onto an extension of the tendon within the anterior half of the muscle. This tendon extension can be seen on MRI.[66] Roh and colleagues found that the physiologic cross section of the anterior muscle belly was much larger than the posterior muscle belly. However, the cross-sectional area of the anterior tendon was slightly smaller than that of the posterior tendon. Thus, a larger anterior muscle belly pulls through a smaller tendon area.[143]

A portion of the coracohumeral ligament runs on the articular surface of the supraspinatus tendon perpendicular to the orientation of the tendon. This creates a laterally based arch that is visible from within the joint and runs all the way to the infraspinatus insertion. Its tendon has an asymptomatic calcium deposit in as many as 2.5% of shoulders.[144] Inferiorly, the muscle portion is bounded by its origin off the bone, the rim of the neck of the glenoid, and the capsule itself, which is not divisible from the deep fibers of the tendon (Fig. 2-40).

The function of the muscle is important because it is active in any motion involving elevation.[145] Its length-tension curve exerts maximal effort at about 30 degrees of elevation.[102] Above this level, the greater tubercle increases its lever arm.[82] Because the muscle circumscribes the humeral head above and its fibers are oriented directly toward the glenoid, it is important for stabilizing the glenohumeral joint. The supraspinatus, together with the other accessory muscles—the infraspinatus, subscapularis, and biceps—contributes equally with the deltoid in the torque of scapular plane elevation and in forward elevation when tested by selective axillary nerve block.[137,146] The supraspinatus has an excursion about two thirds that of the deltoid for the same motion, indicating a shorter lever arm.[147]

Other muscles of the rotator cuff, especially the infraspinatus and subscapularis, provide further downward force on the humeral head to resist shear forces of the deltoid. If these muscles are intact, even with a small rotator cuff tear, enough stabilization may be present for fairly strong abduction of the shoulder by the deltoid muscle, although endurance may be shorter.[12] Some patients externally rotate their shoulder so that they can use their biceps for the same activity. Because the supraspinatus is confined above by the subacromial bursa and the acromion and below by the humeral head, the tendon is at risk for compression and attrition. Because of such compression, Grant and Smith's series and others indicate that 50% of cadaver specimens from persons older than

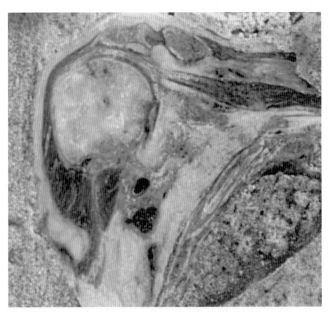

FIGURE 2-40 Cross section of the scapula in the coronal plane showing the important relationships of the supraspinatus muscle. Among these relationships are the course of the tendon that circumscribes the humeral head—essential to its head-depressing effect—and the tendon's course beneath the acromion, the acromioclavicular joint, and the indiscernible subacromial bursa. Inferiorly, it is inseparable from the capsule of the joint. The subacromial bursa above the tendon, being a potential space, is indiscernible. (Compare with Fig. 2-71.)

77 years have rotator cuff tears.[148] A later study by Neer showed a lower incidence.[70]

The boundaries of the path of the supraspinatus tendon are referred to as the *supraspinatus outlet.*[64] This space is decreased by internal rotation and opened by external rotation, thus showing the effect of the greater tubercle.[61] The space is also compromised by use of the shoulder in weight bearing, such as when using crutches and when doing pushups in a wheelchair.[149]

Martin suggested that external rotation of the arm in elevation is produced by the coracoacromial arch acting as an inclined plane on the greater tubercle.[150] Saha and others attribute this limitation of rotation in elevation to ligamentous control.[72,74] More recent data suggest that this external rotation is necessary to eliminate the 45-degree angulation of the humerus from the coronal plane. This adds 45 degrees to the limited elevation allowed by the glenoid (Fig. 2-41).[151] Innervation of the supraspinatus is supplied by the suprascapular nerve (C5 with some C6).

The main arterial supply is the suprascapular artery. The suprascapular vessels enter the muscle near its midpoint at the suprascapular notch at the base of the coracoid process. The nerve goes through the notch and is bounded above by the transverse scapular ligament. The nerve does not have any motion relative to the notch. The artery travels above this ligament. The suprascapular

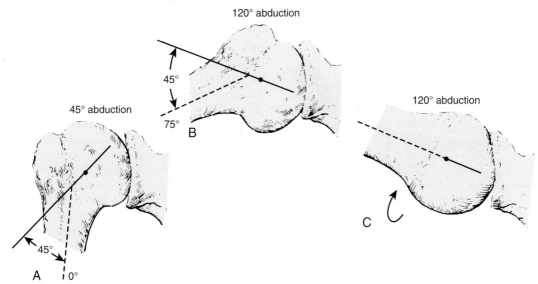

FIGURE 2-41 **A,** The glenohumeral joint. **B,** With some compression of the soft tissues superiorly, this glenohumeral joint allows almost 75 degrees of coronal abduction. **C,** Without changing the orientation of the axis of the head to the glenoid, 90 degrees of upward rotation removes the 135-degree neck-shaft angle from view, thus making the neck-shaft angle appear to be 180 degrees. This adds an additional 45 degrees of apparent elevation in the coronal plane. (From Jobe CM, Iannotti JP: Limits imposed on glenohumeral motion by joint geometry. J Shoulder Elbow Surg 4:281-285, 1995.)

vessels and nerve supply the deep surface of the muscle. A branch also runs between the bone of the scapular spine and the muscle. The medial portion of the muscle receives vessels from the dorsal scapular artery.[76]

Infraspinatus

The infraspinatus is the second most active rotator cuff muscle (Fig. 2-42).[12] It has a fleshy, collagen-poor origin from the infraspinatus fossa of the scapula, the overlying dense fascia, and the spine of the scapula. Its tendinous insertion is in common with the supraspinatus antero-superiorly and the teres minor inferiorly at the greater tuberosity. On its superficial surface it is bounded by an avascular fascial space on the deep surface of the deltoid. The infraspinatus is a pennate muscle with a median raphe, often mistaken at surgery for the gap between the infraspinatus and teres minor muscles.

The infraspinatus is one of the two main external rotators of the humerus and accounts for as much as 60% of external rotation force.[137] It functions as a depressor of the humeral head.[20] Even in the passive (cadaver) state it is an important stabilizer against posterior subluxation.[152,153] An interesting aspect of muscle action at the shoulder is that a muscle can have opposing actions in different positions. The infraspinatus muscle stabilizes the shoulder against posterior subluxation in internal rotation by circumscribing the humeral head and creating a forward force. In contradistinction, it has a line of pull posteriorly and stabilizes against anterior subluxation when the shoulder is in abduction and external rotation.[12,154]

The infraspinatus is innervated by the suprascapular nerve. The nerve tunnels through the spinoglenoid notch, which is not usually spanned by a ligament. Its blood supply is generally described as coming from two large branches of the suprascapular artery.[27] Salmon, however, found in two thirds of his specimens that the subscapular artery through its dorsal or circumflex scapular branch supplied the greater portion of the circulation of the infraspinatus muscle.[76]

Teres Minor

The teres minor has a muscular origin from the middle portion of the lateral border of the scapula and the dense fascia of the infraspinatus (see Fig. 2-42). Rarely are persons found in whom the teres minor overlies the infraspinatus as far as the vertebral border of the scapula.[155] It inserts into the lower portion of the posterior greater tuberosity of the humerus. On its deep surface is the adherent posterior capsule, and on the superficial surface is a fascial plane between it and the deep surface of the deltoid. On the inferior border lie the quadrilateral space laterally and the triangular space medially. In the quadrilateral space, the posterior humeral circumflex artery and the axillary nerve border the teres minor. In the triangular space, the circumflex scapular artery lies just inferior to this muscle. On its deep surface, in the midportion, lies the long head of the triceps tendon, loose alveolar fat, and the subscapularis.

The teres minor is one of the few external rotators of the humerus. It provides up to 45% of the external rotation force and is important in controlling stability in the anterior direction.[137,154] It also probably participates in the short rotator force couple in abduction along with the inferior portion of the subscapularis. The teres minor is

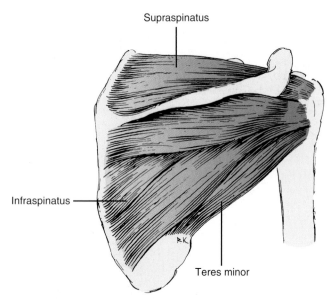

Supraspinatus

Infraspinatus

Teres minor

FIGURE 2-42 The two external rotators of the humerus, the infraspinatus and teres minor muscles, are also the posterior wall of the rotator cuff. Note the median raphe of the infraspinatus, which is often mistaken at surgery for the border between the infraspinatus and the teres minor.

innervated by the posterior branch of the axillary nerve (C5 and C6). Its blood supply is derived from several vessels in the area, but the branch from the posterior humeral scapular circumflex artery is the most constant.[76]

Subscapularis

The subscapularis muscle is the anterior portion of the rotator cuff. The muscle takes a fleshy origin from the subscapularis fossa, which covers most of the anterior surface of the scapula. In its upper 60%, it inserts through a collagen-rich tendon into the lesser tuberosity of the humerus. In its lower 40%, it has a fleshy insertion into the humerus below the lesser tuberosity cupping the head and neck.[156] The internal structure of the muscle is multipennate, and the collagen is so dense in the upper subscapularis that it is considered to be one of the passive stabilizers of the shoulder.[94-96] It is bounded anteriorly by the axillary space and the coracobrachialis bursa.

Superiorly, it passes under the coracoid process and the subscapularis recess, or bursa. The axillary nerve and posterior humeral circumflex artery and veins pass deep below the muscle into the quadrilateral space. The circumflex scapular artery passes into the more medial triangular space. Laterally, the anterior humeral circumflex vessels mark the division between the upper 60% and the lower 40%.[156]

The subscapularis functions as an internal rotator and passive stabilizer to prevent anterior subluxation and, especially in its lower fibers, serves to depress the humeral head (Fig. 2-43).[20] By this last function it resists the shear force of the deltoid to help with elevation. Compression

of the glenohumeral joint also adds to this function. Another aspect of the subscapularis is that its function can vary with the level of training. The function of the subscapularis in acceleration is less in amateur pitchers than in professional pitchers, thus implying that a less-trained pitcher is still adjusting the glenohumeral joint for stability, whereas a professional can use the muscle as an internal rotator.[101]

In common with the insertions of the other rotator cuff muscles, the subscapularis has parallel collagen superficially and more divergent fascicles deep. Such anatomy aids the surgeon by allowing the tendon to hold suture. This divergent structure is probably related to containment of the humeral head and upward and downward rotation of the head on the glenoid. One of the more prominent features of the divergence is an upper group of deep fibers that passes on the deep surface of the biceps and inserts into the floor of the bicipital groove all the way to the supraspinatus insertion.

On its deep surface, in the upper portion, is the glenohumeral joint. The middle glenohumeral ligament lies beneath the upper portion of the tendon. The anterior inferior glenohumeral ligament lies deep to the mid and lower portions. Innervation is generally supplied by two sources: The upper subscapular nerves (C5) supply the upper 50% and the lower subscapular nerves (C5 and C6) supply the lower 20%. The nerve supply to the intervening 30% varies. The upper subscapular nerves, usually two comparatively short nerves in the axilla, come off the posterior cord. Because of the greater relative motion of the lower portion of the scapula, the lower subscapular nerves (also two) are longer in their course.[157]

The blood supply of the subscapularis is usually described as originating from the axillary and subscapular arteries. Bartlett and associates found that 84% of their 50 dissections had no significant vessels off the subscapular artery before the bifurcation into circumflex scapular and thoracodorsal arteries.[158] This finding would increase the importance of the anterior humeral circumflex artery and the "upper subscapular artery" named by Huelke.[119] Salmon also described this latter artery as a constant vessel but stated that it is small in caliber. He found that the major supply was derived from branches of the subscapular artery.[76] Small branches from the dorsal scapular artery reach the medial portion of the muscle after penetrating the serratus anterior. Venous drainage is via two veins to the circumflex scapular vein.[109]

Teres Major

The teres major originates from the posterior surface of the scapula along the inferior portion of the lateral border (Fig. 2-44C). It has a muscular origin and insertion into the humerus posterior to the latissimus dorsi along the medial lip of the bicipital groove, a ridge of bone that is a continuation of the lesser tuberosity and posterior to it. In their course, the latissimus dorsi and teres major undergo a 180-degree spiral; thus, the formerly posterior surface of the muscle is represented by fibers on the

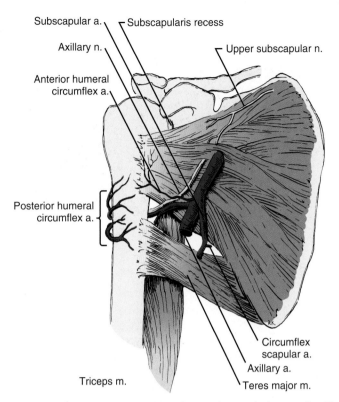

Subscapular a. Subscapularis recess

Axillary n.

Upper subscapular n.

Anterior humeral
circumflex a.

Posterior humeral
circumflex a.

Circumflex
scapular a.
Axillary a.
Teres major m.

Triceps m.

FIGURE 2-43 The anterior and inferior relationships of the subscapularis muscle. The soft tissues not shown are the axillary space fat and the coracobrachialis bursa. The vulnerable structures within the adipose tissue are the axillary nerve, which crosses the fibers of the subscapularis muscle before entering the quadrilateral space, and the posterior humeral circumflex vessels. The size of the quadrilateral space is enlarged in this drawing for illustrative purposes. The anterior humeral circumflex vessels are also vulnerable anteriorly. The triangular space has been enlarged by the illustrator.

anterior surface of the tendon. Moreover, the relationship between the teres major and latissimus dorsi becomes rearranged so that the formerly posterior latissimus dorsi becomes anterior to the teres major. In addition to the boundaries of the latissimus dorsi, it is bounded above by the triangular and quadrilateral spaces, posteriorly by the long head of the triceps, and anteriorly in its medial portion by the axillary space.

The function of the teres major is internal rotation, adduction, and extension of the arm. It is active in these motions only against resistance.[56] It can have an additional function, upward rotation of the scapula, during activities that involve a firmly planted upper limb, such as the iron cross performed by gymnasts. Innervation is supplied by the lower subscapular nerve (C5 and C6), and its blood supply is derived from branches of the subscapular artery, quite regularly a single vessel from the thoracodorsal artery.[76] This branch can originate from the axillary artery directly.

Coracobrachialis

The coracobrachialis has a fleshy and tendinous origin from the coracoid process, in common with and medial to the short head of the biceps, and it inserts on the anteromedial surface in the midportion of the humerus. Laterally it is bounded by its common origin with the biceps. On the deep surface the coracobrachialis bursa lies between the two conjoint muscles and the subscapularis. The deltoid, the deltopectoral groove, and the pectoralis major are on the superficial surface. These surfaces tend to be avascular or are crossed by a few small vessels.

The action of the coracobrachialis is flexion and adduction of the glenohumeral joint, with innervation supplied by small branches from the lateral cord and the musculocutaneous nerve. Most specimens have a direct nerve to the coracobrachialis from the lateral cord, in addition to the larger musculocutaneous (C5 and C6) nerve. This additional nerve enters the coracobrachialis muscle on its deep surface and provides extra innervation.[159] Because the larger musculocutaneous nerve's entrance to the muscle may be situated as high as 1.5 cm from the tip of the coracoid to as low as 7 to 8 cm, it must be located and protected during certain types of repair. The major blood supply is by a single artery, usually off the axillary. This artery can arise in common with the artery to the biceps.[76]

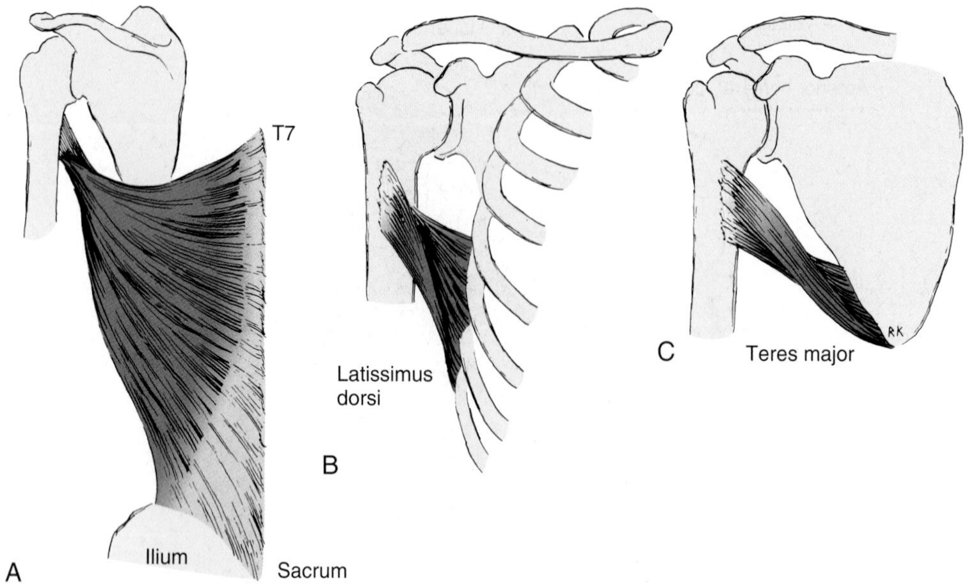

FIGURE 2-44 A, Posterior view of the course of the latissimus dorsi muscle from its origin along the posterior spinous processes from T7 to the sacrum and along the iliac crest. **B,** Anterior view shows that the insertion of the latissimus dorsi muscle is along the medial lip and floor of the bicipital groove. **C,** The accompanying muscle, the teres major, with its similar fiber rotation inserts just medial to the latissimus dorsi.

Multiple Joint Muscles

Multiple joint muscles act on the glenohumeral joint and one other joint, most often the scapulothoracic. When appropriate, the action on both joints is mentioned.

Pectoralis Major

The pectoralis major consists of three portions (Fig. 2-45). The upper portion originates from the medial half to two thirds of the clavicle and inserts along the lateral lip of the bicipital groove. Its fibers maintain a parallel arrangement. The middle portion originates from the manubrium and upper two thirds of the body of the sternum and ribs 2 to 4. It inserts directly behind the clavicular portion and maintains a parallel fiber arrangement. The inferior portion of the pectoralis major originates from the distal body of the sternum, the fifth and sixth ribs, and the external oblique muscle fascia. It has the same insertion as the other two portions, but the fibers rotate 180 degrees so that the inferior fibers insert superiorly on the humerus. Landry noted that when a chondroepitrochlearis muscle anomaly existed, the twisted insertion was not present.[160] A line of separation is often present between the clavicular portion and the lower two portions. The superficial surface of the muscle is bounded by the mammary gland and subcutaneous fat. The inferior border is the border of the axillary fold. The superior lateral border is the deltopectoral groove mentioned earlier. On the deep surface superior to the attachment to the ribs lies the pectoralis minor muscle, which is invested by the clavipectoral fascia.

The action of the pectoralis major depends on its starting position. For example, the clavicular portion participates somewhat in flexion with the anterior portion of the deltoid, whereas the lower fibers are antagonistic. Both these effects are lost in the coronal plane. The muscle is active in internal rotation against resistance and extends the shoulder from flexion until the neutral position is reached.[136] This muscle is also a powerful adductor of the glenohumeral joint and indirectly functions as a depressor of the lateral angle of the scapula. Loss of the sternocostal portion most noticeably affects internal rotation and scapular depression, with some loss of adduction.[161] This loss is significant only for athletics and not for daily activities. The clavicular portion is most active in forward flexion and horizontal adduction.[20] Loss of pectoralis major function seems to be well tolerated.[129,162]

Innervation of the muscle is supplied by two sources. The lateral pectoral nerve (C5, C6, and C7) innervates the clavicular portion of the muscle, probably only with C5 to C6 fibers, and the loop contribution from the lateral to the medial pectoral nerve carrying C7 fibers continues through or around the pectoralis minor into the upper sternal portion. The medial pectoral nerve, which carries fibers from C8 and T1, continues through the pectoralis minor into the remaining portion of the pectoralis major. Klepps and colleagues[163] found that the pectoral nerves innervate the pectoralis major quite medially, far from the humeral insertion. These nerves are safe from surgical dissection as long as one remains lateral to the pectoralis minor and less than 8.5 cm from the humeral insertion point.[163]

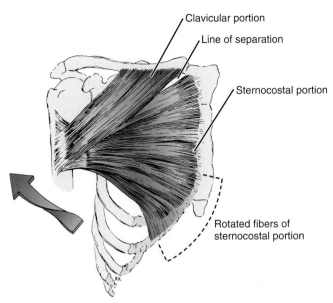

Clavicular portion

Line of separation

Sternocostal portion

Rotated fibers of
sternocostal portion

FIGURE 2-45 Two major divisions of the pectoralis major
muscle. The separation is often readily discernible. Note the
180-degree rotation of the fibers of the lower portion of the
sternocostal division.

The major blood supply is derived from two sources.
The deltoid branch of the thoracoacromial artery supplies
the clavicular portion, and the pectoral artery supplies
the sternocostal portion of the muscle.[128] Additional blood
supply is provided via the internal mammary artery, the
fourth or fifth intercostal artery, and other anastomoses
from the lateral thoracic artery.[76,128] The vessel to the
fourth rib area is within an additional deep origin that
comes off this rib in the midclavicular line. Venous drainage laterally is through two veins to the axillary vein and
medially to the internal mammary system.[128] In a literature
review performed in 1902, Bing found that absence of a
portion or all of the pectoralis major was the most commonly reported muscle defect, and such defects accounted
for 28% of the cases cited.[130]

Latissimus Dorsi

The latissimus dorsi (see Fig. 2-44A and B) originates via
the large and broad aponeurosis from the dorsal spines
of T7 through L5, a portion of the sacrum, and the crest
of the ilium. It often has origins on the lowest three or
four ribs and the inferior angle of the scapula as well.[158]
This muscle wraps around the teres major and inserts into
the medial crest and floor of the bicipital or intertubercular groove.

On its superficial surface the muscle is bounded by
subcutaneous fat and fascia, and along the inferior border,
it forms the posterior axillary fold. Anteriorly, it is bounded
by the axillary space, and its deep surface is bounded by
ribs and the teres major. Actions of the muscle are inward
rotation and adduction of the humerus, shoulder extension, and, indirectly through its pull on the humerus,
downward rotation of the scapula. Scheving and Pauly
found that this muscle is more important than the pecto-

ralis major as an internal rotator.[120] Ekholm and colleagues found its most powerful action in the oblique
motions: extension, adduction, and abduction and internal rotation.[99]

Innervation is through the thoracodorsal nerve (C6 and
C7), and blood supply is derived from the thoracodorsal
artery, with additional supply from the intercostal and
lumbar perforators. The neurovascular hilum is on the
inferior anterior surface of the muscle, about 2 cm medial
to the muscular border.[158] Two investigators have found
that this neurovascular pedicle splits inside the muscle
fascia into superomedial and inferolateral branches.[158,164]
They found that such splits are quite predictable and
suggested that the muscle could be split into two separate
island flaps, or free flaps. The venous drainage mirrors
the arterial supply.[109]

Biceps Brachii

The biceps has its main action at the elbow rather than
the shoulder. It is considered primarily an elbow muscle,
but it is listed here with the shoulder muscles because of
its frequent involvement in shoulder pathology and its
use in substitutional motions.

The biceps muscle has two origins in the shoulder,
both of which are rich in collagen. The long head originates from the bicipital tubercle at the superior rim of the
glenoid and along the posterior superior rim of the
glenoid and labrum, and the short head originates from
the coracoid tip lateral to and in common with the coracobrachialis. Meyer[84] noted that much of the origin of the
long head is via the superior labrum and that the size of
the bicipital tubercle does not reflect the size of the
biceps tendon.

The muscle has two distal tendinous insertions. The
lateral insertion is to the posterior part of the tuberosity
of the radius, and the medial insertion is aponeurotic and
passes medially across and into the deep fascia of the
muscles of the volar forearm. Loss of the long head
attachment is manifested mainly as loss of supination
strength (20%) and with a smaller loss (8%) of elbow
flexion strength.[165]

The relationships of the biceps tendon are most important in its role in shoulder pathology. The long head of
the biceps exits the shoulder through a defect in the
capsule between the greater and lesser tuberosities and
passes distally in the bicipital groove. This portion of the
tendon is most often involved in pathology. Many studies
have been performed in an attempt to correlate construction of the groove with bicipital pathology (see Fig.
2-23).[84,166] It was thought that a shallow bicipital groove
and a supratubercular ridge above the lesser tubercle,
which is the trochlea of the tendon, would predispose
the biceps tendon to dislocation, with subsequent tendon
pathology. It was also noted that the intra-articular tendon
is broader than that in the groove.[84] Other early authors
reported no rupture of the biceps tendon in the absence
of supraspinatus rupture. Recent opinion is that pathology of the tendon is related to impingement. If a correla-

tion exists between bicipital groove morphology and the biceps tendon, it may be that a shallower groove is more likely to expose the long head of the biceps to impingement.[70] The bicipital tendon does not move up and down in the groove. Rather, the humerus moves down and up with adduction and abduction relative to the tendon. The bicipital tendon is retained within the groove by a pulley made up of fibers from the coracohumeral and superior glenohumeral ligaments, with some reinforcement from adjacent tendons.[139,167]

Under normal conditions, the action of the biceps is flexion and supination at the elbow. In certain conditions, particularly paralysis or rupture of the supraspinatus, patients have a hypertrophied long head of the biceps, probably because they are using the muscle as a depressor of the humeral head by placing the shoulder in external rotation.[12] One patient with a large rotator cuff tear reportedly was employed as a waiter and carried trays on the involved side, a substitution maneuver commonly seen in the days of poliomyelitis.[20,168] Lucas reported a 20% loss of elevation strength in external rotation with rupture of the long head of the biceps.[23] Mariani and coauthors, on the other hand, reported that loss of this head depressor effect is unlikely to worsen impingement.[165] In internal rotation, no loss of strength was evident, and we must remember that impingement occurs in internal rotation.[23] In one study involving cadaver specimens it was found that the long head could contribute to joint stability and that this stability is increased in external rotation and decreased in internal rotation.[169] These are *not* the usual activities of the biceps in a person without shoulder pathology studied by electromyography.

Innervation of the biceps is supplied by branches of the musculocutaneous nerve (C5 and C6), and the blood supply is derived from a single large bicipital artery from the brachial artery (35%), multiple very small arteries (40%), or a combination of the two types.[76]

Triceps Brachii

The triceps is another muscle that is not usually considered a shoulder muscle but may be involved in shoulder pathology, particularly the long head. The long head originates from the infraglenoid tubercle. Although this tendon is not intra-articular like the long head of the biceps, the insertion is intimately related to the labrum over a distance of 2 cm centered on the tubercle. The fibers of the tendon adjacent to the capsule radiate into the inferior capsule and reinforce it. The remaining fibers insert into bone. This reinforced capsule, a portion of the inferior glenohumeral ligament, inserts through the labrum and radiates fibers into the circular portion of the labrum.

The origin of the long head is bounded laterally by the quadrilateral space, which contains the axillary nerve and posterior humeral circumflex artery, and medially by the triangular space, which contains the circumflex scapular artery. The teres major muscle passes anteriorly, and the teres minor passes posteriorly. Innervation is supplied by the radial nerve, with root innervation through C6 to C8.[27] The arterial supply is derived mainly from the profunda brachii artery and the superior ulnar collateral artery. However, near its origin, the long head receives branches from the brachial and posterior humeral circumflex arteries.

The major action of the muscle is extension at the elbow. In addition, the long head is believed to function in shoulder adduction against resistance to offset the shear forces generated by the primary adductors. In more violent activities, such as throwing, the muscle can demonstrate electromyographic activity up to 200% of that generated by a maximal muscle test.[170] A portion of the force is transmitted to the origin of the scapula.

Landmark Muscles

Some muscles are important to surgeons as landmarks for shoulder dissection, although these muscles are not shoulder muscles in the sense of producing shoulder motion.

Sternocleidomastoid

The most obvious of these landmarks is the sternocleidomastoid muscle, which, with the superior fibers of the trapezius, forms the borders of the posterior triangle of the neck. It originates via a tendinous head from the sternum and a broader, but thin, muscular head from the medial part of the clavicle.[28] The two heads unite and progress superiorly, obliquely posteriorly, and laterally to insert on the mastoid process. This muscle shares the same innervation with the trapezius: the spinal accessory nerve (cranial nerve XI). The blood supply is derived from two vascular pedicles, the superior from the occipital artery and the lower from the superior thyroid artery.

Scalenus Anterior and Scalenus Medius

The anterior scalene muscle originates from the anterior tubercles of vertebrae C3 through C6 and has a tendinous insertion on the first rib. The middle scalene muscle, largest of the scalenes, originates from all of the transverse processes in the cervical spine and also inserts into the first rib. The first rib and the two scalene muscles form a triangle (Fig. 2-46) through which the entire brachial plexus and the subclavian artery pass. The subclavian vein passes anterior to the anterior scalene and posterior to the clavicle. Innervation of these muscles is supplied by deep branches of the cervical nerves. Variations in the muscles and their relationships are believed to predispose a person to thoracic outlet syndrome.[76]

Omohyoid

The omohyoid muscle is seldom mentioned in a description of surgical procedures, but it divides the posterior

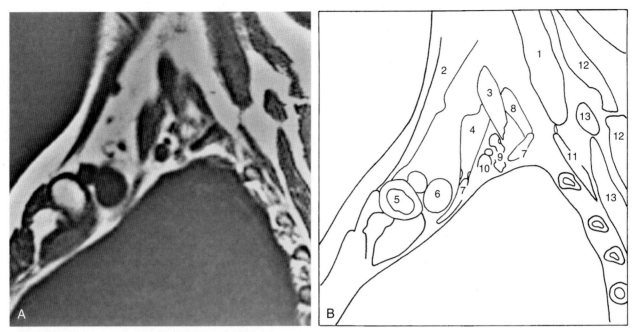

FIGURE 2-46 MRI scan (**A**) and diagram (**B**) of the scalene triangle showing its boundaries and the relationships of the important structures. Note that the anterior tilt of the first rib places the more posterior structures at a more caudad level. Note also the greater thickness of the levator scapulae (*1*) in comparison to the trapezius (*12*). The labeled structures are: *1*, levator scapulae; *2*, sternocleidomastoid; *3*, middle scalene; *4*, anterior scalene; *5*, clavicle; *6*, subclavian vein; *7*, rib 1; *8*, posterior scalene; *9*, brachial plexus; *10*, subclavian artery; *11*, serratus posterior superior; *12*, trapezius; and *13*, rhomboids.

cervical triangle into the upper occipital and lower sub-clavian triangles. It attaches to the superior border of the scapula just medial to the scapular notch and runs ante-riorly, medially, and superiorly across the posterior cervical triangle. Deep to the sternocleidomastoid muscle is a tendon in the midportion of the muscle belly. The muscle continues on above to an insertion on the hyoid.

NERVES

Our discussion of nerves of the shoulder includes the brachial plexus and its branches, the sympathetic nervous system, the nerves that come off the roots that form the brachial plexus, cranial nerve XI, and the supraclavicular nerves. The brachial plexus is unique in the human nervous system because of the great amount of motion involved relative to the adjacent tissues. By way of intro-duction we first discuss the internal anatomy of the nerves. Roots, trunks, and cords of the brachial plexus are also peripheral nerves in their cross-sectional anatomy.[171-173] We then discuss the arrangement of the peripheral nervous system relative to other structures of the limbs. As an overview, we note a uniqueness of the brachial plexus in comparison to the rest of the nervous system; this uniqueness is a product of the increased motion of the shoulder.

We describe the standard brachial plexus and its normal relationships and then discuss nonpathologic variants, variations that do not affect its function but can compli-cate diagnosis and surgical approaches. We also discuss cranial nerve XI, the supraclavicular nerves, and the inter-costal brachial nerve.

Function and Microanatomy

The principal function of nerves is to maintain and support axons of the efferent and afferent nerve cells. Cell bodies of these fibers are located in the dorsal root and autonomic ganglia and in the gray matter of the spinal cord. The axons are maintained somewhat by axoplasmic flow, but conduction of the nerve and its continued function have been found to depend on the layers surrounding the axons and their blood supply.[173-175] These layers in turn depend on an adequate blood supply.[176,177]

The axons in large nerves are contained within Schwann cells either 1:1 or, for smaller nerve fibers, on a multiaxon-to-one Schwann cell ratio. These in turn are embedded in the endoneurium. A basal lamina separates the endoneurium from the myelin sheaths and Schwann cells.

Endoneurial tissue is mainly collagen that is closely arranged and contains capillaries and lymphatics.[173,175,178] The next outer tissue, referred to as the *perineurium*, surrounds groups of axons and serves primarily as a dif-fusion barrier. It also maintains intraneural pressure. The integrity of this layer is essential to function of the nerve and is the tissue most important to the surgeon. The perineurium is divided into multiple layers. The innermost layer has flat cells with tight junctions and appears to maintain the diffusion barrier. The outer layers are lamellated with interspersed collagen. The external layer of perineurium is a proven barrier to infection, whereas the outer layer of the nerve, the epineurium, is not.

The portion of the nerve enclosed in perineurium is referred to as a *fascicle* and is really the functioning portion of the nerve. All axons are contained in fascicles, and fascicles produce the necessary environment for nerve function. The size and number of fascicles vary. Fascicles tend to be larger and fewer in the spinal nerves and smaller and more numerous around branch points.[171] As a branch point is approached, fascicles bound for the branch nerve are gathered into *fascicle groups*.[171,175] The variability in fascicle number and size is further complicated because fascicles travel an average distance of only 5 mm before branching or merging. This arrangement results in a plexiform internal anatomy rather than the cable form that would be more convenient for repair and grafting.[171]

The epineurium is loose areolar tissue that is richly supplied with blood vessels and lymphatics.[175] It can compose more than 80% of the cross-sectional area of the nerve or as little as 25%,[172,175] with an average of about 40% to 50% in peripheral nerves and 65% to 70% in the plexus.[171]

The blood supply to the nerves has been divided into extrinsic and intrinsic vessels.[179] Intrinsic vessels are those contained within the epineurium itself, and such vessels constitute the arterial supply of the nerve. Terzis and Breidenbach further classified the nerves and extrinsic circulation in terms of whether all the extrinsic vessels connected to the same source artery and veins for purposes of free transfer of nerve tissue.[180] The blood vessels within the nerves are redundant and often have a convoluted course. Lundborg found that an average change of 8% in length by stretching had to occur before the development of venous occlusion in the nerves and an average 15% strain for complete cessation of arterial flow. Interestingly, function was normal in laboratory animals in which blood clots and blockage in some of the capillaries persisted even after release of tension on the nerve.[178]

Even the internal arrangement of nerves is designed to accommodate motion (Fig. 2-47). Layers slide past each other and allow almost a laminar motion of the layers relative to their surroundings.

The 15% strain limit also has implications for the anatomic relationships of nerves, particularly in the shoulder. The closer a nerve is positioned to a center of joint rotation, the less the nerve changes in length with motion.

There seem to be two strategies in the arrangement of the brachial plexus that protect the nerve against overstretch. First, the location of the nerves directly behind the sternoclavicular joint protects them against stretch during elevation of the clavicle in the coronal plane. The second crucial arrangement is that the brachial plexus in the axilla is not fixed to surrounding structures but instead floats freely in a quantity of fat. This design allows the plexus to slide superiorly with elevation of the arm so that it moves closer to the center of rotation and is subject to less strain. The implication of this arrangement is that disruption of the biomechanics of the shoulder can produce neurologic symptoms even when the original trauma or disease does not directly affect the nerves themselves. An additional protective arrangement in a joint that is so highly mobile is that most human motion is conducted forward, thus putting less stretch on most of the plexus. One exception to this tendency would be nerves tightly attached to the scapula, which would be stretched by scapular protraction.[181]

The extrinsic vessels to the nerve tend to have an inverse relationship between their size and number. They have a short length of 5 to 15 mm from the adjacent artery. Redundancy of the blood supply is such that a nerve, when stripped of its extrinsic blood supply, continues to function up to 8 cm from the nearest arteria nervorum.[178,182] This redundancy in blood supply is advantageous to tumor surgeons, who find the epineurium to be an effective boundary in certain tumor dissections. The epineurium is sometimes sacrificed in surgery with good preservation of nerve function. Moreover, radiotherapy can be applied to the axilla without loss of function. The redundancy can be overcome, however, with a combination of epineurial stripping and radiation or an excessive dose of radiotherapy alone, with an adverse effect on nerve function.[183,184]

Brachial Plexus

While studying the circulation of blood to the skin, Taylor and Palmer identified some common elements in the distribution of blood vessels in the body that we would also apply to the arrangement of peripheral nerves.[108] First, nerves tend to travel adjacent to bone, in intermuscular septa or other connective tissue structures. Second, the nerves travel from relatively fixed positions to relatively mobile positions. Nerves rarely cross planes in which motion is involved, but when they do, they cross in an oblique fashion in an area of less motion. This arrangement decreases the relative strain incurred by the nerve while crossing a mobile plane even though the actual total motion is not changed.[108]

The brachial plexus seems to contradict these tendencies. It travels from an area where it is relatively fixed at the cervical spine to an area of high mobility in the axilla, and then it returns to normal bone and intermuscular septum relationships in the arm. This pattern is unique in the human body and is necessitated by the highly mobile nature of the shoulder and the motion of the brachial plexus nerves on their way to innervate structures in the arm and forearm. This seeming contradiction is understood when we picture the axillary sheath as the connective tissue framework for the nerves and vessels

FIGURE 2-47 Internal anatomy of peripheral nerves and how it facilitates motion. *A* and *B* are the inner and outer layers of the perineurium; *C* and *D* are the inner and outer layers of the epineurium. *E* is a blood vessel within the epineurium, and *F* is the blood vessel of the nerve on the outside of the epineurium. Much of the cross section of the nerve is epineurium. The various components of the soft tissue of the nerve accommodate nerve motion. (From Lundborg G: Intraneural microcirculation. Orthop Clin North Am 19:1-12, 1988.)

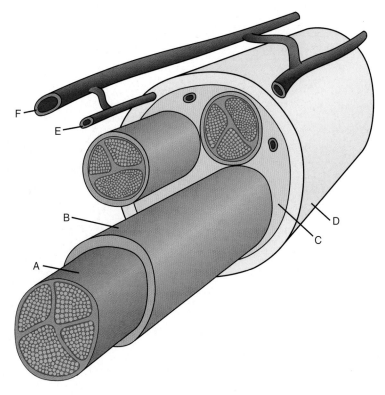

and note that it is the sheath that moves in the axillary space.[185] An excellent review of brachial plexus injury treatment and anatomy has been published by Shin and colleagues.[186]

Roots

The standard brachial plexus (Fig. 2-48) is made up of the distal distribution of the anterior rami of the spinal nerves or roots C5, C6, C7, C8, and T1. The plexus sometimes has contributions from C4 and T2. A plexus with C4 contributions is called *prefixed.* When contributions from T2 occur, the term is *postfixed.*[186] For C4, this contribution appears in 28% to 62% of specimens,[187] although in terms of neural tissue it contributes very little.[171] The incidence of postfixed plexuses reportedly ranges from 16% to 73%.[186,188] The dorsal root ganglion holds the cell bodies. A *preganglionic* injury is one where the roots are avulsed from the spinal cord. An injury distal to the dorsal root ganglion is termed *postganglionic.* Distinguishing between the two has treatment implications because there is little recovery potential for a preganglionic injury.[186]

The roots that form the spinal nerves lack a fibrous sheath[183] and obtain a significant amount of soft tissue support only when they exit the intervertebral foramina, at which point they gain a dural sleeve. Herzberg and colleagues found a posterosuperior semiconic ligament at C5, C6, and C7 that attaches the spinal nerves to the transverse processes.[189] The spinal nerves C8 and T1 lack this additional protection. In most brachial plexus literature the anterior divisions of these spinal nerves are called the *roots of the brachial plexus.* Herzberg and coworkers

found that the C5 and C6 roots could be followed proximally but failed to find a safe surgical approach to spinal nerves C8 and T1 because dissection involved damage to the osseous structures.[189] Other authors mention the difficulty in exposing the lower two nerves.[190]

Trunks, Divisions, and Cords

The roots combine to form trunks: C5 and C6 form the upper trunk, C7 the middle trunk, and C8 and T1 the lower trunk.[186] The trunks then separate into anterior and posterior divisions. The posterior divisions combine to form the posterior cord, the anterior division of the lower trunk forms the medial cord, and the anterior divisions of the upper and middle trunks form the lateral cord. These cords give off the remaining and largest number of terminal nerves of the brachial plexus, with branches from the lateral and medial cords coming together to form the median nerve.

The brachial plexus leaves the cervical spine and progresses into the arm through the interval between the anterior and middle scalene muscles (Fig. 2-49). The subclavian artery follows the same course. Because of the inferior tilt of the first rib, the brachial plexus is posterior and superior to the artery at this point; only the lower trunk is directly posterior to the artery on the rib. It is in this triangle made up of the two scalenes that nerve or vessel can be compromised by any number of abnormalities.[191] The inferior trunk forms high behind the clavicle, directly above the pleura, over a connective tissue layer referred to as *Sibson's fascia.* The upper two roots join to form the upper trunk at Erb's point, located

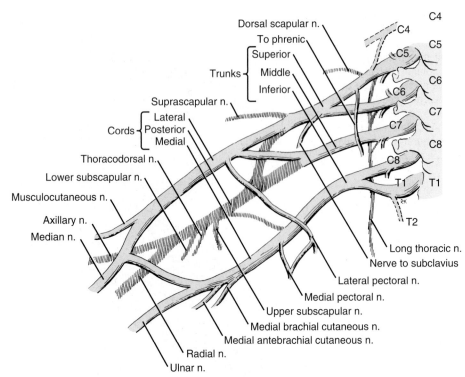

FIGURE 2-48 Standard arrangement of the brachial plexus and its trunks, cords, and terminal branches.

2 to 3 cm above the clavicle, just behind the posterior edge of the sternocleidomastoid muscle. The majority of plexuses are penetrated by a vessel off the subclavian artery, most commonly the dorsal scapular artery, between two of the trunks.[118] The nerves between the scalene muscles become enclosed in the fascia of the scalenes, the prevertebral fascia. This interscalene sheath is important for containing and permitting the dispersal of local anesthetic about the nerves.[192]

The plexus splits into cords at or before it passes below the clavicle. As the cords enter the axilla, they become closely related to the axillary artery and attain positions relative to the artery indicated by their names: lateral, posterior, and medial. The prevertebral fascia invests the plexus and vessels and forms the axillary sheath. Two other landmark arteries are the transverse cervical artery, which crosses anterior to the level of the upper two trunks, and the suprascapular artery at the level of the middle trunk and the clavicle.[184]

Terminal Branches

The plexus gives off some terminal branches above the clavicle. The dorsal scapular nerve comes off C5, with some C4 fibers, and penetrates the scalenus medius and levator scapulae, sometimes contributing C4 fibers to the latter.[189] In the remaining cases, the nerve to the levator is a separate nerve. The dorsal scapular nerve accompanies the deep branch of the transverse cervical artery or the dorsal scapular artery on the undersurface of the rhomboids and innervates them.

Rootlets come off nerves C5, C6, and C7 directly adjacent to the intervertebral foramina and contribute to formation of the long thoracic nerve, which immediately passes between the middle and posterior scalenes[187] or penetrates the middle scalene.[125,193] Horwitz and Tocantins reported the nerve forming after the rootlets exit the muscle, with the C7 contribution not passing through muscle. They also mentioned that the nerve becomes more tightly fixed to muscle by branches near the distal end of the nerve. This nerve might not receive a contribution from C7, but its composition is fairly regular.[125,193] The nerve passes behind the plexus over the prominence caused by the second rib.[194] It is thought that this nerve may be stretched by depression of the shoulder with lateral flexion of the neck in the opposite direction. Prescott and Zollinger reported two cases of injury with abduction; several mechanisms of injury may be responsible.[194]

The small nerve to the subclavius also comes off the upper trunk. Kopell and Thompson pointed out an interesting relationship of the suprascapular nerve. Protraction of the scapula increases the distance between the cervical spine and the notch because the scapula must move laterally around the thorax to travel forward.[181] This location also predisposes the suprascapular nerve to injury in scapular fractures.[195]

The lateral cord generally contains fibers of C5, C6, and C7 and gives off three terminal branches: the musculocutaneous, the lateral pectoral, and the lateral root of the median nerve. The first branch coming off the lateral cord

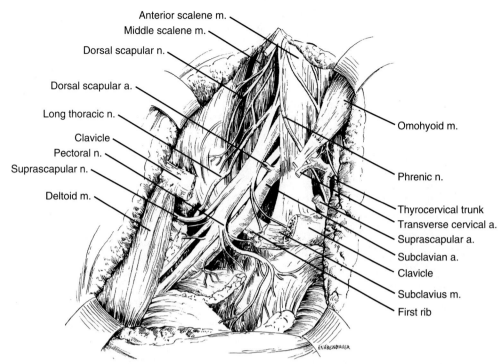

Anterior scalene m.
Middle scalene m.
Dorsal scapular n.
Dorsal scapular a.
Long thoracic n.
Clavicle
Pectoral n.
Suprascapular n.
Deltoid m.

Omohyoid m.
Phrenic n.
Thyrocervical trunk
Transverse cervical a.
Suprascapular a.
Subclavian a.
Clavicle
Subclavius m.
First rib

FIGURE 2-49 The more compressed form of the brachial plexus, found at the time of surgery, and its important anatomic relationships. (From Strohm BR, Colachis SC Jr: Shoulder joint dysfunction following injury to the suprascapular nerve. Phys Ther 45:106-111, 1965.)

is the lateral anterior thoracic or lateral pectoral nerve (C5-C7), which, after leaving the lateral cord, passes anterior to the first part of the axillary artery. It penetrates the clavipectoral fascia above the pectoralis minor at about the midpoint of the clavicle and innervates the clavicular portion and some of the sternal portion of the pectoralis major muscle. This nerve is 4 to 6 cm in length.[98] The nerve also sends a communication to the medial pectoral nerve, which carries its contribution to the remaining portion of the pectoralis major. This loop usually passes over the axillary artery just proximal to the thoracoacromial trunk.[128] Miller,[196] however, showed the artery to be more proximal. The lateral pectoral nerve also innervates the acromioclavicular joint, along with the suprascapular nerve.[197]

The final lateral cord nerve is the lateral root (C5-C7) to the median nerve. The median nerve is formed anterior to the third portion of the axillary artery and accompanies the brachial artery and vein into the arm.

The posterior cord supplies most of the innervation to the muscles of the shoulder in the following order: upper subscapular, thoracodorsal, lower subscapular, axillary, and radial. Because of the great range of motion of the muscles relative to the brachial plexus, nerves to muscles in the shoulder tend to be quite long and come off quite high in relation to their destination. For this reason and because nerves tend to segregate in neural tissue into groups of fascicles,[175] several authors report that the posterior cord is poorly formed and may be a discrete structure in only 25% of cadavers.[188,192]

The next distal nerve, the thoracodorsal nerve (C7 and C8), is the longest (12-18 cm)[98] of the terminal nerves coming off the brachial plexus in the axilla and is referred to as the *long subscapular nerve*. It is also sometimes called the *long thoracic or nerve of Bell*. The nerve follows the subscapular and then the thoracodorsal artery along the posterior wall of the axilla to the latissimus dorsi.[184,188] In the latissimus dorsi muscle the nerve splits into two branches, as does the blood supply.[158]

The final continuation of the posterior cord is the radial nerve (C5-C8), which continues posterior to the axillary artery and, shortly after exiting the axilla, disappears into the space deep to the long head of the triceps. The nerves to the long and medial heads of the triceps arise when the nerve is still in the axilla. The posterior cutaneous branch also arises in the axilla. A branch that comes off medially, referred to as the ulnar collateral nerve because of its proximity to the ulnar nerve, innervates the medial head of the triceps.

The medial cord has five branches in the following order: medial pectoral nerve, medial brachial cutaneous nerve, medial antebrachial cutaneous nerve, medial root of the median nerve, and ulnar nerve. The medial pectoral nerve (C8 and T1) comes off the medial cord, which at this point has finally attained its position medial to the artery. Anteriorly, it passes between the artery and vein (the vein is the more medial structure) and enters the deep surface of the pectoralis minor. Some fibers come out anterior to the muscle to supply the more caudal portions of the pectoralis major. The nerve varies from 8

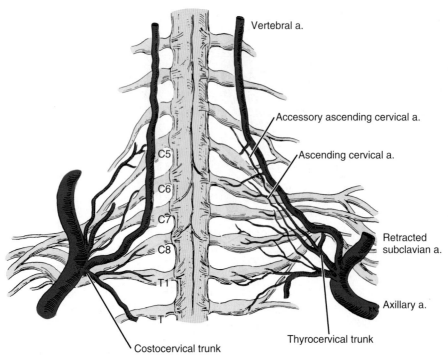

Vertebral a.

Accessory ascending cervical a.

Ascending cervical a.

C5

C6

C7

Retracted
subclavian a.

C8

T1

Axillary a.

T

Thyrocervical trunk

Costocervical trunk

FIGURE 2-50 Blood supply of the proximal brachial plexus and the spinal cord. In the more distal portion of the brachial plexus, the blood supply originates from accompanying arteries and veins. (Redrawn from Abdullah S, Bowden REM: The blood supply of the brachial plexus. Proc R Soc Med 53:203-205, 1960.)

to 14 cm in length.[98] A communicating branch from the lateral pectoral nerve joins the medial pectoral before it enters the pectoralis minor muscle.

The medial brachial cutaneous nerve contains fibers from T1 and is followed in order by the medial antebrachial cutaneous nerves from T1 and C8. Both are cutaneous nerves that supply the area of skin indicated by their names. The medial brachial cutaneous nerve often receives a communication from the intercostal brachial nerve. The medial root of the median nerve (C8 and T1) passes in front of the third portion of the axillary artery to join the lateral root.

The ulnar nerve is the terminal extension of the medial cord. We would expect it to have fibers of C8 and T1 alone, but researchers have found that 50% of specimens have a contribution carrying fibers of C7 from the lateral cord to the ulnar nerve, generally via a nerve off the median nerve.[187,188] The C7 fibers are usually destined for the flexor carpi ulnaris.[184] The ulnar nerve has no important branches in the shoulder area; its first branches appear as it approaches the elbow.

Like all nerves, the brachial plexus receives its blood supply from adjacent arteries. Because there is little motion relative to the vessels, the arteries are short and direct. The blood supply to the brachial plexus proximally was mapped out by Abdullah and Bowden and found to originate from the subclavian artery and its branches (Fig. 2-50).[198] The vertebral artery supplies the proximal plexus along with the ascending and deep cervical arteries and the superior intercostal artery. The

autonomic ganglia lying anterior near the spinal column are supplied by branches of the intercostal vessels in the thorax and branches of the vertebral artery in the cervical area. Distally, adjacent arteries provide contributions. The relationship between the plexus and vessels is abnormal in 8% of shoulders[196] (see Chapter 3), with nerves penetrated by vessels.

Specific Terminal Branches

Because of their importance in surgical dissection in approaches to the shoulder, the following specific terminal nerve branches of the brachial plexus are mentioned separately.

Subscapular Nerves. The upper subscapular nerves (C5) originate from the posterior cord and enter the subscapularis muscle quite high because of the less relative motion here. They are the shortest of the nerves originating from this cord. They supply two thirds to four fifths of the upper portion of the subscapularis muscle. The lower subscapular nerves (C5 and C6) follow a long course from their origin before entering the muscles. They innervate the lower portion of the subscapularis muscle and the teres major.

Yung, Lazarus, and Harryman[199] specifically dissected out the upper and lower subscapular nerves in relation to their innervation of the subscapularis muscle. They described a safe zone for surgical dissection. They found that the palpable anterior border of the glenoid rim deep to the subscapularis along with the medial border of the conjoint tendon could serve as safe landmarks because all neural branches were at least 1.5 cm medial to the conjoint tendon and all neural branches to the subscapularis were on the anterior surface. The lower subscapular nerve muscle insertion site was close to the axillary nerve, and the branches were very small. They thus concluded that the location and protection of the axillary nerve could serve as a guide to the insertion point of the lower subscapular nerve.[199]

Axillary Nerve. The last branch coming off the posterior cord in the shoulder area is the axillary nerve (C5 and C6), which, as it disappears into the gap between the subscapularis and teres major, is accompanied by the posterior circumflex humeral artery. It passes laterally to the inferolateral border of the subscapularis, where it winds 3 to 5 mm medial to the musculotendinous junction. It then passes lateral to the long head of the triceps and is in intimate contact with the capsule.[200] The quadrilateral shape of this space cannot be visualized from the front; when viewed from behind, it is formed by the teres minor superiorly and the teres major inferiorly (Fig. 2-51; see also Fig. 2-43). The medial border is the long head of the triceps, and the lateral border is the shaft of the humerus. Nerve entrapment has also been described in this space.[201]

The axillary nerve divides in the space and sends a posterior branch to the teres minor and the posterior third of the deltoid and an anterior branch to the anterior two thirds of the deltoid. Ball and colleagues[202] performed cadaveric dissection of the posterior branch of the axillary nerve. They found that the posterior branch divided from the anterior branch just anterior to the origin of the long head of the triceps at the 6-o'clock position. The branch to the teres minor and the superior-lateral brachial cutaneous nerve arose from the posterior branch of the axillary nerve in all specimens dissected. In most specimens, a branch from the posterior branch supplied the posterior aspect of the deltoid. In all specimens there was an additional branch from the anterior branch to the posterior deltoid.[202]

The lateral brachial cutaneous nerve supplies the area of skin corresponding in shape and overlying the deltoid muscle, after wrapping around the posterior border of the deltoid.[133] The anterior branch comes to lie approximately 2 inches below the edge of the acromion as the nerve passes anteriorly to innervate the anterior two thirds of the muscle. One or more small branches attach to the lower border of the posterior deltoid muscle and, unlike the anterior branch, do not proceed vertically toward the spine of the scapula but follow the inferior fibers of the muscle.

The axillary nerve also supplies sensory innervation to the lower portion of the glenohumeral joint through two articular branches. The anterior articular branch comes off before the nerve enters the quadrilateral space. The second branch comes off in the space. Together they are the major nerve supply of the joint.[197] Often, another branch accompanies part of the anterior humeral circumflex artery toward the long head of the biceps.

Surgeons worry about axillary nerve safety with deltoid-splitting incisions. Cetik and colleagues[203] performed cadaveric dissection to determine a safe area for the axillary nerve in the deltoid muscle. They found that the average distance from the anterior edge of the acromion to the course of the axillary nerve is 6.08 cm, and 5.2 cm was the closest distance. The average distance from the posterior edge of the acromion to the axillary nerve was 4.87 cm.[203] This distance varies with abduction.

Musculocutaneous Nerve. The musculocutaneous nerve (C5-C7) (Fig. 2-52) originates high in the axilla. It is commonly thought that the musculocutaneous nerve enters the coracobrachialis muscle 5 to 8 cm distal to the coracoid process.[204] Flatow and colleagues found that the nerve did indeed pierce the coracobrachialis at an average of 5.6 cm from the coracoid process.[159] However, they found that the nerve pierced the muscle at a range from 3.1 cm to 8.2 cm. They also found that small nerve twigs from the musculocutaneous nerve pierced the coracobrachialis even more proximally, averaging 3.1 cm from the coracoid process, with some as close as 1.7 cm. They concluded that the frequently cited 5- to 8-cm range could not be relied upon because in 29% of cases the main nerve entered the muscle proximal to the 5 cm mark. If one includes the smaller branches, one or more nerves entering the muscle in the proximal 5 cm were found in 74% of shoulders.[159] This entry point is critical because of the number of procedures that can put traction on the nerve. Kerr found nerve branches from the lateral cord or musculocutaneous nerve in slightly more than half of his specimens.[191] The musculocutaneous nerve appears distally in the forearm as the lateral antebrachial cutaneous nerve.

Suprascapular Nerve. The suprascapular nerve arises from the superior lateral aspect of the upper trunk shortly after its formation at Erb's point. It follows a long oblique course to its next fixed point, the suprascapular notch. This course is parallel to the inferior belly of the omohyoid. The nerve does not move relative to the notch.[205-207] The nerve passes below the transverse scapular or suprascapular ligament and enters the supraspinatus muscle, which it innervates through two branches. Both the origin from the upper trunk and the muscle attachments lie cephalad to the ligament, which forces the nerve to angle around the ligament.[205]

The suprascapular nerve innervates the infraspinatus muscle through two branches after passing inferiorly around the base of the spine of the scapula.[208] It also provides two articular branches: one in the supraspinatus fossa to the acromioclavicular and superior glenohumeral joints and one in the infraspinatus fossa to the posterior superior glenohumeral joint.[197] It is accompanied by the suprascapular artery, which passes over the transverse scapular ligament.

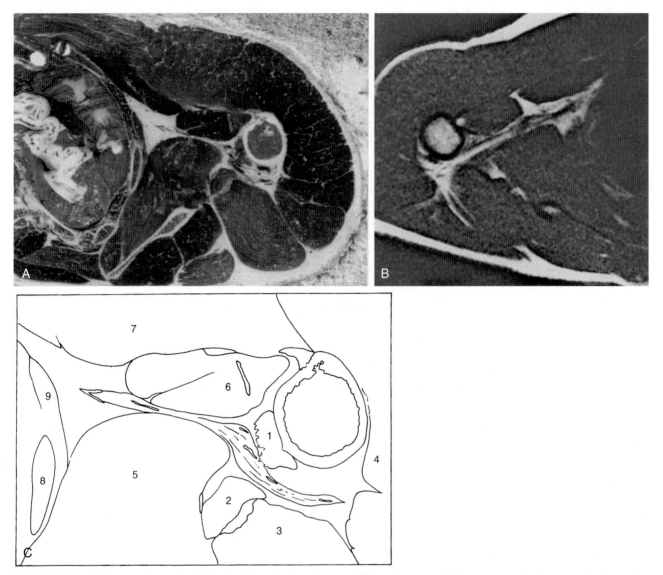

FIGURE 2-51 A, Cross section of a right shoulder showing the quadrilateral space with the nerve and artery coming from the axillary space and passing between the conjoint and subscapularis muscles and then between the triceps and the humerus. Note how small the quadrilateral space is in comparison to the usual representations. **B,** Left shoulder MRI axial cut showing the quadrilateral space. **C,** Diagram labeling the structures shown in **A:** *1,* teres major; *2,* teres minor; *3,* long head of the triceps; *4,* deltoid; *5,* infraspinatus; *6,* coracobrachialis and short head of the biceps; *7,* pectoralis major and minor; *8,* rib 3; and *9,* serratus anterior.

The surrounding bone and ligament form a foramen that can entrap the nerve. Variations in the suprascapular notch anatomy can contribute to nerve entrapment in this area. They include an osseous clavicular tunnel,[209] an ossified transverse scapular ligament, an anterior coracoscapular ligament, and superiorly orientated subscapularis fibers.[210] Paralysis of the nerve has profound effects on shoulder function.[211]

Bigliani and colleagues[212] performed 90 cadaveric dissections to study the course of the suprascapular nerve. The motor branch to the supraspinatus branched within 1 cm of the base of the scapular spine in nearly 90% of

cases. They further found that the nerve courses close to the posterior glenoid rim. The distance from the midline of the posterior glenoid rim to the suprascapular nerve at the base of the scapular spine averaged 1.8 cm, and some were as close as 1.4 cm.[212] Compression of the nerve by the spinoglenoid ligament near the base of the spine has been reported.[213-215]

Autonomic Supply

All nerves of the brachial plexus carry postganglionic autonomic fibers, with the largest portion (27%-44%) at C8 and the smallest portion (1%-9%) at C5.[216] A review

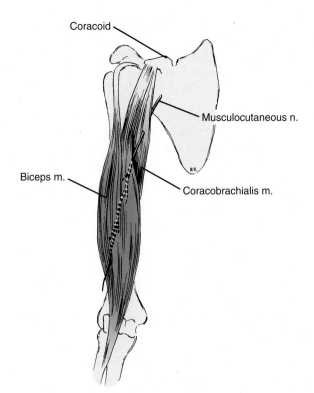

Coracoid

Musculocutaneous n.

Biceps m.

Coracobrachialis m.

FIGURE 2-52 Course of the musculocutaneous nerve. This nerve originates from the lateral cord and penetrates the conjoint muscle–tendon on its deep surface. The point of penetration varies; it may be as close to the coracoid tip as 1.5 cm or as far away as 9 cm (the average is 5 cm). The nerve continues distally, innervates the long head of the biceps brachii and the brachialis muscle, and appears in the forearm as the lateral antebrachial cutaneous nerve.

of the common structure of the sympathetic nervous system indicates that fibers coming from the spinal cord are myelinated and are collected in what is called the *white rami communicantes*, or *type I ramus*. Fibers that leave the ganglion, or postganglionic fibers, are not myelinated and tend to be collected in the gray ramus. Type II rami are gray rami with few myelinated (preganglionic) fibers. Type III rami are mixtures of gray and white fibers. Gray or white rami can also be multiple.[217]

The sympathetic supply to C5 and C6 comes through the gray rami from the middle cervical ganglion, the superior cervical ganglion, and the intervening trunks connecting these ganglia. A sympathetic plexus is located on the vertebral artery. Gray rami from the stellate ganglion are received by the C7, C8, and T1 spinal nerves. The autonomic fibers mix immediately with the somatic fibers and do not travel in separate fasciculi.[217] They enter either at the convergence of the roots or proximal to them.

Determination of whether a lesion is preganglionic or postganglionic is useful in localizing damage to the brachial plexus. The T2 nerve root is often cited as the cephalad limit of the spinal origin of preganglionic fibers

of the sympathetic nervous system, but data indicate that it can arise as high as T1 or C8.[217,218] The caudad limit of preganglionic fibers is T8 or T9.[218] The distribution of sympathetic fibers to vessels is much more prevalent in the hand than in the shoulder. The distribution of sweat and erector pili function is probably different but is still decreased in the C5 and C6 areas.[219]

Nonpathologic Variants

Although most plexuses basically follow the classic formation, they often differ in some small detail. For example, the axon that supplies sensation to an area of skin or stimulus to a particular muscle can take an alternate route from the spinal cord to its destination. There are no physiologic means of determining this variant. Such variants are changes in three-dimensional arrangements, not in the physiology of the brachial plexus. Because it is unlikely that a physiologic test will be developed to determine their existence, preoperative evaluation of these anomalies must await further refinement in imaging techniques (Fig. 2-53).[220] On computed tomography (CT), the nerves and vessels appear as one single structure. MRI can generate a much more brachial plexus–like picture, but the detail is still not sufficient.

Awareness of possible plexus variants is important for several reasons. The existence of a structural anomaly can hinder diagnostic evaluation of pathologic processes or complicate dissection when one attempts to find or avoid branches of the brachial plexus. An example in which accurate diagnosis is confusing occurs with a prefixed brachial plexus. A myelogram or CT scan can reveal an avulsed nerve root at a level one spinal nerve higher than that indicated by physical examination. It is helpful for the diagnostician to know that this anomaly is common and that the myelographic finding is not inconsistent with the physical examination. A prodigious number of patterns have been documented in the published series of brachial plexus dissections. To simplify matters, we have grouped the more common variants together for ease in understanding anomalies.

The existence of anomalies is understandable when one considers the embryology of the limb. In the fourth week of fetal development, the limb develops adjacent to the level at which the relative cervical vertebrae (C5-T1) will appear. The nerves have reached the base of the limb, which is now only condensed connective tissue. By the end of the fifth week, the nerves have reached the hand, but muscle differentiation has not yet occurred. As the limb migrates caudally, the muscles develop and migrate while taking their nerves with them.[221] This muscle differentiation precedes the growth of vessels, whose interposition can also affect the internal arrangement of the plexus.[196] The finding of alternate routes for functioning axons is not unexpected. As they develop, they tend to reach their destination before much of the intervening connective tissues mature. Walsh went so far as to state that there was only one plexus arrangement and that the variants were connective tissue artifacts.[222]

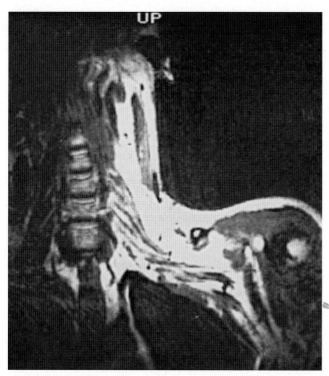

FIGURE 2-53 MRI visualization of the author's brachial plexus. The current level of imaging techniques does not yet allow visualization of nonpathologic variants. (From Kellman GM, Kneeland JB, Middleton WD, et al: MR imaging of the supraclavicular region: Normal anatomy. AJR Am J Roentgenol 148:77-82, 1987.)

Returning to our example, a prefixed brachial plexus is the most commonly cited example of what we will call a *proximal takeoff*. In this pattern, a nerve, or nerves, leaves the parent neural structure more cephalad or proximal than usual. Although a proximal takeoff is defined in various ways, each definition indicates that some neural tissue is exiting at a higher intervertebral foramen than usual for those particular axons. This might not be a strict ratcheting up of the brachial plexus, with all axons moving cephalad, but might indicate a partial shift relative to normal. Although authors disagree about whether this condition actually exists or simply represents an expansion of the plexus in the proximal direction, they do agree that the nerve tissue in the spinal cord maintains the same cephalocaudad relationship from cord to cord. Such agreement helps in evaluating the patient. If one group of axons has a tendency to be prefixed, the other axons will be prefixed, or at least not shifted in the opposite direction.[171]

By studying the amount of neural tissue contained in the spinal nerves that make up the brachial plexus, Slingluff and associates[171] produced much more convincing evidence for the type of prefixation in which all the axons move together. If confirmed by larger series of the same detailed work, it would add another dimension of predictability to brachial plexus anatomy in several ways. First, a cephalad shift of one group would mean a cepha-

lad shift in all axons. Second (a corollary of the first point), this cephalad shift would necessitate certain predictable shifts in the paths that axons would take to their respective end organs. Some of the more important shifts predicted by prefixation are as follows:

- The thoracic spinal nerve has less neural tissue.
- The upper trunk supplies more than half the posterior cord and the median nerve.
- The upper trunk supplies more than a third of the pectoral nerve supply.
- There is no C8 contribution to the lateral cord (loop from the lower trunk to the lateral cord).
- The ulnar nerve carries C7 fibers.

The converse would be predicted by postfixation; that is, T1 and the lower trunk and its contributions are correspondingly larger, and C8 contributes to the lateral cord. In this study, prefixation and postfixation are circumscribed by the content of neural tissue as defined by cross-sectional biopsy.

Because a prefixed brachial plexus can lead to diagnostic confusion, it would be helpful to find an alternative to biopsy of the plexus to determine the presence of the abnormality. For instance, when shifting the nerves into the higher foramina, some nerve tissue destined for an ulnar nerve distribution might exit by the C7 spinal nerve, and a higher correlation of prefixation with a C7 contribution to the ulnar nerve could be predicted.[184] Such information would be helpful before extensive dissection of the brachial plexus, which requires a search for the small contribution from the lateral cord.

Consider the variants that can occur with a single nerve. The fasciculi that form a nerve are grouped together in the source nerve structure (e.g., cords for nerves, trunks for divisions) and often depart the source nerve at a more proximal level (Fig. 2-54A and B). For example, the subscapular nerve usually originates off the upper trunk but can originate more proximally. This arrangement is the peripheral counterpart of the prefixed brachial plexus. The medial pectoral nerve is found to come off the lower trunk in 24% of specimens rather than the medial cord. The medial brachial cutaneous nerve comes off the trunk in 10% of cases.

Conversely, a distal takeoff (see Fig. 2-54A and C) would not be unexpected. The most commonly cited example is the postfixed brachial plexus, which, regardless of how it is defined, is relatively uncommon in comparison to the prefixed plexus. It is often found when the first thoracic rib is rudimentary.[27] Another common distal takeoff is the suprascapular nerve, which in 20% of cadavers took off from the anterior division rather than the upper trunk itself.

In some cases, fasciculi can leave the parent nerve before being joined together and thus result in a multiple origin (see Fig. 2-54A and D) of a nerve from its parent nerve. The most common example is the lateral pectoral nerve, which had a multiple origin in 76% of the specimens examined by Kerr.[188] Conversely, substitutions or a common origin can also occur (see Fig. 2-54A and E). In 55% of specimens, no lower subscapular nerve was found, and its function was assumed by a small branch off the axillary nerve. In addition, the thoracodorsal nerve was a smaller branch off the axillary or radial nerve in 11% of specimens. The brachial and antebrachial cutaneous nerves originated as a single nerve and split later in their course in 27% of specimens.[188]

Another variant is duplication of the nerve (see Fig. 2-54A and F), in which case axons might travel in separate nerves to a common destination. The most common example occurs when at least one other nerve from the lateral cord to the coracobrachialis is found in addition to the musculocutaneous nerve, which occurs in 56% of cadavers.

Finally, loops and collaterals (see Fig. 2-54A and G) can occur. These anomalies are more complex in that the nerves involved might not have the same parent nerve. An example is a loop from the lateral pectoral nerve to the medial pectoral nerve. This finding is so common that it is the rule rather than the exception. The important large loops are the contribution from the lateral cord to the ulnar nerve, which Kerr found in 60% of specimens, and an additional root to the median nerve coming off the musculocutaneous nerve, which occurred in 24% of specimens.[188] In the latter report, a relative decrease in the size of the original lateral root to the median nerve was present and helped indicate the existence of a musculocutaneous contribution. Slingluff and associates found a C8 contribution to the lateral cord in 14% to 29% of their specimens.[171] In 60% of cadavers, the medial brachial cutaneous nerve and the intercostal brachial nerve formed a common nerve, and in 20% of specimens, a radial nerve was formed from two roots.[188]

An interesting source of loops occurs as a result of an abnormal relationship with the axillary vessels and their branches. An abnormal relationship between nerves and arteries was found by Miller[196] in 5% of dissections and between nerves and veins in 4%. One of the more common anomalies was the presence of a vessel that is splitting or diverting axons that should belong to a single structure; this anomaly occurred with the nerve cord levels.[196] Some of these altered relationships can produce pathology (see Chapter 3). Another, rarer source of plexus anomalies is an aberrant accessory muscle that entraps a portion of the plexus.[159,223]

In summary, most anomalies are understandable as alternate routes, created by variations in formation of the intervening connective tissue, for axons to reach their normal destination. Unexpected anomalies such as a single cord plexus[224] or a complete absence of C8 and T1[225] contributions to the plexus can occur, but these variations are extremely rare. Even these less-common anomalies would be considered normal until encountered at surgery because they do not affect physiology. Because they cannot be predicted preoperatively, awareness of the possible existence of these nonpathologic variants should aid dissection and facilitate diagnosis.

Cranial Nerve XI

The spinal accessory nerve, or 11th cranial nerve, originates from the medulla and upper spinal cord through multiple rootlets. It then ascends back through the foramen magnum and exits in the middle compartment of the jugular foramen. The nerve descends between the internal jugular vein and internal carotid artery for a short distance and then descends laterally as it passes posteriorly to supply the sternocleidomastoid muscle. After exiting the sternocleidomastoid, it continues in an inferior posterior direction across the posterior triangle of the neck and then supplies the trapezius muscle. In the posterior triangle (Fig. 2-55), it receives afferent fibers from C2, C3, and sometimes C4.[226] Some upper fibers distribute to the sternocleidomastoid and the lower fibers to the trapezius. Because it lies so superficially in the posterior triangle, the nerve is at maximal risk for injury.

Intercostal Brachial Nerve

The intercostal brachial nerve is a cutaneous branch of T2. It leaves the thorax from the second intercostal space and crosses over the dome of the axillary fossa. It sends a communication to the medial brachial cutaneous nerve (60%)[188] and can supply sensation on the medial side of the arm as far as the elbow.[192,227] Like many of the cutaneous nerves of the upper part of the arm, it is outside the axillary sheath and is not anesthetized by axillary sheath injection.[192]

Supraclavicular Nerves

The supraclavicular nerves (see Fig. 2-55) originate from the spinal nerves C3 and C4. They are important to the shoulder surgeon because they supply sensation to the shoulder in the area described by their name, the area above the clavicle, in addition to the first two intercostal spaces anteriorly and much of the skin overlying the acromion and deltoid. The ventral rami of C3 to C4 emerge between the longi (colli and capitis) and scalenus medius.[28] The contributions to the supraclavicular nerves join and enter the posterior triangle of the neck around the posterior border of the sternocleidomastoid. They descend on the superficial surface of the platysma in three groups. The medial supraclavicular nerves go to the base of the neck and the medial portion of the first two intercostal spaces. The intermediate supraclavicular nerves go to the middle of the base of the posterior cervical triangle and the upper portion of the thorax in this area. The lateral supraclavicular nerves cross the anterior border of the trapezius muscle and go to the tip of the shoulder.[28] The medial nerves can have an anomalous pattern in which they pass through foramina in the clavicle on their way to the anterior of the chest.[209,228,229]

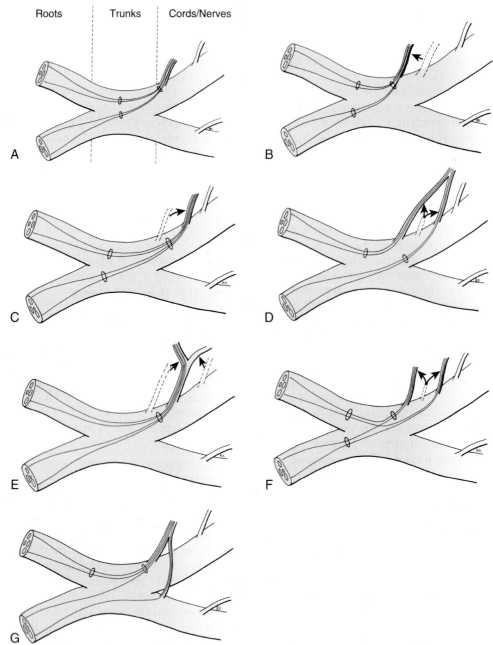

Roots   Trunks   Cords/Nerves

A

B

C

D

E

F

G

FIGURE 2-54 A, A fictitious nerve in its usual relationship to its parent structures and other nerves. The *thin black lines* represent axons that are normally distributed via this nerve. **B,** The *circles* represent fascicles, with the axons coalescing into a nerve at the more proximal level so that the nerve originates from the trunk. **C,** The axons leave this nerve more distally. **D,** The axons in their fascicles depart the parent nerve before joining to form the nerve, thereby resulting in a multiple origin. **E,** The axons of this nerve leave together with the neural material of an adjacent nerve, thereby resulting in a common origin. When the common origin involves two nerves of greatly different size, the smaller nerve may be referred to as absent and its function assumed by a branch of the larger nerve. **F,** The neural material leaves via two separate nerves, which remain separate all the way to the distal structure. This situation is referred to as a *duplication of the nerve.* **G,** Some of the neural material travels to the nerve via a small origin off different parent nerve structures, thereby resulting in a loop.

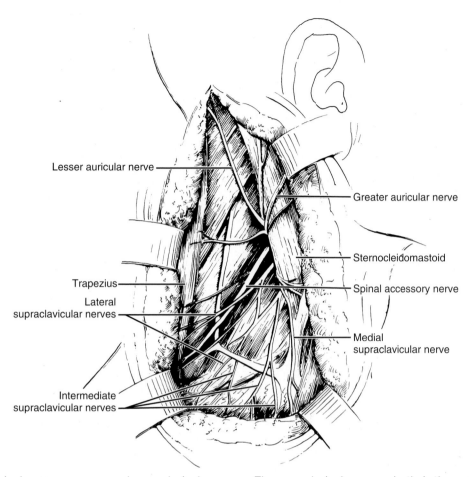

Lesser auricular nerve

Greater auricular nerve

Sternocleidomastoid

Trapezius

Spinal accessory nerve

Lateral
supraclavicular nerves

Medial
supraclavicular nerve

Intermediate
supraclavicular nerves

FIGURE 2-55 Spinal accessory nerve and supraclavicular nerves. The supraclavicular nerves in their three groups account for much of the cutaneous innervation of the shoulder. In the posterior triangle, the spinal accessory nerve runs from the sternocleidomastoid to the trapezius, the two superficial muscles of the neck. The spinal accessory nerve lies adjacent to the most superficial layer of deep fascia in the neck.

BLOOD VESSELS

The surgeon's interest in the anatomy of blood vessels is based on the treatment of blood vessel injury and avoidance of injury to these structures in the course of dissection. The main focus in the shoulder area is the axillary artery and its accompanying veins and lymphatics. These structures are more variable in their formation than the brachial plexus is, but the order of their formation and arrangement makes them easy to understand. Nonpathologic anomalies are more common here than in the brachial plexus. Nonpathologic anomalies are arrangements that have no physiologic significance but are important to the surgeon because their presence can change the diagnostic picture after an injury. In addition, they can affect the collateral circulation pattern or complicate a dissection by altering the position of arteries in relation to bone and tendon landmarks (see the section "Nerves").

Taylor and Palmer,[108] in their extensive studies of circulation of the skin and their literature review, noted basic tendencies in the distribution of blood vessels throughout the body. Blood vessel distribution follows the angiosome concept, or the idea that the body is an intricate jigsaw puzzle, each piece of which is supplied by a dominant artery and its accompanying veins. Muscles provide a vital anastomotic detour. The arteries link to form a continuous unbroken network, intramuscular watersheds of arteries and veins match, vessels travel with the nerves, vessels follow the connective tissue framework, and vessels radiate from fixed to mobile areas. Muscle mobility is directly related to the size and density of the supplying vessels (i.e., more-mobile muscles have fewer but larger-caliber vessels). The watersheds of vessels are constant, but their origin may be variable. The territory of intramuscular arteries obeys the *law of equilibrium* (e.g., if one vessel to a structure is larger than the normal surrounding vessels, its neighbors tend to be smaller). Vessel size and orientation are the product of tissue differentiation and growth in the area. Muscles are the primary force of venous return.[76,108] We would add here the tendency for vessels to cross joints close to the axis of rotation so that less relative change in length occurs (Fig. 2-56), particularly at the very mobile shoulder. The arteries supplying these blocks of tissue are also responsible for supplying the skin and underlying tissue. These blocks and overlying skin are called *angiosomes* in reference to the dominant arterial axes.

Elaborating on these themes, they pointed out that vessels rarely cross planes where a great deal of movement takes place.[108] Their illustrations showed that when vessels do cross these planes, they have a tendency to cross at the periphery of motion planes or at the ends of muscles where less relative motion occurs.[108] Moreover, in cases in which the vessel must cross an area of high mobility, it does so in an oblique fashion (Fig. 2-57). Such an oblique crossing is desirable because the strain (strain being deformation expressed as a percentage of the length of the artery) is greatly reduced and yet the absolute motion between the two sides of the plane does not change.

The axillary artery and its branches might seem to be an exception to such tendencies. It comes from a fixed position adjacent to the first rib and proceeds through a very mobile area within the axilla. It returns to another connective tissue framework adjacent to the humerus, where it becomes the brachial artery continuing into the arm. This apparent exception comes about only because of the highly mobile nature of the shoulder. The axillary artery can be thought of as fixed in a connective tissue structure, the axillary sheath, which has some highly mobile adjacent tissue planes, particularly so in relation to the anterior and posterior walls of the axilla. Given this relationship and the tendencies and formation of the vascular system noted earlier, it has been predicted and found that branches off the axillary artery going to shoulder structures come off more proximal than they would if they followed a direct course to their destination. They tend to be long and oblique in the course of their entrance into the muscles and lie outside the axillary sheath.

Because structures in the shoulder move relative to each other, one would predict a number of hypovascular fascial planes.[76,108,230] These planes are crossed at the periphery by a few large named vessels rather than directly by a large number of small vessels. These hypovascular planes are commonly found between the pectoralis major and pectoralis minor, between the trapezius and rhomboids, and on the deep surface of the rhomboids (see the section "Bursae, Compartments, and Potential Spaces"). Taylor and Palmer mention five angiosomes of the shoulder that have cutaneous representation: the transverse cervical artery, the thoracoacromial artery, the suprascapular artery, the posterior humeral circumflex artery, and the circumflex scapular artery.[108]

Arteries and veins are hollow structures with abundant collagen, some elastin, and layers that contain some smooth muscle. They are under control of the autonomic nervous system. Woollard and Weddell found that the distribution of sympathetic nerves to vessels appears to

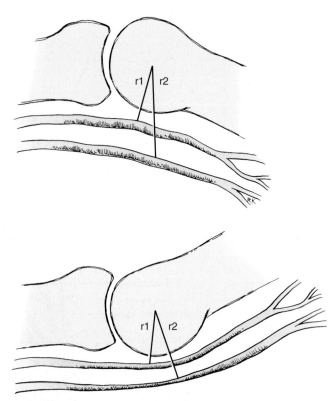

FIGURE 2-56 The strain on a vessel in movement is proportional to its distance from the center of rotation. r, radius.

be more abundant in the more distal part of the limb than in the proximal part.[219] In addition, larger arteries and veins have their own blood supply from the base of the vasa vasorum.[27]

Arteries

Arteries (Fig. 2-58) tend to be named by the watershed of the artery rather than by the main structure that comes off the axillary or subclavian artery.[231] For example, when the blood supply to the lateral wall of the axillary fossa comes from the pectoral branch of the thoracoacromial artery, it is said that the lateral thoracic artery originates from the pectoral artery rather than the lateral thoracic artery being supplanted by the pectoral artery. Huelke has reported a fairly high occurrence of branches of the axillary artery coming off in common trunks that seem to supplant each other. An interesting exception to the naming rule in the area of the subclavian artery is the dorsal scapular artery, which, when it originates from the thyrocervical trunk, is named the *deep transverse cervical artery*, although Huelke has tried to correct this nomenclature.[118] *Dorsal scapular artery* is the preferred name.

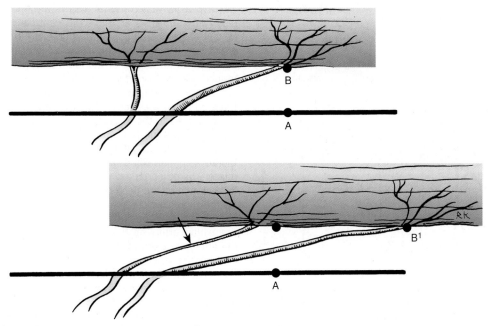

FIGURE 2-57 *A* and *B* are two spots that are across from each other in a fascial plane. *A* is the part on the fascia and *B* is the part directly across from it, which coincidentally is the attachment point of the blood vessel. The muscle is displaced relative to the fascial plane. The point that was at *B* is now at *B1*. All this represents the same linear displacement for both points of vessel attachment. The blood vessel that crosses the interfascial plane at a right angle has a much greater percentage strain (*arrow*) than the vessel that was attached at *B* and now is attached at *B1*.

Subclavian Artery

The blood supply to the limb begins with the subclavian artery, which ends at the lateral border of the first rib. It is divided into three portions in relation to the insertion of the scalenus anterior muscle.[232] The vertebral artery originates in the first portion, and the costocervical trunk and thyrocervical trunk originate in the second portion. Usually, no branches are found in the third portion of the artery. The artery is fairly well protected by the presence of surrounding structures. Rich and Spencer,[233] in their review of the world's literature on vascular injuries, did not find any large series in which injury to the subclavian artery made up more than 1% of the total arterial injuries. Because they are protected, injuries affecting these arteries signify more serious trauma than do injuries to other arteries remote to the great vessels.

The first important branch of the subclavian artery, rarely encountered by shoulder surgeons, is the vertebral artery, which provides the proximal blood supply to the brachial plexus. The internal mammary artery is always a branch of the vertebral artery.[108] Two vessels encountered more often by shoulder surgeons are the transverse cervical artery and the suprascapular artery, which come off the thyrocervical trunk in 70% of cases.[234] In the remaining cases they can come off directly or in common from the subclavian artery. The transverse cervical artery can divide into a superficial branch that sup-

plies the trapezius and a deep branch (when present) that supplies the rhomboids. The suprascapular artery is somewhat more inferior and traverses the soft tissues to enter the supraspinatus muscle just superior to the transverse scapular ligament and the suprascapular nerve.

The superior of the two arteries, the transverse cervical, lies anterior to the upper and middle trunks of the brachial plexus, whereas the suprascapular artery lies anterior to the middle trunk just above the level of the clavicle.[184] The origin of these branch arteries is relatively highly variable, but the subclavian arteries themselves are rarely anomalous. The textbook arrangement of branches of the subclavian is present in only 46% or less of dissections.[118,235]

The dorsal scapular artery is the normal artery to the rhomboids and usually comes off the subclavian but can come off the transverse cervical artery.[28,233] Branches off the first portion of the subclavian artery, the portion between its origin and the medial border of the scalenus anterior muscle, are the vertebral artery, the internal mammary artery, and the thyrocervical trunk. The second portion of the subclavian artery gives rise to the costocervical trunk.[233] A common anomaly that occurs in 30% of persons is a variation in which the transverse cervical artery, the suprascapular artery, or both originate from the subclavian artery rather than the thyrocervical trunk.[236] In most cases, one of these arteries travels between trunks of the brachial plexus to its destination.[119]

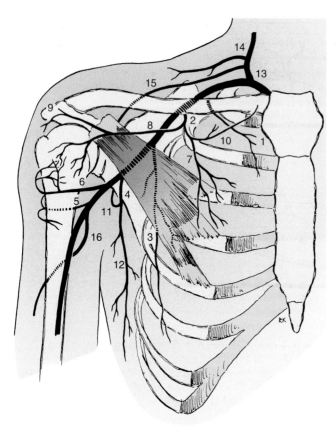

FIGURE 2-58 Major arterial axes of the upper limb. The major arterial axis bears three different names in its course. Medial to the lateral edge of the first rib, it is called the *subclavian artery*. From the lateral edge of the first rib just proximal to the takeoff of the profunda brachii artery, it is termed the *axillary artery*, and distal to that it is known as the *brachial artery*. The axillary artery is divided into three portions: superior to the pectoralis minor muscle (as shown), deep to the muscle, and distal to the muscle. This drawing shows the thoracoacromial axis *(2)* coming off in the first part of the artery, a very common variation. The thoracoacromial axis usually comes off deep to the pectoralis minor. The other variant is the clavicular branch *(10)*, shown as a branch of the pectoral artery. Most commonly it comes off the thoracoacromial axis as a trifurcation, but it can arise from any of the branches of the thoracoacromial axis or from the axillary artery itself. Note that most of the branches of the artery are deep to the pectoralis minor and its superior continuation, the clavipectoral fascia, except for the thoracoacromial axis and its branches, which lie anterior to the clavipectoral fascia. The labeled branches are as follows: *1*, superior thoracic artery; *2*, thoracoacromial artery; *3*, lateral thoracic artery; *4*, subscapular artery; *5*, posterior humeral circumflex artery; *6*, anterior humeral circumflex artery; *7*, pectoral artery; *8*, deltoid artery; *9*, acromial artery; *10*, clavicular artery; *11*, circumflex scapular artery; *12*, thoracodorsal artery; *13*, thyrocervical trunk; *14*, transverse cervical artery; *15*, suprascapular artery; and *16*, profunda brachii artery.

Axillary Artery

The axillary artery is the continuation of the subclavian artery. It begins at the lateral border of the first rib and continues to the inferior border of the latissimus dorsi, at which point it becomes the brachial artery. This artery is traditionally divided into three portions. The first portion is above the superior border of the pectoralis minor, the second portion is deep to the pectoralis minor, and the third portion is distal to the lateral border of the pectoralis minor. The usual number of branches for each of the three sections corresponds to the name of the section: The first portion has one branch, the second has two, and the third has three.

First Portion

The first section of the axillary artery gives off only the superior thoracic artery, which supplies vessels to the first, second, and sometimes the third intercostal spaces.

Second Portion

The first branch given off in the second portion of the axillary artery is the thoracoacromial artery, one of the suppliers of a major angiosome, as defined by Taylor and Palmer.[108] The artery has two very large branches, the deltoid and the pectoral, and two smaller branches, the acromial and clavicular. The acromial branch regularly comes off the deltoid, whereas the clavicular branch has a much more variable origin and can come off any of the other branches, the trunk, or the axillary artery.[128] The thoracoacromial artery pierces the clavipectoral fascia and gives off its four branches.[28] The pectoral branch travels in the space between the pectoralis minor and pectoralis major. In their injections series, Reid and Taylor reported that the pectoral artery supplied the sternocostal portion of the pectoralis major muscles in every case. They found no arterial supply from the pectoral artery to the pectoralis minor in 46% of dissections and reported that the pectoralis minor received a contribution from the pectoral artery in only 14% of dissections. In 34% of dissections, it appeared that the pectoralis minor received a direct supply from the thoracoacromial trunk.[128]

The arterial supply to the pectoralis major coincided closely with the unique nerve supply of the pectoralis major: The deltoid artery supplied the clavicular head and the pectoral artery supplied the sternocostal portion.[128] The authors also found that the plane between the pectoralis major and minor was relatively avascular but had a rich layer of anastomoses, with the lateral thoracic artery at the lateral edges of the pectoralis major origin. When the pectoralis major was attached over the fourth and fifth ribs, an anastomotic connection around the fourth rib area was noted. The pectoral branch also supplied most of the skin anterior to the pectoralis major through vessels that came around the lateral edge of the pectoralis major.[128]

The deltoid artery is directed laterally and supplies the clavicular head of the pectoralis major and much of the anterior deltoid. It also supplies an area of skin over the deltopectoral groove through vessels that emerge from the deltopectoral groove, including usually one large fasciocutaneous or musculocutaneous perforator.

The acromial artery is generally a branch of the deltoid artery that proceeds up to the acromioclavicular joint. It has an anastomotic network with other portions of the deltoid, the suprascapular, and the posterior humeral circumflex arteries and often has an important cutaneous branch.[128]

The clavicular artery often comes off the trunk or the pectoral artery and runs up to the sternoclavicular joint. Reid and Taylor noticed that when the clavicular artery was injected, there was staining of the periosteum in the medial half of the clavicle and the skin in this area.[128] The clavicular artery also has anastomotic connections with the superior thoracic artery, the first perforator of the inferior mammary, and the suprascapular artery.

The second artery that comes off the second portion of the axillary artery is the lateral thoracic, the artery in the axilla with the most variable origin.[119,231] In approximately 25% of specimens it originates from the subscapular artery.[231] At other times it originates from the pectoral branch of the thoracoacromial artery. The lateral thoracic artery runs deep to the pectoralis minor and supplies blood to the pectoralis minor, serratus anterior, and intercostal spaces 3 to 5. It forms a rich anastomotic pattern with intercostal arteries 2 to 5, the pectoral artery, and the thoracodorsal branch of the subscapular artery. In some cases the thoracodorsal artery gives origin to the vessels of the lateral thoracic distribution. A variation of the second portion of the axillary artery that Huelke found in 86% of cadavers is an upper subscapular artery whose course parallels the upper subscapular nerve.[119] This vessel might prove to be an important artery to the subscapularis because of the absence of important branches off the subscapular artery before the circumflex scapular.[158]

Third Portion

The largest branch of the axillary artery, the subscapular, originates in the third part of the axillary artery. This artery runs caudally on the subscapularis muscle, which it reportedly supplies.[27] However, Bartlett and colleagues found no important branches of the subscapular artery before the origin of the circumflex scapular artery.[158] It gives off a branch to the posterior portion of the shoulder, the circumflex scapular artery, which passes posteriorly under the inferior edge of the subscapularis and then medial to the long head of the triceps through the triangular space, where it supplies a branch to the inferior angle of the scapula and a branch to the infraspinatus fossa.[237] These two branches anastomose with the supra-

scapular and the transverse cervical arteries. The circumflex scapular artery has an additional large cutaneous branch that is used in an axial free flap.[237]

The continuation of the subscapular is the thoracodorsal artery, which runs with the thoracodorsal nerve toward the latissimus dorsi on the subscapularis, teres major, and latissimus dorsi. It also has branches to the lateral thoracic wall.

The posterior humeral circumflex comes off posteriorly in the third portion and descends into the quadrilateral space with the axillary nerve. After emerging on the posterior side of the shoulder beneath the teres minor, the artery divides in a fashion similar to the nerve. The anterior branch travels with the axillary nerve, approximately 5 cm below the level of the acromion, and supplies the anterior two thirds of the deltoid. It has a small communicating branch over the acromion with the acromial branch of the thoracoacromial axis and has a communicating branch posteriorly with the deltoid branch of the profunda brachii. It also has small branches to the glenohumeral joint. This artery supplies an area of skin over the deltoid, particularly the middle third of that muscle, through connecting vessels that travel directly to the overlying skin that is firmly attached to the underlying deltoid. The posterior branch corresponds to and accompanies the posterior axillary nerve.

The next branch is the anterior humeral circumflex artery, which is smaller than the posterior humeral circumflex. It is an important surgical landmark because it travels laterally at the inferior border of the subscapularis tendon, where it marks the border between the upper tendinous insertion of the subscapularis and the lower muscular insertion. The artery has anastomoses deep to the deltoid with a posterior humeral circumflex artery. It supplies some branches to the subscapularis muscle. One branch of the anterior humeral circumflex artery crosses the subscapularis tendon anteriorly, where it is regularly encountered during anterior glenohumeral reconstruction.[20] Another branch runs superiorly with the long head of the biceps and supplies most of the humeral head.

Gerber[91] and colleagues found that the anterolateral ascending branch of the anterior humeral circumflex artery supplied the majority of the humeral head. This branch runs parallel to the lateral aspect of the long head of the biceps tendon and has a constant insertion point where the intertubercular groove meets the greater tuberosity.

The terminal end branch is called the *arcuate artery*. Although the main arterial blood supply to the humeral head is via this terminal branch, Brooks[238] found there were significant intraosseous anastomoses between the arcuate artery and posterior medial vessel branches from the posterior humeral circumflex. They concluded that some perfusion of the humeral head persists if the head fragment in a fracture extends distally below the articular surface. This has been confirmed clinically in a new proximal humerus fracture classification scheme.[239]

Nonpathologic Anomalies

The function of arteries, the delivery of blood, is related to the cross-sectional area of the delivering artery rather than the particular route that the artery takes because the arterioles are the resistance vessels.[240,241] Arteries therefore depend less on straight line continuity for their function than nerves do. Among the vessels, one would expect a higher rate of deviance from the anatomic norm without any physiologic consequence than one would expect along nerves, and such turns out to be the case.[190,231] This concept is even more understandable when we recall that contiguous watersheds are connected by choke arteries and that when the vessels in one area are large, those in the adjacent area are small.[108,230] The types of arterial anomalies are similar to those of nerves: a change in the position of origin of the artery; duplication or reduction in the number of stem arteries; and total absence of the artery, with its function taken over by another artery.

The oblique route of the arteries as they course to their destination is necessitated by motion in the shoulder. As one might expect, a proximal displacement of arterial origin is more common than distal displacement. The most common example is proximal displacement of the thoracoacromial axis, which is found in at least a third of cadavers.[119,242]

The next most commonly displaced arterial stem is the subscapular artery, which in 16% to 29% of cases[119,235] originates in the second part of the axillary artery.[242] In a small percentage of cases, the superior thoracic artery was moved proximally to originate off the subscapular artery. Few cases of arteries being moved distally have been reported.

Another common variation is an increase or decrease in the number of direct branches from the axillary artery.[119,231,235,242] For example, in addition to the branches discussed earlier, Huelke described a seventh branch that he found in 86% of his dissections.[119] It is a short, direct branch accompanying the short upper subscapular nerve (and similar in anatomy), thus suggesting the name *upper subscapular artery.*

A change in number occurs when a branch of one of the six named arterial stems coming off the axillary artery originates directly from another artery or when two or more are joined in a common stem. In Huelke's series of dissections, he found seven branches in only 26.7% of dissections, six branches in 37%, five branches in 16%, and fewer than five in 11%. De Garis and Swartley reported as many as 11 separate branches from the axillary artery.[242] The most frequent common stem is that of the transverse cervical and suprascapular arteries, which form a common stem off the thyrocervical trunk in as many as 28% of cadavers.[236] The next most common origin is the posterior humeral circumflex artery with the anterior humeral circumflex (11%) or the subscapular artery (15%). The opposite of consolidation can also occur when major branches of these six or seven named branches originate directly from the axillary artery. This anomaly is seen most often in the thoracoacromial axis,

where the various branches can come off separately from the axillary artery, although only a small percentage of cases have been reported.

The final nonpathologic anomaly is total absence of an artery, with its function performed by one of the other branches. The lateral thoracic is most commonly absent, and its function is supplanted by branches off the subscapular, the pectoral branch of the thoracoacromial, or both. This variant has been seen in as many as 25% of specimens.[119,231,242]

Collateral Circulation

A number of significant anastomoses contribute to good collateral circulation around the shoulder (Figs. 2-59 and 2-60). The subclavian artery communicates with the third portion of the axillary artery through anastomosis with the transverse cervical, dorsal scapular, and suprascapular arteries and branches of the subscapular artery. Moreover, communications can be found between the posterior humeral circumflex artery and the anterior circumflex, deltoid, suprascapular, and profunda brachii arteries. Communications might also be found between the thoracoacromial artery and the intercostal arteries, particularly the fourth intercostal.

This abundant collateral circulation is both an asset to tissue viability and a disadvantage to assessment of possible arterial injury. Collateral circulation ameliorates some of the effects of an injury or sudden blockage of the axillary artery. A limb can survive on a flow pressure as low as 20 mm Hg, which would be fatal to the brain or heart.[240] In the Vietnam War, axillary artery injury had the lowest amputation rate of any of the regions of the arterial tree.[243] These anastomoses can on occasion obscure the diagnosis. Although the collateral circulation can transmit a pulse wave (13-17 mL/sec), it might not be sufficient to allow a flow wave (40-50 mL/sec) because flow varies with the fourth power of the radius of the vessels. Even though the collaterals can have a total cross-sectional area close to that of the axillary artery, resistance is greatly increased.[46,240] Furthermore, the same injury that interrupts flow in the axillary or subclavian artery can injure the collateral circulation.[233,244]

The seriousness of a missed diagnosis in injury is demonstrated by reports on arterial ligation. Ferguson and Holt quote Bailey as showing a 9% amputation rate for subclavian artery ligation and a 9% amputation rate for ligation of the axillary artery in World War I.[245] Battlefield statistics from DeBakey and Simeon[246] in World War II and Rich and colleagues[243] in the Vietnam War reveal a much higher amputation rate: about 28.6% for subclavian artery injury in Vietnam and 43% for axillary artery injury in World War II.[246] An outstanding exception to this dismal report is the treatment of arteriovenous fistula and false aneurysm, where ligation has very low morbidity, perhaps because of enlarged collateral vessels.[247] Interestingly, in the 10 cases of subclavian artery ligation found in the Vietnam War registry, no subsequent amputations

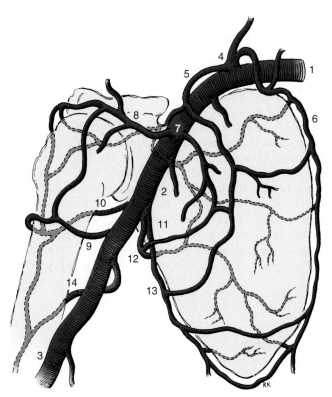

FIGURE 2-59 Diagram demonstrating the large amount of collateral circulation around the shoulder. Some license has been taken in depicting the dorsal scapular and suprascapular collaterals anterior to the major arterial axis. The labeled arteries are as follows: *1*, subclavian; *2*, axillary; *3*, brachial; *4*, thyrocervical trunk; *5*, suprascapular; *6*, dorsal scapular; *7*, thoracoacromial trunk; *8*, deltoid; *9*, anterior humeral circumflex; *10*, posterior humeral circumflex; *11*, subscapular; *12*, circumflex scapular; *13*, thoracodorsal; and *14*, profunda brachii. (Redrawn from Rich NM, Spencer F: Vascular Trauma. Philadelphia: WB Saunders, 1978.)

were needed, as opposed to an overall rate of 28% with subclavian wounds. Conversely, both of the two axillary artery ligations ended in amputation.[233] Radke points out that collateral vessels are fewer when compact and mobile tissues span the joint.[235]

The percentages of amputation reflect the rate of gangrene necessitating amputation after ligation and ignore the severe nerve pain syndromes that often occur with inadequate circulation.[233] Rich and Spencer believe that the increased gangrene rates among the military in World War II and Vietnam over World War I reflect the increasing severity of war wounds. In any event, neither the old nor the modern gangrene rate is acceptable. Axillary or subclavian artery injuries need repair, if possible, not ligation, and therefore require early diagnosis.[233]

Veins

Axillary

The axillary vein begins at the inferior border of the latissimus dorsi as a continuation of the basilic vein, continues to the lateral border of the first rib, and becomes the subclavian vein.[27,248] It is a single structure, in contradistinction to many venae comitantes, which are often double. The subscapular vein is also a single vessel.[158] The axillary and subclavian veins usually have only one valve each,[249] whereas most muscle veins have many valves.[109] Each vein lies anterior to its artery and, especially in its proximal portion, medial or inferior to the artery. Most of the venous drainage is to the axillary vein, except for branches that accompany the thoracoacromial artery, where more than half empty into the cephalic vein rather than continuing all the way to the axillary vein.[128] The relationships of the axillary vein are the artery, which tends to be posterior and lateral, and the brachial plexus.

FIGURE 2-60 Diagram of the collateral circulation. The number of collaterals decreases in areas where dense collagenous structures must move adjacent to each other (e.g., near the glenohumeral joint). (Adapted from Radke HM: Arterial circulation of the upper extremity. In Strandness DE Jr [ed]: Collateral Circulation in Clinical Surgery. Philadelphia: WB Saunders, 1969, pp 294-307.)

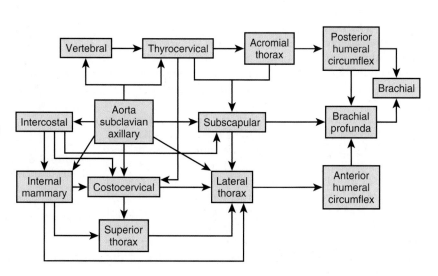

The medial pectoral nerve emerges from the brachial plexus between the artery and the vein. The ulnar nerve comes to lie directly behind the vein as it courses down the arm. The upper limb is similar to the lower limb, which uses a muscle pump action to aid venous return. In the upper limb, the deltoid and triceps muscles receive afferent veins from adjacent muscle and subcutaneous tissue.[109]

Cephalic

The cephalic vein is a superficial vein in the arm that lies deep to the deep fascia after reaching the deltopectoral groove and finally pierces the clavipectoral fascia and empties into the axillary vein.[27] The cephalic vein may be absent in 4% of cases. It receives no branches from the pectoralis major muscle in the groove.[128] Thus, it drains primarily the deltoid muscle and is often preserved laterally when using a deltopectoral approach. It is an important landmark in identifying the deltopectoral interval. It is covered by a constant fat stripe in the deltopectoral groove, which can be helpful in identifying the vein and persons who do not have a cephalic vein.

The lymph nodes of the axilla lie on the surface of the venous structures. The axillary vein often needs to be excised to obtain adequate node dissection in mastectomy. Lymphatic occlusion, rather than removal of the vein, is believed to be the cause of edema in the arm.[250-252] Such a mechanism might mitigate against venous repair, but Rich and associates report that disruption of venous return in the lower extremity results in a higher rate of amputation.[247] Preservation of the cephalic vein during surgery is thought to potentially reduce postoperative discomfort.

Lymphatic Drainage

Lymph drainage in the limbs is more highly developed superficially, where the lymph channels follow the superficial veins, than in the deep portion of the limb, where the lymph channels follow the arteries.[27,28] Lymphatics in the arm generally flow to the axillary nodes (Fig. 2-61). The more radially located lymphatics in the arm can cross to the ulnar side and, hence, to the axilla or can drain consistently with the cephalic vein and deltopectoral node, in which case they bypass the axilla and drain into the cervical nodes.[250]

The lymph nodes are named by the area of the axillary fossa in which they lie rather than by the area that they drain. The areas that they drain are rather constant, and each group of nodes receives one to three large afferents.[234] The nodes are richly supplied with arterial blood and seem to have a constant relationship to their arteries.[253] Drainage from the breast area and anterior chest wall passes into the pectoral nodes (thoracic nodes), which lie on the lateral surface of ribs 2 to 6, deep to or within the serratus anterior fascia on both sides of the

lateral thoracic artery. This group is almost contiguous with the central group. On the posterior wall of the axillary fossa are subscapular nodes that lie on the wall of the subscapularis muscle. They are adjacent to the thoracodorsal artery and nerve, and they drain lymph from this area and from the posterior surface of the shoulder, back, and neck.

These two groups drain into the central, or largest, nodes and higher nodes. The central nodes also receive drainage from the lateral nodes (or brachial nodes) on the medial surface of the great vessels in the axilla and are related to the lateral thoracic and thoracodorsal arteries. All these nodes drain into the apical nodes (subpectoral nodes), which can produce an afferent into the subclavian lymphatic trunk. They then join the thoracic duct on the left side or flow directly into the vein on the right. Some afferents drain into the deep cervical nodes and have a separate entrance into the venous system through the jugular vein.

Relationships

The axillary artery lies in the axillary space, well cushioned by fat, and is relatively well protected from compression damage. As previously mentioned, relatively few injuries occur to the subclavian artery. It is not usually

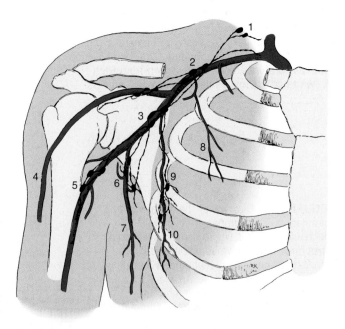

FIGURE 2-61 Diagram of the location of groups of lymph glands or nodes in the axilla and some of their major interconnections. The main drainage is into the vein, but they also have connections to the deep cervical nodes. Labeled nodes and vessels are as follows: *1*, deep cervical; *2*, apical; *3*, central; *4*, cephalic vein; *5*, lateral; *6*, subscapular; *7*, thoracodorsal artery; *8*, pectoral artery; *9*, pectoral nodes; and *10*, lateral thoracic artery.

involved in thoracic outlet syndrome. A case in which a normal artery is involved in a compression syndrome is in the quadrilateral space, where the posterior humeral circumflex may become compressed. Although the arteries in the shoulder are arranged around normal mechanics, one would predict that alterations in joint mechanics might endanger the arteries, but such is not often the case. Most indirect arterial damage involves cases of diseased arteries, as occurs in glenohumeral dislocation.[254,255]

BURSAE, COMPARTMENTS, AND POTENTIAL SPACES

With any study of regional anatomy, structures that allow or restrain the spread of substances into or from that part of the body are an important concept. The substances may be local anesthetics, edema from trauma, infection, or tumor. Surgeons are able to extend their surgical exposure or are prevented from doing so by similar spaces and barriers. Sufficiency of the barrier is related to the speed with which the substance can spread. For example, we prefer that local anesthetics act within a few minutes. A fascial barrier that prevents such spread may be insufficient to prevent the propagation of postinjury trauma that proliferates over a period of hours. Similarly, a barrier that can contain edema, thus causing a compartment syndrome, may be insufficient to act as a compartment barrier against the propagation of a tumor that enlarges over a period of weeks or months. We first discuss tumor compartments and then move on to compartments where more rapidly spreading substances are a concern.

Tumor Compartments

Musculoskeletal tumor surgeons have emphasized the concept of an anatomic compartment for many years. They point out that tumors grow centrifugally until they encounter a collagen barrier of fascia, tendon, or bone that limits their growth. Tumors tend to spread more rapidly in the direction in which no anatomic barriers are encountered. Therefore, a compartment is an anatomic space bounded on all sides by a dense collagen barrier.[256]

Enneking[256] lists four compartments in the shoulder: the scapula and its muscular envelope, the clavicle, the proximal end of the humerus, and the deltoid. The axillary space is a primary example of a space that is, by definition, extracompartmental. It is bounded by fascia posteriorly, medially, and anteriorly and has bone along its lateral border, but it does not provide any anatomic barrier to the spread of tumor in the proximal or distal direction.

Infection

Fortunately, infections in the shoulder area are rare in comparison to the hand, probably because of less exposure to trauma and foreign bodies in the shoulder area. Crandon pointed out that a potentiating anatomic feature for the development of infection in the hands is a closed space, which is infrequent in the shoulder.[257]

The shoulder has three diarthrodial joints: the sternoclavicular, the acromioclavicular, and the glenohumeral. In the absence of penetrating trauma or osteomyelitis, these areas are the most likely to become infected, especially in persons who are predisposed by a systemic disease.

Compartment Syndromes

Gelberman reported that shoulder-area compartment syndromes are found in the biceps, triceps, and deltoid. These syndromes are most often secondary to drug-overdose compression syndromes,[258] which occur when a person has been lying in one position and does not move to relieve this compression because of a low level of consciousness as a result of a drug overdose. The compression occurs in the most topographically prominent muscles that it is possible to lie on. Compartment syndromes can also develop after severe trauma in which compression occurs. Gelberman[258] pointed out that the middle deltoid, because of its multipennate nature, actually consists of many small compartments with regard to the containment of edema, whereas with the spread of tumor, the deltoid is a single compartment (Fig. 2-62). Therefore, decompression of the deltoid requires multiple epimysiotomies in the middle third to adequately release the edema (see Fig. 2-38).

Regional Anesthesia Compartments

The area of the shoulder most closely relevant to anesthesia is the axillary sheath, which begins in the neck as the prevertebral layer of the cervical fascia. This layer of fascia originates in the posterior midline and passes laterally deep to the trapezius. It covers the superficial surfaces of the muscles of the neck and, as it passes forward, forms the floor of the posterior triangle of the neck. It passes lateral to the scalene muscles and lateral to the upper portion of the brachial plexus and then just anterior to the anterior scalene, the longus colli, and the longus capitis muscles. In this anterior position it is truly prevertebral. This layer of fascia continues laterally and distally to surround the brachial plexus and the axillary artery and nerve. The sheath serves the purpose of confining injected material and keeping it in contact with the nerves. In combination with the adjacent brachial fascia, it is also capable of containing the pressure of a postarteriogram hematoma enough to produce nerve compression.[259]

The interscalene position (Fig. 2-63) of the brachial plexus is quite spacious, and the appropriate anesthetic technique requires adequate volume.[260,261] As the sheath proceeds laterally toward the axilla, it is most dense proximally. Thompson and Rorie found septa between

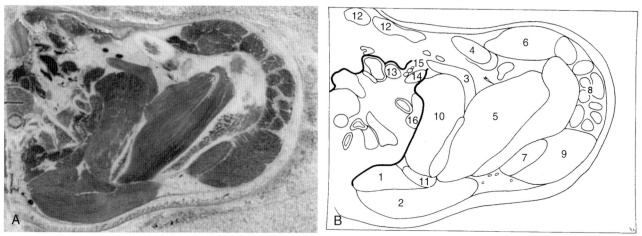

FIGURE 2-62 Photograph (**A**) and diagram (**B**) of a cross section of the shoulder at the level of the acromion. Several important spaces within the shoulder are demonstrated, beginning with the *heavy line* in **B** showing the prevertebral fascia, which contributes to formation of the axillary sheath. In the middle portion anteriorly is a deposit of adipose tissue that is the upper end of the axillary space. Posteriorly, at the base of the spine of the scapula, a body of adipose tissue is located between the trapezius and the deltoid, wherein lie the ramifications of the cutaneous branch of the circumflex scapular artery. At the most lateral extent can be seen the multipennate formation of the middle third of the deltoid, which demonstrates why this portion of the muscle should be considered multiple compartments when treating compartment syndrome. The labeled structures are as follows: *1*, rhomboid major; *2*, trapezius; *3*, omohyoid; *4*, clavicle; *5*, supraspinatus; *6*, anterior third of the deltoid; *7*, infraspinatus; *8*, middle third of the deltoid; *9*, posterior third of the deltoid; *10*, serratus anterior; *11*, rhomboid minor; *12*, sternocleidomastoid; *13*, scalenus anterior; *14*, scalenus medius; *15*, brachial plexus; and *16*, scalenus posterior.

the various components in the sheath in anatomic dissections and by tomography (Fig. 2-64).[262] At least three compartments were present, which might account for the need for multiple injections into the axillary sheath to achieve adequate brachial plexus anesthesia and might explain why axillary hematoma does not affect the entire brachial plexus at once. As we continue without pictures of the sheath as a connective tissue structure moving in relation to the adjacent structures, we should not be surprised to learn that the nerves to the shoulder and upper part of the arm already lie outside the sheath in the arm where axillary block is performed, thus necessitating the use of a distal tourniquet to force the proximal migration of anesthetic solutions.

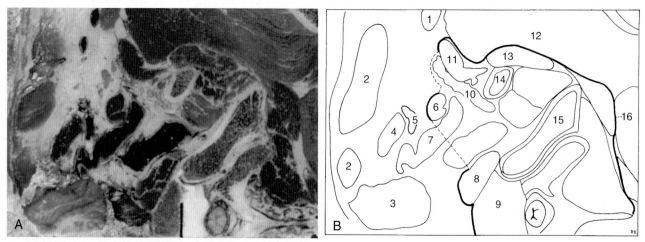

FIGURE 2-63 Photograph (**A**) and diagram (**B**) of a horizontal cross section of the interscalene interval at the level where the subclavian artery is just beginning to pass behind the scalenus anterior. The *heavy line* (*16*) is the prevertebral fascia, which goes on to constitute the proximal axillary sheath at the proximal end. This space is so capacious that anesthesia in this area requires a dose of at least 40 mL. The labeled structures are as follows: *1*, omohyoid; *2*, sternocleidomastoid; *3*, lung; *4*, sternohyoid; *5*, subclavian vein; *6*, scalenus anterior; *7*, subclavian artery; *8*, longus colli; *9*, T2 vertebra; *10*, brachial plexus; *11*, scalenus medius; *12*, serratus anterior; *13*, scalenus posterior; *14*, rib 1; *15*, rib 2; and *16*, prevertebral fascia.

Fascial Spaces and Surgical Planes

The dissection by surgeons through the body is greatly facilitated by planes or areas of the body that are relatively avascular and aneural (see the sections "Nerves" and "Blood Vessels" for discussion.) The crossing of planes by nerve or vessel is greatly discouraged by movement across that plane. This does not mean that no vessels cross such planes, but when these planes are crossed, the vessels tend to be fewer and larger, are named, and cross in an oblique fashion to accommodate the motion. They tend to enter muscles near the points of origin or insertion and thus decrease the effect of excursion of the muscle. Collateral vessels between adjacent watersheds also cross at the periphery of the planes of motion (Fig. 2-65). The shoulder is the most mobile part of the human body and, as one would expect, contains the greatest number of accommodations for that motion. Three structures specifically allow motion: bursae, loose areolar tissue, and adipose tissue.

In loose areolar tissue, the fibers and cellular elements are widely spaced. The purpose of this type of tissue is to facilitate motion between structures in relation to each other: usually muscle and muscle or muscle and underlying bone. These fascial spaces (Figs. 2-66 to 2-68; see also Fig. 2-65) can be easily penetrated by pus or other unwanted fluid and yet are also useful to surgeons because of the paucity of small vessels and nerves traversing them.[108] Again, this is not to say that no vessels are present. Crossing vessels and nerves tend to be large, are named, and are usually well known and easily avoided. These fascial spaces therefore provide useful passages for dissection. The most commonly observed fascial space is seen deep to the deltopectoral groove, beneath the deltoid and pectoralis major muscles, and superficial to the underlying pectoralis minor muscle and conjoint tendon. This space deep to the pectoralis major and deltoid muscles is crossed by branches of the thoracoacromial artery close to the clavicle, with no other vessels of note crossing.

When a deltoid-splitting incision is used in a posterior approach to the shoulder, a space is encountered between the deep surface of the deltoid and the outer surface of the infraspinatus and teres minor. The crossing structures are the axillary nerve and posterior circumflex artery at the inferior border of the teres minor. Deep on the costal surface of the serratus anterior, posterior to its origins, is a fascial space continuous with the loose areolar tissue lying deep to the rhomboids. This avascular plane is used by tumor surgeons when performing a forequarter amputation and by pediatric orthopaedists when correcting an elevated scapula in a fashion that results in a less-bloody dissection. Note in the illustrations that these spaces are thinner than the ink that the artist used to depict them. Their existence must be borne in mind when interpreting tomograms and planning tumor margins that may be compromised by this loose tissue. This same caveat applies to bursae.

Another way to analyze surgical planes is to think of dissection in layers. Cooper and colleagues[140] found four consistent supporting anatomic layers over the glenohumeral joint. Layer 1 consists of the deltoid and pectoralis major muscles. Layer 2 contains the clavipectoral fascia, coracoid process, conjoint tendon, and the coracoacromial ligament. Posteriorly, the posterior scapular fascia is continuous with the clavipectoral fascia. Layer 3 contains the rotator cuff muscles. Layer 4 is the glenohumeral capsule.

Adipose Tissue

Adipose tissue provides the double function of cushioning nerves and vessels and allowing pulsation of arteries and dilation of veins.[108] It also allows movement of tissues in relation to each other. The shoulder has three deposits of adipose tissue that indicate the position of an enclosed nerve or artery. The largest is the axillary space, which contains the brachial plexus and its branches, the axillary artery and vein, and the major lymphatic drainage from the anterior chest wall, upper limb, and back.

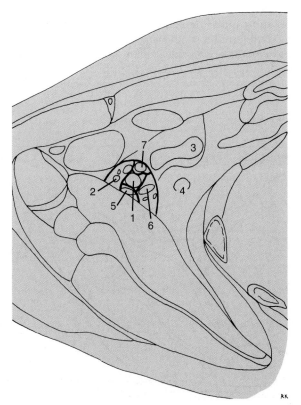

FIGURE 2-64 Cross-sectional diagram of the axillary sheath demonstrating the septa between the structures contained within the sheath. The labeled structures are: *1*, axillary artery; *2*, musculocutaneous nerve; *3*, vein; *4*, lymph node; *5*, axillary nerve; and *6*, median nerve.

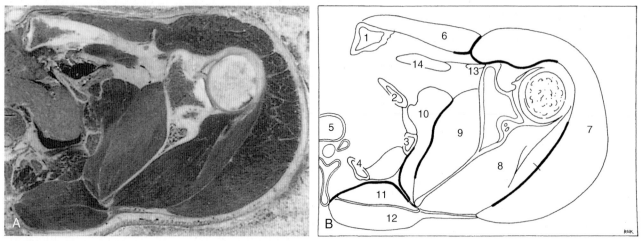

FIGURE 2-65 Transverse section (**A**) and diagram (**B**) showing the relationships at the level of the coracoid process. The planes where most of the motion occurs and that are most likely to be hypovascular are indicated by the *heavy lines* in **B**. The vessels that cross these planes are likely to be found at the edges of the planes of motion. For example, in the plane between the serratus anterior and the subscapularis, the vessels crossing are likely to be found close to the border of the scapula where the relative motion between these two structures is less. Also shown on this section is the proximity of the suprascapular nerve and artery to the posterior rim of the glenoid. Labeled structures are as follows: *1*, clavicle; *2*, rib 1; *3*, rib 2; *4*, rib 3; *5*, T3 vertebra; *6*, pectoralis major muscle; *7*, deltoid muscle; *8*, infraspinatus muscle; *9*, subscapularis muscle; *10*, serratus anterior muscle; *11*, rhomboid muscle; *12*, trapezius muscle; *13*, pectoralis minor muscle; and *14*, subclavius muscle.

The axillary space (Fig. 2-69; see also Figs. 2-62 to 2-67) is bounded posteriorly by a wall of muscle, which, from top to bottom, consists of the subscapularis, the teres major, and the latissimus dorsi muscles. The latissimus dorsi forms the muscle undergirding the posterior axillary fold. These three muscles are innervated by the upper and lower subscapular nerve and by the thoracodorsal nerve, formerly referred to as the *middle subscapular nerve*. The anterior boundary of the axillary space is the pectoralis minor muscle and the clavipectoral fascia (see Fig. 2-69).

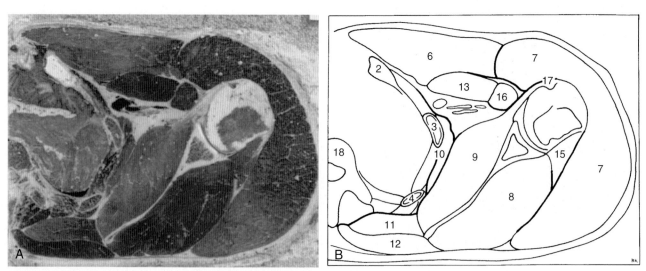

FIGURE 2-66 Cross section (**A**) and diagram (**B**) slightly below the equator of the glenoid. Tissue planes that are likely to be hypovascular are shown by the *heavy lines* in **B**. Labeled structures are as follows: *2*, rib 1; *3*, rib 2; *4*, rib 3; *6*, pectoralis major muscle; *7*, deltoid muscle; *8*, infraspinatus muscle; *9*, subscapularis muscle; *10*, serratus anterior muscle; *11*, rhomboid muscle; *12*, trapezius muscle; *13*, pectoralis minor muscle; *15*, teres minor muscle; *16*, coracobrachialis muscle; *17*, biceps muscle; and *18*, T5 vertebra.

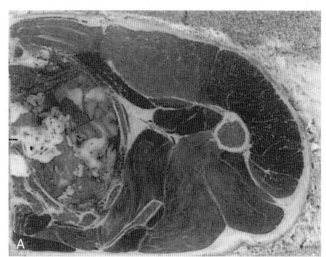
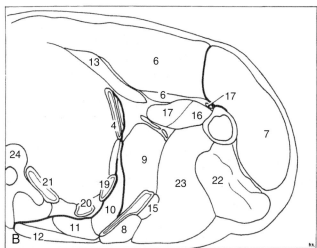

FIGURE 2-67 Cross section (**A**) and diagram (**B**) below the level of the quadrilateral space. Careful examination of **A** shows the two layers of the pectoralis major inserting onto the lateral border of the bicipital groove. At the anterior border of the teres major, the fibers of the teres major and the latissimus dorsi can be seen to insert on the medial lip and floor of the bicipital groove. The position of the brachial plexus is well demarcated. Labeled structures are as follows: *4,* rib 3; *6,* pectoralis major muscle; *7,* deltoid muscle; *8,* infraspinatus muscle; *9,* subscapularis muscle; *10,* serratus anterior muscle; *11,* rhomboid muscle; *12,* trapezius muscle; *13,* pectoralis minor muscle; *15,* teres minor muscle; *16,* coracobrachialis muscle; *17,* biceps muscle; *19,* rib 4; *20,* rib 5; *21,* rib 6; *22,* triceps muscle; *23,* teres major and latissimus dorsi; and *24,* T6 vertebra.

Superior to the pectoralis minor is a dense layer of fascia, referred to as the *clavipectoral fascia,* that continues medially and superiorly from the pectoralis minor. It continues medially to the first rib as the costocoracoid membrane. The pectoralis major muscle and tendon form

the more definitive anterior boundary at the inferior extent of the axillary space, although the clavipectoral fascia continues to the axilla. The medial boundary of the space is the serratus anterior muscle and the ribs. The lateral boundary is the portion of the humerus between

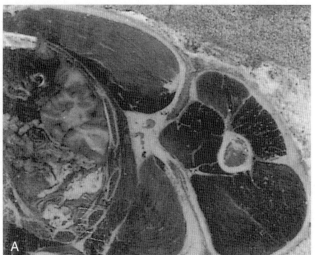
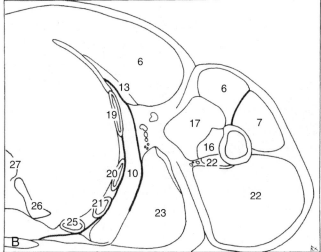

FIGURE 2-68 Cross section (**A**) and diagram (**B**) only a few millimeters superior to the skin of the axillary fossa. The hypovascular planes are again emphasized. Note the large pectoral lymph nodes and the large thoracodorsal vessels. On the lateral side of the teres major, the tendon and a few remaining muscle fibers from the latissimus dorsi can be seen. Labeled structures are as follows: *6,* pectoralis major muscle; *7,* deltoid muscle; *10,* serratus anterior muscle; *13,* pectoralis minor muscle; *16,* coracobrachialis muscle; *17,* biceps muscle; *19,* rib 4; *20,* rib 5; *21,* rib 6; *22,* triceps muscle; *23,* teres major and latissimus dorsi; *25,* rib 7; *26,* rib 8; and *27,* T8 vertebra.

the insertions of the teres major and latissimus dorsi and the insertion of the pectoralis major, which defines the lower extent of the intertubercular groove. In the anatomic position, the axillary space resembles a warped pyramid; its lateral border actually lies on the anterior surface of the humerus.

The next important body of adipose tissue lies posteriorly, deep to the deep fascia (Fig. 2-70). It is inferomedial to the medial border of the posterior deltoid, lateral to the trapezius, and superior to the latissimus dorsi. It might be considered a continuation of the triangular space because this tissue contains the cutaneous continuations of the circumflex scapular artery, and it is here that the microvascular surgeon seeks the artery and veins of the "scapular" cutaneous flap.[237]

The third deep deposit of adipose tissue in the shoulder lies between the supraspinatus tendon and the overlying clavicle and acromioclavicular joint (see Fig. 2-40). The tissue cushions and protects the branches of the acromial artery, which is often encountered in dissections below the acromioclavicular joint.

In summary, for the purpose of dissection, adipose tissue serves to indicate the presence of vessels or nerves.

Bursae

The last structures that facilitate motion are the bursae. Apparently, bursae form in development as a coalescence of fascial spaces.[28] Bursae tend to have incomplete linings in their normal state, but they can become quite thickened in the pathologic states often encountered at surgery. The bursae, being hollow spaces, are totally avascular and can be used as spaces for dissection. Because they are the most complete of the lubricating spaces, they are encountered between the most unyielding tissues: between tendon and bone or skin and bone and occasionally between muscle and bone near a tendon insertion.

The human body has approximately 50 named bursae, and several quite important ones are located in the shoulder.[27,28] The subacromial bursa and the closely related subdeltoid bursa are the most important. These bursae serve to lubricate motion between the rotator cuff and the overlying acromion and acromioclavicular joints. These two bursae are usually coalesced into one (Fig. 2-71). They are the most important bursae in pathologic processes of the shoulder and the ones that cause the most pain when they are inflamed. Although the subacromial bursa is normally only a potential space and therefore not seen on cross section (see Fig. 2-40) or with imaging techniques, it has a capacity of 5 to 10 mL when not compromised by adhesions or edema.[263] It does not normally communicate with the glenohumeral joint.[264]

Another often-encountered bursa is the subscapularis bursa, which develops between the upper portion of the subscapularis tendon and the neck of the glenoid and, in most cases, actually connects with the glenohumeral joint. Therefore, it is usually a recess of the glenohumeral joint rather than a separate bursa. Fairly constant bursae can be found near tendinous insertions: between the muscle and bony insertion of several muscles, including the trapezius, near the base of the scapular spine; the infraspinatus and the teres major near their attachments to the humerus; and an intermuscular bursa between the tendons of the latissimus dorsi and teres major.

A less-constant bursa can occur between the coracoid process and the coracobrachialis muscle and the underly-

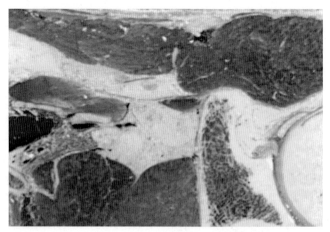

FIGURE 2-69 A close-up view of the axillary space demonstrates a rather prominent clavipectoral fascia starting from the tip of the coracoid and running to the left across the photograph. Just deep to this location and adjacent to the coracoid lies the insertion of the pectoralis minor. The muscle to the left is the subclavius. Immediately posterior to the subclavius can be seen the brachial plexus and axillary vessels.

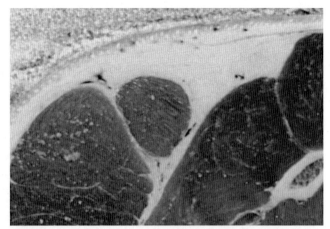

FIGURE 2-70 This cross-sectional view of the back of the shoulder demonstrates the fat pad within which the cutaneous branches of the circumflex scapular artery are located. The muscles on the *left* are the deltoid and the lateral head of the triceps. The teres minor is anterior, and the infraspinatus is lateral. This adipose tissue might be considered a continuation of the triangular space. The presence of a body of adipose tissue indicates an artery or nerve.

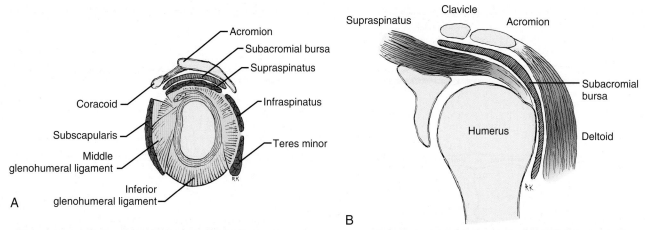

FIGURE 2-71 Relationships and area of distribution of the subacromial bursa. Compare these drawings with the cross-sectional photograph shown in Figure 2-40. In the natural state, the bursa is a potential space and exists only when it is filled—for example, with air from a surgical procedure or with saline from arthroscopy.

ing subscapularis muscle. We have seen such bursae inflamed by subcoracoid impingement processes, most often iatrogenic or post-traumatic, but two of them did not result from antecedent surgery or trauma. The coracobrachialis bursa is often (11% of specimens) an extension of the subacromial bursa.[125] In such cases, the coracoid tip may be visualized through an arthroscope placed in the subacromial bursa.

SKIN

Three requirements with regard to the skin need to be considered in surgical planning:

1. Continued viability of the skin postoperatively
2. Maintenance of sensibility of the skin
3. Cosmesis

Circulation

The skin has several layers of blood vessels. A plexus of interconnecting vessels lies within the dermis itself. The largest dermal vessels lie in the rete cutaneum, a plexus of vessels on the deep surface of the dermis.[265] Another larger layer of vessels is located in the tela subcutanea, or superficial fascia.[27] The blood supply to these layers varies in different areas. Several factors relate to the arrangement of the circulation. The first is the relative growth of the area of the body under consideration. The number of cutaneous arteries that a person has remains constant throughout life.[108] Growth increases the distance between the skin vessels by placing greater demand on them, which then leads to an increase in the size of the vessels.

The second factor is the path taken by direct vessels to the skin. Direct vessels are those whose main destina-

tion is the skin. Indirect vessels are those whose main destination is some other tissue, such as bone or muscle, but that reinforce the cutaneous vessels. The paths of direct vessels are affected by motion among tissues, with a great deal of motion taking place between subcutaneous fat and the deep fascia (Fig. 2-72). With the pectoralis major, for example, the dominant vessels cross at the edge of the plane of motion (i.e., the axilla). Some of these vessels can take direct origin off the axillary artery near its junction with the brachial artery, but they mainly originate from the pectoral area.[108] The vessel travels in the subdermal plexus in the subcutaneous fascia and sends vessels to the rete cutaneum. The plane between deep fascia and subcutaneous fat is an almost bloodless field; dissection can be performed without endangering the primary skin circulation.[108]

When the skin is more fixed, the dominant vessels can lie on the superficial surface of the deep fascia, and vessels to the dermal plexus can run more vertically than obliquely. In these areas, common on the upper part of the arm, retaining a layer of deep fascia with skin flaps maintains another layer of circulation.[266] The perforators to this plexus on the deep fascia travel in the intermuscular septa rather than through muscle, where there is motion between muscle and the deep fascia, including muscle in a flap that offers no additional circulation.[108] A number of classifications of fasciocutaneous flaps have been devised on the basis of how the vessels reach the deep fascia.[267-270]

On the surface, vessels tend to course from concave surfaces of the body toward convexities. Thus, they are likely to be found originating in rich supply adjacent to the borders of the axilla and less commonly on convexities such as the breast or outer prominence of the shoulder, which are distal watersheds. As growth increases the length of limbs and the height of convexities, vessels become longer and of greater diameter because of increased demand.[108]

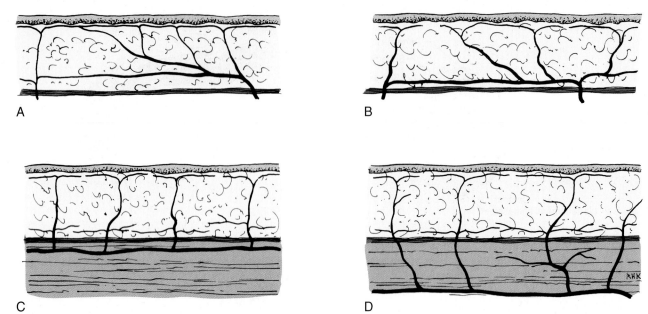

FIGURE 2-72 The four different types of direct circulation to the skin. **A,** Type A is found anterior to the pectoralis major, where considerable motion between the subcutaneous fascia of the skin and the deep fascia of the muscle takes place. The blood supply adapts to this motion by crossing obliquely at the edge of the plane of motion and sending a dominant vessel just deep to the tela subcutanea (subcutaneous fascia). From there the vessel sends branches to the dermal plexus. **B,** Type B circulation occurs in situations with less motion between the subcutaneous fascia and the deep fascia. In fact, there may be relative motion between the overlying deep fascia and the underlying muscle. Direct vessels branch out on the surface of the deep fascia and from there send branches to the dermal plexus. In the shoulder area, such branching occurs over the fascia of the biceps. **C,** In type C, the skin is very tightly attached to the underlying deep fascia, which has an artery running just below it. This specialized situation occurs at the palmar and plantar fascia. **D,** In type D, the dominant vessel supplying this area of skin lies deep to the muscle and sends direct perforators to the dermal plexus. As expected, this type of circulation also occurs in locations with very little motion between the skin and underlying muscle. (Redrawn from Taylor GI, Palmer JH: The vascular territories [angiosomes] of the body; experimental study and clinical applications. Br J Plast Surg 40:133-137, 1930.)

In specialized areas of the body where dominant vessels lie just beneath the deep fascia and the skin is very well fixed, such as the palmar and plantar surfaces, the dermal vessels run straight vertically. In other areas of the body such as over the middle third of the deltoid, the skin is extremely well fixed to underlying muscle. The dominant vessels, here the posterior humeral circumflex artery and veins,[108] actually course on the deep surface of the muscles, with direct vessels running vertically through the intramuscular septa of the deltoid muscle to the skin. Dissection on either side of the deep fascia will divide these vessels. Only a myocutaneous flap would offer additional vessels to the skin.[271]

These types of skin circulation are not mutually exclusive and can reinforce each other. Over the pectoralis major muscle, for example, direct vessels from the internal mammary vessels reinforce the type A vessels from the axilla.[272] Over the deltopectoral groove, perforator vessels from the deltoid artery reinforce the skin circulation. Many of the deltoid muscle vessels in the tela subcutanea are reinforced by type D vessels from the posterior humeral circumflex. Over the middle third of the deltoid,

less overlap is likely; therefore, flap development in this area is less extensive.

Sensation

Sensation related to shoulder surgery is of less concern to the surgeon and the patient than is sensation in other areas of the body. The incidence of postoperative neuroma of the shoulder is low (Fig. 2-73).

The most cephalad of nerves that innervate the skin of the shoulder and lower part of the neck are the supraclavicular nerves. They branch from the third and fourth cervical nerve roots and then descend from the cervical plexus into the posterior triangle of the neck. They penetrate superficial fascia anterior to the platysma, descend over the clavicle, and innervate the skin over the first two intercostal spaces anteriorly.[27] Interestingly, the medial supraclavicular nerves can pass through the clavicle.

The posterior portion of the shoulder and neck is innervated from cutaneous branches off the dorsal rami of the spinal nerves. In the dorsal spine, the area of skin that is innervated is usually caudad to the intervertebral foramen through which the nerve exits. For example, the C8 cutaneous representation is in line with the spine of the scapula, which is at the same height as the third or fourth thoracic vertebra.[27]

Much of the anterior of the chest is innervated by the anterior intercostal nerves. The first branches come forward near the midline adjacent to the sternum and innervate the anterior portion of the chest, somewhat overlapping with the lateral intercostal cutaneous branches. The first intercostal nerve does not have any anterior cutaneous branch.

The lateral cutaneous branches of the intercostal nerve emerge on the lateral aspect of the thorax between the slips of the serratus anterior muscle and innervate the skin in this area. They also supply the larger portion of the chest anteriorly, including the breast.[28]

Only three nerves of the brachial plexus have cutaneous representation in the shoulder, the most proximal of which is the upper lateral brachial cutaneous nerve, a branch of the axillary nerve that innervates the lateral

side of the shoulder and the skin overlying the deltoid. The upper medial side of the arm is innervated by the medial brachial cutaneous and the intercostal brachial nerves combined. In the anterior portion of the arm over the biceps muscle, skin is innervated by the medial antebrachial cutaneous nerve.[27]

Relaxed Skin Tension Lines

Although numerous attempts have been made over the past 200 years—and in recent years—to outline the optimal lines for incision, the best description of the basic principles is Langer's. He found that tension in the skin is determined by the prominence of underlying structures and by motion, with the underlying topography being the predominant influence.[273,274] Langer performed two classic experiments. In the first experiment, he punctured cadavers with a round awl and observed the linear splits that developed because of the orientation of underlying collagen. This he called the *cleavability of the skin*. In the

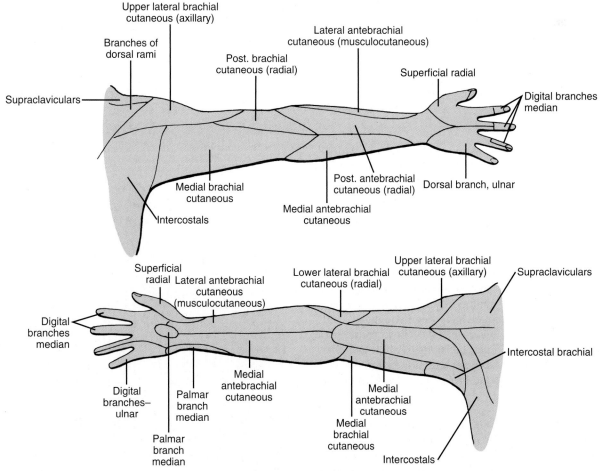

FIGURE 2-73 Representation of the cutaneous sensitivity of the nerves of the upper extremity. Note that of all the nerves to the shoulder, only the axillary nerve has a cutaneous representation. The remainder of the shoulder area is innervated by the supraclavicular nerves and the dorsal rami of the spinal nerves. No sharp demarcation is seen between the area of skin innervated by the intercostal brachial and medial brachial cutaneous nerves because of communication from the former. Intercostal brachial numbness following radical mastectomy is the only cutaneous nerve sensitivity problem common in the shoulder. (Redrawn from Hollinshead WH: Anatomy for Surgeons, vol 3, 3rd ed. Philadelphia: Harper & Row, 1982.)

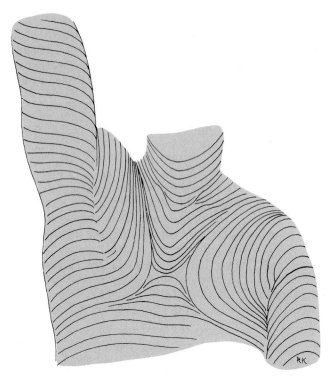

FIGURE 2-74 The usual locations of relaxed skin tension lines in a man. The position of these lines varies among individuals; they need to be sought at each operation. (Redrawn from Kraissel CJ: Selection of appropriate lines for elective surgical incisions. Plast Reconstr Surg 8:1-28, 1951.)

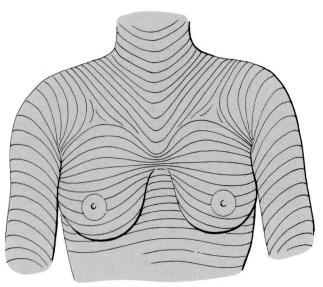

FIGURE 2-75 Because of the different underlying topography, the lines of skin tension in women differ in several respects from those in men. (Redrawn from Kraissel CJ: Selection of appropriate lines for elective surgical incisions. Plast Reconstr Surg 8:1-28, 1951.)

second experiment, he measured skin tension in various ways. In cadavers he made circular incisions and observed wound retraction. He then moved the limb to look for changes in retraction. In living patients, such as women in the delivery room who were about to experience a sudden change in underlying topography, he drew a circle on the skin with ink and observed postpartum changes.

In the 20th century, cosmetic surgeons found Langer's lines to be incorrect in certain areas of the body.[275,276] Although the principles outlined by Langer are still held to be valid, newer techniques have been sought to local-ize the optimal lines in living persons. These techniques have included further circular incisions, wrinkle patterns, and chemical imprints. All these techniques agreed with the incisions empirically found to be best in some regions and not in others.

Plastic surgeons now speak of *relaxed skin tension lines* (Figs. 2-74 to 2-76), which refers to their technique of relaxing the tension on the skin between the thumb and the forefinger of the surgeon and observing the pattern of fine lines in the skin. When the relationship is exactly perpendicular to the optimal incision, the fine lines that form are straight and parallel. The skin is then pinched in other directions. The line pattern is rhomboid or obscured.[277,278] This technique allows the surgeon to compensate for individual variability.

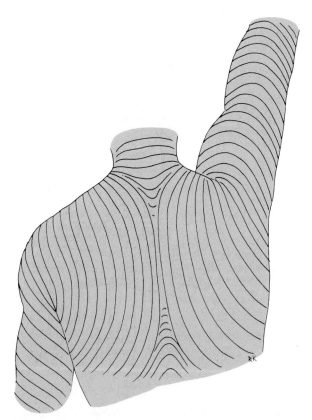

FIGURE 2-76 The usual position of relaxed skin tension lines on the posterior surfaces of the shoulder region. (Redrawn from Kraissel CJ: Selection of appropriate lines for elective surgical incisions. Plast Reconstr Surg 8:1-28, 1951.)

REFERENCES

1. Hsieh ET: A review of ancient Chinese anatomy. Anat Rec 20:97-127, 1921.
2. Huang-Ti N, Wen CS: The Yellow Emperor's Classic of Internal Medicine. Los Angeles: University of California Press, 1966.
3. McGrew R: Encyclopedia of Medical History. New York: McGraw-Hill, 1985.
4. Dung HC: Acupuncture points of the brachial plexus. Am J Chin Med 13:49-64, 1985.
5. Hoernle AFR: Studies in the Medicine of Ancient India. Part I. Osteology or the Bones of the Human Body. Oxford: Clarendon Press, 1907.
6. Persaud TVN: Early History of Human Anatomy. From Antiquity to the Beginning of the Modern Era. Springfield, Ill: Charles C Thomas, 1984.
7. Rasch PJ, Burke RK: Kinesiology and Applied Anatomy. Philadelphia: Lea & Febiger, 1959.
8. Hippocrates: Hippocratic Writings. In Hutchins RM (ed): Great Books of the Western World. Chicago: Encyclopedia Britannica, 1955.
9. Galen: On the Usefulness of the Parts of the Body. Ithaca, NY: Cornell University Press, 1967.
10. Clark K, Pedretti C: The Drawings of Leonardo da Vinci at Windsor Castle, 3 vols. London: Phaidon, 1968-1969.
11. Vesalius A: The Illustrations from the Works of Andreas Vesalius of Brussels. New York: World Publishing Company, 1950.
12. Perry J: Biomechanics of the shoulder. In Rowe C (ed): The Shoulder. New York: Churchill Livingstone, 1988.
13. Duchenne GB: Physiology of Movement: Demonstrated by Means of Electrical Stimulation and Clinical Observation and Applied to the Study of Paralysis and Deformities. Philadelphia: WB Saunders, 1959.
14. Basmajian JV: Muscles Alive: Their Functions Revealed by Electromyography, 4th ed. Baltimore: Williams & Wilkins, 1979.
15. Muybridge E: Animals in Motion. New York: Dover Publications, 1957.
16. Lockhart RD: Movements of the normal shoulder joint and of a case with trapezius paralysis studied by radiogram and experiment in the living. J Anat 64:288-302, 1930.
17. Braune W, Fischer O: The Human Gait. New York: Springer-Verlag, 1987.
18. Braune W, Fischer O: On the Centre of Gravity of the Human Body. New York: Springer-Verlag, 1988.
19. Meyer AW: Chronic functional lesions of the shoulder. Arch Surg 35:646-674, 1937.
20. Inman VT, Saunders JB, Abbott LC: Observations of the function of the shoulder joint. 1944. Clin Orthop Relat Res (330):3-12, 1996.
21. Detrisac DA, Johnson LL: Arthroscopic Shoulder Anatomy: Pathologic and Surgical Implications. Thorofare, NJ: Slack, 1986.
22. Rockwood CA, Green DP: Fractures in Adults, 6th ed. Philadelphia: Lippincott Williams & Wilkins, 2006.
23. Lucas DB: Biomechanics of the shoulder joint. Arch Surg 107:425-432, 1973.
24. Radin E: Biomechanics and functional anatomy. In Post M (ed): The Shoulder. Surgical and Nonsurgical Management. Philadelphia: Lea & Febiger, 1978, pp 44-49.
25. Kaltsas DS: Comparative study of the properties of the shoulder joint capsule with those of other joint capsules. Clin Orthop Relat Res (173):20-26, 1983.
26. Reeves B: Experiments on the tensile strength of the anterior capsular structures of the shoulder in man. J Bone Joint Surg Br 50:858-865, 1968.
27. Hollinshead WH: Anatomy for Surgeons, 3rd ed. Philadelphia: Harper & Row, 1982.
28. Rosse C, Gaddum-Rosse P, Hollinshead WH (eds): Hollinshead's Textbook of Anatomy, 5th ed. Philadelphia: Lippincott-Raven, 1997.
29. DePalma AF: Surgical anatomy of acromioclavicular and sternoclavicular joints. Surg Clin North Am 43:1541-1550, 1963.
30. DePalma AF, Callery G, Bennett GA: Variational anatomy and degenerative lesions of the shoulder joint. Instr Course Lect 6:255-281, 1949.
31. Duggan N: Recurrent dislocation of the sternoclavicular cartilage. J Bone Joint Surg 13:365, 1931.
32. Bearn JG: Direct observations on the function of the capsule of the sternoclavicular joint in clavicular support. J Anat 101:159-170, 1967.
33. Acus RW 3rd, Bell RH, Fisher DL: Proximal clavicle excision: An analysis of results. J Shoulder Elbow Surg 4:182-187, 1995.
34. Cave AJ: The nature and morphology of the costoclavicular ligament. J Anat 95:170-179, 1961.
35. Kennedy JC: Retrosternal dislocation of the clavicle. J Bone Joint Surg Br 31:74-75, 1949.
36. Wirth MA Rockwood CA Jr: Acute and chronic traumatic injuries of the sternoclavicular joint. J Am Acad Orthop Surg 4:268-278, 1996.
37. Cyriax E: A second brief note on the floating clavicle. Anat Rec 52:97, 1932.
38. DePalma A: Surgery of the Shoulder, 3rd ed. Philadelphia: JB Lippincott, 1983.
39. Abbott LLD: The function of the clavicle: Its surgical significance. Ann Surg 140:583-597, 1954.
40. Lewis MM, Ballet FL, Kroll PG, et al: En bloc clavicular resection: operative procedure and postoperative testing of function. Case reports. Clin Orthop Relat Res (193):214-220, 1985.
41. McCally WC, Kelly DA: Treatment of fractures of the clavicle, ribs and scapula. Am J Surg 50:558-562, 1940.
42. Taylor S: Clavicular dysostosis: A case report. J Bone Joint Surg 27:710-711, 1945.
43. Wood VE, Marchinski LM, Congenital anomalies of the shoulder. In Rockwood CA, Matsen FA (ed): The Shoulder. Philadelphia: WB Sanders, 1990, pp 98-148.
44. Borges JL, Shah A, Torres BC, et al: Modified Woodward procedure for Sprengel deformity of the shoulder: Long-term results. J Pediatr Orthop 16:508-513, 1996.
45. Carson WG, Lovell WW, Whitesides TE Jr: Congenital elevation of the scapula. Surgical correction by the Woodward procedure. J Bone Joint Surg Am 63:1199-1207, 1981.
46. Perry MO: Vascular trauma. In Moore W (ed): Vascular Surgery. Orlando: Grune & Stratton, 1986.
47. Johnson EW Jr, Collins HR: Nonunion of the clavicle. Arch Surg 87:963-966, 1963.
48. Howard FM, Shafer SJ: Injuries to the clavicle with neurovascular complications. A study of fourteen cases. J Bone Joint Surg Am 47:1335-1346, 1965.
49. Nutter PD: Coracoclavicular articulations. J Bone Joint Surg 23:177-179, 1941.
50. Lewis OJ: The coraco-clavicular joint. J Anat 93:296-303, 1959.
51. Urist MR: Complete dislocation of the acromioclavicular joint. J Bone Joint Surg Am 45:1750-1753, 1963.
52. Fukuda K, Craig EV, An KN, et al: Biomechanical study of the ligamentous system of the acromioclavicular joint. J Bone Joint Surg Am 68:434-440, 1986.
53. Gagey O, Bonfait H, Gillot C, et al: Anatomic basis of ligamentous control of elevation of the shoulder (reference position of the shoulder joint). Surg Radiol Anat 9:19-26, 1987.
54. Todd TW, D'Errico JJ: The clavicular epiphyses. Am J Anat 41:25-50, 1928.
55. Weinstabl R, Hertz H, Firbas W: [Connection of the ligamentum coracoglenoidale with the muscular pectoralis minor]. Acta Anat (Basel) 125:126-131, 1986.
56. Dines DM, Warren RF, Inglis AE, et al: The coracoid impingement syndrome. J Bone Joint Surg Br 72:314-316, 1990.
57. Gerber C, Terrier F, Ganz R: The role of the coracoid process in the chronic impingement syndrome. J Bone Joint Surg Br 67:703-708, 1985.
58. Gerber C, Terrier F, Zehnder R, et al: The subcoracoid space. An anatomic study. Clin Orthop Relat Res:132-138, 1987.
59. Maves MD, Philippsen LP: Surgical anatomy of the scapular spine in the trapezius-osteomuscular flap. Arch Otolaryngol Head Neck Surg 112:173-175, 1986.
60. Panje W, Cutting C: Trapezius osteomyocutaneous island flap for reconstruction of the anterior floor of the mouth and the mandible. Head Neck Surg 3:66-71, 1980.
61. Neer CS 2nd: Anterior acromioplasty for the chronic impingement syndrome in the shoulder: A preliminary report. J Bone Joint Surg Am 54:41-50, 1972.
62. Nicholson GP, Goodman DA, Flatow EL, et al: The acromion: Morphologic condition and age-related changes. A study of 420 scapulas. J Shoulder Elbow Surg 5:1-11, 1996.
63. Petersson CJ, Redlund-Johnell I: The subacromial space in normal shoulder radiographs. Acta Orthop Scand 55:57-58, 1984.
64. Neer CS, Poppen NK: Supraspinatus outlet. Orthop Transactions 11:234, 1987.
65. Aoki M, Ishii S, Usui M: The slope of the acromion in the rotator cuff impingement. Orthop Trans 10:228, 1986.
66. Bigliani LU, Ticker JB, Flatow EL, et al: The relationship of acromial architecture to rotator cuff disease. Clin Sports Med 10:823-838, 1991.
67. Banas MP, Miller RJ, Totterman S: Relationship between the lateral acromion angle and rotator cuff disease. J Shoulder Elbow Surg 4:454-461, 1995.
68. Holt EM, Allibone RO: Anatomic variants of the coracoacromial ligament. J Shoulder Elbow Surg 4:370-375, 1995.
69. Mudge MK, Wood VE, Frykman GK: Rotator cuff tears associated with os acromiale. J Bone Joint Surg Am 66:427-429, 1984.
70. Neer CS 2nd: Impingement lesions. Clin Orthop Relat Res (173):70-77, 1983.
71. Liberson F: Os acromiale—a contested anomaly. J Bone Joint Surg 19:683-689, 1937.
72. Saha AK: Dynamic stability of the glenohumeral joint. Acta Orthop Scand 42:491-505, 1971.
73. Deutsch AL, Resnick D, Mink JH: Computed tomography of the glenohumeral and sternoclavicular joints. Orthop Clin North Am 16:497-511, 1985.
74. Saha AK: The classic. Mechanism of shoulder movements and a plea for the recognition of "zero position" of glenohumeral joint. Clin Orthop Relat Res (173):3-10, 1983.
75. Brookes M: The blood supply of irregular and flat bones. In Brookes MB (ed): Blood Supply of the Bone. New York: Appleton-Century-Crofts, 1971, pp 47-66.

76. Salmon M: Anatomic Studies: Arteries of the Muscles of the Extremities and the Trunk and Arterial Anastomotic Pathways of the Extremities. St. Louis: Quality Medical Publishing, 1994.

77. Iannotti JP, Gabriel JP, Schneck SL, et al: The normal glenohumeral relationships. An anatomical study of one hundred and forty shoulders. J Bone Joint Surg Am 74:491-500, 1992.

78. Ito N, Eto M, Maeda K, et al: Ultrasonographic measurement of humeral torsion. J Shoulder Elbow Surg 4:157-161, 1995.

79. Boileau P, Walch G: The three-dimensional geometry of the proximal humerus. Implications for surgical technique and prosthetic design. J Bone Joint Surg Br 79:857-865, 1997.

80. Cyprien JM, Vasey HM, Burdet A, et al: Humeral retrotorsion and glenohumeral relationship in the normal shoulder and in recurrent anterior dislocation (scapulometry). Clin Orthop Relat Res (175):8-17, 1983.

81. Tillet E, Smith M, Fulcher M, et al: Anatomic determination of humeral head retorversion: The relationship of the central axis of the humeral head to the bicipital groove. J Shoulder Elbow Surg 2:255-256, 1993.

82. Rietveld AB, Daanen HA, Rozing PM, et al: The lever arm in glenohumeral abduction after hemiarthroplasty. J Bone Joint Surg Br 70:561-565, 1988.

83. Gagey O, Hue E: Mechanics of the deltoid muscle. A new approach. Clin Orthop Relat Res (375):250-257, 2000.

84. Meyer A: Spontaneous dislocation and destruction of tendon of long head of biceps brachii. Fifty-nine instances. Arch Surg 17:493-506, 1928.

85. Paavolainen P Slatis A, Aalto K: Surgical pathology in chronic shoulder pain. In Bateman JE, Welsh HP (eds): Surgery of the Shoulder. St. Louis: CV Mosby, 1984, pp 313-318.

86. Petersson CJ: Spontaneous medial dislocation of the tendon of the long biceps brachii. An anatomic study of prevalence and pathomechanics. Clin Orthop Relat Res (211):224-227, 1986.

87. Slatis P, Aalto K: Medial dislocation of the tendon of the long head of the biceps brachii. Acta Orthop Scand 50:73-77, 1979.

88. Cooper D, O'Brien S, Arnoczky S, et al: The structure and function of the coracohumeral ligament: An anatomic and microscopic study. J Shoulder Elbow Surg 2:70-77, 1993.

89. Walch G, Nove-Josserand L, Boileau P, et al: Subluxations and dislocations of the tendon of the long head of the biceps. J Shoulder Elbow Surg 7:100-108, 1998.

90. Laing PG: The arterial supply of the adult humerus. J Bone Joint Surg Am 38:1105-1116, 1956.

91. Gerber C, Schneeberger AG, Vinh TS: The arterial vascularization of the humeral head. An anatomical study. J Bone Joint Surg Am 72:1486-1494, 1990.

92. Lucas L, Gill J: Humerus varus following birth injury to the proximal humeral epiphysis. J Bone Joint Surg 29:367-369, 1947.

93. Tang T: Humerus varus: A report of 7 cases. Chin J Orthop 3:165-170, 1983.

94. Ovesen J, Nielsen S: Stability of the shoulder joint. Cadaver study of stabilizing structures. Acta Orthop Scand 56:149-151, 1985.

95. Symeonides PP: The significance of the subscapularis muscle in the pathogenesis of recurrent anterior dislocation of the shoulder. J Bone Joint Surg Br 54:476-483, 1972.

96. Turkel SJ, Panio MW, Marshall JL, et al: Stabilizing mechanisms preventing anterior dislocation of the glenohumeral joint. J Bone Joint Surg Am 63:1208-1217, 1981.

97. Franklin JL, Barrett WP, Jackins SE, et al: Glenoid loosening in total shoulder arthroplasty. Association with rotator cuff deficiency. J Arthroplasty 3:39-46, 1988.

98. Harmon PH: Surgical reconstruction of the paralytic shoulder by multiple muscle transplantations. J Bone Joint Surg Am 32:583-595, 1950.

99. Ekholm J, Arborelius UP, Hillered L, et al: Shoulder muscle EMG and resisting moment during diagonal exercise movements resisted by weight-and-pulley-circuit. Scand J Rehabil Med 10:179-185, 1978.

100. Matsen F: Biomechanics of the shoulder. In Frankel VH (ed): Basic Biomechanics of the Skeletal System. Philadelphia: Lea & Febiger, 1980, pp 221-242.

101. Gowan ID, Jobe FW, Tibone JE, et al: A comparative electromyographic analysis of the shoulder during pitching. Professional versus amateur pitchers. Am J Sports Med 15:586-590, 1987.

102. Atwater AE: Biomechanics of overarm throwing movements and of throwing injuries. Exerc Sport Sci Rev 7:43-85, 1979.

103. Doody SG, Freedman L, Waterland JC: Shoulder movements during abduction in the scapular plane. Arch Phys Med Rehabil 51:595-604, 1970.

104. Broome HL, Basmajian JV: The function of the teres major muscle: An electromyographic study. Anat Rec 170:309-310, 1971.

105. Woo SL, Maynard J, Butler D: Ligament, tendon, and joint capsule insertions to bone. In Woo SL, Buckwalter JA (eds): Injury and Repair of the Musculoskeletal Soft Tissues. Park Ridge, Ill: American Academy of Orthopaedic Surgeons, 1988, pp 133-166.

106. Jobe CM, Kropp WE, Wood VE: Spinal accessory nerve in a trapezius-splitting surgical approach. J Shoulder Elbow Surg 5:206-208, 1996.

107. Mathes SJ, Nahai F: Classification of the vascular anatomy of muscles: Experimental and clinical correlation. Plast Reconstr Surg 67:177-187, 1981.

108. Taylor GI, Palmer JH: The vascular territories (angiosomes) of the body: Experimental study and clinical applications. Br J Plast Surg 40:113-141, 1987.

109. Watterson PA, Taylor GI, Crock JG: The venous territories of muscles: Anatomical study and clinical implications. Br J Plast Surg 41:569-585, 1988.

110. Beaton LE, Anson BJ: Variation of the origin of the m. trapezius. Anat Rec 83:41-46, 1942.

111. Mortensen OA, Wiedenbauer MM: An electromyographic study of the trapezius muscle. Anat Rec 112:366-367, 1952.

112. Dewar FP, Harris RI: Restoration of function of the shoulder following paralysis of the trapezius by fascial sling fixation and transplantation of the levator scapulae. Ann Surg 132:1111-1115, 1950.

113. Horan FT, Bonafede RP: Bilateral absence of the trapezius and sternal head of the pectoralis major muscles. A case report. J Bone Joint Surg Am 59:133, 1977.

114. Saunders WH, Johnson EW: Rehabilitation of the shoulder after radical neck dissection. Ann Otol Rhinol Laryngol 84:812-816, 1975.

115. Selden BR: Congenital absence of trapezius and rhomboideus major muscles. J Bone Joint Surg 17:1058-1061, 1935.

116. Sakellarides H: Injury to spinal accessory nerve with paralysis of trapezius muscle and treatment by tendon transfer. Orthop Transactions 10:449, 1986.

117. Teboul F, Bizot P, Kakkar R, et al: Surgical management of trapezius palsy. J Bone Joint Surg Am 86:1884-1890, 2004.

118. Huelke DF: A study of the transverse cervical and dorsal scapular arteries. Anat Rec 132:233-245, 1958.

119. Huelke DF: Variation in the origins of the branches of the axillary artery. Anat Rec 135:33-41, 1959.

120. Scheving LE, Pauly JE: An electromyographic study of some muscles acting on the upper extremity of man. Anat Rec 135:239-245, 1959.

121. Nuber GW, Jobe FW, Perry J, et al: Fine wire electromyography analysis of muscles of the shoulder during swimming. Am J Sports Med 14:7-11, 1986.

122. Kuhn JE, Plancher KD, Hawkins RJ: Scapular winging. J Am Acad Orthop Surg 3:319-325, 1995.

123. Lorhan PH: Isolated paralysis of the serratus magnus following surgical procedures. Report of a case. Arch Surg 54:656-659, 1947.

124. Connor PM, Yamaguchi K, Manifold SG, et al: Split pectoralis major transfer for serratus anterior palsy. Clin Orthop Relat Res (341):134-142, 1997.

125. Horwitz MT, Tocantins LM: Isolated paralysis of the serratus anterior (magnus) muscle. J Bone Joint Surg 20:720-725, 1938.

126. Lambert AE: A rare variation in the pectoralis minor muscle. Anat Rec 31:193-200, 1925.

127. Vare AM, Indurkar GM: Some anomalous findings in the axillary musculature. J Anat Soc India 14:34-36, 1965.

128. Reid CD, Taylor GI: The vascular territory of the acromiothoracic axis. Br J Plast Surg 37:194-212, 1984.

129. Williams GA: Pectoral muscle defects: Cases illustrating 3 varieties. J Bone Joint Surg 12:417, 1930.

130. Bing R: Über Angeborene Muskel-Defecte. Virchows Arch B Cell Pathol 170:175-228, 1902.

131. Cave AJ, Brown RW: On the tendon of the subclavius muscle. J Bone Joint Surg Br 34:466-469, 1952.

132. Reiss FP, DeCarmago AM, Vitti M, et al: Electromyographic study of subclavius muscle. Acta Anat 105:284-290, 1979.

133. Abbott LC, Lucas DB: The tripartite deltoid and its surgical significance in exposure of the scapulohumeral joint. Ann Surg 136:392-403, 1952.

134. Klepps S, Auerbach J, Calhon O, et al: A cadaveric study on the anatomy of the deltoid insertion and its relationship to the deltopectoral approach to the proximal humerus. J Shoulder Elbow Surg 13:322-327, 2004.

135. Bhattacharyya S: Abduction contracture of the shoulder from contracture of the intermediate part of the deltoid. Report of three cases. J Bone Joint Surg Br 48:127-131, 1966.

136. Shevlin MG, Lehmann JF, Lucci JA: Electromyographic study of the function of some muscles crossing the glenohumeral joint. Arch Phys Med Rehabil 50:264-270, 1969.

137. Colachis SC Jr, Strohm BR, Brechner VL: Effects of axillary nerve block on muscle force in the upper extremity. Arch Phys Med Rehabil 50:647-654, 1969.

138. Groh GI, Simoni M, Rolla P, et al: Loss of the deltoid after shoulder operations: An operative disaster. J Shoulder Elbow Surg 3:243-253, 1994.

139. Clark JM, Harryman DT 2nd: Tendons, ligaments, and capsule of the rotator cuff. Gross and microscopic anatomy. J Bone Joint Surg Am 74:713-725, 1992.

140. Cooper DE, O'Brien SJ, Warren RF: Supporting layers of the glenohumeral joint. An anatomic study. Clin Orthop Relat Res (289):144-155, 1993.

141. Staples OS, Watkins AL: Full active abduction in traumatic paralysis of the deltoid. J Bone Joint Surg 25:85-89, 1943.

142. Burkhart SS, Esch JC, Jolson RS: The rotator crescent and rotator cable: An anatomic description of the shoulder's "suspension bridge." Arthroscopy 9:611-616, 1993.

143. Roh MS, Wang VM, April EW, et al: Anterior and posterior musculotendinous anatomy of the supraspinatus. J Shoulder Elbow Surg 9:436-440, 2000.
144. McLaughlin HL: Lesions of the musculotendinous cuff of the shoulder: III. Observations on the pathology, course and treatment of calcific deposits. Ann Surg 124:354-362, 1946.
145. Howell SM, Imobersteg AM, Seger DH, et al: Clarification of the role of the supraspinatus muscle in shoulder function. J Bone Joint Surg Am 68:398-404, 1986.
146. Colachis SC Jr, Strohm BR: Effect of suprascauular and axillary nerve blocks on muscle force in upper extremity. Arch Phys Med Rehabil 52:22-29, 1971.
147. McMahon PJ, Debski RE, Thompson WO, et al: Shoulder muscle forces and tendon excursions during glenohumeral abduction in the scapular plane. J Shoulder Elbow Surg 4:199-208, 1995.
148. Grant JCB, Smith CG: Age incidence of rupture of the supraspinatus tendon. Anat Rec 100:666, 1948.
149. Bayley JC, Cochran TP, Sledge CB: The weight-bearing shoulder. The impingement syndrome in paraplegics. J Bone Joint Surg Am 69:676-678, 1987.
150. Martin CP: The movements of the shoulder-joint, with special reference to rupture of the supraspinatus tendon. Am J Anat 66:213-234, 1940.
151. Jobe CM, Iannotti JP: Limits imposed on glenohumeral motion by joint geometry. J Shoulder Elbow Surg 4:281-285, 1995.
152. Ovesen J, Nielsen S: Posterior instability of the shoulder. A cadaver study. Acta Orthop Scand 57:436-439, 1986.
153. Ovesen J, Nielsen S: Anterior and posterior shoulder instability. A cadaver study. Acta Orthop Scand 57:324-327, 1986.
154. Cain PR, Mutschler TA, Fu FH, et al: Anterior stability of the glenohumeral joint. A dynamic model. Am J Sports Med 15:144-148, 1987.
155. Waterston D: Variations in the teres minor muscle. Anat Anz 32:331-333, 1908.
156. Hinton MA, Parker AW, Drez D, Altchek D: An anatomic study of the subscapularis tendon and myotendinous junction. J Shoulder Elbow Surg 3:224-229, 1994.
157. McCann PD, Cordasco FA, Ticker JB, et al: An anatomic study of the subscapular nerves: A grid for electromyographic analysis of the subscapularis muscle. J Shoulder Elbow Surg 3:94-99, 1994.
158. Bartlett SP, May JW Jr, Yaremchuk MJ: The latissimus dorsi muscle: A fresh cadaver study of the primary neurovascular pedicle. Plast Reconstr Surg 67:631-636, 1981.
159. Flatow EL, Bigliani LU, April EW: An anatomic study of the musculocutaneous nerve and its relationship to the coracoid process. Clin Orthop Relat Res (244):166-171, 1989.
160. Landry SO Jr: The phylogenetic significance of the chondro-epitrochlearis muscle and its accompanying pectoral abnormalities. J Anat 92:57-61, 1958.
161. Marmor L, Bechtol CO, Hall CB: Pectoralis major muscle. J Bone Joint Surg Am 43:81-87, 1961.
162. Hayes WM: Rupture of the pectoralis major muscle: Review of the literature and report of two cases. J Int Coll Surg 14:82-88, 1950.
163. Klepps SJ, Goldfarb C, Flatow E, et al: Anatomic evaluation of the subcoracoid pectoralis major transfer in human cadavers. J Shoulder Elbow Surg 10:453-459, 2001.
164. Tobin GR, Schusterman M, Peterson GH, et al: The intramuscular neurovascular anatomy of the latissimus dorsi muscle: The basis for splitting the flap. Plast Reconstr Surg 67:637-641, 1981.
165. Mariani EM, Cofield RH, Askew LJ, et al: Rupture of the tendon of the long head of the biceps brachii. Surgical versus nonsurgical treatment. Clin Orthop Relat Res (228):233-239, 1988.
166. Hitchcock HH, Bechtol CO: Painful shoulder. Observations of the role of the tendon of the long head of the biceps brachii in its causation. J Bone Joint Surg Am 30:263-273, 1948.
167. Walch G, Nove-Josserand J, Levigne C, et al: Tears of the supraspinatus tendon associated with "hidden" lesions of the rotator interval. J Shoulder Elbow Surg 3:353-360, 1994.
168. Ting A, Jobe FW, Barto P, et al: An EMG analysis of the lateral biceps in shoulders with rotator cuff tears. Presented at the Third Open Meeting of the Society of American Shoulder and Elbow Surgeons, San Francisco, California, January 21-22, 1987.
169. Itoi E, Motzkin ME, Morrey BF, et al: Stabilizing function of the long head of the biceps in the hanging arm position. J Shoulder Elbow Surg 3:135-142, 1994.
170. Jobe FW, Moynes DR, Tibone JE, et al: An EMG analysis of the shoulder in pitching. A second report. Am J Sports Med 12:218-220, 1984.
171. Slingluff CL, Terzis JK, Edgerton MT, The quantitative microanatomy of the brachial plexus in man: Reconstructive relevance. In Terzis JK (ed): Microreconstruction of Nerve Injuries. Philadelphia: WB Saunders, 1987, pp 285-324.
172. Sunderland S, Bradley KC: The cross-sectional area of peripheral nerve trunks devoted to nerve fibers. Brain 72:428-449, 1949.
173. Sunderland S: Nerve and Nerve Injuries, 2nd ed. New York: Churchill Livingstone, 1978.
174. Sunderland S: The anatomic foundation of peripheral nerve repair techniques. Orthop Clin North Am 12:245-266, 1981.
175. Williams HB, Jabaley ME: The importance of internal anatomy of the peripheral nerves to nerve repair in the forearm and hand. Hand Clin 2:689-707, 1986.
176. Seddon HJ: Nerve grafting. J Bone Joint Surg Br 45:447-461, 1963.
177. Tarlov IM, Epstein JA: Nerve grafts: The importance of an adequate blood supply. J Neurosurg 2:49-71, 1945.
178. Lundborg G: Ischemic nerve injury. Experimental studies on intraneural microvascular pathophysiology and nerve function in a limb subjected to temporary circulatory arrest. Scand J Plast Reconstr Surg Suppl 6:3-113, 1970.
179. Lundborg G: Intraneural microcirculation. Orthop Clin North Am 19:1-12, 1988.
180. Terzis JK, Breidenbach W: The anatomy of free vascularized nerve grafts. In Terzis JK (ed): Microreconstruction of Nerve Injuries. Philadelphia: WB Saunders, 1987, pp 101-111.
181. Kopell HP, Thompson WA: Pain and the frozen shoulder. Surg Gynecol Obstet 109:92-96, 1959.
182. Lundborg G, Rydevik B: Effects of stretching the tibial nerve of the rabbit. A preliminary study of the intraneural circulation and the barrier function of the perineurium. J Bone Joint Surg Br 55:390-401, 1973.
183. Enneking WF: Musculoskeletal Tumor Surgery. New York: Churchill Livingstone, 1983.
184. Leffert RD: Brachial Plexus Injuries. New York: Churchill Livingstone, 1985.
185. Gebarski KS, Glazer GM, Gebarski SS: Brachial plexus: Anatomic, radiologic, and pathologic correlation using computed tomography. J Comput Assist Tomogr 6:1058-1063, 1982.
186. Shin AY, Spinner RJ, Steinmann SP, et al: Adult traumatic brachial plexus injuries. J Am Acad Orthop Surg 13:382-396, 2005.
187. Bonnel F: Microscopic anatomy of the adult human brachial plexus: An anatomical and histological basis for microsurgery. Microsurgery 5:107-118, 1984.
188. Kerr AT: The brachial plexus of nerves in man, the variations in its formation and branches. Am J Anat 23:285-395, 1918.
189. Herzberg G, Narakas A, Comtet JJ: Microsurgical relations of the roots of the brachial plexus. Practical applications. Ann Chir Main 4:120-133, 1985.
190. MacCarty CS: Surgical exposure of the brachial plexus. Surg Neurol 21:593-596, 1984.
191. Telford ED, Mottershead S: Pressure at the cervico-brachial junction: An operative and anatomical study. J Bone Joint Surg Br 30:249-265, 1948.
192. Bonica JJ: Regional Anesthesia. Clinical Anesthesia Series. Philadelphia: FA Davis, 1969.
193. Horwitz MT, Tocantins LM: An anatomical study of the role of the long thoracic nerve and the related scapular bursae in the pathogenesis of local paralysis of the serratus anterior muscle. Anat Rec 71:375-385, 1938.
194. Prescott MU, Zollinger RW: Alara scapula: An unusual sugical complication. Am J Surg 65:98-103, 1944.
195. Edeland HG, Zachrisson BE: Fracture of the scapular notch associated with lesion of the suprascapular nerve. Acta Orthop Scand 46:758-763, 1975.
196. Miller RA: Observations upon the arrangement of the axillary artery and brachial plexus. Am J Anat 64:143-159, 1939.
197. Gardner E: The innervation of the shoulder joint. Anat Rec 102:1-18, 1948.
198. Abdullah S, Bowden RE: The blood supply of the brachial plexus. Proc R Soc Med 53:203-205, 1960.
199. Yung SW, Lazarus MD, Harryman DT 2nd: Practical guidelines to safe surgery about the subscapularis. J Shoulder Elbow Surg 5:467-470, 1996.
200. Loomer R, Graham B: Anatomy of the axillary nerve and its relation to inferior capsular shift. Clin Orthop Relat Res (243):100-105, 1989.
201. Cahill BR, Palmer RE: Quadrilateral space syndrome. J Hand Surg [Am] 8:65-69, 1983.
202. Ball CM, Steger T, Galatz LM, et al: The posterior branch of the axillary nerve: An anatomic study. J Bone Joint Surg Am 85:1497-1501, 2003.
203. Cetik O, Uslu M, Acar HI, et al: Is there a safe area for the axillary nerve in the deltoid muscle? A cadaveric study. J Bone Joint Surg Am 88:2395-2399, 2006.
204. Hoppenfeld S, DeBoer P: The shoulder. In Hoppenfeld S, DeBoer P (eds): Surgical Exposures in Orthopaedics: The Anatomic Approach. Philadelphia: Lippincott Williams & Wilkins, 2003, pp 1-49.
205. Rengachary SS, Neff JP, Singer PA, et al: Suprascapular entrapment neuropathy: A clinical, anatomical, and comparative study. Part 1: Clinical study. Neurosurgery 5:441-446, 1979.
206. Rengachary SS, Burr D, Lucas S, et al: Suprascapular entrapment neuropathy: A clinical, anatomical, and comparative study. Part 2: Anatomical study. Neurosurgery 5:447-451, 1979.
207. Rengachary SS, Burr D, Lucas S, et al: Suprascapular entrapment neuropathy: A clinical, anatomical, and comparative study. Part 3: Comparative study. Neurosurgery 5:452-455, 1979.
208. Clein LJ: Suprascapular entrapment neuropathy. J Neurosurg 43:337-342, 1975.
209. Omokawa S, Tanaka Y, Miyauchi Y, et al: Traction neuropathy of the supraclavicular nerve attributable to an osseous tunnel of the clavicle. Clin Orthop Relat Res (431):238-240, 2005.

210. Bayramoglu A, Demiryurek D, Tuccar E, et al: Variations in anatomy at the suprascapular notch possibly causing suprascapular nerve entrapment: An anatomical study. Knee Surg Sports Traumatol Arthrosc 11:393-398, 2003.

211. Strohm BR, Colachis SC Jr: Shoulder joint dysfunction following injury to the suprascapular nerve. Phys Ther 45:106-111, 1965.

212. Bigliani LU, Dalsey RM, McCann PD, et al: An anatomical study of the suprascapular nerve. Arthroscopy 6:301-305, 1990.

213. Thompson RC Jr, Schneider W, Kennedy T: Entrapment neuropathy of the inferior branch of the suprascapular nerve by ganglia. Clin Orthop Relat Res (166):185-187, 1982.

214. Fehrman DA, Orwin JF, Jennings RM: Suprascapular nerve entrapment by ganglion cysts: A report of six cases with arthroscopic findings and review of the literature. Arthroscopy 11:727-734, 1995.

215. Plancher KD, Peterson RK, Johnston JC, et al: The spinoglenoid ligament. Anatomy, morphology, and histological findings. J Bone Joint Surg Am 87:361-365, 2005.

216. Sunderland S, Bedbrook GM: The relative sympathetic contribution to individual roots of the brachial plexus in man. Brain 72:297-301, 1949.

217. Sunderland S: The distribution of sympathetic fibers in the brachial plexus in man. Brain 71:88-102, 1948.

218. Bronson SR, Hinsey JC, Geohegan WA: Observations on the distribution of the sympathetic nerves to the pupil and upper extremity as determined by stimulation of the anterior roots in man. Ann Surg 118:647-655, 1943.

219. Woollard HH, Weddell G: The composition and distri-bution of vascular nerves in the extremities. J Anat 69(Pt 2):165-176, 1935.

220. Kellman GM, Kneeland JB, Middleton WD, et al: MR imaging of the supraclavicular region: Normal anatomy. AJR Am J Roentgenol 148:77-82, 1987.

221. Lewis WH: The development of the arm in man. Am J Anat 1:145-183, 1902.

222. Walsh JF: The anatomy of the brachial plexus. Am J Med Sci 74:387-399, 1987.

223. Breisch EA: A rare human variation: The relationship of the axillary and inferior subscapular nerves to an accessory subscapularis muscle. Anat Rec 216:440-442, 1986.

224. Hasan M, Narayan D: The single cord human brachial plexus. J Anat Soc India 64:103-104, 1964.

225. Tsikaras PD, Agiabasis AS, Hytiroglou PM: A variation in the formation of the brachial plexus characterized by the absence of C8 and T1 fibers in the trunk of the median nerve. Bull Assoc Anat (Nancy) 67:501-505, 1983.

226. Corbin KB, Harrison F: The sensory innervation of the spinal accessory and tongue musculature in the rhesus monkey. Brain 62:191-197, 1939.

227. Ellis H, Feldman ST: Anatomy for Anesthetists, 3rd ed. Oxford: Blackwell Scientific, 1977.

228. Tubbs RS, Salter EG, Oakes WJ: Anomaly of the supraclavicular nerve: Case report and review of the literature. Clin Anat 19:599-601, 2006.

229. Gelberman RH, Verdeck WN, Brodhead WT: Supraclavicular nerve-entrapment syndrome. J Bone Joint Surg Am 57:119, 1975.

230. Palmer JH, Taylor GI: The vascular territories of the anterior chest wall. Br J Plast Surg 39:287-299, 1986.

231. Trotter M, Henderson JL, Gass H: The origins of the branches of the axillary artery in whites and American Negroes. Anat Rec 46:133-137, 1930.

232. Daseler EH, Anson BJ: Surgical anatomy of the subclavian artery and its branches. Surg Gynecol Obstet 108:149-174, 1959.

233. Rich NM, Spencer F: Vascular Trauma. Philadelphia: WB Saunders, 1978.

234. Chepelenko GV: [Lymphatic vessels of the upper extremity and their relation to nodes in the axillary area in healthy subjects and lymph flow blockade]. Arkh Anat Gistol Embriol 89:74-81, 1985.

235. Radke HM: Arterial circulation of the upper extremity. In Strandness DE (ed): Collateral Circulation in Clinical Surgery. Philadelphia: WB Saunders, 1969, pp 294-307.

236. Read WT, Trotter M: The origins of transverse cervical and of transverse scapular arteries in American whites and negroes. Am J Physiol Anthropol 28:239-247, 1941.

237. Mayou BJ, Whitby D, Jones BM: The scapular flap—an anatomical and clinical study. Br J Plast Surg 35:8-13, 1982.

238. Brooks CH, Revell WJ, Heatley FW: Vascularity of the humeral head after proximal humeral fractures. An anatomical cadaver study. J Bone Joint Surg Br 75:132-136, 1993.

239. Hertel R, Hempfing A, Stiehler M, et al: Predictors of humeral head ischemia after intracapsular fracture of the proximal humerus. J Shoulder Elbow Surg 13:427-433, 2004.

240. Strandness DE (ed): Collateral Circulation in Clinical Surgery. Philadelphia: WB Saunders, 1969.

241. Strandness DE: Functional characteristics of normal and collateral circulation. In Strandness DE (ed): Collateral Circulation in Clinical Surgery. Philadelphia: WB Saunders, 1969, pp 2-25.

242. DeGaris CF, Swartley WB: The axillary artery in white and negro stocks. Am J Anat 41:353-397, 1928.

243. Rich NM, Baugh JH, Hughes CW: Acute arterial injuries in Vietnam: 1,000 cases. J Trauma 10:359-369, 1970.

244. McKenzie AD, Sinclair AM: Axillary artery occlusion complicating shoulder dislocation: A report of two cases. Ann Surg 148:139-141, 1958.

245. Ferguson LK, Holt JH: Successful anastomosis of severed brachial artery. Am J Surg 79:344-347, 1950.

246. DeBakey ME, Simeon FA: Battle injuries of the arteries in World War II. Ann Surg 123:534-579, 1946.

247. Rich NM, Hughes CW, Baugh JH: Management of venous injuries. Ann Surg 171:724-730, 1970.

248. Nickalls RW: A new percutaneous infraclavicular approach to the axillary vein. Anaesthesia 42:151-154, 1987.

249. Weathersby HT: The valves of the axillary, subclavian and internal jugular veins. Anat Rec 124:379-380, 1956.

250. Danese C, Howard JM: Postmastectomy lymphedema. Surg Gynecol Obstet 120:797-802, 1965.

251. Kaplan T, Katz A: Thrombosis of the axillary vein. Case report with comments on etiology, pathology, and diagnosis. Am J Surg 37:326-333, 1937.

252. Neuhof H: Excision of the axillary vein in the radical operation for carcinoma of the breast. Ann Surg 108:15-20, 1938.

253. Buschmakin N: Die Lymphdrüsen der Achselhöhle, ihre Einteilung und Blutversorgung. Anat Anz 41:3-30, 1912.

254. Gibson JMC: Rupture of the axillary artery. J Bone Joint Surg Br 44:114-115, 1962.

255. Johnston GW, Lowry JH: Rupture of the axillary artery complicating anterior dislocation of the shoulder. J Bone Joint Surg Br 44:116-118, 1962.

256. Enneking WF: Shoulder girdle. In Enneking WF (ed): Musculoskeletal Tumor Surgery. New York: Churchill Livingstone, 1983 pp 355-410.

257. Crandon JH: Infections of the hand. In Simmons RL (ed): Surgical Infectious Diseases. Norwalk, Conn: Appleton & Lange, 1987.

258. Gelberman RH, Upper extremity compartment syndromes: Treatment. In Mubarak SJ, Hargens AR (eds): Compartment Syndromes and Volkmann's Contracture. Philadelphia: WB Saunders, 1981, pp 133-146.

259. Smith DC, Mitchell DA, Peterson GW, et al: Medial brachial fascial compartment syndrome: Anatomic basis of neuropathy after transaxillary arteriography. Radiology 173:149-154, 1989.

260. Evenepoel MC, Blomme A: Interscalenic approach to the cervico-brachial plexus. Acta Anaesthesiol Belg 32:317-322, 1981.

261. Moore DC, Bridenbaugh LD, Eather KF: Block of the upper extremity. Arch Surg 90:68-72, 1965.

262. Thompson GE, Rorie DK: Functional anatomy of the brachial plexus sheaths. Anesthesiology 59:117-122, 1983.

263. Strizak AM, Danzig L, Jackson DW, et al: Subacromial bursography. An anatomical and clinical study. J Bone Joint Surg Am 64:196-201, 1982.

264. Ellis VH: The diagnosis of shoulder lesions due to injuries of the rotator cuff. J Bone Joint Surg Br 35:72-74, 1953.

265. Leeson T, Leeson CR: Histology, 2nd ed. Philadelphia: WB Saunders, 1970.

266. McCormack LJ, Cauldwell EW, Anson BJ: Brachial and antebrachial arterial patterns: A study of 750 extremities. Surg Gynecol Obstet 96:43-54, 1953.

267. Cormack GC, Lamberty BGH: A classification of fascio-cutaneous flaps according to their patterns of vascularisation. Br J Plast Surg 37:80-87, 1984.

268. Lamberty BGH, Cormack GC: The forearm angiotomes. Br J Plast Surg 35:420-429, 1982.

269. McCraw JB, Dibbell DG, Carraway JH: Clinical definition of independent myocutaneous vascular territories. Plast Reconstr Surg 60:341-352, 1977.

270. Nakajima H, Fujino T, Adachi S: A new concept of vascular supply to the skin and classification of skin flaps according to their vascularization. Ann Plast Surg 16:1-19, 1986.

271. Orticochea M: The musculo-cutaneous flap method: An immediate and heroic substitute for the method of delay. Br J Plast Surg 25:106-110, 1972.

272. Taylor GI: Personal communication, 1988.

273. Langer K: On the anatomy and physiology of the skin. I. The cleavibility of the skin. Br J Plast Surg 31:3-8, 1978.

274. Langer K: On the anatomy and physiology of the skin. II. Skin tension. Br J Plast Surg 31:93-106, 1978.

275. Courtiss EH, Longarcre JJ, Destefano GA, et al: The placement of elective skin incisions. Plast Reconstr Surg 31:31-44, 1963.

276. Kraissl CJ: The selection of appropriate lines for elective surgical incisions. Plast Reconstr Surg 8:1-28, 1951.

277. Borges AF: Relaxed skin tension lines. Dermatol Clin 7:169-177, 1989.

278. Borges AF: Relaxed skin tension lines (RSTL) versus other skin lines. Plast Reconstr Surg 73:144-150, 1984.

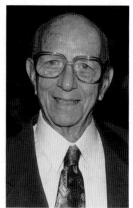

Much of the modern knowledge of shoulder anatomy can be attributed to the work of Anthony DePalma. As an intern at the now-defunct Philadelphia General Hospital, he would purchase cadavers weekly to perform the surgeries he had seen the previous week. He completed his orthopaedic training at New Jersey Orthopaedic Hospital and served as a commander and surgeon in the U.S. Navy during World War II. Following the war, he returned to Philadelphia as the chief of the U.S. Naval Hospital. It was during that period that he resumed cadaveric dissection, this time with an emphasis on recording the anatomy of the shoulder and its degenerative changes.

Subsequently, he became chairman of the Department of Orthopaedic Surgery at Thomas Jefferson University Hospital in Philadelphia and continued his work. He published the landmark Surgery of the Shoulder *in 1950, which went on to three editions. In 1957,* Degenerative Changes in the Sternoclavicular and Acromioclavicular Joints in Various Decades *was published.*

DePalma passed away on April 6, 2005 at the age of 100. His works form the basis of much of the knowledge of variational and degenerative anatomy of the shoulder that is considered today's standard. This chapter draws heavily on these works and is dedicated to the gentleman who has made numerous contributions to the study of shoulder surgery.

This chapter is divided into three sections, each with a different focus. The first section highlights important variations in the shoulder. DePalma's findings from a large volume of dissections in the 1940s and 1950s are used as the framework for this section. The second section is a description of the most common shoulder abnormalities that carry clinical significance. Concluding the chapter is a brief description of rare anomalies and common asymptomatic variations, with an emphasis on the appearance of each abnormality. We attempted to keep the text length of this chapter reasonable and therefore have an extensive reference list for further information.

CHAPTER 3

Congenital Anomalies and Variational Anatomy of the Shoulder

Jennifer L. Vanderbeck, MD, John M. Fenlin, Jr, MD, Charles L. Getz, MD, and Anthony F. DePalma, MD

VARIATIONAL ANATOMY OF THE SHOULDER

The anatomy of the shoulder has a wide range of normal arrangements. Some can play a role in the development of shoulder pathology, but most go completely unnoticed.

Clavicle

The clavicle serves as a strut between the scapula and the thorax. It possesses a unique double curve that accommodates the two very different motions of the sternal and acromial ends. The sternal end is essentially fixed but does rotate on its axis. The acromial end must match scapular motion by elevating 60 degrees with the arm fully abducted. The matched motion of the acromion and clavicle provides bony congruency and stability and thereby prevents internal rotation of the scapula throughout humeral elevation. Only 5 to 8 degrees of rotation occurs at the acromioclavicular joint with the arm moving through a full range of motion.[1,2] In addition, the clavicle is the origin of one of the heads of the pectoralis major and the anterior head of the deltoid, which are essential in elevation of the arm.

The work of DePalma in 1957, in which variations in 150 clavicles were examined, found no two clavicles to have all the same characteristics.[3] He described a definite relationship between the length of the clavicle and the amount of curvature. Within each curve of the clavicle, a circle can be drawn that uses the arc as part of the circle's circumference. DePalma divided the length of the clavicle in inches by the summed radii of the circles in inches (Fig. 3-1) to produce a unitless index that he named the clavicle curve index. The range of values fell between 0.40 and 1.29. He divided the range into groups of 0.10, which resulted in nine groups (e.g., 0.40-0.49 for group 1 and 1.20-1.29 for group 9). Contrary to the work

of Fich,[4] who reported more severe curves in the dominant arm's clavicle, the two groups showed similar curve characteristics.

Of more interest was the variation in anterior torsion of the lateral aspect of the clavicle. DePalma observed 66 specimens with their sternoclavicular and acromioclavicular joints intact and the sternum in a vertical position.[3]

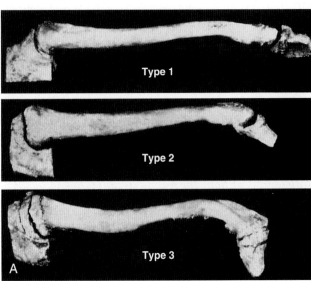

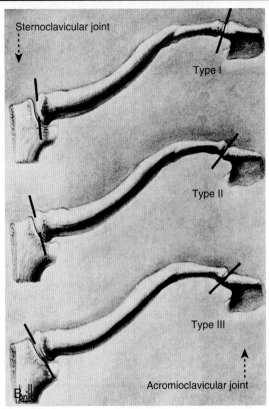

FIGURE 3-1 The clavicle index is determined by dividing the arcs formed by the two curves of the clavicle. R, radius. (From DePalma AF: Degenerative Changes in the Sternoclavicular Joints in Various Decades. Springfield, Ill: Charles C Thomas, 1957, p 116.)

$$\frac{\text{Radius lateral anterior} + \text{Radius medial posterior}}{\text{Length of clavicle}} = \frac{(1.6 + 3.8)}{6.1} = .88$$

= Index

i.e., $\frac{\text{Sum of radii}}{\text{Length}}$ = Index

R = 3.8″

Medial posterior curve

L = 6.1″ — Lateral anterior curve

R = 1.6″

FIGURE 3-2 Torsion (**A**) and inclination (**B**) of the lateral aspect of the clavicle is highly variable and has three major patterns. (From DePalma AF: Degenerative Changes in the Sternoclavicular Joints in Various Decades. Springfield, Ill: Charles C Thomas, 1957.)

The clavicles fell into three categories: type I, type II, and type III (Fig. 3-2).

Type I clavicles show the greatest amount of anterior torsion in their lateral third. The acromial end is flat and thin, with a small articular surface. The plane of the acromioclavicular joint is directed downward and inward; the angle ranges from 10 to 22 degrees with an average of 16 degrees. The plane of the sternoclavicular end is nearly vertical and slopes slightly downward and outward. The angle ranges from 0 to 10 degrees, with the average being 7.5 degrees.

The anterior torsion of the lateral third of the type II clavicle is less than in type I. The acromial end is stouter and slightly more rounded. The plane of the acromioclavicular joint is more horizontal than in type I, the average being 26.1 degrees. The configuration of the lateral aspect of the clavicle describes a smaller curve than the lateral curve of type I. The angle of the sternoclavicular joint is also more horizontal, with the average being 10.9 degrees from the vertical.

In type III clavicles, the outer third of the clavicle has the least amount of anterior torsion. Its acromial end is stout and rounded, with an almost complete circular articular surface. The arc of the lateral curve is also the smallest of all three types. The sternoclavicular and acromioclavicular joints are the most horizontal, with an average of 36.1 and 13.9 degrees from the vertical, respectively.

From this study, it was observed that as the curve of the lateral part of the clavicle decreased, the distal end of the clavicle became thicker, with a more circular acromial end. Of the 66 specimens studied, 27 (41%) were type I, 32 (48%) were type II, and 7 (11%) were type III. Type I distal clavicles have the highest rate of degenerative changes.[3] Either the decrease in surface area of the articulation or the vertical alignment producing higher shearing forces can lead to increased degeneration.

The sternoclavicular joint is stabilized by the strong costoclavicular ligaments and the articulation with the fibrocartilaginous first rib in the anteroposterior plane. The subclavius muscle functions as a depressor on the medial end of the clavicle. The contributions of the sternocleidomastoid, pectoralis major, deltoid, and trapezius are difficult to estimate, but they play roles as dynamic stabilizers of the clavicle.

The acromioclavicular joint is in a plane that allows motion in all directions, including rotation. It is formed by the lateral edge of the clavicle and the acromion and contains a fibrocartilage disk. The ends of the bones are enveloped by a loose articular capsule that is reinforced by an inferior acromioclavicular ligament and a stronger superior acromioclavicular ligament (Fig. 3-3).

Acromioclavicular Joint

The acromioclavicular joint is supported by the acromioclavicular ligaments in the anteroposterior plane and the superoinferior plane. The undersurface of the lateral aspect of the clavicle serves as the attachment point for

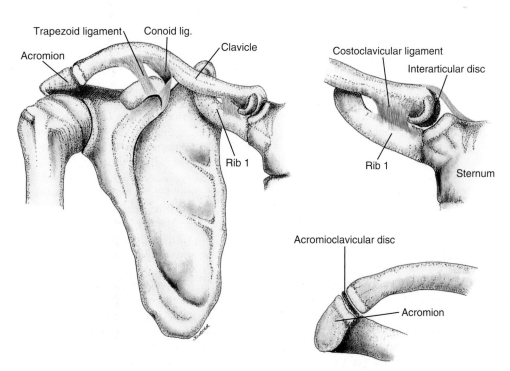

FIGURE 3-3 Major anatomic landmarks of the clavicle. (From DePalma AF: Surgery of the Shoulder, 3rd ed. Philadelphia: JB Lippincott, 1983, p 36.)

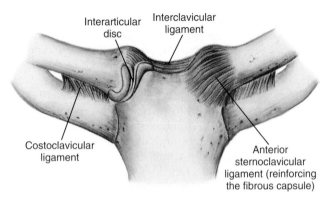

FIGURE 3-4 The sternoclavicular joint has an intra-articular disk, capsular stability, and extracapsular ligamentous support. (From DePalma AF: Surgery of the Shoulder, 3rd ed. Philadelphia: JB Lippincott, 1983, p 40.)

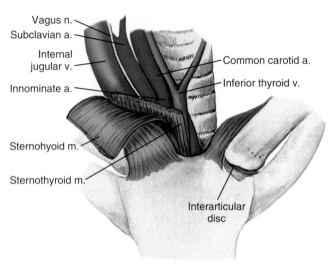

FIGURE 3-5 Major nervous and vascular structures lie in close proximity to the sternoclavicular joint. (From DePalma AF: Surgery of the Shoulder, 3rd ed. Philadelphia: JB Lippincott, 1983, p 41.)

the strong coracoclavicular ligaments. These ligaments can be thought to serve two distinct functions. The first is to prevent superior migration of the clavicle as seen in acromioclavicular separations. The second is to suspend the scapula from the distal end of the clavicle as the shoulder elevates.

Although the coracoclavicular ligament complex functions as a single ligament, it is composed of two distinct ligaments. Posterior and medial is the conoid ligament. Its nearly vertical short, stout fibers form an inverted cone whose base is on the clavicle, extending posteriorly to the conoid tubercle of the clavicle. Its tapered apex is on the posteromedial aspect of the coracoid process. In a cadaveric study, Harris and colleagues reported three anatomic variants of the conoid ligament with differing characteristics at its coracoid insertion.[5] The anterior and lateral segment of the coracoclavicular ligament, the trapezoid ligament, assumes a trapezoid shape. The fibers originate on the superior aspect of the coracoid process, just anterior to the fibers of the conoid ligament. These fibers course anterolaterally and insert on the inferior surface of the clavicle. The trapezoid ligament inserts at the mid arc of the lateral curve of the clavicle, with its most lateral attachment on the trapezoid ridge of the clavicle, averaging 15.3 mm from the distal end of the clavicle.[5]

This manner of attachment provides a mechanism for producing increased outward rotation of the scapula. As the humerus elevates, the scapula rotates to displace the coracoid inferiorly. The resulting tension in the coracoclavicular ligaments acts on the posterior (lateral) curve to rotate the clavicle on its long axis. Without the cranklike phenomenon made possible by the coracoclavicular ligaments and the S shape of the clavicle, abduction of the arm would be restricted.

The coracoacromial ligament originates on the anterior margin of the acromion and inserts on the posterior-lateral aspect of the coracoid. Pieper and colleagues reported variations in the coracoacromial ligament in 124

shoulders.[6] Their findings were two distinct ligaments in 59.7% and one ligament in 25.8% of shoulders. They were also able to identify a third band located more posterior and medial than the conoid in 14.5% of shoulders. Very little variation was found in the dominant and nondominant shoulders of the same cadaver with regard to number of bands.

Over all specimens, the different types of coracoacromial ligament morphology had no side predilection. In a smaller cadaveric study, Holt and Allibone identified four anatomic variants of the coracoacromial ligament.[7,8] A quadrangular variant was seen in 48% of shoulders and a broad band variant in 8%. A Y-shaped variant seen in 42% of shoulders was composed of two distinct ligaments. A multiple-banded variant was seen in 2% of shoulders containing a third band.[8] Fealy and colleagues further described the two-banded ligament as being composed of an anterolateral and posteromedial band.[9] In their study, three distinct bands were seen in 3% of shoulders, two distinct bands in 75%, and only one in 20%. The coracoacromial ligament was completely absent in 2% of shoulders. A lateral extension of the anterolateral band, termed the *falx*, is continuous with fibers of the conjoined tendon on its lateral aspect.

The presumed function of the coracoacromial arch has undergone much change in the past 60 years. Codman described it as a fulcrum that guided the head during abduction.[10] It was subsequently found that the coracoacromial ligament could be sacrificed in the face of normal shoulder musculature without compromising shoulder function.[3] However, in patients with massive rotator cuff tears, the presence of the coracoacromial arch limits superior migration of the humeral head. Thus, the coracoacromial ligament is not to be sacrificed without consideration.

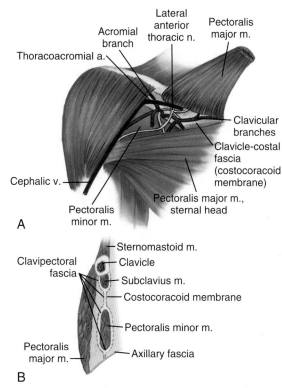

A

B

FIGURE 3-6 The cephalic vein lies in the deltopectoral interval (**A**) anterior to the clavipectoral fascia and the costocoracoid membrane (**B**). (From DePalma AF: Surgery of the Shoulder, 3rd ed. Philadelphia: JB Lippincott, 1983, p 44.)

Sternoclavicular Joint

The sternal end of the clavicle is roughly prismatic in shape. It is concave anteroposteriorly and convex vertically, creating a diarthrodial joint. It is larger than the posterolateral facet of the manubrium sterni and the cartilage of the first rib, and less than half of the medial clavicle articulates with the sternum.[11,12] The clavicle therefore protrudes superiorly from its medial articulation. In addition to the size mismatch, a great deal of incongruence exists between the two surfaces. Nature has compensated by interposing a fibrocartilage disk to buffer the stress and strains of the joint (Fig. 3-4).

The intra-articular disk is slightly thicker at its periphery than at the center. It is also thicker superiorly than at its inferior pole. The disk takes its origin from a circular area on the posterior-superior portion of the medial part of the clavicle. It then inserts inferiorly into the junction of the sternum and the cartilage of the first rib. This orientation makes the disk a strong stabilizer of the medial part of the clavicle to elevation. The disk also divides the sternoclavicular joint into two compartments: the smaller diskosternal (inferomedial) and the larger diskoclavicular (superolateral).[13] Perforation of the disk and resultant communication between the compartments occurs in 2.6% of shoulders.[3] There also appears to be a degenerative pattern of increasing thinning of the inferior pole as one ages.

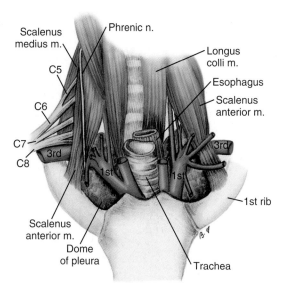

FIGURE 3-7 The subclavian artery and brachial plexus enter the axilla by crossing the first rib together. (From DePalma AF: Surgery of the Shoulder, 3rd ed. Philadelphia: JB Lippincott, 1983, p 41.)

The joint is enclosed in a synovial capsule that also has attachment to the disk periphery. The surface of the capsule is reinforced by strong oblique fibrous bands, the anterior and the posterior sternoclavicular ligaments. These capsular ligaments are the most important structures in preventing superior displacement of the medial clavicle.[14] The interclavicular ligament and the costoclavicular ligaments act to further stabilize the medial part of the clavicle. Along the superior aspect of the manubrium sterni courses the intersternal ligament, which links the clavicles. The costoclavicular or rhomboid ligaments are extracapsular and consist of an anterior and a posterior fasciculus. The anterior and posterior components of this ligament cross and run from the inferior medial portion of the clavicle to the cartilage of the first rib.

Structures lying immediately behind the sternoclavicular joint require familiarity for safe surgery in this area. Important vital structures include the dome of the parietal lung pleura, the esophagus, and the trachea. The sternohyoid and sternothyroid muscles lie directly behind the sternoclavicular joint. These muscles are much thicker and thus a more effective protective layer on the right. A sheath of fascia encompassing the omohyoid is continuous with the clavipectoral fascia, which encloses the subclavius and pectoralis minor muscles. This myofascial layer is anterior to the vessels as they travel from the base of the neck to the axilla (Fig. 3-5).

Coracoid Process and Adjacent Structures

The coracoid process is readily palpable in the infraclavicular region just under the anterior head of the deltoid. The coracoid is a landmark for surgeons and a reminder of the important structures in its vicinity. The process is a

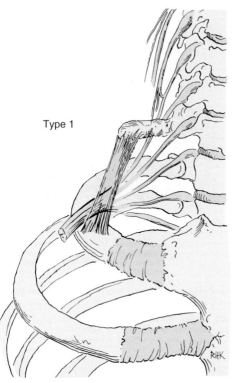

FIGURE 3-8 Type 1 fibrous band. (Modified from Wood VE, Twito RS, Verska JM: Thoracic outlet syndrome: The results of first rib resection in 100 patients. Orthop Clin North Am 19:131-146, 1988.)

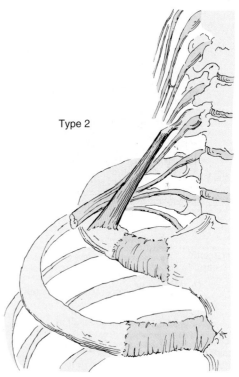

FIGURE 3-9 Type 2 fibrous band. (Modified from Wood VE, Twito RS, Verska JM: Thoracic outlet syndrome: The results of first rib resection in 100 patients. Orthop Clin North Am 19:131-146, 1988.)

short, fat, crooked projection from the anterior neck of the scapula. It is directed anteriorly, laterally, and inferiorly from its origin. The process serves as an origin for the medial and proximal coracoclavicular ligaments and the anterior and lateral coracoacromial ligaments. The short head of the biceps, the coracobrachialis, and the pectoralis minor muscles all attach to the coracoid process.

The clavipectoral fascia, which is an offshoot of the axillary fascia, first envelops the pectoralis minor and then continues superiorly to surround the subclavius muscle and clavicle (Fig. 3-6). The pectoralis minor muscle runs in an inferior-to-medial direction to insert on the second through fifth ribs. The brachiocephalic veins exit the thorax behind the sternoclavicular joint and immediately divide into the internal jugular and subclavian veins. The internal jugular continues cranially within the carotid sheath. The subclavian vein curves laterally and inferiorly atop the anterior scalene muscle, then it ducks under the clavicle and subclavius muscle and over the first rib to become the axillary vein.

The arterial structures are the brachiocephalic trunk on the right and the left common carotid and left subclavian arteries (Fig. 3-7). These arteries are the first three major vessels off the aorta. The course of the arteries is similar to that of the veins. On the right, the brachiocephalic trunk divides posterior to the sternoclavicular joint and becomes the common carotid and subclavian arteries.

The subclavian arteries also exit between the clavicle and first rib but course posterior to the anterior scalene muscle. The subclavian vessels become the axillary vessels as they emerge beneath the clavicle. The axillary vessels travel together with the brachial plexus anterior to the chest wall and posterior to the clavipectoral fascia.

It is the relationship to the pectoralis minor that divides the axillary artery into its three sections. The first part of the axillary artery is medial to the pectoralis minor muscle and has one branch, the thoracoacromial artery. The thoracoacromial artery and vein and the lateral pectoral nerve exit anteriorly through a defect in the clavipectoral fascia just medial to the pectoralis minor. Posterior to the pectoralis minor, the second part of the axillary artery has two branches, the thoracoacromial and the lateral thoracic arteries. Lateral to the pectoralis minor, the third section has three branches, the subscapular artery and the anterior and posterior circumflex humeral arteries.

The posterior aspect of the clavipectoral fascia, the costocoracoid membrane, is continuous with the axillary fascia. It can compress the vessels and brachial plexus if it becomes thickened. It can also compress the neurovascular structures on the humerus with the arm abducted and externally rotated. With the shoulder extended and distracted inferiorly, the neurovascular structures are compressed between the clavicle and first rib.

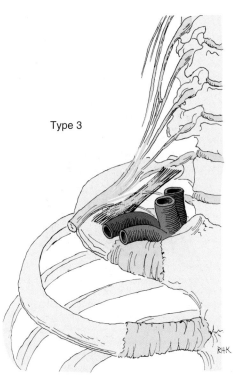

FIGURE 3-10 A type 3 fibrous band is the most common band in thoracic outlet syndrome. (Modified from Wood VE, Twito RS, Verska JM: Thoracic outlet syndrome: The results of first rib resection in 100 patients. Orthop Clin North Am 19:131-146, 1988.)

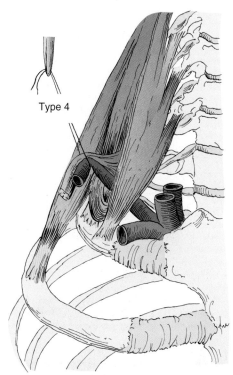

FIGURE 3-11 A type 4 fibrous band forms a sling. (Modified from Wood VE, Twito RS, Verska JM: Thoracic outlet syndrome: The results of first rib resection in 100 patients. Orthop Clin North Am 19:131-146, 1988.)

The interscalene triangle is bordered anteriorly by the anterior scalene muscle, posteriorly by the middle scalene muscle and inferiorly by the medial surface of the first rib. The costoclavicular triangle is bordered anteriorly by the middle third of the clavicle, posteriorly by the first rib, medially by the costoclavicular ligament, and laterally by the edge of the middle scalene muscle. The tight confines of these spaces enclose the contents of the major nervous and vascular supply to the upper extremity.

Any anomalous muscle or band predisposes the patient to the development of thoracic outlet syndrome. Several anomalies have been identified (Figs. 3-8 to 3-16).[15]

One variation consists of the brachial plexus exiting through the fibers of the anterior scalene. Roos[16-18] identified nine types of anomalous fibrous or muscular band arrangements associated with thoracic outlet syndrome. Each anomaly is associated with a different type of compressive pathology.

In addition to the previous nine types identified, Roos also identified five patterns of bands associated with high cervical and median nerve neuropathy (Figs. 3-17 to 3-21).[18] We make this distinction because the presence or absence of upper brachial plexus involvement can aid in the operative approach if the patient requires surgery for brachial plexus entrapment.[18-20]

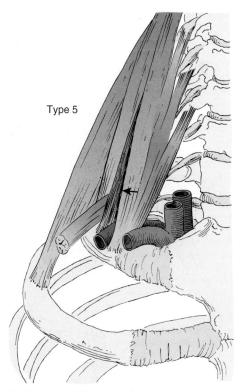

FIGURE 3-12 A type 5 band *(arrow)* is an abnormal scalenus minimus. (Modified from Wood VE, Twito RS, Verska JM: Thoracic outlet syndrome: The results of first rib resection in 100 patients. Orthop Clin North Am 19:131-146, 1988.)

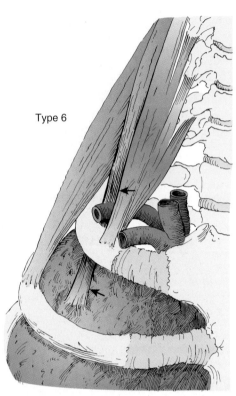

FIGURE 3-13 A type 6 band (*arrows*) inserts on Sibson's fascia. (Modified from Wood VE, Twito RS, Verska JM: Thoracic outlet syndrome: The results of first rib resection in 100 patients. Orthop Clin North Am 19:131-146, 1988.)

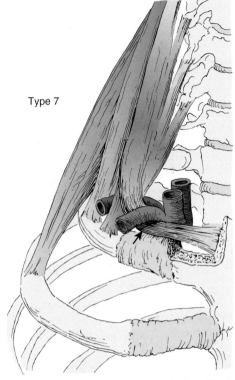

FIGURE 3-14 Type 7 fascial band (*arrow*). (Modified from Wood VE, Twito RS, Verska JM: Thoracic outlet syndrome: The results of first rib resection in 100 patients. Orthop Clin North Am 19:131-146, 1988.)

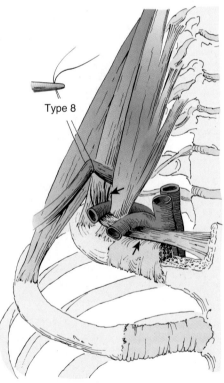

FIGURE 3-15 Type 8 fascial band (*arrows*). (Modified from Wood VE, Twito RS, Verska JM: Thoracic outlet syndrome: The results of first rib resection in 100 patients. Orthop Clin North Am 19:131-146, 1988.)

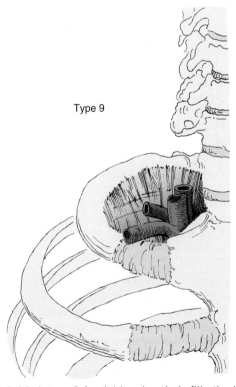

FIGURE 3-16 A type 9 fascial band entirely fills the inside of the first rib. (Modified from Wood VE, Twito RS, Verska JM: Thoracic outlet syndrome: The results of first rib resection in 100 patients. Orthop Clin North Am 19:131-146, 1988.)

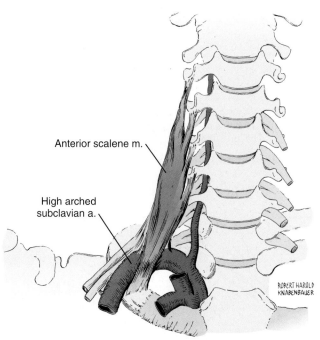

FIGURE 3-17 A type I upper brachial plexus anomaly has the anterior scalene fibers fused to the perineurium. (Modified and reprinted with permission from the Society of Thoracic Surgeons: Wood VE, Ellison DW: Results of upper plexus thoracic outlet syndrome operation. Ann Thorac Surg 58:458-461, 1994.)

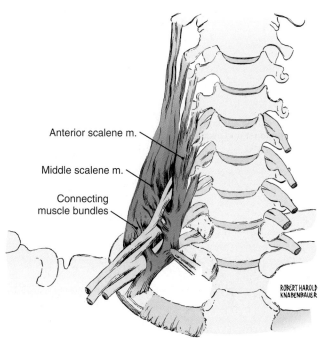

FIGURE 3-18 A type II upper plexus anomaly has connecting muscle bellies of the anterior and middle scalene. (Modified and reprinted with permission from the Society of Thoracic Surgeons: Wood VE, Ellison DW: Results of upper plexus thoracic outlet syndrome operation. Ann Thorac Surg 58:458-461, 1994.)

Large Muscles of the Infraclavicular Region

The two large muscles in the infraclavicular region are the clavicular head of the deltoid and the clavicular portion of the pectoralis major. Below the distal end of the clavicle they form the deltopectoral triangle, which is traversed by the cephalic vein. The cephalic vein can be identified and traced medially, where it empties into the thoracoacromial vein and then into the axillary vein. The cephalic vein can therefore be used as a helpful landmark to identify the division of the pectoralis major and deltoid muscles, as well as to locate the great vessels in the infraclavicular region.

Posterior Deltoid Region

The infraspinatus muscle and the posterior head of the deltoid take their origin from the spine of the scapula and are covered by the trapezius muscle (Fig. 3-22). In the superior lateral region, the suprascapular nerve and artery enter into the infraspinous fossa through the spinoglenoid notch. Here, the suprascapular nerve supplies innervation to the infraspinatus muscle and the fibers of the shoulder joint capsule.

The quadrangular space is another important area of this region. It is formed by the humerus laterally, the long head of the triceps medially, the teres minor superiorly, and the teres major inferiorly. This space is traversed by

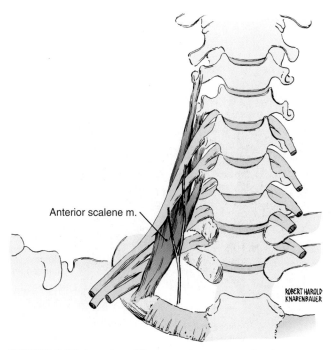

FIGURE 3-19 In a type III upper plexus anomaly, the anterior scalene muscle traverses the brachial plexus. (Modified and reprinted with permission from the Society of Thoracic Surgeons: Wood VE, Ellison DW: Results of upper plexus thoracic outlet syndrome operation. Ann Thorac Surg 58:458-461, 1994.)

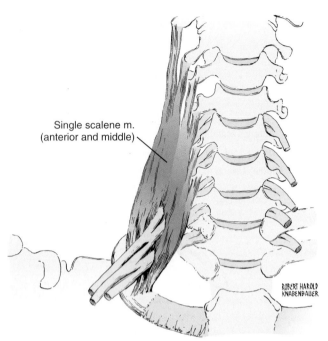

FIGURE 3-20 In a type IV upper plexus anomaly, the brachial plexus traverses the anterior scalene muscle. (Modified and reprinted with permission from the Society of Thoracic Surgeons: Wood VE, Ellison DW: Results of upper plexus thoracic outlet syndrome operation. Ann Thorac Surg 58:458-461, 1994.)

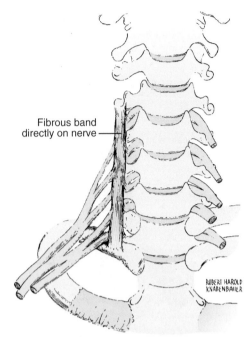

FIGURE 3-21 A type V upper plexus anomaly has a vertical fibrous band posterior to the anterior scalene muscle. (Modified and reprinted with permission from the Society of Thoracic Surgeons: Wood VE, Ellison DW: Results of upper plexus thoracic outlet syndrome operation. Ann Thorac Surg 58:458-461, 1994.)

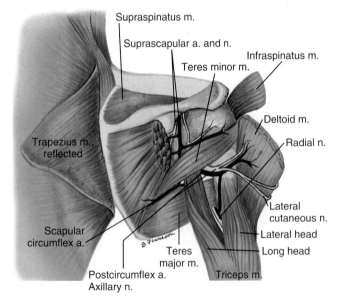

FIGURE 3-22 The posterior deltoid has several potential spaces containing neurovascular structures. (Modified from DePalma AF: Surgery of the Shoulder, 3rd ed. Philadelphia: JB Lippincott, 1983, p 48.)

the axillary nerve and the posterior circumflex humeral artery. Soon after it leaves the quadrangular space, the axillary nerve divides into anterior and posterior branches. The posterior branch innervates the teres minor and posterior deltoid muscles. The posterior branch continues laterally to become the lateral brachial cutaneous nerve, which innervates the lower posterior and lateral portion of the deltoid.

The anterior branch of the axillary nerve continues with the posterior circumflex humeral artery as they wind around the surgical neck of the humerus to reach the anterior aspect of the shoulder. The nerve diminishes in size as it progresses anteriorly and gives off numerous branches that travel vertically to enter the substance of the deltoid. Through the entire course, the axillary nerve runs 5 cm from the lateral edge of the acromion, thus providing a safe zone for the surgeon to operate. Burkhead and associates demonstrated considerable variation in this safe zone. They found the axillary nerve as close as 3.5 cm from the lateral acromion.[21] Cetik and colleagues defined a safe area for surgical dissection as a quadrangular space with differing anterior and posterior lengths depending on arm length.[22] The average distance of the axillary nerve from the anterior acromion was 6.08 cm (range, 5.2-6.9 cm), and the posterior acromion was 4.87 cm (range, 4.3-5.5 cm). Women and persons with small arms tend to have a smaller safe zone and need special consideration when planning for surgery.

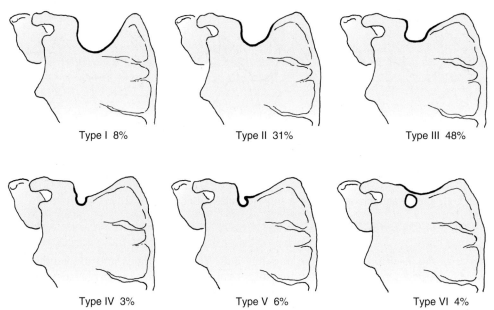

Type I 8%   Type II 31%   Type III 48%

Type IV 3%   Type V 6%   Type VI 4%

FIGURE 3-23 The six types of suprascapular notch configuration as described by Rengachary.

Variations of the Suprascapular Notch and Suprascapular Ligament

The suprascapular nerve is responsible for innervation of the supraspinatus and infraspinatus muscles. It reaches these muscles by way of the suprascapular notch under the suprascapular ligament. Several cases of nerve compression at this site resulting in denervation of the supraspinatus and infraspinatus muscles have been reported.

The morphology of the suprascapular notch is a result of congenital and developmental changes in the area.[23-25] Rengachary and colleagues described six types (Fig. 3-23)[23-25]:

Type I: Wide depression in the superior border of the scapula in 8% of samples
Type II: Wide blunted V shape in 31%
Type III: Symmetric U shape in 48%
Type IV: Very small V shape, often with a shallow groove for the suprascapular nerve, in 3%
Type V: Partial ossified medial portion of the suprascapular ligament in 6%
Type VI: Completely ossified suprascapular ligament in 4%

Congenital duplication of the suprascapular ligament, which is typically manifested as bilateral suprascapular nerve palsy, has also been reported (Fig. 3-24).[26] In a more recent cadaveric study of 79 shoulders by Ticker and colleagues, one bifid and one trifid suprascapular ligament was identified.[27] Partial ossification of the suprascapular ligament has been described in 6% to 18% of cadaveric specimens.[24,27,28] Complete ossification has been reported in 3.7 to 5% of specimens.[24,27-29] A familial association to suprascapular ligament calcification has also been reported.[30]

Subacromial and Anterolateral Subdeltoid Region

Deltoid Muscle

The deltoid is a massive triangular-shaped muscle that drapes itself around the outer third of the clavicle, the acromion process, and the inferior aspect of the spine of the scapula. Its fibers converge distally into a single tendon that inserts onto the deltoid tubercle of the humerus.

The lateral head of the deltoid is formed from obliquely arranged fibers that arise in pennate fashion from either side of five or six tendinous bands whose proximal fibers are attached to the lateral acromion. In addition, three or four similar tendinous bands whose origins are from the

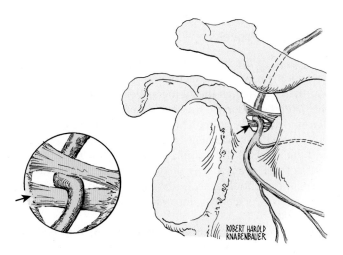

Anomalous ligament

FIGURE 3-24 A duplicated transverse scapular ligament (*arrow*) can compress the suprascapular nerve.

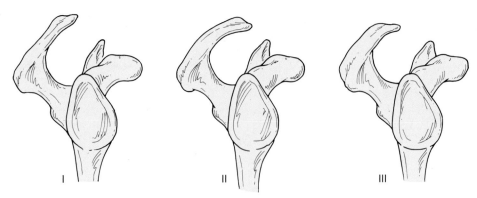

FIGURE 3-25 Types I, II, and III acromia as seen on a suprascapular outlet view.

deltoid tendon serve as the insertion point of the muscle fibers. This complex arrangement provides a powerful contraction that does not require a significant change in length, as would be needed with fibers arranged in parallel.

The anterior and posterior heads of the deltoid are arranged in a simple parallel fashion. All three heads have a fibrous origin that is continuous with the periosteum of the clavicle, the acromion, and the spine of the scapula. Such morphology allows for surgical detachment of part or all of the deltoid and facilitates its repair.

Cephalic Vein

The deltoid lies adjacent to the pectoralis major muscle in the anterior aspect of the shoulder. This border widens superiorly to form the deltopectoral triangle, within which lies the cephalic vein. As the vein progresses superiorly, it receives tributaries from the lateral side and proceeds deeper to lie adjacent to the clavipectoral fascia. Medial to the pectoralis minor and inferior to the clavicle, the cephalic vein pierces the clavipectoral fascia and the costocoracoid membrane to empty into the axillary vein anterior to the axillary artery.

Acromion Process

The spine of the scapula ends laterally as the prominent acromion process. The acromion is a massive flat structure that overhangs the humeral head from behind. It is the lateral border of the coracoacromial arch and the acromioclavicular joint. Therefore, the acromion plays a critical role in movement of the shoulder. The acromion and the spine of the scapula provide a moving origin for most of the deltoid. It is this dynamic arrangement that permits the shoulder to be powerful in an innumerable number of positions, including elevation above the horizontal.

The acromion has an important role in degenerative changes around the shoulder with regard to the rotator cuff, the subacromial bursa, the acromioclavicular joint, and the head of the humerus. In addition, it plays a role in protecting the head of the humerus and the tendinous

cuff. The tuberosities and myotendinous cuff must pass beneath the acromion in elevation. It is difficult to traumatize the humeral head with a blow unless the arm is at the side and extended and the blow is directly anterior on the shoulder.

In a cadaveric study, Bigliani and coworkers identified three types of acromial morphology, with types I, II, and III corresponding to flat, curved, or hooked, respectively, as viewed in sagittal cross section.[31] They found an association between type III acromion morphology and rotator cuff tears (Fig. 3-25).

Nicholson and colleagues examined the morphology of the acromion in 402 shoulder specimens. They found a consistent distribution of type I (27%-37%), type II (33%-52%), and type III (17%-31%) acromion processes across age, gender, and race.[32] However, a significant increase in spur formation was noted at the insertion site of the coracoacromial ligaments when specimens from cadavers younger than 50 years (7%) were compared with specimens older than 50 years (30%). Other authors have also noted this phenomenon.[33-36]

Subacromial Bursa

The musculature of the shoulder is arranged in two layers, an outer layer composed of the deltoid and teres major and an inner layer composed of the rotator cuff. The structure that allows smooth gliding of these muscles is the subacromial bursa. The mechanism works so well that it is sometimes referred to as a secondary scapulohumeral joint.

The subacromial bursa is attached to the outer surface of the greater tuberosity and the rotator cuff muscles. Its roof is adherent to the undersurface of the acromion and the coracoacromial ligament. Its walls are loosely configured to billow laterally and posteriorly under the acromion, medially under the coracoid, and anteriorly under the deltoid. The subacromial bursa has no communication with the glenohumeral joint in a normal shoulder, but with a full-thickness tear of the rotator cuff, fluid will communicate freely.

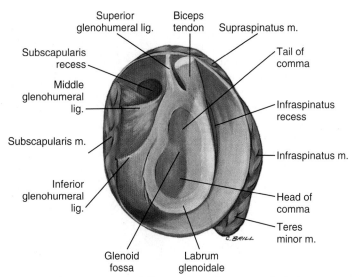

FIGURE 3-26 The glenoid has a general arrangement of ligaments and recesses that show a great deal of variation. Also note that the synovial membrane adheres closely to all the underlying structures. (Modified from DePalma AF: Surgery of the Shoulder, 3rd ed. Philadelphia: JB Lippincott, 1983, p 57.)

Rotator Cuff and Coracohumeral Ligament

The four muscles of the rotator cuff lie immediately below the subacromial bursa. A fibrous capsule is formed from the confluence of the supraspinatus, infraspinatus, teres minor, and subscapularis tendons. The capsular fibers blend indistinguishably into its insertion into the anatomic neck of the humerus and completely fill the sulcus.

An important component of the rotator cuff is the coracohumeral ligament. It originates on the lateral border of the coracoid and lies in the rotator interval between the fibers of the supraspinatus and subscapularis. The fibers of the coracohumeral ligament interlace with the fibers of the underlying capsule and insert with them into both tuberosities to bridge the bicipital groove. It is the position of the coracohumeral ligament that makes it an important stabilizer of the biceps tendon and a secondary suspensory ligament. The fibers are also arranged to unwind as the arm externally rotates and act as a checkrein to external rotation with the arm at the side.

Glenohumeral Ligaments and Recesses

The fibrous capsule is a large redundant structure with twice the surface area of the humeral head. Inferiorly and posteriorly, the capsule is continuous with the labrum and adjacent bone (Fig. 3-26). Anteriorly, the capsule varies in relation to the labrum, the glenohumeral ligaments, and the synovial recesses.[37] Three capsular thickenings are present in the anterior portion of the capsule and are named the *inferior, middle,* and *superior glenohumeral ligaments.* These structures act to reinforce the anterior capsule and serve as a static checkrein to external rotation of the humeral head. From the humeral head, they converge toward the anterior border of the labrum. The superior ligament blends with the superior portion

of the labrum and the biceps tendon, whereas the middle and inferior ligaments blend with the labrum inferior to the superior ligament. In the region of the glenohumeral ligaments are the synovial recesses of the capsule.

DePalma's study of 96 shoulders in 1950 revealed six variations in the relationship of the glenohumeral ligaments and the synovial recesses[3]:

Type 1 (30.2%) has one synovial recess above the middle ligament.
Type 2 (2.04%) has one synovial recess below the middle ligament.
Type 3 (40.6%) has one recess above and one recess below the middle ligament.
Type 4 (9.03%) has one large recess above the inferior ligament with the middle ligament absent.
Type 5 (5.1%) presents the middle ligament as two small synovial folds.
Type 6 (11.4%) has no synovial recesses, but all three ligaments are well defined.

Steinbeck and associates reported similar results in the dissection of 104 shoulders in 1998 (Fig. 3-27)[38]: type 1, 38.5%; type 2, 0%; type 3: 46.2%, type 4, 0.8%; type 5, 0%; type 6, 9.6%.

Study of specimens with large synovial recesses emphasizes that when such recesses are present, the fibrous capsule is not directly continuous with the anterior portion of the labrum. The capsule extends past the labrum toward the coracoid and then returns along the anterior glenoid neck as a thin fibrous sheet attached to the labrum. Within the six variations, the recesses exhibit a great range in size, and they may be very large or small.

DePalma observed that the glenohumeral ligaments have a great amount of variation as well. The middle glenohumeral ligament was found to be a well-defined structure in 68% of specimens; it was poorly defined in 16% and absent in 12%.[3] When present, it arises from the anterior portion of the labrum immediately below the superior ligament. In 4% to 5% of specimens it appears as a double structure. Furthermore, its width, length, and thickness vary considerably.

The superior glenohumeral ligament is the most constant of the three ligaments; it existed in 94 of 96 specimens and was absent in 2. It arises from the upper pole of the glenoid fossa and the root of the coracoid process. In 73 specimens it attached to the middle ligament, the biceps tendon, and the labrum; in 20 specimens it attached to the biceps tendon and the labrum; and in 1 specimen it attached to the biceps only. It inserts into the fovea capitis adjacent to the lesser tuberosity. Although its position varies little, its visibility from within the capsule and its size vary considerably.

The inferior glenohumeral ligament is a triangular structure whose apex is at the labrum and whose base is between the subscapularis and the triceps tendon. It was a well-defined structure in 54 of the 96 specimens, poorly defined in 18, and absent in 24.

Steinbeck and colleagues also examined arrangements of the glenohumeral ligament complex in 104 shoulders.[38] The superior glenohumeral ligament was again found to be the most consistent ligament in that it was present in 98.2% of specimens, although it was less than 2 mm thick in 28.8%. The middle glenohumeral ligament was present in 84.6% of specimens and, when present, consistently crossed the tendon of subscapularis. The inferior glenohumeral ligament was the most variable in existence and arrangement. It was a discrete structure in 72.1% of specimens and present only as a thickening of the capsule in 21.1%.

An anterosuperior foramen has also been identified between the glenoid and the labrum during arthroscopy.[39,40] Williams reported a similar variant with an absent anterior superior labrum and the addition of a cord-like middle glenohumeral ligament that attaches to the superior labrum. Along with his coauthors, he named this arrangement the *Buford complex* (Fig. 3-28). In a review of 200 shoulder arthroscopy tapes, 1.5% had a Buford complex and 12% had a sublabral foramen.[41] Of the patients with sublabral foramina, 75% had cord-like middle glenohumeral ligaments and 25% had normal glenohumeral ligaments. The authors warned against treatment of this lesion by attachment to the glenoid because of the possibility that postoperative range of motion would be restricted.

Glenoid Fossa and Labrum

The glenoid fossa is shaped like an inverted comma, with the superior portion of the glenoid thin like the tail and the base broad like the body. The glenoid is covered with hyaline cartilage that is thinner in the center and thicker at the edges.

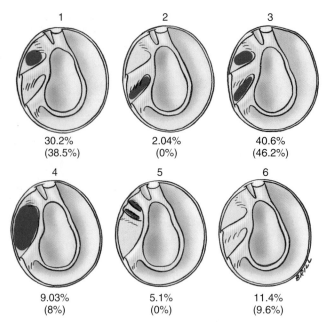

FIGURE 3-27 The six types of arrangement of synovial recesses and their incidence as reported by DePalma and Steinbeck. Steinbeck's results are in parentheses. (Modified from DePalma AF: Surgery of the Shoulder, 3rd ed. Philadelphia: JB Lippincott, 1983, p 58.)

Das and coworkers reported the anatomic finding of glenoid version in 50 shoulders. Their values ranged from 12 degrees of retroversion to 10 degrees of anteversion. The average version for the entire sample was 1.1 degrees of retroversion.[42]

Churchill and colleagues attempted the largest study to identify variations in size, inclination, and version of the glenoid by examining 344 human scapular bones.[43] The size of the glenoid varied between sexes but not among races, with a mean female glenoid height of 32.6 ± 1.8 mm (range, 29.4-37.0 mm) and width of 23.0 ± 1.5 mm (range, 19.7-26.3 mm). Male glenoid size was reported as a mean height of 37.5 ± 2.2 mm (range, 30.4-42.6 mm) and width of 27.8 ± 1.6 mm (range, 24.3-32.5 mm). Iannotti and associates examined 140 fresh shoulders and recorded the average height of the glenoid to be 39.5 ± 3.5 mm (range, 30-48 mm) and the width to be 29 ± 3.2 mm (range, 21-35 mm).[44] The average height of the donors in the study of Iannotti and colleagues was 181 cm, and 60% to 67% were male (cadaveric and living, respectively). The average height in the study of Churchill and associates was 173.0 cm for male patients and 161.3 cm for female patients. These differences might account for the variation in findings.

Churchill and coauthors reported version to be considerably different among races but not between genders. Black female subjects and black male subjects were found to have a transverse axis retroversion of 0.30 degrees (−6 to +6 degrees) and 0.11 degrees (−8.8 to +10.3 degrees), respectively. Glenoid retroversion in white female subjects averaged 2.16 degrees (−2.8 to +10.5 degrees), and

SUBLABRAL HOLE

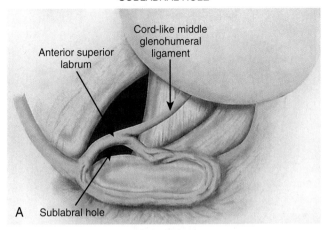

A

BUFORD COMPLEX

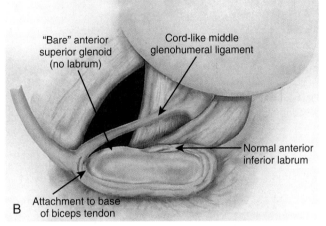

B

FIGURE 3-28 A cord-like middle glenohumeral ligament can insert into the anterior superior labrum (**A**) or directly into the superior glenoid (**B**). Both are associated with an intracapsular foramen and are considered normal variants. (From Williams SM, Snyder SJ, Buford D Jr: The Buford complex—the "cord-like" middle glenohumeral ligament and absent centrosuperior labrum: A normal anatomic capsulolabral variant. Arthroscopy 10:244-245, 1994.)

in white male subjects the average was 2.87 degrees (range, −9.5 to +10.5 degrees). Churchill and associates also studied glenoid inclination and reported a wide variation in results (−7 to +15.8 degrees). Despite the variability in inclination, the majority of shoulders fell between 0 and 9.8 degrees of inclination.

The labrum is a fibrous structure that surrounds the glenoid. In an infant, the fibers of the labrum are continuous with the hyaline cartilage, but as aging occurs, the labrum assumes a looser position and resembles a knee meniscus with a free intra-articular edge.

The long head of the biceps inserts into the superior glenoid tubercle and is continuous with the superior labrum. Variations in the long head of the biceps tendon are discussed later.

Proximal Humerus

The massive humeral head lies beneath the coracoacromial arch and articulates with the glenoid of the scapula. The humeral head has 134 to 160 degrees of internal torsion as reported by DePalma, which corresponds to 44 to 70 degrees of retroversion.[3,45-49] Edelson extensively studied the remains of fetal, child, and adult humeri in an attempt to elucidate the amount and development of humeral head retroversion. He defined retroversion as the angle subtended by the intercondylar axis of the elbow and a line bisecting the humeral head.[50] Fetal retroversion averaged 78 degrees.[51] The adult specimens averaged significantly less, with a range of −8 to +74 degrees; most, however, fell into the range of 25 to 35 degrees of retroversion. Edelson found that the change from fetal to adult retroversion of the humerus can be completed as early as 4.5 years and almost certainly by 11 years. In addition, he hypothesized that further torsion takes place after 11 years of age but occurs in the distal two thirds of the humerus.

Biceps Tendon

The bicipital groove lies 30 degrees medial of center between the tuberosities. The greater tuberosity and the lesser tuberosity form the lateral and medial walls of the bicipital groove, respectively. Between the proximal edge of the tuberosities and the articular surface is a broad sulcus into which the rotator cuff tendons insert.

The tendon of the long head of the biceps is continuous at its insertion with the superior-posterior labrum. Its relationship to the glenohumeral ligaments varies greatly. In most specimens, it blends with the fibers of the superior glenohumeral ligament. In others, it is continuous with the middle glenohumeral ligament, and rarely, it is continuous with all three ligaments.

The biceps tendon has a partially intracapsular position. However, developmental anomalies sometimes occur. The tendon can be attached to a mesentery, can be entirely intracapsular, or can be absent.[3] The tendon can also exist as a double structure.

The synovial lining of the glenohumeral capsule continues distally between the greater and lesser tuberosities. The synovial lining then reflects onto the tendon itself to form an important gliding mechanism within the bicipital groove. The motion of the tendon is minimal, but the amount of contact between the humerus and the tendon changes with arm position and thus does the function of the gliding mechanism.[52-54] Contraction of the biceps under local anesthesia in the operating room produces no movement of the tendon, nor does movement of the arm through a full range of motion.

The bicipital groove has a great deal of anatomic variation. A supratubercle ridge can sometimes extend proximally from the superior aspect of the lesser tuberosity on the medial aspect of the groove (Fig. 3-29). DePalma's study in 1950 found this structure to be well developed in 23.9% of specimens, moderately developed in 31.5%, and absent in 43.4%. Hitchcock and Bechtol observed this feature in 59 of 100 humeri.[55] In Meyer's series of 200 shoulders, the tubercle was present in 17.5% of specimens.[56] It is postulated that a well-developed supratubercle ridge predisposes the biceps tendon to instability by potentially levering it out of the groove.[56] A well-developed ridge can also increase the contact force between the biceps tendon and the transverse humeral ligament and thereby predispose to tendinitis.

The medial wall of the groove varies greatly in height, and such variation defines the obliquity of the groove. When a supratubercle ridge is present, the depth of the groove diminishes further. Hitchcock and Bechtol defined six variations of the angle of the medial wall of the bicipital groove (Fig. 3-30)[55]:

Type 1 grooves had an angle of the medial wall of 90 degrees.
Type 2 grooves had an angle of 75 degrees.
Type 3 grooves had an angle of 60 degrees.
Type 4 grooves had an angle of 45 degrees.
Type 5 grooves had an angle of 30 degrees.
Type 6 grooves had an angle of 15 degrees.

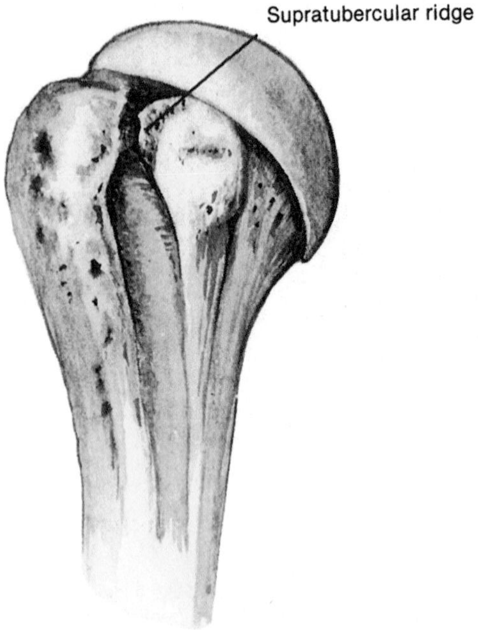

Supratubercular ridge

FIGURE 3-29 Schematic drawing of a supratubercular ridge that can facilitate displacement of the biceps tendon. (From DePalma AF: Surgery of the Shoulder, 3rd ed. Philadelphia: JB Lippincott, 1983, p 54.)

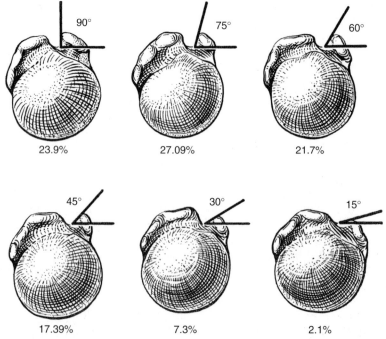

90°	75°	60°
23.9%	27.09%	21.7%
45°	30°	15°
17.39%	7.3%	2.1%

FIGURE 3-30 Six variations of the medial wall of the bicipital groove and their incidence. (Redrawn from Hitchcock HH, Bechtol CO: Painful shoulder. J Bone Joint Surg Am 30:263-273, 1948.)

COMMON MALFORMATIONS OF THE SHOULDER

Cleidocranial Dysostosis

Cleidocranial dysostosis is a hereditary disorder that affects bones formed by intramembranous ossification.[57-66] The skull, clavicles, ribs, teeth, and pubic symphysis are most commonly affected. Normal intelligence, an enlarged head, and forward-sloping shoulders are the typical clinical features (Fig. 3-31). If other malformations are associated with these findings, the condition is known as *mutational dysostosis*.[59,65,67]

The range of shoulder function in this condition is vast.[68] Patients with this syndrome have been reported to work as heavy laborers without shoulder complaints, whereas others report glenohumeral instability.[69] The outer third of the clavicle is the most commonly affected portion, and the medial aspect is usually normal.[70,71] The middle part of the clavicle can also be absent, with spared medial and lateral portions.[70] In either scenario, the missing portion of clavicle is replaced by fibrous tissue. Bilateral shoulder involvement is found in 82% to 90% of patients.[71,72] Although uncommon, normal clavicles do not exclude this diagnosis.[73] Two separate reports of families with this condition included members with normal clavicles.[73,74]

Associated Findings
Craniofacial
Frontal bossing and an enlarged forehead is common. The sutures of the skull remain unfused and are said to be *metopic*.[75] An arched palate with multiple dental abnormalities is common, and consultation with a dentist is necessary. Eustachian tube dysfunction is common as well as both conductive and sensorineural hearing loss.[76,77] Periodic audiologic testing is therefore recommended.

Pelvis, Hip, and Spine
Patients with cleidocranial dysostosis can have the pelvic manifestations of a widened symphysis pubis or sacroiliac joint.[78] These abnormalities are not symptomatic, and their prevalence is therefore uncertain and their clinical relevance limited. Congenital coxa vara is reported to occur in 50% of patients.[79] Neural tube defects can also be associated with this condition. Sacral agenesis, scoliosis, meningomyelocele, and vertebral body defects have all been reported.

Hands and Feet
The metacarpals and metatarsals can have both proximal and distal epiphyseal elongation. A resultant overgrowth of one or several metacarpals is common. Although the other bones of the hands and feet can be involved, the distal phalanx of the thumb and hallux are most greatly

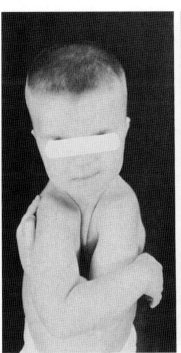
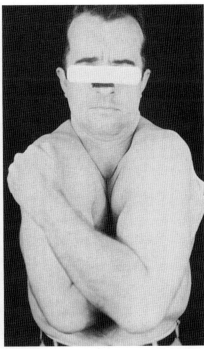

FIGURE 3-31 A, This child with cleidocranial dysostosis can almost touch the tips of his shoulders. **B,** His father performs the same maneuver. (From DePalma AF: Surgery of the Shoulder, 3rd ed. Philadelphia: JB Lippincott, 1983, p 27.)

affected. The tarsal, carpal, and phalangeal bones may be small and irregular.

Inheritance

Approximately half of cases occur de novo, whereas the other 50% of patients have a family history. An autosomal dominant pattern with variable penetration is thought to be the responsible mechanism of transmission; thus, sexes are affected without predilection.[4,65]

Treatment

Patients do well with this condition and rarely require other than dental treatment. Surgery is indicated for those with neurologic or vascular compression secondary to the clavicular malformation or to prevent skin breakdown.[68]

Congenital Pseudarthrosis of the Clavicle

Easily mistaken for a fracture of the clavicle, this anomaly does not show evidence of callus formation (Fig. 3-32).[72,80-83] The entities that need to be ruled out are cleidocranial dysostosis, neurofibromatosis, and trauma.[84] No or minimal resulting loss of function is thought to occur.[85] Overwhelmingly, the abnormality occurs unilaterally on the right side; however, left-sided and bilateral pseudarthrosis have been reported.[86-95] A bump in the midclavicular region is palpable or grossly seen, and smooth ends are apparent on radiographs.[96] Thoracic outlet syndrome has been reported to be secondary to the pseudarthrosis.[97-101]

Inheritance

A familial association has been reported, but a true pattern of genetic transmission has not been documented.[102-105]

Associated Abnormalities

Dextrocardia and the presence of cervical ribs have been associated with a left-sided pseudarthrosis.[89,102] No other abnormalities are associated with this condition. If some are found, either cleidocranial dysostosis or neurofibromatosis needs to be investigated, and perhaps the patient should be referred to a geneticist.[65]

Treatment

Benign neglect has generally been accepted as treatment of this entity.[106,107] Because of reports of thoracic outlet syndrome, some authors have proposed early excision and bone grafting in younger patients.[80,90,91,99,108,109] Evidence that the risks of surgery outweigh the perceived benefits of intervention is sparse.[110]

Sprengel's Deformity

The scapula is formed near the cervical spine in the developing fetus.[40,111-113] Failure of the scapula to descend from its origin causes the scapula to appear small and high riding.[114-120] The resulting deformity causes a wide range of disfigurement and dysfunction of the shoulder (Fig. 3-33). A fibrous connection between the cervical spine and the superior angle of the scapula is often present.[121] When ossified, the connection is known as the *omovertebral bone* and is present in 20% to 40% of cases.[40,122-124] The cause of this malformation is not known (Fig. 3-34).[120,125-128]

Cavendish extensively studied the appearance and dysfunction of 100 affected shoulders. He proposed a grading system to divide shoulders into groups by their appearance[122]:

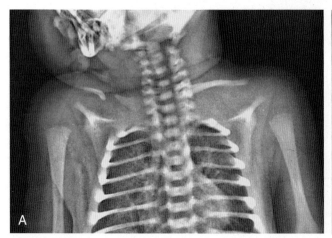
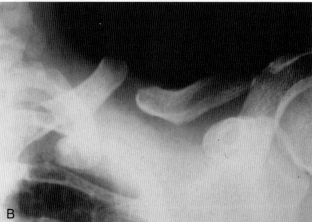

FIGURE 3-32 A, The right side is most commonly involved in congenital pseudarthrosis of the clavicle. **B,** Note the anterosuperiorly displaced sternal fragment that can manifest as a palpable lump and has been described as a *lanceolate deformity.*

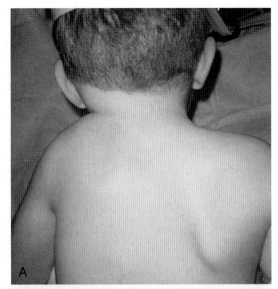

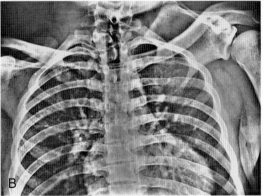

FIGURE 3-33 Typical gross (**A**) and radiographic (**B**) appearance of Sprengel's deformity.

Grade 1 (very mild): The shoulders are level and the deformity is minimally noticeable with the patient dressed.

Grade 2 (mild): The shoulders are level or nearly level, but a lump in the neck is noticeable with the patient dressed.

Grade 3 (moderate): The shoulder is elevated 2 to 5 cm and is easily noticeable.

Grade 4 (severe): The shoulder is elevated more than 5 cm so that the superior angle is at the level of the occiput.

In addition to elevation of the scapula, the scapula is misshapen and rotated. The glenoid is directed inferiorly, and the height of the scapula is reduced in comparison to the unaffected shoulder (Fig. 3-35). This phenomenon can make evaluation of the amount of elevation difficult. The inferior angle of the scapula is easily identified on radiographs, but because of the differences in the shape of the scapulae, elevation in comparison to the contralateral scapula is exaggerated. Likewise, if measurement is carried out to compare the height of the glenoids, the amount of elevation will be underestimated because of the rotatory deformity. Despite the theoretical disadvantage of measuring glenoid height, it seems to be the most accurate and reproducible method of evaluation.

Patients initially have a complaint of prominence of the shoulder or neck. Range of motion is limited and does not respond to physical therapy. Hamner and Hall reported two patients who suffered from multidirectional instability on examination, but because of the young age of the patients (both younger than 9 years), the clinical significance of this condition is unclear.[129]

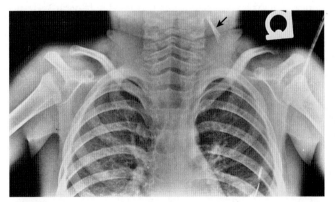

FIGURE 3-34 On the left side of this patient, an omovertebral bone (*arrow*) connects the transverse process of the lower cervical spine of C6 with the superomedial angle of the scapula.

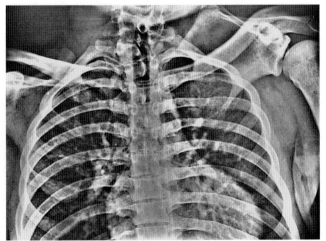

FIGURE 3-35 In Sprengel's deformity, the inferior angle of the scapula is rotated medially and the glenoid is facing inferiorly to decrease the normal arc of motion.

TABLE 3-1 Abnormalities Associated With Congenital Elevation of the Scapula (Sprengel's Deformity)

Abnormalities	Carson[1]	Cavendish[2]	Grogan[3]	Pinsky[4]	All Series	Percentage
Total subjects	11	100	20	48	179	100
Scoliosis, idiopathic	3	23	1	—	27	16
Scoliosis, congenital	4	16	8	25	53	31
Spinal dysraphism	3	28	1	—	32	19
Diastematomyelia	—	3	2	—	5	3
Klippel–Feil syndrome	2	20	9	18	49	29
Rib cage	6	25	9	24	64	38
Muscular	1	14	—	—	15	9
Congenital diaphragmatic hernia	—	1	2	—	3	2
Hand	1	4	1	—	6	4
Foot	—	6	—	—	6	4
Renal	2	0	—	8	10	6
Total associated anomalies	**11**	**98**	**20**	**41**	**170**	**—**

[1]Carson WG, Lovell WW, Whitesides TE: Congenital elevation of the scapula. J Bone Joint Surg Am 63:1199-1207, 1981.
[2]Cavendish ME: Congenital elevation of the scapula. J Bone Joint Surg Br 54:395-408, 1972.
[3]Grogan DP, Stanley EA, Bobechko WP: The congenital undescended scapula. Surgical correction by the Woodward procedure. J Bone Joint Surg Br 65:598-605, 1983.
[4]Pinsky HA, Pizzutillo PD, MacEwen GD: Congenital elevation of the scapula. Orthop Trans 4:288-289, 1980.

Inheritance

Reports of familial Sprengel's deformity are scattered. Overwhelmingly, most cases arise de novo, with a 3:1 preponderance of female to male patients.[122,130]

Associated Anomalies

Sprengel's deformity rarely occurs in isolation. Several large series have reported rates of concurrent deformities of 50% to 100% (Table 3-1).[112,122,131-134] The impact of concurrent anomalies is multiple when planning surgery. The possible renal complications need to be investigated with ultrasound, renal function blood tests, and possibly intravenous pyelography before considering any surgery. Midline dissection must be avoided if thoracic spinal dysraphism is present.[135] Additionally, thoracic malformation can predispose to traction injuries of the brachial plexus when the scapula is lowered.

Treatment

Treatment of Sprengel's deformity is directed at improving the appearance and function of the child.[122,132,136] As regards the appearance of the child, it is important to distinguish the amount of disfigurement that is secondary to the Sprengel's deformity as opposed to the associated scoliosis, Klippel-Feil syndrome, thoracic wall malformation, and other conditions. Otherwise, the results may be disappointing to the patient, surgeon, and family. Similarly, the postsurgical function of the reconstructed shoulder will probably improve but the shoulder will not be at the level of the unaffected shoulder. Surgery is optimally reserved for patients with a moderate to severe appearance and dysfunction.

The patient is best treated before 8 years of age. After this age, the soft tissues are less pliable and the rate of brachial plexus injuries has been reported to increase. Most authors also agree that the surgery is technically difficult to accomplish in children younger than 2 years. Therefore, the preferred age range for surgery is between the ages of 2 and 8 years. However, there have been successful reports of surgical management in adolescence. Grogan and colleagues reported a 15-year-old and McMurtry and colleagues reported a 17-year-old who underwent relocation without complication.[124,137] Borges and colleagues reported surgical management of a 17-year-old without complication but noted no improvement in function.[131]

Many surgeries have been proposed to treat this condition; they fall into four basic categories. The first category is resection of the elevated corner of the scapula and omovertebral bone.[138] Such treatment does nothing to improve function but can have a role in an older patient with mild disfigurement. The second class of surgery consists of releasing the medial muscle attachments, resecting the omovertebral connections, lowering the scapula, and securing the inferior pole to either the rib or surrounding muscles. The Green, Putti, and Petrie

FIGURE 3-36 Essential steps of the Woodward procedure. **A,** Position of the scapula in Sprengel's deformity as it relates to the unaffected side. There is tethering of the superior angle of the scapula to the cervical vertebrae. **B,** The trapezius, rhomboids, and levator scapulae origins are sharply elevated from the spinous processes and retracted laterally. The superior angle of the scapula (A) is carefully exposed, and all tethers to the cervical vertebrae are resected. The scapula is reduced into its anatomic position (B). **C,** The free fascial edge is sutured distal to proximal, holding the reduction (*arrow*).

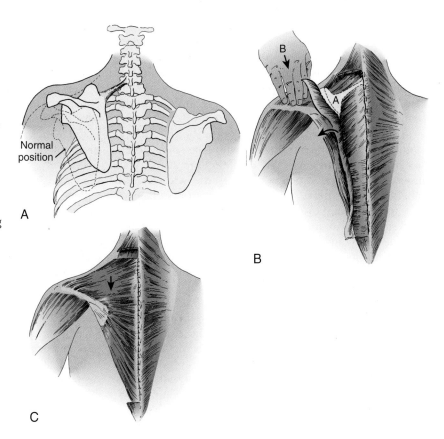

procedures are the best known of this group.[47,113,122,139-141] A third class of procedures attempts to correct the deformity by performing a vertical osteotomy parallel to the medial border. The free medial segment is reattached in a lower position. The best known of these procedures is the Konig-Wittek.[142,143] The last group consists of placing the scapula in an inferiorly located pocket, as well as transferring the muscular attachments of the trapezius, rhomboideus major and minor, and levator scapulae inferiorly.[20] Woodward first described the use of muscle transfers,[144] and several modifications have been reported since.[131,145] Other surgical techniques have been attempted, but none have succeeded to the extent of the Woodward procedure.

The advantage of the Woodward procedure is a more powerful correction that is sustained better over time. It is not at all uncommon for a postsurgical patient to have some degree of recurrence of the deformity. Leibovic and associates, Jeannopoulous, and Ross and Cruess reported recurrence of the rotational deformity when Green's procedure was used and patients were monitored long term (3-14 years).[130,146,147] These results can be compared with the long-term results of Borges and colleagues,[131] who found a sustained 2.7-cm correction, improvement of at least one Cavendish class in all 16 patients who underwent a Woodward procedure, and satisfaction in 14 of 16 patients at 3 to 14 years of follow-up.

Robinson proposed the use of clavicular osteotomy to prevent brachial plexus injury with the Woodward procedure.[148] For older patients (older than 8 years) and those requiring large correction (Cavendish class 4), clavicular osteotomy may be necessary. Several authors question its necessity, however, because no permanent brachial plexus injuries have been reported with translocation of the scapula without clavicular osteotomy.

Authors' Preferred Treatment

The patient is positioned in the lateral decubitus position with use of a beanbag. The entire upper extremity is prepared into the field. The hand is left uncovered during the procedure to facilitate vascular assessment. If a clavicular osteotomy is to be performed, it is carried out first with an incision placed in Langer's lines over the midportion of the clavicle. The clavicle is then dissected subperiosteally, and a 2-cm portion of clavicle is removed from the central third. The bone is morselized and returned to the periosteal tube. The periosteum and skin are then closed.

Attention is next turned to the dorsum. A long midline incision is carried out from the occiput distal to the level of the inferior angle of the unaffected scapula (Fig. 3-36). The dissection is made sharply to the level of the deep fascia. An effort to identify the muscles is facilitated by developing a plane between the fascia and the subcutaneous tissue. The trapezius is identified distally and separated bluntly from the underlying latissimus dorsi. The trapezius, rhomboids, and levator scapulae origins are sharply released from the spinous processes by moving cranially with the releases. The trapezius superior to the fourth cervical vertebra is transected.

Despite the hazards at the superior border of the scapula, any tethering must be resected. The spinal accessory nerve and transverse cervical artery are at risk with surgery around the superior angle of the scapula. The spinal accessory nerve lies on the anterior surface of the trapezius along the medial edge of the scapula. The transverse cervical artery courses posterior to the levator scapulae. If an omovertebral bone is present, it is resected along with its periosteum to prevent regrowth. The scapula is inspected for any curvature at its superior angle that might prevent normal gliding. If such a deformity exists, it is excised extraperiosteally as well. Use of sharp bone biters facilitates this portion of the procedure.

The free fascial edge is sutured distally to lower the scapula into place. To judge the correct height, the levels of the scapular spine and glenoids should be equal, but not the inferior angles. Equalizing the inferior angles would result in over-reduction and possibly neurovascular injury. The hand is checked intermittently for vascular changes after relocation of the scapula. If vascular embarrassment is present, the amount of correction must be reduced. Caudally, the trapezius becomes redundant and is split transversely, folded over, and incorporated into the reattachment.

The incision has a tendency to spread while it heals. A two-layer closure consisting of an interrupted dermal stitch and a running subcuticular stitch is used. No drains are placed. After the application of dressings, the arm is placed in a Velpeau splint for 2 weeks.

Complications of Surgery

Complications result in lower patient and family satisfaction.[130] Brachial plexus traction has been reported in nearly all studies, but all were temporary and did not diminish the results.[40,122,130-132,144,145] Scapular winging is possibly the greatest complication. Patients are dissatisfied with the appearance, and function does not improve. Borges and coworkers noted this complication in 1 of 16 patients.[131] Ross and Cruess reported 3 cases in 17 patients after the Woodward procedure.[130] Carson and associates noted winging in one patient preoperatively and were disappointed with the function and aesthetic results postoperatively.[132] They recommend avoidance of surgery if winging is present preoperatively.

Regrowth of the superior pole has been reported by several authors.[40,130,139] Care in excising the bone extraperiosteally theoretically reduces this risk.

Spreading of the surgical scar, especially the superior portion, was a common complication in early reports.[40,122,132] The rates have decreased with increased attention to closure.

Results

Several studies have found an average range of preoperative motion of 90 to 120 degrees of scapulohumeral combined abduction that improved to 143 to 150 degrees postoperatively.[40,122,130,131,149-151] Nearly every patient improved at least one Cavendish grade. Patients who started with scapular winging or a Cavendish grade 4 appearance had the least improvement and satisfaction.

Os Acromiale

Failure of the acromion process to fuse occurs relatively often, with an average of 8% and a reported range of 1.4% to 15% in study populations.[152-159] It is more common in black patients and in male patients.[159] The acromion forms from three ossification centers, and failure of any of these centers to unite causes an os acromiale (Fig. 3-37).[154] The most common site of persistent cartilage is between the meta-acromion and the meso-acromion.[32,160,161] It has been suggested that a more posteriorly situated acromioclavicular joint in relation to the anterior acromial

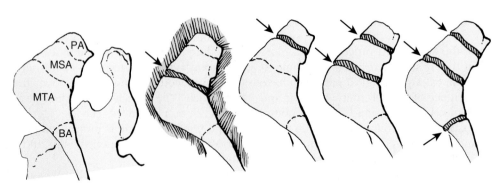

FIGURE 3-37 The acromion has three separate ossification centers. The most common site of os acromiale is between the meso-acromion and the meta-acromion. BA, basi-acromion; MSA, meso-acromion; MTA, meta-acromion; PA, pre-acromion. (From Mudge MK, Wood VE, Frykman GK: Rotator cuff tears associated with os acromiale. J Bone Joint Surg Am 66:427-429, 1984.)

edge is a predisposing factor to the development of an os acromiale.[160] The acromion process should be fully ossified by 25 years of age.[162] Os acromiale is bilateral in 33% to 62% of cases.[32,159,162,163] Most often the abnormality is asymptomatic and is an incidental discovery.[161]

Os acromiale can contribute to shoulder pain as an area of impingement. Neer hypothesized that the presence of unfused nuclei could predispose a patient to impingement.[164,165] Warner and colleagues noted that the anterior-most portion of the unfused segment is more inferiorly slanted than in an unaffected shoulder, a finding that we have also seen at surgery.[166] Such slanting would indeed lead to a decrease in subacromial volume and contribute to impingement.

An unstable acromion can be painful at the nonunion site itself. Warner and coauthors reported several patients who complained of pain at an unstable segment after trauma despite prolonged nonoperative treatment.[166] These patients improved when bony union was achieved. The inferiorly directed pull of the deltoid is thought to contribute to symptoms of the painful mobile segment.

Axillary radiographs are useful as an aid in diagnosis (Fig. 3-38), as are computed tomography and magnetic resonance imaging.[167] We recommend an axillary view as a standard component of all shoulder evaluations.

Treatment

Symptomatic os acromiale falls into two categories[166,168-170]: those associated with pain at the unstable segment and those associated with symptoms of impingement. The first group of patients must be managed conservatively with a sling if seen acutely after trauma, followed by early mobilization. Persistent pain that lasts longer than 3 months and limits work or activities of daily living is an indication for surgery.

The second group of patients, those with impingement and os acromiale, has a more complex treatment protocol. Initially, treatment of the impingement does not vary from that in patients without this finding. Nonsteroidal antiinflammatory medication and tendon-gliding exercises are used. If the patient has evidence of a rotator cuff tear or does not have pain relief, surgical intervention is considered.

A small pre-acromion is excised and the deltoid is repaired. For larger pieces, a decision to perform fusion or subacromial decompression must be made. We perform all acromioplasties and rotator cuff repairs via an open approach and evaluate the stability of the os. If the os acromiale is stable to palpation, a standard acromioplasty is performed. If the segment has motion with palpation, a fusion operation is undertaken.

Surgical Technique

The patient is positioned in a beach chair position, and the operative shoulder and ipsilateral hip are prepared and draped. An incision is made in the direction of the axillary crease and based anteriorly over the lateral acromion. The incision is carried down sharply to but does not enter the deltoid fascia. After obtaining meticulous hemostasis, full-thickness flaps are developed to aid in exposure and closure.

The raphe between the anterior and lateral head of the deltoid is identified and divided in line with its fibers. At this point, either a double-footed Gelpie retractor or two Army–Navy retractors are placed between the divided heads of the deltoid to expose the acromion. The os acromiale can now be inspected for instability. If none is present, subacromial decompression in standard fashion follows.

In patients with a mobile segment, care is taken to leave the anterior deltoid attached to the acromion. The fusion defect is exposed and opened with curets. Several keys aid in reducing the fragment: the inferior soft tissue structures are left intact, all interposed cartilage is completely removed, and bone is removed from the superior corners of the opening (Fig. 3-39). After all cartilage is removed, guidewires for two 4.0-mm cannulated screws are placed in the free fragment in an anterior-to-posterior direction. The fragment is reduced and the guidewires are advanced across the nonunion site. Two distally threaded screws are inserted to compress the reduction. Cancellous bone graft obtained from the hip is placed on the superior surface of the acromion. Large nonabsorbable suture is placed through each screw and secured in a figure-of-eight manner. The wounds are closed and the arm is placed in a sling.

Passive range of motion is begun at the first postoperative visit. Active use of the arm begins at 2 months, but it is restricted to 1 lb with no active overhead activity. Full activity is allowed starting at 3 months.

Results

Our operative technique is similar to that reported by Warner and colleagues and Satterlee.[166,170] Both groups

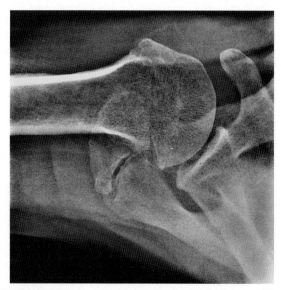

FIGURE 3-38 An os acromiale is best seen on an axillary radiograph.

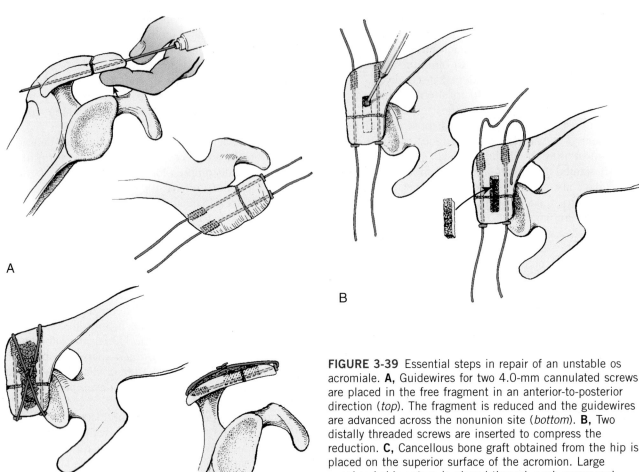

A

B

C

FIGURE 3-39 Essential steps in repair of an unstable os acromiale. **A,** Guidewires for two 4.0-mm cannulated screws are placed in the free fragment in an anterior-to-posterior direction (*top*). The fragment is reduced and the guidewires are advanced across the nonunion site (*bottom*). **B,** Two distally threaded screws are inserted to compress the reduction. **C,** Cancellous bone graft obtained from the hip is placed on the superior surface of the acromion. Large nonabsorbable suture is placed through each screw and secured in a figure-of-eight manner. (From Warner JJP: The treatment of symptomatic os acromiale. J Bone Joint Surg Am 80:1324, 1998.)

used a screw-and-tension-band construct, and both reported results in a small number of patients. Satterlee reported good results in six of six patients, whereas Warner and associates reported good results in five of seven. In Warner and colleagues' series, six of eight patients had poor results with tension banding alone. Despite the small numbers, the evidence appears to favor the combined use of screw-and-tension-band fixation when attempting to fuse an unstable os acromiale.

Hertel reported improved fusion rates when he maintained the anterior deltoid attachments: In three of seven patients the os consolidated when the anterior deltoid was removed versus seven of eight when the deltoid was maintained.[171] Removing the blood supply to the free fragment by soft tissue stripping appears to have deleterious affects on achieving union and thus needs to be minimized.

The results of subacromial decompression in the presence of os acromiale have been mixed. Until recently, the importance of instability as an indication for surgery was not addressed. Perhaps the mixed outcomes from decompression are due to a heterogeneous group being treated and further investigation is warranted. Hutchinson

and Veenstra reported recurrence of impingement at 1 year in three of three shoulders treated arthroscopically.[172] However, Wright and colleagues reported good to excellent results in 11 of 13 shoulders with an os acromiale at the meso-acromion level treated with an extended arthroscopic acromioplasty.[173] Pagnani and colleagues reported successful results of arthroscopic excision of a symptomatic os in 11 shoulders of athletes aged 18 to 25 years with a minimum 2-year follow-up.[174] Although these reports are encouraging for arthroscopic treatment, long-term data are lacking.

Glenoid Hypoplasia

Glenoid hypoplasia results from failure of the inferior glenoid to develop (Fig. 3-40).[61,175-178] The true incidence is uncertain, and the diagnosis is often made on routine chest radiographs. However, patients might complain of pain and limited abduction in the second through fifth decades of life.[177-179] Instability of the glenohumeral joint is reported to be found in a subgroup of patients.[178] Glenoid hypoplasia is most commonly bilateral and noted in men.[178,180] Several reports of familial associations have

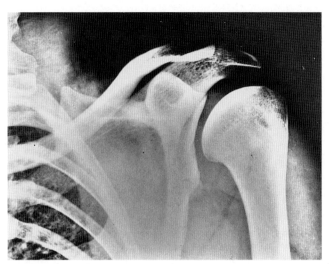

FIGURE 3-40 Varying degrees of glenoid flattening are seen in glenoid hypoplasia.

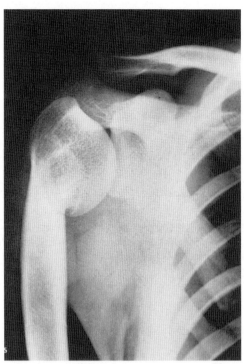

FIGURE 3-41 Typical appearance of humerus varus. (From DePalma AF: Surgery of the Shoulder, 3rd ed. Philadelphia: JB Lippincott, 1983, p 30.)

led to a proposed autosomal dominant mechanism of inheritance.[179,181-183]

The radiographic appearance of a hypoplastic scapular neck with an irregular joint surface is seen in patients with glenoid hypoplasia.[121,184] The proximal end of the humerus is influenced to develop abnormally, similar to developmental dysplasia of the hip. The humeral neck angle decreases to form a humerus varus, and the head flattens. Arthrograms have shown the inferior cartilage to be thickened and fissured and the capsular volume decreased.[184]

Associated Anomalies

Congenital spine, hip, and rib abnormalities can be found in association with glenoid dysplasia.[177,185] Involvement of multiple joints should make the clinician suspicious of an underlying epiphyseal dysplasia, scurvy, or rickets. Conversely, unilateral shoulder joint involvement should alert the physician to rule out brachial plexus injuries and avascular necrosis.

Treatment

Early reports of this entity did little to address treatment. Several authors suggested avoidance of manual labor and overhead activities by those affected.[178,186] Arthroscopic débridement of the ragged articular cartilage in a single patient did little to alter his symptoms.[180] Wirth and coauthors reported successful treatment consisting of organized physical therapy in 16 patients with this disorder.[178] Both patients with and without instability of the shoulder benefited from this intervention.

The results of arthroplasty as treatment of the secondary degenerative arthritis are limited. Sperling and colleagues reported the results in seven patients.[187] Three of four patients treated by hemiarthroplasty required revision to total shoulder or bipolar arthroplasty because of pain. Two of three total shoulder replacements had excellent outcomes, with one prosthesis requiring resection

and reimplantation for infection. These very limited results suggest a trend toward better results with total shoulder replacement. However, the high complication rate should make the standard treatment regimen one that relies mainly on physical therapy.

When nonoperative treatment has failed, total shoulder replacement is fraught with technical challenges. The inferior glenoid and posterior glenoid bone stock is deficient. These deficiencies must be addressed at the time of surgery or the glenoid will be malpositioned and poorly seated. Glenoid osteotomy, bone grafting, or metal augments will be required. Insertion of the humeral component with decreased retroversion is recommended by Sperling and colleagues to improve stability.[187] However, we do not believe that humeral retroversion should be substituted for proper soft tissue tensioning.

Humerus Varus

The humeral neck-to-shaft angle is generally considered to be 140 degrees in a normal shoulder.[3] When the proximal humeral growth plate is disturbed during growth or development, the neck and shaft can be dramatically reduced. Premature closure of the medial growth plate results in a differential growth of the lateral and medial humeral lengths. Köhler defined a neck-to-shaft angle less than 90 degrees, elevation of the greater tuberosity above the top of the humeral head, and reduction of the distance between the articular surface and the lateral cortex as the radiographic criteria for diagnosis (Fig. 3-41).[188]

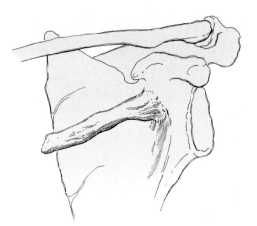

FIGURE 3-42 Duplication of the clavicle is an extremely rare abnormality. The lateral end of the extra clavicle attaches to the base of the coracoid process.

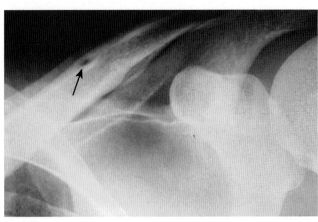

FIGURE 3-43 This clavicle has a large foramen (*arrow*) through which passes the supraclavicular nerve.

Patients have either a decreased ability to perform overhead activities or pain from impingement. Gill and Waters hypothesized that compensation by the unaffected shoulder can result in overuse tendinitis as another complaint.[189]

Trauma during birth or early life may be the underlying cause of idiopathic humerus varus.[190] Idiopathic humerus varus occurs unilaterally and is not associated with other anomalies. Several other processes can be responsible for humerus varus, including thalassemia, skeletal dysplasia, neoplasm, osteomyelitis, cerebral palsy, arthrogryposis, and brachial plexus injuries.[191] Therefore, the underlying cause of humerus varus must be investigated before treating the deformity.

Treatment of idiopathic humerus varus has not been reported very often. Acromionectomy has historically been proposed as treatment, but it has been abandoned because of its disappointing cosmetic and functional outcome.[192] Wedge osteotomy followed by spica cast immobilization for up to 3 months has been reported as well.[193] The prolonged immobilization is difficult for both the patient and family to endure. Complications related to the spica cast include elbow stiffness, skin breakdown, and brachial plexus injury.

Because of the complications of immobilization, Gill and Waters proposed a lateral closing wedge osteotomy secured by tension band wiring.[189] The case report shows a dramatic increase in abduction from 85 to 130 degrees, in forward flexion from 110 to 160 degrees, and in internal rotation from T12 to T4. The neck-shaft angle was corrected from 90 to 140 degrees. At a 5-year follow-up, the patient, who was a 12-year-old boy at the time of surgery, had no recurrence of deformity. These results are very promising and might become the recommended treatment with further evidence of success.

RARE ANOMALIES

Duplicated and Bifurcated Clavicle

Duplication of the clavicle has been described in the literature with some variation. Complete duplication of the clavicle (Fig. 3-42) has been described once and caused no symptoms in that patient.[121,194] In a few cases, bifurcation of the clavicle has also been described in which there is duplication of either the lateral or medial side.[195-199]

Middle Suprascapular Nerve Foramen

A branch from the middle suprascapular nerve might pass through a foramen in the clavicle (Fig. 3-43). No treatment is required unless the patient has neurogenic pain in this area. Treatment involves freeing the nerve from its bony entrapment.[199,200]

Clasp-like Cranial Margin of the Scapula

The superior margin of the scapula can look like the handle of a bucket (Fig. 3-44), but this anomaly has no clinical significance.[121,199,201,202]

Double Acromion and Coracoid Process

Reported only once, this malformation (Fig. 3-45) restricted motion of the shoulder but required no treatment.[203]

Triple Coracoid Process

This anomaly has been reported only once and was in association with a bifurcated clavicle.[197] The patient was asymptomatic and required no treatment.

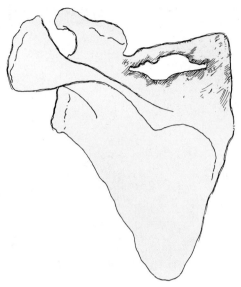

FIGURE 3-44 Clasp-like cranial margin of the scapula.

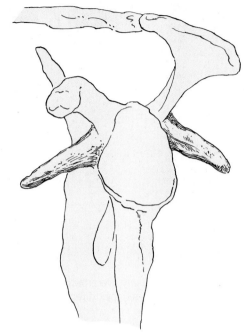

FIGURE 3-45 The double acromion and coracoid processes shown here have been identified only once, by McClure and Raney.

Elongated Acromion

An elongated acromion has been described covering the superior and lateral aspects of the humeral head and extending to the level of the surgical neck.[204]

Duplicated Scapula

Multiple humeri and forearm bones are commonly associated (Fig. 3-46). Fusion of the two scapulae has been reported to be successful in patients whose motion is restricted.[205-207]

Coracoclavicular Joint or Bar

The coracoclavicular ligaments may be replaced by an articulation or a bony bar (Figs. 3-47 to 3-49). Symptomatic patients might complain of neurovascular compression, restriction in range of motion, or pain from arthritis of the joint. When symptomatic, the articulation or bar may be excised.[121,208-217]

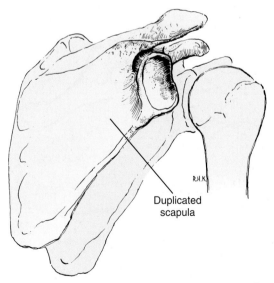

Duplicated
scapula

FIGURE 3-46 A duplicated scapula has been reported only three times.

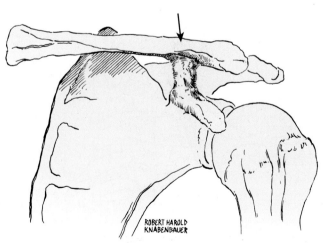

ROBERT HAROLD
KNABENBAUER

FIGURE 3-47 Rarely, a solid bony strut (arrow) connects the coracoid to the clavicle.

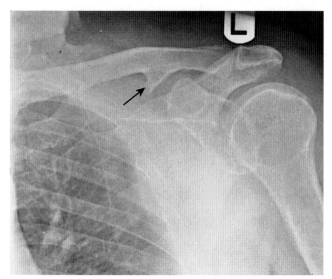

FIGURE 3-48 A triangular bony overgrowth under the clavicle (*arrow*) may be present with its apex directed down toward the coracoid.

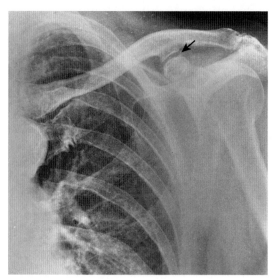

FIGURE 3-49 Both the coracoid and the clavicular projections may be covered with cartilage and form a true diarthrodial joint (*arrow*) with an articular capsule.

Coracosternal Bone

A bony bridge originating from the base of the coracoid and extending cephalad and medially has been reported in one patient with Sprengel's deformity.[218] It was thought to be the persistence of a mesenchymal coracosternal connection normally seen in an early embryologic stage.

Ligamentous Connecting Bands: Costocoracoid, Costosternal, Costovertebral

The three abnormal costocoracoid, costosternal, and costovertebral fibrous connections can lead to progressive deformity and dysfunction of the upper extremity (Fig.

3-50). Excision of the offending structure can provide improved function and prevent further deformity.[218-221]

Osseous Bridge From Clavicle to Spine of Scapula

Compression of neurovascular structures and restriction of motion require excision of this structure (Fig. 3-51).[222,223]

Infrascapular Bone

The infrascapular bone, a normal variant of scapula ossification, represents the attachment of the teres major

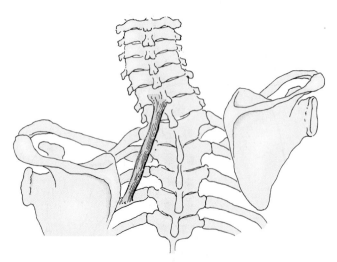

FIGURE 3-50 The costovertebral bone ties together the bifid spinous process of the sixth cervical vertebra and the fourth rib.

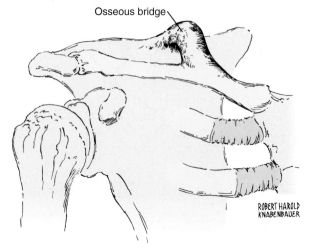

FIGURE 3-51 An osseous bridge can extend from the midportion of the clavicle to the spine of the scapula.

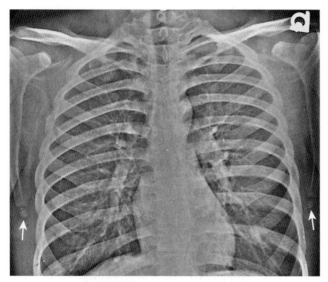

FIGURE 3-52 An infrascapular bone (*arrows*) is present bilaterally in this patient.

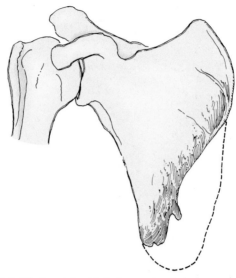

FIGURE 3-53 A notched inferior angle of the scapula probably represents an absence of the ossification nucleus of the inferior angle of the scapula.

muscle and may be misinterpreted as a fracture (Fig. 3-52).[199,224-226]

Notched Inferior Angle of the Scapula

Incomplete development of the inferior scapula results in a misshapen scapula (Fig. 3-53).[29,121,141,199,227]

Dentated Glenoid

Incomplete development of the inferior glenoid results in a rippled appearance of the glenoid (Fig. 3-54). Fusion

of the growth plates usually resolves this appearance, but it can continue into adulthood.[186,199]

Phocomelia

Absence of the entire upper extremity or severe shortening of the limb with absent portions (Figs. 3-55 to 3-60)

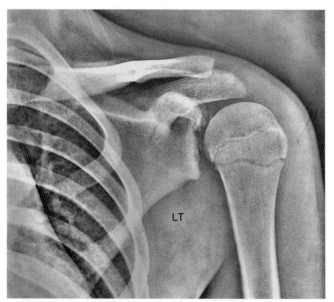

FIGURE 3-54 The epiphyseal annular ring of the glenoid in this patient has not fused and appears to be rippled or dentated (*arrow*). (The letters *LT* indicate that the radiograph is of the left shoulder.)

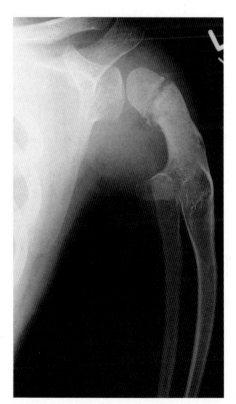

FIGURE 3-55 This child with phocomelia has a fairly well developed shoulder with a small humerus and fused elbow.

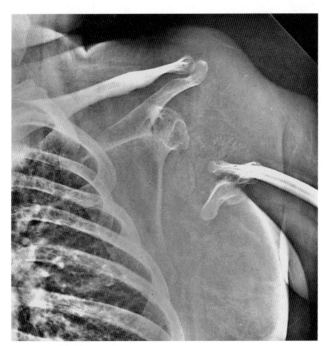

FIGURE 3-56 An abnormal glenoid articulates with only a deformed, short distal end of the humerus and a one-bone forearm in this patient with phocomelia.

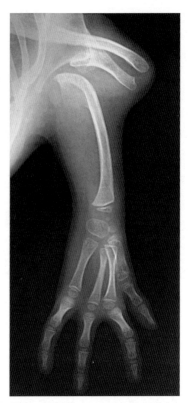

FIGURE 3-57 This child has a poorly formed scapula with part of an elbow articulating inside the shoulder joint and only a radius in the forearm.

was a major health catastrophe during the 1950s with the use of thalidomide in pregnant women. Currently, phocomelia is rare. The function of the remnant limb dictates intervention. Preservation of functional fingers can allow improved prosthetic use. Unsightly and nonfunctioning limbs may be candidates for amputation. Bone transport has been used to lengthen the affected limb, as have vascularized fibula and clavicle grafts.[54,109,121,200,213,228-238]

Absence of the Acromion or Humeral Head

Bilateral absence of the acromion has been reported in a few cases, and a familial association has been identified.[239,240] The coracoacromial ligament is absent and the deltoid origin and the trapezius insertion are found both on the lateral clavicle and on the scapular spine. The lateral end of the clavicle is blunted, and both the clavicle and coracoid process are hypertrophied. Clinical appearance and range of motion of the shoulders were normal, although mild superior translation of the humeral head was noted in one patient.[240] Congenital absence of the humeral head has been reported twice.[241]

Holt–Oram Syndrome

The condition involving multigenerational cardiac and upper extremity congenital anomalies is termed *Holt–Oram syndrome*. Scapular abnormalities similar to Sprengel's deformity are the most common shoulder

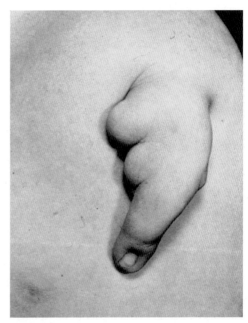

FIGURE 3-58 In an extreme case of phocomelia, sometimes only a finger attaches to the trunk.

FIGURE 3-59 The fibula may be transplanted to the upper part of the arm by placing the epiphysis in the glenoid fossa and attaching the distal end to the humeral remnant.

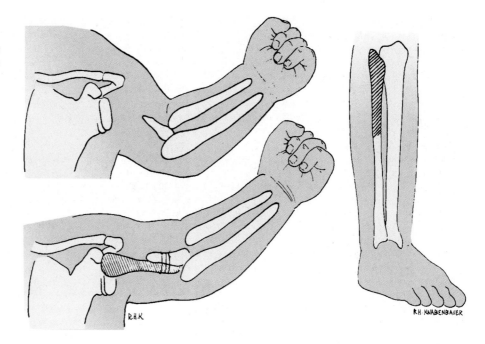

manifestation. Misshapen clavicles, acromia, and humeral heads have also been reported. Inheritance is autosomal dominant.[242-251]

Nail–Patella Syndrome

This autosomal dominant syndrome is a relatively common entity in England, estimated at 22 per 100,000.[252-255] The main features of nail–patella syndrome (also known as *onycho-osteodysplasia*) are absent or hypoplastic nails, typically more severe on the radial side of the hand; dysplasia of the patella and lateral femoral condyle of the knee; dysplasia of the capitellum and radial head of the elbow; and dysplasia of the iliac crests.

Although not the main abnormality of the disease, the scapula and the humerus are often misshapen. The proximal end of the humerus is often small and directed superiorly. The glenoid is often small and directed laterally or inferiorly. A small acromion, a prominent lateral clavicle, and a small coracoid complete the bony abnormalities often found (Fig. 3-61). Some patients complain of impingement-like pain with use of the extremity.[256-258] On examination, the glenohumeral joint is prominent anteriorly and unstable. Loomer described a double osteotomy of the scapula that successfully relieved the pain of a patient who failed nonoperative treatment.[259] However, the vast majority of patients do not require operative intervention.

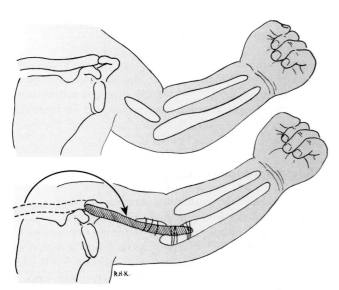

FIGURE 3-60 Transposition of the clavicle is accomplished by exposing it subperiosteally and using the sternal end to lengthen the humerus.

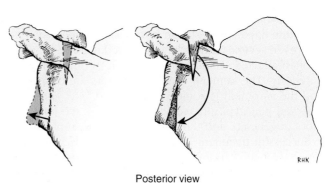

Posterior view

FIGURE 3-61 For correction of the shoulder deformity in the nail–patella syndrome, an opening wedge osteotomy of the inferior glenoid with bone from the spine of the scapula works well. (From Wood VE, Sauser DD, O'Hara RC: The shoulder and elbow in Apert's syndrome. J Pediatr Orthop 15:648-651, 1995.)

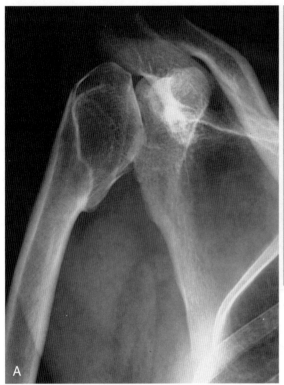

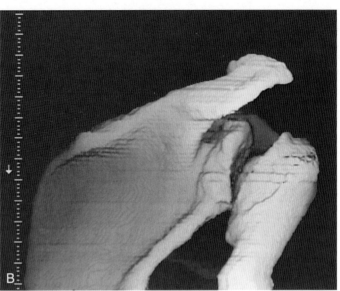

FIGURE 3-62 A, This 23-year-old man with Apert's syndrome has flattening of the humeral head with arthropathy. **B,** A CT scan with three-dimensional reconstruction shows the abnormalities even more dramatically.

Oto–Onycho–Peroneal Syndrome

This rare syndrome characterized by dysmorphic facial features with characteristic ear abnormalities, nail hypoplasia, absent or hypoplastic fibulae, and shoulder anomalies is thought to be an autonomic recessive disorder. Shoulder abnormalities include straight clavicles, fibrous fusion of the distal clavicle and the scapular spine, and an abnormal acromioclavicular joint.[260-262]

Apert's Syndrome

Apert's syndrome (Figs. 3-62 and 3-63) is typically thought of for the hand manifestation acrocephalosyndactyly.[263,264] However, several authors have reported that the shoulder is often affected. The shoulder is reduced but subluxates anteriorly. The humeral head and glenoid are dysplastic, and the acromion is sometimes enlarged.[265,266] The function and pain typically worsen with age as the joint surfaces degenerate and the joint continues to subluxate.

Successful treatment by acromioplasty or acromionectomy has been reported in patients with large acromion processes. The injudicious use of acromionectomy can compromise the patient's results if arthroplasty is necessary to treat the glenohumeral arthritis. In patients with severe pain and motion loss, treatment options include arthrodesis, hemiarthroplasty, and total shoulder arthroplasty. No results comparing these interventions have been published.[267-273]

Multiple Epiphyseal Dysplasia

A defect in the ossification centers of the epiphysis results in multiple joint involvement with this disease (Fig. 3-64).[274] Patients commonly have shoulder manifestations that fall into two categories: mild abnormalities that lead to glenohumeral arthritis and severe failure of epiphyseal development. Both groups typically have pain in the fifth and sixth decades of life.[275] The range of motion and function of the two groups are vastly different. Mildly affected shoulders have nearly normal motion initially but lose motion and become painful over time. Severely deformed shoulders lack motion from an early age but are not painful until later in life. The ideal treatment has not been established.[116,276-281] Total shoulder arthroplasty and hemiarthroplasty have been proposed to treat the glenohumeral arthritis. Fusion can play a role in the treatment of severely affected patients.

Pelvis–Shoulder Dysplasia

Pelvis–shoulder dysplasia, also known as *scapuloiliac dysostosis* or *Kosenow's syndrome,* is an autosomal dominant condition characterized by extreme hypoplasia of the scapulae and ilia.[282-286] The scapular body and glenoid display severe hypoplasia, and the acromion and coracoid may be normal. The clavicles many times appear elongated but can also be hypoplastic. Cases without shoulder girdle involvement have been reported.[287] Anomalies of the eyes, ears, vertebrae, ribs, and upper

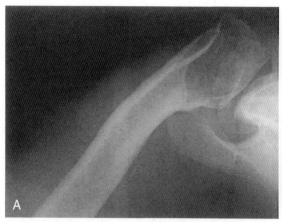
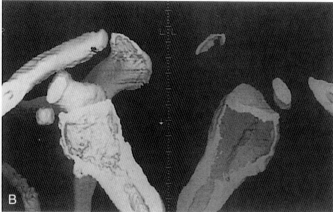

FIGURE 3-63 **A,** The left shoulder of a man with Apert's syndrome. **B,** CT scan with three-dimensional reconstruction.

and lower limbs, along with severe lumbar lordosis and hip dislocation, have been reported.

Congenital Dislocation of the Shoulder

Whether congenital dislocation of the shoulder is a real entity is controversial. The presence of a dislocated shoulder in a child is often associated with brachial plexus injury or arthrogryposis multiplex congenita. If a congenital shoulder dislocation is confirmed, closed reduction is the preferred treatment. Failure of closed reduction can necessitate open reduction.[123,182,288-298]

Chondroepitrochlear Muscle

Reports of this muscle have come mainly from examining the remains of fetuses that died of multiple anomalies. The muscle arises from the pectoralis major fascia and inserts into the medial brachial fascia (Fig. 3-65). The chondroepitrochlear muscle is thought to represent an abnormal insertion of the pectoralis major muscle because of its innervation by the pectoral nerves. In those rare patients who have this muscle and suffer from restricted range of motion, excision is warranted. As a secondary gain, improved appearance of the axilla should also occur.[153,299-316]

Subscapularis–Teres–Latissimus Muscle

This anomalous muscle arises from the lateral border of the scapula, subscapularis, or latissimus dorsi and inserts into the lesser tuberosity with the tendon of the subscapularis (Fig. 3-66). The muscle may be responsible for compression of the brachial plexus in the axilla. However, no reports of the clinical importance of this muscle have been published.[317]

Coracoclaviculosternal Muscle

A single report describes a muscle originating at the tip of the coracoid and inserting into the anterior clavicular facet (Fig. 3-67). The patient was asymptomatic.[318]

Deltoid Muscle Contracture

Fibrosis and subsequent contracture of the deltoid most commonly follow intramuscular injection. Numerous drugs have been implicated. A rarer condition is development of a deltoid contraction without an antecedent history of injection. In either case, range of motion does not improve greatly with physical therapy. Surgery is

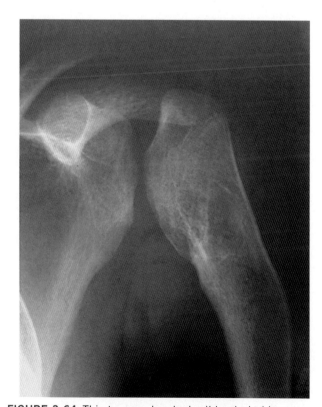

FIGURE 3-64 This teenage boy had mild pain in his shoulders but minimal glenohumeral movement. He demonstrates the typical hatchet head shoulder.

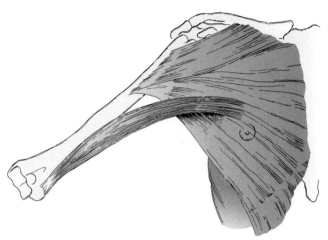

FIGURE 3-65 The chondroepitrochlear muscle originates on the anterior chest wall and inserts along the medial epicondyle.

indicated for patients who have an abduction contracture greater than 25 degrees and have experienced progressive deformity. Release of the fibrotic bands with or without transfer of the posterior deltoid has been recommended.[52,319-339]

Congenital Fossa

The skin over the acromion, clavicle, and supraspinatus can sometimes contain pits or fossae from lack of subcutaneous fat (Fig. 3-68). The fossae may be associated with a syndrome (18q deletion, trisomy 9p, or Russell–Silver syndrome); however, most are asymptomatic and resolve with growth.[208,340-349]

Poland's Syndrome

Absence of the pectoralis major muscle causes relatively little disability.[181,271,301,322,336,350-363] The remnant pectoralis

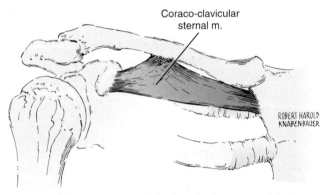

Coraco-clavicular sternal m.

ROBERT HAROLD KNABENBAUER

FIGURE 3-67 The coracoclaviculosternal muscle originates from the anterior margin of the coracoid process and inserts into the clavicular facet of the sternum.

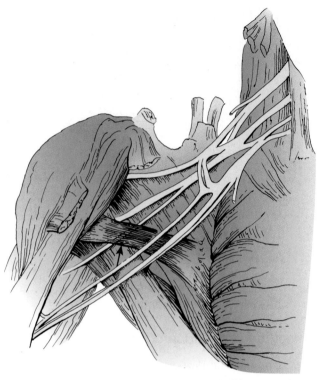

FIGURE 3-66 The subscapularis–teres–latissimus muscle *(arrow)* penetrates the brachial plexus and can lie on top of the axillary, lower subscapular, thoracodorsal, or radial nerves.

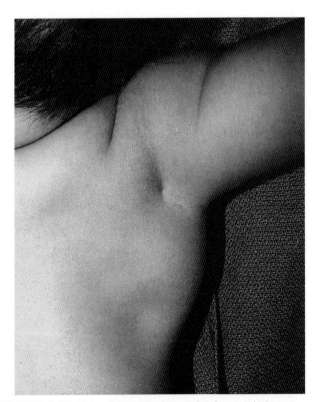

FIGURE 3-68 This child with a scapular fossa cried every time her arm was abducted from her side. (From Wood VE: Congenital skin fossae about the shoulder. Plast Reconstr Surg 85:798-800. 1990.)

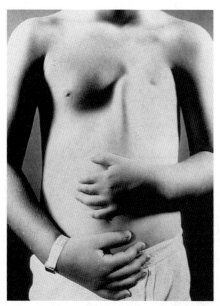

FIGURE 3-69 A typical patient with Poland's syndrome.

major tendon can form an axillary web[364] that can limit shoulder motion. Excision of the aberrant tendon and Z-plasty lengthening can greatly benefit a patient in this instance.

The term *Poland's syndrome* should be reserved for patients with an absent pectoralis major and ipsilateral syndactyly (Figs. 3-69 and 3-70).[365,366] The underlying ribs, fascia, or breast might also be abnormally formed.[342,358,361,367-369] Breast reconstruction may be of cosmetic benefit for female patients. Shoulder dysfunction is unusual unless it is associated with an axillary web, but associated conditions are common.

Associated anomalies[370-373] can be musculoskeletal, genitourinary, gastrointestinal, or hematopoietic. Musculoskeletal anomalies include contralateral syndactyly, ipsilateral upper extremity hypoplasia, clubfoot, toe syndactyly, hemivertebrae, and scoliosis. Genitourinary anomalies include renal aplasia, hypospadias, and inguinal hernia. The gastrointestinal anomaly is situs inversus. Hematopoietic anomalies include spherocytosis, acute lymphoblastic leukemia, and acute myelogenous leukemia.

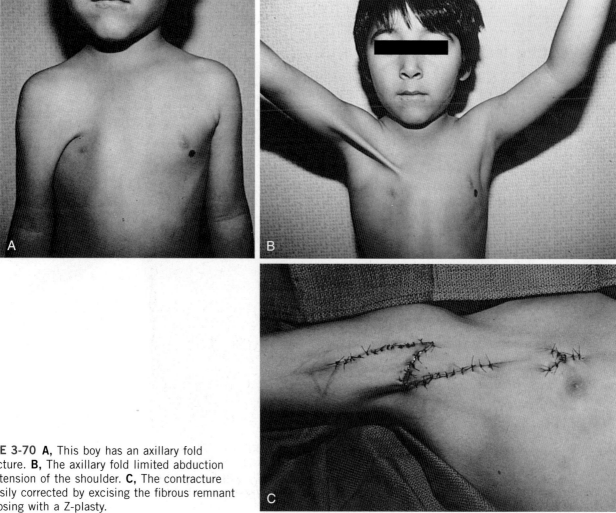

FIGURE 3-70 A, This boy has an axillary fold contracture. **B,** The axillary fold limited abduction and extension of the shoulder. **C,** The contracture was easily corrected by excising the fibrous remnant and closing with a Z-plasty.

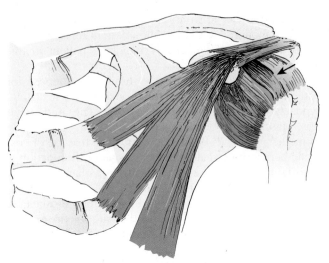

FIGURE 3-71 The tendon of the pectoralis minor can pass over the coracoid process and insert into the humeral head *(arrow)*. A bursa can form under the tendon and cause an impingement syndrome.

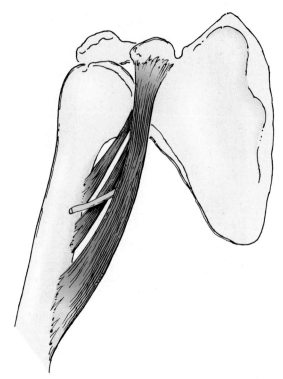

FIGURE 3-72 The coracobrachialis can contain two or three muscle bellies through which the musculocutaneous nerve must pass.

Möbius Syndrome

Möbius syndrome consists of facial paralysis and other cranial nerve involvement with musculoskeletal manifestations similar to Poland's syndrome.[374-376]

Absence of the Trapezius and Rhomboideus

Patients with this entity learn adaptive behavior to overcome the lack of musculature, and they therefore require no treatment.[368,377-380]

Pectoralis Minor Insertion Into the Humerus

The pectoralis minor usually inserts onto the coracoid process. However, it occasionally passes the coracoid process, travels with the coracohumeral ligament, and inserts onto the humeral head (Fig. 3-71). The abnormal slip has been identified as a site of compression for neurovascular structures, as well as a possible cause of impingement. When the pectoralis minor inserts abnormally and causes dysfunction, excision or transfer of the tendon to the coracoid process may be warranted.[209,364,381-389]

Multiple Insertions of the Coracobrachialis

The coracobrachialis is usually composed of a single muscle belly; however, up to three separate muscle bellies may be present (Fig. 3-72). No clinical significance is attached to this variation.[390]

Dorsal Epitrochlearis Muscle

The latissimus dorsi muscle often has an associated muscle that originates from the tendon of the latissimus

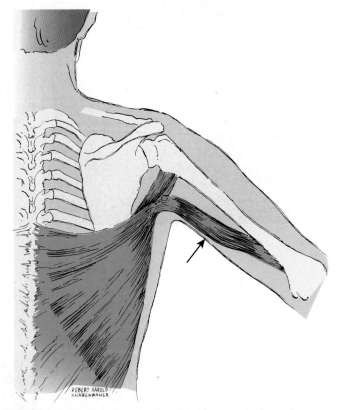

FIGURE 3-73 The dorsal epitrochlearis muscle *(arrow)* originates from the tendon of the latissimus dorsi and inserts onto the brachial and forearm fascia, the humerus, the lateral epicondyle, and the olecranon.

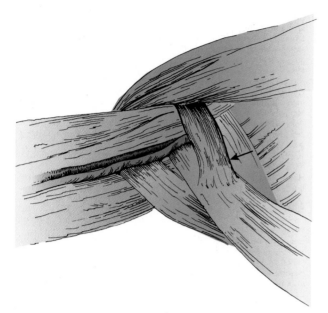

FIGURE 3-74 The axillopectoral muscle *(arrow)* extends from the latissimus dorsi and inserts into the pectoralis major. It overlies the neurovascular bundle in the axilla.

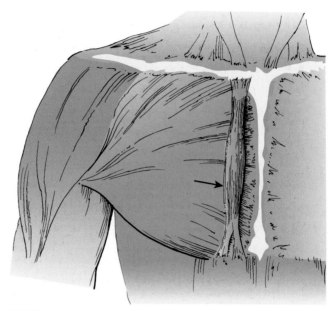

FIGURE 3-75 The sternalis muscle *(arrow).*

dorsi and inserts into the brachial and forearm fascia, the humerus, and the lateral epicondyle. In contrast to the chondroepitrochlearis muscle, the dorsal epitrochlearis muscle (Fig. 3-73) is innervated by the radial nerve and occurs in 18% to 20% of people.[390,391] No clinical significance has been identified for this muscle.[392-394]

Axillopectoral Muscle

Langer's armbogen, Langer's arm arch, and *axillopectoral muscle* are names attributed to the anomalous portion of the latissimus dorsi (Fig. 3-74).[305,395-397] The slip of the latissimus dorsi courses along the inferior border of the axilla and inserts into the pectoralis major muscle. The muscle, which becomes tight with abduction and external rotation, overlies the neurovascular structures in the axilla.[208,398-405] The muscle is innervated by the pectoral nerve. The anomaly occurs in 4% to 7.7% of the population[406] and is usually asymptomatic.

Patients might have complaints related to axillary vein obstruction, specifically, swelling, discomfort, and discoloration of the upper extremity.[395,407,408] The axillopectoral muscle has also been reported to manifest as a painless axillary mass.[409]

Treatment is incision of the muscle. For those concerned with possible malignancy, a specimen must be sent to confirm the presence of normal muscle tissue.

Sternalis Muscle

The sternalis is a long thin muscle that extends from the sternocleidomastoid to the rectus abdominis along the sternum (Fig. 3-75). The muscle is superficial and medial to the pectoralis major muscle.[258,410,411] Barlow reported on 535 cadavers that he dissected and used information on an additional 4805 to report the incidence of the sternalis muscle.[412] He found a 2% rate in persons of European descent, an 8% rate in persons of African descent, and an 11% rate in persons of Asian descent. The sternalis is twice as commonly unilateral as bilateral and occurs equally in male and female patients.

The sternalis has not been reported to cause any pathology. Unfamiliarity with the muscle can cause concern when seen on a mammogram and has even led to biopsy.

REFERENCES

1. Kennedy JC, Cameron H: Complete dislocation of the acromioclavicular joint. J Bone Joint Surg Br 36:202-208, 1954.
2. Rockwood CA Jr, Williams GR Jr, Young DC: Disorders of the acromioclavicular joint. In Rockwood CA Jr, Matsen FA III, Wirth MA, Lippitt SB (eds): The Shoulder, 3rd ed. Philadelphia: WB Saunders, 2004, pp 521-595.
3. DePalma AF: Regional, variational, and surgical anatomy. In DePalma AF (ed): Surgery of the Shoulder, 3rd ed. Philadelphia: JB Lippincott, 1983, pp 35-64.
4. Fich R: In Bardelen V (ed): Handbuch der Anatomie des Menchen, vol 2. Jena, Switzerland, Gustav Disher, 1910, pp 163-187.
5. Harris RI, Vu DH, Sonnabend DH, et al: Anatomic variance of the coracoclavicular ligaments. J Shoulder Elbow Surg 10:585-588, 2001.
6. Pieper HG, Radas CB, Krahl H, Blank M: Anatomic variation of the coracoacromial ligament: A macroscopic and microscopic cadaveric study. J Shoulder Elbow Surg 6:291-296, 1997.
7. Holt EM, Allibone RO: The clinical and surgical implications of the anatomical variants of the coraco-acromial ligament. J Bone Joint Surg Br 76(Suppl 1):40, 1994.
8. Holt EM, Allibone RO: Anatomic variants of the coraco-acromial ligament. J Shoulder Elbow Surg 4:370-375, 1995.
9. Fealy S, April EW, Khazzam M, et al: The coracoacromial ligament: Morphology and study of acromial enthesopathy. J Shoulder Elbow Surg 14:542-548, 2005.

10. Codman EA: The Shoulder: Rupture of the Supraspinatous Tendon and Other Lesions in or about the Subacromial Bursa, 2nd ed. Boston: Thomas Todd, 1934.

11. Renfree KJ, Wright TW: Anatomy and biomechanics of the acromioclavicular and sternoclavicular joints. Clin Sports Med 22:219-237, 2003.

12. Wirth MA, Rockwood CA Jr: Acute and chronic traumatic injuries of the sternoclavicular joint. J Am Acad Orthop Surg 4:268-278, 1996.

13. Brossmann J, Stabler A, Preidler KW, et al: Sternoclavicular joint: MR imaging—anatomic correlation. Radiology 198:193-198, 1996.

14. Bearn JG: Direct observations on the function of the capsule of the sternoclavicular joint in clavicular support. J Anat 101:159-170, 1967.

15. Gage M, Parnell H: Scalenus anticus syndrome. Am J Surg 73:252-268, 1947.

16. Roos DB: Congenital anomalies associated with thoracic outlet syndrome: Anatomy, symptoms, diagnosis, and treatment. Am J Surg 132:771-778, 1976.

17. Roos DB: New concepts of thoracic outlet syndrome that explain etiology and symptoms, diagnosis, and treatment. Vasc Surg 13:313-321, 1979.

18. Roos DB: The place for scalenectomy and first rib resection in thoracic outlet syndrome. Surgery 92:1077-1085, 1982.

19. Wood VE, Ellison DW: Results of upper plexus thoracic outlet syndrome operation. Ann Thoracic Surg 58:458-461, 1994.

20. Wood VE, Twito RS, Verka JM: Thoracic outlet syndrome: The results of first rib resection in 100 patients. Orthop Clin North Am 19:131-146, 1988.

21. Burkhead W, Scheinberg R, Box G: Surgical anatomy of the axillary nerve. J Shoulder Elbow Surg 1:31-36, 1992.

22. Cetik O, Uslu M, Acar HI, et al: Is there a safe area for the axillary nerve in the deltoid muscle? A cadaveric study. J Bone Joint Surg Am 88:2395-2399, 2006.

23. Rengachary SS, Burr D, Lucas S, Brackett CE: Suprascapular entrapment neuropathy: A clinical, anatomical, and comparative study. Part 3: Comparative study. Neurosurgery 5:452-455, 1979.

24. Rengachary SS, Burr D, Lucas S, et al: Suprascapular entrapment neuropathy: A clinical, anatomical, and comparative study. Part 2: Anatomical study. Neurosurgery 5:447-451, 1979.

25. Rengachary SS, Neff JP, Singer PA, Brackett CE: Suprascapular entrapment neuropathy: A clinical, anatomical, and comparative study. Part 1: Clinical study. Neurosurgery 5:441-446, 1979.

26. Alon M, Weiss S, Fishel B, Dekel S: Bilateral suprascapular nerve entrapment syndrome due to an anomalous transverse scapular ligament. Clin Orthop Relat Res (234):31-33, 1988.

27. Ticker JB, Djurasovic M, Strauch RJ, et al: The incidence of ganglion cysts and other variations in anatomy along the course of the suprascapular nerve. J Shoulder Elbow Surg 7:472-478, 1998.

28. Edelson JG: Bony bridges and other variations of the suprascapular notch. J Bone Joint Surg Br 77:505-506, 1995.

29. Hrdlicka A: The scapula: Visual observations. Am J Physiol Anthropol 29:73-94, 287-310, 363-415, 1942.

30. Cohen SB, Dines DM, Moorman CT: Familial calcification of the superior transverse scapular ligament causing neuropathy. Clin Orthop Relat Res (334):131-135, 1997.

31. Bigliani LU, Morrison DS, April EW: Morphology of the acromion and its relation to rotator cuff tears [abstract]. Orthop Trans 10:228, 1986.

32. Nicholson GP, Goodman DA, Flatow EL, Bigliani LU: The acromion: Morphologic condition and age-related changes. A study of 420 scapulas. J Shoulder Elbow Surg 5:1-11, 1996.

33. Edelson JG: The "hooked" acromion revisited. J Bone Joint Surg Br 77:284-287, 1995.

34. Harris JE, Blackney M: The anatomy and function of the coracoacromial ligament [abstract]. J Shoulder Elbow Surg 2(Suppl):S6, 1993.

35. Ogata S, Uhthoff HK: Acromial enthesopathy and rotator cuff tear. A radiologic and histologic postmortem investigation of the coracoacromial arch. Clin Orthop Relat Res (254):39-48, 1990.

36. Ozaki J, Fujimoto S, Nakagawa Y, et al: Tears of the rotator cuff of the shoulder associated with pathologic changes in the acromion. J Bone Joint Surg Am 70:1224-1230, 1988.

37. Yeh L, Kwak S, Kim YS, et al: Anterior labroligamentous structures of the glenohumeral joint: Correlation of MR arthrography and anatomic dissection in cadavers. AJR Am J Roentgenol 171:1229-1236, 1998.

38. Steinbeck J, Liljenquist U, Jerosch J: The anatomy of the glenohumeral ligamentous complex and its contribution to anterior shoulder stability. J Shoulder Elbow Surg 7:122-126, 1998.

39. Cooper DE, Arnoczky SP, O'Brien SJ, et al: Anatomy, histology, and vascularity of the glenoid labrum. An anatomical study. J Bone Joint Surg Am 74:46-52, 1992.

40. Johnson LL: Arthroscopy Surgery: Principles and Practice, 3rd ed. St. Louis: CV Mosby, 1986.

41. Williams MM, Snyder SJ, Buford D Jr: The Buford complex—the "cord-like" middle glenohumeral ligament and absent anterosuperior labrum complex: A normal anatomic capsulolabral variant. Arthroscopy 10:241-247, 1994.

42. Das SP, Ray GS, Saha AK: Observations on the tilt of the glenoid cavity of scapula. J Anat Soc India 15:114-118, 1966.

43. Churchill RS, Brems JJ, Kotschi H: Glenoid size, inclination, and version: An anatomic study. J Shoulder Elbow Surg 10:327-332, 2001.

44. Iannotti JP, Gabriel JP, Schneck SL, et al: The normal glenohumeral relationships. An anatomic study of one hundred and forty shoulders. J Bone Joint Surg Am 74:491-500, 1992.

45. Debevoise NT, Hyatt GW, Townsend GB: Humeral torsion in recurrent shoulder dislocations. Clin Orthop Relat Res 76:87-93, 1971.

46. Farrokh D, Fabeck L, Descamps PY, et al: Computed tomography measurement of humeral head retroversion: Influence of patient positioning. J Shoulder Elbow Surg 10:550-553, 2001.

47. Putti V: Beitrag zur Ätiologie, Pathogenese und Behandlung des angeborenen Hochstandes des Schulterblattes. Fortschr Geb Röntgenstr 12:328-349, 1908.

48. Scaglietti O: The obstetrical shoulder trauma. Surg Gynecol Obstet 66:868-877, 1938.

49. Waters PM, Smith GR, Jaramillo D: Glenohumeral deformity secondary to brachial plexus birth palsy. J Bone Joint Surg Am 80:668-677, 1998.

50. Edelson G: Variations in the retroversion of the humeral head. J Shoulder Elbow Surg 8:142-145, 1999.

51. Edelson G: The development of humeral head retroversion. J Shoulder Elbow Surg 9:316-318, 2000.

52. Crenshaw AH, Kilgore WE: Surgical treatment of bicipital tenosynovitis. J Bone Joint Surg Am 48:1496-1502, 1966.

53. Dines D, Warren RF, Inglis AE: Surgical treatment of lesions of the long head of the biceps. Clin Orthop Relat Res (164):165-171, 1982.

54. O'Donoghue DH: Subluxing biceps tendon in the athlete. Clin Orthop Relat Res (164):26-29, 1982.

55. Hitchcock HH, Bechtol CO: Painful shoulder. Observations on the role of the tendon of the long head of the biceps brachii in its causation. J Bone Joint Surg Am 30:263-273, 1948.

56. Meyer AW: Spontaneous dislocation and destruction of tendon of long head of biceps brachii: Fifty-nine instances. Arch Surg 17:493-506, 1928.

57. Cutter E: Descriptive catalogue of the Warren Anatomical Museum. In Jackson JBS (ed): Descriptive Catalogue, vol 217. Boston: A Williams, 1870, p 21.

58. Fawcett: The development and ossification of the human clavicle. J Anat 47:225-234, 1913.

59. Fitchet SM: Cleidocranial dysostosis: Hereditary and familial. J Bone Joint Surg 11:838-866, 1929.

60. Gardner E: The embryology of the clavicle. Clin Orthop Relat Res (58):9-16, 1968.

61. Gardner E, Gray DJ: Prenatal development of the human shoulder and acromioclavicular joint. Am J Anat 92:219-276, 1953.

62. Hultkrantz JW: Über congenitalen Schlusselbeindefect und damit verbunden Schädelanomalien. Anat Anz 15:237, 1898.

63. Jansen M: Feebleness of Growth and Congenital Dwarfism. London: H Froude, Hodder, and Stoughton, 1921.

64. Marie P, Sainton P: On hereditary cleido-cranial dysostosis. Clin Orthop Relat Res (58):5-7, 1968.

65. Soule AB: Mutational dysostosis (cleidocranial dysostosis). J Bone Joint Surg Am 28:81-102, 1946.

66. Terry RJ: Rudimentary clavicles and other abnormalities of the skeleton of a white woman. Anat Physiol 33:413-422, 1899.

67. Rhinehart BA: Cleidocranial dysostosis (mutational dysostosis) with a case report. Radiology 26:741-748, 1936.

68. Lewis MM, Ballet FL, Kroll PG, Bloom N: En bloc clavicular resection: Operative procedure and postoperative testing of function: Case reports. Clin Orthop Relat Res (193):214-220, 1985.

69. Gross A: Über angeborenen Mangel der Schlüsselbeine. Munch Med Wochenschr 1:1151, 1903.

70. Jones HW: Cleido-cranial dysostosis. St Thomas Hosp Gazette 36:193-201, 1937.

71. Stocks P, Barrington A: Treasury of Human Inheritance, vol 3. London: Cambridge University Press, 1925, p 121.

72. Fitzwilliams DCL: Hereditary cranio-cleido-dysostosis. Lancet 2:1466, 1910.

73. Flynn DM: Family with cleido-cranial dysostosis showing normal and abnormal clavicles. Proc R Soc Med 6:491-492, 1966.

74. Eventov I, Reider-Grosswasser I, Weiss S, et al: Cleidocranial dysplasia: A family study. Clin Radiol 30:323-328, 1979.

75. Crouzon O, Buttier H: Sur une forme particulière, de la dysostosis cleidocranienine de Pierre Marie et Sainton (forme cleido-cranio-pelvienne). Bull Mem Soc Dilale Hop 45:972, 1099, 1921.

76. Dhooge I, Lantsoght B, Lemmerling M, et al: Hearing loss as a presenting symptom of cleidocranial dysplasia. Otol Neurotol 22:855-857, 2001.

77. Visosky AMB, Johnson J, Bingea B, et al: Otolaryngological manifestations of cleidocranial dysplasia, concentrating on audiological findings. Laryngoscope 113:1508-1514, 2003.

78. Paltauf R: Demonstration eines Skelettes von einem Falle von Dysostosis cleidocranialis. Verh Dtsch Ges Pathol 15:337, 1912.

79. Fairbank HAT: Cranio-cleido-dysostosis. J Bone Joint Surg Br 31:608-617, 1949.

80. Alldred AJ: Congenital pseudarthrosis of the clavicle. J Bone Joint Surg Br 45:312-319, 1963.

81. Kite JH: Congenital pseudarthrosis of the clavicle. South Med J 61:703-710, 1968.
82. Saint-Pierre L: Pseudarthrose congénitale de la clavicule droite. Ann Anat Pathol 7:466, 1930.
83. Schoenecker PL, Johnson GE, Howard B, Capelli AM: Congenital pseudarthrosis. Orthop Rev 21:855-860, 1992.
84. Carpenter EB, Garrett RG: Congenital pseudarthrosis of the clavicle. J Bone Joint Surg Am 42:337-340, 1960.
85. Shalom A, Khermosh O, Weintroub S: The natural history of congenital pseudarthrosis of the clavicle. J Bone Joint Surg Br 76:846-847, 1994.
86. Ahmadi B, Steel HH: Congenital pseudarthrosis of the clavicle. Clin Orthop Relat Res (126):130-134, 1977.
87. Ghormley RK, Black JR, Cherry JH: Ununited fractures of the clavicle. Am J Surg 51:343-349, 1941.
88. Herman S: Congenital bilateral pseudarthrosis of the clavicle. Clin Orthop Relat Res (91):162-163, 1973.
89. Lloyd-Roberts GC, Apley AG, Owen R: Reflections upon the aetiology of congenital pseudarthrosis of the clavicle. J Bone Joint Surg Br 57:24-29, 1975.
90. Lorente Molto FJ, Bonete Lluch DJ, Garrido IM: Congenital pseudarthrosis of the clavicle: A proposal for early surgical treatment. J Pediatr Orthop 21:689-693, 2001.
91. Owen R: Congenital pseudarthrosis of the clavicle. J Bone Joint Surg Br 52:644-652, 1970.
92. Padua R, Romanini E, Conti C, et al: Bilateral congenital pseudarthrosis of the clavicle: Report of a case with clinical, radiological and neurophysiological evaluation. Acta Orthop Belg 65:372-375, 1999.
93. Quinlan WR, Brady PG, Regan BF: Congenital pseudar-throsis of the clavicle. Acta Orthop Scand 51:489-492, 1980.
94. Russo MTP, Maffulli N: Bilateral congenital pseudarthrosis of the clavicle. Arch Orthop Trauma Surg 109:177-178, 1990.
95. Sakkers RJ, Tjin a Ton E, Bos CF: Left-sided congenital pseudarthrosis of the clavicula. J Pediatr Orthop B 8:45-47, 1999.
96. Jinkins WJ: Congenital pseudarthrosis of the clavicle. Clin Orthop Relat Res 62:183-186, 1969.
97. Bargar WL, Marcus RE, Ittleman FP: Late thoracic outlet syndrome secondary to pseudarthrosis of the clavicle. J Trauma 24:857-859, 1984.
98. Hahn K, Shah R, Shalev Y, et al: Congenital clavicular pseudoarthrosis associated with vascular thoracic outlet syndrome: Case presentation and review of the literature. Cathet Cardiovasc Diagn 35:321-327, 1995.
99. Sales de Gauzey J, Baunin C, Puget C, et al: Congenital pseudarthrosis of the clavicle and thoracic outlet syndrome in adolescence. J Pediatr Orthop B 8:299-301, 1999.
100. Valette H: Pseudarthrose congénitale de la clavicule et syndrome de la traversée thoraco-brachiale. Revue de la literature à propos d'un cas. J Mal Vasc 20:51-52, 1995.
101. Young MC, Richards RR, Hudson AR: Thoracic outlet syndrome with congenital pseudarthrosis of the clavicle: Treatment by brachial plexus decompression, plate fixation and bone grafting. Can J Surg 31:131-133, 1988.
102. Gibson DA, Carroll N: Congenital pseudarthrosis of the clavicle. J Bone Joint Surg Br 52:629-643, 1970.
103. Gruenberg H: The Genesis of Skeletal Abnormalities. Second International Conference on Congenital Malformations. New York: International Medical Congress, 1963, p 219.
104. Mooney JF, Koman LA: Bilateral pseudarthrosis of the clavicle associated with trisomy 12. Orthopedics 14:171-172, 1991.
105. Price BD, Price CT: Familial congenital pseudoarthrosis of the clavicle: Case report and literature review. Iowa Orthop J 16:153-156, 1996.
106. Tachdjian MO: Pediatric Orthopedics, vol 1, 2nd ed. Philadelphia: WB Saunders, 1990, pp 136-179.
107. Wall JJ: Congenital pseudarthrosis of the clavicle. J Bone Joint Surg Am 52:1003-1009, 1970.
108. Marmor L: Repair of congenital pseudarthrosis of the clavicle. Clin Orthop Relat Res 46:111-113, 1966.
109. Nogi J, Heckman JD, Hakala M, Sweet DE: Non-union of the clavicle in a child. Clin Orthop Relat Res (110):19-21, 1975.
110. Toledo LC, MacEwen GD: Severe complication of surgical treatment of congenital pseudarthrosis of the clavicle. Clin Orthop Relat Res (139):64-67, 1979.
111. Engel D: The etiology of the undescended scapula and related syndromes. J Bone Joint Surg 25:613-625, 1943.
112. Horwitz AE: Congenital elevation of the scapula—Sprengel's deformity. Am J Orthop Surg 6:260-311, 1908.
113. Petrie JG: Congenital elevation of the scapula. J Bone Joint Surg Br 55:441, 1973.
114. Eulenburg M: Beitrag zur Dislocation der Scapula. Amtlicher Bericht über die Versammlung deutscher Naturforscher und Artze 37:291-294, 1863.
115. Eulenburg M: Casuistische Mittheilungen aus dem Gebiete der Orthopädie. Arch Klin Chir 4:301, 1863.
116. Eulenburg M: Hochgradige Dislocation der Scapula, bedingt durch Retraction des M. levator anguli, und des oberen Theiles des M. cucullaris. Heilung mittelst subcutaner Durchschneidung beider Muskeln und entsprechender Nachbehandlung. Arch Klin Chir 4:304-311, 1863.
117. Kolliker T: Mittheilungen aus der chirurgische Casuistik und kleinere Mittheilunge. Bemerkungen zum Aufsatze von Dr. Sprengel. "Die angeborene Vershiebung dies schulter Blattes nach Oben." Arch Klin Chir 42:925, 1891.
118. Sprengel RD: Die angeborene Verschiebung des Schulterblattes nach Oben. Arch Klin Chir 42:545-549, 1891.
119. Willet A, Walsham WJ: An account of the dissection of the parts removed after death from the body of a woman: The subject of congenital malformations of the spinal column, bony thorax, and left scapular arch. Proc R Med Chir Soc 8:503-506, 1880.
120. Willet A, Walsham WJ: A second case of malformation of the left shoulder girdle, with remarks on the probable nature of the deformity. BMJ 1:513-514, 1883.
121. McClure JG, Raney RB: Anomalies of the scapula. Clin Orthop Relat Res (110):22-31, 1975.
122. Cavendish ME: Congenital elevation of the scapula. J Bone Joint Surg Br 54:395-408, 1972.
123. Frosch L: Congenital subluxation of shoulders. Klin Wochenschr 4:701-702, 1923.
124. McMurtry I, Bennet GC, Bradish C: Osteotomy for congenital elevation of the scapula (Sprengel's deformity). J Bone Joint Surg Br 87:986-989, 2005.
125. Bagg HJ, Halter CR: Further studies on the inheritance of structural defects in the descendants of mice exposed to roentgen-ray irradiation [abstract]. Anat Rec 37:183, 1927.
126. Blair JD, Wells PO: Bilateral undescended scapula associated with omovertebral bone. J Bone Joint Surg Am 39:201-206, 1957.
127. Bonnevie K: Embryological analysis of gene manifestation in Little and Bagg's abnormal mouse tribe. J Exp Zool 67:443, 1934.
128. Weed LH: The Development of the Cerebrospinal Spaces (Contribution to Embryology No. 14), Publication 225. Washington, DC: Carnegie Institute, 1916.
129. Hamner DL, Hall JE: Sprengel's deformity associated with multidirectional shoulder instability. J Pediatr Orthop 15:641-643, 1995.
130. Ross DM, Cruess RL: The surgical correction of congenital elevation of the scapula: A review of seventy-seven cases. Clin Orthop Relat Res (125):17-23, 1977.
131. Borges JL, Shah A, Torres BC, Bowen JR: Modified Woodward procedure for Sprengel deformity of the shoulder: Long-term results. J Pediatr Orthop 16:508-513, 1996.
132. Carson WG, Lovell WW, Whitesides TE: Congenital elevation of the scapula. J Bone Joint Surg Am 63:1199-1207, 1981.
133. Farsetti P, Weinstein SL, Caterini R, et al: Sprengel's deformity: Long-term follow-up study of 22 cases. J Pediatr Orthop B 12:202-210, 2003.
134. Pinsky HA, Pizzutillo PD, MacEwen GD: Congenital elevation of the scapula. Orthop Trans 4:288-289, 1980.
135. Banniza von Bazan U: The association between congenital elevation of the scapula and diastematomyelia: A preliminary report. J Bone Joint Surg Br 61:59-63, 1979.
136. Duthie RB, Bentley G: Congenital malformations. In Duthie RB, Bentley G (eds): Mercer's Orthopaedic Surgery, 8th ed. Baltimore: University Park Press, 1983, pp 118-199.
137. Grogan DP, Stanley EA, Bobechko WP: The congenital undescended scapula. Surgical correction by the Woodward procedure. J Bone Joint Surg Br 65:598-605, 1983.
138. McBurney S: Congenital deformity due to malposition of the scapula. N Y Med J 47:582-583, 1888.
139. Green WT: The surgical correction of congenital elevation of the scapula (Sprengel's deformity). J Bone Joint Surg Am 39:1439, 1957.
140. Inclan A: Congenital elevation of the scapula or Sprengel's deformity: Two clinical cases treated with Ober's operation. Circ Ortop Traum (Habana) 15:1, 1949.
141. Khoo FY, Kuo CL: An unusual anomaly of the inferior portion of the scapula. J Bone Joint Surg Am 30:1010-1011, 1948.
142. Konig F: Eine neue Operation des angeborenen Schulterblatthochstandes. Beitr Klin Chir 94:530-537, 1914.
143. Wilkinson JA, Campbell D: Scapular osteotomy for Sprengel's shoulder. J Bone Joint Surg Br 62:486-490, 1980.
144. Woodward JW: Congenital elevation of the scapula: Correction by release and transplantation of muscle origins—a preliminary report. J Bone Joint Surg Am 43:219-228, 1961.
145. Khairouni A, Bensahel H, Csukonyi Z, et al: Congenital high scapula. J Pediatr Orthop B 11:85-88, 2002.
146. Jeannopoulos CL: Congenital elevation of the scapula. J Bone Joint Surg Am 34:883-892, 1952.
147. Leibovic SJ, Ehrlich MG, Zaleske DJ: Sprengel deformity. J Bone Joint Surg Am 72:192-197, 1990.
148. Robinson A, Braun RM, Mack P, Zadek R: The surgical importance of the clavicular component of Sprengel's deformity. J Bone Joint Surg Am 49:1481, 1967.
149. Galpin RD, Birch JG: Congenital elevation of the scapula (Sprengel's deformity). Pediatr Orthop 10:965-970, 1987.

150. Grietemann B, Rondhuis JJ, Karbowski A: Treatment of congenital elevation of the scapula. 10 (2-18) year follow-up of 37 cases of Sprengel's deformity. Acta Orthop Scand 64:365-368, 1993.

151. Klisic P, Filipovic M, Uzelac O, Milinkovic Z: Relocation of congenitally elevated scapula. J Pediatr Orthop 1:43-45, 1981.

152. Anson BJ (ed): Morris' Human Anatomy, 12th ed. New York: Blakiston, 1966.

153. Chiba S, Suzuki T, Kasi T: A rare anomaly of the pectoralis major—the chondroepitrochlearis. Folia Anat (Japan) 60:175-186, 1983.

154. Folliasson A: Un cas d'os acromial. Rev Orthop 20:533-538, 1933.

155. Grant BJC: Grant's Atlas of Anatomy, 6th ed. Baltimore: Williams & Wilkins, 1972.

156. Köhler A: Roentgenology: The Borderlands of the Normal and Early Pathological in the Skiagram, 5th ed, ed and trans A Turnbull. New York: William Wood, 1928.

157. Lewis WH (ed): Gray's Anatomy of the Human Body, 22nd ed. Philadelphia: Lea & Febiger, 1930.

158. Liberson F: Os acromiale—a contested anomaly. J Bone Joint Surg 19:683-689, 1937.

159. Sammarco VJ: Os acromiale: Frequency, anatomy, and clinical implications. J Bone Joint Surg Am 82:394-400, 2000.

160. Gumina S, De Santis P, Salvatore M, Postacchini, F: Relationship between os acromiale and acromioclavicular joint anatomic position. J Shoulder Elbow Surg 12:6-8, 2003.

161. Mudge MK, Wood VE, Frykman GK: Rotator cuff tears associated with os acromiale. J Bone Joint Surg Am 66:427-429, 1984.

162. Neumann W: Über das "Os acromiale." Fortschr Geb Röntgenstr 25:180-191, 1918.

163. Schar W, Zweifel C: Das Os acromiale und seine klinische Bedeutung. Bruns Beitr Klin Chir 164:101-124, 1936.

164. Neer CS: Impingement lesions. Clin Orthop Relat Res (173):70-77, 1983.

165. Bigliani LU, Norris TR, Fischer J, Neer CS 2nd: The relationship between the unfused acromial epiphysis and subacromial impingement lesions. Orthop Trans 7:138, 1983.

166. Warner JJ, Beim GM, Higgins SL: The treatment of symptomatic os acromiale. J Bone Joint Surg Am 80:1320-1326, 1998.

167. Edelson JG, Zuckerman J, Hershkovitz I: Os acromiale: Anatomy and surgical implications. J Bone Joint Surg Br 75:551-555, 1993.

168. Ryu RK, Fan RS, Dunbar WH: The treatment of symptomatic os acromiale. Orthopedics 22:325-328, 1999.

169. Salamon PB: The treatment of symptomatic os acromiale [comment]. J Bone Joint Surg Am 81:1198, 1999.

170. Satterlee CC: Successful osteosynthesis of an unstable mesoacromion in 6 shoulders: A new technique. J Shoulder Elbow Surg 8:125-129, 1999.

171. Hertel R, Windisch W, Schuster A, Ballmer FT: Transacromial approach to obtain fusion of unstable os acromiale. J Shoulder Elbow Surg 7:606-609, 1998.

172. Hutchinson MR, Veenstra MA: Arthroscopic decompression of shoulder impingement secondary to os acromiale. Arthroscopy 9:28-32, 1993.

173. Wright RW, Heller MA, Quick DC, Buss DD: Arthroscopic decompression for impingement syndrome secondary to an unstable os acromiale. Arthroscopy 16:595-599, 2000.

174. Pagnani MJ, Mathis CE, Solman CG: Painful os acromiale (or unfused acromial apophysis) in athletes. J Shoulder Elbow Surg 15:432-435, 2006.

175. Kozlowski K, Colavita N, Morris L, Little KE: Bilateral glenoid dysplasia (report of 8 cases). Australas Radiol 29:174-177, 1985.

176. Kozlowski K, Scougall J: Congenital bilateral glenoid hypoplasia: A report of four cases. Br J Radiol 60:705-706, 1987.

177. Owen R: Bilateral glenoid hypoplasia: Report of five cases. J Bone Joint Surg Br 35:262-267, 1953.

178. Wirth MA, Lyons FR, Rockwood CA: Hypoplasia of the glenoid: A review of sixteen patients. J Bone Joint Surg Am 75:1175-1184, 1993.

179. Samilson RL: Congenital and developmental anomalies of the shoulder girdle. Orthop Clin North Am Relat Res (11):219-231, 1980.

180. Lintner DM, Sebastianelli WJ, Hanks GA, Kalenak A: Glenoid dysplasia: A case report and review of the literature. Clin Orthop Relat Res (283):145-148, 1992.

181. Fuhrmann W, Koch F, Rauterberg K: Dominant erbliche Hypolplasie und Bewegungseinschrankung bei der Schultergelenke. Z Orthop 104:584-588, 1968.

182. Pettersson H: Bilateral dysplasia of the neck of the scapula and associated anomalies. Acta Radiol 22:81-84, 1981.

183. Stanciu C, Morin B: Congenital glenoid dysplasia: Case report in two consecutive generations. J Pediatr Orthop 14:389-391, 1994.

184. Curriano G, Sheffield E, Twickler D: Congenital glenoid dysplasia. Pediatr Radiol 28:30-37, 1998.

185. Brailsford JE: The Radiology of Bones and Joints, 5th ed. Baltimore: Williams & Wilkins, 1953, pp 133, 135-137.

186. Sutro CJ: Dentated articular surface of the glenoid—an anomaly. Bull Hosp Joint Dis 27:104-108, 1967.

187. Sperling JW, Cofield RH, Steinmann SP: Shoulder arthroplasty for osteoarthritis secondary to glenoid dysplasia. J Bone Joint Surg Am 84:541-546, 2002.

188. Köhler A: Röntgenology, 2nd ed. London: Baillière, Tindall & Cox, 1935.

189. Gill TJ, Waters P: Valgus osteotomy of the humeral neck: A technique for treatment of humerus varus. J Shoulder Elbow Surg 6:306-310, 1997.

190. Ellefsen BK, Frierson MA, Raney EM, Ogden JA: Humerus varus: A complication of neonatal, infantile, and child-hood injury and infection. J Pediatr Orthop 14:479-486, 1994.

191. Ogden JA, Weil UH, Hempton RF: Developmental humerus varus. Clin Orthop Relat Res (116):158-165, 1976.

192. Lloyd-Roberts GC: Humerus varus: Report of a case treated by excision of the acromion. J Bone Joint Surg Br Relat Res (35):268-269, 1953.

193. Lucas LS, Gill JH: Humerus varus following birth injury to the proximal humeral epiphysis. J Bone Joint Surg 29:367-369, 1947.

194. Golthamer CR: Duplication of the clavicle ("os subclaviculare"). Radiology 68:576-578, 1957.

195. Reinhardt K: Eine doppelseitige Anomalie am lateralen Klavikuladrittel, bestehend aus einer bogenförmigen Duplikatur des Knochens in Richtung auf das Caracoid und aus akzessorischen Knochenelementen. Fortschr Geb Röntgenstr Nuklearmed 113:527-530, 1970.

196. Rutherford H: Bifurcate clavicle. J Anat 55:286-287, 1921.

197. Sharma BG: Duplication of the clavicle with triplication of the coracoid process. Skeletal Radiol 32:661-664, 2003.

198. Twigg HL, Rosenbaum RC: Duplication of the clavicle. Skeletal Radiol 6:281, 1981.

199. Köhler A, Wilk S: Borderlands of the Normal and Early Pathologic in Skeletal Roentgenology, 3rd ed. New York: Grune & Stratton, 1968, p 163.

200. Sharrard WJW: Paediatric Orthopaedics and Fractures. Oxford: Blackwell Scientific, 1971.

201. Birkner R: Fortschr Röntgenstr 82:695, 1935.

202. Pate D, Kursunoglu S, Resnick D, Resnik CS: Scapular foramina. Skeletal Radiol 14:270-275, 1985.

203. McClure JG, Raney RB: Double acromion and coracoid processes: Case report of an anomaly of the scapula. J Bone Joint Surg Am 56:830-832, 1974.

204. Arens W: Eine seltene angeborene Missbildung des Schultergelenkes. Fortschr Geb Röntgenstr Nuklearmed 75:365-367, 1951.

205. Martini AK, Neusel E: Duplication of the scapula. Int Orthop 11:361-366, 1987.

206. Stacy GS, Yousefzadeh DK: Scapular duplication. Pediatr Radiol 30:412-414, 2000.

207. Stein HC, Bettmann EH: Rare malformation of the arm. Double humerus with three hands and sixteen fingers. Am J Surg 1:336-343, 1940.

208. Bateman JE: Evolution, Embryology and Congenital Anomalies. Philadelphia: WB Saunders, 1972, pp 5-38.

209. DePalma AF: Congenital abnormalities of the neck–shoulder region. In DePalma AF (ed): Surgery of the Shoulder, 3rd ed. Philadelphia: JB Lippincott, 1983, pp 24-34.

210. Frasseto F: Tre casi di articolazione coraco-clavicolare osservati radiograficamente sul vivente. Nota antropologica e clinica. Chir Organi Mov 5:116-124, 1921.

211. Hall FJS: Coracoclavicular joint: A rare condition treated successfully by operation. BMJ 1:766-768, 1950.

212. Hama H, Matsusue Y, Ito H, Yamamuro T: Thoracic outlet syndrome associated with an anomalous coracoclavicular joint. A case report. J Bone Joint Surg Am 75:1368-1369, 1993.

213. Nutter PD: Coracoclavicular articulations. J Bone Joint Surg 23:177-179, 1941.

214. Poirer P: La clavicle et ses articulations: Bourses séreuses des ligaments costo-claviculaire. J Anat Physiol 26:81-103, 1890.

215. Ponde A, Silveira J: Estudos radiológicos da articulacao coraco-clavicular. J Clin 22:325-328, 1930.

216. Schlyvitch B: Über den Articulus coracoclavicularis. Anat Anz 85:89-93, 1937.

217. Wertheimer LG: Coracoclavicular joint. J Bone Joint Surg Am 30:570-578, 1948.

218. Finder JG: Congenital anomaly of the coracoid. Os coracocosternale vestigiale. J Bone Joint Surg 18:148-152, 1936.

219. Bamforth JS, Bell MH, Hall JG, Salter RB: Congenital shortness of the costocoracoid ligament. Am J Med Genet 33:444-446, 1989.

220. Goodwin CB, Simmons EH, Taylor I: Cervical vertebral-costal process (costovertebral bone)—a previously unreported anomaly. J Bone Joint Surg Am 66:1477-1479, 1984.

221. Subkowitsch EM: Zur Frage der Morphologie des Schultergurtels. I. Entwicklung und Morphologie des Processus coracoides bei Mensch und Fledermaus. Morphol Jahrb 65:517-538, 1931.

222. Mikawa Y, Watanabe R, Yamano Y: Omoclavicular bar in congenital elevation of the scapula: A new finding. Spine 16:376-377, 1991.

223. Orrell KG, Bell DF: Structural abnormality of the clavicle associated with Sprengel's deformity: A case report. Clin Orthop Relat Res (258):157-159, 1990.

224. Adler KJ: Verwechslung der Apophyse des Angulus inferior Scapulae mit linem Rundschalten. Röntgenpraxis 13:188, 1941.

225. Edelson JG: Variations in the anatomy of the scapula with reference to the snapping scapula. Clin Orthop Relat Res (322):111-115, 1996.

226. Lossen H, Wegner RN: Die Knockenkene der scapula, röntgenodogisch und verglerchend-anatomish Behachtet. Fortschr Geb Röntgenstr 53:443, 1936.

227. Gray DJ: Variations in human scapulae. Am J Physiol Anthropol 29:57-72, 1942.

228. Brown LM, Robson MJ, Sharrard WJW: The pathophysiology of arthrogryposis multiplex congenita neurologica. J Bone Joint Surg Br 62:291-296, 1980.

229. Dick HM, Tietjen R: Humeral lengthening for septic neonatal growth arrest. Case report. J Bone Joint Surg Am 60:1138, 1978.

230. Dobyns JH: Phocomelia. In Green DP (ed): Operative Hand Surgery, vol 1. New York: Churchill Livingstone, 1982, pp 216-219.

231. Flatt AE: The Care of Congenital Hand Anomalies. St. Louis: CV Mosby, 1977, p 51.

232. Frantz CH, O'Rahilly R: Congenital skeletal limb deficiencies. J Bone Joint Surg Am 43:1202-1224, 1961.

233. Neviaser RJ: Injuries to and developmental deformities of the shoulder. In Bora FW (ed): The Pediatric Upper Extremity: Diagnosis and Management. Philadelphia: WB Saunders, 1986, pp 235-246.

234. Sulamaa M: Autotransplantation of epiphysis in neonates. Acta Chir Scand 119:194, 1960.

235. Sulamaa M: Treatment of some skeletal deformities. Postgrad Med J 39:67-82, 1963.

236. Sulamaa M: Upper extremity phocomelia: A contribution to its operative treatment. Clin Pediatr (Phila) 2:251-257, 1963.

237. Swanson AB: A classification for congenital limb malformations. J Hand Surg 1:8-22, 1976.

238. Taussig HB: A study of the German outbreak of phocomelia: The thalidomide syndrome. JAMA 180:1106-1114, 1962.

239. Hermans JJ, Mooyaart EL, Hendriks JG, Diercks RL: Familial congenital bilateral agenesis of the acromion: A radiologically illustrated case report. Surg Radiol Anat 21:337-339, 1999.

240. Kim SJ, Min BH: Congenital bilateral absence of the acromion. A case report. Clin Orthop Relat Res (300):117-119, 1994.

241. Andreasen AT: Congenital absence of the humeral head: Report of two cases. J Bone Joint Surg Br 30:333-337, 1948.

242. Chang CJ: Holt–Oram syndrome. Radiology 88:479-483, 1967.

243. Ferrell RL, Jones B, Lucas RV: Simultaneous occurrence of the Holt–Oram and the Duane syndromes. J Pediatr 69:630-634, 1966.

244. Gall JC Jr, Stern AM, Cohen MM, et al: Holt–Oram syndrome: Clinical and genetic study of a large family. Am J Hum Genet 18:187-200, 1966.

245. Gellis SS, Feingold M: Denouement and discussion. Holt–Oram syndrome. Am J Dis Child 112:465-466, 1966.

246. Gibson S, Clifton WM: Congenital heart disease: Clinical and postmortem study of 105 cases. Am J Dis Child 55:761-767, 1938.

247. Holmes LB: Congenital heart disease and upper-extremity deformities: A report of two families. N Engl J Med 272:437-444, 1965.

248. Holt M, Oram S: Familial heart disease with skeletal malformations. Br Heart J 22:236-242, 1960.

249. MacMahon B, McKeown T, Record RG: Incidence and life expectation of children with congenital heart disease. Br Heart J 15:121-129, 1953.

250. Poznanski AK, Gall JC, Stern AM: Skeletal manifestations of the Holt–Oram syndrome. Radiology 94:45-53, 1970.

251. Wiland OK: Extracardiac anomalies in association with congenital heart disease: Analysis of 200 necropsy cases. Lab Invest 5:380-388, 1956.

252. Beals RK, Crawford S: Congenital absence of the pectoral muscles: A review of twenty-five patients. Clin Orthop Relat Res (119):166-171, 1976.

253. Duncan JG, Souter WA: Hereditary onycho-osteodysplasia: The nail patella syndrome. J Bone Joint Surg Br 45:242-258, 1963.

254. Jameson RJ, Lawler SD, Renwick JH: Nail patella syndrome: Clinical and linkage data on family G. Ann Hum Genet 20:348-360, 1956.

255. Renwick JH: Nail–patella syndrome: Evidence for modification by alleles at the main locus. Ann Hum Genet 21:159-169, 1956.

256. Duthie RB, Hecht F: The inheritance and development of the nail patella syndrome. J Bone Joint Surg Br 45:259-267, 1963.

257. McCluskey KA: The nail patella syndrome (hereditary onycho-osteodysplasia.) Can J Surg 4:192-204, 1961.

258. Turner JW: An hereditary arthrodysplasia associated with hereditary dystrophy of the nails. JAMA 100:882-884, 1933.

259. Loomer RL: Shoulder girdle dysplasia associated with nail patella syndrome: A case report and literature review. Clin Orthop Relat Res (238):112-116, 1989.

260. Bessieres-Grattagliano B, Brodaty G, Martinovic J, et al: Oto-onycho-peroneal syndrome: Further delineation and first fetal report. Am J Med Genet A 128:316-319, 2004.

261. Devriendt K, Stoffelen D, Pfeiffer R, et al: Oto-onycho-peroneal syndrome: confirmation of a syndrome. J Med Genet 35:508-509, 1998.

262. Pfeiffer RA: The oto-onycho-peroneal syndrome. A probably new genetic entity. Eur J Pediatr 138:317-320, 1982.

263. Apert E: De l'acrocephalosyndactylie. Bull Mem Soc Med Hop Paris 23:1310-1330, 1906.

264. Upton J: Classification and pathologic anatomy of limb anomalies. Clin Plast Surg 18:321-355, 1991.

265. Cuthbert R: Acrocephalosyndactyly with case report illustrating some of the radiological features. Glasgow Med J 35:349-356, 1954.

266. Wood VE, Sauser DD, O'Hara RC: The shoulder and elbow in Apert's syndrome. J Pediatr Orthop 15:648-651, 1995.

267. Blank CE: Apert's syndrome (a type of acrocephalosyndactyly): Observations of a British series of thirty-nine cases. Ann Hum Genet 24:151-164, 1960.

268. Bosley RC: Total acromionectomy: A twenty-year review. J Bone Joint Surg Am 73:961-968, 1991.

269. Hoover GH, Flatt AE, Weiss MW: The hand and Apert's syndrome. J Bone Joint Surg Am 52:878-895, 1970.

270. Park AE, Powers EF: Acrocephaly and scaphocephaly with symmetrically distributed malformation of the extremities: Study of so-called "acrocephalosyndactylism." Am J Dis Child 20:255-315, 1920.

271. Senrui H, Egawa T, Horiki A: Anatomical findings in the hands of patients with Poland's syndrome. J Bone Joint Surg Am 64:1079-1082, 1982.

272. Weech AA: Combined acrocephaly and syndactylism occurring in mother and daughter: A case report. Bull Johns Hopkins Hosp 40:73-74, 1927.

273. Yonenobu K, Tada K, Tsuyuguchi Y: Apert's syndrome—a report of five cases. Hand 14:317-325, 1982.

274. Rubin P: Dynamic Classification of Bone Dysplasias. Chicago: Year Book Medical Publishers, 1964, p 146.

275. Ingram RR: The shoulder in multiple epiphyseal dysplasia. J Bone Joint Surg Br 73:277-279, 1991.

276. Barrie H, Carter C, Sutcliffe J: Multiple epiphyseal dysplasia. BMJ 2(5089):133-137, 1958.

277. Hoefnagel D, Sycamore LK, Russell SW, Bucknall WE: Hereditary multiple epiphyseal dysplasia. Ann Hum Genet 30:201-210, 1967.

278. Juberg RC, Holt JF: Inheritance of multiple epiphyseal dysplasia tarda. Am J Hum Genet 20:549-563, 1968.

279. Kozlowski K, Lipska E: Hereditary dysplasia epiphysealis multiplex. Clin Radiol 18:330-336, 1967.

280. Ribbing S: Studien über hereditäre multiple epiphysenstörungen. Acta Radiol 1-107, 1937.

281. Wynne-Davies R, Hall CM, Apley AG: Multiple epiphyseal dysplasia. In Wynne-Davies R, Hall CM, Apley AG (eds): Atlas of Skeletal Dysplasias. New York: Churchill Livingstone, 1985, pp 19-35.

282. Amor DJ, Savarirayan R, Bankier A, et al: Autosomal dominant inheritance of scapuloiliac dysostosis. Am J Med Genet 95:507-509, 2000.

283. Blane CE, Holt JF, Vine AK: Scapuloiliac dysostosis. Br J Radiol 57:526-528, 1984.

284. Kosenow W, Niederle J, Sinios A: Becken-Schuler-Dysplasie. Fortschr Geb Röntgenstr Nuklearmed 113:39-48, 1970.

285. Thomas PS, Reid M, McCurdy A: Pelvis–shoulder dysplasia. Pediatr Radiol 5:219-223, 1977.

286. Walbaum R, Titran M, Durieux Y, Crepin G: Tetradactylie des deux mains, hypoplasie des deux perones et hypoplasie scapulo-iliaque: Un nouveau syndrome? J Genet Hum 30:309-312, 1982.

287. Hauser SE, Chemke JM, Bankier A: Pelvis-shoulder dysplasia. Pediatr Radiol 28:681-682, 1998.

288. Cozen L: Congenital dislocation of the shoulder and other anomalies. Report of a case and review of the literature. Arch Surg 35:956-966, 1937.

289. Edwards H: Congenital displacement of shoulder joint. J Anat 62:177-182, 1928.

290. Greig DM: True congenital dislocation of shoulder. Edinburgh Med J 30:157-175, 1923.

291. Heilbronner DM: True congenital dislocation of the shoulder. J Pediatr Orthop 10:408-410, 1990.

292. Kuhn D, Rosman M: Traumatic, nonparalytic dislocation of the shoulder in a newborn infant. J Pediatr Orthop 4:121-122, 1984.

293. Roberts J: Quoted in Rockwood CA: Fractures and dislocations of the ends of the clavicle, scapula, and glenohumeral joint. In Rockwood CA, Wilkins KE, King RE (eds): Fractures in Children, vol 3, 2nd ed. Philadelphia: JB Lippincott, 1984, pp 624-682.

294. Roberts JB: A case of excision of the head of the humerus for congenital subacromial dislocation of the humerus. Am J Med Sci 130:1001-1007, 1905.

295. Robinson D, Aghasi M, Halperin N, Kopilowicz L: Congenital dislocation of the shoulder: Case report and review of the literature. Contemp Orthop 18:595-598, 1989.

296. Valentin B: Die kongenitale Schulterluxation, Bericht über drei Falle in einer Familie. Z Orthop Chir 55:229-240, 1931.

297. Whitman R: The treatment of congenital and acquired luxations at the shoulder in childhood. Ann Surg 42:110-115, 1905.

298. Wolff G: Über einen Fall von kongenitaler Schulterluxation. Z Orthop Chir 51:199-209, 1929.

299. Aziz MA: Anatomical defects in a case of trisomy 13 with a D/D translocation. Teratology 22:217-237, 1980.

300. Bersu ET, Ramirez-Castro JJ: Anatomical analysis of the developmental effect of aneuploidy in man. The 18 trisomy syndrome: Anomalies of the head and neck. Am J Med Genet 1:173-193, 1977.

301. Brash JC: Upper limb. In Brash JC (ed): Cunningham's Manual of Practical Anatomy, 11th ed. London: Oxford University Press, 1948, pp 19-182.

302. Bryce T: Note on a group of varieties of the pectoral sheet of muscle. J Anat 34:75-83, 1899.

303. Clemente C (ed): Gray's Anatomy: Anatomy of the Human Body, 13th ed. Philadelphia: Lea & Febiger, 1985, p 520.

304. Landry SO: The phylogenetic significance of the chondroepitrochlearis muscle and its accompanying pectoral abnormalities. J Anat 92:57-61, 1958.

305. Langer-Oester: Med Wochenschr 15:6, 1846.

306. Ledouble AF: Muscles des Parois de la Poitrine. Traite des Variations du Système Musculaire de l'Homme, vol 1. Paris: Schleicher Freres, 1897, pp 243-258.

307. Macalister A: Additional observations on muscular anomalies in human anatomy (3rd series), with a catalogue of the principal muscular variations hitherto published. Trans R Ir Acad 25:1-134, 1875.

308. Mortenson OA, Pettersen JC: The musculature. In Anson BJ (ed): Morris' Human Anatomy, 12th ed. New York: McGraw-Hill, 1966, pp 421-611.

309. Perrin JB: Notes on some variations of the pectoralis major, with its associate muscles seen during sessions 1866-69, 1869-70, at King's College, London. J Anat Physiol 5:233-240, 1871.

310. Ruge G: Ein Rest des Haut-rumpf-muskels in der Achselgegend des Meschen-Achselbogen. Morphol Jahrb 41:519-538, 1910.

311. Spinner RJ, Carmichael SW, Spinner M: Infraclavicular ulnar nerve entrapment due to a chondroepitrochlearis muscle. J Hand Surg [Br] 16:315-317, 1991.

312. Tachendorf F: Einige seltenere atypische Brustmuskeln des Menschen und ihre Beurteilung. Z Anat Ent 114:216-229, 1949.

313. Testut L: Les Anomalies Musculaires Chez L'Homme Expliquées par L'Anatomie Comparée, Leur Importance en Anthropologie. Paris: Doin, 1884.

314. Tobler L: Der Achsiebogen des Menschen, ein Rudiment des Panniculus Cornosus der Mannaliev. Morphol Jahrb 30:453-507, 1902.

315. Voto SJ, Weiner DS: The chondroepitrochlearis muscle: Case report. J Pediatr Orthop 7:213-214, 1987.

316. Wood J: Variations in human myology observed during the winter session of 1865-66 at King's College, London. Proc R Soc 15:229-244, 1866.

317. Kameda Y: An anomalous muscle (accessory subscapularis teres latissimus muscle) in the axilla penetrating the brachial plexus in man. Acta Anat 96:513-533, 1976.

318. Lane WA: A coraco-clavicular sternal muscle. J Anat Physiol 21(Pt 4):673-674, 1887.

319. Bhattacharyya S: Abduction contracture of the shoulder from contracture of the intermediate part of the deltoid. J Bone Joint Surg Br 48:127-131, 1966.

320. Branick RL, Roberts JL, Glynn JJ, Beatre JC: Talwin-induced deltoid contracture. J Bone Joint Surg Am 58:279-286, 1976.

321. Chatterjee P, Gupta SK: Deltoid contracture in children of central Calcutta. J Pediatr Orthop 3:380-383, 1983.

322. Chiari PR, Rao VY, Rao BK: Congenital abduction contracture with dislocation of the shoulder in children: A report of two cases. Aust N Z J Surg 49:105-106, 1979.

323. Cozen LN: Pentazocine injections as a causative factor in dislocation of the shoulder: A case report. J Bone Joint Surg Am 59:979, 1977.

324. Enna CD: Bilateral abduction contracture of shoulder girdle, case report. Orthop Rev 2:111-113, 1982.

325. Goodfellow JW, Nade S: Flexion contracture of the shoulder joint from fibrosis of the anterior part of the deltoid muscle. J Bone Joint Surg Br 51:356-358, 1969.

326. Groves J, Goldner JL: Contracture of the deltoid muscle in the adult after intramuscular injections. J Bone Joint Surg Am 56:817-820, 1974.

327. Hang YS: Contracture of the hip secondary to fibrosis of the gluteus maximus muscle. J Bone Joint Surg Am 61:52-55, 1979.

328. Hashimoto M: A case of the congenital deltoid contracture. Orthop Surg (Tokyo) 19:1259-1260, 1968.

329. Hayashi T, Sugiura Y: Three cases of the deltoid contracture. Arch Orthop Trauma Surg 15:383-390, 1971.

330. Hill NA, Liebler WA, Wilson HJ, Rosenthal E: Abduction contractures of both glenohumeral joints and extension contracture of one knee secondary to partial muscle fibrosis: A case report. J Bone Joint Surg Am 49:961-964, 1967.

331. Jhunjhunwala HR: Abduction contracture of the deltoid muscle in children. Int Orthop 19:289-290, 1995.

332. Kitano K, Tada K, Oka S: Congenital contracture of the infraspinous muscle: A case report. Arch Orthop Trauma Surg 107:54-57, 1988.

333. Minami M, Ishii S, Usui M, Terashima Y: The deltoid contracture. Clin Orthop Surg (Tokyo) 11:493-501, 1976.

334. Minami M, Yamazaki J, Minami A, Ishii S: A postoperative long-term study of the deltoid contracture in children. J Pediatr Orthop 4:609-613, 1984.

335. Nakaya M, Kumon Y, Fujiwara M: Two cases of the congenital deltoid contracture. Orthop Surg (Tokyo) 22:814-818, 1971.

336. Pizzutillo PD: Congenital anomalies of the shoulder. In Post M (ed): The Shoulder: Surgical and Nonsurgical Management, 2nd ed. Philadelphia: Lea & Febiger, 1988, pp 644-653.

337. Roldan R, Warren D: Abduction deformity of the shoulder secondary to fibrosis of the central portion of the deltoid muscle [abstract]. J Bone Joint Surg Am 54:1332, 1972.

338. Sato M, Hondo S, Inoue H: Three cases of abduction contracture of the shoulder joint caused by fibrosis of the deltoid muscle. Orthop Surg (Tokyo) 16:1052-1056, 1965.

339. Wolbrink AJ, Hsu Z, Bianco AJ: Abduction contracture of the shoulders and hips secondary to fibrous bands. J Bone Joint Surg Am 55:844-846, 1973.

340. Bianchine JW: Acromial dimples: A benign familial trait. Am J Hum Genet 26:412-413, 1974.

341. Browne D: Congenital deformities of mechanical origin. Proc R Soc Med 29:1409-1431, 1936.

342. De Grouchy J, Royer P, Salmon C, Lamy M: Deletion partielle du bras long du chromosome 18. Pathol Biol (Paris) 12:579-582, 1964.

343. Halal F: Dominant inheritance of acromion skin dimples. Am J Med Genet 6:259, 1980.

344. Insley J: Syndrome associated with a deficiency of part of the long arm of chromosome No. 18. Arch Dis Child 42:140-146, 1967.

345. Lejeune J, Berger R, Lafourcade J, Rethore MO: La deletion partielle du bras long du chromosome 18: Individualisation d'un nouvel état morbide. Ann Genet (Paris) 9:32-38, 1966.

346. Mehes K, Meggyessy V: Autosomal dominant inheritance of benign bilateral acromial dimples. Hum Genet 76:206, 1987.

347. Smith DW: Recognizable patterns of malformation. In Jones KL (ed): Smith's Recognizable Patterns of Human Malformation, 4th ed. Philadelphia: WB Saunders, 1988, pp 10-613.

348. Thieffry S, Arthuis M, De Grouchy J, et al: Deletion des bras courts d'un chromosome 17-18: Dysmorphies complexes avec oligophrenie. Arch Fr Pediatr 20:740-745, 1963.

349. Wood VE: Congenital skin fossae about the shoulder. Plast Reconstr Surg 85:798-800, 1990.

350. Baudine P, Bovy GL, Wasterlain A: Un cas de syndrome de Poland. Acta Paediatr Belg 32:407-410, 1967.

351. Bing R: Über angeborene Muskeldefekte. Virchows Arch Path Anat 170:175-228, 1902.

352. Brooksaler FS, Graivier L: Poland's syndrome. Am J Dis Child 121:263-264, 1971.

353. David TJ: Nature and etiology of the Poland anomaly. N Engl J Med 287:487-489, 1972.

354. Engber WD: Cleft hand and pectoral aplasia. J Hand Surg 6:574-577, 1981.

355. Freire-Maia N, Chautard EA, Opitz JM, et al: The Poland syndrome—clinical and genealogical data, dermatoglyphic analysis, and incidence. Hum Hered 23:97-104, 1973.

356. Ireland DC, Takayama N, Flatt AE: Poland's syndrome: A review of forty-three cases. J Bone Joint Surg Am 58:52-58, 1976.

357. Lanzkowsky P: Absence of pectoralis major muscle in association with acute leukemia [letter]. J Pediatr 86:817-818, 1975.

358. Lewis WH: Observations on the pectoralis major muscle in man. Johns Hopkins Bull 12:172-177, 1901.

359. Mace JW, Kaplan JM, Schanberger JE, Gotlin RW: Poland's syndrome: Report of seven cases and review of the literature. Clin Pediatr (Phila) 11:98-102, 1972.

360. Miller RA, Miller DR: Congenital absence of the pectoralis major muscle with acute lymphoblastic leukemia and genitourinary anomalies. J Pediatr 87:146-147, 1975.

361. Opitz JM, Herrmann J, Dieker H: The study of malformation syndromes in man. Birth Defects 5:1-10, 1969.

362. Resnick E: Congenital unilateral absence of the pectoral muscles often associated with syndactylism. J Bone Joint Surg 24:925-928, 1942.

363. Soderberg BN: Congenital absence of the pectoral muscle and syndactylism: A deformity association sometimes overlooked. Plast Reconstr Surg 4:434-436, 1949.

364. Gantzer CJ: Dissertatio anatomica musculorum varietatis. Cited by Hecker, 1923, 1813.

365. Clarkson P: Poland's syndactyly. Guys Hosp Rep 111:335-346, 1962.

366. Poland A: Deficiency of the pectoralis muscles. Guys Hosp Rep 6:191-193, 1841.

367. Bouvet JP, Leveque D, Bernetieres F, Gros JJ: Vascular origin of Poland syndrome? Eur J Pediatr 128:17-26, 1978.

368. Castilla EE, Paz JE, Orioli IM: Pectoralis major muscle defect and Poland complex. Am J Med Genet 4:263-269, 1979.

369. Ehrenhaft JL, Rossi NP, Lawrence MS: Developmental chest wall defects. Ann Thorac Surg 2:384-398, 1966.

370. Armendares S: Absence of pectoralis major muscle in two sisters associated with leukemia in one of them [letter]. J Pediatr 85:436-437, 1974.

371. Beals RK, Eckhardt AL: Hereditary onycho-osteodysplasia (nail–patella syndrome). A report of nine kindreds. J Bone Joint Surg Am 51:505-516, 1969.

372. Boaz D, Mace JW, Gotlin RW: Poland's syndrome and leukemia. Lancet 1:349-350, 1971.

373. Gausewitz SH, Meals RA, Setoguchi Y: Severe limb deficiency in Poland's syndrome. Clin Orthop Relat Res (185):9-13, 1984.

374. Bouwes Bavinck JN, Weaver DD: Subclavian artery supply disruption sequence: Hypothesis of a vascular etiology for Poland, Klippel-Feil, and Möbius anomalies. Am J Med Genet 23:903-918, 1986.

375. Gorlin RJ, Sedano H: Moebius syndrome. Mod Med Sept:110-111, 1972.

376. Jorgenson RJ: Moebius syndrome, ectrodactyly, hypoplasia of tongue and pectoral muscles. Birth Defects 7:283-284, 1971.

377. Gross-Kieselstein E, Shalev RS: Familial absence of the trapezius muscle with associated shoulder girdle abnormalities. Clin Genet 32:145-147, 1987.

378. Schulze-Gocht W: Über den Trapeziusdefekt. Zugleich ein Beitrag zur Frage der Skoliosenentstehung. Arch Orthop Chir 26:302-307, 1928.

379. Selden BR: Congenital absence of trapezius and rhomboideus major muscles. J Bone Joint Surg 17:1058-1059, 1935.

380. Sheehan D: Bilateral absence of trapezius. J Anat 67:180, 1932.

381. Daskalakis E, Bouhoutsos J: Subclavian and axillary vein compression of musculoskeletal origin. Br J Surg 67:573-576, 1980.

382. Foltz: Homologie des membres pelviens et thoraciques de l'homme. J Physiol Homme Animaux 6:48-81, 1863.

383. Grant BJC: An Atlas of Anatomy, 5th ed. Baltimore: Williams & Wilkins, 1962.

384. Hewitt RL: Acute axillary-vein obstruction by the pectoralis-minor muscle. N Engl J Med 279:595, 1968.

385. Lord JW Jr, Stone PW: Pectoralis minor tenotomy and anterior scalenotomy with special reference to hyperabduction syndrome and "effort thrombosis" of subclavian vein. Circulation 13:537-542, 1956.

386. Rowe CR: Unusual Shoulder Conditions. New York: Churchill Livingstone, 1988, pp 639-646.

387. Seib GA: The musculus pectoralis minor in American whites and American Negroes. Am J Physiol Anthropol 4:389, 1938.

388. Wright IS: Neurovascular syndrome produced by hyperabduction of arms: Immediate changes produced in 150 normal controls, and effects on some persons of prolonged hyperabduction of arms as in sleeping, and in certain occupations. Am Heart J 29:1-19, 1945.

389. Evans SRT, Nauta RJ, Walsh DB: An unusual case of intermittent venous obstruction of the upper extremity. Am Surg 58:455-457, 1992.

390. Bergman RA, Thompson SA, Afifi AK: Catalog of Human Variation. Baltimore: Urban & Schwarzenberg, 1984, pp 26-27.

391. Dwight T, McMurrich JP, Hamann CA, et al: Piersol GA (ed): Historical Title Page. First Edition (1907) Through the Eighth Edition (1923) of Human Anatomy, Including Structure and Development and Practical Considerations. London: JB Lippincott, 1930, p 574.

392. Bartlett SP, May JW, Yaremchuk MJ: The latissimus dorsi muscle: A fresh cadaver study of the primary neurovascular pedicle. Plast Reconstr Surg 67:631-636, 1981.

393. Bostwick J, Nahai F, Wallace JG, Vasconez LO: Sixty latissimus dorsi flaps. Plast Reconstr Surg 63:31-41, 1979.

394. Schottstaedt ER, Larsen LJ, Bost FC: Complete muscle transposition. J Bone Joint Surg Am 37:897-918, 1955.

395. Boontje AH: Axillary vein entrapment. Br J Surg 66:331-332, 1979.

396. Corning HK: Lehrbuch der topographischen Anatomie, 24th ed. Munich: Bergmann, 1949, p 635.

397. Testut L: Traite d'Anatomie Humaine. Paris: Gaston Doin & Cie, 1928, p 879.

398. Campbell CB, Chandler JG, Tegtmeyer CJ, et al: Axillary, subclavian and brachiocephalic vein obstruction. Surgery 82:816-826, 1977.

399. Dodd H, Cockett FB: The Pathology and Surgery of the Veins of the Lower Limb, 2nd ed. Edinburgh: Churchill Livingstone, 1976, pp 206-207.

400. Kaplan EB: Surgical anatomy: Langer's muscles of the axilla. Bull Hosp Jt Dis 6:78-79, 1945.

401. Karacagil S, Eriksson I: Entrapment of the axillary artery by anomalous muscle: Case report. Acta Chir Scand 153:633-634, 1987.

402. Migeul M, Llusa M, Ortiz JC, et al: The axillopectoral muscle (of Langer): Report of three cases. Surg Radiol Anat 23:341-343, 2001.

403. Rob C, May AG: Neurovascular compression syndromes. Adv Surg 9:211-234, 1975.

404. Roos DB: Transaxillary approach for first rib resection to relieve thoracic outlet syndrome. Ann Surg 163:354-358, 1966.

405. Sisley JF: The axillopectoral muscle. Surg Gynecol Obstet 165:73, 1987.

406. Haagenson CD: Diseases of the Breast. Philadelphia: WB Saunders, 1953, p 607.

407. Sachatello CR: The axillopectoral muscle (Langer's axillary arch): A cause of axillary vein obstruction. Surgery 81:610-612, 1977.

408. Tilney NL, Griffiths HJG, Edwards EA: Natural history of major venous thrombosis of upper extremity. Arch Surg 101:792-796, 1970.

409. Saitta GF, Baum V: Langer's axillary arch, an unusual cause of axillary mass. JAMA 180:122, 1962.

410. Cunningham DJ: The musculus sternalis. J Anat Physiol 22:391-407, 1888.

411. Hollinshead WH: The back and limbs. In Hollinshead WH: Anatomy for Surgeons, vol 3, 2nd ed. New York: Harper & Row, 1969, pp 231, 286-288.

412. Barlow RN: The sternalis muscle in American whites and Negroes. Anat Rec 61:413-426, 1935.

Clinical Evaluation of Shoulder Problems

Michael Codsi, MD, Jesse McCarron, MD, and John J. Brems, MD

From our first days in medical school, we are taught that establishing a correct diagnosis depends on obtaining a meaningful and detailed medical history from the patient. This requires the physician to ask specific questions while at the same time actively listening to the responses from the patient. Often physicians formulate their next question without listening to and interpreting the answer to the previous inquiry. Obtaining a good patient history is, in itself, an art that requires experience and patience. I vividly recall one of my mentors stating that all patients come to your office and tell you exactly what is wrong with them when they answer but four or five questions. Our task is to decipher their answers to those few questions.

Time is perhaps the most valuable—and least available—commodity in our medical lives in the 21st century. We employ physician extenders to help our efficiency and we ask patients to fill out reams of paperwork with numerous questions while we are seeing another patient. We thus lose the advantage of directly listening to our patient, observing their expressions and interpreting their body language. Each of these facets can offer valuable information about the diagnosis of their shoulder problem. We must recognize that often the answer to one question leads to the formation of the next question. This valuable opportunity is lost in the hustle of managing medical care in this era, and it is indeed a lost opportunity. Our duty to our patients is to inquire, listen, examine, test, and then formulate a diagnosis. When performed in this logical fashion, the diagnosis is nearly always straightforward and the treatment then easily rendered.

In evaluating the patient we also must bear in mind that we really are assessing *the patient* not just interpreting radiographic studies or laboratory values. In this increasingly technological world, it is often easy to lose sight and begin treating magnetic resonance imaging (MRI) scans without treating the patient. For example, nearly every MRI of the shoulder we have seen in a patient older than 30 years suggests acromioclavicular joint pathology. Perhaps it is then not surprising that the most overdiagnosed and overtreated condition about the shoulder relates to the acromioclavicular joint.

As clinicians we must evaluate the patient's history and perform a thorough physical examination to establish a strong correlation in the features of each pathologic process. Our confidence rises when the patient's history of the complaint is consistent with the majority of the physical findings. This confidence rises even more when radiographic and laboratory studies are also consistent with the initial diagnosis. When each of these features of the patient evaluation point to the same diagnosis, our certainty of the correct diagnosis becomes assured. It is obviously much more disconcerting when a patient's history suggests impingement syndrome, the physical examination is more consistent with instability, the radiographs document osteoarthritis and the laboratory values suggest gout.

We hope the methods described in this chapter for taking a history and performing a physical examination allow any clinician to determine which pathology is primarily responsible for the patient's complaints.

PATIENT HISTORY

Taking a history from a patient is an art. We must ask specific questions, actively listen to the response, and only *then* formulate the next question. The answer to each successive question should ultimately lead the physician to a correct diagnosis. It is important not to get tunnel vision and lead the patient toward the diagnosis that *you* think is present.

Recall that many widely varying diagnoses manifest with similar symptoms and only after a complete history and examination can differentiation of diagnoses be made. For example, if a patient presents complaining of an inability to elevate or externally rotate the arm, the physician might immediately diagnose a frozen shoulder. Sending that patient, who really has advanced osteoarthritis, to physical therapy to increase the range of motion (ROM) ensures a therapeutic failure. A diagnosis is only established after each phase of the evaluation is complete. Anything else in the name of expedience and efficiency does a disservice to our patients.

Age

Most, if not all, disease processes occur in specific patient age ranges. Although malignancies and traumas can occur at any chronologic age, even these processes tend to stratify by age. Surgical neck fractures of the humerus are typical of a postmenopausal woman with osteoporosis rather than an 18-year-old male football player. Osteosarcomas of the proximal humerus are more common in a 20-year-old than in a geriatric patient. The younger, athletic person in the second or third decade of life more likely has instability, whereas the 60-year-old golfer with a painful shoulder more likely has rotator cuff disease.

Though not fully studied or accurately analyzed, the perception is that osteoarthritis of the shoulder is occurring at ever-younger ages. Not only is it in the domain of the 70- and 80-year-old patient; often patients present in their 50s and younger with osteoarthritis. Avascular necrosis, infections, and rheumatoid arthritis can occur at any age, and thus age is a poor discriminator. Spontaneous hematogenous septic arthritis may be slightly more common in youth, but its clinical presentation is usually so specific that age of the patient need not be considered.

Shoulder instability and its subsets of pathology are much more common in the youthful years. Labral tears, superior labrum anterior and posterior (SLAP) tears, and biceps tendinitis are commonly seen in patients younger than 30 years. However, some activities that span the entire age range, such as downhill skiing, offer much opportunity for acute shoulder dislocations. Nevertheless, the implications of a traumatic shoulder dislocation are age specific. In the younger patient who sustains a glenohumeral dislocation, the more likely associated injury involves the labrum or biceps anchor. Conversely, in the older patient, the acute glenohumeral dislocation is more commonly associated with a rotator cuff tear. Similarly, trauma to the shoulder can afflict the acromioclavicular joint. In the younger patient, disruption of the joint is more common, whereas in the older person, clavicular fracture may be more common.

Less-common conditions afflicting the shoulder still display a predilection for certain age groups. Gout and symptomatic calcific tendinitis usually occur in middle age. Adhesive capsulitis appears in midlife (more commonly in women), and diabetic neuropathic disease is more common in the older person. Cuff tear arthropathy clearly favors women in their mid-70s.

Sex

Most pathologic processes that afflict the shoulder know no gender boundaries. Trauma can occur to anyone; arthritis, infection, cuff tears, avascular necrosis, calcific tendinitis, and gout can likewise occur with equal frequency in male and female patients. However, three conditions have a significantly higher prevalence in female patients. Although none of these maladies is exclusive to women, their prevalence strongly favors them.

Multidirectional shoulder instability is seen many times more often in young female patients between the ages of 15 and 25 years than in male patients of the same age. Why this occurs remains unclear. Male patients might present with clinical evidence of multidirectional laxity, but perhaps because of stronger and better-conditioned muscles they are better able to compensate for their ligamentous laxity in ways female patients cannot or do not. In this condition, it remains doubtful that there is a difference between sexes in the pathophysiology of the condition, but the positive biological response to the process seems to favor the male patients. A teenage female athlete who presents with shoulder complaints likely has some type of instability pathology. However, the clinician must remain open to other diagnoses and never forget to distinguish patient symptoms from clinical signs. The young person might present with *symptoms* of cuff tendinitis that are caused by underlying shoulder instability.

Female patients also tend to present in far greater numbers than males with adhesive capsulitis.[1] This is in contrast to the idiopathic stiff and painful frozen shoulder, which is equally prevalent among male and female patients and describes restricted shoulder ROM associated with pain. A frozen shoulder can result from any number of pathologic processes such as post-traumatic stiffness, immobilization, and tendinitis. Adhesive capsulitis is a specific diagnosis most prevalent in women 40 to 60 years of age. It is associated with an idiopathic inflammatory process involving the glenohumeral joint capsule and synovium that results in capsular contraction and adhesion formation.

Although massive rotator cuff tears probably occur in greater numbers in men, it is the women, classically older than 70 years, who develop the sequelae of these massive cuff tears. The diagnosis of cuff tear arthropathy as defined by painful collapse of the humeral head with superior migration (not iatrogenically provoked by prior release of the coracoacromial ligament) favors geriatric women much more than men for unclear reasons.

Presenting Complaint

When the physician inquires about a patient's chief complaint during the initial visit, the response is most commonly one of pain. Subsequent questioning is directed toward better understanding the characteristics of that pain; a presumptive diagnosis will follow from this. Most presenting complaints related to the shoulder are defined by patients as pain, stiffness, loss of smooth motion, instability, neurologic symptoms, or combinations of these.

With respect to shoulder pathology, another chief complaint may be one of joint instability. In this case, the patient might have no pain and is only concerned by the sense that the shoulder joint is loose, sloppy, or recurrently dislocating. The patient might initially complain of numbness or tingling down the limb, which may be caused by neurologic pathology unrelated to the shoulder. Dissection of this symptom may be more challenging because pathology in the neck might have to be distinguished from shoulder pathology.

Weakness is rarely a singular presenting complaint. Painless weakness nearly always defines a significant neurologic event or pathologic process. If stiffness of the shoulder is a presenting complaint, it is nearly always accompanied by some element of pain. A patient might present with a complaint of crepitus or popping in and about the shoulder associated with activity or a specific arm motion. An isolated awareness of crepitus without pain is very rare.

Pain

The discussion of pain is challenging because it is, by definition, a completely subjective complaint. In our vast armamentarium of technology and laboratory analyses, we cannot objectify pain. Pain is a perception of data presenting to our brains. We have all experienced the reality of injuring ourselves with minor scrapes and scratches in our daily lives but been fully unaware of any event until hours later. Have we all not jumped into a pool of water only to feel cold initially? Within minutes, the initial discomfort fades as we rapidly become conditioned to the water temperature. The water temperature obviously does not change; it is our *perception* of the same data input to our brain that changes.

So too it is with other painful stimuli. Psychologists (and perhaps our own experience) tell us that mood can have a dramatic effect on pain perceptions. People who are depressed or sullen by nature tend to experience more discomfort and be more disabled for a given amount of noxious stimuli, and the opposite is likewise true. Energetic, optimistic, and happy patients tend to discount even significant amounts of otherwise painful stimuli.

Other societal issues are also known to affect a patient's perception and response to pain. Specifically, issues that relate to secondary gain can have significant influence on patients' responses to treatment of their pain. Active litigation where contested remuneration is involved can lead to perpetuation of symptoms. In much the same way, patients with workers' compensation claims might have little incentive to report improvement in their symptoms. Yet we have no pain meter to substantiate or dispute a person's claims.

Despite these limitations, obtaining a history related to pain is critically important and valuable. Such features as its character, onset, radiating patterns, aggravating factors, and alleviating features nearly always assist the clinician in discerning a diagnosis.

Character of the Pain

Despite our inability to *measure* pain, patients use similar adjectives to *describe* their pain. These descriptions can offer much insight into its cause. Pain associated with an acute fracture understandably causes a severe and disabling pain, often remaining for days minimally responsive to narcotic analgesics. By contrast, the pain of impingement and rotator cuff pathology is commonly described as dull, boring, and toothache-like in quality. The pain of a frozen shoulder is typified as all or none. When it is present at the endpoint of available motion, the pain is truly disabling, whereas when the arm is functioning within its available arcs of motion, pain does not exist. Patients with painful osteoarthritis describe pain that frequently alternates between a sharp stabbing pain under high compressive joint loads and a chronic lower level of pain with less-demanding activities. Patients with severely destructive rheumatoid disease are often so conditioned by the chronicity of their disease that description of their pain appears inconsistent with the degree of joint destruction. These patients tend to be more disabled by their functional loss than by their perceived pain.

Acute calcium deposition in the cuff tendons provides a characteristic type of pain. The pain is so acute and so severe that calcium deposit in the shoulder has been likened to a kidney stone of the shoulder. The pain associated with a kidney stone seems so well understood by the population at large that the pain in the shoulder associated with acute calcific deposit is easily understood as well. Patients seek a dark, quiet room with minimal competing stimulation. The pain can be nauseating and disabling enough that many patients find their way to an emergency department (ED). The clinical picture is so evident and the radiographs so predictable that the diagnosis is rarely in doubt.

Onset of the Pain

The clinician asks about the onset of the symptoms because this feature has implications in the diagnosis of shoulder pathology. Understandably, with an acute onset of severe pain following a traumatic event, the diagnosis of fracture on an x-ray is not challenging. Other diagnoses may be discerned by inquiring about the circumstances of the onset of their pain. Impingement and rotator cuff disease more commonly lack a specific date or time of onset; the patient recalls an insidious onset of the pain, often dating its initiation many weeks or months in the past without a clearly identifiable event. Even if the patient presents with a recent onset of pain in the absence of trauma, inquiry needs to be made regarding a history of pain predating the more recent traumatic event.

Radicular pain of cervical origin likely has an insidious onset. Patients might acknowledge that turning the head provokes symptoms. Arm pain while driving is often a tip-off to pain of a cervical origin. Pain described as sharp and stabbing and occurring intermittently in the scapular muscles and around the top of the shoulder nearly always finds its source in the cervical spine.

Location of Pain Perception

Pain is poorly localized around the shoulder girdle. The specific location where the patient perceives the pain is rarely the site of origin of the pain. The most common location for the perception of rotator cuff disease and the associated bursitis is down the arm toward the deltoid muscle insertion. The pain and inflammation associated with bicipital tendinitis is typically down the anterior arm, although the site of pathology is proximal to the intertubercular groove.

The pain pattern of most intrinsic shoulder pathology is one that radiates down the arm to the level of the elbow. It is distinctly rare for intrinsic shoulder maladies to result in pain perceived to extend below the elbow joint. Conversely, pain of cervical origin usually radiates from the base of the ipsilateral ear toward the posterior shoulder and into the scapular region. A true cervical radiculopathy, which most commonly involves the fifth and sixth cervical nerve roots, provokes symptoms that are perceived to radiate into the forearm and hand in a dermatomal pattern. In contrast to pain derived from cervical radiculopathy, pain from adhesive capsulitis does not follow a dermatomal pattern. The pain often radiates along the trapezius muscle and periscapular muscles because these muscles become strained and fatigued by the excessive scapular rotation that must compensate for the decreased glenohumeral motion.

Pain associated with an acromioclavicular injury usually radiates medially and results in perceived pain along the mid and medial clavicle. Intra-articular processes such as osteoarthritis, avascular necrosis, and rheumatoid disease rarely result in perceived radiation of pain. Patients report that their pain is poorly localized and remains centered around the shoulder without associated arm pain.

The pain of an intra-articular infection is not unlike that associated with any joint. The pain is severe, exquisite, and maximally disabling. The clinical picture is so specific that the clinical suspicion is exceedingly high until a definitive laboratory diagnosis is confirmed.

Aggravating Factors of Pain

As a part of the history of pain, the clinician needs to elicit circumstances that seem to make the pain worse. Often the pain is influenced by arm position, which can provide insight into its cause. Patients might state that the pain is worse or aggravated when the arm is positioned above shoulder level, such as occurs when washing or combing their hair. Activities that result in a long lever arm with the elbow extended, such as reaching across the car seat or reaching out the window to use an auto-matic teller machine, increase the pain of a weak or torn rotator cuff. Increasing pain in the shoulder that occurs while pulling bed covers up at night is strongly associated with impingement and cuff disease. The occurrence of pain at night needs to be elicited.

There appear to be two distinct types of night pain, each associated with a different shoulder condition. The more severe and disabling type of night pain strongly suggests a rotator cuff tear. The pain is described as gnawing, incessant, and unremitting, and it not only awakens patients from sleep but it often precludes any meaningful sleep at all. Patients often relate that the only way to obtain sleep is to rest semirecumbent in a chair. In a different circumstance, patients might acknowledge night pain that is *positional*. They can typically fall asleep but they are awakened if they roll onto or away from the affected shoulder.

Patients with positional night pain rarely convey the degree of frustration with sleep interruption that occurs with a cuff tear. Although patients with positional night pain may be annoyed by the sleep interruption, they generally can fall back to sleep easily and don't develop that deep sense of misery associated with persistent sleep deprivation. Positional night pain is most often associated with loss of shoulder internal rotation through muscle stiffness or loss of capsular compliance. Painful arthritis of the acromioclavicular joint can also result in positional night pain and is caused by the compressive loads borne by that joint when lying on the affected side. The pain of these conditions might also be aggravated by lying on the unaffected shoulder. While lying on the unaffected shoulder, the weight of the arm falling across the chest in adduction also results in acromioclavicular joint compression and posterior capsular stretch.

Patients with adhesive capsulitis describe pain that is characterized by its sudden severity aggravated by clearly reproducible arm positions. They have no pain until they reach the endpoint of their available motion, when their pain becomes immediate and severe. As their condition progresses they note an increasing inability to perform their activities of daily living, including reaching overhead or reaching behind their back for dressing or personal hygiene.

With an intra-articular process such as glenohumeral arthritis, patients usually note that aggravation of symptoms comes with activities associated with repetition of a similar motion. Painting, sweeping, polishing, vacuuming, ironing, and washing a car are activities that predictably aggravate the pain of arthritis and impingement. Loading of the joint while at the same time performing a repetitive act is particularly aggravating to joint maladies that result from incongruent joint surfaces such as avascular necrosis, osteoarthritis, and rheumatoid arthritis.

Although inquiry about and analysis of aggravating factors in the assessment of shoulder pain is rarely in itself fully diagnostic, it remains a very important consideration as the history taking progresses.

Factors That Alleviate Pain

In the same way that analysis of aggravating factors provides insight into the etiology of the shoulder problem, so too does inquiry into those features and factors that alleviate or improve the symptoms. Many times the alleviating factor provides the best information in arriving at the correct diagnosis. Whereas there is much overlap in diagnoses with respect to aggravating factors, it would be unusual to find one factor that solves several different problems. For example, if a patient finds that an over-the-counter antiinflammatory truly improves the symptoms, it would logically follow that the patient has an inflammatory condition. Certainly an antiinflammatory does not solve the apprehension of a shoulder instability problem, nor would it likely manage the pain of an acute fracture. Patients with a frozen shoulder characteristically state that there is absolutely no improvement in their pain with nonsteroidal antiinflammatories.

Patients with rotator cuff tears and impingement often note that in placing the affected arm over their head, they find significant improvement in their pain. Often this arm position is the only way they can find meaningful sleep. This is called the *Saha position* (Fig. 4-1), named for the Indian orthopaedic surgeon who recognized this phenomenon. He postulated that with the arm resting overhead, there is a balance of tension of the cuff muscles in their least tense state. When the arm is passively elevated overhead in the supine patient, the supraspinatus is subject to its least tension, and pain diminishes in many patients.

Alleviating factors can include activity modification, medications, narcotics, antiinflammatories, injections, and physical therapy. Physical therapy for stretching over long time spans usually improves symptoms and needs to be assessed during history taking.

The response to local anesthetic injections when placed in specific anatomic locations around the shoulder can be very instructive and diagnostic. In a patient with chronic subacromial impingement, 5 mL of 1% lidocaine placed in the subacromial space provides immediate and dramatic relief of pain (Fig. 4-2). This response becomes diagnostic of a subacromial process, and it becomes especially valuable when trying to discern whether the patient's perceived pain is originating in the shoulder or whether it is referred pain from the neck. A similar local injection test is useful in evaluating the acromioclavicular joint as a source of the patient's pain. Alleviation of pain with arm adduction following an injection directly into the acromioclavicular joint strongly suggests pathology at this joint. Intra-articular injections can provide similar supporting information regarding the source of a patient's symptoms.

These specific injection tests are valuable in defining the pathologic process, and in the case of subacromial impingement, the response to the local anesthetic can predict response to surgical treatment. Moreover, a negative response to a subacromial local anesthetic can predict a negative response to subacromial surgical treatment.

Response of Symptoms to Self-Prescribed Treatment

With the advent and ubiquity of the Internet, patients have now become more involved in their health care decisions. There are countless websites dedicated to patient information, and these help them self-diagnose, although not always with great clarity or accuracy. There are likely even more websites from which patients can receive a wide variety of treatment recommendations for their self-diagnosed shoulder malady. Searching for "physical therapy" brings up millions of hits, and searching for shoulder-specific physical therapy brings up well more than 1 million websites. No doubt then that it is the rare patient who arrives at your office without some knowledge, opinion, and effort at self-management of shoulder pain.

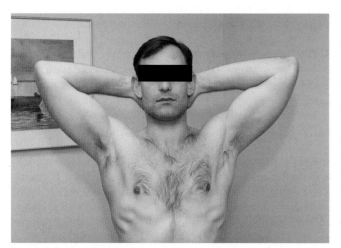

FIGURE 4-1 The Saha position often provides relief from pain related to rotator cuff pathology.

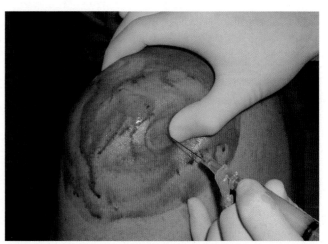

FIGURE 4-2 Subacromial injection technique from the posterior aspect of the shoulder. The thumb is resting on the inferior border of the spine of the scapula.

It is important to take time to explore what methods, medications, and modalities the patient might have tried before coming to the physician. Explore the realm of nutraceuticals and ask specifically about the common ones, including glucosamine, chondroitin, shark cartilage, and methylsulfonylmethane (MSM), because many patients do not consider these to be medicines and do not include them in their medication lists. Patients consume seemingly countless vitamins and vitamin combinations in their effort to improve their physical well-being. With the exception of glucosamine and chondroitin, which themselves have not been subjected to the rigors of the scientific method to prove their efficacy, there is little published objective information to make recommendations to patients. Nevertheless, we have all seen patients who are certain that some combination of these herbs, vitamins, and supplements have affected their medical condition in some way or another. It is important to query and document these treatments in the overall evaluation of the patient with a shoulder problem.

Box 4-1 lists the facets of pain that need to be explored during a patient history.

Instability

In this discussion, it is imperative that the concept of instability is understood to mean the *patient has symptoms* of some shoulder problem. Many asymptomatic shoulders exhibit increased joint translation and are clearly loose during a physical examination. Such asymptomatic shoulders are defined as *lax*, not unstable. To have shoulder instability, by definition, means the shoulder is symptomatic for the patient.

In the younger and active age groups, the symptom of shoulder instability may be the patient's presenting complaint. Although there is often a history of acute traumatic event resulting in the initial well-defined onset, in many cases no such traumatic event occurred. Indeed, it has only been since the 1980s that genetic factors in ligamentous laxity have been recognized as significant factors in patient perceptions of shoulder instability.

The diagnosis of shoulder instability can be very easy when the patient presents with an appropriate history of trauma. Nearly always there has been a trip to the ED and radiographs to document the events. However, with the increasing availability of sports trainers at most of the high school, college, and professional competitions, reduction of a dislocation by those personnel results in a history only; there are no ED records or radiographs. Although the history in these situations is still strong, an examination and radiographs even a few days following the event makes this a less-than-challenging diagnosis.

The more challenging problem occurs in the patient with a sense of slipping and looseness in their shoulder without a history of macrotrauma. More often than not, this more subtle instability pattern is associated with a nondescript level of discomfort and diffuse pain around the shoulder girdle. The discomfort is poorly localized and may be more scapular in location. The association of such symptoms with paresthesias down the arm is nearly always related to shoulder instability. A history of repetitive microtrauma is elicited. Such activities might include frequent swimming, gymnastics, and ballet. Although these activities would not appear to be highly stressful to the joint, they do demand muscle function defined by high endurance. Conventional thought suggests that when the ligament quality and integrity do not contribute to joint stability, the surrounding muscle activity and appropriate proprioceptive activity become more important to maintaining a functioning joint.

The sense of instability might occur with the arm only in certain positions or it may be present regardless of arm placement or position. True symptomatic multidirectional instability is typically symptomatic in midrange positions before ligament tension reaches the end of the range. The physician must carefully inquire about which activities and arm positions provoke the symptoms. Patients with this type of instability might have symptoms that are incapacitating enough that they tend to avoid extremes of glenohumeral motion. Pain is the more common symptom with a shoulder instability based on ligamentous laxity (AMBRI), and apprehension is more common with unidirectional traumatic instability (TUBS). (TUBS stands for *t*raumatic etiology, *u*nidirectional instability, *B*ankart ligamentous detachment, and *s*urgical repair. AMBRI stands for *a*traumatic etiology, *m*ultidirectional instability, *b*ilateral shoulders, *r*ehabilitation with rotational strengthening, and *i*nferior capsular tightening [surgery performed when conservative therapy fails].)

The classic patient with traumatic instability is a male athlete who sustained an identifiable traumatic event during the course of a violent activity. Football tackling, a high-speed fall or collision while downhill skiing, and a hyperextension force on an extended arm (basketball blocking shot) are very common scenarios that result in an acute traumatic shoulder dislocation. Conversely, the classic patient with multidirectional shoulder instability is the young asthenic female ballet dancer, swimmer, or volleyball player with nondescript shoulder pain that also involves the scapula and provokes paresthesias down the arm occurring in the absence of a defined traumatic event.

BOX 4-1 Aspects of Pain to Be Evaluated

Severity (scale, 1-10)

Character (dull, sharp, ache, lancinating)

Onset (acute, chronic, insidious, defining moment)

Location (e.g., superior, posterior, anterior)

Patterns of radiation (neck, arm, below elbow, deltoid insertion)

Aggravating factors (e.g., arm position, time of day)

Alleviating factors (e.g., arm position, medications)

Prior treatment

Isolated symptomatic posterior shoulder instability is most often associated with a very specific event or process. Although falling on the outstretched arm is a common scenario, because the arm is most often placed in the scapular plane to brace the fall and protect the head, a posterior force is only placed on the hand. As the body continues to fall to the ground, the arm is extended at the shoulder, placing an anterior force on the shoulder. This results in the much more common anterior dislocation under such circumstances; posterior shoulder dislocations are rarely associated with traumatic events that include falls.

Posterior shoulder instability is seen most often in the scenario of electric shocks and epilepsy. It appears that electrical stimulation to the muscles around the shoulder, when provided in a pathologic setting, can result in posterior shoulder dislocations. Severe electrical discharges, whether from within (major grand mal seizure) or extrinsically provided (such as an electric shock), appear to result in the posterior shoulder musculature actually *pulling* the shoulder out of joint. Historically, there is an associated increase in posterior dislocations of the shoulder associated with excessive use of ethanol and the social activities that can follow. Falling asleep on a park bench with the arms over the back of the bench while inebriated has been associated with posterior shoulder dislocations.

Box 4-2 lists the queries that should accompany a history that suggests instability.

Paresthesias

The most common shoulder-related pathology associated with a perception of numbness, tingling, or paresthesias down the arm is instability. The patient's perception of the neurologic symptom is usually nondermatomal if the process occurs in the shoulder girdle. A person with multidirectional instability might note a tingling all the way down the arm involving several peripheral nerve dermatomes. By contrast, a cervical root irritation of a herniated cervical disc predictably results in a known dermatomal pattern of symptoms. An intrinsic shoulder problem such as a rotator cuff tear can result in secondary neurologic symptoms. In an effort to support the painful arm, the patient might rest it on an armrest for a prolonged time and develop a cubital tunnel syndrome. Similarly, a patient who is protecting the arm and minimizing functional elevation can develop carpal tunnel symptoms from inadequate fluid mobilization and prolonged dependency of the limb.

Weakness

Common causes of weakness include cerebral dysfunction, nerve transmission dysfunction, musculotendinous deficiency, pain, and biochemical causes. With cerebral dysfunction, the patient is not generating the electrical signal (malingering). Nerve transmission dysfunction can result from primary neuronal injury (Parsonage-Turner syndrome). Biochemical problems result from synaptic biochemical pathology as in myasthenia gravis, polymyalgia rheumatica, and dystrophies.

In a clinical setting, the most common cause of weakness is likely a rotator cuff tear, and although some tears are pain free, most patients have some complaint of pain associated with the weak arm. Nevertheless, it is important to ascertain other potential causes of weakness in the complete evaluation of a shoulder-related complaint.

Crepitus

A patient's perception of crepitus around the shoulder is rarely seen without other associated symptoms. Chronic rotator cuff tendinitis and chronic inflammation of the subacromial bursa can result in a crunching sensation and cause the patient to report a noise coming from the shoulder. Because these are inflammatory conditions, they are nearly always associated with some perception and complaint of pain as well. Scapulothoracic bursitis and snapping scapula syndrome can cause a painful crunching sensation in the patient's upper chest posteriorly when the patient elevates the arm. This usually is also associated with some pain.

Following surgery for rotator cuff repair, patients often become aware of painless crepitus in the subacromial space. Although the exact etiology remains unclear, it is likely related to the regeneration of the bursa that had been excised as part of the initial surgical procedure. It seems to become most apparent during physical therapy rehabilitation at about the sixth week and can linger for several months. Although patients predictably hear the crepitus and perceive the vibrato, only rarely is there an accompanying complaint of pain.

Other intra-articular processes can cause noise to be perceived in the shoulder. Minor subluxations may be perceived as a *thunk;* labral tears similarly can cause a low-frequency noise that a patient either hears or feels. Chasing down noises and their specific causes can be frustrating and elusive. Fortunately, many other history and physical examination features offer substantive clues as to a correct diagnosis.

BOX 4-2 History Related to Instability

Nature of onset (traumatic or atraumatic)

Perceived direction (anterior, posterior, inferior, or combination)

Degree (subluxation or dislocation)

Method of reduction (spontaneous or manipulative)

Character of symptoms (apprehension, pain, paresthesias)

Frequency (daily or intermittently)

Volition (voluntary, involuntary, obligatory)

Ease of dislocation (significant energy or minimal energy)

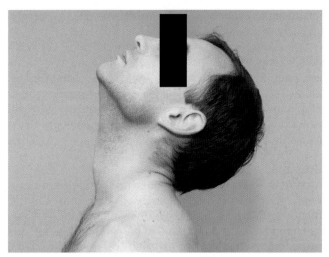

FIGURE 4-3 Neck extension is measured by imagining a line drawn from the occiput to the mentum of the chin and estimating the angle subtended between this line and a horizontal plane.

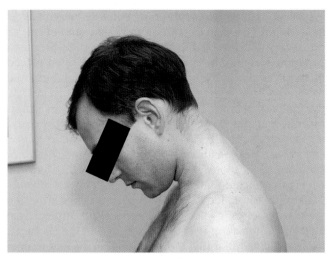

FIGURE 4-4 Neck flexion is measured by imagining a line drawn from the occiput to the mentum of the chin and estimating the angle subtended between this line and a horizontal plane.

PHYSICAL EXAMINATION

Cervical Spine (Neck)

The physical examination of the shoulder begins at the neck. Pathology within the cervical spine can manifest with arm pain and nerve symptoms that radiate down the arm. The patient might believe the source of the problem is somewhere other than the neck. The examiner begins by standing behind the patient and observing the neck and shoulder girdle for symmetry, muscle mass, scars, and deformity. The examiner assesses the ROM including extension, flexion, rotation, and bending. This is best done while standing behind the patient. Because it is difficult to use a goniometer to make measurements, surface relationships are commonly substituted.

Neck extension (Fig. 4-3) is recorded by noting that the imaginary line from the occiput to the mentum of the chin extends beyond the horizontal. Flexion is recorded by noting how many fingerbreadths the chin is from the chest when the patient flexes the neck as much as possible (Fig. 4-4). The patient leans the head to the side while looking forward (Fig. 4-5), and the distance from the shoulder to the ear is recorded for lateral flexion. Lastly, the patient turns the head from side to side and the examiner notes the degree of rotation. These cervical spine motions are made actively (by the patient) rather than passively (by the examiner).

The Spurling test (Fig. 4-6) is performed by placing the cervical spine in extension and rotating the head toward the affected shoulder. An axial load is then placed on the spine. Reproduction of the patient's shoulder or arm pain is considered a positive response.

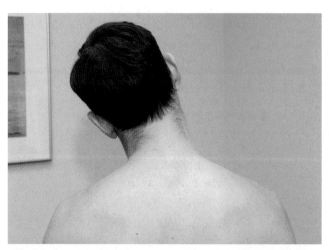

FIGURE 4-5 Lateral bending of the cervical spine is assessed by estimating the distance between the ear and the shoulder.

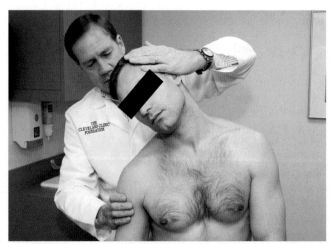

FIGURE 4-6 The Spurling test is performed by axially loading the top of the head with the cervical spine extended and the head rotated toward the affected shoulder. A positive test reproduces the shoulder pain.

Although a detailed neurologic examination is beyond the purview of most shoulder examinations, clinical judgment determines the degree of peripheral nerve assessment necessary to establish a correct and complete diagnosis. Examining the strength of the trapezius, deltoid, spinati, and biceps and triceps muscles suffices for most general shoulder examinations. However, in some situations a more thorough examination needs to be completed, which includes assessment of motor and sensory distributions of each peripheral nerve of the upper extremity or extremities.

Shoulder

Inspection

Inspection of both shoulders can reveal pathology that would otherwise go unnoticed if the examiner relied solely on the patient history or physical examination. Both shoulders need to be exposed (Fig. 4-7). First, observe the clavicles for deformity at both the sternoclavicular joint and acromioclavicular joint. A prominent sternoclavicular joint can be due to an anterior dislocation, inflammation of the synovium, osteoarthritis, infection, or condensing osteitis. A loss of sternoclavicular joint contour is consistent with a posterior dislocation of the medial clavicle, which is worked up urgently to confirm the diagnosis. The acromioclavicular joint is often prominent secondary to osteoarthritis and needs to be compared to the opposite side for symmetry.

The relative height of each shoulder is noted as the patient sits with arms by the sides. Small differences in shoulder height are often found in normal patients and can be confirmed by asking whether their shirt sleeves seem longer on one side than the other. Pathologic causes of a difference in shoulder height can be explained by problems with the articulation of the scapula and thorax or glenohumeral joint. Drooping of the scapula

can be caused by trapezius paralysis, scapular winging, scoliosis, pain that results in splinting of the scapula, fractures of the scapula, or disruption of the scapula–clavicular suspensory complex. Deltoid dysfunction can cause the humerus to hang lower than on the normal side.

Muscle inspection begins with the three portions of the deltoid muscle. Marked atrophy is easy to identify, but deficiencies in the posterior or middle deltoid are more difficult to appreciate until active shoulder motion is initiated (Fig. 4-8). In patients with a large amount of subcutaneous tissue, palpation of the muscle belly may be the only way to distinguish a pathologic muscle contraction from the normal side. Inspection from the back reveals the muscle bulk of the supraspinatus and infraspinatus muscles, as well as the trapezius muscle (Fig. 4-9).

Once the muscle bulk has been assessed, the static position of the scapulae must be noted. If the soft tissue obscures the view of the medial border or the scapular spine, palpation of these landmarks can help visualize the attitude of the scapula at rest. Excessive lateral rotation of the scapula or an increased distance between the

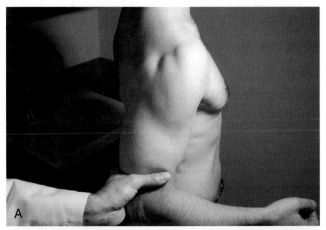

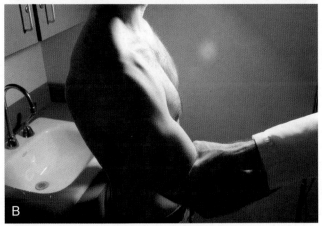

FIGURE 4-8 A, Active muscle contraction against resistance allows the raphe between the middle and posterior bundles of the deltoid muscle to be more easily visualized. **B,** Resisted forward flexion accentuates the raphe between anterior and middle deltoid muscle bundles.

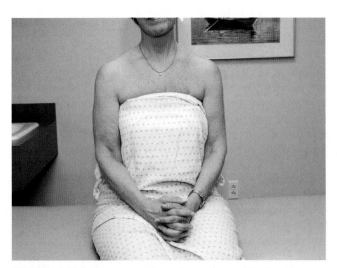

FIGURE 4-7 Proper evaluation of a patient with shoulder complaints requires that both shoulders can be visually inspected simultaneously.

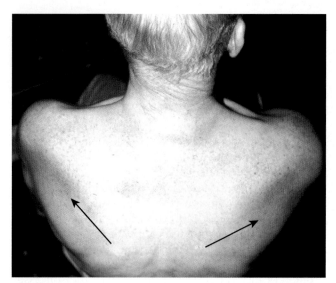

FIGURE 4-9 Bilateral infraspinatus muscle wasting (*arrows*).

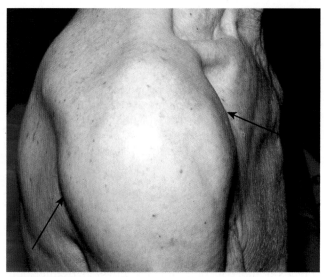

FIGURE 4-10 The fluid bulge (*arrows*) seen here can be an obvious sign of a large or massive rotator cuff tear.

medial border of the scapula and the spine could be caused by trapezius palsy. This can also be accompanied by a prominent inferior tip of the scapula. A laterally prominent inferior scapula tip can be caused by serratus anterior muscle weakness related to a long thoracic nerve injury, but this might only be recognized during active shoulder motion.

The most common skin manifestations of shoulder pathology are ecchymosis, which occurs after fractures, dislocations, or traumatic tendon ruptures, and erythema, which occurs with infection and systemic inflammatory conditions. Less commonly, the skin around the anterior shoulder is swollen and enlarged due to a subacromial effusion and a chronic rotator cuff tear (Fig. 4-10). The examiner notes the presence of scars and their location and character. A widened scar can indicate a collagenopathy often seen in association with shoulder instability.

Palpation

All joints around the shoulder girdle and potentially pathologic tissue is palpated for deformity, tenderness, or asymmetry with the normal side. These locations include the sternoclavicular and acromioclavicular joints, the acromion, the greater tuberosity, the bicipital groove, the trapezius, the superior-medial tip of the scapula, and the posterior glenohumeral joint line. The sternoclavicular joint should not be tender, nor should it move in relation to the manubrium.

Localization of the acromioclavicular joint is easy in thin patients, but many patients require the identification of other more easily palpable landmarks. The examiner can start on the medial clavicle and continue laterally until the acromioclavicular joint is felt. Also, the soft spot where the spine of the scapula meets the clavicle can usually be palpated even in obese patients. Just anterior to the soft spot is the acromioclavicular joint (Fig. 4-11). Lateral to the soft spot is the acromion. The acromiocla-

vicular joint should not be mobile in relation to the acromion and it should not be tender to palpation. The posterior edge of the acromion is palpated as an easy landmark to distinguish the lateral edge of the acromion. This is especially useful in obese patients who do not have easily identifiable landmarks. Knowing where the lateral acromion ends allows palpation of the greater tuberosity and the insertion of the supraspinatus. Any crepitus with passive motion of the shoulder is noted because it can be felt in patients with a rotator cuff tear or calcific tendinitis. Crepitus is difficult to palpate during active motion because the contracted deltoid masks this finding.

Palpation of the deltoid muscle may be necessary to ensure that the muscle belly contracts when visualization is obscured by the subcutaneous tissue. Where a fracture is present, small movements in the anterior, lateral, and posterior directions can allow the examiner to quickly assess all three muscle bellies of the deltoid while minimizing patient discomfort.

The bicipital groove is palpated with the forearm rotated in neutral position or directed straight in front of the patient. The groove is in line with the forearm and approximately a centimeter lateral to the coracoid process when the arm is in neutral rotation. Moving the arm in short arcs of internal and external rotation with the arm at the patient's side allows the examiner to palpate the ridge of the lesser and greater tuberosities, thereby revealing the location of the groove. Many patients have tenderness in this location, especially near the acromion, because of the proximity of the rotator cuff and the subacromial bursa, any of which may be inflamed and tender.

Joint Motion

In measuring and recording the ROM, it is important that *both* affected and normal shoulders be examined passively and actively. Furthermore, the active elevation

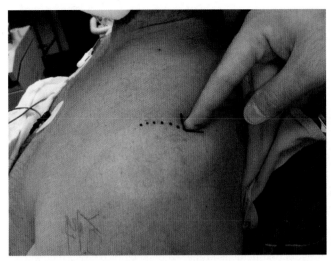

FIGURE 4-11 The soft spot where the spine of the scapula meets the clavicle is easily palpable. Anterior to the soft spot is the acromioclavicular joint, marked here with a *dotted line*.

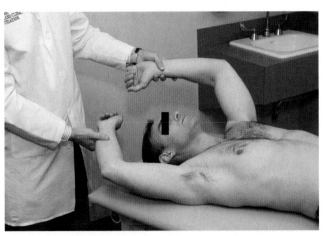

FIGURE 4-12 Passive supine elevation prevents the patient from arching the back, which can mislead the examiner into thinking the patient has better elevation. This examination demonstrates 170 degrees of elevation on the right and 130 degrees of elevation on the left shoulder.

is recorded both while the patient is supine and while sitting against the force of gravity.

Many years ago, the American Shoulder and Elbow Surgeons Society agreed to measure and record the three cardinal planes of motion: elevation in the scapular plane, external rotation with the elbow near the side, and internal rotation using spinal segments as the reference points. Abduction (elevation with the arm in the coronal plane) is not considered a cardinal plane of shoulder motion. Instability assessment does record both internal and external rotation with the arm in 90 degrees of abduction.

Because shoulder motion is the result of four separate articulations (glenohumeral, scapulothoracic, acromioclavicular, and sternoclavicular), only the *total* motions are recorded, not those occurring at the individual joints. The examination begins by measuring the motion of the unaffected arm initially.

Passive Shoulder Elevation

The patient is placed supine on the examination table without a pillow (unless severe kyphosis or cervical spine diseases necessitates one). The examiner passively lifts the arm over the head and records the highest part of the arc that the *elbow* makes while the axis of the humerus generally points to the opposite hip (Fig. 4-12). Because the elbow begins at the patient's side (0 degrees), as the arm is passively elevated, the elbow traverses an angle (in the sagittal plane) as the arm is brought overhead. One standard point is the patient's forehead, which typically represents 160 degrees. If the arm can only be brought up so it points to the ceiling, the elbow has traversed 90 degrees. Motion is *not* measured along the axillary crease. The elevation angle is ideally recorded in increments of 10 degrees.

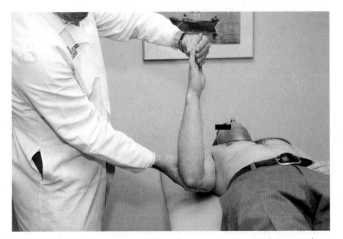

FIGURE 4-13 Starting position for measuring supine passive external rotation. Note the arm is slightly away from the side of the body and the elbow is off the table and parallel with the torso.

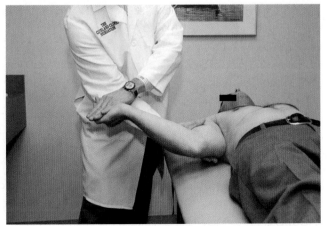

FIGURE 4-14 Ending position for testing supine passive external rotation, demonstrating 70 degrees of passive motion.

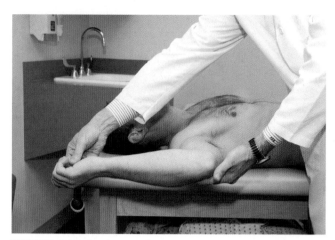

FIGURE 4-15 Supine passive external rotation in 90 degrees of abduction demonstrating 90 degrees of passive motion.

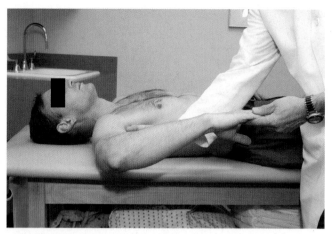

FIGURE 4-16 Supine passive internal rotation in 90 degrees of abduction demonstrating 70 degrees of passive motion.

Active Elevation (Supine)

After the passive motion is recorded, the patient elevates the arm under his or her own power in the same fashion as it was passively examined. Once again, the arc of motion recorded is the arc the elbow makes relative to a sagittal plane. The elevation angle is measured to the nearest 10 degrees.

Passive External Rotation

While the patient remains supine, passive external rotation is measured. The elbow is flexed to 90 degrees and the elbow is moved away from the side (slight shoulder abduction) about the width of the examiner's fist (Fig. 4-13). This establishes an orthogonal angle between the long axis of the humerus and the central axis of the glenoid, which relaxes the superior glenohumeral ligament and the coracohumeral ligament. The examiner

cradles the humerus to hold the humeral shaft parallel to the long axis of the spine and prevent the arm from being in relative shoulder extension (Fig. 4-14). The arm is externally rotated by using the forearm as the handle. The arc of motion is recorded from 0 degrees to 90 degrees (or potentially greater with multidirectional instability). The motion is recorded to the nearest 10 degrees.

Passive External Rotation in 90 Degrees of Abduction

The patient is positioned supine, with the humerus abducted in the coronal plane to 90 degrees. With the elbow flexed to 90 degrees, the forearm is rotated toward the patient's head and the degree of motion is recorded. Zero degrees is the starting point with the forearm pointed toward the ceiling. Motion is recorded to the nearest 10 degrees (Fig. 4-15).

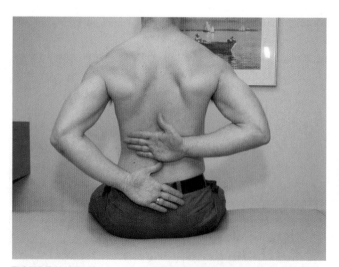

FIGURE 4-17 Measurement of internal rotation by spinal level, demonstrating L3 internal rotation on the left and T7 internal rotation on the right shoulder.

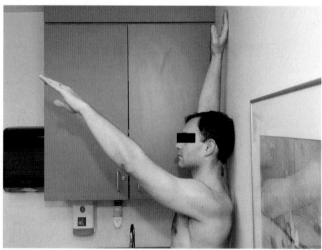

FIGURE 4-18 Active shoulder elevation performed with the patient's back against a wall prevents back extension and the false perception of improved ROM. The patient demonstrates 170 degrees on the right and 140 degrees on the left.

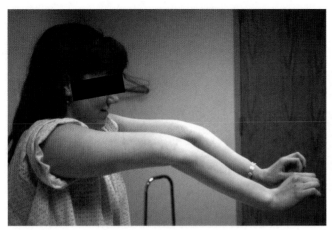

FIGURE 4-19 Hyperlaxity of the elbows.

Passive Internal Rotation in 90 Degrees of Abduction

With the patient remaining supine, the humerus is abducted in the coronal plane to 90 degrees. The elbow remains flexed to 90 degrees as the forearm is rotated toward the patient's foot, and the degree of motion is recorded. Zero degrees is the starting point with the patient's forearm pointed toward the ceiling. Motion is recorded to the nearest 10 degrees (Fig. 4-16).

Passive Internal Rotation

The patient reaches behind his or her back and then reaches up between the scapulae (in the fashion of passing a belt or fastening a bra). The tip of the thumb is pulled up the back, and the tip of the thumb determines the level along the spine, which is recorded as the degree of internal rotation. The position of the scapula of the arm that is not being examined provides the proper levels to interpolate. The superior angle *of the nonmeasured side* is opposite T4, the inferior angle is opposite T7. The iliac crest is at the L4 level (Fig. 4-17). Occasionally the shoulder is so stiff that the patient can only reach the sacrum or greater trochanter of the ipsilateral hip. Severe scoliosis or a stiff elbow on the affected side invalidates the measurements.

Active Total Shoulder Elevation

The patient is positioned standing with his or her back against a wall; this prevents hyperextension of the back. The patient lifts the arm toward the ceiling, and the arc of motion is recorded to the nearest 10 degrees. The patient is observed from the lateral perspective, and the arc of motion that the elbow has traversed is recorded as the active elevation of the arm (Fig. 4-18).

Active Cross-Body Adduction

The patient may be either standing or sitting. The patient elevates the arm to shoulder level, with the upper arm in the scapular plane (0 degrees). The patient brings the arm across the front of the chest while maintaining the arm at shoulder level. The arc of motion is recorded.

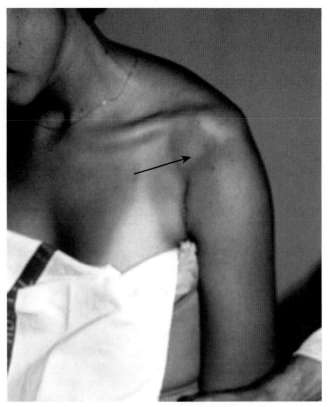

FIGURE 4-20 The sulcus sign *(arrow)*.

Stability Assessment

Stability of the glenohumeral joint is conferred by the passive restraints of the glenohumeral ligaments and by the dynamic restraints of the rotator cuff muscles and the scapular stabilizers. To assess the amount of ligamentous laxity in the shoulder, an examination of the patient's other joints should first be made. Hyperextension of the metacarpophalangeal joints, elbow joints, and knee joints is often found in patients with general ligamentous laxity, and if laxity is found, the examiner can expect more laxity in both shoulders as well (Fig. 4-19). A history of frequent ankle sprains or patella–femur problems can also be associated with ligamentous laxity of the shoulder. Even if the patient does not exhibit signs of ligamentous laxity in other joints, the shoulders might have excessive laxity. The best way to distinguish between pathologic instability and laxity is to always compare the symptomatic shoulder with the opposite shoulder for all of the following tests.

The sulcus test can be performed with the patient sitting or supine. The examiner pulls the adducted arm at the side toward the foot and measures the amount of translation between the acromion and the humeral head (Fig. 4-20). The translation of the humeral head in centimeters is documented as a 1+ for 1 cm and 2+ for 2 cm.

Glenohumeral translation can be measured while the patient's arms are resting at the patient's side in neutral rotation. The examiner stabilizes the scapula with one hand and translates the humeral head with the other

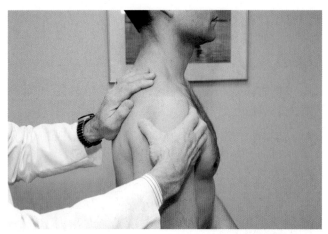

FIGURE 4-21 Assessment of humeral head translation on the glenoid, performed by stabilizing the scapula and grasping the humeral head between thumb and fingers, then applying anterior and posterior translation force.

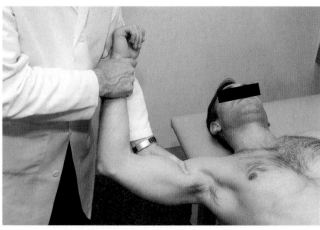

FIGURE 4-22 Assessment of stability conferred by differing aspects of the glenohumeral ligaments. In 90 degrees of abduction and neutral rotation, the inferior glenohumeral ligaments and inferior capsule become taut, providing the majority of ligamentous stability.

hand (Fig. 4-21). The translation of the head is documented as a percentage of the humeral head that can be subluxed anterior to the glenoid rim. The same is done to assess posterior translation. To assess the passive stability that is conferred by the glenohumeral ligaments, the glenohumeral translation is assessed in varying degrees of internal and external rotation as well as varying degrees of abduction. The patient is positioned supine and placed at the edge of the table so that the arm can be taken through a full ROM. With one arm, the examiner holds the patient's forearm to control rotation. The examiner's other hand is placed around the patient's upper arm to control translation. An axial load is placed at the distal humerus so that the examiner can gain a tactile feeling of the humeral head as it articulates with the glenoid. The arm is abducted and rotated into the desired position, and then a gentle anterior shift is made with the hand at the upper arm (Fig. 4-22). Translation of the head is recorded as a percentage of the humeral head that moves out of the glenoid. This maneuver is repeated with a posteriorly directed force. The amount of translation varies with different amounts of arm rotation, so the examiner must repeat the examination on the opposite shoulder using the same arm positions.

The anterior and posterior drawer tests as described by Gerber and Ganz[2] are alternative methods used to assess laxity in the shoulder. The patient is placed supine and the arm is abducted 60 degrees. The examiner applies an axial force to the humeral head while holding the arm in neutral rotation. The examiner's other hand is used to translate the humeral head both anteriorly and posteriorly. Translation of the head to the glenoid rim is grade I, translation over the rim that spontaneously reduces is grade II, and dislocation without spontaneous reduction is grade III.

Apprehension Tests

The apprehension test as described by Rowe and Zarins[3] is performed while the patient is supine. The examiner abducts the patient's arm 90 degrees and then slowly externally rotates the arm to 90 degrees (Fig. 4-23). The patient is asked if the shoulder feels like it is about to dislocate. Many patients complain of a vague uncomfortable feeling in the shoulder. Others only show their discomfort with a grimace, or the shoulder muscles involuntarily contract to prevent further shoulder rotation. Any elicitation of apprehension during this maneuver is a positive test. Some patients also complain of pain during this maneuver, and the location of the pain can help the examiner localize the pathology, but pain alone is a poor predictor of traumatic anterior instability. Posterior and superior pain can be caused by posterosuperior labral

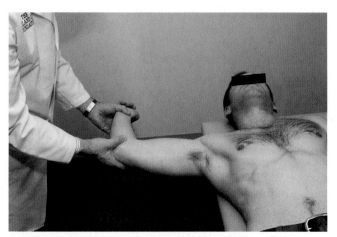

FIGURE 4-23 The position of apprehension for patients with anterior instability as described by Rowe and Zarins is 90 degrees of abduction and 90 degrees of external rotation.

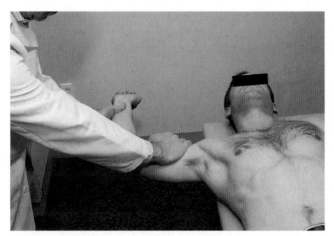

FIGURE 4-24 The relocation test.

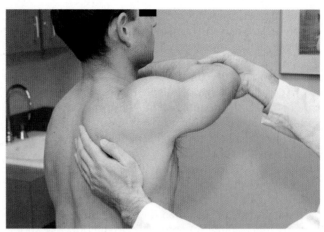

FIGURE 4-25 In patients with posterior instability, the humeral head can be subluxed posteriorly by placing the arm in 90 degrees of flexion and 90 degrees of internal rotation and slight adduction and then applying a posterior load.

tears or internal impingement, whereas anterior pain is more likely caused by an anteroinferior labral tear.

The relocation test as described by Jobe and colleagues[4] is performed in conjunction with the apprehension test. If the patient feels apprehension while the shoulder is externally rotated and abducted 90 degrees, then the examiner applies a posterior force against the proximal arm, which moves the humeral head from an anteriorly subluxed position to a centered position in the glenoid. If the patient no longer has apprehension, then the relocation test is positive (Fig. 4-24). The patient's apprehension should return once the examiner stops applying the posterior force. Patients with posterosuperior labral tears or internal impingement usually experience an increase in pain during this maneuver because the examiner's posterior force loads the humeral head against the torn labrum.

The diagnostic accuracy of the apprehension test and the relocation test were studied by Farber and colleagues.[5] A physical examination and subsequent arthroscopy were performed on 363 patients. Of those patients, 46 had a Bankart tear, a Hill-Sachs lesion, a humeral avulsion of the glenohumeral ligament by arthroscopy, or an x-ray with a documented anterior dislocation, and they made up the study group. The other patients were used as a comparison group. When apprehension was used as the criterion for a positive test, the sensitivity and specificity of the apprehension test were 72% and 96%, respectively, compared to 50% and 56% when pain was used as the criterion for a positive test. When apprehension was used as the criterion for a positive test, the sensitivity and specificity of the relocation test were 81% and 92%, respectively, compared to 30% and 90% when pain was used as the criterion for a positive test.

Posterior Instability Testing

Posterior instability is best tested while the patient is sitting or standing for easy visualization of the entire scapula and the posterior muscle contours that often change when the humeral head subluxes or dislocates

posteriorly. In patients with severe posterior instability, active forward flexion to 90 degrees, internal rotation, and adduction across the front of the body can cause a posterior dislocation that is easily seen by the examiner. Most patients, however, experience posterior instability during exertional activities, so the examiner needs to reproduce those conditions to demonstrate posterior instability.

In contrast to anterior instability testing, posterior instability testing begins when the examiner moves the humeral head into a dislocated or subluxated position. This is accomplished by grasping the patient's elbow with one hand and stabilizing the scapula with the other hand. The humerus is brought to 90 degrees of flexion, is internally rotated, and is adducted across the chest (Fig. 4-25). The examiner then applies a posterior load to the humeral head and maintains that load while slowly abducting the arm. The humerus is kept parallel to the floor and the patient relaxes the shoulder muscles as much as possible. If a clunk is felt when the humeral head relocates into the glenoid, then this is a positive test. This test has been called the *jerk test* because the shoulder jerks back into the glenoid during a positive test. It has also been called the *Jahnke test* or simply a *posterior load test*.

Rotator Cuff Examination

The rotator cuff examination begins with a visual inspection of the supraspinatus and infraspinatus muscle bulk. Patients with chronic rotator cuff tears often have atrophy of the muscle in the supraspinatus fossa or below the spine of the scapula when compared to the asymptomatic side (see Fig. 4-9). An assessment of the passive and active motion arcs is the second step of the rotator cuff examination, with the expectation that only the active motion is affected in patients with isolated rotator cuff pathology. It is often the case, however, that patients have a small loss of passive motion secondary to disuse and pain at the extremes of motion.

The subscapularis muscle is difficult to isolate with one specific test because so many other muscles around the shoulder girdle contribute to internal rotation. The lift-off test can be used if the patient does not have an internal rotation contracture that prevents the patient from passively placing the hand behind the patient's back. The patient places the hand behind the back at waist level and then pushes the hand away from the body. The elbow should not move as the patient pushes the hand away from the body. If the patient does not have the strength to push the hand away from the waist, the examiner can pull the hand away from the waist and ask the patient to hold the hand in that position (Fig. 4-26). If the patient can do this, then the subscapularis muscle is partially functioning. A comparison to the opposite shoulder is always made if the test is abnormal in any way.

Another test specific to the subscapularis muscle is the belly-press test (Fig. 4-27).[6] This test requires slightly less internal rotation than the lift-off test and is often less painful for the patient to perform because the hand is not rotated behind the back. The patient must place the hand on the belly, keeping the wrist extended so that the elbow is in front of the body. Then the patient presses against the belly without flexing the wrist. If the wrist and elbow are locked, this motion can only be done if

the shoulder internally rotates, which is done primarily by the subscapularis. A positive test is when the patient must flex the wrist to push against their belly.

A modification of the belly-press test is the Napoleon test. The patient places the hand on the belly with the elbows resting at the patient's side. Then the patient pushes the elbow in front of the patient while keeping the hand on the belly (Fig. 4-28). A positive test is recorded when the patient is unable to bring the elbow anteriorly without moving the entire shoulder girdle forward. The examiner can also grade muscle strength by holding resistance against the elbow as the patient attempts to push the elbow forward.

A third test recently described is called the *bear hug test*.[7] The patient brings the hand over the opposite shoulder. The examiner holds the elbow to prevent elbow flexion during the test. The patient pushes the hand down against the opposite shoulder or down against the examiner's other hand. The patient who has a subscapularis tendon tear or muscle weakness experiences pain during this maneuver, or he or she cannot push down (Fig. 4-29).

The supraspinatus muscle-tendon unit is difficult to isolate from the activity of the deltoid because they both elevate the humerus. Rotator cuff muscle testing can also

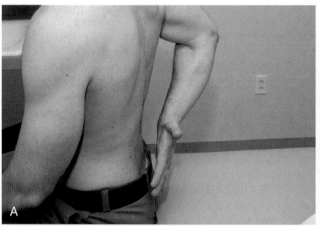

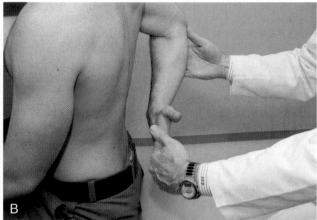

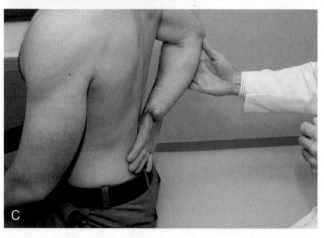

FIGURE 4-26 The lift-off test. **A,** Patients with a functional subscapularis muscle and adequate internal rotation should be able to hold their hand away from the small of their back. **B,** Patients with a weak but functioning subscapularis can keep their hand off of their back if the examiner positions it there. **C,** Absent subscapularis function results in the inability to bring the hand off the back or maintain it there if it is lifted off by the examiner.

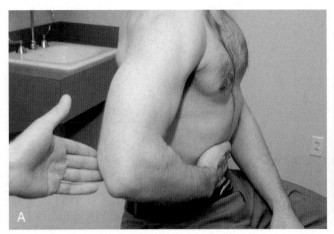
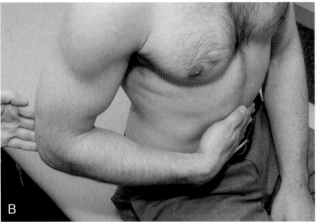

FIGURE 4-27 The belly-press test. **A,** The test is negative when the patient can press against the abdomen while keeping the wrist straight and the elbow in front of the plane of the body. **B,** The test is positive when the patient must flex the wrist to press against the abdomen.

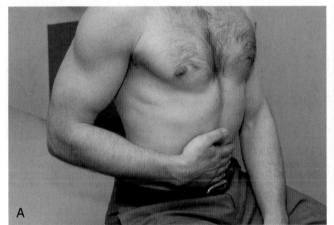
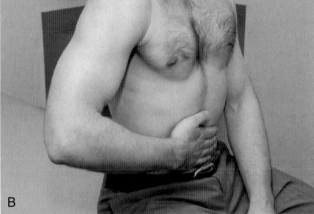

FIGURE 4-28 The Napoleon test. **A,** Starting position from which the patient is asked to bring the elbow forward. **B,** Ending position indicating a negative test and a functional subscapularis.

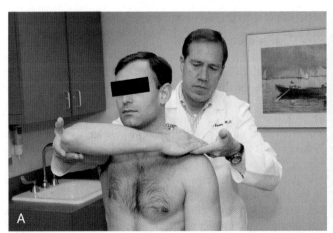
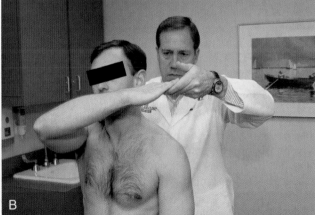

FIGURE 4-29 The bear hug test. **A,** Patients with a functional subscapularis can resist the examiner's attempt to raise the patient's hand off the contralateral shoulder without pain. **B,** The ability to lift the hand off the contralateral shoulder indicates a weak or nonfunctional subscapularis.

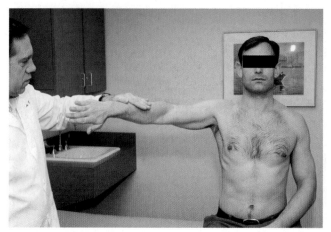

FIGURE 4-30 Supraspinatus strength testing. Ninety degrees of elevation in the scapular plane and full internal rotation of the arm.

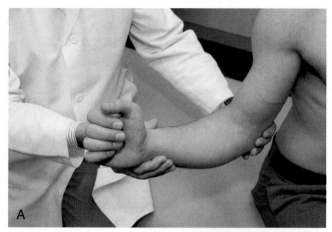

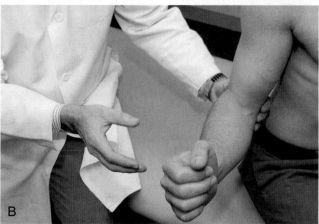

FIGURE 4-31 Infraspinatus and teres minor testing. **A,** The arm is passively maximally externally rotated. **B,** Inability to maintain that position when the examiner releases the arm indicates a positive lag sign and weak or absent infraspinatus and teres minor function.

be difficult to perform in patients who have significant pain that compromises their effort. If the examiner believes pain is a significant factor in the patient's weakness, then a subacromial lidocaine injection may be used to eliminate pain as a factor.

To best isolate the supraspinatus muscle, the arm is internally rotated and elevated 90 degrees so that the muscle-tendon unit is parallel to the floor (Fig. 4-30). Testing both arms simultaneously makes it easy for the examiner to detect subtle differences in strength. The examiner pushes both arms toward the floor while the patient resists. Any difference in strength can be attributed to the supraspinatus muscle if the deltoid is not injured. According to a study by Itoi and colleagues, internal or external rotation of the humerus during supraspinatus testing did not improve the accuracy of detecting a torn tendon.[8]

The infraspinatus and teres minor muscles are more easily isolated from action of the deltoid because the deltoid has very limited ability to externally rotate the humerus. Any loss of strength to external rotation can be attributed to an abnormality in these muscles. Patients with large or massive rotator cuff tears often have a lag sign (Fig. 4-31). This is found when the patient holds the arms by the patient's sides with the elbows flexed 90 degrees.

The examiner externally rotates the arm as far as it will go passively, and then the patient holds the arm in that position when the examiner releases it. If the patient's arm internally rotates from where the examiner held it, then that patient has a lag sign that can be documented in degrees. For instance, if the patient has passive external rotation to 45 degrees and the patient can only hold the arm externally rotated to 20 degrees, then that patient has a 25-degree lag sign. In effect, the lag sign is just another way of documenting the difference between the patient's active and passive external rotation.

SPECIAL TESTS

Impingement Tests

Neer Impingement Sign

This maneuver, first reported by Neer in 1972 and later fully described by Neer in 1983,[9] attempts to reproduce compression of the inflamed rotator cuff and subacromial bursa between the humeral head and the undersurface of the acromion and coracoacromial arch. In the classic version of this maneuver, the examiner stands behind the patient and stabilizes the scapula with one hand on the acromion. With the other hand, the examiner elevates the patient's arm in the plane of the scapula. As the arm is brought into full elevation, the examiner holds down the scapula to prevent it from rotating superiorly, bringing the greater tuberosity into contact with the acromion, compressing the inflamed supraspinatus tendon and bursa. In a positive Neer impingement sign, this maneuver reproduces the patient's anterior shoulder pain.

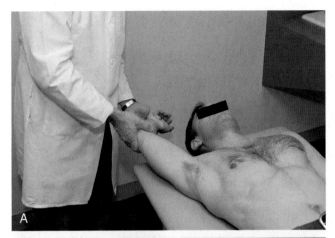

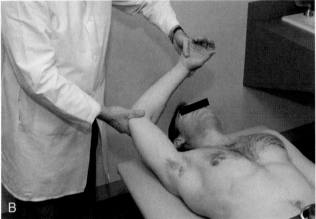

FIGURE 4-32 Modified Neer impingement sign. **A,** With the patient supine, the arm is brought into full forward flexion, which can reproduce anterior shoulder pain related to subacromial impingement. **B,** Internal rotation of the arm from this position further accentuates supraspinatus impingement underneath the coracoacromial arch.

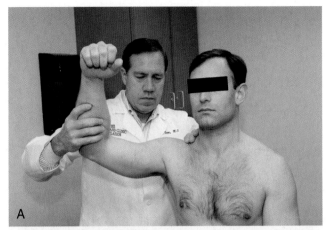

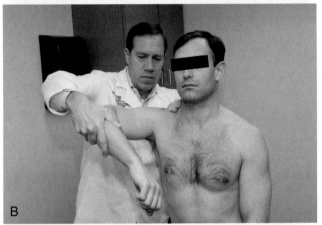

FIGURE 4-33 The Hawkins-Kennedy impingement sign. **A,** Starting position in 90 degrees of flexion. **B,** From here the arm is forcibly internally rotated, reproducing pain in patients with subacromial impingement.

In a modification of this technique, which one of us has seen Dr. Neer use, the patient lies supine on the examination table and the examiner stands at the patient's head. The examiner brings the patient's arm into full elevation and then, with the elbow flexed, applies an internal rotation torque to the arm similar to that described by Hawkins and Kennedy[10] (Fig. 4-32). Performing this maneuver with the patient supine minimizes scapular rotation, eliminating the need for manual stabilization of the scapula by the examiner.

Neer noted in his original work, and others have confirmed,[11] that other shoulder pathology, especially Bankart lesions, SLAP lesions, and acromioclavicular joint arthritis, often cause pain with this maneuver. Anatomic studies[12] have shown that in addition to rotator cuff and bursal impingement, the greater tuberosity itself or the biceps tendon can directly impinge underneath the acromion when the arm is placed in the Neer position. This likely explains the good sensitivity but limited specificity of the Neer impingement sign.

Neer Impingement Test

This test is performed after the patient demonstrates a positive Neer impingement sign. Approximately 5 mL of 1% lidocaine is injected into the subacromial space. After several minutes the Neer impingement maneuver is again performed. A Neer impingement test is considered positive when the pain associated with the preinjection Neer impingement sign is significantly reduced or absent, indicating that the injected subacromial space was the source of pain.

Hawkins-Kennedy Impingement Test

This Hawkins-Kennedy impingement test was first described by Hawkins and Kennedy in 1980.[10] For this maneuver, the examiner stands at the patient's side. The patient's shoulder is placed in 90 degrees of forward flexion with the elbow bent 90 degrees, and the examiner then forcibly internally rotates the arm (Fig. 4-33). A positive Hawkins impingement sign is pain as the greater tuberosity rotates under the acromion and coracoacromial arch, compressing the inflamed bursa and supraspinatus tendon. In one anatomic study,[12] all specimens showed direct contact between the coracoacromial ligament and

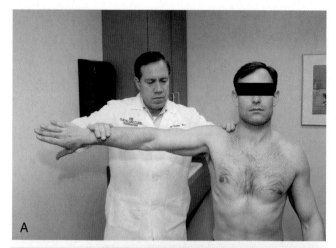

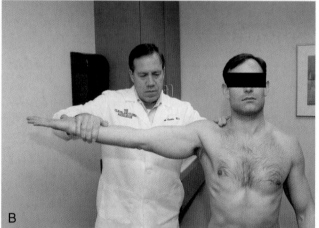

FIGURE 4-34 Jobe-Yocum test. **A,** The patient is asked to resist a downward force at the wrist with the arm in 90 degrees of scapular elevation and full internal rotation. **B,** The maneuver is repeated with the hand fully supinated. Pain against resistance in internal rotation that improves with full hand supination indicates supraspinatus tendinitis.

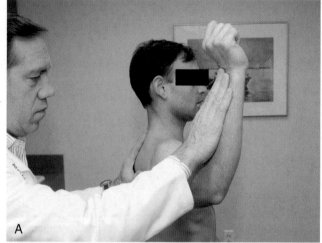

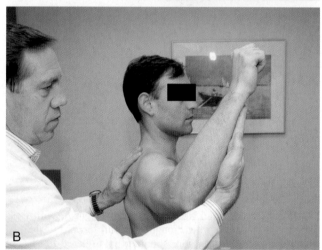

FIGURE 4-35 The internal rotation resistance stress test. **A,** Weakness with resisted external rotation indicates classic subacromial impingement. **B,** Weakness in resisted internal rotation indicates internal impingement.

rotator cuff or biceps tendon with this maneuver. As with the Neer impingement sign, this test is sensitive but lacks specificity.

Jobe-Yocum Test

Supraspinatus tendinitis is assessed using this test, which was first described separately by Jobe and colleagues and by Yocum in 1983.[13,14] With the patient maintaining the arm in 90 degrees of elevation in the plane of the scapula, the arm is placed in internal rotation with the thumb pointing straight down. The patient resists a downward force applied by the examiner to the patient's wrist. The test is positive for supraspinatus pathology if this maneuver is painful. Repeating the same maneuver with the arm in full external rotation should decrease or eliminate the pain (Fig. 4-34). Although a positive test is classically described as pain associated with resistance of the downward force, weakness resulting in the inability to resist the examiner may be present as well, due to pain-generated muscle inhibition.

Internal Rotation Resistance Stress Test

This test was first described by Zaslav[15] to differentiate between intra-articular and subacromial impingement in patients with a positive Neer impingement sign. The test is performed with the patient standing and the arm positioned in 90 degrees of abduction in the coronal plane and 80 degrees of external rotation. With the examiner standing behind the patient, stabilizing the patient's elbow with one hand and holding the patient's wrist with the other hand, isometric external rotation strength is tested, followed by isometric internal rotation strength (Fig. 4-35). Relative weakness of internal rotation compared to external rotation is considered a positive sign, suggesting internal impingement. Conversely, relative weakness in external rotation suggests classic subacromial impingement.

Relative strength of internal versus external rotation in the affected extremity is the important determinant for this examination, and for this reason comparison to the unaffected contralateral shoulder is not performed with this

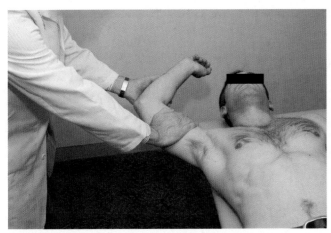

FIGURE 4-36 The modified relocation test. Pain with an anteriorly directed force that is relieved by a posteriorly directed force in 90, 110, or 120 degrees of abduction suggests internal impingement of the undersurface of the rotator cuff against the posterosuperior glenoid labrum.

test. The utility of this test was investigated only in patients who already had an established diagnosis of impingement as defined by a positive Neer impingement sign.

Modified Relocation Test

This modification of Jobe's relocation test was reported by Hamner and colleagues in 2000[16] as a method for testing for internal impingement. To perform this test, the patient lies supine on the examination table with the affected shoulder off the edge of the table. The arm is examined in a position of maximal external rotation and 90, 110, and 120 degrees of abduction. In each of these three positions, an anterior load followed by a posterior load is placed on the shoulder (Fig. 4-36). Pain that is caused by an anteriorly directed force and is alleviated by a posteriorly directed force is considered a positive sign. Contact between the undersurface of the rotator cuff and the posterosuperior labrum was documented arthroscopically in 79% of patients with a positive test. Fraying and undersurface partial thickness cuff tears have been identified in conjunction with a positive test, but the specificity and sensitivity of this test are unknown.

Painful Arc Test

For this test the patient elevates the arm in the scapular plane with the elbow straight, making sure that the arm is kept in neutral rotation. Conversely, the arm can be placed in full elevation and the patient slowly brings the arm down to the side. A positive painful arc test is documented when the patient experiences pain between 60 and 100 degrees of abduction during the maneuver (Fig. 4-37). Attention to arm rotation is important when performing this test because patients might minimize or avoid pain by performing the test with the arm in external rotation, thereby rotating the greater tuberosity out from under the acromion and preventing impingement of the involved portion of the rotator cuff.

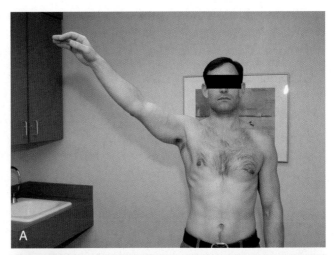

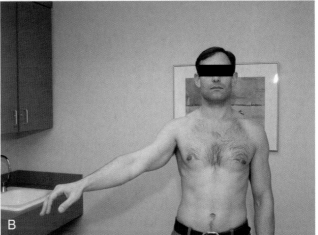

FIGURE 4-37 The painful arc test. Pain with attempted controlled descent of the arm between 100 degrees (**A**) and 60 degrees (**B**) indicates subacromial impingement.

Combining Tests for Rotator Cuff Pathology

Park and colleagues[17] studied eight physical examination tests to determine their diagnostic accuracy of rotator cuff tears and impingement syndrome. The Neer test was the only test that could predict bursitis or partial rotator cuff tears. The best combination of tests to diagnose a full-thickness rotator cuff tear were the drop-arm sign, the painful arc sign, and weakness in external rotation with the arm at the side. If all three tests were positive in the study cohort, then the patient had a 91% chance of having a rotator cuff tear. If all three tests were negative, then the patient had a 9% chance of having a rotator cuff tear. Table 4-1 lists the reported sensitivity and specificity of these tests for diagnosing rotator cuff pathology and subacromial impingement.

Acromioclavicular Joint Tests

The acromioclavicular joint is tested with the cross-body adduction maneuver. To perform this maneuver, the

TABLE 4-1 Subacromial Impingement

Test	Sensitivity (%)	Specificity (%)	Positive Predictive Value (%)	Negative Predictive Value (%)
Neer sign[1]	68.0	68.7	80.4	53.2
Hawkins-Kennedy test[1]	71.5	66.3	79.7	55.7
Painful arc test[1]	73.5	81.1	88.2	61.5
Jobe test[1]	44.1	89.5	88.4	46.8
Internal rotation resistance stress test[2]	96	88	88	94

[1]Park HB, Yokota A, Gill HS, et al: Diagnostic accuracy of clinical tests for the different degrees of subacromial impingement syndrome. J Bone Joint Surg Am 87:1146-1155, 2005.
[2]Zaslav KR: Internal rotation resistance strength test: A new diagnostic test to differentiate intra-articular pathology from outlet (Neer) impingement syndrome in the shoulder. J Shoulder Elbow Surg 10(1):23-27, 2001.

examiner stands beside or behind the patient. The patient's arm is held forward flexed to 90 degrees, and the examiner adducts the arm across the body toward the opposite shoulder (Fig. 4-38). This maneuver attempts to generate compression across the acromioclavicular joint, causing pain and a positive test.

It is important to be clear with the patient about the location of any reported pain because this maneuver can produce pain in the posterior shoulder due to posterior capsular tightness or in the anterior shoulder due to subcoracoid impingement. To be considered positive for acromioclavicular joint pathology, this test must reproduce pain located on the top of the shoulder at the acromioclavicular joint.

Further confirmation of primary acromioclavicular joint pathology can be obtained by injecting the acromioclavicular joint with 1% lidocaine after a positive cross-body adduction maneuver. Repeating the maneuver with reso-lution of pain after the injection establishes the acromioclavicular joint as the source of pain.

Biceps Tendon Tests

Yergason's Test

This test is performed with the arm at the patient's side, the elbow flexed 90 degrees, and the hand in full pronation. In this position, the examiner grasps the patient's hand and asks the patient to attempt to supinate the hand against resistance (Fig. 4-39). Reproduction of pain in the anterior shoulder or bicipital groove is a positive sign suggesting pathology in the long head of the biceps tendon.

Speed's Test

Crenshaw and Kilgore first described Speed's test in 1966.[18] With the elbow extended and the hand in full supination, the arm is placed in 60 to 90 degrees of forward flexion, and the patient resists a downward force at the wrist. A positive test produces anterior shoulder pain or pain in the bicipital groove. Bennett[19] reported a specificity of 14%, sensitivity of 90%, positive predictive value of 23%, and negative predictive value of 83% based on correlations of a positive Speed's test with arthroscopic findings of biceps pathology.

Ludington's Test

For this test, the patient places the hands on top of the head with palms down and fingers interlocked. The patient contracts and relaxes the biceps. Pain in the bicipital groove with this test indicates a positive test and pathology of the long head of the biceps.

Superior Labrum Tests

Table 4-2 lists the sensitivity and specificity of biceps and SLAP tests.

O'Brien Test (Active Compression Test)

In 1998, O'Brien and colleagues[20] reported on use of the active compression test to differentiate between acromio-

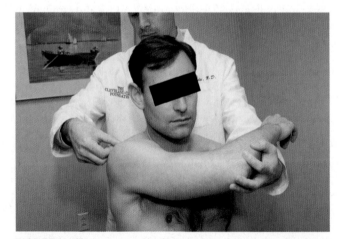

FIGURE 4-38 The cross-body adduction maneuver. With the arm forward flexed 90 degrees and in 90 degrees of internal rotation, the examiner adducts the arm across the body. Acromioclavicular joint pathology reproduces pain over the superior aspect of the shoulder at the acromioclavicular joint.

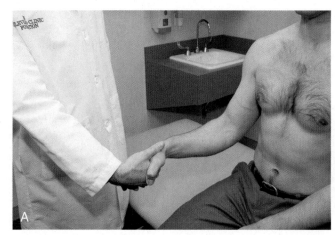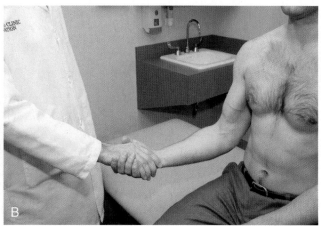

FIGURE 4-39 The Yergason test. **A,** Starting from full pronation, the patient is asked to supinate the hand against resistance (**B**). Pain anteriorly along the bicipital groove or in the anterior shoulder suggests biceps tendinitis.

clavicular joint pathology and superior labral pathology. This test is performed with the examiner standing behind the patient. The affected shoulder is forward flexed to 90 degrees and adducted 15 degrees toward the midline. In this position, the patient resists a downward force first with the arm internally rotated so that the thumb points to the floor, then with the arm in full supination and external rotation (Fig. 4-40). Anterior shoulder pain with the arm internally rotated that is then relieved when the maneuver is performed with the arm in full supination and external rotation is a positive test indicating superior labral pathology. The location of the pain is also important because pain produced over the top of the shoulder or acromioclavicular joint indicates acromioclavicular joint pathology.

SLAP-rehension Test

This is a modification of the O'Brien test. The arm is brought into 45 degrees of adduction instead of 15 degrees. The same resisted maneuvers are performed as with the O'Brien test. This different arm position attempts to place more stress on the biceps origin and superior labrum, but it is also more likely to cause acromioclavicular joint abutment and pain.

Biceps Tension Test

In 1990, Snyder and colleagues[21] described use of the biceps tension test as an effective means of identifying SLAP tears. The biceps tension test is described as resisted shoulder flexion with the elbow fully extended and the hand in supination. This test maneuver is nearly identical

TABLE 4-2 Biceps Tendon and SLAP Lesions

Test	Sensitivity (%)	Specificity (%)	Positive Predictive Value (%)	Negative Predictive Value (%)
Speed's test[1]	14	90	23	83
O'Brien test[2]	100	99	89	89
Anterior slide test[3]	78	91	NA	NA
Crank test[4]	91	93	94	90
Pain provocation test[5]	100	90	NA	NA
Biceps load test I[6]	91	97	83	98
Biceps load test II[7]	90	97	92	96

[1]Bennett WF: Specificity of the Speed's test: Arthroscopic technique for evaluating the biceps tendon at the level of the bicipital groove. Arthroscopy 14(8):789-796, 1998.
[2]O'Brien SJ, Pagnani MJ, Fealy S, et al: The active compression test: A new and effective test for diagnosing labral tears and acromioclavicular joint abnormality. Am J Sports Med 26:610-613, 1998.
[3]Kibler WB: Sensitivity and specificity of the anterior slide test in throwing athletes with superior glenoid labral tears. Arthroscopy 14(2):447-457, 1995.
[4]Liu SH, Henry MH, Nuccion SL: A prospective evaluation of a new physical examination in predicting glenoid labral tears. Am J Sports Med 24(6):721-725, 1996.
[5]Mimori K, Muneta T, Nakagawa T: A new pain provocation test for superior labral tears of the shoulder. Am J Sports Med 27(2):137-142, 1999.
[6]Kim SH, Ha KI, Han KY: Biceps load test: A clinical test for superior labrum anterior and posterior lesions in shoulders with recurrent anterior dislocations. Am J Sports Med 27:300-303, 1999.
[7]Kim SH, Ha KI, Ahn JH, et al: Biceps load test II: A clinical test for SLAP lesions of the shoulder. Arthroscopy 17:160-164, 2001.
NA, not available; SLAP, superior labrum anterior and posterior.

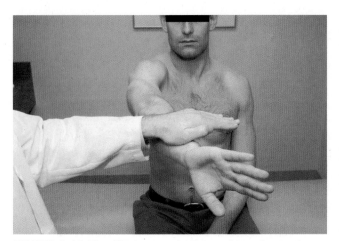

FIGURE 4-40 The O'Brien test (active compression test). Pain in the anterior shoulder with resistance against downward pressure with the arm in 90 degrees of flexion, 15 degrees of adduction, and full internal rotation indicates biceps pathology.

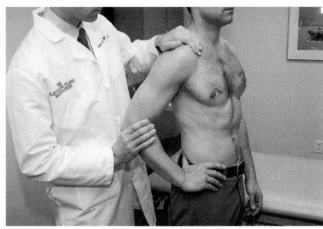

FIGURE 4-41 Anterior slide test. Pain or a click felt over the anterior shoulder with resistance to an anterosuperior directed force at the elbow suggests a SLAP lesion.

to the Speed test for biceps pathology but is applied as a method of generating tension on the biceps anchor and superior labrum.

Anterior Slide Test

Kibler described the anterior slide test is 1995[22] as a method to assess superior labral pathology. To perform this test, the patient stands with arms akimbo (hands on hips, thumbs along the posterior iliac crests). The examiner stands behind the patient with one hand over the top of the acromion, with the tips of the examiner's fingers just off the anterior edge of the acromion and the other hand on the patient's elbow. The examiner pushes the arm forward and slightly superior at the elbow while the patient resists this anterior-superior force (Fig. 4-41). Pain or a click over the anterior shoulder is considered a positive sign indicating a SLAP lesion.

Crank Test

This test for superior labral pathology is similar to the McMurray test for the knee. The crank test attempts to catch labrum tears between the two joint surfaces. This test is performed in approximately 160 degrees of forward flexion (Fig. 4-42) in either the sitting or supine position.[23] Glenohumeral joint compression is created by axial loading through the humeral shaft with the arm in extreme forward flexion and abduction. The arm is then internally and externally rotated. Reproduction of symptoms of pain, catching, or a click indicates a positive test.

Pain Provocation Test

This test is performed with the patient sitting up and the examiner standing behind the patient. In the original description of this test, Mimori's group[24] positioned the arm in 90 degrees of abduction and full external rotation. The patient's hand is then placed in two different positions, first in full supination then in full pronation (Fig.

4-43). The patient is asked which hand position provokes more pain, supination or pronation. The test is considered positive for a SLAP lesion if the patient reports more pain while the hand is in pronation. In the Minori group's report, the test was 100% sensitive and 90% specific when comparing to MR arthrography as the gold standard.

Biceps Load Test I

This test for SLAP lesions in patients with a history of recurrent anterior instability was first described by Kim and colleagues in 1999.[25] The test is performed by placing the patient's arm in 90 degrees of abduction and full external rotation (as if performing the apprehension test). With the patient's forearm supinated, the examiner externally rotates the patient's arm until the patient begins to feel apprehension. The examiner holds the patient's arm at that position and the patient flexes the elbow against

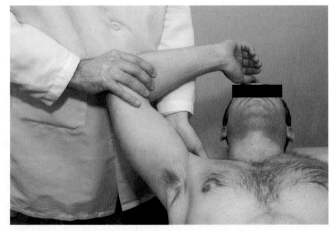

FIGURE 4-42 The crank test. With the patient either supine or sitting, the arm is axially loaded in 160 degrees of flexion and then internally and externally rotated with glenohumeral joint compression.

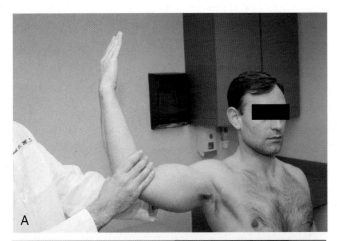

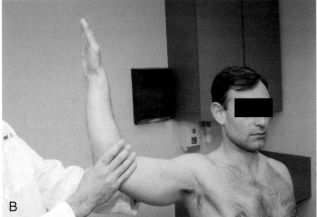

FIGURE 4-43 The pain provocation test. With the arm in 90 degrees of abduction and full external rotation, the hand is placed in full supination (**A**), and then full pronation (**B**). Increased pain in full pronation suggests a SLAP lesion.

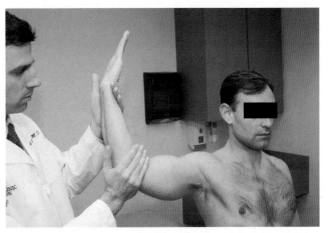

FIGURE 4-44 The biceps load test I. The patient is placed into the position of apprehension, with the hand supinated, and then asked to flex the elbow against resistance. Decreased pain and apprehension indicates a negative test and the absence of a SLAP lesion.

resistance (Fig. 4-44). A decrease in the patient's apprehension with active biceps contraction indicates a negative test and the absence of a SLAP lesion. No change or worsening of the patient's pain and apprehension with active biceps contraction against resistance indicates a positive test and the presence of a SLAP lesion.

Biceps Load Test II

In 2001, Kim and colleagues described a SLAP test for patients who lack a history of anterior instability.[26] For this maneuver, the patient is lies supine and the examiner stands at the patient's side by the affected shoulder. The patient's arm is placed into 120 degrees of elevation, with full external rotation, the elbow flexed to 90 degrees, and the forearm in full supination. The patient then flexes the elbow against resistance (Fig. 4-45). The test is considered positive if the patient has increased pain with resisted elbow flexion, indicating the presence of a SLAP lesion.

Posteroinferior Labral Pathology

The Kim test is a provocative maneuver similar to the clunk test that is used to diagnose posterior-inferior

labrum tears. While the patient is sitting on the examination table, the examiner holds the patient's arm parallel to the floor (90 degrees of forward flexion) with the arm internally rotated 90 degrees. With one of the examiner's hands holding the elbow to control internal rotation, an axial force is directed toward the humeral head. The other hand is used to direct a posterior load on the proximal humerus. Then the hand on the elbow is used to forward flex the humerus 45 degrees. Pain in the posterior shoulder is a positive Kim test result. In the only study conducted by the inventor of the test, the sensitivity and specificity for the diagnosis of posteroinferior labral lesions was 80% and 94%, respectively, using arthroscopic evaluation of the posterior labrum as the gold standard. If the test was combined with the results of the jerk test, then the sensitivity increased to 97% for detecting posteroinferior labral lesions.[27]

Subcoracoid Impingement Test

Gerber and colleagues first reported on subcoracoid impingement of the supraspinatus tendon between the coracoid tip and lesser tuberosity in a cohort of postsurgical patients in 1985.[28] This report was subsequently followed by one by Dines and colleagues,[29] who performed coracoid tip resections in eight shoulders for idiopathic subcoracoid impingement. Through variations in normal anatomy, trauma, or iatrogenic causes such as proximal humeral osteotomies, there is potential for entrapment of the rotator cuff and other structures between the coracoid and proximal humerus, resulting in pain, weakness, and degenerative tendon injuries.

The subcoracoid impingement test was first described by Gerber and colleagues[28] and consists of two variations designed to reproduce subscapularis impingement between the humeral head and coracoid. In the first technique, the arm is elevated to 90 degrees in the scapu-

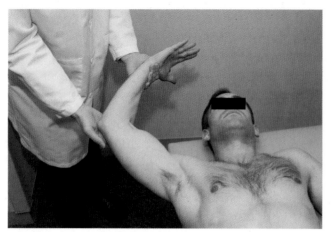

FIGURE 4-45 The biceps load test II. The arm is placed in 120 degrees of elevation, full external rotation, 90 degrees of elbow flexion, and forearm supination. Increased pain with resisted elbow flexion indicates the presence of a SLAP lesion.

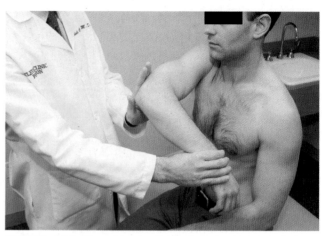

FIGURE 4-46 The subcoracoid impingement test. A positive finding of anterior shoulder pain is produced with the arm flexed to 90 degrees, maximally internally rotated, and adducted toward the midline.

lar plane combined with medial (internal) rotation of the extremity, reproducing the patient's impingement symptoms and radiation of pain into the upper arm and forearm when the test is positive. The second method involves forward flexion of the arm instead of elevation in the scapular plane, again with medial (internal) rotation of the arm reproducing impingement symptoms and radiation of pain into the arm.

Dines and colleagues describe their own version of the subcoracoid impingement test.[29] For this maneuver, the patient's arm is forward flexed to 90 degrees, adducted toward the midline, and internally rotated (Fig. 4-46). A positive finding produces anterior shoulder pain or a click in the anterior shoulder.

Scapular Dyskinesis Tests

Weakness or poorly coordinated muscle activation in the trapezius, levator scapulae, serratus anterior, or rhomboid muscles can lead to malpositioning of the scapula or scapular dyskinesis. The appropriate function of these muscles serves to decrease shoulder load and facilitate effective rotator cuff function. Provocative and stabilization maneuvers can be used to elicit evidence of scapulothoracic dysfunction.

Observed Repetitive Forward Elevation
The patient's shoulders and back must be exposed to allow a full view of both scapulae. The examiner stands behind the patient while the patient repetitively elevates and lowers both arms slowly in the plane of the scapula. The examiner observes for asymmetry along the medial border of the scapulae and lack of the normally fluid movement of the scapula as it is protracted and rotates superiorly on the chest wall with arm elevation. Subtle presentations of scapular dyskinesis often manifest during the lowering phase of arm motion as a hitch or jump.

This method of evaluation allows assessment of the resting position of the scapulae and the best view of the pattern of motion that occurs with active use of the shoulder girdle. Scapular dyskinesis that can be observed with this method is classified as type I (prominence of the inferomedial border of scapula), type II (prominence of the entire medial border of the scapula), or type III (prominence of the superomedial border of the scapula).[30]

Push-up Test
For most patients, this test is easily done by asking the patient to do a push-up while standing by leaning into a wall. For more muscular, well-conditioned patients who can do a regular push-up with ease, it is best to have them perform the test in the classic fashion on the floor. As the patient does a push-up, the examiner observes the exposed scapulae for asymmetry of movement or scapular winging along the medial border of the scapula.

Resisted Forward Elevation
The patient's arms are placed in 30 degrees of forward flexion, and the patient elevates the arms while the examiner applies resistance at the wrist. The examiner looks for winging along the medial border of the scapula.

Scapular Stabilization Test
In patients with shoulder dysfunction and evidence of scapular winging, this test is used to evaluate the improvement of symptoms and function that can result from stabilization of the scapula. To perform the maneuver, the examiner stands behind the patient and places the palm of one hand on the patient's sternum anteriorly, and the other hand on the medial border of the scapula. With the clinician applying a compressive force to prevent the medial border of the scapula from lifting off of the chest wall, the patient elevates the arm in the

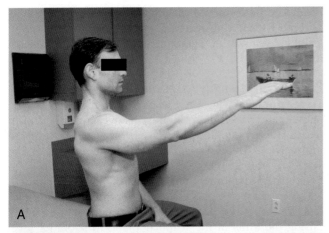

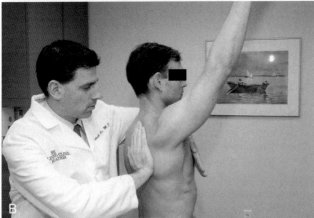

FIGURE 4-47 The scapular stabilization test. **A,** Significant scapular winging can limit a patient's ability to get full shoulder elevation secondary to pain or weakness and dysfunction. **B,** Elimination of the winging by stabilizing the medial border of the scapula improves active ROM and decreases pain.

scapular plane. Improved overhead active ROM or a decrease in symptoms while the scapular border is being stabilized is a positive test (Fig. 4-47). A positive test result indicates that the scapular winging is a significant source of the shoulder girdle dysfunction. It also suggests a higher likelihood of improved shoulder function with rehabilitation or surgical stabilization of the scapular winging.

Scapular Assistance Test
As opposed to simply stabilizing the scapula, this test allows the examiner to manually recreate more normal scapular motion, thereby reducing subacromial impingement during arm elevation and improving dynamic glenohumeral function.[31] For this test, the examiner stands behind the patient and manually stabilizes the medial border of the upper part of the scapula with one hand. With the thumb and fingers of the other hand, the examiner assists the inferomedial border of the scapula in superior rotation and protraction around the chest wall as the patient actively elevates the arm. Reduced pain

and weakness with scapular assistance is a positive finding suggesting that abnormal scapular kinematics is contributing to the shoulder dysfunction.

Resting Scapular Positional Measurements
The examiner uses a tape measure to measure the distance between the inferomedial border of the scapulae and the spinous processes in three positions: arms resting at the patient's side, hands on hips, and arms at 90 degrees of abduction and full internal rotation. Measurement can also demonstrate side-to-side differences due to scapular malposition. A side-to-side difference of 1.5 cm or greater is considered a pathologic finding.

Crepitus Testing

Crepitus detected on physical examination or reported by a patient can result from bursal pathology or abnormal bone-on-bone contact and can be asymptomatic or associated with pain. Both auscultation and palpation are used to evaluate the location and character of the crepitus. Subacromial crepitus is best assessed by placing one hand over the top of the shoulder and using the other hand to passively range the glenohumeral joint. Passive ROM is often more effective in reproducing crepitus than active ROM because the rotator cuff is not depressing the humeral head, which allows the humeral head to be brought up into the undersurface of the acromion, where the subacromial bursa can be compressed. In addition, a firm, actively contracting deltoid muscle can prevent palpation of crepitus occurring in the deeper tissues.

Scapulothoracic crepitus usually results from bursitis or bursal scarring at the superomedial, inferomedial, or deep surface of the body of the scapula. Crepitus involving the scapulothoracic articulation is usually best elicited by active scapular motion performed by the patient who usually knows how to reliably reproduce the finding. Although more subtle crepitus may only be palpable, scapulothoracic crepitus is often audible because the air-filled thoracic cavity resonates with the crepitus, amplifying the sound.

Glenohumeral crepitus, most often related to articular cartilage loss and bone-on-bone arthritis, is best reproduced by active shoulder ROM against resistance. Assessment with active resisted ROM is better than with passive motion because of the increased compressive contact forces that are generated across the glenohumeral joint with active muscle contraction compared to those seen during passive joint motion. When palpating over the superior or anterior shoulder, the crepitus produced by bone-on-bone arthritis is usually coarser than that produced by bursal pathology.

Functional Strength Testing

General Principles of Functional Strength Testing
Strength testing in a patient being evaluated for shoulder problems requires a systematic, bilateral assessment of

TABLE 4-3 Strength Grading

Grade	Description
0	Complete muscle paralysis, absence of muscle fasciculation
1	Visible or palpable muscle contraction that is too weak to move the affected joint even in the absence of gravity
2	Muscle contraction that can move the involved joint when gravity is eliminated but that is too weak to range the joint against gravity
3	Muscle strength is adequate to range the involved joint against gravity but without any added resistance
4	Muscle contraction is adequate to range the joint against gravity with added resistance, but range is less than full compared to the contralateral side
5	Normal and full range compared to the contralateral side

the primary muscles responsible for shoulder ROM. When evaluating patients with more subtle symptoms related to dynamic activities or high levels of athletic performance, a more global assessment of whole-body muscle strength may be needed to identify deficits in lower body or core muscle strength, which may be responsible for kinetic chain problems causing overload and injury to the shoulder.

Functional strength testing in the three cardinal planes of elevation in the plane of the scapula and in external rotation and internal rotation are necessary to understanding a patient's functional limitations and their affect on activities of daily living. Assessment of functional strength is often a good place for the orthopaedic surgeon to start the strength testing because it can direct the clinician to where a more detailed examination of muscle strength

should be performed. Isolated muscle strength testing is covered later in the neurologic testing section.

Table 4-3 lists the grading system of assessment of muscle strength.

Functional Strength Assessment

To test strength with active elevation in the plane of the scapula, the patient raises both arms over his or her head. Because most people naturally perform overhead reaching activities by elevating the arm in the plane of the scapula,[32] this simple maneuver usually results in good demonstration of functional forward elevation strength and the ability to assess grades 0 to 3 functional strength. Muscle strength of grades 4 or 5 is tested by the patient raising the arms in the scapular plane to shoulder level and then resisting a downward force (Fig. 4-48).

To test functional external rotation strength, the patient keeps the elbows flexed to 90 degrees and at the side while rotating the arms out away from the body. Symmetrical external rotation is assessed. Because this movement requires no work against gravity, symmetrical motion might indicate only grade 2 strength of the affected shoulder.

Functional internal rotation strength is assessed by placing the patient's arm in neutral rotation at the patient's side, with the elbow in 90 degrees of flexion. The patient rotates the arm in toward the abdomen as the examiner applies resistance at the wrist.

Patients who can perform these functional ROM and strength tests should then have bilateral isometric strength testing in each cardinal plane to differentiate among grades 3 to 5 strength. This test is performed by positioning the arms in 90 degrees of scapular elevation or in adduction with the arm in neutral rotation. The patient maintains that arm position against the clinician's manual internal or external resistance (Fig. 4-49). An asymmetry in the ability to maintain the arm position against resistance indicates grade 4 functional muscle strength in a given cardinal plane. Symmetrical and full ability to resist the clinician indicates grade 5 muscle strength. Some

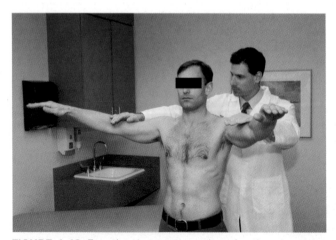

FIGURE 4-48 Functional strength testing of active elevation.

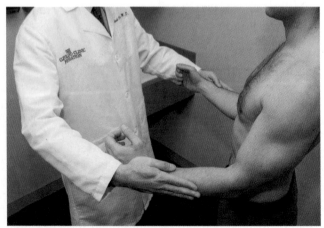

FIGURE 4-49 Testing bilateral external rotation strength.

patients have full and symmetrical strength without being able to maintain the arm position against vigorous resistance.

Neurologic Testing

Shoulder dysfunction can often be associated with subtle or overt neurologic deficits. For this reason, some degree of neurologic testing in the form of isolated muscle strength testing, sensory testing, and reflex testing is needed to fully evaluate most shoulders.

Isolated Muscle Strength Testing

Every assessment of shoulder muscle strength must be performed bilaterally to allow comparison of the relative strength between the involved and uninvolved shoulders. What might be considered pathologic weakness in one person's shoulder can represent full, normal strength in a patient of lesser strength. A comprehensive evaluation of muscle strength can identify weakness resulting from pain-related muscle inhibition, it can reveal weakness not anticipated based on patient history and functional assessments, or it can demonstrate better strength than expected given a patient's level of functional impairment.

Position of testing also is selected to best isolate the function of each individual muscle group so that groups of muscles are not being tested in conjunction with each other. Isometric muscle testing with the involved joint and muscle in a position of optimal mechanical advantage best gives consistent, reproducible assessment of strength. The exception to this guideline is when testing a muscle group with apparently full strength. Full symmetrical muscle strength is assessed with the involved muscle in its position of maximal shortening because this position accentuates subtle weakness within the muscle that might otherwise go undetected in stronger patients.

Deltoid

Muscle strength testing of the deltoid needs to independently assess anterior, middle, and posterior bundles of the deltoid. The anterior bundle is assessed by placing the shoulder in 90 degrees of forward flexion with the elbow extended and the arm in neutral rotation. The patient maintains the arms in this position against a downward force applied by the clinician to the wrist. The middle bundle is assessed by placing the shoulder in 90 degrees of abduction with the elbow extended and the palm of the hand facing up. The patient maintains the arm position against the clinician's downward force applied to the wrist. This position of external rotation in abduction rotates the greater tuberosity out from under the acromion, decreasing the likelihood of supraspinatus impingement within the subacromial space, which can lead to pain and weakness in isometric deltoid strength testing. The posterior bundle of the deltoid is tested by placing the shoulder in extension with the elbow flexed to 90 degrees. The patient resists a forward-directed force applied to the elbow. Applying

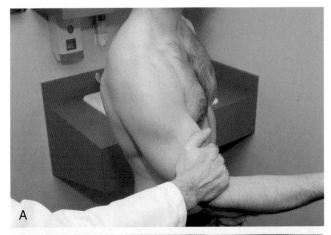

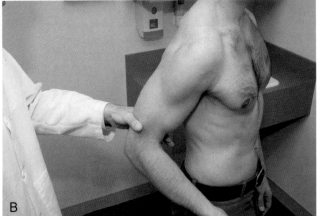

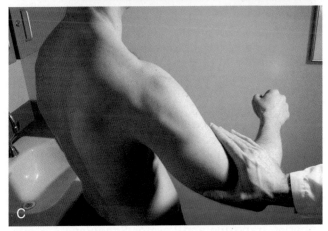

FIGURE 4-50 Deltoid muscle strength testing. **A,** Anterior deltoid. **B,** Posterior deltoid. **C,** Middle deltoid.

force at the flexed elbow eliminates confusion that might arise from pushing at the wrist with the elbow extended, which can lead to breaking of the elbow extension and the misperception that the isometric posterior deltoid is weak (Fig. 4-50).

Biceps

The clinician stands in front of the patient and positions the arm with the shoulder in neutral rotation, the elbow

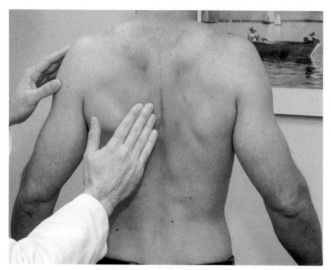

FIGURE 4-51 Assessment of middle trapezius and rhomboids. The patient pinches the shoulder blades together while the physician observes and palpates along the medial border of the scapula. The scapular motion and palpable muscle contraction should be symmetrical.

TABLE 4-4 Reflexes

Location	Peripheral Nerve	Nerve Root
Clavicle	Nonspecific	Nonspecific
Scapula	Dorsal scapular	C5
Scapula	Spinal accessory	Cranial nerve XI
Pectoralis	Medial and lateral pectoral	C5-C8, T1
Biceps	Musculocutaneous	C5, C6
Triceps	Radial	C6, C7
Brachioradialis	Musculocutaneous	C5, C6

flexed fully, and the palm in full supination. The examiner grasps the patient's hand and places the other hand on the patient's shoulder for stabilization. The patient pulls his or her arm into the chest while the examiner applies resistance.

Brachialis

The position and testing of the brachialis is identical to that used for the biceps except that the forearm is placed in full pronation to prevent co-contraction of the biceps, which would bring the forearm into supination.

Triceps

The examiner stands beside the patient and positions the arm in 90 degrees of forward elevation with the elbow fully extended and the hand in full supination. The patient resists elbow flexion while the clinician attempts to flex the elbow by stabilizing the arm with one hand on the biceps and the other hand applying force at the wrist.

Superior Trapezius and Levator Scapulae

The examiner stands behind the patient with both hands on the patient's shoulders. The patient performs a shoulder shrug while the examiner attempts to hold the shoulders in a depressed position.

Middle Trapezius and Rhomboids

The examiner stands behind the patient and places several fingers along the medial border of the scapula. The patient pinches the shoulder blades together. Although absolute strength testing of these muscle groups is not possible with this maneuver, the quality of the contraction can be generally assessed by direct palpation of the involved rhomboids and middle trapezius (Fig. 4-51).

Subscapularis, Supraspinatus, Infraspinatus and Teres Minor Strength Testing

Isolated strength testing of the subscapularis, supraspinatus, infraspinatus, and teres major is covered in the earlier section on rotator cuff testing..

Reflex Testing

Reflexes are tested bilaterally in all patients to allow side-to-side comparison of reflexes. The presence or absence of reflexes is noted, as well as whether they are excessively brisk or sluggish. Table 4-4 gives each reflex and its associated root level and peripheral nerve involved.

Clavicular Reflex

The patient stands with arms hanging at his or her sides, and the examiner taps the lateral aspect of each clavicle with a reflex hammer. This maneuver can produce a reflexive contraction of the trapezius, or, less commonly, other muscles around the shoulder girdle. This reflex does not assess an independent nerve root, but the test can be useful in assessing general irritability of the proximal nerves in the upper extremity.

Scapular Reflex

The patient stands with arms abducted 20 degrees, and the examiner taps the inferior angle of the scapula with a reflex hammer. The reflex response of the rhomboids (dorsal scapular nerve, C5) and middle and lower trapezius (spinal accessory nerve, cranial nerve XI) causes adduction of the arms and medial movement of the scapula.

Pectoralis Reflex

With the patient's arm abducted 20 degrees, the examiner's thumb is placed over the pectoralis major tendon insertion on the proximal humerus. The examiner taps the thumb with a reflex hammer. Adduction or internal rotation of the arm occurs as a reflex response (medial and lateral pectoralis nerves, C5-C8, T1).

TABLE 4-5 Sensory Testing

Vertebra	Anatomic Location	Peripheral Nerve
C4	Superior aspect of shoulder	
C5	Lateral aspect of deltoid	Axillary
C6	Lateral forearm and thumb	Musculocutaneous and median
C7	Dorsal tip of long finger	Median
C8	Medial forearm	Medial antebrachial cutaneous
T1	Medial arm	Medial brachial cutaneous

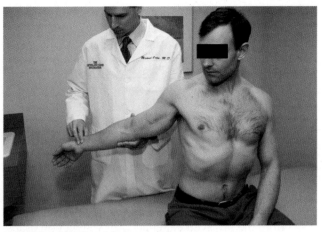

FIGURE 4-52 The Adson maneuver.

Biceps Reflex

With the patient's elbow supported in 90 degrees of flexion, the examiner places his or her thumb over the distal biceps tendon and taps the thumb. The elbow flexes reflexively (musculocutaneous nerve, C5, C6).

Triceps Reflex

With the patient's elbow supported in 90 degrees of flexion, the examiner uses a reflex hammer to tap the distal triceps tendon just proximal to its insertion on the olecranon. Reflexive elbow extension (radial nerve, C7) occurs.

Brachioradialis Reflex

The patient's elbow supported in 90 degrees of flexion, and the wrist in neutral rotation and neutral flexion/extension. The examiner uses a reflex hammer to tap the brachioradialis tendon approximately 2 cm proximal to its insertion on the radial styloid. A normal reflex response results in elbow flexion (musculocutaneous nerve, C5,C6). The inverted radial reflex is an abnormal reflexive wrist extension that can be seen in response to this test. It is a sign of upper motor neuron pathology.

Horner's Syndrome

Complete assessment of the upper extremity neurologic status should include observation for Horner's syndrome, which is a constellation of ipsilateral miosis, ptosis, and anhidrosis. This finding is associated with a lesion involving the sympathetic chain at the C6 cervical level. It can be found with very proximal brachial plexus nerve root injuries or with tumors involving the apex of the lung.

Sensory Testing

Evaluation of the sensation in the upper extremity can be used to identify focal nerve lesions, regional nerve deficits such as those caused by syringomyelia, or systemic problems such as peripheral neuropathy secondary to diabetes. Although dermatomal sensory regions often overlap and are somewhat variable, certain areas on the arm are usually isolated and consistently innervated by a single nerve root level. Light touch or discrimination between sharp and dull can be used to grossly assess sensation in any given area. Sensation is compared bilaterally. Symmetrical alterations in sensation suggest systemic or more proximal pathology than asymmetric alteration in sensation. Table 4-5 gives the location and dermatome associated with each part of the extremity.

Vascular Examination

Complaints of altered sensation (either transient or chronic), changes in temperature, skin changes, or loss of hair on an involved extremity can all be presenting signs of vascular problems that can be contributing factors to a patient's shoulder pathology. Patient history alone can make it difficult to discern whether such complaints are related to and caused by intrinsic shoulder pathology. For example, the sudden onset of radiating paresthesias that are often reported in patients with multidirectional instability may be related to the intrinsic shoulder pathology or they may be related to a vascular problem like thoracic outlet syndrome.

A careful vascular examination is essential in these scenarios to clarify what can otherwise be a confusing clinical scenario. Although the tests described here can be very helpful in identifying significant vascular issues involving the upper extremity, it is important to remember that none of these tests are highly sensitive or specific for vascular compromise. With any of these tests, auscultation over the clavicle, first rib, and axilla might detect a bruit related to partial vascular occlusion that might not be detectable as a palpable decrease in distal pulses.

Adson's Maneuver

This test to assess for thoracic outlet syndrome is best performed with the examiner standing behind the shoulder to be examined. With the examiner palpating the radial pulse at the wrist, the patient extends the shoulder and arm, turns the head toward the involved side, and takes a deep breath in and holds it (Fig. 4-52). Any decrease or obliteration of the radial pulse suggests subclavian artery compression between the anterior and middle scalene muscles or the first rib.

Modified Adson's Maneuver

This test is performed the same way as the traditional Adson's maneuver except that the patient turns the head away from the involved extremity. Any diminution or loss of the pulse at the wrist is considered a positive test, suggesting thoracic outlet syndrome.

Halstead's Test

The patient looks toward the opposite shoulder and extends the neck. Downward traction is then applied to the involved arm while palpating the pulse at the wrist. Loss of the pulse is considered a positive sign, indicating vascular compression.

Hyperabduction Syndrome Test

While palpating bilateral radial arteries at the wrist, the patient brings the arms into full abduction over his or her head. A decrease in pulse may be a normal finding, but asymmetry between the two arms is considered a positive finding. With this maneuver, the axillary artery can be compressed under the coracoid and pectoralis minor.

Wright Test

The patient elevates both arms to head height and rapidly opens and closes the hands 10 to 15 times. Fatigue, cramping, or tingling suggests vascular insufficiency.

REFERENCES

1. Neviaser RJ, Neviaser TJ: The frozen shoulder. Diagnosis and management. Clin Orthop Relat Res (223):59-64, 1987.
2. Gerber C, Ganz R: Clinical assessment of instability of the shoulder with special reference to anterior and posterior drawer tests. J Bone Joint Surg Br 66:551-556, 1984.
3. Rowe CR, Zarins B: Recurrent transient subluxation of the shoulder. J Bone Joint Surg Am 63:863-872, 1981.
4. Jobe FW, Kvitne RS, Giangarra CD: Shoulder pain in the overhand or throwing athlete: The relationship of anterior instability and rotator cuff impingement. Orthop Rev 18:963-975, 1989.
5. Farber AJ, Castillo R, Clough M, et al: Clinical assessment of three common tests for traumatic anterior shoulder instability. J Bone Joint Surg Am 88:1467-1474, 2006.
6. Gerber C, Hersche O, Farron J: Isolated rupture of the subscapularis tendon. J Bone Joint Surg Am 78:1015-1023, 1996.
7. Barth JRH, Burkhead SS, De Beer, JF: The bear hug test. A new and sensitive test for diagnosis of subscapularis tear. Arthroscopy 22(10):1076-1084, 2006.
8. Itoi E, Kido T, Sano A, et al: Which is more useful, the full can test or the empty can test in detecting the torn supraspinatus tendon? Am J Sport Med 27:65-68, 1999.
9. Neer CS: Impingement lesions. Clin Orthop Relat Res (173):70-77, 1983.
10. Hawkins RJ, Kennedy JC: Impingement syndrome in athletes. Am J Sports Med. 8:151-158, 1980.
11. MacDonald PB, Clark P, Sutherland K: An analysis of the diagnostic accuracy of the Hawkins and Neer subacromial impingement signs. J Shoulder Elbow Surg 9(4):299-301, 2000.
12. Valadie AL, Jobe CM, Pink MM: Anatomy of provocative tests for impingement syndrome of the shoulder. J Shoulder Elbow Surg. 9(4):36-46, 2000.
13. Jobe FW, Jobe CM: Painful athletic injuries of the shoulder. Clin Orthop Relat Res (173):117-124, 1983.
14. Yocum LA: Assessing the shoulder. History, physical examination, differential diagnosis and special tests used. Clin Sports Med 2(2):281-289, 1983.
15. Zaslav KR: Internal rotation resistance strength test: A new diagnostic test to differentiate intra-articular pathology from outlet (Neer) impingement syndrome in the shoulder. J Shoulder Elbow Surg 10(1):23-27, 2001.
16. Hamner DL, Pink MM, Jobe FW: A modification of the relocation test: Arthroscopic findings associated with a positive test. J Shoulder Elbow Surg 9(4):263-267, 2000.
17. Park HB, Yokota A, Gill HS, et al: Diagnostic accuracy of clinical tests for the different degrees of subacromial impingement syndrome. J Bone Joint Surg Am 87:1146-1155, 2005.
18. Crenshaw HA, Kilgore WE: Surgical treatment of bicipital tenosynovitis. J Bone Joint Surg Am 48:1496-1502, 1966.
19. Bennett WF: Specificity of the Speed's test: Arthroscopic technique for evaluating the biceps tendon at the level of the bicipital groove. Arthroscopy 14(8):789-796, 1998.
20. O'Brien SJ, Pagnani MJ, Fealy S, et al: The active compression test: A new and effective test for diagnosing labral tears and acromioclavicular joint abnormality. Am J Sports Med 26:610-613, 1998.
21. Snyder SJ, Karzel RP, Del Pizzo W, et al: SLAP lesions of the shoulder. Arthroscopy 6(4):274-279, 1990.
22. Kibler WB: Sensitivity and specificity of the anterior slide test in throwing athletes with superior glenoid labral tears. Arthroscopy 14(2):447-457, 1995.
23. Liu SH, Henry MH, Nuccion SL: A prospective evaluation of a new physical examination in predicting glenoid labral tears. Am J Sports Med 24(6):721-725, 1996.
24. Mimori K, Muneta T, Nakagawa T: A new pain provocation test for superior labral tears of the shoulder. Am J Sports Med 27(2):137-142, 1999.
25. Kim SH, Ha KI, Han KY: Biceps load test: A clinical test for superior labrum anterior and posterior lesions in shoulders with recurrent anterior dislocations. Am J Sports Med 27:300-303, 1999.
26. Kim SH, Ha KI, Ahn JH, et al: Biceps load test II: A clinical test for SLAP lesions of the shoulder. Arthroscopy 17:160-164, 2001.
27. Kim SH, Park JS, Jeong WK, et al: The Kim test. A novel test for posteroinferior labral lesion of the shoulder—a comparison to the jerk test. Am J Sports Med 33(8):1188-1192, 2005.
28. Gerber C, Terrier F: The role of the coracoid process in the chronic impingement syndrome. J Bone Joint Surg Br 67(5):703-708, 1985.
29. Dines DM, Warren RF, Inglis AE, et al: The coracoidimpingement syndrome. J Bone Joint Surg Br 72:314-316, 1990.
30. Kibler WB, Uhl TL, Maddux JW, et al: Qualitative clinical evaluation of scapular dysfunction: A reliability study. J Shoulder Elbow Surg 11:550-556, 2002.
31. Kibler WB, Livingston B: Closed-chain rehabilitation of the upper and lower extremities. J Am Acad Orthop Surg 9:412-421, 2001.
32. Inman VT, Sanders JB, Abbott LC: Observations on the function of the shoulder joint. J Bone Joint Surg 26:1-30, 1944.

Radiographic Evaluation of Shoulder Problems

Kirk L. Jensen, MD, and Charles A. Rockwood, Jr, MD

Radiographic evaluation of the shoulder requires a minimum of two views of the area that are perpendicular to each other. The shoulder is a complicated anatomic unit made up of numerous bony landmarks, projections, and joints. The scapula, which lies on the posterolateral portion of the rib cage, rests at an angle of approximately 45 degrees to the frontal plane of the thorax. Thus, the plane of the glenohumeral joint is not the plane of the thorax, and radiographs taken in the anteroposterior plane of the thorax provide oblique views of the shoulder joint (Fig. 5-1). All too commonly, a radiographic evaluation of the shoulder consists of two anteroposterior views of the rotated proximal humerus, which are taken perpendicular to the frontal axis of the thorax.

Orthopaedists do not diagnose and treat injuries in any other part of the body on the basis of a one-plane radiographic evaluation. With the exception of localizing rotator cuff calcium deposits, the two traditional anteroposterior views of the shoulder in internal and external rotation are, by themselves, inadequate to evaluate injuries and disorders of the shoulder. Rotating the humerus into internal and external rotation does not change the orientation of the scapula to the x-ray beam. Therefore, radiographic evaluation of the shoulder should consist of, at a minimum, both anteroposterior and lateral views. Specific oblique views may be required to further investigate specific pathologic conditions of the shoulder.

FRACTURES OF THE GLENOHUMERAL JOINT

Recommended Views

The recommended views are the trauma series of radiographs, that is, true anteroposterior radiographs in internal and external rotation and an axillary lateral or a scapulolateral view. Modified axillary laterals or a computed tomography (CT) scan may be required.

Radiographs of the injured shoulder in two planes (anteroposterior and axillary lateral or scapular lateral) are absolutely essential to evaluation of an acutely injured shoulder. McLaughlin,[1] Neer,[2,3] Neviaser,[4] DeSmet,[5] Rockwood and Green,[6] Post,[7] Rowe,[8] Bateman,[9] and many others have recognized the shortcomings of the usual two anteroposterior radiographs of the shoulder and have recommended anteroposterior and lateral views to properly assess shoulder problems. The radiographs used to evaluate traumatic shoulder problems have been referred to as the *trauma series*. The trauma series can also be used as baseline radiographs to evaluate many chronic shoulder problems as well.

Recommended radiographs for the trauma series include the following:

- A true anteroposterior view in the plane of the scapula with the arm in internal and external rotation
- An axillary lateral view. If an axillary radiograph cannot be obtained, one of the following views must be obtained:
  - A scapulolateral view
  - One of the modified axillary views
  - A CT scan

Techniques for Taking the Trauma Series

True Anteroposterior Views

Because the scapula lies on the posterolateral aspect of the thoracic cage, the true anteroposterior view of the glenohumeral joint is obtained by angling the x-ray beam 45 degrees from medial to lateral (Fig. 5-2; see also Fig.

177

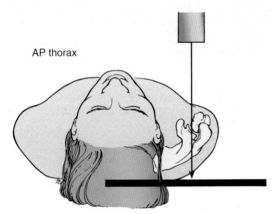

FIGURE 5-1 AP radiograph of the shoulder taken in the plane of the thorax. Note that the film is actually an oblique view of the glenohumeral joint.

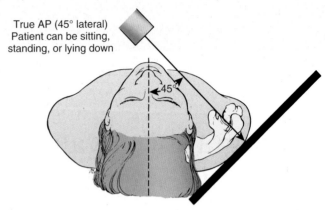

FIGURE 5-2 To obtain a true AP view of the glenohumeral joint, the beam must be angled 45 degrees, or the patient can rotate the body until the scapula is parallel to the x-ray cassette.

5-1). The patient may be supine or erect, with the arm at the side or in the sling position. An alternative technique is to rotate the patient until the scapula is flat against the x-ray cassette and then take the x-ray with the beam perpendicular to the scapula. Sometimes it is difficult for the technician to properly align the patient for the view. A simple technique to assist the technician in positioning the patient correctly consists of using a heavy marking pen to draw a line on the skin along the spine of the scapula. The technician aligns the x-ray beam perpendicular to the line on the skin and directs it at the cassette, which is placed parallel to the line and posterior to the scapula and glenohumeral joint (Fig. 5-3). Although the scapular spine is not exactly parallel to the plane of the scapula, this technique has proved effective in clinical practice.

The advantage of the true anteroposterior views of the scapula over traditional anteroposterior views in the plane of the thorax is that the x-ray demonstrates the glenoid in profile rather than obliquely and, in the normal shoulder, clearly separates the glenoid from the humeral head (Fig. 5-4). In the true anteroposterior x-ray, the coracoid process overlaps the glenohumeral joint. If the true anteroposterior x-ray demonstrates the humeral head to be overlapping with the glenoid, the glenohumeral joint is dislocated either anteriorly or posteriorly.

Axillary Lateral View

Initially described by Lawrence[10,11] in 1915, the axillary lateral x-ray can be taken with the patient supine or erect. Ideally, the arm is positioned in 70 to 90 degrees of abduction. The x-ray beam is directed into the axilla from inferior to superior, and the x-ray cassette is placed superior to the patient's shoulder (Fig. 5-5). To minimize the amount of abduction required to obtain an axillary lateral x-ray, an alternative technique was devised by Cleaves[12] in 1941. In this technique, the patient may be

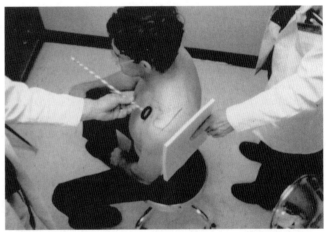

FIGURE 5-3 Position of the patient and the x-ray beam to obtain a true anteroposterior view of the glenohumeral joint.

sitting or supine; the arm is abducted only enough to admit a curved x-ray cassette into the axilla. The x-ray is taken from superior to inferior through the axilla. In some situations when abduction is severely limited to only 20 or 30 degrees, a rolled-up cardboard cassette can be substituted for the curved cassette in the axilla (Fig. 5-6).

Axillary lateral x-rays provide excellent visualization of the glenoid and the humeral head and clearly delineate the spatial relationship of the two structures. Loss of glenohumeral cartilage is clearly revealed when the joint space between the glenoid and the humeral head is decreased or absent. Dislocations are easily identified, as are compression fractures of the humeral head and large fractures of the anterior or posterior glenoid rim (see Fig. 5-17). Some fractures of the coracoid and the acromion and the spatial relationship of the acromioclavicular joint can also be seen on this view.

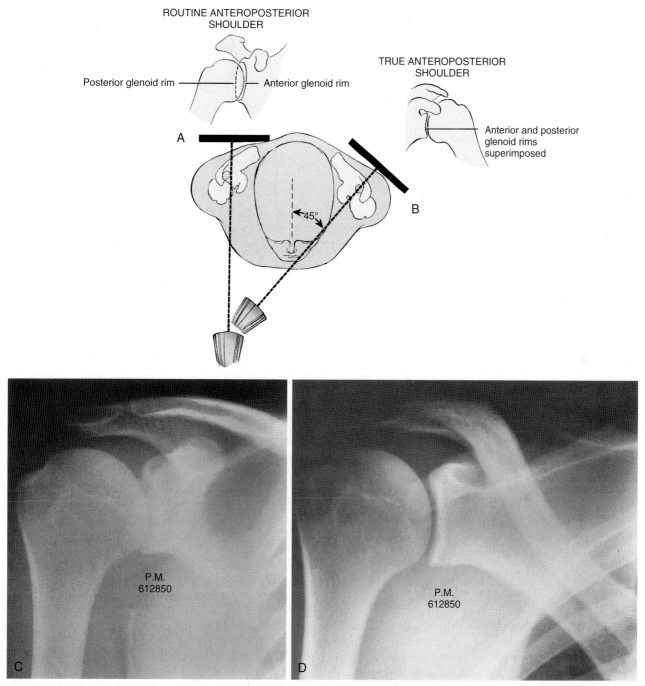

FIGURE 5-4 A and **B,** Note the great difference between the two angles of the x-ray beam, the placement of the cassettes, and the schematic drawings of the glenohumeral joint. **C,** A radiograph of the shoulder in the plane of the thorax. **D,** A radiograph of the shoulder taken in the plane of the scapula. (Modified from Rockwood CA, Green DP [eds]: Fractures [3 vols], 2nd ed. Philadelphia: JB Lippincott, 1984.)

If a good-quality axillary lateral x-ray can be obtained, the true scapulolateral view or the modified axillary lateral views are not necessary. However, if because of pain and muscle spasm the patient does not allow enough abduction to get a good axillary view, the scapulolateral or the modified axillary lateral views *must* be obtained.

Technique for the Scapulolateral Radiograph

The scapulolateral view is sometimes known as the *transscapular*, the *tangential lateral*, or the *Y lateral*.[13] The position of the injured shoulder, which is usually held in internal rotation (the arm having been placed in a sling),

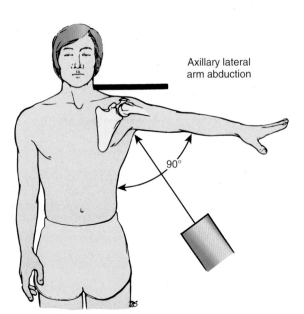

FIGURE 5-5 The axillary lateral radiograph. Ideally, the arm is abducted 70 to 90 degrees and the beam is directed inferiorly up to the x-ray cassette.

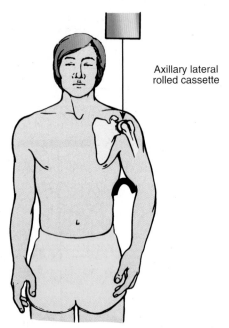

FIGURE 5-6 When the patient cannot fully abduct the arm, a curved cassette can be placed in the axilla and the beam directed inferiorly through the glenohumeral joint onto the cassette.

is left undisturbed. A marking pen is used to draw a heavy line over the spine of the scapula (Fig. 5-7A). The technician then aligns the x-ray beam parallel to the line on the skin, directed to the cassette, which is placed perpendicular to the line at the anterolateral shoulder. The x-ray beam passes tangentially across the posterolateral chest, parallel to and down the spine of the scapula onto the x-ray cassette (see Fig. 5-7A and B). The projected image is a true lateral of the scapula and, hence, a lateral view of the glenohumeral joint (see Fig. 5-7B).

A lateral projection of the scapula forms a Y shape (Fig. 5-8A to C).[14] The upper arms of the Y are formed by the coracoid process anteriorly and by the scapular spine posteriorly. The vertical portion of the Y is formed by the body of the scapula. At the intersection of the three limbs of the Y lies the glenoid fossa. In the normal shoulder, the humeral head is located overlapping the glenoid fossa (see Figs. 5-7B and 5-8D). This view is particularly helpful in determining the anterior or posterior relationship of the humeral head to the glenoid fossa.

In anterior dislocations of the shoulder, the humeral head lies anterior to the glenoid fossa (see Figs. 5-7C and 5-8F); in posterior dislocations, the humeral head lies posterior to the glenoid fossa (see Figs. 5-7D and 5-8E). The scapulolateral view does not define fractures of the anterior or posterior glenoid rim, but it does reveal displaced fractures of the greater tuberosity. When this view is added to the true anteroposterior and the axillary lateral views, they represent three views, all 90 degrees to each other, which maximizes the information available for the clinician to use to make an accurate diagnosis.

Techniques for the Modified Axillary Views

Velpeau Axillary Lateral View

Bloom and Obata's[14] modification of the axillary lateral x-ray of the shoulder is known as the *Velpeau axillary lateral* because it was intended to be taken with the acutely injured shoulder still in a sling without abduction.

With the Velpeau bandage or shoulder sling in place, the patient stands or sits at the end of the x-ray table and leans backwards 20 to 30 degrees over the table. The x-ray cassette is placed on the table directly beneath the shoulder, and the x-ray machine is placed directly over the shoulder so that the beam passes vertically from superior to inferior, through the shoulder joint onto the cassette (Fig. 5-9). On this view, the humeral shaft appears foreshortened and the glenohumeral joint appears magnified, but otherwise, it demonstrates the relationship of the head of the humerus to the scapula.

Apical Oblique View

Garth, Slappey, and Ochs have described an apical oblique projection that reliably demonstrates the pathology of the glenohumeral joint.[15] The patient may be seated or in a supine position, and the arm may remain in a sling. The x-ray cassette is placed posteriorly, parallel to the spine of the scapula. The x-ray beam is directed through the glenohumeral joint toward the cassette at an angle of 45 degrees to the plane of the thorax and is also tipped 45 degrees caudally (Fig. 5-10A and B).

The resultant x-ray demonstrates the relationship of the humeral head to the glenoid and therefore identifies the

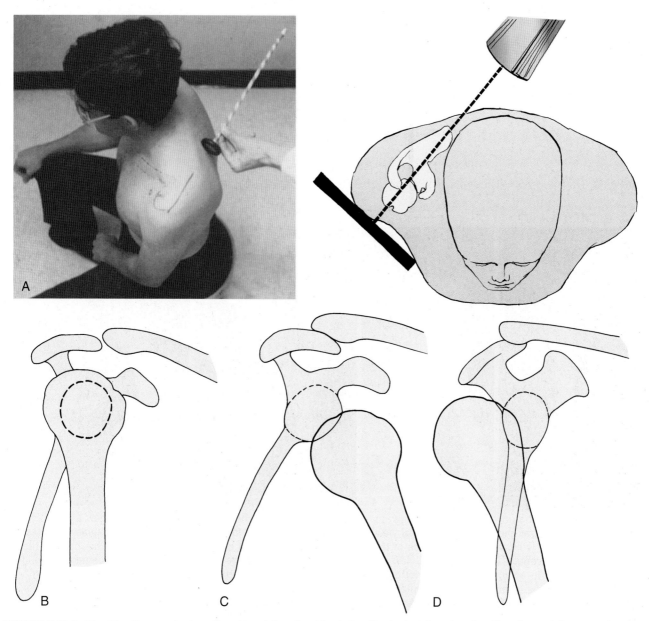

FIGURE 5-7 A, How the line marked on the skin of the shoulder helps the technician visualize the plane of the x-ray for the true scapulolateral radiograph. (Modified from Rockwood CA, Green DP [eds]: Fractures [3 vols], 2nd ed. Philadelphia: JB Lippincott, 1984.) **B,** A schematic drawing illustrates how the humeral head on the true scapulolateral radiograph should be centered around the glenoid fossa. **C,** In anterior dislocations, the humeral head is displaced anterior to the glenoid fossa. **D,** In posterior dislocations of the shoulder, the humeral head sits posterior to the glenoid fossa.

presence and direction of glenohumeral dislocations and subluxations. This view clearly defines the anteroinferior and posterosuperior rims of the glenoid and is useful for detecting calcifications or fractures at the glenoid rim (see Fig. 5-10C and D). Posterolateral and anterior humeral head compression fractures are also revealed by this view.

Kornguth and Salazar[16] reported that this technique is excellent for diagnosis in the acute setting.

Stripp Axial Lateral View

The Stripp axial view, described by Horsfield,[17] is similar to the Velpeau axillary lateral view, except that the beam passes from inferior to superior and the x-ray cassette is positioned above the shoulder.

Trauma Axillary Lateral View

Another modification of the axillary lateral view has been described by Teitge and Ciullo.[18,19] The advantage of this

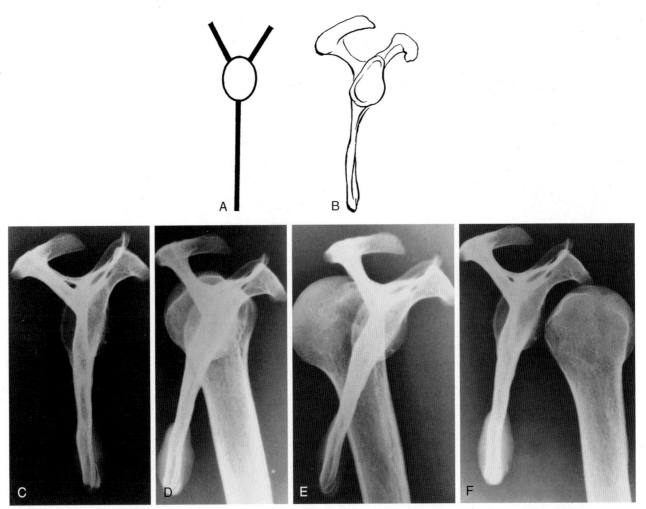

FIGURE 5-8 Interpretation of a true lateral radiograph of the shoulder. **A,** A schematic drawing illustrates how a lateral view of the scapula projects as the letter Y. **B,** Lateral view of the scapula. **C,** A true lateral radiograph of the scapula indicates that the glenoid fossa is located at the junction of the base of the spine and the base of the coracoid with the body of the vertically projecting scapula. **D,** A true lateral view of the glenohumeral joint shows the humeral head well centered around the glenoid fossa. **E,** In a subacromial, posterior dislocation of the shoulder, the articular surface of the humeral head is directed posterior to the glenoid fossa. **F,** In anterior subcoracoid dislocations of the shoulder, the humeral head is anterior to the glenoid fossa. (Modified from Rockwood CA, Green DP [eds]: Fractures [3 vols], 2nd ed. Philadelphia: JB Lippincott, 1984.)

view over the Velpeau and Stripp views is that it can be taken while the patient is supine, as is often necessary in patients with multiple trauma. This view can be taken while the injured shoulder is still immobilized in a shoulder-immobilizer dressing. To obtain this view, the patient is supine on the x-ray table, and the involved arm is supported in 20 degrees of flexion by placing radiolucent material under the elbow. The x-ray beam is directed up through the axilla to a cassette propped up against the superior aspect of the shoulder (Fig. 5-11). This view defines the relationship of the humeral head to the glenoid fossa.

Computed Tomography Scan

A CT scan reliably demonstrates fractures, the number of fracture fragments, and fracture-dislocations of the gleno-

humeral joint. However the addition of a CT scan to the trauma series does not apparently improve the reproducibility of the Neer or AO (Arbeitsgemeinschaft für Osteosynthesefragen) fracture classification.[20,21] The technique should consist of 3-mm-thick contiguous sections with a bone algorithm from the top of the acromion to the inferior pole of the glenoid. It is very important that the scan include both shoulders so that the physician can compare the anatomy of the injured shoulder with that of the normal shoulder. Three-dimensional CT scans can provide additional information in the acute setting to evaluate complex or multiple shoulder girdle fractures.

Magnetic Resonance Imaging

The magnetic resonance imaging (MRI) scan is rarely indicated for managing fractures of the shoulder. Specific

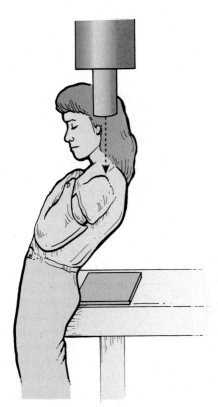

FIGURE 5-9 Positioning of the patient for the Velpeau axillary lateral radiograph, as described by Bloom and Obata. (Modified from Bloom MH, Obata WG: Diagnosis of posterior dislocation of the shoulder with use of the Velpeau axillary and angled up radiographic views. J Bone Joint Surg Am 49:943-949, 1967.)

indications include differentiating nondisplaced greater tuberosity fractures from rotator tendon tears involving a young patient in a post-traumatic situation.[22-24] It might also diagnose the pattern of postfracture avascular necrosis.

ANTERIOR INSTABILITY

Recommended Views

Recommended views are the true anteroposterior x-rays, the West Point axillary lateral, and the apical oblique projection. Arthrograms, arthrotomograms, CT scans, CT arthrography, and MRI scans are discussed in the section "Special Studies to Evaluate Shoulder Instability."

With anterior dislocation or subluxation of the glenohumeral joint, there may be bone damage or soft tissue calcification adjacent to the anterior or, particularly, the anteroinferior rim of the glenoid. The true anteroposterior view can demonstrate a fracture of the inferior glenoid that might not be visualized on the anteroposterior views in the plane of the thorax. Although the axillary lateral may be useful to demonstrate some anterior glenoid

abnormality, the West Point axillary lateral and the apical-oblique x-rays provide more information.[25,26]

Anterior shoulder dislocations may be accompanied by fractures of the anterior glenoid rim, which may be demonstrated on a routine axillary lateral x-ray. However, when evaluating traumatic anterior subluxation, the glenoid defect almost exclusively involves the anteroinferior glenoid, which cannot be seen on routine axillary lateral x-rays. In many cases, the lesions seen on the anteroinferior glenoid rim provide the only x-ray evidence of traumatic anterior shoulder subluxation. Two techniques have been described to evaluate the anteroinferior glenoid rim. They are the West Point and the apical oblique projections.

West Point Axillary Lateral View

This projection was described by Rokous, Feagin, and Abbott when they were stationed at the US Military Academy at West Point, New York.[26] Rockwood has referred to this technique as the *West Point view.*[6] The patient is positioned prone on the x-ray table, with the involved shoulder on a pad raised approximately 8 cm from the top of the table. The head and neck are turned away from the involved side. With the cassette held against the superior aspect of the shoulder, the x-ray beam is centered at the axilla with 25 degrees of downward angulation of the beam from the horizontal and 25 degrees of medial angulation of the beam from the midline (Fig. 5-12A and B). The resultant x-ray is a tangential view of the anteroinferior rim of the glenoid.

The usual finding seen in the traumatic anterior-subluxating shoulder is soft tissue calcification located just anterior to the glenoid rim or anterior-inferior bony fracture avulsions (see Fig. 5-12C and D). A cadaveric study revealed that a 21% glenoid bony defect appeared to be approximately 18% of the intact glenoid on a West Point axillary radiograph.[27] Therefore the West Point axillary view provides decisive information regarding anterior-inferior glenoid rim fractures and operative treatment.

Apical Oblique View

The apical oblique view clearly defines the anteroinferior and posterior superior rims of the glenoid. Pathologic findings of the rim associated with recurrent instability such as displaced malunited rim fractures, glenoid bone loss, or anterior inferior cartilage loss are identified with this view (Fig 5-13). Posterolateral and anterior humeral head defects are also revealed by this view, although CT is necessary to quantify the size of the defect.

Recurrent Anterior Glenohumeral Instability

Radiographic views for recurrent anterior glenohumeral instability include the apical oblique for anterior glenoid erosion, the Stryker notch for a posterior lateral humeral head defect, and MRI arthrography for detachment of the labrum.

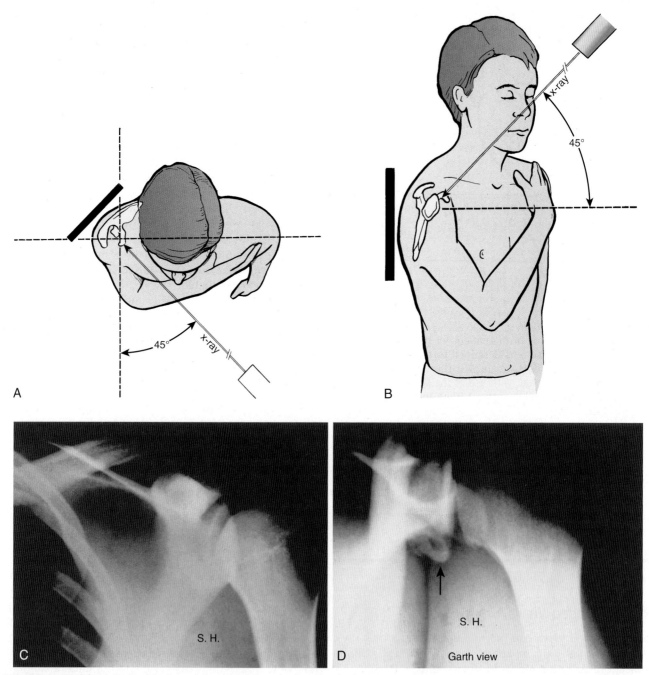

FIGURE 5-10 A and **B,** Positioning of the patient to obtain an apical oblique radiograph. This is a true anteroposterior view of the glenohumeral joint with a 45-degree caudal tilt of the x-ray beam. (Modified from Garth WP Jr, Slappey CE, Ochs CW: Radiographic demonstration of instability of the shoulder: The apical oblique projection, a technical note. J Bone Joint Surg Am 66:1450-1453, 1984.) **C,** Radiograph of the left shoulder in the plane of the thorax does not reveal any significant abnormality. **D,** In the apical oblique view, note the calcification on the anteroinferior glenoid rim (*arrow*). (**C** and **D,** Courtesy of William Garth, MD.)

FIGURE 5-11 Positioning of the patient for the trauma axillary lateral radiograph. The patient is supine. The elbow is elevated by a piece of foam rubber to allow the x-ray beam to pass in an inferior direction up through the glenohumeral joint onto the x-ray cassette, which is superior to the shoulder. (Modified from Teitge RA, Ciullo JV: The CAM axillary x-ray. Exhibit at AAOS Meeting. Orthop Trans 6:451, 1982.)

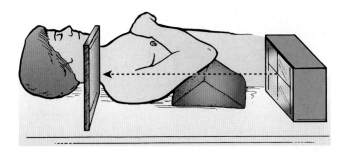

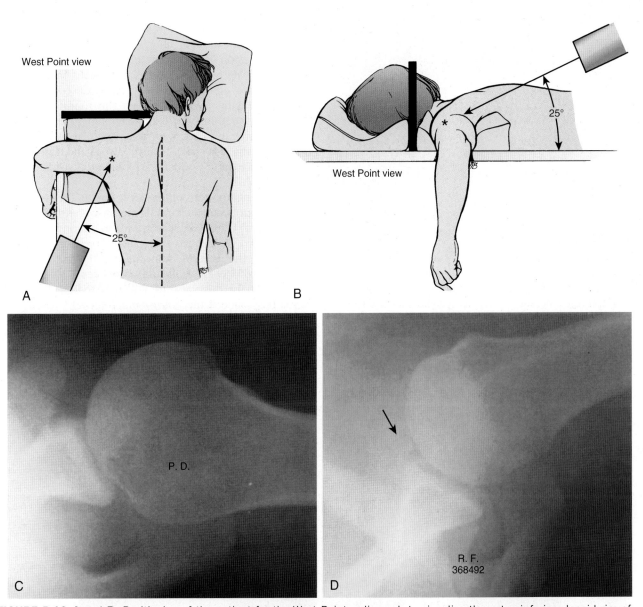

FIGURE 5-12 A and **B,** Positioning of the patient for the West Point radiograph to visualize the anteroinferior glenoid rim of the shoulder. *, beam target. (Modified from the work of Rokous JR, Feagin JA, Abbott HG: Modified axillary roentgenogram. Clin Orthop Relat Res 82:84-86, 1972.) **C** and **D,** Examples of calcification on the anteroinferior glenoid rim as noted on the West Point x-ray view. (Modified from Rockwood CA, Green DP [eds]: Fractures [3 vols], 2nd ed. Philadelphia: JB Lippincott, 1984.)

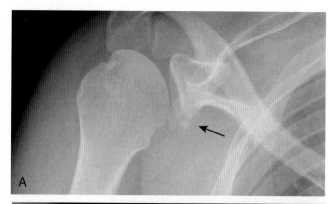

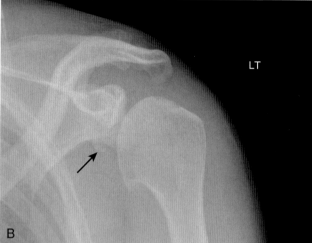

FIGURE 5-13 **A,** Apical oblique radiograph revealing an anterior glenoid rim fracture (*arrow*). **B,** Apical oblique radiograph revealing anterior inferior glenoid cartilage and bone loss (*arrow*).

POSTERIOR HUMERAL HEAD COMPRESSION FRACTURES ASSOCIATED WITH ANTERIOR DISLOCATION: THE HILL–SACHS DEFECT

Recommended Views

The recommended views are the Stryker notch view, the anteroposterior view with arm in full internal rotation, and other views.

A commonly encountered sequela of anterior shoulder dislocation is a compression fracture of the posterolateral humeral head. This fracture can occur during the first traumatic dislocation or after recurrent anterior dislocations. The lesion is commonly referred to as a *Hill–Sachs lesion* and was reported by Hill and Sachs in 1940 (Fig. 5-14).[28] However, the defect was clearly described by Eve in 1880.[29] In the period between the report by Eve in 1880 and the report by Hill and Sachs in 1940, the defect in the humeral head was described by Malgaigne,[30] Kuster,[31] Cramer,[32] Popke,[33] Caird,[34] Broca and Hartman,[35,36] Perthes,[37] Bankart,[38,39] Eden,[40] Hybbinette,[41] Didiee,[42] and Hermodsson.[43]

The indentation, or compression fracture, may be seen on the anteroposterior x-ray if the arm is in full internal rotation, and it may be seen occasionally on the axillary lateral view. We believe that one of the best views for identifying the compression fracture is the technique reported in 1959 by Hall and associates.[44] The authors gave credit for this view to William Stryker, and Rockwood has called it the *Stryker notch view.*[6]

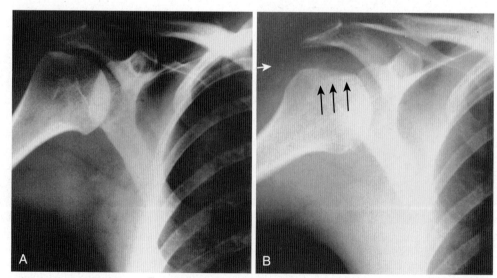

FIGURE 5-14 The Hill–Sachs sign. **A,** Anteroposterior radiograph of the right shoulder in 45 degrees of abduction and external rotation. Note that some sclerosis is present in the superior aspect of the head of the humerus. **B,** In full internal rotation, note the defect in the posterolateral aspect of the humeral head (*white arrow*). Also note the dense line of bone condensation marked by the *black arrows*, the Hill–Sachs sign.

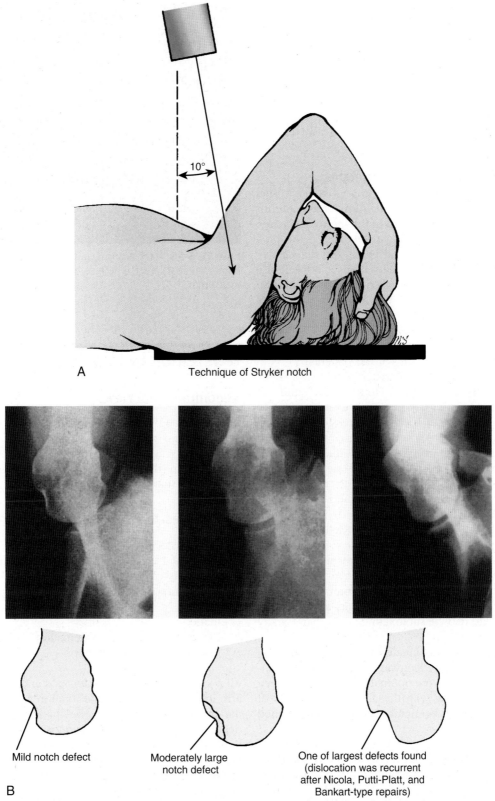

A   Technique of Stryker notch

Mild notch defect

Moderately large
notch defect

One of largest defects found
(dislocation was recurrent
after Nicola, Putti-Platt, and
Bankart-type repairs)

B

FIGURE 5-15 A, Position of the patient for the Stryker notch view. The patient is supine with the cassette posterior to the shoulder. The humerus is flexed approximately 120 degrees so that the hand can be placed on top of the patient's head. Note that the angle of the x-ray tube is 10 degrees superior. **B,** Defects in the posterolateral aspect of the humeral head are seen in three different patients with recurring anterior dislocations of the shoulder. (Modified from the work of Hall RH, Isaac F, Booth CR: Dislocation of the shoulder with special reference to accompanying small fractures. J Bone Joint Surg Am 41:489-494, 1959.)

Stryker Notch View

For the Stryker notch view,[44] the patient is placed supine on the x-ray table with the cassette under the involved shoulder (Fig. 5-15A). The palm of the hand of the affected upper extremity is placed on top of the head, with the fingers toward the back of the head. The x-ray beam is tilted 10 degrees cephalad and is centered over the coracoid process. A positive result is a distinct notch in the posterolateral part of the humeral head (see Fig. 5-15B).

Anteroposterior View in Internal Rotation

Probably the simplest view, but not the most diagnostic, is the one described by Adams.[45] It is an anteroposterior view of the shoulder with the arm in full internal rotation. An indentation or compression can be seen in the posterolateral portion of the humeral head. The defect may simply appear as a vertical condensation of bone. Pring and colleagues[46] compared the Stryker view with the internal (60 degrees) rotation view of Adams in 84 patients with anterior dislocation of the shoulder for evidence of the posterolateral defect in the humeral head. The internal rotation view was positive in 48%, whereas the Stryker notch view was positive in 70% of the patients.

Other views predating the Stryker notch view have been described by Didiee[42] and Hermodsson[43] and are useful in demonstrating the presence and size of the posterolateral humeral head compression fractures. Although these techniques involve views of the proximal humerus with the arm in internal rotation, they are slightly awkward to obtain. The apical oblique view described by Garth and colleagues[15] also demonstrates the compression fracture. Strauss and coworkers[47] and Danzig and colleagues[48] have independently evaluated the efficacy of the various x-rays in revealing the Hill–Sachs lesion and reported that although none of these views always reveals the lesion in question, the Stryker notch view is probably the most effective. The presence of the compression head fracture on the x-ray confirms that the shoulder has been dislocated, whereas its absence suggests that the head may be subluxating rather than frankly dislocating.

After a study of lesions created in the posterolateral humeral head, Danzig, Greenway, and Resnick[48] concluded that three views were optimal to define the defect: the anteroposterior view with the arm in 45 degrees of internal rotation, the Stryker notch view, and the modified Didiee view.

In a study of 120 patients, Strauss and colleagues[49] stated that a special set of x-rays could confirm the diagnosis of anterior shoulder instability with 95% accuracy. The x-rays were the anteroposterior view of the shoulder in internal rotation and the Hermodsson, axillary lateral, Stryker notch, Didiee, and West Point views. Whereas the Stryker notch view can document the presence of the compression fracture, the CT scan can be very helpful in determining the size of the compression defect (Fig 5-16).[50-56]

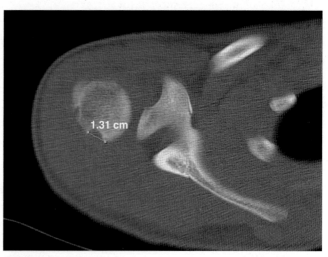

FIGURE 5-16 A CT scan revealing an engaging posterior humeral head defect. The size of the defect can be directly measured.

POSTERIOR INSTABILITY

Recommended Views

Recommended views are the trauma series of radiographs and modified axillary views. Arthrograms, arthrotomograms, CT scans, CT arthrography, and MRI scans are discussed in the section "Special Studies to Evaluate Shoulder Instability."

Techniques to Evaluate Posterior Instability

Posterior dislocation of the shoulder is a rare problem, consisting of 1% to 3% of all dislocations about the shoulder, and it is commonly misdiagnosed.[6] There are three reasons for missing the posterior displacement:

1. Inadequate patient history
2. Inadequate physical examination
3. Inadequate x-ray evaluation

All too often, only two anteroposterior x-rays with the arm in internal and external rotation are made. X-rays of the injured shoulder must be made in two planes, 90 degrees to each other. The diagnosis of posterior dislocation of the shoulder can always be made if the anteroposterior view and one of the previously described lateral views are obtained. Usually, the patient does not allow enough abduction to take the true axillary view, in which case the scapulolateral or modified axillary view or a CT scan must be obtained.

Traumatic posterior glenohumeral instability may be accompanied by either damage to the posterior glenoid rim or impaction fractures on the anteromedial surface of the humeral head, the reverse Hill–Sachs lesion (Fig. 5-

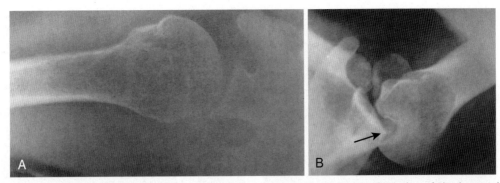

FIGURE 5-17 A, An axillary lateral view of a normal left shoulder shows the normal articulation of the humeral head with the glenoid fossa and the normal relationship of the humeral head to the coracoid process and the acromion process. **B,** An axillary lateral view of the injured right shoulder shows a large anteromedial compression fracture of the humeral head, the reverse Hill–Sachs sign. The *arrow* indicates the posterior glenoid rim that has produced the hatchet-like defect in the humeral head. (From Rockwood CA, Green DP [eds]: Fractures (3 vols), 2nd ed. Philadelphia: JB Lippincott, 1984.)

17). Lesions of the posterior glenoid rim can usually be noted on the axillary x-ray. The CT scan and MRI scan are very helpful in defining the glenoid rim fracture and in determining the size of the compression fracture of the humeral head.

Special Studies to Evaluate Shoulder Instability

Occasionally in patients with recurrent anterior or posterior dislocations and subluxations, bone abnormalities are not visible on the x-rays. Despite the routine, normal radiologic examination, a significant injury to the soft tissues may be present. In anterior dislocations, the anterior capsule and the glenoid labrum may be stripped off the glenoid rim, as originally described by Perthes[37] in 1906 and later by Bankart[38] in 1923.

Although an arthrogram might reveal a displaced labrum with contrast material adjacent to the anterior glenoid rim and neck of the scapula, Albright,[57] Braunstein,[58] Kleinman,[59] and Pappas[60] have each demonstrated that the displaced labrum and capsular stripping can best be documented by arthrotomography of the shoulder joint. Kilcoyne and Matsen[61] and Kleinman and colleagues[62] used pneumotomography to demonstrate injury to the glenoid labrum and the joint capsule. In a report on 33 cases, they reported good correlation between the tomogram and the surgical findings.

The CT scan, combined with arthrography, can further define the condition of the anterior and anteroinferior labrum. Shuman and coworkers[63] used double-contrast CT to study the glenoid labrum with a high degree of accuracy (Fig. 5-18). Various authors[54,56,64-66] have shown

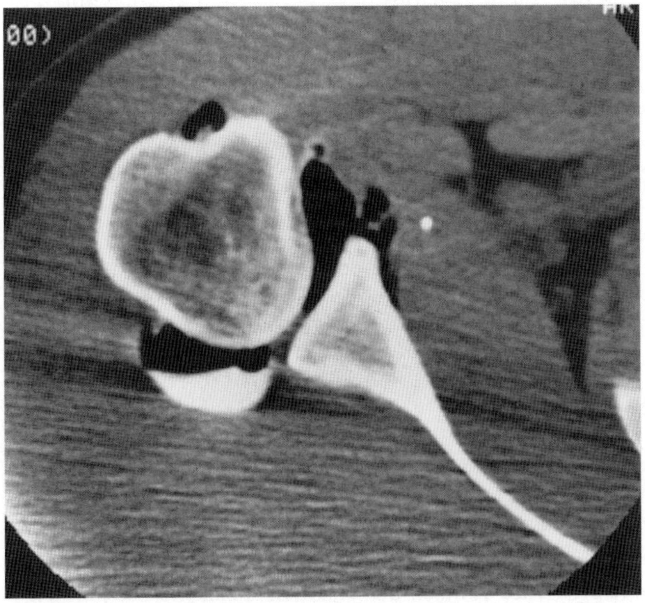

FIGURE 5-18 CT arthrogram of the left shoulder. Note that the labrum and capsular structures have been stripped away from the anterior glenoid rim and neck of the scapula. (Courtesy of Becky Laredo, MD.)

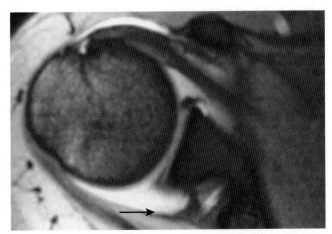

FIGURE 5-19 Axial MRI with intra-articular gadolinium in which the posterior capsule is avulsed from its insertion on the posterior labrum *(arrow).*

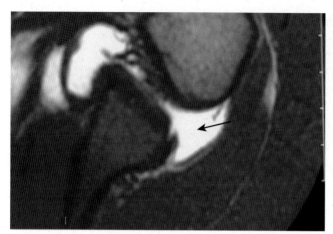

FIGURE 5-20 Posterior labral detachment demonstrated on an axial MRI with intra-articular gadolinium (*arrow*).

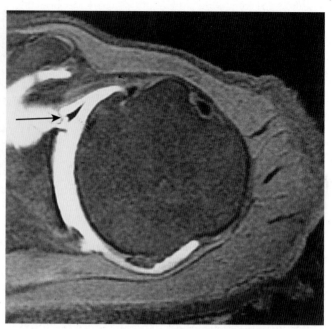

FIGURE 5-21 MRI with gadolinium identifies disruption of the anterior glenoid labrum (*arrow*). Other cuts also demonstrated a deficiency of attachment of the anterior glenohumeral ligament on the rim of the anterior glenoid.

CT arthrography to be sensitive for imaging the anterior-inferior labrum; however, the presence of anatomic variations has affected its accuracy and reliability.[67,68]

The MRI has become popular for imaging a suspected labral and capsular abnormality associated with anterior or posterior instability because it provides anatomic images, is noninvasive, and does not use ionizing radiation. MRI without intra-articular contrast provides limited specific information regarding glenohumeral instability, and a study that is interpreted as normal does not rule out symptomatic glenohumeral instability. Authors have reported the sensitivities of MRI without intra-articular contrast to detect anterior labral tearing to range from 44% to 100%[69-73] and the specificities to range from 68% to 95%.[68,70,71,73-76] Posterior labral abnormalities have been detected with a reported 74% sensitivity and 95% specificity.[71] Superior labral tearing was reported with an 86% sensitivity and a 100% specificity.[77] Capsular laxity and capsular insertion sites cannot be assessed by MRI without intra-articular contrast (Figs. 5-19 and 5-20). The high cost of the MRI and the variability in accuracy of the interpretation of the images should negate its routine use in instability imaging.

MRI combined with intra-articular gadolinium[67] or saline[78] provides images that accurately identify labral and glenohumeral ligament anatomy and injury, as well as associated rotator tendon tearing (Figs. 5-21 and 5-22). Intra-articular injection of gadolinium-DTPA (diethylene-triamine pentaacetate) at 2 mmol/L has been shown to have complete passive diffusion from the joint within 6 to 24 hours, and rapid renal elimination has led to almost no systemic side effects.[79] A study evaluating MR arthrography of normal shoulders accurately revealed anatomic variations concerning anterior labral signal intensity, form, and size, and the authors concluded that only major tears or detachments of the labrum should be diagnosed.[80]

In a prospective study of 30 patients, surgical correlation was used to show MR arthrography to be superior to CT arthrography in detecting anterior labral pathol-

ogy.[67] MR arthrography is also useful in evaluating failed anterior instability surgery with a reported 100% sensitivity and 60% specificity in detecting recurrent anterior labral tears.[81] The addition of the abduction and external rotation (ABER) position has been shown to increase the sensitivity of MR arthrography in revealing tears of the anterior glenoid labrum (Fig. 5-23). Cvitanic and col-

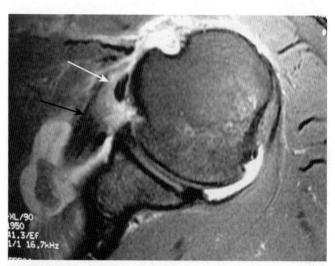

FIGURE 5-22 An MRI demonstrates dislocation of the long head of the biceps tendon into the joint (*white arrow*). The dislocation can occur only with rupture of the subscapularis tendon and the capsule. A *black arrow* identifies the stump of the remaining subscapularis tendon.

FIGURE 5-23 A, An axial, gadolinium-enhanced, MR arthrogram that does not identify an anterior labral tear. **B,** Addition of the oblique axial image in the ABER (abduction and external rotation) position identifies the anterior labral detachment *(arrow).*

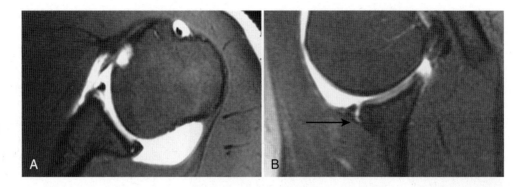

leagues compared conventional axial MR arthrograms to oblique axial MR arthrograms in the ABER position and found the latter to be significantly more sensitive in revealing anterior glenoid labral tears ($P = .005$).[82]

Capsular laxity remains problematic. In one study of 121 patients undergoing surgery for anterior instability, capsular laxity was missed in all shoulders and capsular insertion sites were found to have no role in predicting clinical shoulder instability.[83] In another retrospective review following arthroscopic correlation, MRI and MR arthrography were found by the authors to be limited in providing diagnostic information important to the patient's surgical management.[84] Therefore, routine use of MR arthrography in the diagnosis of glenohumeral instability is not recommended and should be relegated for use as an adjunctive study for special cases. An MR arthrogram study that is perceived as a negative study does not rule out symptomatic clinical glenohumeral instability.

Imaging of the superior labrum may be difficult. However, on coronal fat-suppressed proton-density-weighted MRI, a hyperintense linear fluid signal within the superior labrum creating a 5-mm superior shift of labrum indicates a superior labral tear. Surgical confirmation has shown that MR arthrography reliably and accurately reveals superior labral tears. Sensitivities of 84% to 92% and specificities of 82% to 91% along with substantial interobserver agreement make MR arthrography the gold standard for radiographically evaluating superior labral tears.[85,86]

GLENOHUMERAL ARTHRITIS

Recommended Views

Recommended views are the true anteroposterior views in internal and external rotation and an axillary lateral view. A limited CT scan may be required to assess glenoid erosion.

Loss of articular cartilage leads to the shoulder pain of glenohumeral arthritis. The radiographic views that demonstrate joint space narrowing or articular cartilage loss are the true anteroposterior, the axillary lateral, and the apical oblique (Fig. 5-24). Osteophyte formation and humeral head deformity are revealed by internal and external rotation anteroposterior radiographs of the shoulder. Posterior glenoid erosion and posterior humeral head subluxation can also be shown by the axillary lateral radiograph and apical oblique. However, we do not rely upon the axillary lateral to determine glenoid version because Galinat[87] determined that up to 27 degrees of variation exists, depending on the angle of the x-ray beam and scapular rotation.

Glenohumeral arthritis may be accompanied by various patterns of glenoid erosion (e.g., central or posterior). CT of the glenohumeral joint has been shown to be accurate and reliable in assessing glenoid morphology and version (Fig. 5-25).[88,89] A limited CT scan of both shoulders should be performed, beginning just inferior to the coracoid process (Box 5-1) to determine the glenoid version (Fig. 5-26). The glenoid version is the angle formed by a line between the anterior and posterior rims of the glenoid and a line perpendicular to the axis of the scapular body. The normal glenoid version varies from 0 to 7 degrees

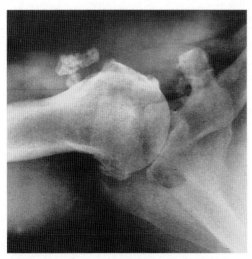

FIGURE 5-24 Axillary lateral radiograph reveals loss of the clear space between the humeral head and glenoid, indicating loss of cartilage.

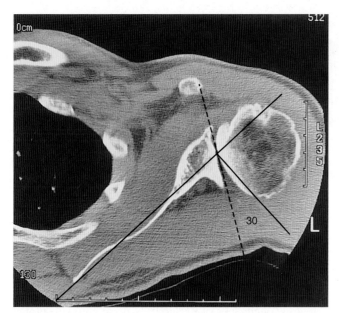

FIGURE 5-25 CT scan revealing posterior subluxation of the head of the humerus along with posterior glenoid erosion of 30 degrees.

of retroversion. The version increases when posterior glenoid erosion is present (Fig. 5-27).[88,90,91]

A preoperative shoulder CT scan to assess glenoid version has been shown to avoid shoulder arthroplasty component malposition and subsequent failure due to unrecognized posterior glenoid wear.[90] A CT scan is recommended before shoulder arthroplasty if the patient has less than 0 degrees of glenohumeral external rotation, has had a previous anterior reconstructive procedure, or has questionable radiographic posterior glenoid erosion or posterior humeral head subluxation. Preoperative three-dimensional CT scans have also been shown to accurately reflect the glenoid vault and surface.[92] This information may be useful in preoperatively evaluating shoulder arthroplasty patients who have significant glenoid bone loss.

GLENOHUMERAL ARTHROPLASTY

Recommended Views

Recommended views are the true anteroposterior views in internal and external rotation and an axillary lateral or apical oblique view. Fluoroscopy is helpful to assess glenoid component fixation. A limited CT scan may be required to assess glenoid erosion.

Evaluation

The routine radiographic evaluation of a glenohumeral arthroplasty should consist of the recommended views to evaluate component position and glenoid articulation. Humeral stem lucencies or migration and humeral head height with respect to the greater tuberosity can easily be followed with anteroposterior views in internal and exter-

---

BOX 5-1 Technique for Limited Computed Tomography Scans of the Shoulders

Purpose
To determine the glenoid version of both shoulders

Scout Scans
Bilateral shoulders in a straight line, symmetrically placed across the top of each acromion
Bilateral shoulders with scan lines

Range
No tilt

Filming
Bone windows only (9 on 1, only 1 sheet)
Bilateral shoulders

Intravenous Contrast
None

Display
Bone algorithm

Technique
Arms: Neutral at the side
Shoulders: Flat, at the *exact* same level or height
kVp: 140 to 160
mAs: 300 or higher
FOV: 28 to 32 cm

Start Location
Inferior *tip* of the coracoid process

End Location
Six images below tip

Mode
Axial or helical

Collimation
3 mm

Increments
No gap

FOV, field of view.
Developed by Becky Laredo, MD, San Antonio, Tex.

---

nal rotation.[93] The axillary lateral and apical oblique views can reveal cartilage wear of the glenoid or instability of the humeral component.

Radiographic evaluation of the glenoid component should routinely consist of a true anteroposterior view of the glenohumeral joint, an axillary lateral, or an apical oblique. The presence of lucent lines about a keeled or pegged component should be noted at the first postoperative visit as well as the seating of the component on the native glenoid.[94] Fluoroscopic positioning of radiographs has been shown to be a more accurate method of identifying glenoid component radiolucent lines,[95] but it exposes the patient to a large amount of radiation and is time consuming for the patient.

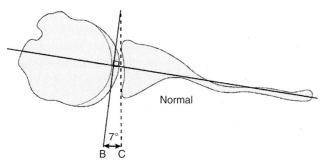

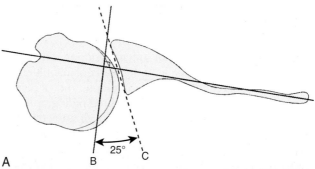

FIGURE 5-26 Normal glenoid version varies from 0 to −7 degrees of retroversion. On a CT scan, measurement of version is accomplished by drawing a line along the axis of the scapular body and then drawing a line perpendicular to it (*B*). A third line is drawn along the anterior and posterior rims of the glenoid (*C*). The angle between *B* and *C* is the glenoid version.

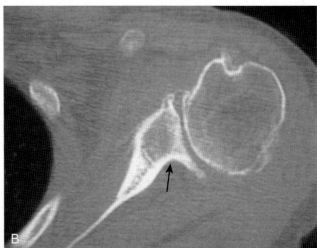

The painful shoulder arthroplasty radiographic evaluation should consist of the recommended views to assess component fixation, position, and stability. Occasionally a limited CT scan provides useful information regarding glenoid wear or humeral component malposition. CT of a cemented pegged polyethylene glenoid component has been shown to be more sensitive than radiography in identifying the size and number of peg lucencies.[96] MRI[97] and ultrasonography[98,99] have been reported as useful for identifying rotator cuff tendon tears in the painful shoulder arthroplasty.

FIGURE 5-27 A, An increase in retroversion to 25 degrees is usually accompanied by posterior subluxation of the head of the humerus. **B,** A CT scan reveals posterior glenoid wear and humeral head posterior subluxation.

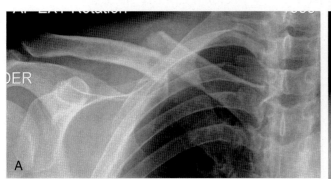

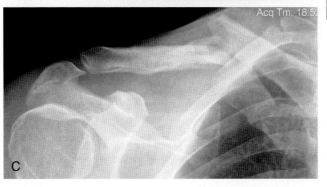

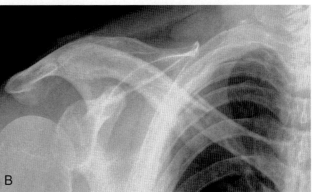

FIGURE 5-28 Clavicle trauma views to delineate fracture pattern and displacement. **A,** A routine anteroposterior view. **B,** A caudal tilt view. **C,** A cephalic tilt view.

CLAVICLE

Recommended views are an anteroposterior radiograph in the plane of the thorax, a 30-degree cephalic tilt radiograph, a 30-degree caudal tilt radiograph, and occasionally a tomogram or CT scan. These three radiographs are useful for delineating the characteristics of an acute fracture (Fig 5-28) and are even more helpful in monitoring progress of the fracture toward union. Tomograms or CT scans are required to assess fracture healing and evaluate fractures of the medial portions of the clavicle.

ACROMIOCLAVICULAR JOINT AND DISTAL CLAVICLE

Recommended Views

Recommended views are an anteroposterior view in the plane of the thorax, a 10-degree cephalic tilt view of the acromioclavicular joint, and an axillary lateral view. A scapulothoracic lateral radiograph, stress views, tomograms, bone scan, CT, or MRI may be required.

Evaluation Techniques

Reduced Voltage

The x-ray technician should be specifically requested to take films of the acromioclavicular joint and not of the shoulder because the technique used for the glenohumeral joint produces a dark, overexposed radiograph of the acromioclavicular joint, which can mask traumatic or degenerative changes (Fig. 5-29A). The acromioclavicular joint can be clearly visualized by using 50% of the x-ray voltage used to expose an anteroposterior radiograph of the glenohumeral joint (see Fig. 5-29B).

Zanca View

Sometimes, fractures about the distal end of the clavicle or the acromion, osteolysis of the distal end of the clavicle, or arthritis of the acromioclavicular joint is obscured on routine anteroposterior radiographs of the joint because the inferior portion of the distal part of the clavicle is obscured by the overlapping shadow of the spine of the scapula. To obtain the clearest unobstructed view of the acromioclavicular joint and distal portion of the clavicle, Zanca has recommended that the x-ray beam be aimed

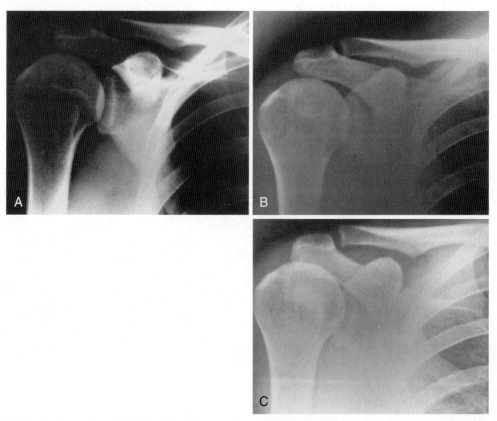

FIGURE 5-29 Routine radiographs of the shoulder often produce a poorly visualized acromioclavicular joint. **A,** A routine anteroposterior view of the shoulder demonstrates good visualization of the glenohumeral joint. However, the acromioclavicular joint is overpenetrated by the x-ray technique. **B,** When the exposure is decreased by 50%, the acromioclavicular joint is much better visualized. However, the inferior aspect of the acromioclavicular joint is superimposed on the spine of the scapula. **C,** With the Zanca view, tipping the tube 10 to 15 degrees superiorly provides a clear view of the acromioclavicular joint. (From Rockwood CA, Green DP [eds]: Fractures [3 vols], 2nd ed. Philadelphia: JB Lippincott, 1984.)

at the acromioclavicular joint with a 10-degree cephalic tilt (Fig. 5-30).[58]

Occasionally, none of the routine radiographs clearly delineate the extent of the pathology in this region, and tomograms, a CT scan, MRI, or a bone scan may be required.

Anteroposterior Views

If the patient has a drooping injured shoulder, it is important to compare radiographs of the injured acromioclavicular joint with those of the normal shoulder. The radiograph may be taken with the patient either standing or sitting and the arms hanging free. If the patient is small, both shoulders may be exposed on a single horizontal 14 × 17 inch x-ray cassette, but for most adults, it is better to use separate 10 × 10 inch cassettes for each shoulder.

To interpret injuries to the acromioclavicular joint, the appearance of the acromioclavicular joint and the coracoclavicular distance in the injured shoulder are compared with those in the normal shoulder[100] (Fig. 5-31).

It is important to determine the degree of injury to the acromioclavicular and coracoclavicular ligaments. If the acromioclavicular and the coracoclavicular ligaments are both disrupted, surgical correction may be indicated. A full description of the various degrees of injury to these ligaments, types I to VI, is given in Chapter 12.

Anteroposterior Stress View

If the original radiographs of a patient with an injury to the acromioclavicular joint demonstrate a complete acromioclavicular dislocation (i.e., types III, IV, V, or VI), stress radiographs are not required. If complete disloca-

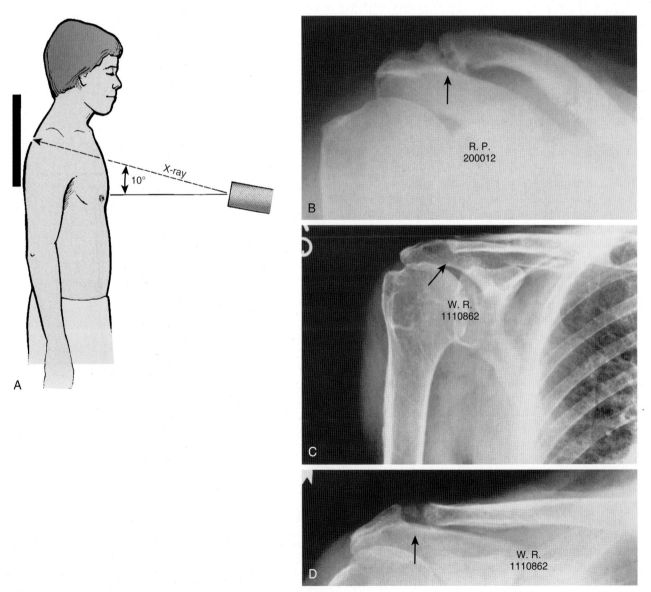

FIGURE 5-30 A, Positioning of the patient to obtain a Zanca view of the acromioclavicular joint. **B,** A Zanca view of the joint reveals significant degenerative changes. **C,** An anteroposterior radiograph of good quality fails to reveal any abnormality of the joint. **D,** With the Zanca view, a loose body is clearly noted within the joint.

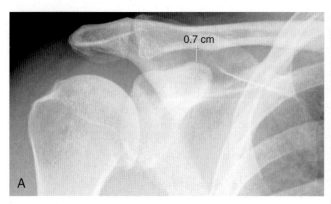
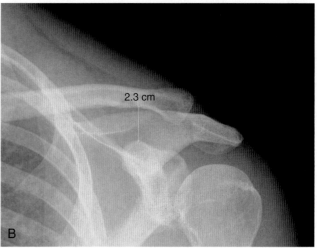

FIGURE 5-31 Comparison of the coracoclavicular interspace in the injured and the normal shoulder. **A,** In the normal shoulder, the distance between the top of the coracoid and the bottom of the clavicle is 7 mm. **B,** In the injured shoulder, the distance between the top of the coracoid and the bottom of the clavicle is 23 mm, which indicates disruption of not only the acromioclavicular but also the coracoclavicular ligament.

tion of the joint is clinically suspected, stress views of both shoulders should be taken. With the patient erect, 10 to 20 lb of weight, depending on the size of the patient, is *strapped* around the patient's wrists while radiographs are taken of both shoulders[6] (Fig. 5-32). Patients should not grip the weights in their hands because the muscle contractions can produce a false-negative radiograph. If stress radiographs demonstrate that the coracoclavicular distance is the same in both shoulders or has a difference of less than 25%, a type III or greater injury can be ruled out.

Axillary Lateral View

With the arm abducted 70 to 90 degrees, the cassette should be placed superior to the shoulder and the x-ray tube placed inferior to the axilla. Obtaining this view is consistent with the basic principle of obtaining at least two x-ray views at 90 degrees to one another for evaluation of musculoskeletal trauma. This view can reveal small intra-articular fractures not visualized on the anteroposterior radiograph, and such findings indicate a worse prognosis.[3,101] This view also demonstrates anterior or posterior (as seen in type IV injuries) displacement of the clavicle and the degree of displacement of fractures of the distal end of the clavicle.

Alexander View

Alexander[102,103] described a modification of the true scapulolateral view that he found useful in evaluating injuries to the acromioclavicular joint. This view is a supplemental projection to demonstrate the posterior displacement of the clavicle that occurs with acromioclavicular injuries. The position of the cassette and the x-ray beam is essentially the same as for the true scapulolateral radiograph. With the patient standing or sitting, the patient shrugs the shoulders forward while the true scapulolateral radio-

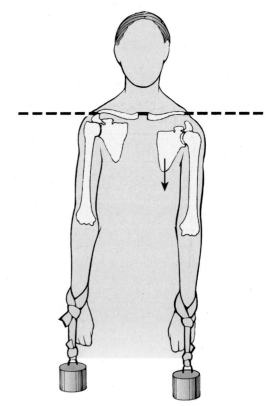

FIGURE 5-32 Technique of obtaining stress radiographs of both acromioclavicular joints with 10 to 15 lb of weight hanging from the patient's wrists. The distance between the superior aspect of the coracoid and the undersurface of the clavicle is measured to determine whether the coracoclavicular ligaments have been disrupted. One large, horizontally placed 14 × 17 inch cassette can be used in smaller patients to visualize both shoulders. In large patients, however, it is better to use two horizontally placed smaller cassettes and take two separate radiographs for the measurements. In disruption of the coracoclavicular ligaments, note that the shoulder is displaced downward rather than the clavicle being displaced upward.

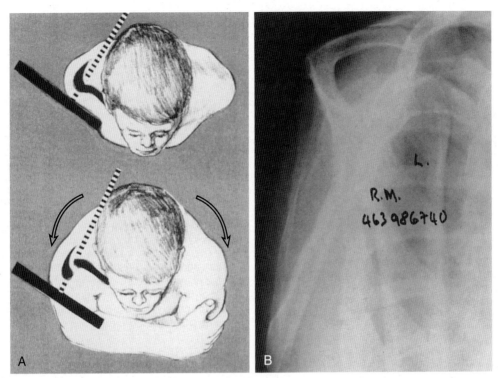

FIGURE 5-33 Technique of obtaining the Alexander or scapulolateral view of the acromioclavicular joint. **A,** A schematic drawing illustrates how the shoulders are thrust forward when the radiograph is taken. (From Rockwood CA, Green DP [eds]: Fractures [3 vols], 2nd ed. Philadelphia: JB Lippincott, 1984.) **B,** With the left shoulder thrust forward, note the gross displacement of the acromioclavicular joint. The clavicle is superior and posterior to the acromion.

graph is taken (Fig. 5-33). If no injury to the acromioclavicular ligament has occurred, no displacement or overlap of the distal end of the clavicle and the acromion will be noted. However, with acromioclavicular ligament disruption, the distal part of the clavicle is superiorly displaced and overlaps the acromion.

Tomogram or Computed Tomography Scan

Occasionally, none of the routine radiographs clearly delineate the extent of the pathology of the distal end of the clavicle or the acromioclavicular joint, and tomograms or a CT scan may be required.

Bone Scan

A bone scan detects early evidence of degenerative arthritis, infection, and traumatic osteolysis of the distal part of the clavicle before x-ray changes are noted on a routine radiograph.[104-106]

Magnetic Resonance Imaging

MRI of the shoulder can reveal abnormalities of the distal end of the clavicle. Increased T2 signal in the distal part of the clavicle is the most common and conspicuous MRI finding in both post-traumatic and stress-induced osteolysis of the distal end of the clavicle.[107-109] However, increased signal is a very common finding, and there appears to be no correlation between the MRI appearance and clinical findings in the acromioclavicular joint.[110] MRI in an asymptomatic population revealed that three fourths had changes consistent with acromioclavicular

joint osteoarthritis that were independent of rotator cuff disease.[111] Therefore, an abnormal MRI finding in the acromioclavicular joint is not a reliable indicator that the acromioclavicular joint is a source of pain or is related to associated rotator cuff tendon changes.

STERNOCLAVICULAR JOINT AND MEDIAL CLAVICLE

Recommended Views

A CT scan of both medial clavicles is recommended. An anteroposterior view in the plane of the thorax with a 40-degree cephalic tilt view of both clavicles or a tomogram or bone scan may be helpful.

Although some authors have reported that injury to the sternoclavicular joint is purely a clinical diagnosis, appropriate use of radiographs is a critical part of the work-up of this problem. Without radiographs, even the most experienced clinicians occasionally misdiagnose injuries to the sternoclavicular joint. One cannot rely only on clinical findings to make the proper diagnosis because severe anterior swelling about the sternoclavicular joint, which clinically appears to be a benign anterior sternoclavicular dislocation, can be either a fracture of the medial part of the clavicle or a very serious and dangerous posterior dislocation of the sternoclavicular joint.

Occasionally, routine anteroposterior or posteroanterior chest radiographs demonstrate asymmetry between

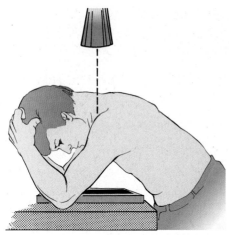

FIGURE 5-34 Positioning of the patient for x-ray evaluation of the sternoclavicular joint, as recommended by Hobbs. (Modified from Hobbs DW: Sternoclavicular joint, a new axial radiographic view. Radiology 90:801, 1968. Reproduced with permission from Rockwood CA, Green DP [eds]: Fractures [3 vols], 2nd ed. Philadelphia: JB Lippincott, 1984.)

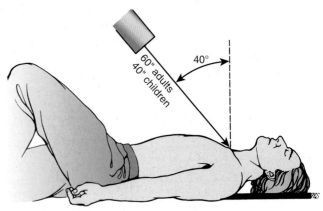

FIGURE 5-35 Positioning of the patient to take the serendipity cephalic tilt radiograph of the sternoclavicular joint. The x-ray tube is tilted 40 degrees from the vertical position and aimed directly at the manubrium. The cassette is large enough to receive the projected images of the medial halves of both clavicles. In children, the tube distance should be approximately 40 inches; in a thicker-chested adult, the distance should be 60 inches.

the sternoclavicular joints, which suggests a dislocation or fracture of the medial part of the clavicle. The ideal view for studying this joint is one taken at 90 degrees to the anteroposterior plane. However, because of our anatomy, it is impossible to take a true 90-degree cephalic-to-caudal view. A lateral radiograph of the chest is difficult to interpret because of the density of the chest and the overlap of the medial ends of the clavicles with the first rib and the sternum. As a result, numerous special projections have been devised by Hobbs,[112] Kattan,[113] Kurzbauer,[114] Ritvo and Ritvo,[115] and Rockwood and Green[6] (Fig. 5-34). Although most of these x-ray views are very helpful, CT offers the best information for evaluating fractures of the medial part of the clavicle and injuries to the sternoclavicular joint. The serendipity view (a 40-degree cephalic tilt view described in 1972) is easy to obtain and is reliable for demonstrating anterior and posterior subluxations and dislocations of the sternoclavicular joint and some fractures of the medial part of the clavicle.[6] This tomographic view is helpful in making the diagnosis if CT scanning is not available.

Evaluation Techniques

Serendipity View (40-Degree Cephalic Tilt View)

When CT scans and tomograms are not available, the serendipity view[6] can be very helpful in determining the type of injury to the region of the sternoclavicular joint. It will certainly distinguish between a benign anterior dislocation and a dangerous posterior dislocation. The patient is positioned supine on the x-ray table with a nongrid 11 × 14 inch cassette placed under the patient's upper chest, shoul-

der, and neck region. The x-ray beam is angled 40 degrees off the vertical and centered directly at the sternum (Fig. 5-35). The distance from the tube to the x-ray cassette should be 60 inches in adults and 40 inches in children. The voltage should be the same as for an anteroposterior chest radiograph. The x-ray beam is adjusted so that it will project *both* clavicles onto the film.

To interpret this radiograph, one compares the relationship of the medial end of the injured clavicle with that of the normal clavicle. In normal shoulders, both clavicles are on the same horizontal plane (Fig. 5-36A). In anterior dislocation, the injured clavicle is more superior than the normal clavicle (see Fig. 5-36B). In a posterior sternoclavicular joint, the medial end of the involved dislocated clavicle appears more inferior on the radiograph than the medial end of the normal clavicle (see Fig. 5-36C). Fractures of the medial part of the clavicle can also be noted on this view.

Tomogram

Tomograms can be very helpful in delineating medial clavicular fractures,[45] in distinguishing fractures from dislocations, and in detecting arthritic problems of the sternoclavicular joint.

Computed Tomography

CT scans offer the best information for demonstrating sternoclavicular subluxations, dislocations, fractures extending into the sternoclavicular joint, fractures of the medial part of the clavicle, arthritis of this joint[6,116-118] (Fig. 5-37A), and irreducible posterior dislocations.[6] CT scans, especially if enhanced with vascular studies, accurately document the intimate juxtaposition of the displaced

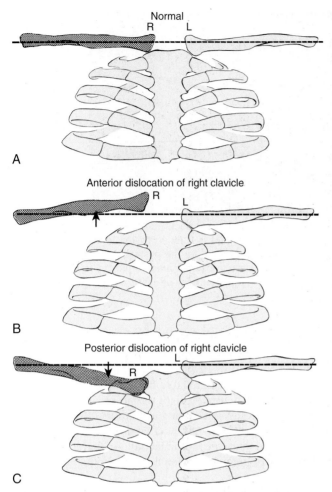

FIGURE 5-36 Interpretation of the cephalic tilt serendipity view of the sternoclavicular joint. **A,** In a normal person, both clavicles appear on the same imaginary line drawn through them. **B,** In a patient with anterior dislocation of the right sternoclavicular joint, the medial end of the right clavicle is projected above an imaginary line drawn through the level of the normal left clavicle. **C,** If the patient has a posterior dislocation of the right sternoclavicular joint, the medial end of the right clavicle is displaced below an imaginary line drawn through the normal left clavicle. L, left; R, right. (Modified from Rockwood CA, Green DP [eds]: Fractures [3 vols], 2nd ed. Philadelphia: JB Lippincott, 1984.)

medial end of the clavicle to the great vessels of the mediastinum. This is an invaluable preoperative study (see Fig. 5-37B).

Magnetic Resonance Imaging

In children and young adults, when the diagnosis is thought to be either dislocation of the sternoclavicular joint or meniscal disk injury, MRI can be used to determine whether the physis has displaced with the clavicle or is still adjacent to the manubrium (Fig. 5-38). MRI may also be useful in the diagnosis of medial clavicular osteomyelitis, metabolic disease, or benign and malignant processes.

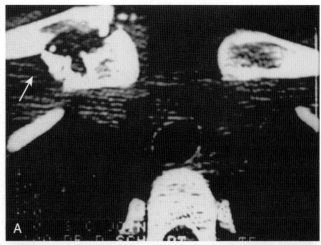

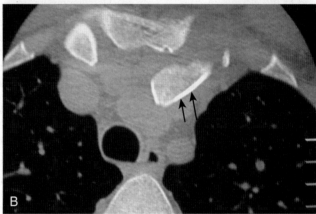

FIGURE 5-37 A, A CT scan clearly demonstrates a fracture of the medial aspect of the clavicle (*arrow*). **B,** A CT scan demonstrates a posterior fracture-dislocation of the left sternoclavicular joint (*arrows*).

Bone Scan

Bone scans are helpful in detecting degenerative changes, inflammatory problems, and tumors of the sternoclavicular joint.[106]

ROTATOR CUFF

Recommended Views

Recommended views are the anteroposterior and axillary lateral views, a 30-degree caudal tilt, or the scapular outlet view. Arthrography, CT arthrography, bursography, ultrasonography, or MRI can be used to evaluate the integrity of the rotator cuff.

Impingement syndrome is a common cause of pain and disability in the adult shoulder. It begins with soft tissue compromise involving the subacromial bursa and the rotator cuff, and radiographs are usually normal. As the impingement problem persists and progresses, a spur can form off the anteroinferior acromion, ossification in the coracoacromial ligament may be noted,[119] or an unusual shape of the acromion may be present.[120]

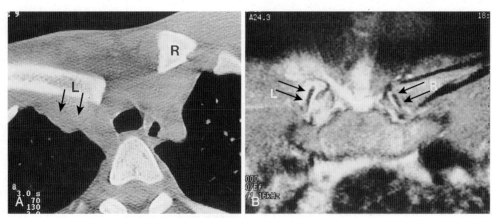

FIGURE 5-38 CT scan of a 15-year-old boy who has a posterior dislocation of the left sternoclavicular joint. Usually, in male patients younger than 22 to 24 years, apparent dislocation of the sternoclavicular joint is truly a physeal injury to the medial end of the clavicle. **A,** The CT scan reveals compression of the lung and trachea (*arrows*) by the posteriorly displaced medial left clavicle. **B,** However, MRI clearly shows that the physis of the left medial clavicle has remained adjacent to the manubrium, just as the physis of the right medial clavicle (*arrows*). L, left; R, right. (Courtesy of Jesse De Lee, MD, San Antonio, Texas.)

Rotator cuff tendon lesions are usually degenerative and associated with overuse or a progressive impingement syndrome; only rarely are they traumatic. Radiographic evaluation should include assessment of the coracoacromial arch[121] and, in a younger patient, assessment of the anteroinferior glenoid for signs of instability.

Techniques to Evaluate Rotator Cuff Tendinitis

Anteroposterior View

Anteroposterior radiographs of the glenohumeral joint with the arm in internal and external rotation can reveal associated calcific tendinitis in the tendons of the cuff and superior migration of the humeral head under the acromion. Cystic and sclerotic changes may be noted in the greater tuberosity.[122] Degenerative changes may also be seen in the acromioclavicular joint. In addition, sclerotic changes secondary to anterior proliferation of the acromion may be present in the anterior acromion. Narrowing of the acromiohumeral interval has often been noted.

Axillary Lateral View

Routine radiologic evaluation of impingement syndrome should include an axillary lateral view to investigate the presence of underlying glenohumeral arthritis.

Thirty-Degree Caudal Tilt View

Routine anteroposterior shoulder radiographs usually do not demonstrate spurs from the acromion, calcification in the coracoacromial ligament, or anteroinferior proliferation of the acromion. However, with the patient in the erect position, an anteroposterior radiograph of the shoulder taken with a 30-degree caudal tilt adequately demonstrates the anterior acromial spur or ossification in the coracoacromial ligament (Fig. 5-39). Anteroinferior subacromial spurs can be noted on the radiographs of

patients with either impingement syndrome or rotator cuff problems. Rockwood has used this technique to define spurs since 1979 because this view is easier to accomplish and more reliable for demonstrating spurring of the anterior acromion than the scapular outlet view is (Fig. 5-40). Kitay and colleagues[59] and Ono, Yamamuro, and Rockwood[123] have shown that this technique is highly reliable and that the acromial image correlates significantly with operative acromial spur length.

Scapular Outlet View

The patient is positioned as for a true scapulolateral radiograph, and the tube is angled caudally 10 degrees. This radiograph offers a view of the outlet of the supraspinatus-tendon unit as it passes under the coracoacromial arch. Deformities of the anteroinferior acromion or the acromioclavicular arch down into the outlet can be noted on this view (see Fig. 5-40D). Bigliani and colleagues[120] identified three distinct acromial shapes on this radiologic view:

Type I: A flat acromion
Type II: A curved acromion
Type III: An anterior downward hook on the acromion

Although this classification of acromial shapes has been shown to have low interobserver reliability,[121,124] the acromial slope measure on the outlet view correlates with acromial thickness.[59]

Techniques to Evaluate Rotator Cuff Integrity

Arthrography, Arthrotomography, and Computed Tomography Arthrography

The shoulder arthrogram, either single contrast with just radiopaque material or double contrast with both air and contrast material, is extremely accurate in diagnosing full-

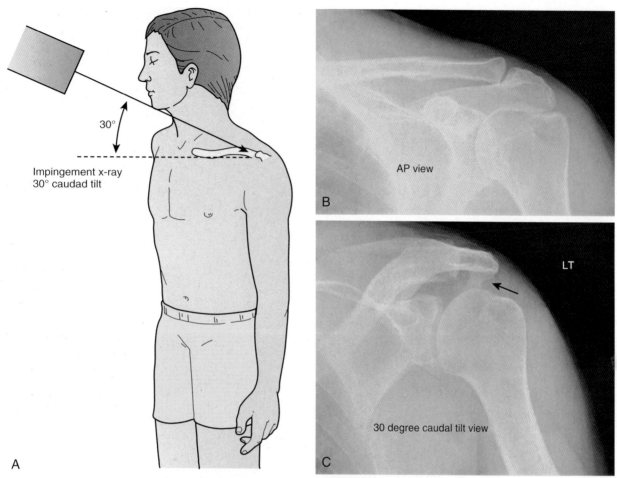

30°

Impingement x-ray
30° caudad tilt

A

AP view

B

LT

30 degree caudal tilt view

C

FIGURE 5-39 A, Positioning of the patient and the x-ray tube to demonstrate spurring or proliferation of the anteroinferior acromion, which is associated with impingement syndrome and lesions of the rotator cuff. The patient should be erect for this evaluation. **B,** Anteroposterior radiograph of a 52-year-old patient with impingement syndrome. The acromion does not appear to be abnormal. **C,** However, when the anteroposterior radiograph is taken with a 30-degree caudal tilt of the x-ray tube, the large, prominent, irregular spurring of the anterior acromion (*arrow*) is easily noted. LT, left shoulder.

thickness tears. Deep surface partial-thickness cuff tears are not always demonstrated. Escape of dye from the glenohumeral joint into the subacromial-subdeltoid bursa is conclusive evidence of a defect in the rotator cuff (Fig. 5-41). The accuracy of the arthrogram is between 95% and 100%. Goldman and Ghelman favor double-contrast studies (i.e., air and contrast media).[125] Although double-contrast studies can offer more information about the size of a given tear, neither technique is considered more sensitive than the other for detecting tears. Hall and colleagues[126] demonstrated less patient discomfort after arthrography with the water-soluble contrast medium metrizamide. Combining arthrography with tomography or CT scans can help in defining the size of the defect in the rotator cuff.[61,65,127]

Subacromial Bursography

Subacromial bursography has been reported by Lie and Mast,[128] Mikasa,[129] and Strizak and coworkers.[130] In 1982, Strizak and coworkers studied the technique in cadavers and in patients. They reported that normal bursae would accept 5 to 10 mL of contrast medium and that patients with impingement syndrome and thickened walls of the subacromial deltoid bursae would accept only 1 to 2 mL of medium.

Ultrasonography

Reliable demonstration of full-thickness rotator cuff tears with an ultrasound scanner has been reported in 92% to 95% of cases.[131-136] In some centers, it has virtually replaced arthrography for cuff evaluation. It is reported to be safe, rapid, noninvasive, and inexpensive and has the advantage of imaging and comparing both shoulders. The accuracy of sonographic evaluation of the cuff depends on the experience of the ultrasonographer and the quality of the high-resolution, linear array sonographic equipment. The spatial resolution of ultrasound images is not as great as that of conventional radiographic techniques (including arthrography). Therefore, the sonographic examination is a hands-on experience; that is, it requires an experienced sonographer, and one may not rely on the recorded images to convey the full diagnostic impact

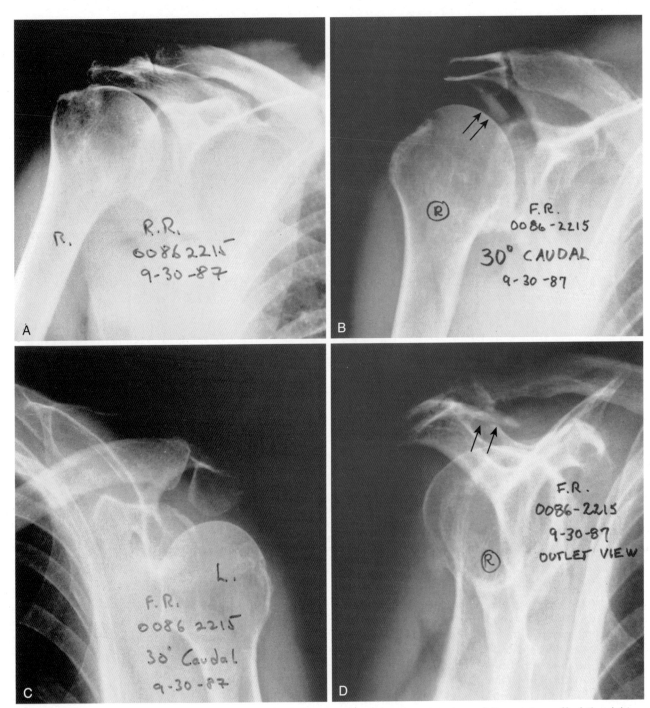

FIGURE 5-40 A, Anteroposterior view of a patient with impingement syndrome and rupture of the rotator cuff of the right shoulder. Minimal changes are noted on the anterior acromion. **B,** On a 30-degree caudal tilt view, note the large, irregularly shaped spike of bone that extends down the coracoacromial ligament into the bursa and the cuff (*arrows*). **C,** A 30-degree caudal tilt radiograph of the normal shoulder shows the normal relationship of the anterior acromion to the distal end of the clavicle. **D,** The scapular outlet view does reveal the spur (*arrows*), but there is considerable overlap with other structures.

of the study. Technologic advances have led to a more portable unit that may be used in the office by the orthopaedic surgeon to evaluate the integrity of the rotator cuff. Ziegler reported surgically confirmed positive and negative predictive values of 96.6% and 93.2%, respectively, for partial thickness tears; and 92.9% and 96.8%, respectively for full-thickness tears.[137]

Mack and colleagues use a technique that depends on the absence of motion in the cuff tissue when studied with real-time ultrasound.[134,138] Secondary signs of cuff tear, such as thinning of the cuff or abnormal echoes in the cuff, are more difficult to interpret. These latter findings might not represent a complete cuff tear but may be due to an incomplete tear, edema, recent steroid injec-

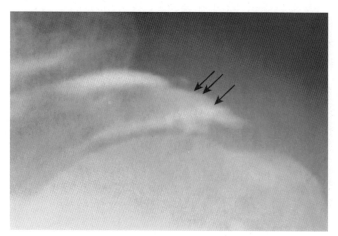

FIGURE 5-41 Positive arthrogram of the left shoulder. The dye is seen not only in the glenohumeral joint but also up into the subacromial-subdeltoid bursa. The size of the tear can also be well visualized (*arrows*).

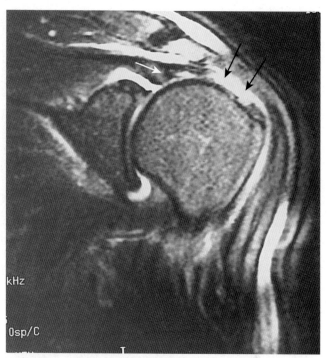

FIGURE 5-42 MRI demonstrating complete rupture of the rotator cuff. The remaining cuff tendon is identified by a *white arrow*, and the cuff defect area is identified by *black arrows*.

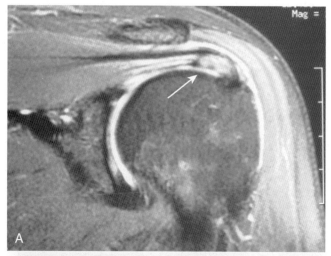

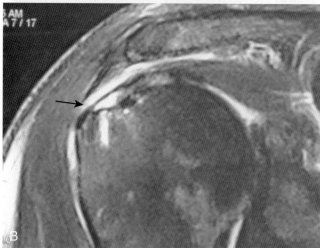

FIGURE 5-43 A, MRI reveals a high-grade articular-sided supraspinatus partial-thickness tendon tear (*arrow*). **B,** MRI reveals an intrasubstance partial-thickness supraspinatus tendon tear (*arrow*).

tion, calcifications in the cuff, surgical scar, or normal tissues in some patients.

Kilcoyne and Matsen believe that for sonography to offer a useful alternative to arthrography or arthroscopy as a screening procedure, certain criteria should be adhered to: The diagnosis of a complete rotator cuff tear depends on the absence of motion in the cuff tissue when studied sonographically, and if the patient continues to have symptoms suggesting a cuff tear, an arthrogram should be performed to determine whether a small cuff tear is present.[61] Using these criteria, Mack and colleagues found that sonography had a sensitivity of 91%, a specificity of 100%, and an overall accuracy of 94%.[138] These results have been duplicated at several other centers,[139-141] and ultrasound can be recommended for screening evaluations if an experienced technician is available.[138,142,143]

Magnetic Resonance Imaging

MRI offers an alternative, noninvasive technique for investigating lesions of the rotator cuff.[144-150] It provides information regarding the tendinous attachments of the rotator cuff as well as the condition of the specific rotator cuff muscle. MRI has been used to categorize acromial morphology, but interobserver agreement has been shown to be poor[151] because of multiple images revealing a variation in acromial shape when progressing from lateral to medial.

Various studies have shown MRI to be very sensitive for detecting lesions of the rotator cuff (Fig. 5-42).[146,150,152-154] Rotator cuff tendinopathy appears as a thickened inho-

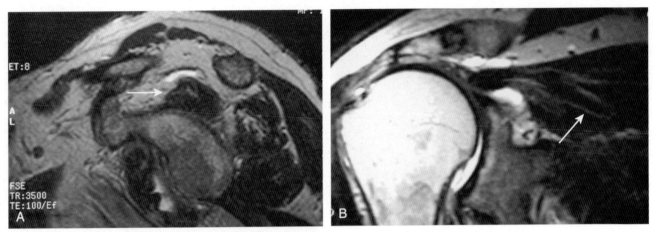

FIGURE 5-44 A, Sagittal MRI reveals supraspinatus muscle atrophy as determined by the diminished cross-sectional area *(arrow).* **B,** Supraspinatus muscle atrophy demonstrated by coronal oblique MRI, with fat striping *(arrow)* indicating replacement of muscle by fat deposition. Superior humeral head migration is also noted.

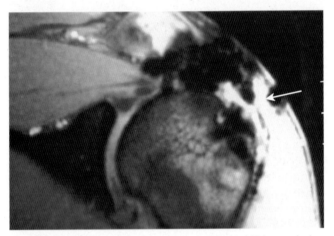

FIGURE 5-45 A T1-weighted coronal oblique MRI reveals low signal artifact from ferrous material; however, retearing of the tendon is apparent *(arrow).*

mogeneous tendon with increased signal intensity on FS PD FSE (fat saturation, proton density–weighted, fast spin echo) or FSE PD. Partial-thickness tendon tearing can involve the articular side, the bursal side, or the intrasubstance portion of the tendon (Fig. 5-43) Partial-thickness tears can be differentiated from tendinosis by the hyperintense signal seen on T2 FSE and FS PD FSE images, whereas tendinosis is hyperintense on FS PD FSE only.

Operative correlation studies[155,156] have shown MRI to be accurate in detecting large, full-thickness tears and less accurate in detecting small (<1 cm) tears or in differentiating tendinitis from partial-thickness tears or small full-thickness tears.[157] Rotator cuff tendon tears are represented by a well-defined high-intensity signal on T2-weighted images, which reflect a discontinuity in the normal tendon signal that is not evident on the PD scan.[158] Increased signal in the supraspinatus on coronal oblique T1-

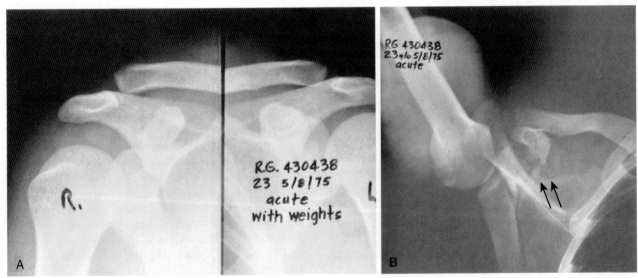

FIGURE 5-46 A, This 23-year-old patient had a traumatic injury to his right acromioclavicular joint. Note the superior displacement of the right clavicle from the acromion when compared with the left; also note that the coracoclavicular distance in both shoulders is approximately the same. The fracture at the base of the coracoid is not well visualized. **B,** The Stryker notch view reveals a fracture through the base of the coracoid *(arrows).*

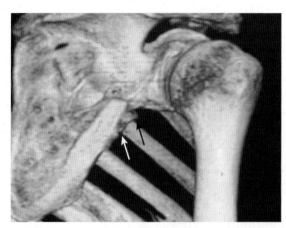

FIGURE 5-47 A three-dimensional CT scan reveals scapular body fractures and lateral border displacement (*arrows*).

weighted images has been shown to have no histologic correlation and may be artifact.[159] The MRI can also be useful in revealing the condition of the muscle belly of a detached rotator cuff tendon.[160] Rotator cuff muscle atrophy is revealed by a reduced cross-sectional area on the sagittal images and the presence of increased signal streaks (fatty infiltrates) within the muscle belly seen best on the coronal oblique images (Fig 5-44).

Some younger patients with a suspected lesion of the rotator cuff, as suggested by weakness and atrophy, might indeed have a ganglion compressing the suprascapular nerve. An MRI can easily detect the ganglion and determine if the cyst has an intra-articular source.

The use of MRI to evaluate the integrity of a rotator cuff tendon that has undergone previous surgery can be problematic.[161] Artifact from small amounts of ferrous material left in the soft tissues following arthroscopic

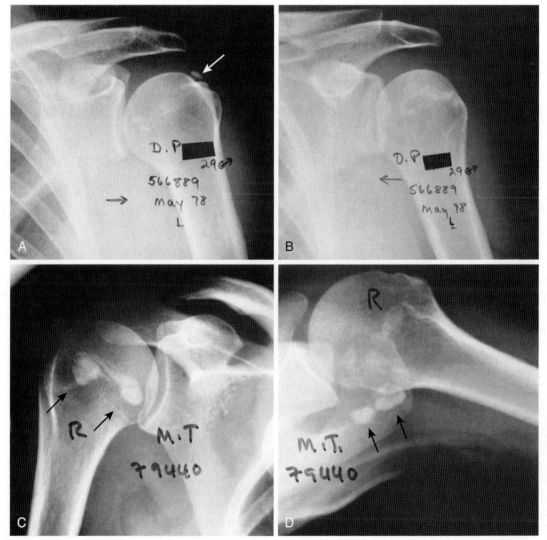

FIGURE 5-48 Calcific tendinitis of the left shoulder. **A,** With the arm in external rotation, the calcium deposit is visible (*arrow*). **B,** With the arm in internal rotation, the calcium deposit is no longer visible, thus indicating that the calcium must be in the anterior aspect of the supraspinatus tendon. **C,** On an anteroposterior radiograph in internal and external rotation, the calcium deposit cannot be accurately localized. **D,** However, on the axillary view, the calcium deposit is quite distinct and localized in either the infraspinatus tendon or the teres minor tendon.

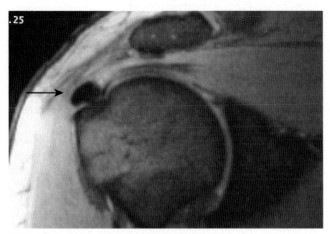

FIGURE 5-49 The presence of a calcific deposit *(arrow)* in the supraspinatus tendon is easily identifiable on a T2-weighted coronal oblique MRI scan.

subacromial burring or shaving causes signal alterations that can obscure the rotator tendon insertion and produce wild-appearing images that suggest infection or other processes. Complete retracted retearing is accurately revealed by MRI; however, the size and delineation between partial-thickness or small full-thickness tears is difficult, and clinical assessment is recommended.[162] Previous suture repair of a tendon can appear as an increased intermediate signal on T2-weighted images (Fig 5-45).

SCAPULA

Recommended Views

Recommended views include true anteroposterior views and an axillary lateral view. Special views such as the Stryker notch and West Point views, tomograms, and CT may be required.

The trauma series of radiographs usually adequately demonstrate fractures of the scapular body, spine, and neck. Fractures located elsewhere might require other

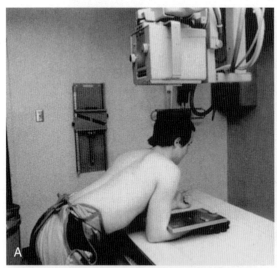

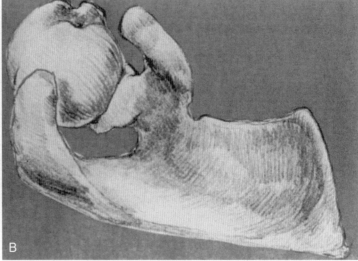

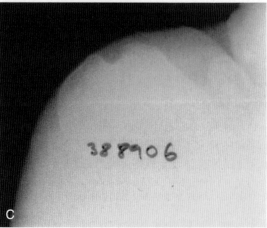

FIGURE 5-50 A, Position of the patient for the Fisk view to visualize the bicipital groove in the proximal end of the humerus. Note that the patient is holding the cassette and leaning forward so that the beam passing down through the bicipital groove will be projected onto the cassette. **B,** Anatomy of the bicipital groove. **C,** Projection of the bicipital groove onto the x-ray film with the Fisk technique. (Modified from Fisk C: Adaptation of the technique for radiography of the bicipital groove. Radiol Technol 37:47-50, 1965.)

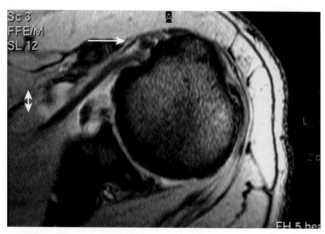

FIGURE 5-51 An axial MRI scan reveals medial subluxation of the long head of the biceps into the substance of the superior part of the subscapularis tendon (*arrow*).

views for optimal visualization. Glenoid rim fractures, although often visualized on the axillary lateral view of the trauma series, may be better visualized on a West Point or apical oblique view of the glenohumeral joint.[15,22] Coracoid fractures may be visible on the axillary lateral view but are much better defined on the Stryker notch view[44] (Fig. 5-46). Acromial fractures can be seen on the axillary lateral view but may be difficult to distinguish from an os acromiale.

When determining the degree of displacement of fractures of the scapula and defining the amount of displacement of glenoid fractures, a CT scan can be of great value (Fig. 5-47).

CALCIFYING TENDINITIS

Calcium deposits in the rotator cuff can be specifically localized in the tendons of the rotator cuff using anteroposterior x-rays of the shoulder in internal and external rotation and an axillary lateral x-ray (Fig. 5-48). MRI is useful in the preoperative evaluation of chronic calcific tendinopathy because it delineates the size of the calcific lesion and can define the amount of rotator cuff tendon involvement (Fig. 5-49).

BICEPS TENDON

Rarely is biceps tendinitis the primary cause of shoulder pain. It is usually secondarily involved as a part of an impingement syndrome or degenerative lesions of the rotator cuff. The anatomy of the groove can be evaluated by the Fisk view.[163,164] In this view, the x-ray machine is superior to the shoulder. The image of the bicipital groove is projected down onto the cassette, which is held by

the patient (Fig. 5-50). Cone and colleagues[165] have extensively studied the x-ray anatomy and pathologic irregularities of the bicipital groove.

Bicipital instability is usually associated with rotator interval injury or subscapularis tendon injury, or both. MRI accurately reveals the varying degrees of instability, from a flat long head of the biceps tendon perched on the lesser tuberosity to dislocation within the glenohumeral joint with complete detachment of the subscapularis tendon (Fig. 5-51; see Fig. 5-22).

ACKNOWLEDGMENTS

The author sincerely thanks Becky Laredo, MD, musculoskeletal radiologist at the University of Texas Health Science Center in San Antonio, for her contributions involving special radiologic evaluations of the shoulder.

REFERENCES

1. McLaughlin HL: Posterior dislocation of the shoulder. J Bone Joint Surg Am 34:584-590, 1952.
2. Neer CS II: Displaced proximal humeral fractures. J Bone Joint Surg Am 52:1077-1089, 1970.
3. Neer CS II: Fractures of the distal clavicle with detachment of the coracoclavicular ligaments in adults. J Trauma 3:99-110, 1963.
4. Neviaser RJ: Radiologic assessment of the shoulder: Plain and arthrographic. Orthop Clin North Am 18:343-349, 1987.
5. DeSmet AA: Axillary projection in radiography of the nontraumatized shoulder. AJR Am J Roentgenol 134:511-514, 1980.
6. Rockwood CA Jr, Green DP (eds): Fractures, 2nd ed. Philadelphia: JB Lippincott, 1984.
7. Post M: The Shoulder. Philadelphia: Lea & Febiger, 1978.
8. Rowe CR: The Shoulder. New York: Churchill Livingstone, 1988.
9. Bateman JE: The Shoulder and Neck, 2nd ed. Philadelphia: WB Saunders, 1978.
10. Lawrence WS: A method of obtaining an accurate lateral roentgenogram of the shoulder joint. AJR Am J Roentgenol 5:193-194, 1918.
11. Lawrence WS: New position in radiographing the shoulder joint. AJR Am J Roentgenol 2:728-730, 1915.
12. Cleaves EN: A new film holder for roentgen examinations of the shoulder. AJR Am J Roentgenol 45:88-90, 1941.
13. Rontgen WK: On a new kind of rays. Nature 53:274-276, 1896.
14. Bloom MH, Obata WG: Diagnosis of posterior dislocation of the shoulder with use of Velpeau axillary and angle up roentgenographic views. J Bone Joint Surg Am 49:943-949, 1967.
15. Garth WP Jr, Slappey CE, Ochs CW: Roentgenographic demonstration of instability of the shoulder: the apical oblique projection technical note. J Bone Joint Surg Am 66:1450-1453, 1984.
16. Kornguth PJ, Salazar AM: The apical oblique view of the shoulder: Its usefulness in acute trauma. AJR Am J Roentgenol 149:113-116, 1987.
17. Horsfield D, Jones SN: A useful projection in radiography of the shoulder. J Bone Joint Surg Br 69:338, 1987.
18. Ciullo JV, Koniuch MP, Teitge RA: Axillary shoulder roentgenography in clinical orthopaedic practice [abstract]. Orthop Trans 6:451, 1982.
19. Teitge RA, Ciullo JV: C.A.M. axillary x-ray: Exhibit to the Academy Meeting of the American Academy of Orthopaedic Surgeons. Orthop Trans 6:451, 1982.
20. Sjödén GO, Movin T, Aspelin P, et al: 3D-radiographic analysis does not improve the Neer and AO classifications of proximal humeral fractures. Acta Orthop Scand 70:325-328, 1999.
21. Sjödén GO, Movin T, Guntner P, et al: Poor reproducibility of classification of proximal humeral fractures. Additional CT of minor value. Acta Orthop Scand 68:239-242,1997.
22. Madler M, Mayr B, Baierl P, et al: [Value of conventional x-ray diagnosis and computerized tomography in the detection of Hill–Sachs defects and bony Bankart lesions in recurrent shoulder dislocations.] Rofo 148:384-389, 1988.
23. Mason BJ, Kier R, Bindleglass DF: Occult fractures of the greater tuberosity of the humerus: Radiographic and MR imaging findings. AJR Am J Roentgenol 172:469-473, 1999.
24. Reinus WR, Hatem SF: Fractures of the greater tuberosity presenting as rotator cuff abnormality: Magnetic resonance demonstration. J Trauma 44:670-675, 1998.

25. Resch H, Benedetto KP, Kadletz R, et al: X-ray examination in recurrent dislocation of the shoulder; value of different techniques. Unfallchirurgie 11:65-69, 1985.

26. Rokous JR, Feagin JA, Abbott HG: Modified axillary roentgenogram. Clin Orthop Relat Res 82:84-86, 1972.

27. Itoi E, Lee SB, Amrami KK, et al: Quantitative assessment of classic antero-inferior bony Bankart lesions by radiography and computed tomography. Am J Sports Med 31:112-118, 2003.

28. Hill HA, Sachs MD: The grooved defect of the humeral head: A frequently unrecognized complication of dislocations of the shoulder joint. Radiology 690-700, 1940.

29. Eve FS: A case of subcoracoid dislocation of the humerus with the formation of an indentation on the posterior surface of the head. Medico-Chir Trans Soc (London) 63:317-321, 1880.

30. Malgaigne JF: Traité des Fractures et des Luxations. Philadelphia: JB Lippincott, 1859.

31. Kuster E: Ueber Habituelle Schulterluxation. Verh Dtsch Ges Chir 11:112-114, 1882.

32. Cramer M: Resection des Oberarmkopfes wegen habitueller Luxation. Klin Wochenschr 19:21-25, 1882.

33. Popke LOA: Zur Kasuistik und Therapie der Habituellen Schulterluxation. Dissertation, Halle, 1882.

34. Caird FM: The shoulder joint in relation to certain dislocations and fractures. Edinburgh Med J 32:708-714, 1887.

35. Broca A, Hartman H: Contribution à l'étude des luxa-tions de l'épaule (luxations dites incomplète, décollements périostiques, luxations directes et luxations indirectes). Bull Soc Anat Paris 65:312-336, 1890.

36. Broca A, Hartman H: Contribution à l'étude des luxations de l'épaule (luxations anciennes, luxations recidivantes). Bull Soc Anat Paris 65:416-423, 1890.

37. Friedman RJ, Hawthorne KB, Genez BM: The use of computerized tomography in the measurement of glenoid version. J Bone Joint Surg Am 74:1032-1037, 1992.

38. Bankart ASB: Recurrent or habitual dislocation of the shoulder joint. Br Med J 2:1132-1133, 1923.

39. Bankart ASB: The pathology and treatment of recurrent dislocation of the shoulder joint. Br J Surg 26:23-29, 1938.

40. Eden R: Zur Operation der habituellen Schulterluxation unter Mitteilung eines nuenen Verfahrens bei Abriss am innren Pfannenrande. Dtsch Z Chir 144:269-280, 1918.

41. Hybbinette S: De la transplantation d'un fragment osseux pour remeádier aux luxations reácidivantes de l'eápaule; constatations et reásultats opeáratonês. Acta Chir Scand 71:411-445, 1932.

42. Didiee J: Le radiodiagnostic dans la luxation reácidivante de l'eápaule. J Radiol Electrologie 14:209-218, 1930.

43. Hermodsson I: Röntgenologischen Studien über die traumatischen und habituellen Schultergelenkverrenkungen nach vorn und nach unten. Acta Radiol 20:1-173, 1940.

44. Hall RH, Isaac F, Booth CR: Dislocations of the shoulder with special reference to accompanying small fractures. J Bone Joint Surg Am 41:489-494, 1959.

45. Adams JC: The humeral head defect in recurrent anterior dislocations of the shoulder. Br J Radiol 23:151-156, 1950.

46. Pring DJ, Constant O, Bayley JIL, et al: Radiology of the humeral head in recurrent anterior shoulder dislocations: Brief report. J Bone Joint Surg Br 71:141-142, 1989.

47. Strauss MB, Wroble LJ, Neff RS, et al: The shrugged-off shoulder: A comparison of patients with recurrent shoulder subluxations and dislocations. Phys Sports Med 12:85-97, 1983.

48. Danzig LA, Greenway G, Resnick D: The Hill–Sachs lesion: An experimental study. Am J Sports Med 8:328-332, 1980.

49. Strauss MB, Wroble LJ, Neff RS, et al: X-ray confirmation of anterior shoulder instability. Orthop Trans 2:225, 1978.

50. Kinnard P, Gordon D, Levesque RY, et al: Computerized arthrotomography in recurring shoulder dislocations and subluxations. Can J Surg 27:487-488, 1984.

51. Kinnard P, Tricoir JL, Levesque RY, et al: Assessment of the unstable shoulder by computed arthrography: A preliminary report. Am J Sports Med 11:157-159, 1983.

52. McMaster WC: Anterior glenoid labrum damage: A painful lesion in swimmers. Am J Sports Med 14:383-387, 1986.

53. McNiesch LM, Callaghan JJ: CT arthrography of the shoulder: Variations of the glenoid labrum. Am J Roentgenol 149:936-966, 1987.

54. Nottage WM, Duge WD, Fields WA: Computed arthrotomography of the glenohumeral joint to evaluate anterior instability: Correlation with arthroscopic findings. Arthroscopy 3:273-276, 1987.

55. Rafii M, Firooznia H, Golimbu C, et al: CT arthrography of capsular structures of the shoulder. AJR Am J Roentgenol 146:361-367, 1986.

56. Rafii M, Minkoff J, Bonamo J, et al: Computed tomography (CT) arthrography of shoulder instabilities in athletes. Am J Sports Med 16:352-361, 1988.

57. Albright J, El Khoury G: Shoulder arthrotomography in the evaluation of the injured throwing arm. In Zarins B, Andrews JR, Carson WG Jr (eds): Injuries to the Throwing Arm. Philadelphia: WB Saunders, 1985, pp 66-75.

58. Braunstein EM, O'Connor G: Double contrast arthrotomography of the shoulder. J Bone Joint Surg Am 64:192-195, 1982.

59. Kitay GS, Iannotti JP, Williams GR, et al: Roentgenographic assessment of acromial morphologic condition in rotator cuff impingement syndrome. J Shoulder Elbow Surg 4:441-448, 1995.

60. Pappas AM, Goss TP, Kleinman PK: Symptomatic shoulder instability due to lesions of the glenoid labrum. Am J Sports Med 11:279-288, 1983.

61. Kilcoyne RF, Matsen FA III: Rotator cuff tear measurement by arthropneumotomography. AJR Am J Roentgenol 140:315-318, 1983.

62. Kleinman PK, Kanzaria PK, Goss TP, Pappas AM: Axillary arthrotomography of the glenoid labrum. AJR Am J Roentgenol 141:993-999, 1984.

63. Shuman WP, Kilcoyne RF, Matsen FA III, et al: Double-contrast computed tomography of the glenoid labrum. AJR Am J Roentgenol 141:581-584, 1983.

64. Jahnke AH, Petersen SA, Neumann C, et al: A prospective comparison of computerized arthrotomography and magnetic resonance imaging of the glenohumeral joint. Am J Sports Med 20:695-701, 1992.

65. Resch H, Helweg G, zur Nedden D, et al: Double contrast computed tomographic examination techniques in habitual and recurrent shoulder dislocation. Eur J Radiol 8:6-12, 1988.

66. Resch H, Kadletz R, Beck E, et al: Simple and double-contrast CT scanning in the examination of recurrent shoulder dislocations. Unfallchirurg 89:441-445, 1986.

67. Chandnani VP, Yeager TD, Deberardino T, et al: Glenoid labral tears: Prospective evaluation with MR imaging, MR arthrography, and CT arthrography. AJR Am J Roentgenol 161:1220-1235, 1993.

68. Coumas JM, Waite RJ, Goss TP, et al: CT and MR evaluation of the labral capsular ligamentous complex of the shoulder. AJR Am J Roentgenol 158:591-597, 1992.

69. Beltran J, Rosenberg ZS, Chandnani VP, et al: Glenohumeral instability: Evaluation with MR arthrography. Radiographics 17:657-673, 1997.

70. Green MR, Christensen KP: Magnetic resonance imaging of the glenoid labrum in anterior shoulder instability. Am J Sports Med 22:493-498,1994.

71. Gusmer PB, Potter HG, Schatz JA, et al: Labral injuries: Accuracy of detection with unenhanced MR imaging of the shoulder. Radiology 200:519-524, 1996.

72. Legan JM, Burkhard TK, Goff WB, et al: Tears of the glenoid labrum: MR imaging of 88 arthroscopically confirmed cases. Radiology 179:241-246, 1991.

73. Liu SH, Henry MH, Nuccion S, et al: Diagnosis of glenoid labral tears. A comparison between magnetic resonance imaging and clinical examinations. Am J Sports Med 24:149-154, 1996.

74. Flannigan B, Kursunoglu-Brahme S, Snyder S, et al: MR arthrography of the shoulder: Comparison with conventional MR imaging. AJR Am J Roentgenol 155:829-832, 1990.

75. Kieft GJ, Bloem JL, Rozing PM, et al: MR imaging of recurrent anterior dislocation of the shoulder: Comparison with CT arthrography. AJR Am J Roentgenol 150:1083-1087, 1988.

76. Neumann CH, Petersen SA, Jahnke AH: MR imaging of the labral-capsular complex: Normal variations. AJR Am J Roentgenol 157:1015-1021, 1991.

77. Griffith JF, Antonio GE, Tong CW, et al. Anterior shoulder dislocation: Quantification of glenoid bone loss with CT. Am J Roentgenol 180:1423-1430, 2003.

78. Tirman PF, Stauffer AE, Crues JV, et al: Saline magnetic resonance arthrography in the evaluation of glenohumeral instability. Arthroscopy 9:550-559, 1993.

79. Schulte-Altedorneburg G, Gebhard M, Wohlgemuth WA, et al: MR arthrography: Pharmacology, efficacy and safety in clinical trials. Skeletal Radiol 32:1-12,2003.

80. Zanetti M, Carstensen T, Weishaupt D, et al: MR arthrographic variability of the arthroscopically normal glenoid labrum: Qualitative and quantitative assessment. Eur Radiol 11:559-566, 2001.

81. Wagner SC, Schweitzer ME, Morrison WB, et al: Shoulder instability: Accuracy of MR imaging performed after surgery in depicting recurrent injury—initial findings. Radiology 222:196-203, 2002.

82. Cvitanic O, Tirman PF, Feller JF, et al: Using abduction and external rotation of the shoulder to increase the sensitivity of MR arthrography in revealing tears of the anterior glenoid labrum. AJR Am J Roentgenol 169:837-844, 1997.

83. Palmer WE, Caslowitz PL: Anterior shoulder instability: Diagnostic criteria determined from prospective analysis of 121 MR arthrograms. Radiology 197:819-825,1995.

84. Davidson JJ, Speer KP: Clinical utility of high resonance imaging and MR arthrography of the shoulder. AAOS Shoulder Meeting, Atlanta, Georgia, February 1996.

85. Bencardino JT, Beltran J, Rosenberg ZS, et al: Superior labrum anterior-posterior lesions: Diagnosis with MR arthro-graphy of the shoulder. Radiology 214:267-271, 2000.

86. Jee WH, McCauley TR, Katz LD, et al: Superior labral anterior posterior (SLAP) lesions of the glenoid labrum: Reliability and accuracy of MR arthrography for diagnosis. Radiology 218:127-132, 2001.

87. Galinat BJ, Howell SM, Kraft, TA: The glenoid posterior acromial angle: An accurate method for evaluating glenoid version [abstract]. Orthop Trans 12:727, 1988.

88. Friedman RJ, Hawthorne KB, Genez BM: The use of computerized tomography in the measurement of glenoid version. J Bone Joint Surg Am 74:1032-1037, 1992.

89. Mullaji AB, Beddow FH, Lamb H: CT measurement of glenoid erosion in arthritis. J Bone Joint Surg Br 76:384-388, 1994.

90. Jensen KL, Jacobs PM, Loredo R, et al: The value of preoperative CT in shoulder arthroplasty [exhibit]. AAOS Shoulder Meeting, Atlanta, Georgia, February 1996.

91. Randelli M, Gambrioli PL: Glenohumeral osteometry by computed tomography in normal and unstable shoulders. Clin Orthop Relat Res (208):151-156, 1986.

92. Kwon YW, Powell KA, Yum JK, et al: Use of three-dimensional tomography for the analysis of the glenoid anatomy. J Shoulder Elbow Surg 14:85-90, 2005.

93. Matsen FA 3rd, Iannotti JP, Rockwood CA Jr: Humeral fixation by press-fitting of a tapered metaphyseal stem: A prospective radiographic study. J Bone Joint Surg Am 85:304-308, 2003.

94. Lazarus MD, Jensen KL, Southworth C, Matsen FA 3rd: The radiographic evaluation of keeled and pegged glenoid component insertion. J Bone Joint Surg Am 84:1174-1182, 2002.

95. Kelleher IM, Cofield RH, Becker DA, Beabout JW: Fluoroscopically positioned radiographs of total shoulder arthroplasty. J Shoulder Elbow Surg 1:306-311, 1992.

96. Yian EH, Werner CM, Nyffeler RW, et al: Radiographic and computed tomography analysis of cemented pegged polyethylene glenoid components in total shoulder replacement. J Bone Joint Surg Am 87:1928-1936, 2005.

97. Sperling JW, Potter HG, Craig EV, et al: Magnetic resonance imaging of painful shoulder arthroplasty. J Shoulder Elbow Surg 11:315-321, 2002.

98. Sofka CM, Adler RS: Sonographic evaluation of shoulder arthroplasty. AJR Am J Roentgenol 180:1117-1120, 2003.

99. Westhoff B, Wild A, Werner A, et al: The value of ultrasound after shoulder arthroplasty. Skeletal Radiol 31:695-701, 2002.

100. Neer CS II: Fractures about the shoulder. In Rockwood CA, Green DP (eds): Fractures, 2nd ed. Philadelphia: JB Lippincott, 1984, pp 679.

101. Neer CS II: Fractures of the distal third of the clavicle. Clin Orthop Relat Res 58:43-50, 1968.

102. Alexander OM: Dislocation of the acromio-clavicular joint. Radiography 15:260, 1949.

103. Waldrop JI, Norwood LA, Alvarez RG: Lateral roentgenographic projections of the acromioclavicular joint. Am J Sports Med 9:337-341, 1981.

104. Richardson JB, Ramsay A, Davidson JK, et al: Radiographs in shoulder trauma. J Bone Joint Surg Br 70:457-460, 1988.

105. Stewart CA, Siegel ME, King D, et al: Radionuclide and radiographic demonstration of condensing osteitis of the clavicle. Clin Nucl Med 13:177-178, 1988.

106. Teates CD, Brower AC, Williamson BRJ, et al: Bone scans in condensing osteitis of the clavicle. South Med J 71:736-738, 1978.

107. DePalma AF: Surgery of the Shoulder, 3rd ed. Philadelphia: JB Lippincott, 1983.

108. Farin PV, Jaroma H: Acute traumatic tears of the rotator cuff the value of sonography. Radiology 197:269-273, 1995.

109. Fiorella D, Helms CA, Speer KP: Increased T2 signal intensity in the distal clavicle: Incidence and clinical implications. Skeletal Radiol 29:697-702, 2000.

110. Jordan LK, Kenter K, Griffiths HL. Relationship between MRI and clinical findings in the acromioclavicular joint. Skeletal Radiol 31:516-521, 2002.

111. Needell SD, Zlatkin MB, Sher JS, et al: MR imaging of the rotator cuff: Peritendinous and bone abnormalities in an asymptomatic population. AJR Am J Roentgenol 166:863-867, 1996.

112. Hobbs DW: Sternoclavicular joint: A new axial radiographic view. Radiology 90:801-802, 1968.

113. Kattan KR: Modified view for use in roentgen examination of the sternoclavicular joints. Radiology 108:8, 1973.

114. Kurzbauer R: The lateral projection in roentgenography of the sternoclavicular articulation. AJR Am J Roentgenol 56:104-105, 1946.

115. Ritvo M, Ritvo M: Roentgen study of the sternoclavicular region. AJR Am J Roentgenol 53:644-650, 1947.

116. Destouet JM, Gilula LA, Murphy WA, et al: Computed tomography of the sternoclavicular joint and sternum. Radiology 138:123-128, 1981.

117. Levinsohn EM, Bunnell WP, Yuan HA: Computed tomography in the diagnosis of dislocations of the sternoclavicular joint. Clin Orthop Relat Res (140):12-16, 1979.

118. Lourie JA: Tomography in the diagnosis of posterior dislocations of the sternoclavicular joint. Acta Orthop Scand 51:579-580, 1980.

119. Neer CS II: Anterior acromioplasty for the chronic impingement syndrome in the shoulder. J Bone Joint Surg Am 54:41-50, 1972.

120. Bigliani LU, Morrison D, April EW: The morphology of the acromion and its relationship to rotator cuff tears. Orthop Trans 10:228, 1986.

121. Zuckerman JD, Kummer FJ, Cuomo F, et al: The influence of coracoacromial arch anatomy on rotator cuff tears. J Shoulder Elbow Surg 1:4-14, 1992.

122. Fritz LB, Oullette HA, O'Hanley TA, et al: Cystic changes at supraspinatus and infraspinatus tendon insertion sites: Association with age and rotator cuff disorders in 238 patients. Radiology 244(1):239-248, 2007.

123. Ono K, Yamamuro T, Rockwood CA Jr: Use of a thirty-degree caudal tilt radiograph in the shoulder impingement syndrome. J Shoulder Elbow Surg 1:246-252, 1992.

124. Jacobsen SR, Speer KP, Moor JT, et al: Reliability of radiographic assessment of acromial morphology. J Shoulder Elbow Surg 4:449-453, 1995.

125. Goldman AB, Ghelman B: The double contrast shoulder arthrogram. Radiology 127:655-663, 1978.

126. Hall FM, Goldberg RP, Wyshak G, et al: Shoulder arthrography: Comparison of morbidity after use of various contrast media. Radiology 154:339-341, 1985.

127. Yoh S: The value of computed tomography in the diagnosis of the rotator cuff tears, and bone and soft tissue tumors. Nippon Seikeigeka Gakkai Zasshi 58:639-658, 1984.

128. Lie S, Mast WA: Subacromial bursography. Radiology 144:626-630, 1982.

129. Mikasa M: Subacromial bursography. Nippon Seikeigeka Gakkai Zasshi 53:225-231, 1979.

130. Strizak AM, Danzig LA, Jackson DW, et al: Subacromial bursography: An anatomical and clinical study. J Bone Joint Surg Am 64:196-201, 1982.

131. Craig EV: Importance of proper radiography in acute shoulder trauma. Minn Med 68:109-112, 1985.

132. Hodler J, Fretz CJ, Terrier F, et al: Rotator cuff tears: Correlation of sonographic and surgical findings. Radiology 169:791-794, 1988.

133. Lind T, Reinmann I, Karstrup S, et al: Ultrasonography in the evaluation of injuries to the shoulder region [abstract]. Acta Orthop Scand 58:328, 1987.

134. Mack LA, Gannon MK, Kilcoyne RF, et al: Sonographic evaluation of the rotator cuff: Accuracy in patients without prior surgery. Clin Orthop Relat Res (234):21-27, 1988.

135. Middleton WD, Edelstein G, Reinus WR, et al: Ultrasonography of the rotator cuff: Technique and normal anatomy. J Ultrasound Med 3:549-551, 1984.

136. Middleton WD, Edelstein G, Reinus WR, et al: Sonographic detection of rotator cuff tears. AJR Am J Roentgenol 144:349-353, 1985.

137. Ziegler DW: The use of in-office, orthopaedist-performed ultrasound of the shoulder to evaluate and manage rotator cuff disorders. J Shoulder Elbow Surg 13:291-297, 2004.

138. Mack LA, Matsen FA III, Kilcoyne RF, et al: Ultrasonographic (US) evaluation of the rotator cuff. Radiology 157:205-209, 1985.

139. Read JW, Perko M: Shoulder ultrasound: Diagnostic accuracy for impingement syndrome, rotator cuff tear, and biceps tendon pathology. J Shoulder Elbow Surg 7:264-271, 1998.

140. Teefey SA, Hasan SA, Middleton WD, et al: Ultrasonography of the rotator cuff. A comparison of ultrasonographic and arthroscopic findings in one hundred consecutive cases. J Bone Joint Surg Am 82:498-504, 2000.

141. Zehetgruber H, Lang T, Wurnig C: Distinction between supraspinatus, infraspinatus and subscapularis tendon tears with ultrasound in 332 surgically confirmed cases. Ultrasound Med Biol 28:711-717, 2002.

142. Bretzke CA, Crass JR, Craig EV et al: Ultrasonography of the rotator cuff: Normal and pathologic anatomy. Invest Radiol 20:311-315, 1985.

143. Fery A, Lenard A: Transsternal sternoclavicular projection: Diagnostic value in sternoclavicular dislocations. J Radiol 62:167-170, 1981.

144. Kieft GJ, Bloem JL, Obermann WR, et al: Normal shoulder: MR imaging. Radiology 159:741-745, 1986.

145. Kieft GJ, Bloem JL, Rozing PM, et al: Rotator cuff im-pingement syndrome: MR imaging. Radiology 166:211-214, 1988.

146. Kneeland JB, Middleton WD, Carrera GF, et al: MR imaging of the shoulder: Diagnosis of rotator cuff tears. AJR Am J Roentgenol 149:333-337, 1987.

147. Reeder JD, Andelman S: The rotator cuff tear: MR evaluation. Magn Reson Imaging 5:331-338, 1987.

148. Reiser M, Erlemann R, Bongartz G, et al: Role of magnetic resonance imaging in the diagnosis of shoulder joint injuries. Radiologe 28:79-83, 1988.

149. Seeger LL, Gold RH, Bassett LW, Ellman H: Shoulder impingement syndrome: MR findings in 53 shoulders. AJR Am J Roentgenol 150:343-347, 1988.

150. Seeger LL, Ruszkowski JT, Bassett LW, et al: MR imaging of the normal shoulder: Anatomic correlation. AJR Am J Roentgenol 148:83-91, 1988.

151. Haywood TM, Langlotz CP, Kneeland JB, et al: Categorization of acromial shape: Interobserver variability with MR imaging and conventional radiography. AJR Am J Roentgenol 162:1377-1382, 1994.

152. Iannotti JP, Zlatkin MB, Esterhai JL, et al: Magnetic resonance imaging of the shoulder. J Bone Joint Surg Am 73:17-29, 1991.

153. Kneeland JB, Carrera GF, Middleton WD, et al: Rotator cuff tears: Preliminary application of high resolution MR imaging with counter rotating current loop-gap resonators. Radiology 160:695-699, 1986.

154. Seeger LL, Gold RH, Bassett LW: Shoulder instability: Evaluation with MR imaging. Radiology 168:695-697, 1988.

155. Hodler J, Kursunoglu-Brahme S, Snyder S, et al: Rotator cuff disease: Assessment with MR arthrography versus standard MR imaging in 36 patients with arthroscopic confirmation. Radiology 182:431-436, 1992.

156. Owen RS, Ianotti JP, Kneeland JB, et al: Shoulder after surgery: MR imaging with surgical validation. Radiology 186:443-447, 1993.

157. Jensen KL, Dickinson J, Helms C, et al: MRI, arthrography, and ultrasound in the diagnosis of rotator cuff pathology [exhibit]. AAOS Shoulder Meeting, Anaheim, California, February 1991.

158. Neumann CH, Holt RG, Steinbach LS, et al: MR imaging of the shoulder: Appearance of the supraspinatus tendon in asymptomatic volunteers. AJR Am J Roentgenol 158:1281-1287, 1992.

159. Speer KP, Paletta GA, Pavlov H, et al: Degenerative supraspinatus: A correlative investigation. Presented at AAOS Shoulder Meeting, Atlanta, Georgia, February 1996.

160. Thomazeau H, Rolland Y, Lucas C, et al: Atrophy of the supraspinatus belly. Assessment by MRI in 55 patients with rotator cuff pathology. Acta Orthop Scand 67:264-268, 1996.

161. Schaefer O, Winterer J, Lohrmann C, et al: Magnetic resonance imaging for supraspinatus muscle atrophy after cuff repair. Clin Orthop Relat Res (403):93-99, 2002.

162. Motamedi AR, Urrea LH, Hancock RE, et al: Accuracy of magnetic resonance imaging in determining the presence and size of recurrent rotator cuff tears. J Shoulder Elbow Surg 11:6-10, 2002.

163. Fisk C: Adaptation of the technique for radiography of the bicipital groove. Radiol Technol 37:47-50, 1965.

164. Merrill V (ed): Shoulder: Anteroposterior projections, posteroanterior views, glenoid fossa, Grashey position, rolled-film axial projection, Cleaves position, superoinferior axial projection, inferosuperior axial projection, Lawrence position. In Merrill V: Atlas of Roentgenographic Positions and Standard Radiologic Procedures, 4th ed. St. Louis: CV Mosby, 1975.

165. Cone RO III, Danzig L, Resnick D, et al: The bicipital groove: Radiographic, anatomic, and pathologic study. AJR Am J Roentgenol 141:781-788, 1983.

BIBLIOGRAPHY

Abel MS: Symmetrical anteroposterior projections of the sternoclavicular joints with motion studies. Radiology 132:757-759, 1979.

Adam P, Escude Alberge Y, Labbe JL, et al: Value of standard computed tomography and computed arthrography for the radiologic evaluation of injuries of the shoulder. Ann Radiol 28:629-635, 1985.

Adams JC: Recurrent dislocation of the shoulder. J Bone Joint Surg Br 30:26-38, 1948.

Alexander OM: Radiography of the acromioclavicular articulation. Med Radiogr Photogr 30:34-39, 1954.

Andren L, Lundbert BJ: Treatment of rigid shoulders by joint distension during arthrography. Acta Orthop Scand 36:45-53, 1965.

Argen RJ, Wilson CH Jr, Wood P: Suppurative arthritis: Clinical features of 42 cases. Arch Intern Med 117:661-666, 1966.

Armbuster TG, Slivka J, Resnick D, et al: Extraarticular manifestations of septic arthritis of the glenohumeral joint. AJR Am J Roentgenol 129:667-672, 1977.

Baker EC: Tomography of the sternoclavicular joint. Ohio State Med J 55:60, 1959.

Baker ME, Martinez S, Kier R, Wain S: High resolution computed tomography of the cadaveric sternoclavicular joint: Findings in degenerative joint disease. J Comput Tomogr 12:13-18, 1988.

Beardon JM, Hughston JC, Whatley GS: Acromioclavicular dislocation: Method of treatment. J Sports Med 1:5-17, 1973.

Beck A, Papacharalampous X, Grosser G, et al: Importance of transthoracic x-ray in arthrography of the shoulder. Radiology 28:69-72, 1988.

Beltran J, Gray LA, Bools JC, et al: Rotator cuff lesions of the shoulder: Evaluation by direct sagittal CT arthrography. Radiology 160:161-165, 1986.

Berman MM, LeMay M: Dislocation of shoulder: X-ray signs [letter]. N Engl J Med 283:600, 1970.

Binz P, Johner R, Haertel M: Computerized axial tomography in patients with traumatic shoulder dislocation. Helv Chir Acta 49:231-234, 1982.

Blackett CW, Healy TR: Roentgen studies of the shoulder. AJR Am J Roentgenol 37:760-766, 1937.

Blazina ME, Satzman JS: Recurrent anterior subluxation of the shoulder in athletics: Distinct entity [proceedings]. J Bone Joint Surg Am 51:1037-1038, 1969.

Blazina ME: The modified axillary roentgenogram; useful adjunct in the diagnosis of recurrent subluxation of the shoulder. Exhibit, US Military Academy, West Point, New York.

Bonavita JA, Dalinka MK: Shoulder erosions in renal osteodystrophy. Skeletal Radiol 5:105-108, 1980.

Bongartz G, Muller-Miny H, Reiser M: Role of computed tomography in the diagnosis of shoulder joint injuries. Radiologe 28:73-78, 1988.

Bongartz G, Peters PE: Problems associated with magnetic resonance imaging of the shoulder [abstract]. Z Rheumatol 47:300-301, 1988.

Bosworth BM: Complete acromioclavicular dislocations. N Engl J Med 241:221-225, 1949.

Boulis ZF, Dick R: The greater tuberosity of the humerus: An area for mis-diagnosis. Australas Radiol 26:267-268, 1982.

Brandt TD, Cardone BW, Grant TH, et al: Rotator cuff sonography: A reassessment. Radiology 173:323-327, 1989.

Brendt TL, Le Clair RG: A tangential projection or a lateral view of the scapula. Radiol Technol 52:631-634, 1986.

Brower AC, Allman RM: Pathogenesis of the neurotrophic joint: Neurotraumatic vs. neurovascular. Radiology 139:349-354, 1981.

Callaghan JJ, McNeish LM, Dehaven JP, et al: A prospective comparison study of double contrast computed tomography (CT), arthrography and arthroscopy of the shoulder. Am J Sports Med 16:13-20, 1988.

Callaghan JJ, York JJ, McNeish LM, et al: Unusual anomaly of the scapula defined by arthroscopy and computerized tomographic arthrography. J Bone Joint Surg Am 70:452-453, 1988.

Calvert PT, Packer NP, Stoker DJ, et al: Arthrography of the shoulder after operative repair of the torn rotator cuff. J Bone Joint Surg Br 68:147-150, 1986.

Castagno AA, Shuman WP, Kilcoyne RF, et al: Complex fractures of the proximal humerus: Role of CT in treatment. Radiology 165:759-762, 1987.

Cisternino SJ, Rogers LF, Stufflebam BC, Kruglik GD: The trough line: A radiographic sign of posterior shoulder dislocation. AJR Am J Roentgenol 130:951-954, 1978.

Clark KC: Positioning in Radiography, 8th ed. New York: Grune & Stratton, 1964.

Cockshott P: The coracoclavicular joint. Radiology 131:313-316, 1979.

Codman EA: The shoulder: Rupture of the Supraspinatus Tendon and Other Lesions in or About the Subacromial Bursa. Boston: Thomas Todd and Company, 1934, pp 18-31, 65-122.

Cone RO III, Resnick D, Danzig L: Shoulder impingement syndrome: Radiographic evaluation. Radiology 150:29-33, 1984.

Connolly J: X-ray defects in recurrent shoulder dislocations [proceedings]. J Bone Joint Surg Am 51:1235-1236, 1969.

Cope R, Riddervold HO: Posterior dislocation of the sternoclavicular joint: Report of two cases, with emphasis on radiologic management and early diagnosis. Skeletal Radiol 17:247-250, 1988.

Craig EV, Crass JR, Bretzke CL: Ultrasonography of the rotator cuff: Normal anatomy and pathologic variation [abstract]. Third Annual Meeting of the American Shoulder and Elbow Surgeons, Boston, November 1-4, 1984.

Crass JR, Craig EV, Thompson RG, et al: Ultrasonography of the rotator cuff: Surgical correlation. J Clin Ultrasound 12:487-492, 1984.

Crass JR, Craig EV: Noninvasive imaging of the rotator cuff. Orthopedics 11:57-64, 1988.

Cyprien JM, Vasey HM, Burdet A, et al: Humeral retrotor-sion and glenohumeral relationship in the normal shoulder and in recurrent anterior dislocation. Clin Orthop Relat Res (175):8-17, 1983.

Danzig LA, Resnick D, Greenway G: Evaluation of unstable shoulders by computed tomography. Am J Sports Med 10:138-141, 1982.

DeAnquin CE, DeAnquin CA: Comparative study of bone lesions in traumatic recurrent dislocation of the shoulder: Their importance and treatment. In DePalma AF: Surgery of the Shoulder, 3rd ed. Philadelphia: JB Lippincott, 1984, p 303.

DeAnquin CE: Recurrent dislocation of the shoulder roentgenographic study [proceedings]. J Bone Joint Surg Am 47:1085, 1965.

DeHaven JP, Callaghan JJ, McNiesh LM, et al: A prospective comparison study of double contrast CT arthrography and shoulder arthroscopy [abstract]. American Orthopedic Society of Sports Medicine, Interim Meeting, San Francisco, January 21, 1987.

De la Puente R, Boutin RD, Theodorou DJ, et al: Post-traumatic and stress-induced osteolysis of the distal clavicle: MR imaging findings in 17 patients. Skeletal Radiol 28:202-208, 1999.

DeSmet AA: Anterior oblique projection in radiography of the traumatized shoulder. AJR Am J Roentgenol 134:515-518, 1980.

DeSmet AA, Ting YM, Weiss JJ: Shoulder arthrography in rheumatoid arthritis. Radiology 116:601-605, 1975.

DeSouza LJ: Shoulder radiography in acute trauma: True anteroposterior and true lateral views make for better reading. Postgrad Med 73:234-236, 1983.

Deichgraber E, Olssen, B: Soft tissue radiography in painful shoulder. Acta Radiol Diagn 16:393-400, 1975.

Delgoffe C, Fery A, Regent D, et al: Computed tomography in anterior instability of the shoulder: A review of 23 cases. J Radiol 65:737-745, 1984.

Demos TC: Radiologic case study: Bilateral posterior shoulder dislocations. Orthopedics 3:887-897, 1980.

Ducrest P Johner R: Die Bedeutung der Ossaren Läsionen für die Prognose der Schulterluxation. Z Unfallchir Versicherungsmed Berufskr 77:85-89, 1984.

Dyson S: Interpreting radiographs. 7: Radiology of the equine shoulder and elbow. Equine Vet J 18:352-361, 1986.

Eaton R, Serletti J: Computerized axial tomography method of localizing Steinmann pin migration: A case report. Orthopedics 4:1357-1360, 1981.

El-Khoury GY, Albright JP, Yousef MM, et al: Arthrotomography of the glenoid labrum. Radiology 131:333-337, 1979.

Faletti C, Clerico P, Indemini E, et al: Standard radiography in "recurrent dislocation of the shoulder." Ital J Sports Med 7:33-40, 1985.

Fedoseev VA: Method of radiographic study of the sternoclavicular joint. Vestn Rentgenol Radiol 3:88-91, 1977.

Feldman F: The radiology of total shoulder prostheses. Semin Roentgenol 2:47-65, 1986.

Fery A, Lenard A, Sommelet J: Shoulder radiographic evaluation: Radiographic examination of shoulder and scapular girdle trauma. J Radiol 62:247-256, 1981.

Fery A, Sommelet J: Os acromiale: Diagnosis, pathology, and clinical significance. Twenty-eight cases including two fracture-separations. Rev Chir Orthop 74:160-172, 1988.

Figiel SJ, Figiel LS, Bardenstein MB, Blodgett WH: Posterior dislocation of the shoulder. Radiology 87:737-740, 1966.

Flinn RM, MacMillan CL Jr, Campbell DR, et al: Optimal radiography of the acutely injured shoulder. J Can Assoc Radiol 34:128-132, 1983.

Garneau RA, Renfrew DL, Moore TE, et al: Glenoid labrum: Evaluation with MR imaging. Radiology 179:519-522, 1991.

Ghelman G, Goldman AB: The double contrast shoulder arthrogram: Evaluation of rotary cuff tears. Radiology 124:251-254, 1979.

Glas K, Mayerhofer K, Obletter N: [Roentgenographic representation of the shoulder girdle in recurrent shoulder dislocation.] Röntgenpraxis 41:116-120, 1988.

Golding FC: Radiology and orthopaedic surgery. J Bone Joint Surg Br 48:320-332, 1966.

Golding FC: The shoulder, the forgotten joint. Br J Radiol 35:149-158, 1962.

Goldstone RA: Dislocation of the shoulder x-ray signs [letter]. N Engl J Med 283:600, 1970.

Gould R, Rosenfield AT, Friedlaender GE: Case report: Loose body within the glenohumeral joint in recurrent anterior dislocation: CT demonstration. J Comput Assist Tomogr 9:404-406, 1985.

Greenway GH, Danzig LA, Resnick D, et al: The painful shoulder. Med Radiogr Photogr 58:22-67, 1982.

Griffiths HJ, Ozer H: Changes in the medial half of the clavicle: New sign in renal osteodystrophy. J Can Assoc Radiol 24:334-336, 1973.

Gunson EF: Radiography of the sternoclavicular articulation. Radiogr Clin Photogr 19:20-24, 1943.

Gutjahr G, Weigand H: Conventional radiographic studies of the proximal humerus. Unfallchirurgie 10:282-287, 1984.

Hardy DC, Vogler JB III, White RH: The shoulder impingement syndrome: Prevalence of radiographic findings and correlation with response to therapy. AJR Am J Roentgenol 147:557-561, 1986.

Hermann G, Yeh HC, Schwartz I: Computed tomography of soft-tissue lesions of the extremities, pelvic and shoulder girdles: Sonographic and pathological correlations. Clin Radiol 35:193-202, 1984.

Hess F, Schnepper E: Success and long-term results of radiotherapy for humeroscapular periarthritis. Radiologe 28:84-86, 1988.

Hill JA, Tkach L: A study of glenohumeral orientation in patients with anterior recurrent shoulder dislocations using computerized axial tomography [abstract]. AAOS Shoulder Meeting, Las Vegas, Nev, January 1985.

Horsfield D, Renton P: The other view in the radiography of shoulder trauma. Radiography 46:213-214, 1980.

Huber DJ, Sauter R, Mueller E, et al: MR imaging of the normal shoulder. Radiology 158:405-408, 1986.

Jelbert M: A pilot study of the incidence and distribution of certain skeletal and soft tissue abnormalities. Cent Afr J Med 16:37-40, 1970.

Johner R, Binz P, Staubli HU: Diagnostic, therapeutic and prognostic aspects of shoulder dislocation. Schweiz Z Sportmed 30:48-52, 1982.

Johner R, Burch HB: Radiologische Diagnostik bei Schulterluxationen. Internationales Symposium Über Spezielle Fragen der Orthopädischen Chirurgie, 1984.

Johner R, Burch HB, Staubli HU, et al: Radiologisches Vorgehen bei der Schulterluxation. Z Unfallchir Versicherungsmed Berufskr 77:79-84, 1984.

Johner R, Ducrest P, Staubli HU, Burch HB: Begleitfrakturen und Prognose der Schulterluxation im Alter. Z Unfallchir Versicherungsmed Berufskr 76:189-193, 1983.

Johner R, Joz-Roland P, Burch HB: Anterior luxation of the shoulder: New diagnostic and therapeutic aspects. Rev Med Suisse Romande 102:1143-1150, 1982.

Jonsson G: A method of obtaining structural pictures of the sternum. Acta Radiol 18:336-340, 1937.

Kalliomäki JL, Viitanen SM, Virtama P: Radiological findings of sternoclavicular joints in rheumatoid arthritis. Acta Rheum Scand 14:233-240, 1968.

Katz SR, Peter JB, Pearson CM, et al: The shoulder-pad and diagnostic feature of amyloid arthropathy. N Engl J Med 288:354-355, 1973.

Keats TE: The emergency x-ray. Emerg Med 19:175-176, 1987.

Keats TE, Pope TL Jr: The acromioclavicular joint: Normal variation and the diagnosis of dislocation. Skeletal Radiol 17:159-162, 1988.

Khizhko II: Supplemental (axial) roentgenography of the clavicle with patient in a sitting position. Ortop Travmatol Protez 9:8-10, 1984.

Kieft GJ, Sartoris DJ, Bloem JL, et al: Magnetic resonance imaging of glenohumeral joint diseases. Skeletal Radiol 16:285-290, 1987.

Killoran PJ, Marcove RC, Freiberger RH: Shoulder arthrography. AJR Am J Roentgenol 103:658-668, 1968.

Kimberlin GE: Radiography of injuries to the region of the shoulder girdle: Revisited. Radiol Technol 46:69-83, 1974.

King JM Jr, Holmes GW: A review of four hundred and fifty roentgen-ray examinations of the shoulder. AJR Am J Roentgenol 17:214-218, 1927.

Kotzen LM: Roentgen diagnosis of rotator cuff tear: Report of 48 surgically proven cases. AJR Am J Roentgenol 112:507-511, 1971.

Kuhlman JE, Fishman ED, Ney DR, et al: Complex shoulder trauma: Three dimensional CT imaging. Orthopedics 11:1561-1563, 1988.

Lahde S, Putkonen M: Positioning of the painful patient for the axial view of the glenohumeral joint. Röntgenblätter 38:380-382, 1985.

Laing PG: The arterial supply of the adult humerus. J Bone Joint Surg Am 38:1105-1116, 1956.

Lams PM, Jolles H: The scapula companion shadow. Radiology 138:19-23, 1981.

Larde D, Benazet JP, Benameur CH, et al: Value of the transscapular view in radiology of shoulder trauma. J Radiol 62:227-282, 1981.

Larde D: Radiological exploration of the shoulder. Rev Prat 34:2957-2969, 1984.

Laumann U: Disorders of the shoulder from the orthopedic point of view. Radiologe 28:49-53, 1988.

Levine AH, Pais MJ, Schwarts EE: Posttraumatic osteolysis of the distal clavicle with emphasis on early radiologic changes. AJR Am J Roentgenol 127:781-784, 1976.

Levy M, Goldberg I, Fischel RE, et al: Friedrich's disease: Aseptic necrosis of the sternal end of the clavicle. J Bone Joint Surg Br 63:539-541, 1981.

Liberson F: Os acromiale: Contested anomaly. J Bone Joint Surg 19:683-689, 1937.

Liberson F: The value and limitation of the oblique view as compared with the ordinary anteroposterior exposure of the shoulder. AJR Am J Roentgenol 37:498-509, 1937.

Lindblom K: Arthrography and roentgenography in ruptures of the tendons of the shoulder joint. Acta Radiol 20:548-562, 1939.

Lippmann RK: Frozen shoulder; periarthritis; bicipital tenosynovitis. Arch Surg 47:283-296, 1943.

Lippmann RK: Observations concerning the calcific cuff deposit. Clin Orthop 20:49-59, 1961.

Lower RF, McNiesh LM, Callaghan JJ: Computed tomographic documentation of intraarticular penetration of a screw after operations on the shoulder. J Bone Joint Surg Am 67:1120-1122, 1985.

Lusted LB, Miller ER: Progress in indirect cineroentgenography. AJR Am J Roentgenol 75:56-62, 1956.

Macdonald W, Thrum CB, Hamilton SGL: Designing an implant by CT scanning and solid modeling. J Bone Joint Surg Br 68:208-212, 1986.

Maki NJ: Cineradiographic studies with shoulder instabilities. Am J Sports Med 16:362-364, 1988.

Matsen FA III: Shoulder roentgenography. AAOS Summer Institute, 1980.

McCauley TR, Disler DG, Tam MK: Bone marrow edema in the greater tuberosity of the humerus at MR imaging: Association with rotator cuff tears and traumatic injury. Magn Reson Imaging 18:979-984, 2000.

Metges PJ, Kleitz C, Tellier P, et al: Arthropneumotomography in recurrent dislocations and subluxations of the shoulder: Methods, results, and indications in 45 cases. J Radiol 60:789-796, 1979.

Middleton WD, Reinus WR, Melson GL, et al: Pitfalls of rotator cuff sonography. AJR Am J Roentgenol 146:555-560, 1986.

Middleton WD, Reinus WR, Totty WG, et al: Ultrasonographic evaluation of the rotator cuff and biceps tendon. J Bone Joint Surg Am 68:440-450, 1986.

Milbradt H, Rosenthal H: Sonography of the shoulder joint: Techniques, sonomorphology and diagnostic significance. Radiologe 28:61-68, 1988.

Mink JH, Richardson A, Grant TT: Evaluation of glenoid labrum by double-contrast shoulder arthrography. AJR Am J Roentgenol 133:883-887, 1979.

Neviaser JS: Adhesive capsulitis of the shoulder: A study of the pathological findings in periarthritis of the shoulder. J Bone Joint Surg 27:211-222, 1945.

Neviaser JS: Adhesive capsulitis and the stiff painful shoulder. Orthop Clin North Am 11:327-331, 1980.

Newhouse KE, El-Khoury GY, Neopola JV, et al: The shoulder impingement view: A fluoroscopic technique for the detection of subacromial spurs. AJR Am J Roentgenol 151:539-541, 1988.

Nixon JD, DiStefano V: Ruptures of the rotator cuff. Orthop Clin North Am 4:423-447, 1975.

Norman A: The use of tomography in the diagnosis of skeletal disorders. Clin Orthop Relat Res (107):139-145, 1975.

Norwood T, Terry GC: Shoulder posterior subluxation. Am J Sports Med 12:25-30, 1984.

Ogawa K: Double contrast arthrography of the shoulder joint. Nippon Seikelgeka Gakka: Zasshi 58:745-759, 1984.

Ogden JA, Conlogue GJ, Bronson ML: Radiology of postnatal skeletal development. III. The clavicle. Skeletal Radiol 4:196-203, 1979.

Ozonoff MB, Ziter FMH Jr: The upper humeral notch: A normal variant in children. Radiology 113:699-701, 1974.

Palmer WE, Brown JH, Rosenthal DI: Labral-ligamentous complex of the shoulder: Evaluation with MR arthrography. Radiology 190:645-651,1994.

Pancoast HK: Importance of careful roentgen-ray investigations of apical chest tumors. JAMA 83:1407, 1924.

Pavlov H, Freibergerger RH: Fractures and dislocations about the shoulder. Semin Roentgenol 13:85-96, 1978.

Pavlov H, Warren RF, Weiss CB Jr, et al: The roentgenographic evaluation of anterior shoulder instability. Clin Orthop Relat Res (194):153-158, 1985.

Pear BL: Bilateral posterior fracture dislocation of the shoulder: An uncommon complication of a convulsive seizure. N Engl J Med 283:135-136, 1970.

Pear BL: Dislocation of the shoulder: X-ray signs [letter]. N Engl J Med 283:1113, 1970.

Percy EC, Birbrager D, Pitt MJ: Snapping scapula: A review of the literature and presentation of 14 patients. Can J Surg 31:248-250, 1988.

Petersson CJ, Redlund-Johnell I: The subacromial space in normal shoulder radiographs. Acta Orthop Scand 55:57-58, 1984.

Preston BJ, Jackson JP: Investigation of shoulder disability by arthrography. Clin Radiol 28:259-266, 1977.

Putkonen M, Lahde S, Puranan J, et al: The value of axial view in the radiography of shoulder girdle: Experiences with a new modification of positioning. Röntgenblätter 41:158-162, 1988.

Quesada F: Technique for the roentgen diagnosis of fractures of the clavicle. Surg Gynecol Obstet 42:424-428, 1926.

Rapf CH, Furtschegger A, Resch H: Sonography as a new diagnostic procedure for investigating abnormalities of the shoulder. Fortschr Geb Rontgenstr Nuklearmed Erganzungsband 145:288-295, 1986.

Reichmann S, Astrand K, Deichgraber E, et al: Soft tissue xeroradiography of the shoulder joint. Acta Radiol Diagn 16:572-576, 1975.

Resnick D: Shoulder arthrography. Radiol Clin North Am 19:243-253, 1981.

Resnick CS, Deutsch AL, Resnick D, et al: Arthrotomography of the shoulder. Radiographics 4:963-976, 1984.

Resnick D, Niwayama G: Anatomy of individual joints. In Resnick D, Niwayama G (eds): Diagnosis of Bone and Joint Disorders, vol 1. Philadelphia: WB Saunders, 1981, pp 69-77.

Resnick D, Niwayama G: Resorption of the undersurface of the distal clavicle in rheumatoid arthritis. Radiology 120:75-77, 1976.

Resnick D, Niwayama G (eds): Diagnosis of Bone and Joint Disorders, 2nd ed. Philadelphia: WB Saunders, 1988.

Rosen PS: A unique shoulder lesion in ankylosing spondylitis: Clinical comment [letter]. J Rheumatol 7:109-110, 1980.

Rosenthal H, Galanski M: Positioning in plain film radiography of the shoulder. Radiologe 28:54-60, 1988.

Rothman RH, Marvel JP Jr, Heppenstall RB: Anatomic considerations in the glenohumeral joint. Orthop Clin North Am 6:341-352, 1975.

Rubin SA, Gray RL, Green WR: The scapular Y: A diagnostic aid in shoulder trauma. Radiology 110:725-726, 1974.

Russell AR (ed): Medical Radiography and Photography, vol 58. Rochester, NY: Eastman Kodak Company, 1982.

Sackellares JC, Swift TR: Shoulder enlargement as the presenting sign in syringomyelia: report of two cases and review of the literature. JAMA 236:2878-2879, 1976.

Saha AK: Dynamic stability of the glenohumeral joint. Acta Orthop Scand 42:491-505, 1971.

Sante LR: Manual of Roentgenological Technique, 9th ed. Ann Arbor, Mich: Edwards Brothers, 1942, pp 160-161.

Schweitzer ME, Magbalon MJ, Frieman BG, et al: Acromioclavicular joint fluid: Determination of clinical significance with MR imaging. Radiology. 192:205-207,1994.

Schweitzer ME, Magbalon MJ, Fenlin JM, et al: Effusion criteria and clinical importance of glenohumeral joint fluid: MR imaging evaluation. Radiology 194:821-824,1995.

Seymour EQ: Osteolysis of the clavicular tip associated with repetitive minor trauma to the shoulder. Radiology 123:56, 1977.

Shai G, Ring H, Costeff H, Solzi P: Glenohumeral malalignment in the hemiplegic shoulder: An early radiologic sign. Scand J Rehabil Med 16:133-136, 1984.

Shenton AF: The modified axial view: An alternative radiograph in shoulder injuries [letter]. Arch Emerg Med 4:201-203, 1987.

Singson RD, Feldman F, Bigliani LU, et al: Recurrent shoulder dislocation after surgical repair: Double-contrast CT arthrography: Work in progress. Radiology 164:425-428, 1987.

Slivka J, Resnick D: An improved radiographic view of the glenohumeral joint. J Can Assoc Radiol 30:83-85, 1979.

Stodell MA, Nicholson R, Scott J, Sturrock RD: Radioisotope scanning in the painful shoulder. Rheumatol Rehabil 19:163-166, 1980.

Tijmes J, Lloyd H, Tullos HS: Arthrography in acute shoulder dislocations. South Med J 72:564-567, 1979.

Treble NJ: Normal variations in radiographs of the clavicle: Brief report. J Bone Joint Surg Br 70:490, 1988.

Uhthoff HK, Hammond DI, Sarkar K, et al: The role of the coracoacromial ligament in the impingement syndrome: A clinical, radiological, and histological study. Int Orthop 12:97-104, 1988.

Usselman JA, Vint VC, Waltz TA: CT demonstration of a brachial plexus neuroma. AJNR Am J Neuroradiol 1:346-347, 1980.

ViGario GD, Keats TE: Localization of calcific deposits in the shoulder. AJR Am J Roentgenol 108:806-811, 1970.

Wallace WA, Johnson F: Dynamic radiography in shoulder kinematics: Problems and their solutions [proceedings]. J Bone Joint Surg Br 62:256, 1980.

Weston WJ: Arthrography of the acromio-clavicular joint. Australas Radiol 18:213-214, 1974.

Widner LA, Riddervold HO: The value of the lordotic view in diagnosis of fractures of the clavicle (a technical note). Rev Interam Radiol 5:69-70, 1980.

Wiener SN, Seitz JR: Sonography of the shoulder in pa-tients with tears of the rotator cuff: Accuracy and value for selecting surgical options. AJR Am J Roentgenol 160:103-107, 1993.

Woolson ST, Fellingham LL, Vassiliadis PDA: Three dimensional images of the elbow and shoulder from computerized tomography data [abstract]. AAOS Shoulder Meeting, Las Vegas, Nev, January 1985.

Wright T, Yoon C, Schmit BP: Shoulder MRI refinements: Differentiation of rotator cuff tear from artifacts and tendinosis, and reassessment of normal findings. Semin Ultrasound CT MRI 22(4):383-395, 2001.

Yang SO, Cho KJ, Kim MJ, Ro IW: Assessment of anterior shoulder instability by CT arthrography. J Korean Med Sci 2:167-171, 1987.

Yu YS, Dardani M, Fischer RA: MR observations of postraumatic osteolysis of the distal clavicle after traumatic separation of the acromioclavicular joint. J Comput Assist Tomogr 24(1):159-164, 2000.

Zachrisson BE, Ejeskar A: Arthrography in dislocation of the acromioclavicular joint. Acta Radiol 20:81-87, 1979.

Zanca P: Shoulder pain: Involvement of the acromioclavicular joint: Analysis of 1000 cases. AJR Am J Roentgenol 112:493-506, 1971.

Zeiger M, Dorr U, Schulz RD: Sonography of slipped humeral epiphysis due to birth injury. Pediatr Radiol 17:425-426, 1987.

Ziegler R: X-ray examination of the shoulder in suspected luxation. Z Orthop 119:31-35, 1981.

Zlatkin MB, Bjorkengren AG, Gylys-Morin V, et al: Cross-sectional imaging of the capsular mechanism of the glenohumeral joint. AJR Am J Roentgenol 150:151-158, 1988.

Biomechanics of the Shoulder

Eiji Itoi, MD, PhD, Bernard F. Morrey, MD, and Kai-Nan An, PhD

Because of its component parts, a description of the biomechanics of the shoulder complex is rather involved. To make the subject at once comprehensive and relevant to the clinician, the structure and function of the sternoclavicular and acromioclavicular joints are dealt with first. The anatomy and biomechanics of the glenohumeral joint are then discussed in three parts according to an outline familiar to clinicians: motion, constraints, and forces across the joint (Table 6-1). By way of classification, we have adopted the increasingly accepted phrase of *arm elevation* rather than abduction or flexion, when possible. Although this organization is somewhat arbitrary and has some overlap, it does allow a reasonably simple and logical approach to understanding the entire shoulder complex.

SHOULDER COMPLEX

The function of the shoulder girdle requires the integrated motion of the sternoclavicular, acromioclavicular, glenohumeral, and scapulothoracic joints. This motion is created by the delicate interaction of almost 30 muscles that control the total system complex. Discussion of the biomechanics of this complex focuses first on the sternoclavicular and acromioclavicular joints and then on the glenohumeral and scapulothoracic joints.

Sternoclavicular Joint

According to Dempster, six actions occur at the sternoclavicular joint: elevation, depression, protrusion, retraction, and upward and downward rotation.[1] The amount of potential motion present at this articulation has been studied by disarticulating the scapula. Anteroposterior rotation exceeds superoinferior motion by about 2:1.[2] In an intact and functioning extremity, the actual amount of

displacement is of course limited by the attachment to the scapula; this motion is described later. At the extremes, motion is limited by tension developed in the ligamentous complex on the opposite side of the joint. This constraint occurs in concert with increased contact pressure at the articulation and the intra-articular disk ligament (Fig. 6-1). Approximately 35 degrees of upward rotation occurs at the sternoclavicular joint.[3,4] A similar 35 degrees of anterior and posterior rotation and up to 45 to 50 degrees of axial rotation also occur at this joint.

Anterior displacement of the distal end of the clavicle is not affected by release of the interclavicular or costoclavicular ligaments or by the intra-articular disk.[5] Release of the capsular ligament is followed by downward displacement of the lateral aspect of the clavicle.

Inferior displacement of the clavicle at the sternum is resisted by articular contact at the inferior aspect of the joint and by tautness developed in the interclavicular ligament and the posterior expansion of the capsular ligament.[1] Superior translation of the joint is resisted by tension developed in the entire costoclavicular complex. Little, if any, articular constraint assists in resisting this displacement.

Protrusion or anterior displacement of the clavicle is resisted not only by the anterior capsule but also by the posterior portion of the interclavicular ligament and the posterior sternoclavicular ligament. Conversely, posterior displacement or retraction of the medial aspect of the clavicle generates tension in the anterior portion of the inferior capsular ligaments and in the anterior sternoclavicular ligament, as well as in the anterior portion of the costoclavicular ligament. Only a limited amount of articular contact resists such displacement; this contact is on the posterior vertical ridge of the sternal articulation and the posterior portion of the clavicle. Spencer and colleagues demonstrated that the posterior capsule was the most important stabilizer for both the anterior and posterior translations of the medial end of the clavicle, whereas the anterior capsule was also important for anterior translation.[6] According to them, the costoclavicular and interclavicular ligaments had little effect on the anterior-to-posterior stability of this joint.

Clavicular rotation causes twisting of the capsular ligaments. Only about 10 degrees of downward (forward) rotation occurs before the ligaments become taut and limit further motion. With upward (backward) rotation of the clavicle, up to 45 degrees of rotation occurs before the entire complex again becomes taut and resists further rotatory displacement.[7] Both these actions increase compression across the sternoclavicular joint. The costoclavicular ligament is thought to be the most important single constraint in limiting motion at this joint.[8]

TABLE 6-1 Relationship of Joint Function and Biomechanical Measurements	
Clinical Function	**Biomechanical Description**
Motion	Kinematics
Stability	Constraints
Strength	Force transmission

Acromioclavicular Joint

Motion and Constraint

The amount of possible acromioclavicular motion that is independent of the sternoclavicular link has been found to be limited by the complex arrangement of the coracoclavicular and acromioclavicular ligaments. According to most investigators, rotation of the acromioclavicular joint takes place about three axes.[1,3,8,9] These motions are variously described but can simply be termed *anteroposterior rotation* of the clavicle on the scapula, *superoinferior rotation*, and *anterior (inferior) and posterior (superior) axial rotation*. Of these three, anteroposterior rotation of the clavicle with respect to the acromion is approximately three times as great as superoinferior rotation of an intact specimen.[10] Sahara and colleagues quantified anterior-to-posterior and superior-to-inferior translations of the distal end of the clavicle on the acromion using open MRI. They reported that the distal end of the clavicle translated most posteriorly (average 1.9 mm) at 90 degrees of abduction and most anteriorly (average 1.6 mm) at maximum abduction. The superior-to-inferior translation was much smaller, with the distal end of the clavicle shifted slightly superiorly (average 0.9 mm) during arm elevation.

Regarding the constraints of the acromioclavicular joint, Dempster noted that the conoid and trapezoid became taut with anteroposterior scapular rotation, thus serving as the constraint of this motion.[1] In a subsequent study by Fukuda and coworkers, however, the acromioclavicu-

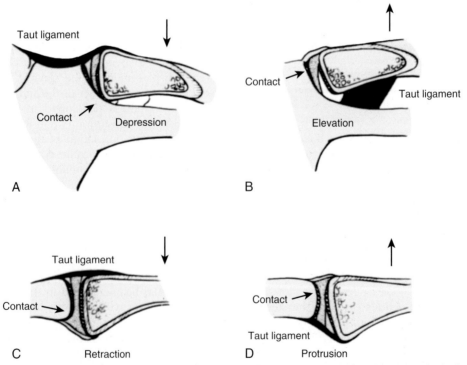

FIGURE 6-1 Superior (**A**), inferior (**B**), anterior (**C**), and posterior (**D**) ligaments stabilize the sternoclavicular joint by enhancing the contact force at certain joint positions. (Redrawn from Dempster WT: Mechanisms of shoulder movement. Arch Phys Med Rehabil 46A:49-70, 1965.)

lar ligament was noted to be taut in its anterior component with posterior rotation and taught in its posterior component with anterior rotation.[9] Anterior rotation of the clavicle with regard to the scapula was also found to cause some tightness in the conoid and trapezoid ligaments, but this tightness was of a magnitude approximately equal to the stretch observed in the posterior acromioclavicular ligament. Thus, the limiting factor to this motion is the posterior component of the acromioclavicular ligament. On the other hand, posterior rotation of the clavicle is restrained only by the anterior fibers of the acromioclavicular ligament, with virtually no contribution from the other structures.

Superoinferior rotation of the clavicle is quite limited at the acromioclavicular joint. Both Dempster and Kapandji noted virtually no ligamentous contribution to resisting inferior displacement (Fig. 6-2).[1,8] However, superior rotation of the clavicle with respect to the acromion is limited primarily by the medial aspect of the conoid ligament, with subsequent tightening of the lateral portion of this structure (Fig. 6-3). The trapezoid provides approximately the same degree of constraint as do the anterior and posterior portions of the acromioclavicular ligament complex. Once again, the magnitude of this displacement is not reported by either investigator but is said to be limited.

Anterior and posterior axial rotation (inferior to superior) was reported by Dempster to be about 60 degrees in cadaveric shoulders without the thorax.[1] In live shoulders, Rockwood and Green demonstrated only 5 to 8 degrees of motion at the acromioclavicular joint using two Kirschner wires inserted into the acromion and the clavicle.[7] According to the recent three-dimensional kinematic analysis using open MRI, Sahara and colleagues demonstrated in volunteer shoulders that the anterior axial rotation of the clavicle at the acromioclavicular joint increased linearly with abduction and reached 35 degrees on average at maximum abduction of the arm.[11]

Both anterior and posterior axial rotations are limited by the conoid ligament. Posterior axial rotation is accompanied by tightening of the trapezoid ligament, with some contribution from the medial and anterior conoid as well as from the acromioclavicular ligament complex.[9] Dempster, however, indicates that the acromioclavicular ligament is taut in the extreme of anterior and posterior axial rotation and is a limiting factor of this motion.[1] Fukuda and colleagues have quantified the displacement as a function of the ligamentous constraints.[9] Slight displacement is limited by the acromioclavicular ligament, but large displacements are resisted by the coracoclavicular ligaments (Fig. 6-4).

Relative contributions of the individual capsular ligaments (anterior, posterior, superior, and inferior) were studied by Klimkiewicz and colleagues, who demonstrated that the superior and posterior acromioclavicular ligaments were the most important contributors to the acromioclavicular restraint against posterior translation of the distal end of the clavicle (56% and 25%, respectively).[12]

Debski and coworkers also investigated the capsular contribution to stability of the acromioclavicular joint. When the capsule was released, significant anterior-to-posterior instability was observed but not superior-to-inferior instability.[13] Capsular release increased loading

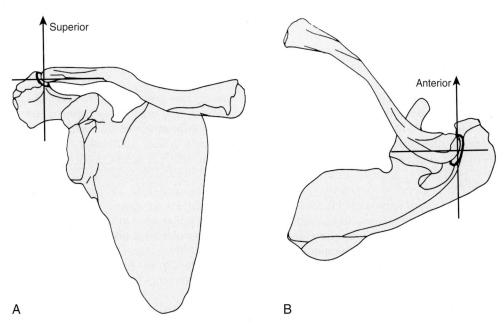

FIGURE 6-2 Superior orientation (**A**) and anterior orientation (**B**) of the acromioclavicular joint. It is considered a plane type of joint.

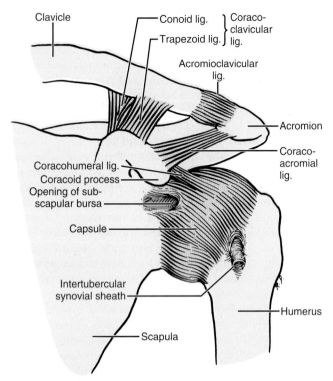

FIGURE 6-3 The coracoclavicular ligament complex consists of the larger and heavier trapezoid ligament, which is oriented laterally, and the smaller conoid ligament, which is situated more medially. (Modified from Hollinshead WH: Anatomy for Surgeons, vol 3. New York: Harper & Row, 1969.)

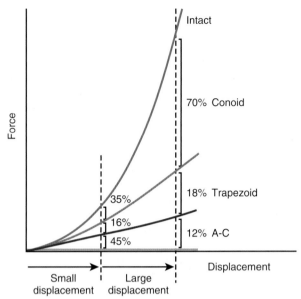

FIGURE 6-4 All displacements are resisted by the force generated in the acromioclavicular ligament, and large displacements are also resisted by the conoid and trapezoid structures. A-C, acromioclavicular. (Redrawn from Fukuda K, Craig EV, An K-N, et al: Biomechanical study of the ligamentous system of the acromioclavicular joint. J Bone Joint Surg Am 68:434-440, 1986.)

on the coracoclavicular ligaments: Anterior load increased tension in the conoid ligament, and posterior load increased tension in the trapezoid ligament. Thus, the trapezoid and conoid ligaments have different functions.

Motion of the Clavicle

The potential motion present at the sternoclavicular and acromioclavicular joints exceeds that actually attained during active motion of the shoulder complex. Current data indicate that accurate demonstration of the phasic three-dimensional motion of the sternoclavicular and acromioclavicular joints that occurs with arm elevation is a complex problem.[14] During elevation of the extremity, clavicular elevation of about 30 degrees occurs, with the maximum at about 130 degrees of elevation (Fig. 6-5).[3] The clavicle also rotates forward approximately 10 degrees during the first 40 degrees of elevation. No change takes place during the next 90 degrees of elevation, but an additional 15 to 20 degrees of forward rotation subsequently occurs during the terminal arc. Forward elevation (flexion) demonstrates virtually an identical pattern of clavicular motion.

Axial rotation of the clavicle is reported by Inman and coworkers to be an essential and fundamental feature of shoulder motion, particularly arm elevation (Fig. 6-6). If the clavicle is not allowed to rotate, elevation of only about 110 degrees is said to be possible.[3] Superior (posterior) rotation of the clavicle begins after the arm has attained an arc of about 90 degrees of elevation and then progresses in a rather linear fashion, with approximately 40 degrees of rotation attained at full elevation (see Fig. 6-6).[3] These findings have been challenged by Rockwood and Green. Placement of pins in the clavicle and acromion shows less than 10 degrees of rotation with full arm elevation.[7] This discrepancy suggests that more than 30 degrees of axial rotation occurs at the sternoclavicular joint.

Sahara and coworkers, in contrast, reported that 35 degrees of axial rotation occurred at the acromioclavicular joint, indicating that less rotation occurred at the sternoclavicular joint.[11] Clinically, fixation of the clavicle to the coracoid by a screw does not greatly limit shoulder elevation and ankylosis caused by ectopic bone also causes minimal loss of arm elevation (Fig. 6-7). The patient shown in Figure 6-7 could elevate his arm to about 160 degrees. On the other hand, ankylosis of the sternoclavicular joint allows only 90 degrees of shoulder elevation.[7] Thus, loss of motion at the acromioclavicular joint appears to be better tolerated than loss of motion at the sternoclavicular joint.

Clinical Relevance

Acromioclavicular instability is one of the most important and controversial topics clinically relevant to the shoul-

FIGURE 6-5 Clavicular elevation during abduction and forward flexion of the arm. (Redrawn from Inman VT, Saunders JR, Abbott LC: Observations on the function of the shoulder joint. J Bone Joint Surg 26:1-30, 1944.)

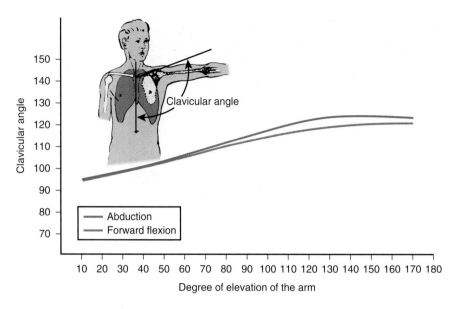

der. The acromioclavicular capsular ligament complex is the primary constraint for small rotational displacements at this joint. Downward force applied to the end of the scapula causes inferior displacement of the acromion (grade III injury) and thus violates the constraint provided by the conoid and trapezoid ligaments. Lesser degrees of ligamentous disruption, such as occur with grade I or II acromioclavicular sprains, demonstrate minimal or no inferior migration of the acromion. Biomechanical data have explained this finding by showing that the conoid ligament must be intact to prevent even slight displacement.

Resection of the distal clavicle is commonly performed in patients with osteoarthritis of the acromioclavicular joint. Debski and colleagues reported that acromioplasty did not affect kinematics of this joint, but acromioplasty together with distal clavicle resection increased posterior translation by 30% during posterior loading and increased the in situ force in the trapezoid and conoid ligaments almost three times greater than in the intact shoulder during anterior loading.[15] Corteen and Teitge also reported that resection of the distal clavicle increased

posterior translation by 32%.[16] Reconstruction using the coracoacromial ligament significantly stabilized the acromioclavicular joint. Thus, the significant effect of distal clavicle resection on motion and ligament forces should be taken into consideration when this procedure is to be used.

GLENOHUMERAL AND SCAPULOTHORACIC JOINT MOTION

The motion of the shoulder complex is probably greater than that of any other joint in the body. The arm can move through an angle of approximately 0 to 180 degrees in elevation, internal and external rotation of approximately 150 degrees is possible, and flexion and extension—or anterior and posterior rotation in the horizontal plane—is approximately 170 degrees.[17] This motion, which represents the composite motion of several joints, occurs primarily in the glenohumeral and scapulothoracic joints; extreme positions require rotation at the sternoclavicular and acromioclavicular joints.

FIGURE 6-6 Axial rotation of the clavicle during arm elevation. (Redrawn from Inman VT, Saunders JR, Abbott LC: Observations on the function of the shoulder joint. J Bone Joint Surg 26:1-30, 1944.)

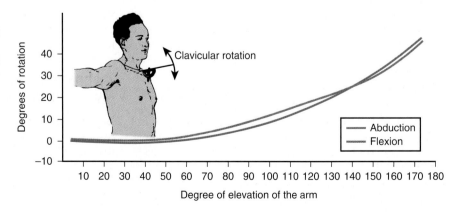

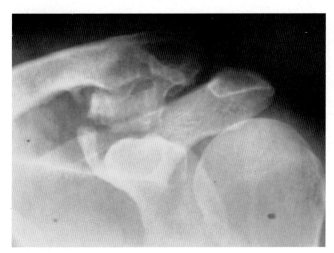

FIGURE 6-7 Extensive ectopic ossification of the coracoclavicular ligaments. By limiting clavicular motion, only a small portion of the full range of motion of the shoulder complex is limited.

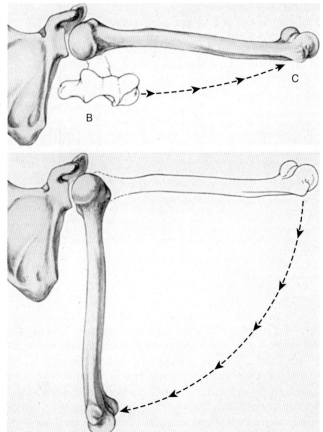

FIGURE 6-8 Codman's paradox. *Top,* The humerus is flexed to a right angle *(B)* and swung backward to the plane of the scapula *(C). Bottom,* It is then brought back to the vertical. An axial rotation position change has occurred without actual axial rotation taking place. (From Johnston TB: The movements of the shoulder joint. A plea for the use of the "plane of the scapula" as the plane of reference for movements occurring at the humero-scapular joint. Br J Surg 25:252-260, 1937.)

Motion of the shoulder complex has been a topic of concern and controversy for more than 100 years. Reasons for this debate are numerous and include imperfect devices or means of measurement because the soft tissue envelope makes it difficult to actually observe the skeletal motion, confusion with respect to terminology, inconsistency in defining the reference system, and an early lack of understanding of the concept of sequence-dependent serial rotation. Early investigations focused on arm motion about the sagittal, coronal, and transverse planes. However, because the sequence-dependent nature of rotation about orthogonal axes was not appreciated, years of debate and discussion centered on understanding and explaining Codman's paradox.

Codman's Paradox

Codman's paradox may be demonstrated easily (Fig. 6-8). From the resting position in the anatomic posture with the medial epicondyle pointing toward the midline of the body, the arm is brought forward to 90 degrees of flexion and abducted 90 degrees. The epicondyle is now pointing perpendicular to the coronal plane. The arm is then brought back to the side to its apparent initial position, but the medial epicondyle is now observed to be rotated anteriorly away from the body instead of medially toward the midline of the body. The humerus, however, was never axially rotated.[18]

The difficulty in understanding this phenomenon has prompted numerous discussions.[18-21] The simplest explanation is that serial angular rotations are not additive but are sequence dependent, which means that 90 degrees of rotation about the z-axis and then the x-axis results in a different final position than does rotation about the x-axis and then the z-axis (Fig. 6-9). Multiple rotations about orthogonal axes must therefore be defined by the sequence of the rotation. In aerospace terms, these rotations are called the *Eulerian angles:* yaw, pitch, and roll.

The confusion is significantly resolved by the use of two reference systems. First, scapular motion is best defined in reference to the classic anatomic system of the trunk. Second, humeral motion is described in reference to the scapula. This issue is discussed in detail later.

Techniques to Observe and Describe Motion of the Shoulder Complex

Because of the complexity of this issue and the conflicting results, it is appropriate to describe various techniques that have been used to measure upper extremity motion. Methods of observing and describing motion of the upper extremities may be broadly categorized into research and clinical effort.

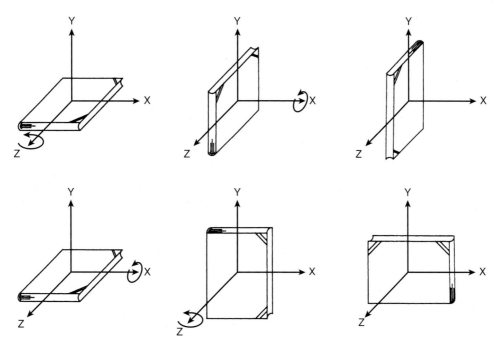

FIGURE 6-9 Final orientation depends on the sequence of serial rotations around the orthogonal axes.

The early research effort to describe shoulder joint (complex) motion consisted of simple (but careful) observation of cadaveric material and thus often included observation of the ligamentous constraints.[18,22-24] A gross description of motion and displacement has proved to be accurate even today because of the careful nature of these early observations. With the advent of the roentgenogram, uniplanar[25] and biplanar cineradiographic studies are the more common techniques used today for active and passive investigations. These techniques are particularly attractive because they can be used in vivo. By implanting metal markers, very accurate three-dimensional rotation may be measured from these radiographs.[26] With the advent of computer data manipulation, replication of motion by using a complex system involving an interactive microcomputer for analyzing images with real-time graphic display has been developed. This method and other modeling techniques are much too complex for routine use but can serve as valuable research tools.[27,28]

Clinical measurement techniques include simple and complex goniometers. Doody and associates designed a goniometer to be used in vivo that measures glenohumeral and scapulothoracic motion simultaneously.[24,29] Electrogoniometers have not been of routine clinical value but have been used extensively for basic science investigations. Unfortunately, the anatomy constraints at the shoulder limit the value of electrogoniometers. A stereometric method has also been used for three-dimensional kinematic analysis. Basically, when three non-colinear points fixed to a rigid body are defined within an inertial reference frame, the position and orientation of that rigid body can be specified and the rela-

tive rotation and translation occurring at a joint can be determined. Numerous commercial systems using light-emitting diodes, reflecting dots, and ultrasonic transducer techniques are available for such an application.

Aerospace technology has provided a device that uses three mutually orthogonal magnetic fields[30]; it has proved useful as both a research and a clinical tool. This instrument has been applied to in vivo and in vitro studies and measures simultaneous three-dimensional rotational motion.[31,32] In addition, translation displacement has also been calculated, thus allowing determination of the screw axis, which defines the complete displacement characteristics of the system.

More recently, Sahara and colleagues used magnetic resonance images to measure three-dimensional kinematics of the glenohumeral joint.[33] Magnetic resonance images were obtained with volunteers in a seated position and in seven static positions of the arm from 0 degrees to maximum abduction using vertically open magnetic resonance imaging. Three-dimensional surface models were created and three-dimensional movements of each bone in the glenohumeral joint were calculated using a computer algorithm. This is a noninvasive method, and in vivo kinematics of the bony structures can be precisely measured.

Description of Joint Motion

The aforementioned techniques permit joint motion to be described with varying degrees of sophistication. In general, joint kinematics may be divided into two-dimensional planar motion and three-dimensional spatial motion. With planar motion, the moving segment both

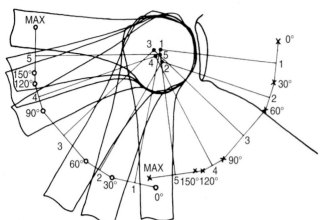

FIGURE 6-10 Measurement of the center of rotation of the humeral head as defined by the Rouleaux technique. MAX, maximum. (From Walker PS: Human Joints and Their Artificial Replacements. Springfield, Ill: Charles C Thomas, 1977.)

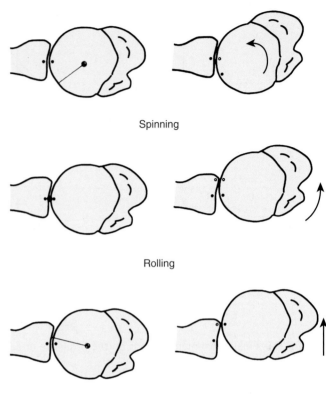

FIGURE 6-11 All three types of motion (spinning, rolling, and sliding) occur at the glenohumeral articulation.

translates and rotates around the fixed segment. A more distinctive description of planar motion, however, can be based on rotation around a point or axis, which is defined as the instantaneous center of rotation (ICR). Theoretically, the ICR could be determined accurately if the velocities of points on the rigid body are measurable. In practice, an alternative technique based on the method of Rouleaux is commonly adopted. In this method, the instantaneous locations of two points on the moving segment are identified from two consecutive positions within a short period of time, and the intersection of the bisectors of the lines joining the same points at the two positions defines the ICR (Fig. 6-10).

Occasionally it is useful to describe the planar joint articulating motion.[34] For general planar or gliding motion of the articular surface, the terms *sliding, spinning,* and *rolling* are commonly used (Fig. 6-11).

Sliding motion is defined as pure translation of a moving segment against the surface of a fixed segment. The contact point of the moving segment does not change, but its mating surface has a constantly changing contact point. If the surface of the fixed segment is flat, the ICR is located at infinity; otherwise, it is at the center of the curvature of the fixed surface.

Spinning motion is the exact opposite of sliding motion; the moving segment rotates and the contact point on the fixed surface does not change. The ICR, in this case, is located at the center of curvature of the spinning body that is undergoing pure rotation.

Rolling motion is motion between moving and fixed segments in which the contact points on each surface are constantly changing. However, the arc length of the moving surface matches the path on the fixed surface so that the two surfaces have point-to-point contact without slippage. The relative motion of rolling is a combination of translation and rotation. The ICR is located at the contact point.

Most planar articulating motion can be described by using a combination of any two of these three basic types of motion.

Three-Dimensional Glenohumeral Joint Motion

Three-dimensional analysis of motion of a rigid body requires three linear and three angular coordinates to specify the location and orientation of a rigid body in space. In other words, any rigid body with unconstrained motion has six degrees of freedom in space. Numerous methods are available to describe spatial rigid body motion, two of the most commonly used of which are description of the Eulerian angle and the screw displacement axis.

If the glenohumeral joint is stable and the motion can be assumed to be that of a ball-and-socket joint, it is sufficient to consider only rotation of the joint and neglect small amounts of translation. In this case, description of three-dimensional rotation by using the Eulerian angle system is most appropriate (Fig. 6-12). It should be remembered, as emphasized earlier, that general three-dimensional rotation is sequence dependent. In other words, with the same specified amount of rotation around

1–3'–1" ROTATION SEQUENCE
[LEFT SHOULDER (PA VIEW)]

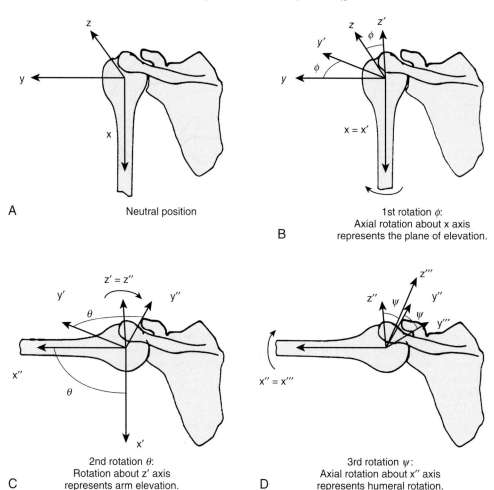

A Neutral position

B 1st rotation ϕ:
Axial rotation about x axis
represents the plane of elevation.

C 2nd rotation θ:
Rotation about z' axis
represents arm elevation.

D 3rd rotation ψ:
Axial rotation about x" axis
represents humeral rotation.

FIGURE 6-12 Three-dimensional rotation around each of the orthogonal axes is most accurately described by using the Eulerian angle system. Glenohumeral motion is defined by the sequence-dependent Eulerian angles. PA, posteroanterior.

three axes, the final result will be different if the sequence of the axes of rotation is different, which is one of the explanations for Codman's paradox.

With the arm hanging at the side of the body, the z-axis is defined to be perpendicular to the scapular plane. The y-axis points out laterally and the x-axis points distally along the humeral shaft axis. The rotational sequence for the Eulerian description of glenohumeral joint rotation or the orientation of the humerus relative to the scapula is as follows: First rotate the humerus around the x-axis by an amount f to define the plane of elevation. Then rotate the arm around the rotated z (z')-axis by an amount q to define the arm elevation. Finally, axial rotation of the humerus around the rotated x (x")-axis by an amount ψ completes the process.

During circumduction motion of the humerus, for example, the corresponding Eulerian angle could be measured as shown in Figure 6-12. This description could be used clinically to describe the range of joint motion as well as the specification of joint position at which any abnormality or pathologic process should be documented.

In instances in which a more general description of glenohumeral joint displacement is required, the screw displacement axis (SDA) description is most appropriate. The rotation and translation components of displacement of the humerus relative to the glenoid or scapula are defined by rotation around and translation along a unique *screw axis* (Fig. 6-13). In addition to incorporating a description of translation, the advantage of using the SDA method is that the orientation of the SDA remains invariant regardless of the reference coordinate axes used. The SDA can be determined experimentally with various methods. With a rotational matrix describing the orientation and a positional vector from a reference point known for the rigid body, the SDA can be calculated.[35] If the coordinates of at least three reference points on the rigid body are measured, the SDA can also be calculated.[36]

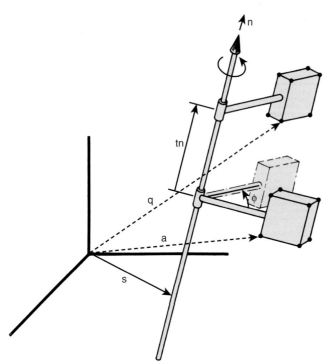

FIGURE 6-13 Both rotational (ϕ) and translational (*tn*) components of displacement of a rigid body may be expressed by the concept of the screw axis (*n*), which represents the shortest path from position *a* to position *q* around or along which the displacement can be described. s, shortest distance from the center of coordinate system to the screw axis.

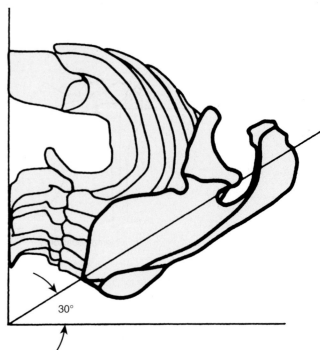

FIGURE 6-14 The resting position of the scapula is about 30 degrees forward with respect to the coronal plane as viewed in the transverse plane.

SHOULDER MOTION

Resting Posture

Scapula

The resting position of the scapula relative to the trunk is anteriorly rotated about 30 degrees with respect to the frontal plane as viewed from above (Fig. 6-14). The scapula is also rotated upward about 3 degrees with respect to the sagittal plane as viewed from the back (Fig. 6-15).[17,37] Finally, it is tilted forward (anteflexed) about 20 degrees with respect to the frontal plane when viewed from the side.[14] This posture of the scapula is not influenced by an external load (up to 20 kg) applied to the extremity.[14]

McClure and colleagues measured the three-dimensional kinematics of the scapula during dynamic movement of the shoulder. A three-dimensional motion sensor was firmly fixed to the scapula with a Kirschner wire.[38] During arm elevation in the scapular plane, the scapula upwardly rotated (average of 50 degrees), tilted posteriorly around a medial-lateral axis (30 degrees), and externally rotated around a vertical axis (24 degrees). Lowering of the arm resulted in reversal of these motions in a slightly different pattern. The mean ratio of gleno-

humeral to scapulothoracic motion was 1.7:1. The researchers concluded that normal scapular motion consists of substantial rotation around three axes, not simply upward rotation. Using the same method, Bourne and colleagues reported similar results.[39]

Fung and associates measured scapular and clavicular kinematics during passive humeral motion.[40] Scapular and clavicular rotation was relatively small until the humerus reached approximately 90 degrees of elevation. The glenohumeral-to-scapulothoracic ratio was approximately 2 for the entire range of elevation for each elevation plane, but it was dramatically larger during early elevation than during late elevation.

Humerus

The humeral head rests in the center of the glenoid when viewed in the plane of the glenoid surface.[18,41] Fick referred to this relationship as *Nullmeridianebene*, or dead meridian plane.[41] The humeral head and shaft are thought to lie in the plane of the scapula. The 30-degree retroversion of the articular orientation is complemented by the 30-degree anterior rotation of the scapula on the trunk.

Articular Surface and Orientation

Humerus

The articular surface of the humerus constitutes approximately one third the surface of a sphere with an arc of about 120 degrees. This articular surface is oriented with

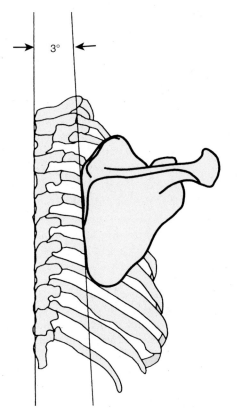

FIGURE 6-15 The resting position of the scapula is rotated about 3 degrees superior as viewed in the frontal plane.

an upward tilt of approximately 45 degrees and is retroverted approximately 30 degrees with respect to the condylar line of the distal end of the humerus (Fig. 6-16).[1,17,41,42] Retroversion of the humerus is much greater in children.[43] The average retroversion is 65 degrees

between 4 months and 4 years of age and 38 degrees between 10 and 12 years of age. Most of the derotation process takes place by the age of 8 years, with the remainder developing gradually until adulthood. This derotation process seems to be restricted in young throwing athletes,[44] resulting in increased retroversion in dominant arms.[45,46]

Glenoid

In the coronal plane, the articular surface of the glenoid comprises an arc of approximately 75 degrees. The shape of the articulation is that of an inverted comma. The typical long-axis dimension is about 3.5 to 4 cm. In the transverse plane, the arc of curvature of the glenoid is only about 50 degrees, with a linear dimension of approximately 2.5 to 3 cm.[41] The relationship of the articular surface to the body of the scapula is difficult to define precisely because of the difficulty in defining a frame of reference. Typically, it is accepted that the glenoid has a slight upward tilt of about 5 degrees[47] with respect to the medial border of the scapula and is retroverted a mean of approximately 7 degrees, although individual variation in these measurements is considerable (Fig. 6-17).[48]

Saha has defined the relationship of the dimensions of the humeral head and the glenoid as the *glenohumeral ratio*. This relationship is approximately 0.8 in the coronal plane and 0.6 in the horizontal or transverse plane.[48] These values are consistent with several observations that have estimated that only about one third of the surface of the humeral head is in contact with the glenoid at any given time.[17] Hertz[49] measured the surface area of the glenoid with and without the labrum and compared it with that of the humeral head. The surface ratio of the glenoid and humeral head was 1:4.3 without the labrum and 1:2.8 with the labrum. In other words, the glenoid

FIGURE 6-16 Two-dimensional orientation of the articular surface of the humerus with respect to the bicondylar axis. (Modified from Mayo Clinic © 1984.)

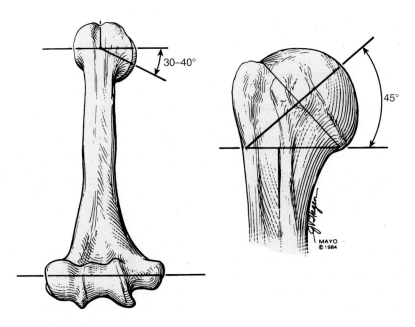

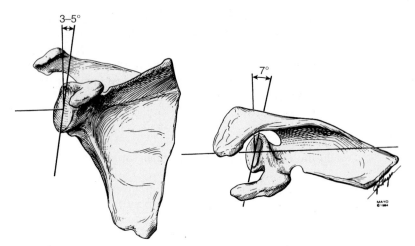

FIGURE 6-17 The glenoid faces slightly superior and posterior (retroverted) with respect to the body of the scapula. (Modified from Mayo Clinic © 1984.)

surface with the labrum attached is approximately one third the humeral head surface, and it is approximately one fourth the humeral head surface without the labrum.

Arm Elevation

The most important function of the shoulder—arm elevation—has been extensively studied to determine the relationship and contribution of the glenohumeral and scapulothoracic joints, the *scapulohumeral rhythm*.[3,24,25,42,48,50-55] Although early descriptions of scapulohumeral rhythm were based on motion with respect to the coronal (frontal) plane, recent discussion has defined this motion with respect to the scapular plane. Neither reference system is completely adequate to fully describe the complex rotational sequences involved in elevation of the arm because the changes in scapular position during elevation usually have not been considered.

Early descriptions of this motion defined the glenohumeral contribution as the first 90 degrees, followed by scapulothoracic rotation.[17] Subsequent discussions place the overall glenohumeral-to-scapulothoracic motion ratio at 2:1.[3,14] This ratio is inconsistent during the first 30 degrees of elevation, with variation by person and even by sex.[21,29,52]

Poppen and Walker reported a 4:1 glenohumeral-to-scapulothoracic motion ratio during the first 25 degrees of arm elevation.[25] Thereafter, an almost equal 5:4 rotation ratio occurs during subsequent elevation. The average overall ratio is about 2:1.

The lack of linearity of this motion complex has also been observed by Doody and coworkers, who showed a 7:1 ratio of scapulothoracic-to-glenohumeral motion during the first 30 degrees of elevation and an approximately 1:1 ratio from 90 to 150 degrees of arm elevation.[29] Others have also shown nonlinear variation during elevation.[55] Further evaluation of the arm against resistance elicits scapulothoracic motion earlier than with passive motion alone.[29]

The various studies have been simply summarized by Bergmann.[56] During the first 30 degrees of elevation, variably greater motion occurs at the glenohumeral joint. The last 60 degrees occurs with about an equal contribution of glenohumeral and scapulothoracic motion. The overall ratio throughout the entire arc of elevation is about 2:1 (Fig. 6-18).

Harryman and associates confirmed this ratio for planes other than the scapular or coronal plane.[57] After measuring the three-dimensional kinematics of the glenohumeral and scapulothoracic joints in various planes of elevation, they concluded that the relative contribution of glenohumeral and scapulothoracic motion to the total arc of elevation was consistent and essentially 2:1. The scapulohumeral rhythm is affected by the speed of arm elevation.[58] At high speed, glenohumeral motion is more dominant at the beginning of motion. The rhythm remains the same, although the total range of motion is reduced with age.[59]

With upward movement of the arm, a complex rotational motion of the scapula occurs (Fig. 6-19). In addition to the upward rotation described earlier, about 6 degrees of anterior rotation with respect to the thorax occurs during the first 90 degrees of arm elevation. Posterior rotation of about 16 degrees occurs next, with the scapula coming to rest about 10 degrees posteriorly rotated in comparison to the original resting position.[50] Thus, an arc of about 15 degrees of anteroposterior rotation of the scapula occurs with elevation of the arm; about 20 degrees of forward tilt with respect to the thorax also occurs during elevation.[14] Scapulohumeral rhythm is affected by various pathologic conditions of the shoulder. In stiff shoulders with anterior capsular tightness, a more excessive scapular upward rotation is observed.[60] On the other hand, shoulders with instability show delay in retraction and posterior tilt of the scapula during arm elevation, which can contribute to shoulder instability.[61] Scapulohumeral rhythm changes after total shoulder arthroplasty, with the 2:1 ratio changed to 1:2 after nonconstrained total shoulder arthroplasty.[62]

FIGURE 6-18 A, The classic study by Inman and colleagues shows the relationship between glenohumeral and scapulothoracic motion. The *blue line* indicates the regression line. The *red lines* indicate the range of ±2 SD. **B,** Angular changes of the glenohumeral joint with respect to arm elevation were determined by several investigators. *1,* Nobuhara K: The Shoulder: Its Function and Clinical Aspects. Tokyo: Igaku-Shoin, 1987. *2,* Poppen NK, Walker PS: Normal and abnormal motion of the shoulder. J Bone Joint Surg Am 58:195-201, 1976. *3,* Inman VT, Saunders JR, Abbott LC: Observations on the function of the shoulder joint. J Bone Joint Surg 26:1-30, 1944. *4,* Freedman L, Munro RH: Abduction of the arm in scapular plane: Scapular and glenohumeral movements. J Bone Joint Surg Am 18:1503-1510, 1966. *5,* Reeves B, Jobbins B, Flowers M: Biomechanical problems in the development of a total shoulder endoprosthesis. (Proc Br Orthop Res Soc) J Bone Joint Surg [Br] 54:193, 1972. (**A,** Redrawn from Inman VT, Saunders JR, Abbott LC: Observations on the function of the shoulder joint. J Bone Joint Surg 26:1-30, 1944. **B,** Redrawn from Bergmann G: Biomechanics and pathomechanics of the shoulder joint with reference to prosthetic joint replacement. In Koelbel R, Helbig B, Blauth W [eds]: Shoulder Replacement. Berlin: Springer-Verlag, 1987, pp 33-43.)

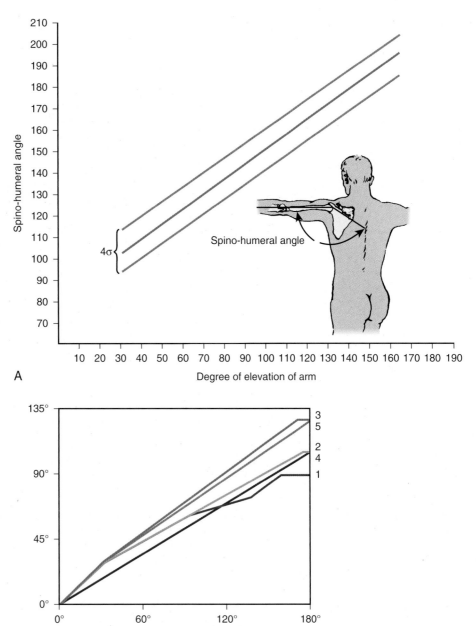

External Rotation of the Humerus

Early observers noted that "obligatory" external rotation of the humerus was necessary for maximal elevation.[18] Impingement of the tuberosity on the coracoacromial arch was assumed to be the mechanical constraint. External rotation clears the tuberosity posteriorly, thereby allowing full arm elevation (Fig. 6-20).[18] We have observed in our laboratory that external rotation of the humerus also loosens the inferior ligaments of the glenohumeral joint. This mechanism thus releases the inferior checkrein effect and allows full elevation of the arm. Full elevation with maximal external rotation has also been shown to be a position of greater stability of the shoulder than the elevated position.[51]

Browne and associates[63] quantified the relationship between elevation and rotation of the humerus with respect to the fixed scapula by using a three-dimensional magnetic tracking device. The plane of maximal arm elevation was shown to occur 23 degrees anterior to the plane of the scapula. Elevation in any plane anterior to the scapular plane required external rotation of the humerus, and maximal elevation was associated with approximately 35 degrees of external rotation. Conversely, maximal glenohumeral elevation with the arm in full internal rotation occurs in a plane about 20 to 30 degrees posterior to that of the scapula and is limited to only about 115 degrees.[63] They reported that the observed effects of this rotation were to clear the humeral

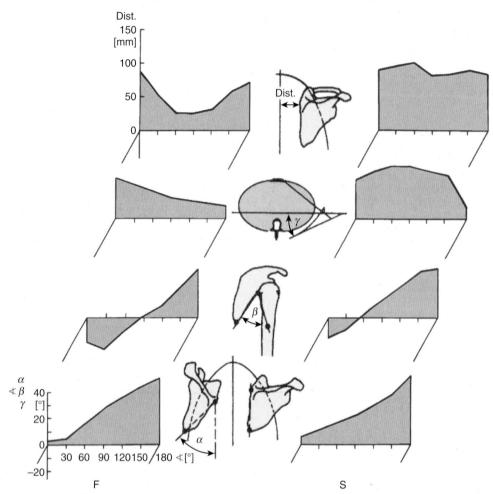

FIGURE 6-19 Complex three-dimensional rotation and translation of the scapula during arm elevation from 0 to 180 degrees in the frontal plane (F) and sagittal plane (S). α, scapular rotation in the frontal plane; β, scapular rotation in the sagittal plane; γ, scapular rotation in the horizontal plane; Dist, distance between the vertical at C7 and the medial border of the scapular spine. (Modified from Laumann U: Kinesiology of the shoulder joint. In Koelbel R, Helbig B, Blauth W [eds]: Shoulder Replacement. Berlin: Springer-Verlag, 1987, pp 23-31.)

tuberosity from abutting beneath the acromion and to relax the inferior capsuloligamentous constraints. Gagey and Boisrenoult also reported that the inferior capsule determines the maximum abduction angle.[64] On the other hand, Jobe and Iannotti reported that obligatory external rotation occurs not because of abutment between the greater tuberosity and the acromion but because of abutment between the greater tuberosity and the superior posterior glenoid rim.[65] This concept was first described by Walch and colleagues as posterosuperior impingement[66] and was later known as *internal impingement*.

In vivo measurements of maximal elevation by Pearl and colleagues[67] revealed a slight difference from these cadaver studies. According to them, maximal elevation was achieved with the humerus just behind the scapular plane (−4 degrees). A difference in definition of the scapular plane and a difference between in vivo behavior and that of the cadaver might explain the discrepancy.

The complex sequence of events in combined motion of the glenohumeral and scapulothoracic joints has been

divided into four stages. Glenohumeral motion occurs first; next, sternoclavicular and then acromioclavicular rotation is observed with elevation of the scapula; and finally, the scapula pivots upward around the acromioclavicular joint. This simplified analytic description is, in general, consistent with the observations of Laumann, Nobuhara, and others.[14,55]

Center of Rotation

An accurate calculation of the ICR of the humeral head is a complex problem that is much simplified if the motion is limited to a single plane.[68,69] Such has been the assumption of most analyses. Hence, the center of rotation of the glenohumeral joint has been defined as a locus of points situated within 6 ± 2 mm of the geometric center of the humeral head (see Fig. 6-10).[25] This definition, generated by the Rouleaux technique, is considered reasonably accurate.[70] However, this particular technique for defining the center of rotation is accurate only for pure

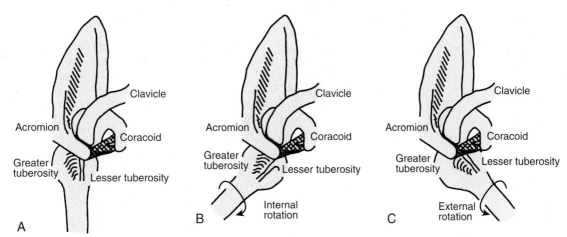

FIGURE 6-20 Upward elevation of the arm requires obligatory external rotation to avoid impingement of the tuberosity under the acromial process. **A,** Neutral position. **B,** Internal rotation. **C,** External rotation.

spinning motion, is subject to input-type error,[71] and is not accurate in pathologic conditions in which translation is a significant component of the displacement or in which a significant amount of nonplanar motion is present. These limitations might explain why other authors have found the center to lie 8 mm behind and 6 mm below the intersection of the shaft and head axes.[72] Still others have reported that multiple centers of rotation occur during abduction.[73]

The relatively small dimension of this locus as well as the relative consistency of its definition as lying in the geometric center of the humeral head reflects the small

amount of translation that normally occurs at this joint and is consistent with the aforementioned observations. A small amount (~3 mm) of upward translation has been reported in the intact shoulder during the first 30 degrees of elevation; only about 1 mm of additional excursion occurs with elevation measured at greater than 30 degrees.[25] A small amount of translation has also been confirmed in cadaver models. During passive elevation without force to the muscles, the humeral head shifted superiorly by 0.35 to 1.2 mm.[31,74] By using simulated muscle force to the deltoid and rotator cuff muscles, greater superior-to-inferior translation of the humeral

FIGURE 6-21 The center of rotation of the scapula for arm elevation is focused in the tip of the acromion. *Left,* Anterposterior view. *Right,* Lateral view. Os, reference point of the scapula (center of the glenoid). (Redrawn from Poppen NK, Walker PS: Normal and abnormal motion of the shoulder. J Bone Joint Surg Am 58:195-201, 1976.)

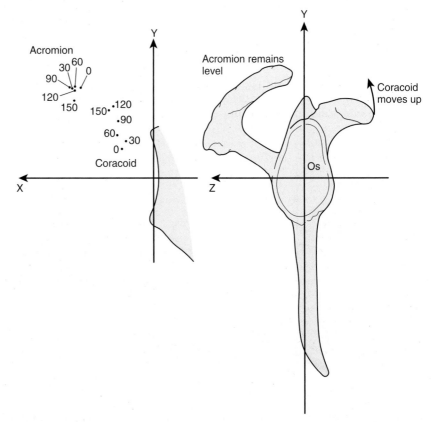

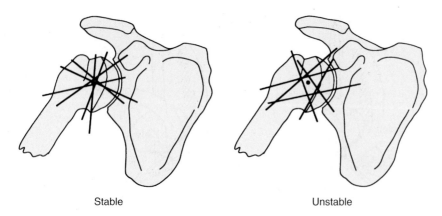

Stable   Unstable

FIGURE 6-22 The common intersection of the screw axes creates a perfect ball-and-socket joint (*left*). When significant translation occurs, the axes do not intersect at a single point (*right*).

head was recorded (2.0-9.0 mm).[75,76] Furthermore, an increase in translation occurs with certain pathologic processes such as rotator cuff deficiency[25] and tendon rupture of the long head of the biceps (LHB).[77]

The center of rotation of the scapula for arm elevation is situated at the tip of the acromion as viewed edge on (Fig. 6-21).[78]

Screw Axis

Application of the SDA for glenohumeral joint motion has one specific advantage. By using the concept of the intersection or the middle point of the common perpendicular between two instantaneous screw axes as the measurement of the three-dimensional ICR, the stability or laxity of the joint can be described. If the joint is tight and stable, the points of intersection of all the screw axes will be confined within a small sphere (Fig. 6-22). On the other hand, when the joint is becoming unstable because of disease of either the capsuloligamentous structures or the rotator cuff, the points of intersection of the screw axes will be more dispersed and confined in a larger sphere. Stokdijk and colleagues compared different methods in determining the glenohumeral joint rotation center in vivo, and they prefer the screw axes method as a reliable and valid method in movement registration.[79]

The concept had also been used to measure the anterior instability of the shoulder at the end of the late preparatory phase of throwing.[80]

Clinical Relevance

Understanding of the biomechanical features discussed earlier has several clinically relevant applications. The orientation of the scapula and humerus with respect to the thorax and to each other has been important in designing the optimal radiographic studies to best visualize the scapulohumeral relationship. Thus, the true anteroposterior radiograph of the glenohumeral joint is taken 30 degrees oblique to the sagittal plane. Some think that this orientation is closer to 45 degrees because this angle produces a better true anteroposterior radiographic study.[7] The scapular view is taken at a 30-degree angle to the frontal plane; thus, the anteroposterior radiograph (Fig. 6-23) that is perpendicular to this view is taken at an angle of about 60 degrees to the thorax.[81]

The relationship of coupled external rotation with maximal arm elevation helps explain, to some extent, the limitation in elevation that is seen with a frozen shoulder. To the extent that this condition results in limitation of external rotation, an even more severe restriction of arm elevation is likely to occur. In fact, any simple movement

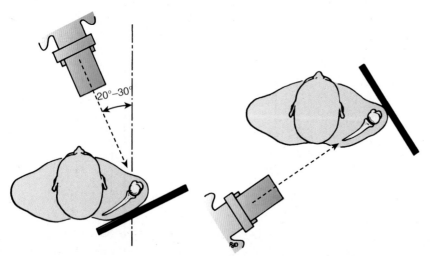

20°–30°

FIGURE 6-23 The anterior (*left*) and lateral (*right*) views of the glenohumeral joint were defined by Neer based on knowledge of the scapulothoracic orientation. (Modified from Neer CS II: Displaced proximal humeral fractures. I. Classification and evaluation. J Bone Joint Surg Am 52:1077-1089, 1970.)

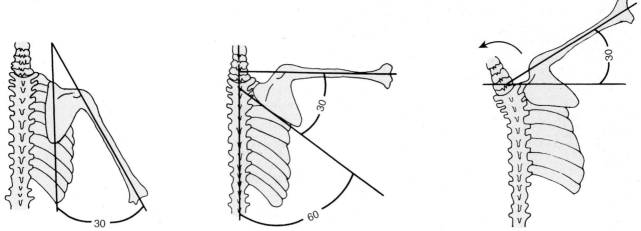

FIGURE 6-24 Arthrodesis of the glenohumeral joint in the optimal position (*left*) allows arm elevation to and above the horizontal by scapulothoracic motion (*center*) as well as by tilting the trunk (*right*).

of the glenohumeral joint results in coupled motion in two additional planes. By using a universal full-circle goniometer to determine the relationship between flexion and rotation at the glenohumeral joint it was found that flexion was accomplished by internal rotation.[82] It has also been demonstrated that certain passive motions of the glenohumeral joint were reproducibly accompanied by translation of the humeral head on the glenoid.[31] Knowledge of this coupling effect is also important with

respect to prescribing the appropriate physical therapy after certain surgical procedures or pathologic states.

Arthrodesis of the shoulder is an effective procedure but is most efficacious if the fusion is performed in the appropriate position.[83] Although the optimal position is debated, the basis of the selection depends on normal scapulothoracic motion (Fig. 6-24). This knowledge, combined with an understanding of the motion required for activities of daily living, dictates the position of the fusion.

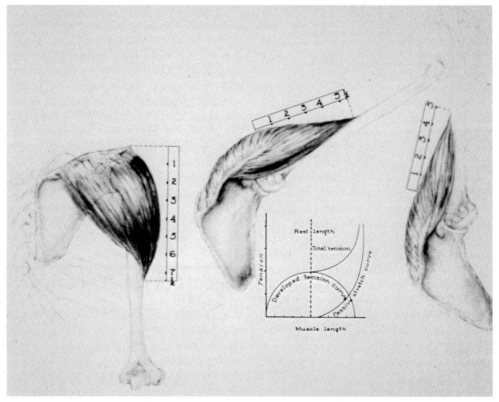

FIGURE 6-25 Scapulothoracic motion allows the deltoid to remain in the optimal position for effective contraction throughout the arc of arm elevation. (From Lucas DB: Biomechanics of the shoulder joint. Arch Surg 107:425-432, 1973. © 1973, American Medical Association.)

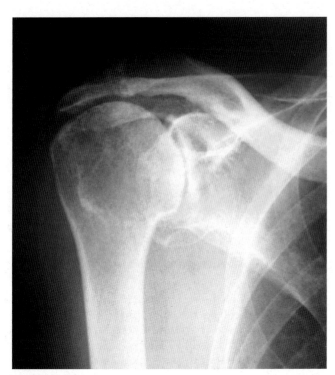

FIGURE 6-26 Superior migration of the humeral head in a rotator cuff–deficient shoulder is due in part to pull of the deltoid muscle.

BOX 6-1 Static and Dynamic Contributions to Shoulder Stability

Static

Soft Tissue
Coracohumeral ligament
Glenohumeral ligaments
Labrum
Capsule

Articular Surface
Joint contact
Scapular inclination
Intra-articular pressure

Dynamic
Rotator cuff muscles
Biceps
Deltoid

The potential for scapulothoracic motion provides an explanation for the remaining motion of the shoulder girdle present with a frozen shoulder and after arthrodesis. In addition, rotation of the scapula may be viewed as a means of providing a glenohumeral relationship that allows the deltoid muscle to remain effective even with the arm fully elevated (Fig. 6-25).

Understanding the axis of rotation is important for prosthetic replacement of the glenohumeral joint. The relative lack of translation in an intact shoulder justifies the design of an unconstrained glenoid surface. Karduna and associates[84] reported a significant increase in superoinferior and anteroposterior translation with increased radial mismatch of the prosthesis. The mean translation for natural joints was best reproduced by implant joints with a 3- to 4-mm radial mismatch. To the extent that the cuff musculature is deficient, a greater amount of translation is anticipated, which places additional requirements on the optimal glenoid design to accommodate the increased translation.[85] As is discussed later, probably more important is that the initiation of shoulder abduction results in forces directed toward the superior rim of the glenoid; this has implications regarding the stability, force, and optimal prosthetic design and surgical implantation technique.

Finally, the well-recognized superior translation of the humeral head in a rotator cuff–deficient shoulder is explained in part by the superiorly directed resultant vector that occurs with initiation of abduction by the intact deltoid, the lack of soft tissue interposition of the rotator cuff (Fig. 6-26),[86] and the lack of centralizing force to the humeral head against the glenoid socket produced by the rotator cuff. Yamaguchi and colleagues measured the kinematics of the glenohumeral joint with symptomatic and asymptomatic rotator cuff tears.[87] They found similar superior migration of the humeral head during arm elevation in both symptomatic and asymptomatic rotator cuff tears. Symptoms in shoulders with a rotator cuff tear may be related to factors other than superior migration of the humeral head. In addition to the size of the tear and the duration of symptoms, the important factor that influences superior migration of the humeral head is fatty degeneration of the infraspinatus muscle.[88]

Thus, knowledge of the motion of the glenohumeral and scapulothoracic joints has numerous current clinical applications. A clear understanding of these factors is important for proper diagnosis and management of many shoulder conditions.

SHOULDER CONSTRAINTS

It is convenient to consider the constraints of any joint as consisting of static and dynamic elements. The static contribution may be further subdivided into articular and capsuloligamentous components (Box 6-1). Knowledge of the shoulder constraints is of particular clinical interest because it pertains to anterior dislocation as well as to posterior and multidirectional instability of the shoulder.[23,89]

Early investigators focused on one element or the other. Hence, Saha emphasized the articular component of shoulder stability,[48,90] Moseley and Overgaard[91] and Townley[70] focused on the capsuloligamentous complex, and DePalma and others emphasized the dynamic contribution of the interrelationship between the dynamic and the static capsuloligamentous constraints.[92-94] Since the 1990s, the static and dynamic components have been extensively investigated. In addition, the interrelationship between these components has become clarified in both experimental and clinical settings.

The shoulder stability is easy to understand if we think about it in two different conditions: the mid range of motion and the end range of motion. The mid range of motion is the position of the arm when the capsuloligamentous structures are all lax, for example, with the arm in the hanging position or at 60 degrees of abduction. The end range of motion is defined as the position of the arm when the capsuloligamentous structures become tight, such as at 90 degrees of abduction and maximum external rotation or at 90 degrees of flexion and maximum horizontal adduction.

In the mid range of motion, the capsuloligamentous structures are lax and the humeral head is movable anteriorly, posteriorly, or inferiorly by applying force. This mobility is called *laxity*. There is a great variety in the midrange laxity: Some patients are very stiff, but others can dislocate their shoulders voluntarily without any symptoms. The midrange stabilizers are the intra-articular pressure when all the muscles are relaxed; when the muscles are in contraction, the midrange stabilizer is the concavity of the glenoid. On the other hand, translation of the humeral head at the end range of motion is quite limited because the capsuloligamentous structures are tight and prevent further movement of the arm. At this limit of motion, an excessive force can cause failure of the capsuloligamentous structures, which results in traumatic dislocation of the shoulder.

The end-range stabilizers are the capsuloligamentous structures. The midrange stabilizers and the end-range stabilizers are independent. For example, a shoulder with hyperlaxity can reveal an inferior dislocation of the shoulder with the arm in hanging position (midrange laxity), but it might not be dislocated with the arm in an apprehension position of abduction and maximum external rotation (end-range stability). Conversely, a shoulder with recurrent anterior dislocation does not show inferior subluxation or dislocation with the arm in hanging position because the end-range stabilizers are not intact but the midrange stabilizers are intact.

Static Constraints

Articular Contribution to Glenohumeral Stability

The humeral articular surface is not inherently stable. The 30-degree retroversion is obviously necessary for proper balance of the soft tissues and normal kinematics. Most studies of the articular contribution to shoulder stability

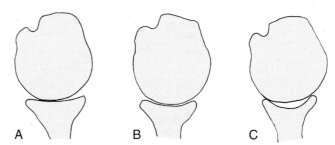

FIGURE 6-27 Articular stability of the glenohumeral joint is enhanced or lessened according to the variation in articular congruence. **A,** Shallow glenoid surface. **B,** Conforming surfaces. **C,** Excessively deepened glenoid surface. (Modified from Saha AK: Dynamic stability of the glenohumeral joint. Acta Orthop Scand 42:491-505, 1971.)

have focused on the glenoid. The glenoid articulation demonstrates a slight, but definite posterior or retroverted orientation averaging about 7 degrees with regard to the body of the scapula (see Fig. 6-17). Saha has emphasized that this orientation is an important contribution to stability of the joint.[48] Recent biomechanical studies have revealed that an anteverted glenoid component results in increased anterior translation of the humeral head and a retroverted glenoid component increases posterior translation of the humeral head,[95] whereas compensatory anteversion of the humeral component does not increase shoulder stability.[96] Theoretically, version of the glenoid could be a predisposing factor for instability. In the clinical setting, however, anterior shoulder instability often observed as a result of traumatic dislocation is not associated with anteversion of the glenoid,[97] whereas posterior shoulder instability often observed as a symptom of atraumatic multidirectional instability is associated with increased retroversion of the glenoid.[98]

Only 25% to 30% of the humeral head is covered by the glenoid surface in any given anatomic position.[17,42,49,92] The dimensional relationship between the humeral head and the glenoid reflects the inherent instability of the joint and has been referred to as the *glenohumeral index,* which is calculated as the maximal diameter of the glenoid divided by the maximal diameter of the humeral head. Saha reported this ratio to be approximately 0.75 in the sagittal plane and approximately 0.6 in the more critical transverse plane.[48] Later, this relationship was redetermined, with similar values of 0.86 and 0.58, respectively.[99] Developmental hypoplasia of the glenoid can alter this ratio and might play some role in recurrent dislocation of the shoulder, but such observations have been rather limited in the clinical literature.[100,101] Subtle variation in articular anatomy of the glenoid has also been described and has been advocated as an explanation for inherent instability of the joint (Fig. 6-27).

The glenoid labrum has three layers of collagen fibers.[102] The thin superficial layer (articular side) is composed of reticulated collagen fibers, the second layer is composed

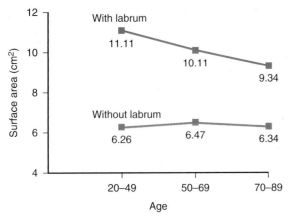

FIGURE 6-28 The labral area decreases with age, but the osseous glenoid area remains unchanged. (Redrawn from Hertz H: Hertz H: Die Bedeutung des Limbus glenoidalis für die Stabilität des Schultergelenks. Wien Klin Wochenschr Suppl 152:1-23, 1984.)

of stratified collagen fibers, and the third is composed of dense collagen fibers running parallel to each other and oblique to the glenoid rim. The glenoid labrum increases the area and depth of the glenoid cavity. The area of the glenoid with the labrum attached is approximately one third the humeral articular surface, and it is one quarter without the labrum.[49] The area of the labrum decreases with age, but the area of the osseous glenoid does not change (Fig. 6-28). The depth of the glenoid is also functionally deepened by the presence of the glenoid labrum.

The early literature placed little emphasis on this anatomic structure as increasing the stability offered by the glenoid articular surface. Townley[70] removed the labrum of cadaveric shoulders through a posterior approach but could not create anterior dislocation until he resected the anterior capsule. Moseley and Overgaard demonstrated that the labrum was a specialized portion of the anterior capsule.[91] With external rotation, this structure flattens and thus serves only as a source of attachment for the inferior glenohumeral ligament (IGHL); hence, they concluded that the labrum itself seems to offer little to the inherent stability of the joint. However, other studies have attributed additional importance to the labrum.[94] Howell and coworkers measured an average depth of 9 mm in the superior-to-inferior direction of the glenoid.[103] This depth is equivalent to approximately 40% of the radius of a typical 44-mm humeral replacement prosthesis. The anteroposterior depth of the glenoid measured an average of only 2.5 mm. However, these investigators thought that the anterior and posterior glenoid labrum added an additional 2.5 mm of depth. These data suggest that the labrum may be effective in increasing the depth of the glenoid and therefore has some contribution to articular stability. The humeral head needs to override the rim of the glenoid to dislocate. In other words, midrange stability depends on the depth of the glenoid to some extent.

A cadaveric study revealed that removal of the entire anterior labrum without damaging the capsule resulted in increased translation of the humeral head in adduction (midrange instability) but did not alter the degree of stability in the anterior apprehension position (end-range stability).[104]

Fukuda and associates[105] were the first to evaluate the relationship between the glenoid depth and stability in various kinds of shoulder prostheses. They used a ratio of a force necessary to dislocate the humeral component out of the glenoid socket to a force compressing the humeral component against the glenoid component to assess the inherent stability of the shoulder prosthesis. This ratio was constant in each type of prosthesis, and the deeper the glenoid socket, the greater the ratio. Later, Lippitt and associates[106] termed this ratio the *stability ratio*. In normal shoulders, the stability ratio is 50% to 60% in the superior-to-inferior direction and 30% to 35% in the anterior-to-posterior direction. The stability ratio increases with an increase in glenoid depth. After the labrum is removed, the stability ratio decreases by approximately 20%. The stability ratio further decreases after creating a chondrolabral defect.[37] According to Halder and colleagues,[107] the stability ratio was greatest in the inferior direction (Fig. 6-29), and it was greater with the arm in adduction than in abduction. In shoulders with multidirectional instability, the stability ratio is decreased due to glenoid dysplasia. In surgical procedures, the stability ratio can be increased by 25% with use of capsulolabral augmentation[78] and by 34% with use of glenoid osteotomy.[108]

Detachment of the superior aspect of the labrum from anterior and posterior is called a type II SLAP lesion. The pathogenesis of this lesion has been studied in the literature. Grauer and coworkers applied a 20-N force to the LHB and measured the strain in the anterior and posterior portions of the labrum.[109] They found that strain was the greatest with the arm in full abduction and the smallest in adduction. Bey and colleagues applied a failure load to the LHB with the shoulder reduced and subluxated inferiorly.[110] In reduced shoulders, the load created a type II SLAP lesion in two of eight shoulders, whereas in subluxated shoulders, the lesion developed in seven of eight shoulders.

Pradhan and associates simulated a throwing motion and measured strain on the anterosuperior and posterosuperior portions of the labrum in cadaveric shoulders.[111] They found that the strain was greatest at the posterosuperior portion of the labrum when the arm was in abduction and external rotation (late cocking phase). Repetitive throwing motion can bring the superior labrum under constant strain and various degrees of shear force created by the cuff tendons during internal impingement, which can eventually result in detachment of the superior labrum from the glenoid. Once a type II SLAP lesion is created, a cadaveric study has shown that range of motion increases and the translation of the humeral head also increases.[112,113]

FIGURE 6-29 The average stability ratios of the shoulders, with and without the labrum, in eight tested directions. The ratios are defined as the peak translational force divided by the applied compressive force. The values are given as the average (and standard deviation). (From Halder AM, Kuhl SG, Zobitz ME, et al: Effects of the glenoid labrum and glenohumeral abduction on stability of the shoulder joint through concavity-compression: An in vitro study. J Bone Joint Surg Am 7:1062-1069, 2001.)

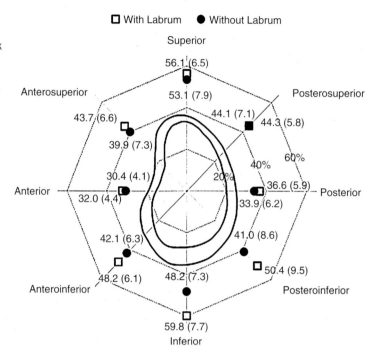

The joint contact area and position change during various glenohumeral motions are difficult to accurately measure by direct techniques. The contact point moves forward and inferior during internal rotation.[14,48] With external rotation, the contact is just posteroinferior (Fig. 6-30). Saha reported that with elevation, the contact area moves superiorly. If elevation is combined with internal and external rotation, however, the humeral head remains centered in the glenoid as viewed in the axillary plane.[53] The joint surface geometry and contact area have been measured with either stereophotogrammetry[114] or electromagnetic tracking devices.[115] In one study, the maximal contact area was obtained at 120 degrees of elevation. With an increase in arm elevation, the contact area shifted from an inferior region to a superocentral-posterior region, whereas the glenoid contact area shifted posteriorly (Fig. 6-31).[114] Glenohumeral contact is maximal at functional positions (60-120 degrees of elevation) that provide stability to this joint.

Warner and colleagues measured the contact area by using Fuji prescale film. In adduction, the contact area of the humeral head on the glenoid was limited to the anatomic region of the central glenoid known as the *bare area*, whereas in abduction, the contact area as well as the congruity increased.[116] They concluded that there was a slight articular mismatch in adduction but that it became more congruent and stable in abduction. Sahara and colleagues used open MRI to describe three-dimensional motion of the glenoid on the articular surface of the humeral head (Fig. 6-32).[11] The glenoid was initially

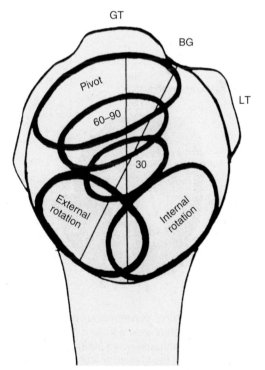

FIGURE 6-30 Humeral contact positions as a function of glenohumeral motion and positions. BG, bicipital groove; GT, greater tuberosity; LT, lesser tuberosity. (Colorized from Nobuhara K: The Shoulder: Its Function and Clinical Aspects. Tokyo: Igaku-Shoin, 1987.)

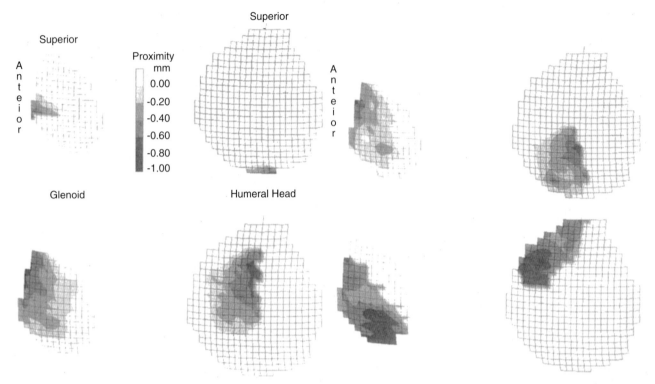

FIGURE 6-31 The contact area of the humeral head shifts from the inferior to the superocentral-posterior region with an increase in arm elevation, whereas the glenoid contact area shifts posteriorly. (From Soslowsky LJ, Flatow EL, Bigliani LU, et al: Quantitation of in situ contact areas at the glenohumeral joint: A biomechanical study. J Orthop Res 10:524-534, 1992.)

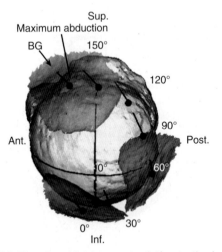

FIGURE 6-32 The glenoid movement relative to the humeral head. The semitransparent *gray ellipse* is the glenoid at 0 degrees, 60 degrees, and maximum abduction. The *black dots* are the centers of the glenoid at each abducted position. The *bars* indicate the superior directions of the long axis of the glenoid. Ant, anterior; BG, bicipital groove; Inf, inferior; Post, posterior; Sup, superior. (From Sahara W, Sugamoto K, Murai M, Tanaka H: Yoshikawa H: The three-dimensional motions of glenohumeral joint under semi-loaded condition during arm abduction using vertically open MRI. Clin Biomech 22:304-312, 2007.)

located at the inferior portion of the humeral head at 0 degrees of abduction. The glenoid shifted posteriorly from 0 to 60 degrees of abduction, moved up to the posterior-superior part of the humeral head from 60 to 120 degrees of abduction, and then moved anteriorly close to the bicipital groove at maximum abduction.

The slight 5-degree superior tilt of the articular surface has been offered by Basmajian and Bazant as a factor in preventing inferior subluxation of the humerus when combined with the effect of the superior capsule and superior glenohumeral ligament (SGHL) (Fig. 6-33).[47] Clinically, glenoid dysplasia with the glenoid facing downward is related to multidirectional instability of the shoulder.[117] Glenoid osteotomy or pectoralis major transfer can be performed in shoulders with multidirectional instability to increase scapular inclination.[55] A biomechanical study by Itoi and associates[118] has clarified the relationship between scapular inclination and inferior stability of the shoulder. As the scapula was adducted (glenoid facing downward), all the vented shoulders dislocated inferiorly, whereas they were reduced with an increase in scapular abduction (Fig. 6-34). They further studied the bulk effect of the rotator cuff muscles on the stability provided by scapular inclination.[119] After removal of the cuff muscles, the stability provided by scapular inclination did not change. Thus, the mechanism of scapular inclination seems to be a cam effect determined by the geometry of the glenoid and humerus and also by the length and orientation of the superior capsuloliga-

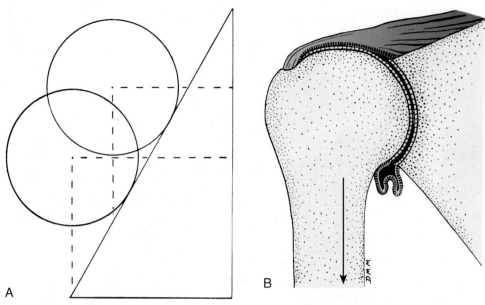

FIGURE 6-33 The upward tilt of the glenoid, coupled with the superior glenohumeral ligament and the coracohumeral ligament, resists passive downward displacement of the humeral head. **A,** Plane geometric diagram. **B,** Anatomic diagram. (Modified from Basmajian JV, Bazant FJ: Factors preventing downward dislocation of the adducted shoulder joint. J Bone Joint Surg Am 41:1182-1186, 1959.)

mentous structures. Later, Metcalf and colleagues demonstrated that glenoid osteotomy and a 5-mm bone graft increased the stability ratio from 0.47 to 0.81 in the posteroinferior direction.[108]

Intra-articular pressure is another important stabilizer. An intensive study by Kumar and Balasubramaniam has shown that a negative pressure normally exists in the glenohumeral joint.[120] If this pressure is equalized by an arthrotomy or even by a small puncture, inferior subluxation of the shoulder readily occurs (Fig. 6-35). This effect is greater when the cuff musculature has been removed but is present in muscle-intact specimens as well. A similar observation was also reported in 1930 by Lockhart.[54] The intra-articular pressure stabilizes the shoulder not only in the inferior direction but also in all the other directions.[121] Intra-articular pressure changes with the application of inferior translation load. Strong correlations have been found among load, pressure, and displacement.[122] However, intra-articular pressure does not correlate with the external load in shoulders with recurrent anterior instability.[123]

The change in intra-articular pressure with shoulder motion was analyzed by Hashimoto and associates.[124] According to their study, intra-articular pressure was minimal with the arm in slight elevation and maximal with the arm in full elevation. In shoulders with multidirectional instability, the joint capsule is enlarged and the joint volume is increased.[89,125] Enlarged joint volume makes the intra-articular pressure less sensitive to the external load.[126] The mechanism of the inferior capsular shift procedure is that reducing the joint volume and increasing the capsular thickness increase the responsiveness of the intra-articular pressure.

Capsular and Ligamentous Contributions to Static Shoulder Stability

Little is known of the biochemical constitution of the capsule of the shoulder joint except that it consists of types I, III, and V collagen. In this respect (not surprisingly), its composition is qualitatively similar to that of the elbow and other joints.[127]

The force required to dislocate the shoulder and elbow was studied by Kaltsas. A markedly greater force of up to 2000 N was needed to disrupt the shoulder complex, in contrast to the 1500 N required for the elbow in persons younger than 40 years.[127] The force needed to dislocate both these joints decreases with increasing age, but the decrease is more drastic in the shoulder (Fig. 6-36).

The tensile strength of the anterior capsular complex has been investigated by Reeves.[128] Cadaver specimens demonstrated a maximal tensile failure load in bodies between 30 and 40 years of age: Mean tensile strength was 56.5 kg and ranged from 40 to 70 kg. Considerable variation exists with age and from one cadaver to another. Less tensile resistance was noted in those younger than 20 and older than 50 years (Fig. 6-37). The anterior shear force has been calculated to be 42 kg if the arm is abducted and externally rotated (Fig. 6-38). Hence, the static constraints might potentially be exceeded in some persons under certain muscle activity or loading conditions.[129]

The shoulder capsule itself is thin and redundant. In some persons, this redundancy may be a congenital variation and hence might explain the great variation in laxity in normal shoulders.[130] Hyperlaxity can predispose to shoulder instability.[131] The capsule–ligament complex

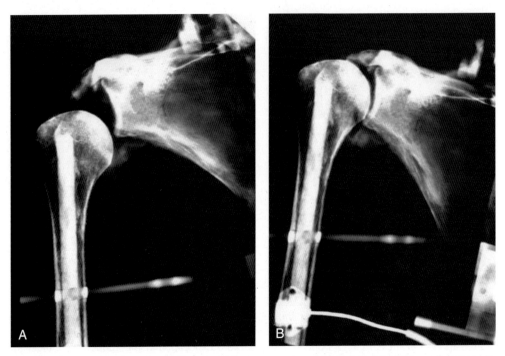

FIGURE 6-34 A, The humeral head dislocates inferiorly with the scapula adducted in 15 degrees. **B,** When the scapula is abducted in 15 degrees, the humeral head becomes reduced. (From Itoi E, Motzkin NE, Morrey BF, An KN: Scapular inclination and inferior stability of the shoulder. J Shoulder Elbow Surg 1:131-139, 1992.)

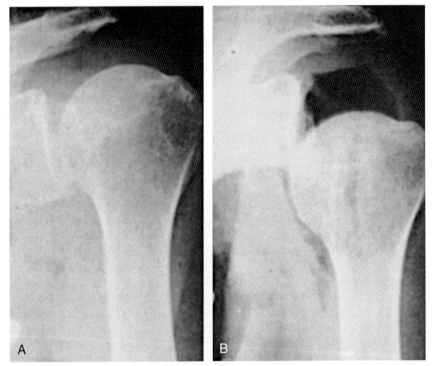

FIGURE 6-35 A, An intact shoulder joint. **B,** Inferior displacement of the humeral head occurs with loss of hydrostatic pressure of the glenohumeral joint. (From Kumar VP, Balasubramaniam P: The role of atmospheric pressure in stabilizing the shoulder: An experimental study. J Bone Joint Surg Br 67:719-721, 1985.)

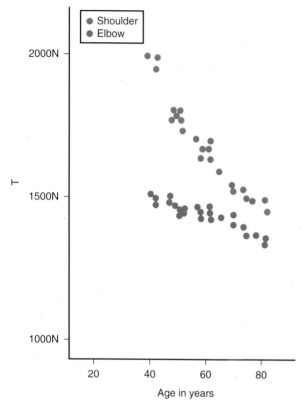

FIGURE 6-36 Comparison of dislocation forces at the shoulder and the elbow. (Redrawn from Kaltsas DS: Comparative study of the properties of the shoulder joint capsules with those of other joint capsules. Clin Orthop Relat Res [173]:20-26, 1973.)

consists of superior, middle, and inferior portions, which together with the coracohumeral ligament (CHL), constitute the defined ligamentous structures of the anterior and superior shoulder joint (Fig. 6-39). These structures were defined and carefully depicted by Flood in 1829.[132]

Coracoacromial Ligament

The coracoacromial ligament connects two portions of the scapula: the coracoid process and the acromion. The function of this ligament had not been of interest until Flatow and colleagues focused on this ligament as a superior stabilizer of the shoulder.[133] They reported the results of coracoacromial ligament reconstruction for anterosuperior subluxation after failed rotator cuff repair.[134] In a cadaveric study, Lee and coworkers measured translation of the humeral head after release of the coracoacromial ligament.[135] After releasing the ligament, anterior and inferior translation increased at 0 and 30 degrees of abduction. They warned that release of the coracoacromial ligament should be performed carefully because this ligament is a stabilizer.

The coracoacromial ligament forms a part of the coracoacromial arch, which is in close contact with the upper surface of the rotator cuff. If impingement of the rotator cuff against the coracoacromial arch causes a rotator cuff tear, the material properties of the coracoacromial ligament are likely to be altered in shoulders with rotator cuff tears because of repetitive stress and friction between the rotator cuff and the ligament.

FIGURE 6-37 Tensile strength of attachment of the glenoid labrum and the rotator cuff (subscapularis tendon) as a function of age. (Redrawn from Reeves B: Experiments on the tensile strength of the anterior capsular structures of the shoulder region. J Bone Joint Surg Br 50:858-865, 1968.)

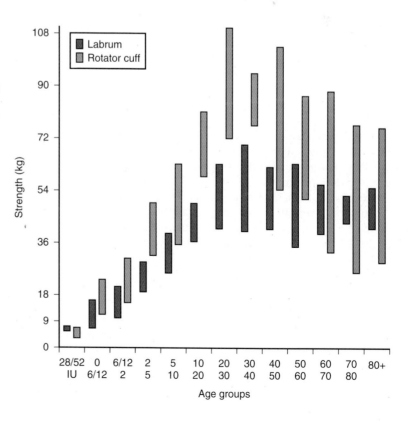

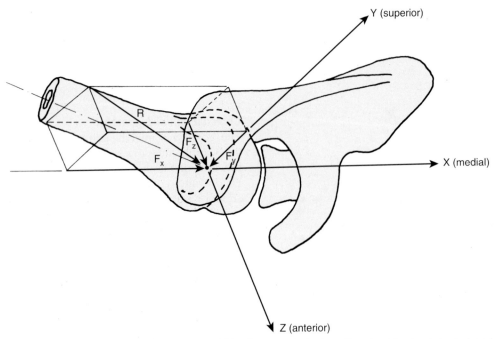

FIGURE 6-38 A significant anterior shear force of up to 40 kg is generated when the shoulder is abducted and externally rotated and all muscles are contracting. F_x, medial contact force, 210 kg; F_y, inferior shear force, 58 kg; F_z, anterior shear force, 42 kg; R, joint resultant force, 221.8 kg. (Modified from Morrey BF, Chao EYS: Recurrent anterior dislocation of the shoulder. In Dumbleton J, Black JH [eds]: Clinical Biomechanics. London: Churchill Livingstone, 1981, pp 24-46.)

Soslowsky and associates measured the tensile properties of this ligament in shoulders with and without rotator cuff tears.[136] They observed no difference in strength and stress relaxation response in those with and without rotator cuff tears. The only difference was that strength decreased more in shoulders with rotator cuff tears after cyclic loading. This study reveals that little change in material properties occurs in this ligament, which suggests that a cuff tear is not likely to be the result of subacromial impingement. Fremerey and colleagues[137] reported that shoulders with rotator cuff tears showed less failure stress than shoulders with intact rotator cuffs, but this change in material property was observed only in the older specimens. This indicates that the change is the result, not the cause, of rotator cuff tears. Hansen and coworkers[138] reported that regenerated ligament after partial resection regained normal mechanical properties of the ligament, but it took more than 3 years. This indicates that the ligament has an essential function for our body, which needs to be clarified.

Coracohumeral Ligament

The CHL originates from the anterior lateral base of the coracoid process and extends as two bands over the top of the shoulder to blend with the capsule and attach to the greater and lesser tuberosities.[8] This ligament is a constant finding and is considered the most consistent of the ligaments of the fibrous capsule.[139] The function of

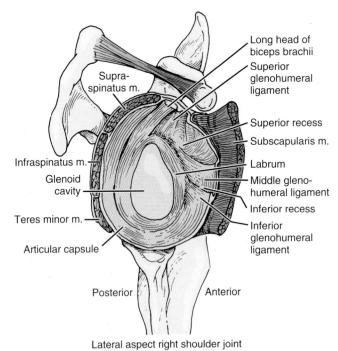

Lateral aspect right shoulder joint

FIGURE 6-39 Schematic representation of the glenohumeral ligaments and the rotator cuff stabilizers of the glenohumeral joint. Ant, anterior; Inf, inferior; Post, posterior; Sup, superior. (Modified from Morrey BF, Chao EYS: Recurrent anterior dislocation of the shoulder. In Dumbleton J, Black JH [eds]: Clinical Biomechanics. London: Churchill Livingstone, 1981, pp 21-46.)

FIGURE 6-40 Humeral attachment of the glenohumeral ligaments. *Left,* Posterior view. *Right,* Anterior view. (Redrawn from Turkel SJ, Panio MW, Marshall JL, Girgis FG: Stabilizing mechanisms preventing anterior dislocation of the glenohumeral joint. J Bone Joint Surg Am 63:1208-1217, 1981.)

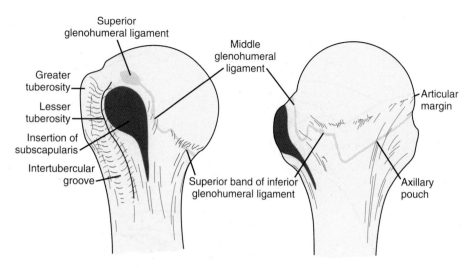

this ligament has been studied by several investigators but is very controversial.

Terry and coworkers[140] and Basmajian and Bazant[47] have demonstrated that the CHL becomes taut in external rotation and also that it appears to contribute to resisting inferior subluxation of the joint (see Fig. 6-33). This function was confirmed by a so-called load control study done by Ovesen and Nielsen,[141] who showed that the most important inferior stabilizer was the CHL. However, Warner and associates[142] observed no suspensory role of the CHL, and Kuboyama[143] reported that the main stabilizing function of the CHL was not in external rotation but in neutral and internal rotation. Strain of the CHL increases in external rotation,[144] which suggests that this ligament is expected to function in external rotation. Another study revealed that the CHL is an inferior stabilizer with the arm in external rotation but not in neutral and internal rotation.[145] Furthermore, the anterior portion of the CHL that attaches to the lesser tuberosity has a more important function than does the posterior portion that attaches to the greater tuberosity.[146] As reported by Jost and colleagues,[147] the CHL is thought to play a key role in limiting external rotation and inferior translation of the humeral head.

Rotator Interval

The rotator interval is a space between the supraspinatus and subscapularis that is covered by the joint capsule and reinforced by the CHL.[19] Shoulders with rotator interval lesions have inferior instability with the arm in internal rotation but not in external rotation.[148]

A cadaveric study by Harryman and associates[149] revealed that sectioning of the rotator interval capsule together with the CHL resulted in inferior and posterior instability and that tightening of the rotator interval capsule increased resistance to inferior and posterior translation. Itoi and colleagues[145] demonstrated that although venting the capsule had a significant effect on inferior stability with the arm in internal and neutral rotation, further sectioning of the capsule with the CHL intact had no effect on inferior stability. They concluded that the rotator interval capsule per se does not have a direct mechanical stabilizing function, but that it stabilizes the shoulder indirectly through maintaining intra-articular pressure. Tamai and colleagues speculated that this ligament may be related to pain during impingement because they observed a rich nerve distribution on the bursal side of the ligament.[150] Wolf and colleagues[151] reported that isolated rotator interval closure decreased glenohumeral laxity in all directions, particularly inferior translation. Plausinis colleagues[152] and Yamamoto and coworkers[153] reported that rotator interval closure produced significant decreases in range of motion and anterior-to-posterior translation.

Superior Glenohumeral Ligament

The SGHL is a constant structure that arises from the tubercle of the glenoid anterior to the origin of the long biceps tendon and runs inferior and lateral to insert on the head of the humerus near the proximal tip of the lesser tuberosity (Fig. 6-40). Basmajian thought that the function of the SGHL was, in conjunction with superior tilt of the glenoid, to provide passive resistance to inferior subluxation or dislocation of the humerus.[154] Previous work supports this concept by showing that if this structure is intact, the shoulder does not translate posteriorly and inferiorly, even in the absence of the inferior ligament and capsule.[155] When this structure is sectioned, however, the lesion created in the posteroinferior aspect of the capsule allows the humeral head to readily dislocate inferiorly.

These observations support Dempster's global concept of stability as being provided by both the anterior and posterior structures because both are observed to force the articular surface of the humeral head against the

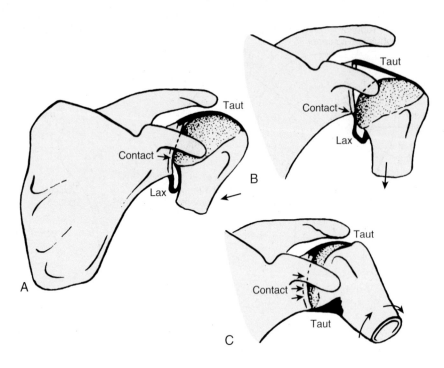

FIGURE 6-41 A-C, Dempster's concept of the shared contribution of the ligaments and articular surface in providing stability to a joint system. (Modified from Dempster WT: Mechanisms of shoulder movement. Arch Phys Med Rehabil 46A:49-70, 1965.)

glenoid (Fig. 6-41). Translation in one direction causes tension in the ligament on the opposite side of the joint; thus, inferior translation causes increased tension in the superior capsule and the SGHL.

Based on selective sectioning of the ligaments via arthroscopy, Warner and associates[142] found that the SGHL was an important inferior stabilizer. A study by Patel and coworkers[146] also revealed that strain on the SGHL and the anterior portion of the CHL was maximal with the arm in adduction and external rotation. The SGHL seems to have a function similar to that of the CHL regarding motion and inferior stability of the glenohumeral joint.

Middle Glenohumeral Ligament

The middle glenohumeral ligament (MGHL) originates from the supraglenoid tubercle at the superior aspect of the glenoid and from the anterosuperior aspect of the labrum and extends laterally and inferiorly to blend with the subscapularis tendon about 2 cm medial to its insertion at the lesser tuberosity (see Figs. 6-39 and 6-40). The MGHL is a substantial structure measuring up to 2 cm wide and 4 mm thick.[156] This ligament is one of the more developed of the glenohumeral ligaments and was reported by DePalma, Moseley, and others to be the major constraint to anterior humeral displacement.[91,139] It is observed to become taut when the shoulder is abducted and externally rotated.[157] Although its origin is from the superior aspect of the labrum, this attachment is probably not disrupted often with recurrent anterior dislocation. Turkel and coworkers also observed that the MGHL tightens in the position of instability when the shoulder is abducted and externally rotated (Fig. 6-42).[157] Selective sectioning of the glenohumeral ligament does allow

increased excursion but does not typically result in instability.[155] Thus, although this structure is not essential to resist anterior translation with abduction and external rotation, in this position it nonetheless contributes to anterior stability of the glenohumeral joint.

Biomechanical studies have shown that with the arm in external rotation, strain of the MGHL was maximal at lower angles of abduction and decreased with an increase in abduction, but it still showed significant tension at 90 degrees of abduction.[144,158] With the arm in neutral and internal rotation, however, the strain became almost zero regardless of the abduction angle. In a displacement control study, Blasier and associates[159] demonstrated that the contribution of the SGHL and MGHL is equal to that of the IGHL with the arm in abduction and external rotation. This observation seems to contradict the previous strain study. The SGHL and MGHL might play a role even though they are relatively lax in neutral rotation, but their role becomes significant when they are taut in external rotation because the IGHL becomes much more important than these ligaments in this position. Thus, the stabilizing function of the MGHL needs to be clearly defined in relation to positions of increasing angles of elevation and external rotation.

Inferior Glenohumeral Ligament

Anatomy. DePalma and colleagues thought that the IGHL was a relatively unimportant stabilizer because in their dissections, about half the specimens lacked a recognizable, discrete IGHL.[93] More recent interpretations of the anatomy of the shoulder have suggested an expanded definition of the ligament that includes the anteroinferior, inferior, and posteroinferior aspects of the capsule,

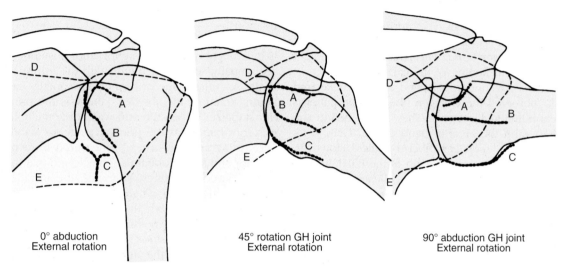

0° abduction
External rotation

45° rotation GH joint
External rotation

90° abduction GH joint
External rotation

FIGURE 6-42 Anteroposterior views of the orientation of the glenohumeral ligaments in external rotation as a function of shoulder position. *A,* Superior glenohumeral ligament. *B,* Middle glenohumeral ligament. *C,* Inferior glenohumeral ligament. *D* and *E,* The capsule. (Modified from Turkel SJ, Panio MW, Marshall JL,, Girgis FG: Stabilizing mechanisms preventing anterior dislocation of the glenohumeral joint. J Bone Joint Surg Am 63:1208-1217, 1981.)

regardless of whether discrete thickening is present (see Figs. 6-40 and 6-41).[157,160]

The origin of the IGHL consists of almost the entire anterior glenoid labrum, as can be seen on careful inspection (Fig. 6-43). The IGHL then courses laterally and

inferiorly to insert on the inferior margin of the humeral articular surface and then down and around the anatomic neck of the humerus (see Fig. 6-40). This anatomic arrangement was further studied by O'Brien and colleagues,[160] who demonstrated that the posterior-inferior

FIGURE 6-43 The inferior glenohumeral ligament inserts onto the glenoid by way of the anterior labrum; it extends more proximally than might be thought. (From Grant JCB: Method of Anatomy, 7th ed. Baltimore: Williams & Wilkins, 1965.)

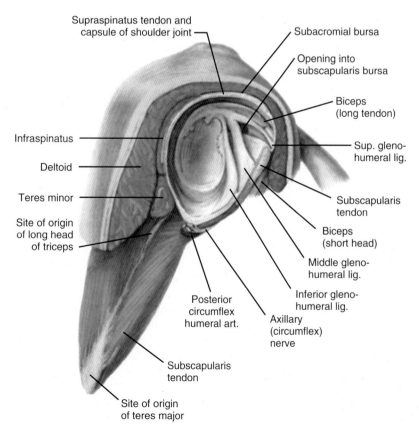

Supraspinatus tendon and capsule of shoulder joint

Subacromial bursa

Opening into subscapularis bursa

Biceps (long tendon)

Infraspinatus

Deltoid

Teres minor

Site of origin of long head of triceps

Sup. gleno-humeral lig.

Subscapularis tendon

Biceps (short head)

Middle gleno-humeral lig.

Inferior gleno-humeral lig.

Posterior circumflex humeral art.

Axillary (circumflex) nerve

Subscapularis tendon

Site of origin of teres major

portion of the capsule contains a thick band composed of dense collagen fibers, which is similar to the anterior-superior margin of the IGHL. They termed this structure the *posterior band* and the anterior-superior structure of the IGHL the *anterior band*. The posterior band might not be a discrete thickening of the capsule.[161,162]

Using microscopy under polarized light, Gohlke and associates[163] observed the collagen fiber bundle patterns of the glenohumeral ligaments. They could define the SGHL, MGHL, and the anterior band of the IGHL in all specimens from the collagen fiber bundles. However, they could define the posterior band of the IGHL in only 62.8% of specimens. Urayama and colleagues demonstrated a thickening in the innermost layer of the inferior capsule at the superior border that corresponds to the anterior band of the IGHL.[164] However, there is no such thickening of the capsule at the posteroinferior portion of the capsule that corresponds to the posterior band. The posterior band is a border between the thick inferior and thin posterior capsule rather than a localized band-like structure like the anterior band. This anatomic arrangement is consistent with emerging data suggesting a central role and function of this ligament in anterior and inferior glenohumeral instability.[89]

Function. The function of the IGHL was described by Delorme in 1910.[156] He noticed that the IGHL became taut in abduction and external rotation, whereas in adduction, the MGHL was taut. This observation was confirmed later by Moseley and Overgaard.[91] Turkel and associates[157] were the first to assess the individual function of the glenohumeral ligaments by sequential sectioning of these ligaments. They found that in 90 degrees of abduction and external rotation, the IGHL was the most important anterior stabilizer.

In a displacement control study, Blasier and colleagues[159] compared the stabilizing function of three components: the SGHL and MGHL, the IGHL, and the posterior-superior portion of the capsule. With the arm in abduction and neutral rotation, the contribution of the SGHL plus the MGHL was equal to that of the IGHL. When the arm was rotated externally, the contribution of the IGHL became more than double, whereas that of the SGHL plus the MGHL became insignificant. It is of particular interest that they pointed out the importance of the posterior-superior capsule as a secondary anterior stabilizer in both neutral and external rotation of the abducted arm.

The function of the anterior and posterior bands of the IGHL has also been studied. Jerosch and associates[144] measured the strain of the anterior and posterior bands of the IGHL and concluded that the anterior band was most tight with the arm in abduction and external rotation, whereas the posterior band was most tight with the arm in abduction and internal rotation. Debski and colleagues[165] also measured the change in length of these ligaments in various arm positions. They showed that the MGHL was the primary anterior stabilizer with the arm in adduction and neutral rotation and that the MGHL and the anterior band of the IGHL were the primary anterior stabilizers with the arm in abduction and neutral rotation.

O'Brien and coworkers[166] directly measured the stabilizing function of the anterior and posterior bands by sequentially sectioning them. With the arm in abduction in the scapular plane or further horizontally extended in neutral rotation, the anterior band was the primary anterior stabilizer. When the arm was horizontally flexed, the posterior band was the primary posterior stabilizer.

Urayama and coworkers[167] measured the strain of the anterior and posterior bands. They found that the anterior band showed the highest strain with the arm in abduction and external rotation, whereas the posterior band showed the highest strain with the arm in flexion and internal rotation. They also measured the strain of the axillary pouch (6-o'clock position) and found that it was an anterior stabilizer with the arm in abduction and external rotation. This biomechanical observation is supported by a clinical finding that 76% of the Bankart lesion extends posteriorly over the axillary pouch.[168]

In terms of posterior stability, Naggar and associates[169] demonstrated that the inferior-posterior portion of the capsule was the primary posterior restraint with the arm in flexion and internal rotation, whereas the superior-posterior portion was the primary posterior restraint in flexion and external rotation. From these studies, the posterior band or the posterior-inferior portion of the capsule seems to be the primary posterior stabilizer with the arm in flexion and internal rotation, which is known to be the position of posterior apprehension.

The entire inferior capsule has traditionally been recognized as one of the contributing factors to limiting elevation of the arm.[18,50,170] The structure also becomes taut with internal or external rotation of the dependent humerus.[157] Release of the IGHL has been further demonstrated to allow anterior and inferior subluxation in an experimental model.[155] A study using a capsular-shrinkage cadaveric model showed that there was a constant relationship between the reduction of a given movement and the area of capsular shrinkage.[64] However, the greatest amount of inferior translation occurs only when the superior-posterior portion of the capsule is also released. Similar observations were made by Ovesen and Nielsen, who studied the entire glenohumeral complex as a unit. Increased anterior translation occurred with posterior capsular release (Fig. 6-44).[171] Conversely, posterior translation was shown to increase with sectioning of the anterior capsule. The overall displacement patterns increased with inferior capsular release.

These observations also pertain to posterior translation of the humeral head.[155,171] Release of the anterior structures increases posterior rotation and translation of the humeral head. The patterns described relate to translation in the neutral position. Different results would be expected if the arm were fully internally or externally rotated.

In summary, the major static stabilizer of the shoulder joint consists of the capsuloligamentous complex, with

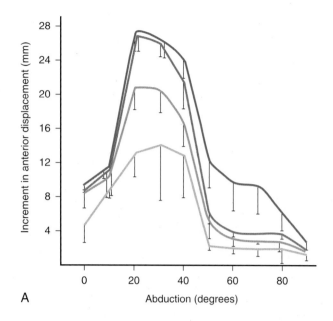

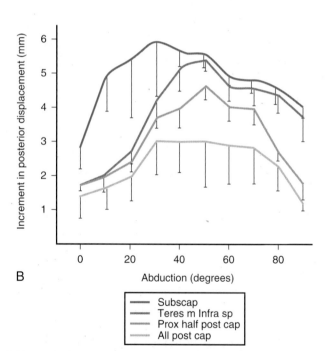

——	Subscap
——	Teres m Infra sp
——	Prox half post cap
——	All post cap

FIGURE 6-44 Contribution of the muscle and the capsule to abduction. Incremental anterior (**A**) and posterior (**B**) displacement of the humeral head in millimeters as a function of serial release of the constraints on glenohumeral joint motion. (Redrawn from Ovesen J, Nielsen S: Anterior and posterior shoulder instability. Acta Orthop Scand 57:324-327, 1986.)

their presence and secondarily by imparting increased joint contact pressure opposite the direction of displacement, which also increases joint stability (see Fig. 6-41).[31]

Dynamic Stabilizers

The suspensory stabilizing function of active or passive muscle activity of the shoulder girdle is surprisingly minimal under resting conditions.[172] Electromyographic (EMG) studies have revealed inactivity of the deltoid, pectoralis major, serratus anterior, and latissimus dorsi muscles when the arm is hanging freely at the side. Subsequent investigations have shown no or minimal EMG activity even when the upper extremity is loaded up to 11 kg.[173] These findings are in concert with and give further credence to the previously discussed theories that negative pressure and the articular ligamentous constraints resist inferior subluxation of the humeral head.

Dynamic shoulder stability during activity occurs by action of the shoulder musculature. The contribution of the cuff muscles to joint stability may be due to passive muscle tension from the bulk effect of the muscle,[63,120,140,174] contraction causing compression of the articular surfaces (concavity-compression effect), joint motion that secondarily tightens the passive ligamentous constraints, or the barrier effect of the contracted muscles.

Mechanisms of Stabilization by Muscles
Passive Muscle Tension
The passive role played by muscle bulk in joint stability is demonstrated by the increased passive arc of motion when the muscle is removed.[63,170] Howell and Kraft demonstrated that when the supraspinatus and infraspinatus were paralyzed by a suprascapular nerve block, normal kinematics were retained in 45 of 47 shoulders.[94] Active contraction of these muscles is not necessary to maintain ball-and-socket kinematics. Ovesen and Nielsen have shown increased translation, both anteriorly and posteriorly, with shoulder muscle release in cadaver specimens (Fig. 6-45).[171] Kumar and Balasubramaniam have shown greater inferior translation as a result of the effect of gravity when the muscles are removed in a cadaver preparation.[120] Motzkin and associates[174] demonstrated that removal of the skin, subcutaneous tissue, and deltoid did not affect inferior translation of the humeral head both in adduction and in abduction, as long as intraarticular pressure was intact. Judging from these results and the results of EMG studies, the bulk effect of these muscles seems to be minimal.

Compression of the Articular Surface (Concavity-Compression Effect)
By simulating active rotator cuff muscle function, an elaborate cadaver experiment has demonstrated that the humeral head is positioned in the center of the glenoid in the horizontal plane.[94] This stabilizing effect may be largely independent of the specific simulated muscle

the IGHL being the most essential component of the complex. Yet, the function of the other components must not be overlooked; hence the concept of *load sharing* of the soft tissue constraints. This concept states that ligaments function in a coordinated manner to resist joint translation, primarily by resisting displacement through

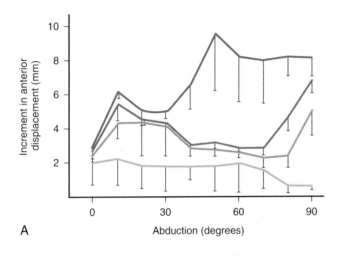

A

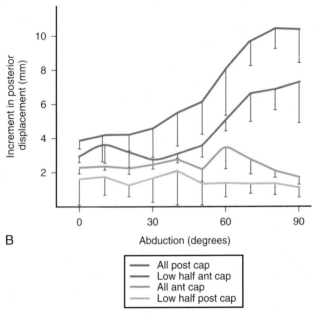

B

Legend:
- All post cap
- Low half ant cap
- All ant cap
- Low half post cap

FIGURE 6-45 Contribution of the capsule to anterior (**A**) and posterior (**B**) translation of the shoulder joint with serial constraint release as a function of glenohumeral position. Removal of the muscle envelope increases the possible displacement. (Redrawn from Ovesen J, Nielsen S: Anterior and posterior shoulder instability. Acta Orthop Scand 57:324-327, 1986.)

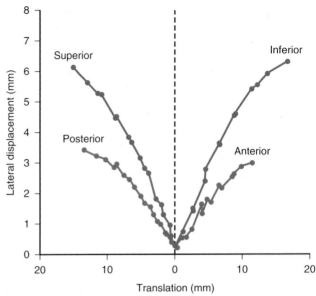

FIGURE 6-46 Lateral displacement of the center of the humeral head necessary for translation to the lip of the glenoid in four different directions (glenoidogram). The glenoid depth for the humeral head to override is much greater in the superior and inferior direction than in the anterior and posterior direction. (Redrawn from Matsen FA III, Lippitt SB, Sidles JA, Harryman DT II: Practical Evaluation and Management of the Shoulder. Philadelphia: WB Saunders, 1994.)

action. Even with unequal (unbalanced) simulated activity of the anterior and posterior cuff musculature, the function of the active cuff still brings about the centering phenomenon. McMahon and colleagues[175] demonstrated in a cadaveric study that humeral head translation was less than 2 mm with and without supraspinatus force. Thus, it has been hypothesized that the centering effect of the humeral head in the glenoid is possible without balanced muscle activity and that the contact area and pressure are mediated by secondary obligatory tightening of the ligaments.

However, some investigators put more emphasis on the function of cuff muscles. Wuelker and colleagues,[76] using cadaver shoulders with simulated constant muscle force to the deltoid and cuff muscles, demonstrated that translation of the humeral head between 20 and 90 degrees of elevation averaged 9 mm superiorly and 4.4 mm anteriorly. Hsu and coworkers[176] observed the shift of the humeral head in a tendon-defective model. They evaluated the stability of the shoulder in three different directions (anterior, posterior, and inferior) with the arm in four different positions (hanging position, flexion, abduction, and abduction–external rotation). Cuff defect was created either anteriorly or superiorly in two different sizes. They found that with the muscles loaded, a large and more anteriorly located defect had the most influence on stability.

The glenoid has a concavity on its articular surface. When the humeral head is compressed against this concavity, the head needs a certain amount of force to override the rim of the glenoid to dislocate. The path of the center of the humeral head when it is translated away from the center of the glenoid is shown in a glenoidogram (Fig. 6-46).[177] The humeral head must be translated laterally to override the glenoid rim, and this translation is resisted by the compressive force applied to the humeral head against the glenoid. The greater the compressive force, the greater the resistance to lateral translation of the humeral head. This stabilization created by the glenoid concavity and the compressive force of the muscles is the *concavity-compression effect.*[177] This stabilizing mechanism is related to the depth of the glenoid and the magnitude of compressive force.

Dynamic Elements Causing Secondary Tightening of Static Constraints

Dempster has pointed out that the supraspinatus muscle simultaneously elevates and externally rotates the arm.[1] As previously shown, external rotation tightens the inferior ligament and thus limits upward elevation. Thus, the cuff musculature rotates the shoulder to a configuration rendered stable, at least in part, by tightening of the ligaments in the direction opposite the rotation (see Fig. 6-41).[1,31,50]

Barrier Effect

The damping effect of the shoulder musculature during active motion and the subsequent limitation in the active arc of motion have long been recognized.[50] Classically, the subscapularis muscle has been shown to be important, if not essential, as an anterior barrier to resist anterior-inferior humeral head displacement. When the subscapularis is lax or stretched, recurrent anterior dislocation occurs; hence, several procedures have been directed toward restoring or strengthening the barrier effect of the subscapularis.[93,178] Furthermore, the cross-sectional areas of the anterior (subscapularis) and posterior (infraspinatus and teres minor) rotators are approximately equal.[179] Therefore, the torques generated by these groups are balanced and represent a force couple that resists both anterior and posterior humeral head translation.

Rotator Cuff
Passive Muscle Tension

The subscapularis muscle was thought to be important as an anterior barrier to resist anterior dislocation of the humeral head.[93,178] However, Turkel and associates,[157] who observed a change in external rotation after sectioning the subscapularis tendon, concluded that the passive muscle tension of the subscapularis was the primary anterior stabilizer at 0 and 45 degrees of abduction, but not at 90 degrees of abduction, at which angle the IGHL played the most important role. Tuoheti and colleagues have demonstrated that the subscapularis tendon undergoes an 18.7% decrease in thickness and a 29.1% decrease in cross-sectional area in shoulders with recurrent anterior dislocation compared with normal controls.[180] These changes may be the result of recurrent dislocations, but once the subscapularis tendon is stretched and lax, it may better be strengthened.[93,178] Shortening of the subscapularis tendon, however, is not commonly performed these days because of poor outcome.[181]

Posterior stability is also provided by passive muscle tension of the rotator cuff. In their consecutive studies,

Ovesen and colleagues demonstrated that both the supraspinatus and the infraspinatus and teres minor were important in stabilizing the shoulder posteriorly.[171,182,183]

Inferior stability and the passive muscle tension of the cuff were investigated by Motzkin and coworkers.[184] They elevated the supraspinatus and the other cuff muscles in different orders and measured the displacement of the humeral head. Because no significant effect was observed after removing the cuff muscles, the static contribution of these muscles to inferior stability seems to be insignificant.

Dynamic Contraction

Basmajian and Bazant[47] reported the importance of the supraspinatus as an inferior stabilizer, and DePalma and associates[93] emphasized that the subscapularis was the most important anterior stabilizer. Saha[48] introduced the concept of a force couple provided by the anterior and posterior cuff muscles. The EMG study showed that both the subscapularis and infraspinatus contracted during the mid range of elevation to provide stability to the shoulder joint.

Glousman and colleagues[185] investigated the EMG activity of the shoulder muscles during throwing motion in stable and unstable shoulders. The EMG activity of the supraspinatus and the biceps increased in anteriorly unstable shoulders. These muscles might have compensated for the anterior instability during throwing motion. Kronberg and associates[186] observed increased EMG activity in the subscapularis and supraspinatus in patients with generalized joint laxity. Increased activity of these muscles likely compensates for the shoulder instability. Chen and coworkers demonstrated that muscle exercises of the deltoid and rotator cuff caused inferior migration of the humeral head at the resting position and superior migration during arm elevation in healthy subjects.[187] This finding indicates that muscle fatigue has an intimate relationship with superior-to-inferior stability of the humeral head.

However, some investigators do not think that the cuff is an important stabilizer. Howell and Kraft[94] performed a suprascapular nerve block in patients with recurrent anterior instability and labral defects. They concluded that a balanced muscle envelope was not necessary to maintain centering of the humerus on the glenoid.

Several in vitro studies have been carried out to clarify the stabilizing function of each of the rotator cuff muscles. Cain and associates[188] applied constant loads to the cuff muscles and measured the strain of the IGHL in the position simulating the cocking phase of throwing. The result showed that the infraspinatus and teres minor were most effective in controlling external rotation of the humerus and in reducing ligamentous strain. Using the same dynamic model, McKernan and associates applied maximal physiologic loads to the rotator cuff muscles.[189] The results revealed that the subscapularis is of primary importance in stabilizing the shoulder anteriorly with the arm in abduction and neutral rotation but becomes less important with external rotation, at which point the posterior cuff muscles become more important. Blasier and colleagues, in a displacement control study, demonstrated that the supraspinatus, infraspinatus and teres minor, and subscapularis equally contributed to anterior stability of the abducted shoulder with the arm both in neutral and in external rotation.[159]

Newman applied both constant and physiologic loads to the rotator cuff muscles and measured anterior displacement of the humeral head with an electromagnetic tracking device.[190] Under constant loading to the cuff, the supraspinatus and infraspinatus were equally important in stable shoulders, whereas the supraspinatus was more important than the other muscles in shoulders with a Bankart lesion. Under physiologic loading, the supraspinatus and infraspinatus were also equally important in stable shoulders, but no significant difference was seen among the rotator cuff muscles in unstable shoulders. However, Hsu and associates observed increased instability after changing the muscle force balance of the rotator cuff, thus suggesting the importance of muscle balance.[191]

In general, the stabilizing function of these muscles depends on the force generated by each muscle and the relative importance of each muscle to the force generated by the entire muscle complex around the shoulder. Lee and colleagues measured the force vector components created by the cuff muscles,[192] as well as the dynamic stability provided by these muscles. The dynamic stability index, a new biomechanical parameter reflecting the shear force component and the compressive force component associated with the concavity-compression mechanism, was defined and calculated. In the midrange, the supraspinatus and the subscapularis provided more stability than the other muscles did. In the end range, the subscapularis, infraspinatus, and teres minor provided more stability than the supraspinatus (Fig. 6-47). They concluded that the rotator cuff muscles provided substantial anterior dynamic stability in the end range of motion as well as in the midrange.

In the superior direction, Halder and coauthors reported that the latissimus dorsi was the most efficient superior stabilizer, followed by the teres major and the subscapularis.[193] The supraspinatus was proved to be less important as a superior stabilizer than previously thought. In vivo contraction of these muscles during various motions and movements needs to be investigated.

Biceps

The LHB has been known to be a depressor of the humeral head.[20,77,194] During arthroscopy, Andrews and associates[195] observed that when the LHB was electrically stimulated, the humeral head was compressed against the glenoid fossa. They speculated that the biceps might contribute to shoulder stability. Habermeyer and coworkers[196] concluded from an EMG study that the effectiveness of the LHB as a stabilizer was greatest in external rotation and least in internal rotation. Glousman and associates[185] observed increased activity of the biceps in throwers with anterior shoulder instability, which suggests the possibility of the biceps as a stabilizer.

In the research field, Rodosky and colleagues[197] simulated a SLAP lesion by detaching the superior labrum along with the origin of the LHB from the superior glenoid rim. With the SLAP lesion, torsional rigidity with the arm in abduction and external rotation decreased 10% in comparison to the normal shoulder. This observation can be interpreted as showing that damage to the superior labrum sacrifices anterior stability of the shoulder directly or by reducing a possible stabilizing function of the LHB. Rodosky and associates[198] further investigated the relationship between torsional rigidity and LHB force and found that torsional rigidity increased and IGHL strain decreased with LHB

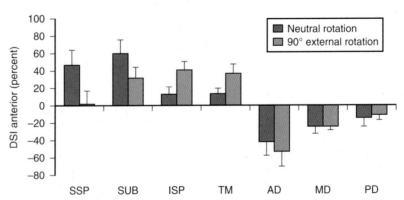

FIGURE 6-47 Mean and standard deviation of the dynamic stability index (DSI) in the anterior direction (percentage compressive force times the stability ratio of 0.35 minus the percentage anterior shear force). Significant differences were found for all four rotator cuff muscles and the three heads of the deltoid muscle when the humerus was in the mid range of motion and the end range of motion. AD, anterior deltoid; ISP, infraspinatus; MD, middle deltoid; PD, posterior deltoid; SSP, supraspinatus; SUB, subscapularis; TM, teres minor. (Redrawn from Lee SB, An KN: Dynamic glenohumeral stability provided by three heads of the deltoid muscle. Clin Orthop Relat Res [400]:40-77, 2002.)

loading. Judging from these results, the LHB seems to contribute to anterior stability of the shoulder by increasing torsional rigidity.

More direct observation of the stabilizing function of the LHB was carried out by Itoi and associates.[199] They measured displacement of the humeral head under a constant translation force in various directions in the hanging arm position with and without loads to the LHB. The results showed that the LHB significantly stabilized the shoulder in the anterior, inferior, and posterior directions. Further study[32] revealed that the LHB in conjunction with the short head of the biceps stabilizes the shoulder anteriorly with the arm in abduction and external rotation. In a displacement control study, Blasier and colleagues[200] also reported the importance of the LHB in anterior stabilization of the abducted shoulder.

Pagnani and coworkers[201] observed that anterior and inferior displacement of the humeral head under constant loading to the LHB increased after creating a SLAP lesion. They thought that one of the mechanisms of destabilization was less-efficient stabilization by the LHB as a result of a lax labrum and elongated tendon of the LHB. This mechanism suggests that a superior labral lesion might result in instability, although this finding was not confirmed in clinical studies.[202]

Levy and colleagues have reported that they did not observe any EMG activity in the biceps during activities of daily living.[203] They concluded that any hypothesis on bicipital function must be based on either a passive role or tension. However, Kim and associates reported that in abduction and external rotation, the EMG activity of the biceps increased in shoulders with recurrent anterior dislocation but did not increase in those without such dislocation.[204] This result indicates that the biceps functions as an anterior stabilizer not in normal shoulders but in shoulders with anterior instability.

Classically, the rotator cuff muscles have been thought to be the most important dynamic stabilizers of the shoulder. Is the biceps as important as the cuff muscles? In a cadaveric study comparing the biceps and the rotator cuff, Itoi and associates[205] observed that in stable shoulders, the biceps was as efficient as the supraspinatus and the infraspinatus and teres minor as a stabilizer. However, the biceps became more important than any of the cuff muscles when the shoulder was unstable. This observation does not mean that the biceps is the most important stabilizer of all because they assessed and compared the individual function of each.

With in vivo stabilization, these muscles work together in various combinations that are not easy to simulate in experimental studies. When the rotator cuff is deficient, active contraction of the biceps prevents superior migration of the humeral head, thus making the kinematics of the glenohumeral joint almost normal.[206] Such biceps contraction produces less impingement between the acromion and the rotator cuff and, as a result, less pain during arm elevation. This finding was also confirmed in cadaveric shoulders by Payne and coworkers, who demonstrated that loading the biceps decreased 10% of the subacromial impingement pressure.[207]

In cuff-deficient shoulders, hypertrophy of the long head of the biceps is often observed. Cross-sectional area is significantly increased in shoulders with rotator cuff tears at the entrance to the bicipital groove compared with those with intact cuffs, whereas the cross-sectional area of the muscle of the long head of the biceps showed no significant difference between those with and without rotator cuff tears.[208] Therefore, hypertrophy of the tendon seems to be the result of localized pathologies such as subacromial impingement rather than the result of compensatory overuse and hypertrophy of the muscle.

Deltoid

The deltoid is a large bulky muscle that accounts for approximately 20% of the shoulder muscles.[179] Thus, the function of the deltoid as a stabilizer is thought to be significant. However, little has been studied about the stabilizing function of this muscle.

Motzkin and associates[174] investigated the static contribution of the deltoid to inferior stability of the shoulder in adduction and abduction of the arm. Because humeral head displacement did not change significantly after removal of the deltoid, they concluded that the passive muscle tension of the deltoid was insignificant in stabilizing the shoulder inferiorly.

Michiels and Bodem[209] carried out an EMG examination of the activity of five different regions of the deltoid muscle during abduction and adduction in various body postures. The results showed that the action of the deltoid was highly differentiated in its different regions and was not restricted solely to generating an abducting moment in the shoulder joint. They mentioned that the spinal and clavicular regions of the deltoid contributed to stabilization of the glenohumeral joint, although this statement was not proved.

Lee and An measured the contribution of the deltoid to shoulder stability by using the dynamic stability ratio.[210] They demonstrated that the deltoid provided dynamic stability in the scapular plane, but not in the coronal plane.

Kido and colleagues demonstrated the stabilizing function of the deltoid more directly in cadaveric shoulders.[211] They concluded that the deltoid was an anterior stabilizer of the glenohumeral joint with the arm in abduction and external rotation and that this function took on more importance as the shoulder became unstable.

The origin of the middle portion of the deltoid is the acromion. Nyffeler and colleagues[212] reported that a large lateral extension of the acromion is associated with full-thickness tears of the rotator cuff. In shoulders with the acromion extending laterally, the deltoid is located more vertically and the resultant force of the deltoid is oriented more superiorly, which can cause superior migration of the humerus and mechanical impingement of the cuff. On the other hand, in shoulders with the acromion located more medially, the resultant force of the deltoid is oriented more medially and helps to stabilize the humeral head. Thus, the deltoid could be a stabilizer or destabilzer of the humeral head depending upon its inherent orientation.

Interrelationship Between Static and Dynamic Stabilizers

Static and dynamic stabilizers do not function separately. Experimentally, Blasier and associates[200] investigated the interrelationship of these stabilizing components in cadaver shoulders. They analyzed the relative importance of the glenohumeral and coracohumeral ligaments as static stabilizers and the rotator cuff and biceps muscles as dynamic stabilizers. According to them, the dynamic stabilizers were more important when displacement of the humeral head was small, whereas the static stabilizers played a more important role in large displacement of the humeral head. This distinction is quite understandable because with a small displacement, the capsuloligamentous components are still lax and thus cannot be expected to function as stabilizers.

Debski and colleagues also compared the stabilizing function of the rotator cuff muscles and the capsule.[213] According to them, the cuff muscles and the capsule have equal function as an anterior stabilizer, but the cuff is more important as a posterior stabilizer.

Hsu and colleagues compared the cuff-defect model with the muscle-unloaded model.[214] The effect on instability of a small tendon defect was less than that of muscle unloading, but with a larger tear, the defect had a greater effect on instability than muscle-unloading because the defect involved the glenohumeral and coracohumeral ligaments in the model. Clinically, a large anterior cuff tear can involve the anterior capsuloligamentous structures and thus affect the anterior stability.

Blasier and coworkers investigated the relative contribution of the static and dynamic stabilizers in a posterior direction with the arm in 90 degrees of flexion.[215] They concluded that the IGHL was the primary posterior stabilizer with the arm in internal rotation, whereas the CHL was the primary stabilizer with the arm in neutral rotation. The subscapularis muscle plays an important role as a dynamic posterior stabilizer.

The capsuloligamentous structures detect position, motion (kinesthesia), and stretching. All these sensory modalities are transmitted from static stabilizers to dynamic stabilizers through a reflex arc. This process is called *proprioception*. Kinesthesia of the normal shoulder was investigated by Hall and McCloskey in 1983.[216] Smith and Brunolli[217] reported that kinesthesia was disturbed in shoulders with recurrent anterior dislocation.

Murakami and coworkers[218] noticed that the EMG activity of the infraspinatus muscle increased when posteriorly directed force was applied to the humerus flexed in 90 degrees. They also found mechanoreceptors in a monkey shoulder capsule. The mechanoreceptors in the human shoulder were found in the coracoacromial ligament,[150,219]

the subacromial bursa,[220] and the capsule and labrum.[221] These anatomic studies prompted Lephart and associates[222] to compare shoulders with recurrent anterior dislocation and those that underwent surgical repair in a cross-sectional study. They found that shoulders with anterior instability showed deteriorated proprioception, but that after surgical repair they showed no difference from the normal shoulders.

Zuckerman and colleagues[223] conducted a longitudinal study to measure the proprioceptive ability of shoulders with recurrent anterior instability before surgery and 6 and 12 months after repair. They observed a decreased ability to detect slow motion before the operation, which eventually returned to normal 12 months after surgical repair. Wallace and associates measured the latency between a sudden external rotation force and reaction of the muscles in shoulders with recurrent anterior dislocation.[224] They observed no significant difference between the involved and uninvolved shoulders. The defect in proprioceptive ability seems to depend on the speed of motion.

Using feline shoulders, Guanche and associates[225] demonstrated a reflex arc from mechanoreceptors within the glenohumeral joint capsule to muscles crossing the joint. Stimulation of the anterior and inferior branches of the axillary nerve caused contraction of the biceps and cuff muscles, and stimulation of the posterior branch caused contraction of the deltoid. Thus, the static and dynamic stabilizers interrelated intimately and responded to any motion or displacement unfavorable to the shoulder.

Lesions of static and dynamic stabilizers can each affect the stabilizing function of the other. According to Pouliart and Gagey,[226] the humeral head dislocates easily with less-extensive capsuloligamentous lesions when rotator cuff lesions are present. Rotator cuff lesions destabilize the glenohumeral joint. This effect is more pronounced when the capsular lesion is on the humeral side (humeral avulsion of the glenohumeral ligament [HAGL lesion]) than on the glenoid side (Bankart lesion).

Clinical Relevance

The topic of shoulder stability is covered extensively in this text, and details of the surgical procedures need not be addressed here. Suffice it to say that shoulder instability is one of the most common clinical problems. As our understanding increases and as patients' expectations expand, the problem takes on an even greater significance and complexity than was once appreciated. An articular defect regularly occurs in the humeral head after anterior dislocation, as has been recognized for more than 100 years.[22,227] Nonetheless, the articular defect of the humeral head is the result of the dislocation, not its cause. Thus, most procedures directed at altering the articular relationship have limited benefit. The exception is posterior instability or cases that relate to osseous deficiency[68,228]; in these circumstances, glenoid osteotomy or augmentation procedures may be an option (Fig. 6-48).

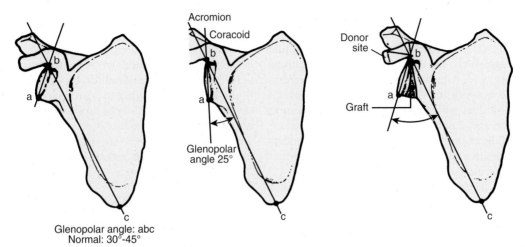

Glenopolar angle: abc
Normal: 30°-45°

FIGURE 6-48 Glenoid osteotomy is the acceptable clinical option for posterior instability but not for typical anterior instability problems. *Left,* Normal glenoid with the glenopolar angle ranging between 30 and 45 degrees. *Center,* Glenoid dysplasia with a decreased glenopolar angle. *Right,* After glenoid osteotomy with an increased glenopolar angle. a, inferior glenoid tubercle; b, superior glenoid tubercle; c, inferior angle of the scapula. (Modified from Bestard EA, Schvene HR, Bestard EH: Glenoplasty in the management of recurrent shoulder dislocation. Contemp Orthop 12:47, 1986.)

However, the significance of these capsular mechanisms has probably not been fully appreciated.[23,89] It is possible that more careful observation will confirm the anterior or anteroposterior capsuloligamentous complex as important in resisting posteroinferior shoulder dislocation.[23]

Muscle-tightening procedures effectively improve stability by intentionally limiting range of motion. Such procedures cause a functional limitation that is no longer an accepted clinical goal. Biomechanical data have clarified the central role of the IGHL complex in providing shoulder stability. With the recognition that this ligament inserts or attaches to the glenoid via the labrum, a rationale is provided for the observation of Bankart lesions and for the more popular current procedures—that is, those directed at restoring capsuloligamentous integrity

(Fig. 6-49).[83,89,101,140,171,229-235] This knowledge now allows restoration of stability and preservation of motion.

Classically, capsular tensile load was less than 20 kg.[128] Investigation by Bigliani and associates[161] revealed that the mean tensile strength of the three portions of the IGHL was 5.5 MPa. The force necessary to rupture the whole ligament complex is calculated to be less than 50 kg (~47 kg). Correlation of the biomechanical data and the anterior shear force from muscle contraction (42 kg)[129] might help explain the spontaneous dislocation seen after some seizure episodes.

A single dislocation stretches the IGHL up to 7.23% until failure occurs[236]; such dislocation produces a permanent deformation averaging 2.3 mm (2.4%).[237] Repetitive subfailure strains on the IGHL cause more permanent

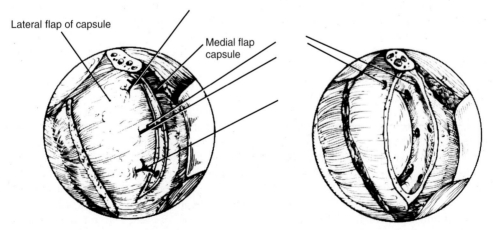

FIGURE 6-49 Anterior capsuloplasty provides excellent clinical results and has a sound rationale based on the biomechanics of this joint. *Left,* A Bankart lesion (detachment of the capsulolabral complex from the glenoid rim) before repair. There are three holes at the rim of the glenoid and one suture passing through the most superior hole of the glenoid. *Right,* After repair. The Bankart lesion is repaired by three sutures. The medial and lateral flaps are also tightly sutured. (From Rowe CR, Patel D, Southmayd WE: The Bankart procedure: A long-term end-result study. J Bone Joint Surg Am 60:1-16, 1978.)

elongation (4.6%-7.1%).[238] Habermeyer and colleagues[239] measured the joint volume of shoulders with and without dislocations. They observed that the joint volume increased progressively as the number of dislocations increased up to five. Urayama and coworkers demonstrated that the anterior-inferior and inferior portions of capsules of shoulders with recurrent anterior dislocation showed an average capsular elongation of 19% when compared with the contralateral shoulder.[240] These reports suggest that measures to reduce this permanent deformation may be necessary during a Bankart procedure.

Molina and colleagues demonstrated in a dislocation model of cadaveric shoulders that the amount of capsular shortening required to return to a stable shoulder was between 16 and 18 mm.[241] However, Novotny and associates[242] demonstrated in cadaveric shoulders that external rotation and extension were significantly reduced after the Bankart repair, thus suggesting that loss of motion during the cocking phase can occur after the Bankart repair. From these studies, the decision to imbricate the capsule during a Bankart procedure needs to be made carefully.

The stabilizing effect of negative pressure in the shoulder is not well recognized, but possibly it helps explain the often-observed phenomenon of inferior humeral head subluxation after proximal humerus fractures (Fig. 6-50). Although this finding has traditionally been thought to be related to muscle atony, this explanation is not supported by the EMG data, which demonstrate a limited role of active muscle contracture in resisting downward displacement of the humeral head. On the other hand, the stabilizing effect of negative pressure, which is lost when a fracture tears the capsule, does provide at least one possible explanation for this phenomenon.

MUSCLE AND JOINT FORCES

Forces across the glenohumeral joint are considered in three parts: the general and specific role of the muscles crossing the joint, idealized calculation of the glenohumeral forces, and the maximal strength characteristics for each motion function.

General Observations

Understanding muscle function with regard to shoulder motion and transmission of force requires consideration of three clinically recognized characteristics of that muscle: size, orientation, and activity.

Muscle Size

The effective size of a muscle, which is related to its ability to generate force, is called the *physiologic cross section*. This parameter is not simply the area of a given muscle cross section; it is the cross section of the muscle fibers calculated by measuring the volume of the muscle and dividing by fiber length. Calculation of this variable is a tedious task because of the difficulty in determining the fiber length of different types of muscles and in accurately demonstrating muscle volume.[243] Nevertheless, it has been performed by several investigators (Table 6-2).[179,244] The proportional force per cross-sectional area of the muscle generating the force has been discussed by several authors but is not known with certainty.[3,245,246] Although estimates have varied considerably from 10 N/cm^2 to 243 N/cm^2,[247-251] our experience in evaluation of muscle force supports values of about 90 N/cm^2.[247]

Orientation

Accurate and precise definition of the orientation of each muscle is an essential variable in determining the forces that act on the shoulder in a given position. However, orientation of shoulder muscles is very difficult to define accurately. Because of the great amount of motion present and because the line of action often crosses close to the axis of rotation, some muscles change their function depending on the position of the joint.[3,14,54,252-254] Hence, the straight-line technique connecting the origin and insertion is only a first estimate that just approximates the effective moment of the muscle for a given position.[3] A more accurate determination consists of calculating the centroid of successive cross-sectional areas of the muscle as it crosses the joint. By connecting these centroids, the orientation and lever arm of the muscle can be accurately determined at a given position (Fig. 6-51).[179] The limitation of this particular technique is that only a single position of the shoulder can be studied for a given specimen.[255]

The effective lever arm of the shoulder muscles and the orientation of the muscle to the glenoid surface have been calculated for different positions by Poppen and Walker with the use of radiographic techniques (Fig. 6-52).[256] A similar technique was used by Howell and colleagues.[53]

The moment arm may be analytically estimated by knowing the excursion of the muscle and the arc of motion that this muscle imparts, as well as the load required for the activity.[257,258] Kuechle and associates[252] measured the moment arms of shoulder muscles with a potentiometer (Fig. 6-53). Overall, during elevation, the anterior deltoid, middle deltoid, and supraspinatus have the largest agonist moment arm. Conversely, the teres major, latissimus dorsi, and pectoralis major tendons were found to have the greatest antagonist or depressor moment arms. The infraspinatus, subscapularis, and posterior deltoid had biphasic function in that they acted as either an elevator or a depressor, depending on joint position.

Regarding rotation, it is well known that the subscapularis is an internal rotator, whereas the infraspinatus and teres minor are external rotators. Kuechle and associates[253] also demonstrated, using the same technique, that the supraspinatus is a weak external rotator with the arm in adduction. Decrease in external rotation strength observed in patients with isolated tears of the supraspinatus tendon may be explained by this finding.

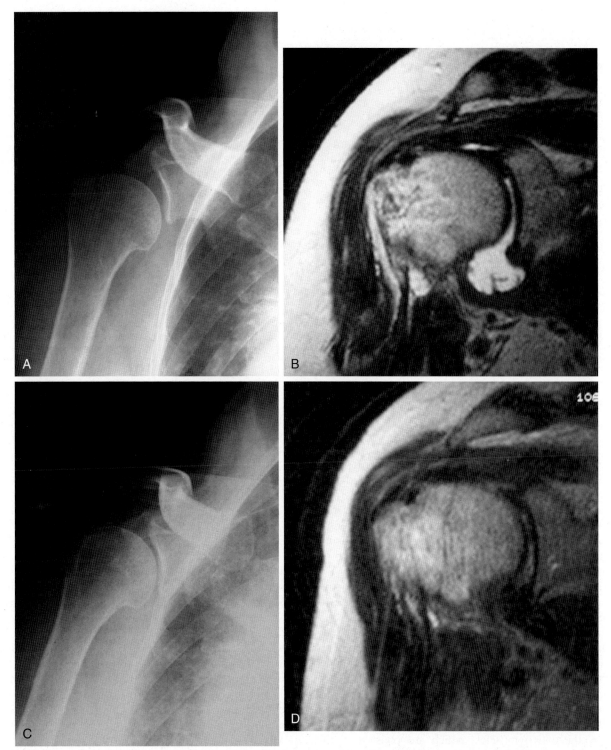

FIGURE 6-50 Transient inferior subluxation of the shoulder after fracture of the greater tuberosity. **A,** Inferior subluxation is observed on a plain x-ray taken on the day of the injury. **B,** Magnetic resonance imaging (MRI) shows a significant amount of joint effusion. **C,** Four weeks after the injury, the humeral head is reduced. **D,** Four weeks after the injury, joint effusion disappeared on MRI. This transient subluxation seems to be related to loss of the hydrostatic pressure of the shoulder joint.

TABLE 6-2 Cross-Sectional Area and Percentage Contribution of Muscles Crossing the Shoulder Joint

Muscle	Area Contribution	
	Mean (cm²)	%
Biceps (long head)	2.01	1.9
Biceps (short head)	2.11	2.0
Coracobrachialis	1.60	1.6
Deltoid	18.17	17.7
Deltoid posterior	5.00	4.9
Infraspinatus and teres minor	13.74	13.4
Latissimus dorsi	12.00	11.7
Pectoralis major	13.34	13.0
Subscapularis	16.30	15.9
Supraspinatus	5.72	5.6
Teres major	8.77	8.5
Triceps (long head)	2.96	3.8

Data from Bassett RW, Browne AO, Morrey BF, An KN: Glenohumeral muscle force and moment mechanics in a position of shoulder instability. J Biomech 23:405-415, 1990

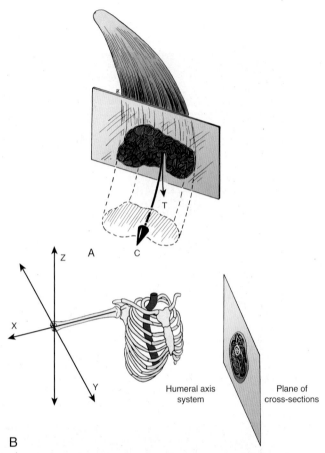

FIGURE 6-51 Cross-sectional studies of muscles allow an estimate of the force contributed by that muscle. **A,** The centroid estimates the location (*C*) and the size and magnitude (*T*) of the force. **B,** The technique is limited by allowing study of a single position per specimen.

Activity

The final variable required to calculate joint force is whether a specific muscle is active during a given function and, if so, the degree of activity at a given joint position. A technique to determine these data for all 26 muscles does not exist. The muscles responsible for shoulder motion were first systematically defined by Duchenne through the use of galvanic stimulation.[259] These early efforts to define which muscles are active for given positions have been refined by EMG studies.[3,154,173,186,260,261]

These studies have demonstrated the important relationship of the integrated activity of the supraspinatus and deltoid muscles (Fig. 6-54).[154,262] This integrated activity is the best-known and most important relationship for active shoulder motion. (In addition to the deltoid and supraspinatus, the rotator cuff musculature is responsible for effective arm elevation.) Although this motion is initiated by these two muscles, which are considered the primary elevators of the glenohumeral joint, their action is made possible by the stabilizing effect of the subscapularis, teres minor, and infraspinatus.[254]

Although both muscles are active in arm elevation, their specific role is debated. The classic functional relationship has been described by Bechtol (Fig. 6-55).[263] Absence of the deltoid causes a uniform decrease in abduction strength that is independent of joint position. Absence of the rotator cuff, on the other hand, allows almost normal initial abduction strength but a rapid drop-off at elevations greater than 30 degrees.

This classic and popularly held relationship has been reassessed. Using dynamometer data and careful dissection to accurately define the physiologic cross-sectional area of the muscles, Howell and coworkers studied abduction torque in subjects who had axillary or supraspinatus nerve palsy that was induced by lidocaine.[255] Contrary to popular clinical belief, both the supraspinatus and the deltoid muscles were found to be equally responsible for generating torque during arm flexion and abduction (Fig. 6-56). Care must be taken to avoid direct clinical correlation inasmuch as Peat and Grahame[262] have shown that the EMG pattern of a muscle is altered in a diseased or pathologic state (Fig. 6-57). The accuracy of the data of Howell and colleagues has been confirmed by additional experimental studies and by the clinical experience

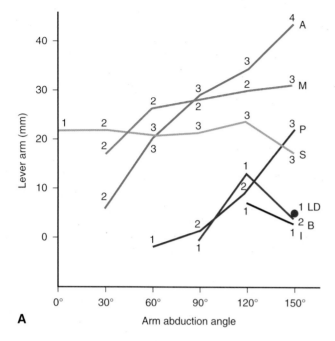

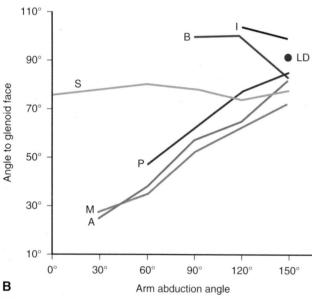

FIGURE 6-52 The moment arm of some of the essential shoulder muscles across the glenohumeral joint. **A,** Change of moment arms (lever arms) with the change of abduction. **B,** Change of orientation of muscle contraction force with the change of abduction. A, anterior deltoid; B, subscapularis; I, infraspinatus; LD, latissimus dorsi; M, middle deltoid; P, posterior deltoid; S, supraspinatus. 1-4, level of muscle activity on electromyogram **(A)**. (Redrawn from Poppen NK, Walker PS: Forces at the glenohumeral joint in abduction. Clin Orthop 135:165-170, 1978.)

of Markhede and associates, who demonstrated surprisingly good function in five patients after deltoid muscle resection.[2,264]

In a cadaveric study, Wuelker and coworkers[76] showed that elimination of supraspinatus force can be compen-

sated by deltoid force, which is one third of the supraspinatus force. Thus, they concluded that the supraspinatus is a less-efficient elevator than the deltoid is. They also found that inferior cuff muscles such as the infraspinatus and teres minor function as depressors, which was confirmed by other investigators.[265]

Thompson and colleagues demonstrated in cadaveric shoulders that paralysis of the supraspinatus necessitated a 101% increase in middle deltoid force to initiate abduction, but it required only a 12% increase for full abduction.[266] Thus, the supraspinatus is an important initiator of abduction.

Itoi and associates[267] evaluated the isokinetic strength of shoulders with isolated tears of the supraspinatus. The decrease in abduction strength ranged from 19% to 33%, which seems to reflect the contribution of the supraspinatus to shoulder abduction. Of particular interest is the contribution of the infraspinatus and teres minor, which is calculated to be almost the same as that of the supraspinatus, given the fact that the deltoid contribution is approximately 50%.

The function of the infraspinatus and teres minor as an elevator has been demonstrated in an experimental study by Sharkey and associates.[268] These investigators showed that the deltoid force needed to elevate the arm decreased to 72% in combination with the supraspinatus force, decreased to 64% when combined with the infraspinatus and teres minor force, and decreased to 41% when all the cuff muscle forces were involved. Even inferiorly positioned cuff muscles function to abduct the arm. Kuechle and colleagues' data also have shown that the infraspinatus and teres minor have biphasic patterns, being an elevator during the early phase of abduction.[252]

Hence, the force-generating activity of a muscle for a given function varies according to its physiologic cross-sectional area, joint position, external load, rate of joint motion, and so on. The impact of these variables may be condensed by further refining the EMG signal through an integration technique.[73,186,255,261] However, many technical difficulties still exist when simultaneously studying the EMG pattern of multiple muscles.[261]

Furthermore, the position of arm elevation has been determined to be the most important factor that influences the amount of shoulder muscle load.[255,269] In addition, loading at the hand produces greater EMG activity in the short rotators than in the deltoid muscle. Thus, motion of the loaded extremity is brought about by the increased activity of the cuff muscles, which stabilize the glenohumeral joint. This activity is even greater than in muscles elevating the arm: the deltoid and the supraspinatus.

Alpert and coworkers examined the EMG activity of the deltoid and rotator cuff muscles under various loading conditions and speed of elevation.[270] According to them, loading the arm increased the EMG activity of these muscles during the first 90 degrees of elevation but decreased it during the last 30 degrees. With doubling of

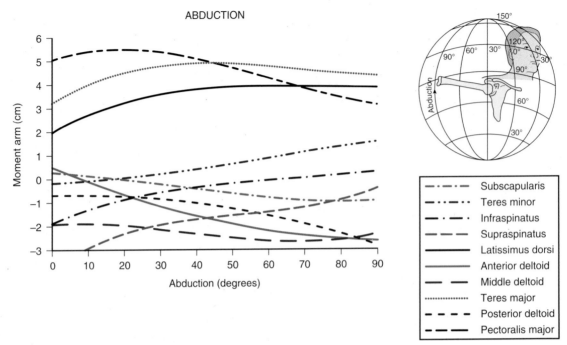

FIGURE 6-53 Moment arm of some of the essential shoulder muscles during elevation in the coronal plane. (Redrawn from Kuechle DK, Newman SR, Itoi E, et al: Shoulder muscle moment arm during horizontal flexion and elevation. J Shoulder Elbow Surg 6: 429-439, 1997.)

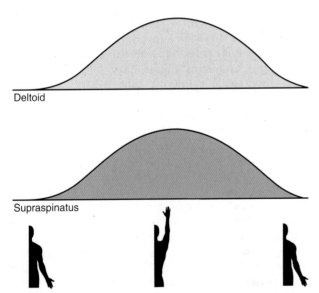

FIGURE 6-54 Simultaneous electromyographic activity of the deltoid and supraspinatus muscles during arm elevation and descent. (Modified from Basmajian JV: Muscles Alive, 2nd ed. Baltimore: Williams & Wilkins, 1967.)

the speed of elevation, EMG activity increased during the first 60 degrees and decreased during the last 60 degrees. It is interesting that both load and speed affect muscle activity during arm elevation.

Laumann has defined what he considers to be the essential shoulder muscles for arm elevation.[14] Muscles are defined as essential if the loss of any two of them renders it impossible to elevate the arm. In addition to the deltoid and supraspinatus muscles, the trapezius and serratus anterior are required for shoulder elevation. These findings are in accord with Duchenne's early studies showing that these muscles are active in concert with the deltoid during arm elevation.[259] The latter two (the serratus anterior and trapezius) are required to stabilize or move the scapula.

The activity of the biceps brachii is still controversial. Some say that it is an abductor, flexor, and external rotator,[271,272] whereas others say that it is only a supplementary muscle.[87] Yamaguchi and colleagues[87] showed that if the elbow was flexed, no significant activity of the biceps was present in either cuff-deficient or intact shoulders. However, Kido and associates measured the EMG activity of the biceps in shoulders with an intact cuff and those with rotator cuff tears and demonstrated that approximately a third of the patients with rotator cuff tears showed increased activity of the biceps during arm elevation.[273] It is likely that under certain circumstances, the biceps functions as an elevator of the arm in cuff-deficient shoulders.

Glenohumeral Force

Forces at the glenohumeral joint during arm elevation have been studied by several investigators. Inman, Saunders, and Abbott, in their classic observation on the func-

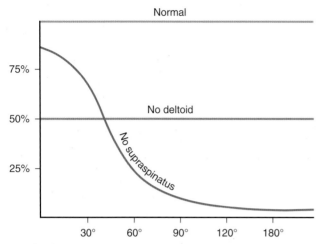

FIGURE 6-55 Classic representation of the relative contributions of the deltoid and supraspinatus muscles to arm elevation. (Redrawn from Bechtol CO: Biomechanics of the shoulder. Clin Orthop Relat Res [146]:37-41, 1980.)

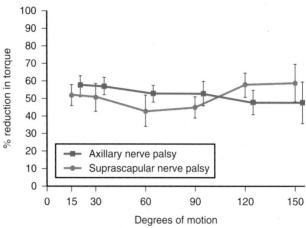

FIGURE 6-56 A nerve block study demonstrates similar contributions of both the supraspinatus and the deltoid muscles during arm forward flexion. (Redrawn from Howell SM, Imobersteg AM, Seger DH, Marone PJ: Clarification of the role of the supraspinatus muscle in shoulder function. J Bone Joint Surg Am 68:398-404, 1986.)

tion of the shoulder joint, analyzed the forces in abduction by considering the deltoid muscle force, a compressive joint force, and a resultant rotator cuff force acting parallel to the lateral border of the scapula.[3] They found a maximal compressive force of 10 times and a deltoid muscle force of 8 times the weight of the extremity at 90 degrees of arm abduction. This value is about half the body weight. They calculated a maximal resultant rotator cuff force of 9 times the weight of the extremity at 60 degrees of arm abduction (Fig. 6-58).

A simplified two-dimensional force analysis across the glenohumeral joint, similar to the model of Poppen and Walker,[256] is presented to illustrate several important concepts (Fig. 6-59). Consider the normal glenohumeral joint to be approximately a ball-and-socket joint with the center of rotation at the center of the humeral head.[274] The muscle and joint forces involved in elevation of the entire upper part of the arm in the coronal plane are analyzed. By using the glenoid surface as the reference for the coordinate system, the direction and location of

FIGURE 6-57 Alteration of the electromyographic pattern in normal persons and in those with a rotator cuff–deficient shoulder. EMG, electromyographic. (Redrawn from Peat M, Grahame RE: Electromyographic analysis of soft tissue lesions affecting shoulder function. Am J Phys Med 56:223-240, 1977.)

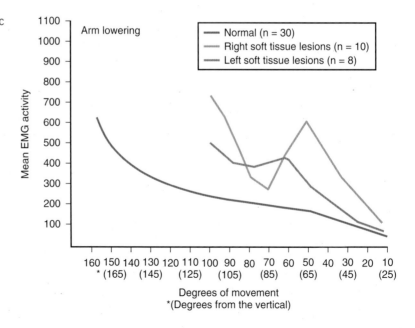

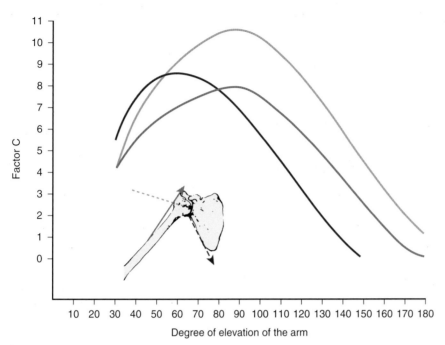

FIGURE 6-58 A simplified two-dimensional model has estimated a compression force (C) of up to about 0.5 times body weight across the joint at 90 degrees of elevation (*green line*). The deltoid force (*blue line*) is about 0.4 times body weight, and an inferior depressive force of about 0.4 times body weight (*red line*) was calculated with the formula C × weight of extremity = force required. The *red curve* shows the inferior depressive force by the infraspinatus. The *green curve* shows the compressive force. The *blue curve* shows the deltoid force.

the muscle forces and the external load on the upper part of the arm can be defined. The x-axis is perpendicular to the joint surface, and the y-axis is parallel to the glenoid surface. A weight of 0.052 body weight is applied at a point 318 mm distal to the glenohumeral joint center.[256]

Free-body analysis of the entire upper arm region, disarticulated at the glenohumeral joint, provides the force and moment equilibrium equations. Three groups of force are applied to the upper part of the arm: the weight of the arm, the muscle forces, and the reactive joint forces. The weight of the arm creates a moment around the joint, which is counterbalanced by the moment generated by the muscle forces. According to the results of EMG studies, the deltoid and supraspinatus muscles are actively involved in arm elevation.[275] Only these two groups of muscles are considered in this example. The frictional force on the joint surface is considered to be negligible, so the reactive joint force must pass through the joint center of rotation and provides no contribution to the balance of the moment. The moment equilibrium around joint center 0 can be expressed as:

$$W \times \sin(\theta_A) \times 1_W - F_d \times r_d - F_s \times r_s = 0$$

where W is the weight of the upper part of the arm (0.052 body weight), θ_A is the arm abduction angle, 1_W is the distance between the joint center and the center of mass of the upper part of the arm (318 mm), F_d is the deltoid muscle force, r_d is the moment arm of the deltoid muscle force, F_s is the supraspinatus muscle force, and r_s is the moment arm of the supraspinatus muscle force. Two force equilibrium equations can be obtained for the force components perpendicular (x) and parallel (y) to the glenoid surface:

$$W \times \sin(\theta_{GT}) + F_d \times \sin(\theta_d) + F_s \times \sin(\theta_s) - R \times \cos(\theta_R) = 0$$

$$W \times \cos(\theta_{GT}) + F_d \times \cos(\theta_d) + F_s \times \cos(\theta_s) - R \times \sin(\theta_R) = 0$$

where θ_{GT} is the glenothoracic angle, θ_d is the angle between the deltoid muscle line of action and the x-axis, θ_s is the angle between the supraspinatus muscle line of action and the x-axis, R is the reactive joint force, and θ_R is the angle between the joint force and the x-axis.

With the data provided in the literature,[3,256] the simplified muscle force and the model resultant force at the

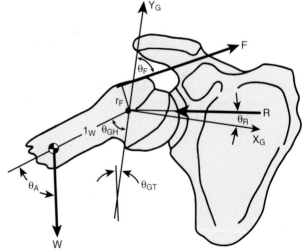

FIGURE 6-59 A more-detailed two-dimensional model representation of the forces that cross the glenohumeral joint. (Modified from Morrey BF, Chao EYS: Recurrent anterior dislocation of the shoulder. In Dumbleton J, Black JH [eds]: Clinical Biomechanics. London: Churchill Livingstone, 1981, pp 24-46.)

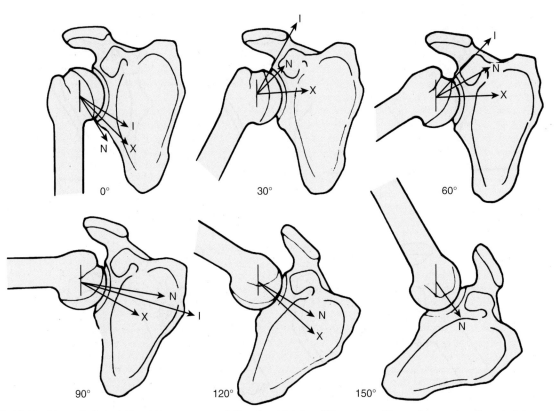

FIGURE 6-60 Position of the resultant force vector of the shoulder for different positions of arm elevation. I, internal rotation; N, neutral rotation, X, external rotation. (Modified from Poppen NK, Walker PS: Forces at the glenohumeral joint in abduction. Clin Orthop Relat Res [135]:165-170, 1978.)

glenohumeral joint could be estimated at various abduction angles. In fact, the number of unknown muscle forces is greater than the number of available equations, so the solution to the problem becomes "indeterminate." To solve such a problem, various methods based on either reducing the number of variables (as earlier) or introducing additional relationships among the unknown variables have been described.[276] An assumption was made by Poppen and Walker[256] that the muscle force was proportional to the product of the integrated EMG activity and the cross-sectional area of the muscles. The resultant joint forces at various positions of arm elevation and rotation are shown in Figure 6-60. The maximal resultant force was about 0.9 times body weight with the arm at 90 degrees of abduction. A great amount of shear force occurred between 30 and 60 degrees of arm abduction.

To further illustrate the importance of the coordinate efforts of muscle action, a more refined set of three solutions was obtained for the following circumstances. First, assume that the deltoid muscle acts alone; second, that the supraspinatus muscle acts alone; and third, that both the deltoid and supraspinatus muscles act together and the relative force generated by each muscle is proportional to its physiologic cross-sectional area.

The results of the joint reaction force expressed as a percentage of body weight and the angle of the reaction

joint force to the x-axis are illustrated in Figure 6-61A. In general, the joint reaction force is highest at about 90 degrees of arm elevation, which is simply because the largest moment generated by the weight of the upper part of the arm must be balanced by the muscle force that induces the large joint reaction force. At lower positions of arm elevation, the supraspinatus muscle has a larger moment arm and thus a greater mechanical advantage than the deltoid muscle has.[252,256] Using the supraspinatus to counterbalance the moment at this position requires less muscle force and thus less joint reaction force. When the arm is elevated at a higher position, the deltoid muscle has a greater mechanical advantage; accordingly, models that use the deltoid muscle show a lower joint force.

Because the shoulder joint is not inherently stable, the orientation and location of the joint reaction force with regard to the glenoid surface is an additional important parameter for consideration. The joint articulating pressure distribution, which is discussed in more detail later, depends not only on the available size of the articulating surface but also on the location of the joint reaction force relative to the joint surface.[277] More centrally located joint reaction forces are associated with supraspinatus activity because the relative orientation of the line of action of the supraspinatus muscle is almost perpendicular to the

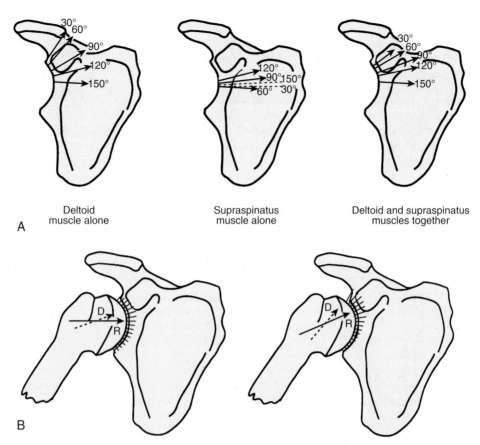

A **Deltoid muscle alone**   **Supraspinatus muscle alone**   **Deltoid and supraspinatus muscles together**

B

FIGURE 6-61 A, Direction of the magnitude of the resultant vector for different glenohumeral joint positions as a function of different muscle activity. **B,** Resultant force across the glenohumeral joint (R) as a function of arm elevation. The direction of the humeral head is attempted displacement as shown (D). When the resultant vector is directed superiorly, the humeral head tends to sublux superiorly and causes increased superior joint pressure.

surface of the glenoid joint throughout the range of arm elevation.[179,256] Hence, if the arm elevation is achieved by the supraspinatus muscle, the joint reaction force will be more or less centrally located. On the other hand, the line of action of the deltoid muscles deviates from the surface of the glenoid joint with elevation of the arm. With the arm at less than 40 degrees of abduction, the line of action is superiorly oriented and more or less parallel to the glenoid surface. The action of the deltoid muscle will therefore result in a more off-center joint reaction force at the glenoid surface.

By considering both the magnitude and the location of the joint reaction force on the glenoid surface, it is possible to explain the EMG pattern and activity of both the supraspinatus and the deltoid muscle at different positions of arm elevation.

Joint Contact Pressure

Conzen and Eckstein measured the joint contact pressure of the glenohumeral joint by using a pressure film in cadavers.[278] Maximal pressure with the arm in 90 degrees of abduction and 90 degrees of external rotation was recorded to be 5.1 MPa for single-arm weight and 10 MPa for double-arm weight. In addition, the joint contact was

more central with the arm in external rotation, thus indicating that the humeral head was not a complete sphere. On the other hand, Apreleva and associates also measured the glenohumeral contact force with a force-moment sensor.[279] The force increased during arm elevation and peaked at about 90 degrees. Moreover, they noticed that the contact force was influenced by the force ratio of the deltoid and the supraspinatus. Parsons and coworkers[280] demonstrated that the joint reaction force was affected by the integrity of the cuff muscles, especially by the transverse force couple formed by the anterior and posterior cuff muscles.

Now let us consider the problem of joint articulating or contact pressure distribution. An analytic model for determining joint pressure was established and based on mechanical consideration of the contact problem. In this model, it is assumed that the bony structures of the articulating joint are relatively rigid, so with the joint reaction force applied, the displacement or deformation takes place predominantly on the joint surface. Reaction forces between adjacent bodies are thus simulated by a series of compressive springs distributed over the possible contact surfaces between the two adjacent bodies. The capsule and ligaments are also modeled with tensile

TABLE 6-3 Maximal Isokinetic Torque of the Shoulder and Position of Occurrence as a Function of Joint Velocity in Men 20 to 40 Years Old

Angular Velocity (Deg/Sec)	Abduction		Adduction	
	Torque (N·m)	Position/Degree	Torque (N·m)	Position/Degree
60	39	27	81	75
180	32	33	73	72
300	26	45	64	74

Data from Cahalan TD, Johnson ME, Chao EYS: Shoulder strength analysis using the Cybex II isokinetic dynamometer. Clin Orthop Relat Res (271):249-257, 1991.

springs. For a given joint reaction load, a system of equations could be formulated. Displacement and force in the spring system, which describe the pressure distribution on articular surfaces, are then determined. Factors such as the available size of the contact area and the relative location of the joint reaction force on the joint surface have been found to be important determinants of not only the magnitude but also the uniformity of the contact pressure distribution.

For the glenohumeral joint, the same magnitude of the resultant joint reaction force R causes more uniform contact pressure when centrally loaded than when loaded toward the rim (see Fig. 6-61). The associated directions of the attempted humeral motion are indicated by D. It has also been hypothesized that if the direction of the attempted displacement of the rigid body is within the arc of the articular surface, the joint will be stable. On the other hand, if the direction of the attempted displacement is located beyond the articulating arc, the joint can become unstable or even dislocated (see Fig. 6-60). Based on this argument, the contribution of rotator cuff muscle

as a kind of musculotendinous glenoid acting in conjunction with the osseous glenoid to maintain humeral head stability has been proposed.[277]

Maximal Torque

The overall and relative working capacity of the shoulder was studied by the early German anatomists.[17,41] Their data revealed a balance between potential flexor and extensor torque.[17] However, internal rotation power exceeds external rotation by 2:1, and the adduction force or power exceeds that of abduction by at least 1:2.

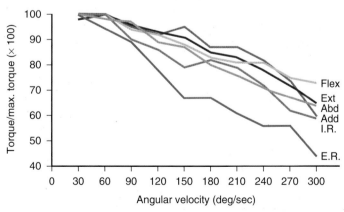

FIGURE 6-62 Torque decreases as the angular velocity of arm elevation increases for all muscle functions studied. Abd, abduction; Add, adduction; E.R., external rotation; Ext, extension; Flex, flexion; I.R., internal rotation. (Redrawn from Cahalan TD, Johnson ME, Chao EYS: Shoulder strength analysis using the Cybex II isokinetic dynamometer. Clin Orthop Relat Res [271]:249-257, 1991.)

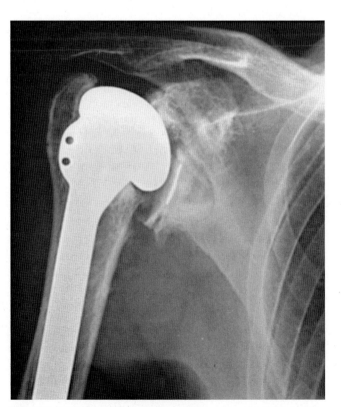

FIGURE 6-63 Glenoid-loosening patterns are consistent with increased superior forces across the glenohumeral joint, noted particularly during the first 60 degrees of elevation.

More detailed information about maximal torque is now available from data generated by the use of variable-resistance isokinetic devices. Using such a device, Ivey and Rusche demonstrated the following torque relationships: flexion-to-extension ratio, 4:5; abduction-to-adduction ratio, 1:2; and internal rotation–to–external rotation ratio, 3:2.[281] On an absolute basis, the greatest strength function is exhibited in adduction, followed by extension, flexion, abduction, internal rotation, and external rotation.[281,282] Otis and associates[283] measured isokinetic shoulder torque to determine the effects of dominance, angular velocity, and joint position. Isometric strength was always greater than isokinetic strength. Torque in each direction (flexion, abduction, internal rotation, and external rotation) was greatest when the arm was at the side, whereas it decreased with an increase in abduction.

The magnitude and position of the maximal torque generated by the shoulder muscles differ according to the strength function studied (Table 6-3). Torque data from our laboratory have revealed that the maximal torque occurs at different positions, with some variation depending on the velocity of the joint.[282] The peak torque is typically greatest at slower speeds—60 degrees per second. The maximal torque decreases for all strength functions with increasing angular test velocity (Fig. 6-62). Our data compare favorably with the relative torque values described by Ivey and Rusche, but slight variations were recorded at faster joint speeds. The maximal torque and the position of the shoulder at the maximal torque are recorded in Table 6-3.

Clinical Relevance

The contributions of the deltoid and supraspinatus muscles to arm elevation are easily observed clinically. In patients without a deltoid muscle, arm elevation with modest strength is possible.[282] However, the laboratory data for supraspinatus deficiency presented by Howell and colleagues[255] and by Colachis and Strohm[2] are contrary to clinical experience. Clinical experience does parallel the observations made by Bechtol, although no experimental details are presented by this author (see Fig. 6-55).[263] The EMG data correlated with various shoulder activities closely support the role of the supraspinatus in stabilizing the humeral head in the glenoid, thus allowing the other muscles to act more effectively across this joint.

When the deltoid becomes weak due to partial rupture or other reasons in cuff-deficient shoulders, the arm can no longer be elevated. This is called *pseudoparalysis*. In 1993, Grammont and Baulot[284] introduced a new concept of reverse shoulder prosthesis to improve the function of the shoulder with pseudoparalysis. Excellent outcome has been reported by other investigators.[285,286] This prosthesis has a unique design: The center of rotation during arm elevation is shifted medially almost on the original surface of the glenoid. This increases the moment arm of the deltoid and helps the muscle to function to the extent of its ability.

The recognition that the resultant force vector is directed superiorly during the first 60 degrees of arm elevation explains the superior migration of the humeral head in a rotator cuff–deficient shoulder (see Fig. 6-26). Recently, Gagey and colleagues[287] proposed a new biomechanical model of the deltoid and stated that the force vector of the deltoid was oriented inferiorly rather than superiorly in most cases. However, Blasier and coauthors[288] did not agree with them. The legitimacy of Gagey's model needs to be further validated. The orientation and magnitude are also consistent with the glenoid-loosening pattern seen in some cases after shoulder joint replacement (Fig. 6-63). These force data may be further correlated with glenoid component fixation. The capacity of the glenoid bone is of limited dimensions. Hence, the fixation technique is critical (see Fig. 6-39). Appropriate design considerations can be incorporated into the glenoid compartment to take advantage of the anatomy and resist the applied force.[289]

Finally, a rotator cuff–deficient shoulder may also be considered to be at risk for glenoid loosening.[10,85,290,291] The basis for this speculation is that arm elevation of greater than 60 degrees is often not possible with this condition. Thus, the elevation that is possible loads the glenoid in a superior, nonstable configuration that exerts a downward, tilting force to the glenoid component. Accordingly, cuff-deficient shoulders tend to show proximal migration and, possibly, increased glenoid component loosening, often called a *rocking horse glenoid*.[290]

REFERENCES

1. Dempster WT: Mechanisms of shoulder movement. Arch Phys Med Rehabil 46A:49-70, 1965.
2. Colachis SC Jr, Strohm BR: Effect of suprascapular and axillary nerve blocks on muscle force in upper extremity. Arch Phys Med Rehabil 52:22-29, 1971.
3. Inman VT, Saunders JR, Abbott LC: Observations on the function of the shoulder joint. J Bone Joint Surg 26:1-30, 1944.
4. Lucas DB: Biomechanics of the shoulder joint. Arch Surg 107:425-432, 1973.
5. Bearn JG: Direct observation on the function of the capsule of the sternoclavicular joint in clavicular support. J Anat 101:159-170, 1967.
6. Spencer EE, Kuhn JE, Huston LJ, et al: Ligamentous restraints to anterior and posterior translation of the sternoclavicular joint. J Shoulder Elbow Surg 11:43-47, 2002.
7. Rockwood CA Jr, Green DP (eds): Fractures in Adults, 2nd ed. Philadelphia: JB Lippincott, 1984.
8. Kapandji I: The Physiology of Joints, vol 1. Baltimore: Williams & Wilkins, 1970.
9. Fukuda K, Craig EV, An K-N, et al: Biomechanical study of the ligamentous system of the acromioclavicular joint. J Bone Joint Surg Am 68:434-440, 1986.
10. Collins D, Tencer A, Sidles J, Matsen F III: Edge displacement and deformation of glenoid components in response to eccentric loading: The effect of preparation of the glenoid bone. J Bone Joint Surg Am 74:501-507, 1992.
11. Sahara W, Sugamoto K, Murai M, et al: 3D kinematic analysis of the acromioclavicular joint during arm abduction using vertically open MRI. J Orthop Res 24:1823-1831, 2006.
12. Klimkiewicz JJ, Williams GR, Sher JS, et al: The acromioclavicular capsule as a restraint to posterior translation of the clavicle: A biomechanical analysis. J Shoulder Elbow Surg 8:119-124, 1999.
13. Debski RE, Parsons IM 4th, Woo SL, Fu FH: Effect of capsular injury on acromioclavicular joint mechanics. J Bone Joint Surg Am 83:1344-1351, 2001.
14. Laumann U: Kinesiology of the shoulder joint. In Koelbel R, Helbig B, Blauth W (eds): Shoulder Replacement. Berlin: Springer-Verlag, 1987, pp 23-31.

15. Debski RE, Fenwick JA, Vangura A Jr, et al: Effect of arthroscopic procedures on the acromioclavicular joint. Clin Orthop Relat Res (406):89-96, 2003.
16. Corteen DP, Teitge RA: Stabilization of the clavicle after distal resection: A biomechanical study. Am J Sports Med 33:61-67, 2005.
17. Steindler A: Kinesiology of the Human Body under Normal and Pathological Conditions. Springfield, Ill: Charles C Thomas, 1955.
18. Johnston TB: The movements of the shoulder joint. A plea for the use of the "plane of the scapula" as the plane of reference for movements occurring at the humero-scapular joint. Br J Surg 25:252-260, 1937.
19. Pearl ML, Sidles JA, Lippitt SB, et al: Codman's paradox: Sixty years later. J Shoulder Elbow Surg 1:219-225, 1992.
20. Saha AK: Mechanism of shoulder movements and a plea for the recognition of "zero position" of glenohumeral joint. Clin Orthop Relat Res (173):3-10, 1983.
21. Walker PS: Human Joints and Their Artificial Replacements. Springfield, Ill: Charles C Thomas, 1977.
22. Cathcart CW: Movements of the shoulder girdle involved in those of the arm on the trunk. Worcester Meeting, British Medical Association, 1882. J Anat Physiol 18:210, 1884.
23. Craig EV: The posterior mechanism of acute anterior shoulder dislocations. Clin Orthop Relat Res (190):212-216, 1984.
24. Doody SG, Waterland JC, Freedman L: Scapulohumeral goniometer. Arch Phys Med Rehabil 51:711-713, 1970.
25. Poppen NK, Walker PS: Normal and abnormal motion of the shoulder. J Bone Joint Surg Am 58:195-201, 1976.
26. Morrey BF, Chao EYS: Passive motion of the elbow joint. J Bone Joint Surg Am 58:501-508, 1976.
27. Hogfors C, Sigholm G, Herberts P: Biomechanical model of the human shoulder. I. Elements. J Biomech 20:157-166, 1987.
28. Ohwovoriole EN, Mekow C: A technique for studying the kinematics of human joints. Part II. The humeroscapular joint. Orthopedics 10:457-462, 1987.
29. Doody SG, Freedman L, Waterland JC: Shoulder movements during abduction in the scapular plane. Arch Phys Med Rehabil 51:595-604, 1970.
30. An K-N, Jacobsen MC, Berglund LJ, Chao EYS: Application of a magnetic tracking device to kinesiologic studies. J Biomech 21:613-620, 1988.
31. Harryman DT, Sidles JA, Clark JM, et al: Translation of the humeral head on the glenoid with passive glenohumeral motion. J Bone Joint Surg Am 72:1334-1343, 1990.
32. Itoi E, Kuechle DK, Newman SR, et al: Stabilising function of the biceps in stable and unstable shoulders. J Bone Joint Surg Br 75:546-550, 1993.
33. Sahara W, Sugamoto K, Murai M, et al: The three-dimensional motions of glenohumeral joint under semi-loaded condition during arm abduction using vertically open MRI. Clin Biomech 22:304-312, 2007.
34. An K-N, Chao EYS: Kinematic analysis of human movement. Ann Biomed Eng 12:585-597, 1984.
35. Chao EYS, An K-N: Perspectives in measurements and modeling of muscu-loskeletal joint dynamics. In Huiskes R, von Campen DH, de Wijn JR (eds): Biomechanics: Principles and Applications. The Hague: Martinus Nijhoff, 1982, pp 1-18.
36. Spoor CW, Veldpaus FE: Rigid body motion calculated from spatial co-ordinates of markers. J Biomech 13:391-393, 1980.
37. Lazarus MD, Sidles JA, Harryman DT, Matsen FA III: Effect of a chondral-labral defect on glenoid concavity and glenohumeral stability. J Bone Joint Surg Am 78:94-102, 1996.
38. McClure PW, Michener LA, Sennett BJ, Karduna AR: Direct 3-dimensional measurement of scapular kinematics during dynamic movements in vivo. J Shoulder Elbow Surg 10:269-277, 2001.
39. Bourne DA, Choo AM, Regan WD, et al: Three-dimensional rotation of the scapula during functional movements: An in vivo study in healthy volunteers. J Shoulder Elbow Surg 16:150-162, 2007.
40. Fung M, Kato S, Barrance PJ, et al: Scapular and clavicular kinematics during humeral elevation: A study with cadavers. J Shoulder Elbow Surg 10:278-285, 2001.
41. Fick R: Handbuch der Anatomie und Mechanik der Gelenke. Part 3: Spezielle Gelenk- and Muskelmechanik. Jena, Germany: Gustaf Fischer Verlag, 1911, p 521.
42. Codman EA: The Shoulder. Boston: Thomas Todd, 1934.
43. Edelson G: The development of humeral head retroversion. J Shoulder Elbow Surg 9:316-318, 2000.
44. Yamamoto N, Itoi E, Minagawa H, et al: Why is the humeral retroversion of throwing athletes greater in dominant shoulders than in nondominant shoulders? J Shoulder Elbow Surg 15:571-575, 2006.
45. Crockett HC, Gross LB, Wilk LE, et al: Osseous adaptation and range of motion at the glenohumeral joint in professional baseball pitchers. Am J Sports Med 30:20-26, 2002.
46. Reagan KM, Meister K, Horodyski MB, et al: Humeral retroversion and its relationship to glenohumeral rotation in the shoulder of college baseball players. Am J Sports Med 30:354-360, 2002.
47. Basmajian JV, Bazant FJ: Factors preventing downward dislocation of the adducted shoulder joint. J Bone Joint Surg Am 41:1182-1186, 1959.
48. Saha AK: Dynamic stability of the glenohumeral joint. Acta Orthop Scand 42:491-505, 1971.

49. Hertz H: Die Bedeutung des Limbus glenoidalis für die Stabilität des Schul-tergelenks. Wien Klin Wochenschr Suppl 152:1-23, 1984.
50. Cleland: Notes on raising the arm. J Anat Physiol 18(pt 3):275-278, 1884.
51. Dvir Z, Berme N: The shoulder complex in elevation of the arm: A mecha-nism approach. J Biomech 11:219-225, 1978.
52. Freedman L, Munro RH: Abduction of the arm in scapular plane: Scapular and glenohumeral movements. J Bone Joint Surg Am 18:1503-1510, 1966.
53. Howell SM, Galinat BJ, Renzi AJ, Marone PJ: Normal and abnormal mechan-ics of the glenohumeral joint in the horizontal plane. J Bone Joint Surg Am 70:227-232, 1988.
54. Lockhart RD: Movements of the normal shoulder joint and of a case with trapezius paralysis studied by radiogram and experiment in the living. J Anat 64:288-302, 1930.
55. Nobuhara K: The Shoulder: Its Function and Clinical Aspects. Tokyo: Igaku-Shoin, 1987.
56. Bergmann G: Biomechanics and pathomechanics of the shoulder joint with reference to prosthetic joint replacement. In Koelbel R, Helbig B, Blauth W (eds): Shoulder Replacement. Berlin: Springer-Verlag, 1987, pp 33-43.
57. Harryman DT II, Walker ED, Harris SL, et al: Residual motion and function after glenohumeral or scapulothoracic arthrodesis. J Shoulder Elbow Surg 2:275-285, 1993.
58. Sugamoto K, Harada T, Machida A, et al: Scapulohumeral rhythm: Relation-ship between motion velocity and rhythm. Clin Orthop Relat Res (401):119-124, 2002.
59. Talkhani IS, Kelly CP: Movement analysis of asymptomatic normal shoulders: A preliminary study. J Shoulder Elbow Surg 10:580-584, 2001.
60. Lin JJ, Lim HK, Yang JL: Effect of shoulder tightness on glenohumeral transla-tion, scapular kinematics, and scapulohumeral rhythm in subjects with stiff shoulders. J Orthop Res 24(5):1044-1051, 2006.
61. Matias R, Pascoal AG: The unstable shoulder in arm elevation: A three-dimensional and electromyographic study in subjects with glenohumeral instability. Clin Biomech 21(Suppl 1):S52-S58, 2006.
62. Friedman RJ: Shoulder biomechanics following total joint arthroplasty. Trans Orthop Res Soc 14:4, 1989.
63. Browne AO, Hoffmeyer P, Tanaka S, et al: Glenohumeral elevation studied in three dimensions. J Bone Joint Surg 72:843-845, 1990.
64. Gagey OJ, Boisrenoult P: Shoulder capsule shrinkage and consequences on shoulder movements. Clin Orthop Relat Res (419):218-222, 2004.
65. Jobe CM, Iannotti JP: Limits imposed on glenohumeral motion by joint geometry. J Shoulder Elbow Surg 4: 281-285, 1995.
66. Walch G, Liotard JP, Boileau P, Noel E: Postero-superior glenoid impinge-ment. Another shoulder impingement. Rev Chir Orthop Reparatrice Appar Mot 1991;77(8):571-574.
67. Pearl ML, Jackins S, Lippitt SB, et al: Humeroscapular positions in a shoulder range-of-motion-examination. J Shoulder Elbow Surg 1:296-305, 1992.
68. Scott DJ: Treatment of recurrent posterior dislocations of the shoulder by glenoplasty. J Bone Joint Surg Am 49:471-476, 1967.
69. Taylor CL, Blaschke AC: Method for kinematic analysis of motions of the shoulder, arm, and hand complex. Ann N Y Acad Sci 51:1251-1265, 1951.
70. Townley CO: The capsular mechanism in recurrent dislocation of the shoul-der. J Bone Joint Surg Am 32:370-380, 1950.
71. Spiegelman JJ, Woo SL-Y: A rigid-body method for finding centers of rotation and angular displacements of planar joint motion. J Biomech 20:715-721, 1987.
72. Jackson KM, Joseph J, Wyard SJ: Sequential muscular contraction. J Biomech 10:97-106, 1977.
73. de Luca CJ, Forrest WJ: Force analysis of individual muscles acting simulta-neously on the shoulder joint during isometric abduction. J Biomech 6:385-393, 1973.
74. Helmig P, S<o/>jbjerg JO, Sneppen O, et al: Glenohumeral movement pat-terns after puncture of the joint capsule: An experimental study. J Shoulder Elbow Surg 2:209-215, 1993.
75. Kelkar R, Wang VM, Flatow EL, et al: Glenohumeral mechanics: A study of articular geometry, contact, and kinematics. J Shoulder Elbow Surg 10:73-84, 2001.
76. Wuelker N, Schmotzer H, Thren K, Korell M: Translation of the glenohu-meral joint with simulated active elevation. Clin Orthop Relat Res (309):193-200, 1994.
77. Warner JJP, McMahon PJ: The role of the long head of the biceps brachii in superior stability of the glenohumeral joint. J Bone Joint Surg Am 77:366-372, 1995.
78. Metcalf MH, Pon JD, Harryman DT 2nd, et al: Capsulolabral augmentation increases glenohumeral stability in the cadaver shoulder. J Shoulder Elbow Surg 10:532-538, 2001.
79. Stokdijk M, Nagels J, Rozing PM: The glenohumeral joint rotation centre in vivo. J Biomech 33(12):1629-1636, 2000.
80. Baeyens JP, van Roy P, De Schepper A, et al: Glenohumeral joint kinematics related to minor anterior instability of the shoulder at the end of the late preparatory phase of throwing. Clin Biomech 16:752-757, 2001.
81. Neer CS II: Displaced proximal humeral fractures. I. Classification and evalu-ation. J Bone Joint Surg Am 52:1077-1089, 1970.
82. Blakely RL, Palmer ML: Analysis of rotation accompanying shoulder flexion. Phys Ther 64:1214-1216, 1984.

83. Rowe CR, Patel D, Southmayd WE: The Bankart procedure: A long-term end-result study. J Bone Joint Surg Am 60:1-16, 1978.

84. Karduna AR, Williams GR, Williams JL, Iannotti JP: Glenohumeral joint translations before and after total shoulder arthroplasty. A study in cadavera. J Bone Joint Surg Am 79:1166-1174, 1997.

85. Pollock RG, Deliz ED, McIlveen SJ, et al: Prosthetic replacement in rotator cuff-deficient shoulders. J Shoulder Elbow Surg 1:173-186, 1992.

86. Weiner DS, MacNab I: Superior migration of the humeral head. J Bone Joint Surg Br 52:524-527, 1970.

87. Yamaguchi K, Sher JS, Andersen WK, et al: Glenohumeral motion in patients with rotator cuff tears: A comparison of asymptomatic and symptomatic shoulders. J Shoulder Elbow Surg 9:6-11, 2000.

88. Nové-Josserand L, Edwards TB, O'Connor DP, Walch G: The acromiohumeral and coracohumeral intervals are abnormal in rotator cuff tears with muscular fatty degeneration. Clin Orthop Relat Res 433:90-96, 2005.

89. Neer CS II, Foster CR: Inferior capsular shift for involuntary inferior and multidirectional instability of the shoulder. J Bone Joint Surg Am 62:897-908, 1980.

90. Das SP, Ray GS, Saha AK: Observation of the tilt of the glenoid cavity of the scapula. J Anat Soc India 15:114-118, 1966.

91. Moseley HE, Overgaard B: The anterior capsular mechanism in recurrent anterior dislocation of the shoulder. J Bone Joint Surg Br 44:913-927, 1962.

92. Bost FC, Inman VTG: The pathological changes in recurrent dislocation of the shoulder. J Bone Joint Surg 24:595-613, 1942.

93. DePalma AF, Cooke AJ, Probhaker M: The role of the subscapularis in recurrent anterior dislocation of the shoulder. Clin Orthop Relat Res 54:35-49, 1969.

94. Howell SM, Kraft TA: The role of the supraspinatus and infraspinatus muscles in glenohumeral kinematics of anterior shoulder instability. Clin Orthop Relat Res (263):128-134, 1991.

95. Nyffeler RW, Sheikh R, Atkinson TS, et al: Effects of glenoid component version on humeral head displacement and joint reaction forces: An experimental study. J Shoulder Elbow Surg 15(5):625-629, 2006.

96. Spencer EE Jr, Valdevit A, Kambic H, et al: The effect of humeral component anteversion on shoulder stability with glenoid component retroversion. J Bone Joint Surg Am 87(4):808-814, 2005.

97. Randelli M, Gambrioli PL: Glenohumeral osteometry by computed tomography in normal and unstable shoulders. Clin Orthop Relat Res (208):151-156, 1986.

98. Kim SH, Noh KC, Park JS, et al: Loss of chondrolabral containment of the glenohumeral joint in atraumatic posteroinferior multidirectional instability. J Bone Joint Surg Am 87(1):92-98, 2005.

99. Maki S, Gruen T: Anthropometric study of the glenohumeral joint. Presented at the 22nd Annual Orthopedic Research Society, New Orleans, January 28-30, 1976.

100. Bergman RA, Thompson SA, Afifi A: Catalog of Human Variation. Baltimore: Urban & Schwarzenberg, 1984.

101. Morrey BF, Janes JJ: Recurrent anterior dislocation of the shoulder. Long-term follow-up of the Putti-Platt and Bankart procedures. J Bone Joint Surg Am 58:252-256, 1976.

102. Nishida K, Hashizume H, Toda K, Inoue H: Histologic and scanning electron microscopic study of the glenoid labrum. J Shoulder Elbow Surg 5:132-138, 1996.

103. Howell SM, Galinat BJ: The glenoid-labral socket. A constrained articular surface. Clin Orthop Relat Res (243):122-125, 1989.

104. Pouliart N, Gagey O: The effect of isolated labrum resection on shoulder stability. Knee Surg Sports Traumatol Arthrosc 14(3):301-308, 2006.

105. Fukuda K, Chen CM, Cofield RH, Chao EY: Biomechanical analysis of stability and fixation strength of total shoulder prostheses. Orthopedics 11(1):141-149, 1988.

106. Lippitt SB, Vanderhooft JE, Harris SL, et al: Glenohumeral stability from concavity-compression: A quantitative analysis. J Shoulder Elbow Surg 2:27-35, 1993.

107. Halder AM, Kuhl SG, Zobitz ME, et al: Effects of the glenoid labrum and glenohumeral abduction on stability of the shoulder joint through concavity-compression: An in vitro study. J Bone Joint Surg Am 83:1062-1069, 2001.

108. Metcalf MH, Duckworth DG, Lee SB, et al: Posteroinferior glenoplasty can change glenoid shape and increase the mechanical stability of the shoulder. J Shoulder Elbow Surg 8:205-213, 1999.

109. Grauer JD, Paulos LE, Smutz WP: Biceps tendon and superior labral injuries. Arthroscopy 8:488-497, 1992.

110. Bey MJ, Elders GJ, Huston LJ, et al: The mechanism of creation of superior labrum, anterior, and posterior lesions in a dynamic biomechanical model of the shoulder: The role of inferior subluxation. J Shoulder Elbow Surg 7:397-401, 1998.

111. Pradhan RL, Itoi E, Hatakeyama Y, et al: Superior labral strain during the throwing motion. A cadaveric study. Am J Sports Med 29:488-492, 2001.

112. McMahon PJ, Burkart A, Musahl V, Debski RE. Glenohumeral translations are increased after a type II superior labrum anterior-posterior lesion: A cadaveric study of severity of passive stabilizer injury. J Shoulder Elbow Surg 13(1):39-44, 2004.

113. Panossian VR, Mihata T, Tibone JE, et al: Biomechanical analysis of isolated type II SLAP lesions and repair. J Shoulder Elbow Surg 14(5):529-534, 2005.

114. Soslowsky LJ, Flatow EL, Bigliani LU, et al: Quantitation of in situ contact areas at the glenohumeral joint: A biomechanical study. J Orthop Res 10:524-534, 1992.

115. Luo ZP, Niebur GL, An KN: Determination of the proximity tolerance for measurement of surface contact areas using a magnetic tracking device. J Biomech 29:367-372, 1996.

116. Warner JJ, Bowen MK, Deng XH, et al: Articular contact patterns of the normal glenohumeral joint. J Shoulder Elbow Surg 10:496-497, 2001.

117. Smith SP, Bunker TD: Primary glenoid dysplasia. A review of 12 patients. J Bone Joint Surg Br 83:868-872, 2001.

118. Itoi E, Motzkin NE, Morrey BF, An KN: Scapular inclination and inferior stability of the shoulder. J Shoulder Elbow Surg 1:131-139, 1992.

119. Itoi E, Motzkin NE, Morrey BF, An KN: Bulk effect of rotator cuff on inferior glenohumeral stability as function of scapular inclination angle: A cadaver study. Tohoku J Exp Med 171:267-276, 1993.

120. Kumar VP, Balasubramaniam P: The role of atmospheric pressure in stabilizing the shoulder: An experimental study. J Bone Joint Surg Br 67:719-721, 1985.

121. Gibb TD, Sidles JA, Harryman DT II, et al: The effect of capsular venting on glenohumeral laxity. Clin Orthop Relat Res (268):120-127, 1991.

122. Itoi E, Motzkin NE, Browne AO: Intraarticular pressure of the shoulder. Arthroscopy 9:406-413, 1993.

123. Habermeyer P, Schuller U, Wiedemann E: The intra-articular pressure of the shoulder: An experimental study on the role of the glenoid labrum in stabilizing the joint. Arthroscopy 8:166-172, 1992.

124. Hashimoto T, Suzuki K, Nobuhara K: Dynamic analysis of intraarticular pressure in the glenohumeral joint. J Shoulder Elbow Surg 4:209-218, 1995.

125. Schenk TJ, Brems JJ: Multidirectional instability of the shoulder: Pathophysiology, diagnosis, and management. J Am Acad Orthop Surg 6:65-72, 1998.

126. Yamamoto N, Itoi E, Tuoheti Y, et al: The effect of the inferior capsular shift on shoulder intra-articular pressure: A cadaveric study. Am J Sports Med 34:939-944, 2006.

127. Kaltsas DS: Comparative study of the properties of the shoulder joint capsules with those of other joint capsules. Clin Orthop Relat Res (173):20-26, 1973.

128. Reeves B: Experiments on the tensile strength of the anterior capsular structures of the shoulder region. J Bone Joint Surg Br 50:858-865, 1968.

129. Morrey BF, Chao EYS: Recurrent anterior dislocation of the shoulder. In Dumbleton J, Black JH (eds): Clinical Biomechanics. London: Churchill Livingstone, 1981, pp 24-46.

130. Harryman DT II, Sidles JA, Harris SL, Matsen FA III: Laxity of the normal glenohumeral joint. A quantitative in vivo assessment. J Shoulder Elbow Surg 1:66-76, 1992.

131. Uhthoff H, Piscopo M: Anterior capsular redundancy of the shoulder: Congenital or traumatic? J Bone Joint Surg Br 67:363-366, 1985.

132. Flood V: Discovery of a new ligament of the shoulder. Lancet 1:672-673, 1829.

133. Flatow EL, Wang VM, Kelkar R, et al: The coracoacromial ligament passively restrains anterosuperior humeral subluxation in the rotator cuff deficient shoulder. Trans Orthop Res Soc 21:229, 1996.

134. Flatow EL, Connor PM, Levine WN, et al: Coracoacromial arch reconstruction for anterosuperior instability. Presented at the 13th Open Meeting of the American Shoulder and Elbow Surgeons, San Francisco, February 16, 1997.

135. Lee TQ, Black AD, Tibone JE, McMahon PJ: Release of the coracoacromial ligament can lead to glenohumeral laxity: A biomechanical study. J Shoulder Elbow Surg 10:68-72, 2001.

136. Soslowsky LJ, An CH, DeBano CM, Carpenter JE: Coracoacromial ligament: In situ load and viscoelastic properties in rotator cuff disease. Clin Orthop Relat Res 330:40-44, 1996.

137. Fremerey R, Bastian L, Siebert WE: The coracoacromial ligament: Anatomical and biomechanical properties with respect to age and rotator cuff disease. Knee Surg Sports Traumatol Arthrosc 8(5):309-313, 2000.

138. Hansen U, Levy O, Even T, Copeland SA: Mechanical properties of regenerated coracoacromial ligament after subacromial decompression. J Shoulder Elbow Surg 13(1):51-56, 2004.

139. DePalma AF, Callery G, Bennett GA: Variational anatomy and degenerative lesions of the shoulder bone. Instr Course Lect 16:255-281, 1949.

140. Terry GC, Hammon D, France P: Stabilizing function of passive shoulder restraints. Unpublished data from the Hughston Orthopaedic Clinic, Columbus, Ga, 1988.

141. Ovesen J Nielsen S: Experimental distal subluxation in the glenohumeral joint. Arch Orthop Trauma Surg 104:78-81, 1985.

142. Warner JJ, Deng XH, Warren RF, Torzilli PA: Static capsuloligamentous restraints to superior–inferior translation of the glenohumeral joint. Am J Sports Med 20:675-680, 1992.

143. Kuboyama M: The role of soft tissues in downward stability of the glenohumeral joint: An experimental study with fresh cadavers [in Japanese with English abstract]. Igaku Kenkyu 61:20-33, 1991.

144. Jerosch J, Moersler M, Castro WH: Über die Funktion der passiven Stabilisatoren des glenohumeralen Gelenkes: Eine biomechanische Untersuchung. Z Orthop Ihre Grenzgeb 128:206-212, 1990.

145. Itoi E, Berglund LJ, Grabowski JJ, et al: Superior–inferior stability of the shoulder: Role of the coracohumeral ligament and the rotator interval capsule. Mayo Clin Proc 73:508-515, 1998.

146. Patel PR, Debski RE, Imhoff AB, et al: Anatomy and biomechanics of the coracohumeral and superior glenohumeral ligaments. Trans Orthop Res Soc 21:702, 1996.

147. Jost B, Koch PP, Gerber C: Anatomy and functional aspects of the rotator interval. J Shoulder Elbow Surg 9(4):336-341, 2000.

148. Nobuhara K, Ikeda H: Rotator interval lesion. Clin Orthop Relat Res (223):44-50, 1987.

149. Harryman DT II, Sidles JA, Harris SL, Matsen FA III: The role of the rotator interval capsule in passive motion and stability of the shoulder. J Bone Joint Surg Am 74:53-66, 1992.

150. Tamai M, Okajima S, Fushiki S, Hirasawa Y: Quantitative analysis of neural distribution in human coracoacromial ligaments. Clin Orthop Relat Res (373):125-134, 2000.

151. Wolf RS, Zheng N, Iero J, Weichel D: The effects of thermal capsulorrhaphy and rotator interval closure on multidirectional laxity in the glenohumeral joint: A cadaveric biomechanical study. Arthroscopy 20(10):1044-1049, 2004.

152. Plausinis D, Bravman JT, Heywood C, et al: Arthroscopic rotator interval closure: Effect of sutures on glenohumeral motion and anterior–posterior translation. Am J Sports Med 34(10):1656-1661, 2006.

153. Yamamoto N, Itoi E, Tuoheti Y, et al: Effect of rotator interval closure on glenohumeral stability and motion: A cadaveric study. J Shoulder Elbow Surg 15:750-758, 2006.

154. Basmajian JV: Muscles Alive, 2nd ed. Baltimore: Williams & Wilkins, 1967.

155. Schwartz E, Warren RF, O'Brien SJ, Fronek J: Posterior shoulder instability. Orthop Clin North Am 18:409-419, 1987.

156. DeLorme D: Die Hemmungsbänder des Schultergelenks und ihre Bedeutung für die Schulterluxationen. Arch Klin Chirurg 92:79-101, 1910.

157. Turkel SJ, Panio MW, Marshall JL, Girgis FG: Stabilizing mechanisms preventing anterior dislocation of the glenohumeral joint. J Bone Joint Surg Am 63:1208-1217, 1981.

158. O'Connell PW, Nuber GW, Mileski RA, Lautenschlager E: The contribution of the glenohumeral ligaments to anterior stability of the shoulder joint. Am J Sports Med 18:579-584, 1990.

159. Blasier RB, Guldberg RE, Rothman ED: Anterior shoulder stability: Contributions of rotator cuff forces and the capsular ligaments in a cadaver model. J Shoulder Elbow Surg 1:140-150, 1992.

160. O'Brien SJ, Neves MC, Arnoczky SP, et al: The anatomy and histology of the inferior glenohumeral ligament complex of the shoulder. Am J Sports Med 18:449-456, 1990.

161. Bigliani LU, Pollock RG, Soslowsky LJ, et al: Tensile properties of the inferior glenohumeral ligament. J Orthop Res 10:187-197, 1992.

162. Ticker JB, Bigliani LU, Soslowsky LJ, et al: Inferior glenohumeral ligament: Geometric and strain-rate dependent properties. J Shoulder Elbow Surg 5:269-279, 1996.

163. Gohlke F, Essigkrug B, Schmitz F: The pattern of the collagen fiber bundles of the capsule of the glenohumeral joint. J Shoulder Elbow Surg 3:111-128, 1994.

164. Urayama M, Itoi E, Shimizu T, Sato K: Morphology of the inferior glenohumeral ligaments. Jpn J Orthop Assoc 73:S1631, 1999.

165. Debski RE, Wong EK, Warner JP, et al: Interrelationships of the capsuloligamentous restraints during translation of the glenohumeral joint. Trans Orthop Res Soc 21:230, 1996.

166. O'Brien SJ, Schwartz RS, Warren RF, Torzilli PA: Capsular restraints to anterior–posterior motion of the abducted shoulder: A biomechanical study. J Shoulder Elbow Surg 4:298-308, 1995.

167. Urayama M, Itoi E, Hatakeyama Y, et al: Function of the 3 portions of the inferior glenohumeral ligament: A cadaveric study. J Shoulder Elbow Surg 10:589-594, 2001.

168. Hart WJ, Kelly CP: Arthroscopic observation of capsulolabral reduction after shoulder dislocation. J Shoulder Elbow Surg 14(2):134-137, 2005.

169. Naggar L, Jenp YN, Malanga G, et al: Major capsuloligamentous restraints to posterior instability of the shoulder. Presented at the 62nd Annual Meeting of the American Academy of Orthopaedic Surgeons, New Orleans, February 16-21, 1995.

170. Partridge MJ: Joints. The limitation of their range of movement, and an explanation of certain surgical conditions. J Anat 108:346, 1923.

171. Ovesen J, Nielsen S: Anterior and posterior shoulder instability. Acta Orthop Scand 57:324-327, 1986.

172. Scheving LE, Pauly JE: An electromyographic study of some muscles acting on the upper extremity of man. Anat Rec 135:239-245, 1959.

173. Bearn JG: An electromyographic study of the trapezius, deltoid, pectoralis major, biceps and triceps muscles during static loading of the upper limb. Anat Rec 140:103-108, 1961.

174. Motzkin NE, Itoi E, Morrey BF, An KN: Contribution of passive bulk tissues and deltoid to static inferior glenohumeral stability. J Shoulder Elbow Surg 3:313-319, 1994.

175. McMahon PJ, Debski RE, Thompson WO, et al: Shoulder muscle forces and tendon excursions during glenohumeral abduction in the scapular plane. J Shoulder Elbow Surg 4:199-208, 1995.

176. Hsu HC, Luo ZP, Cofield RH, An KN: Influence of rotator cuff tearing on glenohumeral stability. J Shoulder Elbow Surg 6:413-422, 1997.

177. Matsen FA III, Lippitt SB, Sidles JA, Harryman DT II: Practical Evaluation and Management of the Shoulder. Philadelphia: WB Saunders, 1994.

178. Symeonides PP: The significance of the subscapularis muscle in the pathogenesis of recurrent anterior dislocation of the shoulder. J Bone Joint Surg Br 54:476-483, 1972.

179. Bassett RW, Browne AO, Morrey BF, An KN: Glenohumeral muscle force and moment mechanics in a position of shoulder instability. J Biomech 23:405-415, 1990.

180. Tuoheti Y, Itoi E, Minagawa H, et al: Quantitative assessment of thinning of the subscapularis tendon in recurrent anterior dislocation of the shoulder by use of magnetic resonance imaging. J Shoulder Elbow Surg 14(1):11-15, 2005.

181. Boss A, Pellegrini L, Hintermann B: Prognostically relevant factors in treatment of the post-traumatic unstable shoulder joint. Unfallchirurg 103(4):289-294, 2000.

182. Ovesen J, Nielsen S: Posterior instability of the shoulder: A cadaver study. Acta Orthop Scand 57:436-439, 1986.

183. Ovesen J, Sojbjerg JO: Posterior shoulder dislocation: Muscle and capsular lesions in cadaver experiments. Acta Orthop Scand 57:535-536, 1986.

184. Motzkin NE, Itoi E, Morrey BF, An KN: Contribution of rotator cuff to inferior shoulder stability. Paper presented at the 5th International Conference on Surgery of the Shoulder, Paris, July 12-15, 1992.

185. Glousman R, Jobe F, Tibone J, et al: Dynamic electromyographic analysis of the throwing shoulder with glenohumeral instability. J Bone Joint Surg Am 70:220-226, 1988.

186. Kronberg M, Broström L-Å, Nemeth G: Differences in shoulder muscle activity between patients with generalized joint laxity and normal controls. Clin Orthop Relat Res (269):181-192, 1991.

187. Chen SK, Simonian PT, Wickiewicz TL, et al: Radiographic evaluation of glenohumeral kinematics: A muscle fatigue model. J Shoulder Elbow Surg 8:49-52, 1999.

188. Cain PR, Mutschler TA, Fu FH, and Lee SK: Anterior stability of the glenohumeral joint: A dynamic model. Am J Sports Med 15:144-148, 1987.

189. McKernan DJ, Mutschler TA, Rudert MJ, et al: The characterization of rotator cuff muscle forces and their effect on glenohumeral joint stability: A biomechanical study. Orthop Trans 14:237-238, 1990.

190. Newman SR: Stabilizing Function of the Rotator Cuff Muscles [master's thesis]. Rochester, Minn, Mayo Graduate School of Medicine, 1993.

191. Hsu HC, Luo ZP, Stone JJS, An KN: Importance of rotator cuff balance to glenohumeral instability and degeneration. Trans Orthop Res Soc 21:232, 1996.

192. Lee SB, Kim KJ, O'Driscoll SW, et al: Dynamic glenohumeral stability provided by the rotator cuff muscles in the mid-range and end-range of motion. A study in cadavera. J Bone Joint Surg Am 82:849-857, 2000.

193. Halder AM, Zhao KD, O'Driscoll SW, et al: Dynamic contributions to superior shoulder stability. J Orthop Res 19:206-212, 2001.

194. Kumar VP, Satku K, Balasubramaniam P: The role of the long head of biceps brachii in the stabilization of the head of the humerus. Clin Orthop Relat Res (244):172-175, 1989.

195. Andrews JR, Carson WG Jr, McLeod WD: Glenoid labrum tears related to the long head of the biceps. Am J Sports Med 13:337-341, 1985.

196. Habermeyer P, Kaiser E, Knappe M, et al: Zur funktionellen Anatomie und Biomechanik der langen Bizepssehne. Unfallchirurgie 90:319-329, 1987.

197. Rodosky MW, Rudert MJ, Harner CD, et al: Significance of a superior labral lesion of the shoulder: A biomechanical study. Trans Orthop Res Soc 15:276, 1990.

198. Rodosky MW, Harner CD, Fu FH: The role of the long head of the biceps muscle and superior glenoid labrum in anterior stability of the shoulder. Am J Sports Med 22:121-130, 1994.

199. Itoi E, Motzkin NE, Morrey BF, An KN: Stabilizing function of the long head of the biceps. With the arm in hanging position. Orthop Trans 16:775, 1992.

200. Malicky DM, Soslowsky LJ, Blasier RB: Anterior glenohumeral stabilization factors: Progressive effects in a biomechanical model. J Orthop Res 14:282-288, 1996.

201. Pagnani MJ, Deng X-H, Warren RF, et al: Effect of lesions of the superior portion of the glenoid labrum on glenohumeral translation. J Bone Joint Surg Am 77:1003-1010, 1995.

202. Funk L, Snow M: SLAP tears of the glenoid labrum in contact athletes. Clin J Sport Med 17(1):1-4, 2007.

203. Levy AS, Kelly BT, Lintner SA, et al: Function of the long head of the biceps at the shoulder: Electromyographic analysis. J Shoulder Elbow Surg 10:250-255, 2001.

204. Kim SH, Ha KI, Kim HS, Kim SW: Electromyographic activity of the biceps brachii muscle in shoulders with anterior instability. Arthroscopy 17:864-868, 2001.

205. Itoi E, Newman SR, Kuechle DK, et al: Dynamic anterior stabilisers of the shoulder with the arm in abduction. J Bone Joint Surg Br 76:834-836, 1994.

206. Kido T, Itoi E, Konno N, et al: The depressor function of biceps on the head of the humerus in shoulders with tears of the rotator cuff. J Bone Joint Surg Br 82:416-419, 2000.

207. Payne LZ, Deng XH, Craig EV, et al: The combined dynamic and static contributions to subacromial impingement. A biomechanical analysis. Am J Sports Med 25:801-808, 1997.

208. Toshiaki A, Itoi E, Minagawa H, et al: Cross-sectional area of the tendon and the muscle of the biceps brachii in shoulders with rotator cuff tears: A study of 14 cadaveric shoulders. Acta Orthop 76(4):509-512, 2005.

209. Michiels I, Bodem F: The deltoid muscle: An electromyographical analysis of its activity in arm abduction in various body postures. Int Orthop 16:268-271, 1992.

210. Lee SB, An KN: Dynamic glenohumeral stability provided by three heads of the deltoid muscle. Clin Orthop Relat Res (400):40-47, 2002.

211. Kido T, Itoi E, Lee SB, et al: Dynamic stabilizing function of the deltoid muscle in shoulders with anterior instability. Am J Sports Med 31:399-403, 2003.

212. Nyffeler RW, Werner CM, Sukthankar A, et al: Association of a large lateral extension of the acromion with rotator cuff tears. J Bone Joint Surg Am 88(4):800-805, 2006.

213. Debski RE, Sakone M, Woo SL, et al: Contribution of the passive properties of the rotator cuff to glenohumeral stability during anterior–posterior loading. J Shoulder Elbow Surg 8:324-329, 1999.

214. Hsu HC, Boardman ND 3rd, Luo ZP, An KN: Tendon-defect and muscle-unloaded models for relating a rotator cuff tear to glenohumeral stability. J Orthop Res 18(6):952-958, 2000.

215. Blasier RB, Soslowsky LJ, Malicky DM, Palmer ML: Posterior glenohumeral subluxation: Active and passive stabilization in a biomechanical model. J Bone Joint Surg Am 79:433-440, 1997.

216. Hall AL, McCloskey DI: Detection of movement imposed on finger, elbow and shoulder joints. J Physiol 335:519-533, 1983.

217. Smith RL, Brunolli J: Shoulder kinesthesia after anterior glenohumeral joint dislocation. Phys Ther 69:106-112, 1989.

218. Murakami M, Hukuda S, Kojima Y: A study of dynamic stabilizing system of the shoulder. Role of the infraspinatus muscle responding to posterior stress and a histochemical study of the sensory nerve endings of the capsule. Katakansetsu 14:187-191, 1990.

219. Morisawa Y, Sadahiro T, Kawakami T, Yamamoto H: Mechanoreceptors in the coracoacromial ligament. A study of its morphology and distribution. Katakansetsu 14:161-165, 1990.

220. Tomita Y, Ozaki J, Nakagawa Y, et al: Pathological changes of the subacromial bursa associated with rotator cuff tears. Katakansetsu 15:62-66, 1991.

221. Vangsness CT Jr, Ennis M, Taylor JG, Atkinson R: Neural anatomy of the glenohumeral ligaments, labrum, and subacromial bursa. Arthroscopy 11:180-184, 1995.

222. Lephart SM, Warner JJP, Borsa PA, Fu FH: Proprioception of the shoulder joint in healthy, unstable, and surgically repaired shoulders. J Shoulder Elbow Surg 3:371-381, 1994.

223. Zuckerman JD, Gallagher MA, Cuomo F, Rokito AS: Effect of instability and subsequent anterior shoulder repair on proprioceptive ability. Paper presented at the 63rd Annual Meeting of the American Academy of Orthopaedic Surgery, Atlanta, February 22-26, 1996.

224. Wallace DA, Beard DJ, Gill RH, et al: Reflex muscle contraction in anterior shoulder instability. J Shoulder Elbow Surg 6:150-155, 1997.

225. Guanche C, Knatt T, Solomonow M, et al: The synergistic action of the capsule and the shoulder muscles. Am J Sports Med 23:301-306, 1995.

226. Pouliart N, Gagey O: Concomitant rotator cuff and capsuloligamentous lesions of the shoulder: A cadaver study. Arthroscopy 22(7):728-735, 2006.

227. Hill HS, Sachs MD: The grooved defect of the humeral head. A frequently unrecognized complication of dislocations of the shoulder joint. Radiology 35:690-700, 1940.

228. Bestard EA, Schvene HR, Bestard EH: Glenoplasty in the management of recurrent shoulder dislocation. Contemp Orthop 12:47, 1986.

229. Altchek DW, Warren RF, Skyhar MJ, Ortiz G: T-plasty modification of the Bankart procedure for multidirectional instability of the anterior and inferior types. J Bone Joint Surg Am 73:105-112, 1991.

230. Bankart ASB: The pathology and treatment of recurrent dislocation of the shoulder joint. Br J Surg 26:23-29, 1938.

231. McLaughlin HL: Primary anterior dislocated shoulder. Morbid anatomy. Am J Surg 99:628-632, 1960.

232. McLaughlin HL, MacLellan DI: Recurrent anterior dislocation of the shoulder. II. A comparative study. J Trauma 7:191-201, 1967.

233. Remmel E, Köckerling F: Anatomical study of the capsular mechanism in dislocation of the shoulder [abstract]. J Biomech 20:807, 1987.

234. Thomas SC, Matsen FA 3rd: An approach to the repair of avulsion of the glenohumeral ligaments in the management of traumatic anterior glenohumeral instability. J Bone Joint Surg Am 71:506-513, 1989.

235. Wirth MA, Blatter G, Rockwood CA Jr: The capsular imbrication procedure for recurrent anterior instability of the shoulder. J Bone Joint Surg Am 78:246-259, 1996.

236. Stefko JM, Tibone JE, Cawley PW, et al: Strain of the anterior band of the inferior glenohumeral ligament during capsule failure. J Shoulder Elbow Surg 6:473-479, 1997.

237. McMahon PJ, Dettling J, Sandusky MD, et al: The anterior band of the inferior glenohumeral ligament. Assessment of its permanent deformation and the anatomy of its glenoid attachment. J Bone Joint Surg Br 81:406-413, 1999.

238. Pollock RG, Wang VM, Bucchieri JS, et al: Effects of repetitive subfailure strains on the mechanical behavior of the inferior glenohumeral ligament. J Shoulder Elbow Surg 9:427-435, 2000.

239. Habermeyer P, Gleyze P, Lehmann M, Schneider M: The intraarticular joint volume in acute and chronic shoulder instability [abstract]. J Shoulder Elbow Surg 4(Suppl):29, 1995.

240. Urayama M, Itoi E, Sashi R, et al: Capsular elongation in shoulders with recurrent anterior dislocation: Quantitative assessment with magnetic resonance arthrography. Am J Sports Med 31:64-67, 2003.

241. Molina V, Pouliart N, Gagey O: Quantitation of ligament laxity in anterior shoulder instability: An experimental cadaver model. Surg Radiol Anat 26(5):349-354, 2004.

242. Novotny JE, Nichols CE, Beynnon BD: Kinematics of the glenohumeral joint with Bankart lesion and repair. J Orthop Res 16:116-121, 1998.

243. An K-N, Hui FC, Morrey BF, et al: Muscle across the elbow joint: A biomechanical analysis. J Biomech 14:659-669, 1981.

244. Veeger HEJ, Van der Woude FCT, Van der Woude LHV, et al: Inertia and muscle contraction parameters for musculoskeletal modelling of the shoulder mechanism. J Biomech 24:615-629, 1991.

245. Ikai M, Fukunaga T: Calculation of muscle strength per unit of cross-sectional area of human muscle. Int Z Angew Physiol 26(1):26-32, 1968.

246. Morris CB: The measurements of the strength of muscle relative to the cross-section. Res Q Am Assoc Health Phys Ed Recreation 19:295-303, 1948.

247. An KN, Kaufman KR, Chao EYS: Physiological consideration of muscle force through the elbow joint. J Biomech 22:1249-1256, 1989.

248. Buchanan TS: Evidence that maximum muscle stress in not a constant: Differences in specific tension in elbow flexors and extensors. Med Eng Phys 17:529-536, 1995.

249. Dowling JJ, Cardone N: Relative cross-sectional areas of upper and lower extremity muscles and implications for force prediction. Int J Sports Med 15:453-459, 1994.

250. Fukunaga T, Roy RR, Shellock FG, et al: Specific tension of human plantar flexors and dorsiflexors. J Appl Physiol 80:158-165, 1996.

251. Wuelker N, Korell M, Thren K: Dynamic glenohumeral joint stability. J Shoulder Elbow Surg 7:45-52, 1998.

252. Kuechle DK, Newman SR, Itoi E, et al: Shoulder muscle moment arm during horizontal flexion and elevation. J Shoulder Elbow Surg 6:429-439, 1997.

253. Kuechle DK, Newman SR, Itoi E, et al: The relevance of the moment arm of shoulder muscles with respect to axial rotation of the glenohumeral joint in four positions. Clin Biomech 15:322-329, 2000.

254. Stevens JH: The action of the short rotators on the normal abduction of the arm, with a consideration of their action in some cases of subacromial bursitis and allied conditions. Am J Med Sci 136:871, 1909.

255. Howell SM, Imobersteg AM, Seger DH, Marone PJ: Clarification of the role of the supraspinatus muscle in shoulder function. J Bone Joint Surg Am 68:398-404, 1986.

256. Poppen NK, Walker PS: Forces at the glenohumeral joint in abduction. Clin Orthop Relat Res (135):165-170, 1978.

257. An KN, Takahashi K, Hanigan TP, Chao EYS: Determination of muscle orientations and moment arms. J Biomech Eng 106:280-282, 1984.

258. Jiang CC, Otis JC, Warren RF, Wickiewicz TL: Muscle excursion measurements and moment arm definitions [abstract]. Presented at the 34th Annual Meeting of the Orthopedic Research Society, Atlanta, February 1-4, 1988.

259. Duchenne GB: Physiology of Movement, ed and trans EB Kaplan. Philadelphia: WB Saunders, 1959.

260. Shevlin MG, Lehmann JF, Lucci JA: Electromyographic study of the function of some muscles crossing the glenohumeral joint. Arch Phys Med Rehabil 50:264-270, 1969.

261. Sigholm G, Herberts P, Almström C, Kadefors R: Electromyographic analysis of shoulder muscle load. J Orthop Res 1:379-386, 1984.

262. Peat M, Grahame RE: Electromyographic analysis of soft tissue lesions affecting shoulder function. Am J Phys Med 56:223-240, 1977.

263. Bechtol CO: Biomechanics of the shoulder. Clin Orthop Relat Res (146):37-41, 1980.

264. Markhede G, Monastyrski J, Stener B: Shoulder function after deltoid muscle removal. Acta Orthop Scand 56:242-244, 1985.

265. Sharkey NA, Marder RA: The rotator cuff opposes superior translation of the humeral head. Am J Sports Med 23:270-275, 1995.

266. Thompson WO, Debski RE, Boardman ND 3rd, et al: A biomechanical analysis of rotator cuff deficiency in a cadaveric model. Am J Sports Med 24:286-292, 1996.

267. Itoi E, Minagawa H, Sato T, et al: Isokinetic strength after tears of the supraspinatus tendon. J Bone Joint Surg Br 79:77-82, 1997.

268. Sharkey NA, Marder RA, Hanson PB: The entire rotator cuff contributes to elevation of the arm. J Orthop Res 12:699-708, 1994.

269. Järvholm U, Palmerud G, Styf J, et al: Intramuscular pressure in the supraspinatus muscle. J Orthop Res 6:230-238, 1988.

270. Alpert SW, Pink MM, Jobe FW, et al: Electromyographic analysis of deltoid and rotator cuff function under varying loads and speeds. J Shoulder Elbow Surg 9:47-58, 2000.

271. Itoi E, An KN, Lee SB, et al: Arm rotation affects the function of arm muscles at the glenohumeral joint. Transactions of the 45th Annual Meeting of the Orthopedic Research Society 24:380, 1999.

272. Sakurai G, Ozaki J, Tomita Y, et al: Electromyographic analysis of shoulder joint function of the biceps brachii muscle during isometric contraction. Clin Orthop Relat Res (354):123-131, 1998.

273. Kido T, Itoi E, Konno N, et al: Electromyographic activities of the biceps during arm elevation in shoulders with rotator cuff tears. Acta Orthop Scand 69:575-579, 1998.

274. Schiffern SC, Rozencwaig R, Antoniou J, et al: Anteroposterior centering of the humeral head on the glenoid in vivo. Am J Sports Med 30:382-387, 2002.

275. Jones DW Jr: The Role of the Shoulder Muscles in the Control of Humeral Position [master's thesis]. Cleveland, Ohio, Case Western Reserve University, 1970.

276. An K-N, Kwak BM, Chao EYS, Morrey BF: Determination of muscle and joint forces: A new technique to solve the indeterminate problem. J Biomech Eng 106(4):364-367, 1984.

277. Himeno S, Tsumura H: The role of the rotator cuff as a stabilizing mechanism of the shoulder. In Bateman J, Welsh RP (eds): Surgery of the Shoulder. St Louis: CV Mosby, 1984, pp 17-21.

278. Conzen A, Eckstein F: Quantitative determination of articular pressure in the human shoulder joint. J Shoulder Elbow Surg 9:196-204, 2000.

279. Apreleva M, Parsons IM 4th, Warner JJ, et al: Experimental investigation of reaction forces at the glenohumeral joint during active abduction. J Shoulder Elbow Surg 9:409-417, 2000.

280. Parsons IM, Apreleva M, Fu FH, Woo SL: The effect of rotator cuff tears on reaction forces at the glenohumeral joint. J Orthop Res 20:439-446, 2002.

281. Ivey FM Jr, Rusche K: Isokinetic testing of shoulder strength: Normal values. Arch Phys Med Rehabil 66:384-386, 1985.

282. Cahalan TD, Johnson ME, Chao EYS: Shoulder strength analysis using the Cybex II isokinetic dynamometer. Clin Orthop Relat Res (271):249-257, 1991.

283. Otis JC, Warren RF, Backus SI, et al: Torque production in the shoulder of the normal young adult male. Am J Sports Med 18:119-123, 1990.

284. Grammont PM, Baulot E: Delta shoulder prosthesis for rotator cuff rupture. Orthopedics 16:65-68, 1993.

285. Boileau P, Watkinson D, Hatzidakis AM, Hovorka I.: The Grammont reverse shoulder prosthesis: Results in cuff tear arthritis, fracture sequelae, and revision arthroplasty. J Shoulder Elbow Surg 15:527-540, 2006.

286. Rittmeister M, Kerschbaumer F: Grammont reverse total shoulder arthroplasty in patients with rheumatoid arthritis and nonreconstructible rotator cuff lesions. J Shoulder Elbow Surg 10:17-22, 2001.

287. Gagey O, Hue E: Mechanics of the deltoid muscle. A new approach. Clin Orthop Relat Res (375):250-257, 2000.

288. Blasier RB, Hughes RE, Carpenter JE, Kuhn JE: A new model for the action of the middle deltoid. Clin Orthop Relat Res (388):258-259, 2001.

289. Batte SWP, Cordy ME, Lee TY, et al: Cancellous bone of the glenoid. Correlation of quantitative CT and mechanical strength. Trans Orthop Res Soc 21:707, 1996.

290. Franklin JL, Barrett WP, Jackins SE, Matsen FA 3rd: Glenoid loosening in total shoulder arthroplasty. Association with rotator cuff deficiency. J Arthroplasty 3(1):39-46, 1988.

291. Hawkins RJ, Bell RH, Jallay B: Total shoulder arthroplasty. Clin Orthop Relat Res (242):188-194, 1989.

Effectiveness Evaluation of the Shoulder

Robin R. Richards, MD, FRCSC

The assessment of outcome following treatment is an important component of providing clinical care to patients. Patients, their relatives, employers, third-party payers, colleagues in other fields of medicine, hospital administrators, and government officials are all stakeholders in the health care system. Stakeholders need to know whether or not the health care interventions that are occurring in the system are effective, the degree to which they are affecting the health of patients, and, in relative terms, the cost-effectiveness of treatment. Duckworth and colleagues[1] demonstrated the wide variability in the clinical expression of patients with full-thickness rotator cuff tears and showed the importance of documenting the clinical expression of shoulder pathology at initial evaluation in individual patients when treatment is being considered.

The concepts of quality assurance and continuous improvement demand that measurements be available to use as yardsticks against which to assess the outcome of treatment. There has been an explosion of interest in the assessment of general health outcome and in the assessment of outcome in the shoulder. This chapter details the history of outcome assessment in the shoulder and the methodology by which outcome measures themselves are assessed, critically analyzes the outcome measures currently available, and makes recommendations regarding the current use of outcome measures in clinical practice.

HISTORY

Codman[2] is credited with introducing the concept of outcome assessment in the early part of the 20th century. He espoused the concept of the "end result idea" wherein the clinician critically evaluates the results of treating all surgical cases in order to identify and understand treat-ment failures so that the care of future patients could be improved.

Until recently, outcome following shoulder reconstruction was usually assessed in terms of treatment efficacy. Observer-based measures such as range of motion, stability, and deformity, together with radiographic assessment of fracture union or prosthesis alignment were used to determine whether or not a procedure had been effective. Such observer-based methodology ignores the consumer of the product when assessing its effectiveness and does not address the larger concept of patient health and the role of the shoulder disorder in affecting the general well-being of the individual.

Scientific analysis has demonstrated that observer-based assessment of shoulder function can be inconsistent. Hayes and coworkers[3] found visual estimation, goniometry, still photography, and reach for six different shoulder motions to have standard errors of measurement of between 14 and 25 degrees between raters and 11 and 23 degrees with the same rater on different occasions. Ostor and colleagues[4] determined the inter-rater reproducibility of clinical tests for rotator cuff function. Fair concordance between assessments was found in 40 of 55 observations, and moderate concordance was found in only 21 of 55 instances. Tzannes and coauthors[5] found some tests of shoulder instability to be reliable among examiners, providing pain was not used as a criterion for a positive test. However, their study involved a small group of 13 patients who were preselected by referral to a shoulder specialist with complaints of instability. Terwee and colleagues[6] found interobserver agreement to be low for assessing active and passive elevation of the shoulder, especially for patients with high pain severity and disability. Rudiger and coworkers[7] found that even "objective" measurements of shoulder mobility by patients and surgeons correlated poorly in a prospective study. Dowrick and colleagues[8] compared self-reported and independently observed disability in an orthopaedic trauma population. They found that disability level ratings varied greatly and that observers consistently rated the disability levels lower than participants. Hickey and associates[9] found that experienced manipulative physiotherapists had difficulty determining the symptomatic status of patients using observational motion analysis.

The comparison of the results of various health care interventions in different fields of medicine is hampered by the absence of a common measurement instrument. Patient-based outcome assessment tools are widely accepted for assessing general health. General health outcome measures have also been used to determine the effect of shoulder conditions on patient well-being, and patient-based outcome instruments have been developed for the shoulder and the upper extremity as a whole. Cook and colleagues[10] assessed four shoulder outcome measures and found them to exhibit good internal consistency across surgical status, in contrast to the inconsistency observed when observer-based systems are assessed.

DEVELOPMENT OF OUTCOME MEASURES

The outcome of treatment is best viewed through the paradigm of a disablement scheme. *Disablement* is a global term that reflects all of the diverse consequences that disease, injury, or congenital abnormalities can have on human function at many different levels. Pathologic conditions can lead to *impairment,* which is an anatomic or physiologic abnormality or loss that may be the direct result or secondary result of pathology. Outcome measures are developed through a process involving identifying a specific patient population, generating items (questions), reducing items (questions), pretesting the outcome instrument, and determining the instrument's measurement properties (validity, reliability, and responsiveness).

TYPES OF OUTCOME MEASURES

The decision about which outcome measure to use should be based on many factors, including the population being studied, the purpose of the assessment (routine assessment vs. clinical research), training required, time required for administration and scoring, and availability of normative data. Generic health instruments, joint-specific instruments, limb-specific instruments, and disease-specific instruments are available for outcome assessment in the shoulder. Beaton and Schemitsch[11] have reviewed the development of measures of health-related quality-of-life and physical-function instruments, noting the development of many outcome measures in the 1990s and reports of their reliability, validity, and responsiveness (see later).

Generic Health Instruments

In the past, the function of the shoulder has traditionally been assessed with measures that reflect the local impact of a disorder rather than the impact of that disorder on the ability of the patient to function in daily life. Generic health instruments provide information regarding the impact of the specific condition of interest and any coexisting conditions on general health that is comparable across different patient groups. The Short Form-36 (SF-36) is a commonly used generic health status instrument that has been found to be a reliable and valid measure of the health of patients with musculoskeletal conditions (see later).

Joint-Specific Outcome Instruments

Joint-specific health instruments have been found to be more responsive than generic health status instruments in assessing conditions of the upper extremity. The increase in responsiveness is probably the result of including specific items that are relevant to the patient group being studied. The disadvantage of joint-specific instruments is the need for numerous scales and the inability to compare outcomes across various conditions, populations, or interventions. Studies of joint-specific instruments have demonstrated lower correlations with generic measures of health than with each other. Joint-specific instruments tend to be less powerful in their ability to discriminate among levels of overall health, a role better fulfilled by generic health measures such as the SF-36.

Limb-Specific Outcome Instruments

Limb-specific outcome instruments are based on the supposition that the upper extremity functions as a kinematic chain. According to this paradigm, the shoulder and the elbow, forearm, and wrist position the hand for grasping and manipulating the environment. Studies of limb-specific instruments have shown close correlation with joint-specific and disease-specific measures, although they tend not to have the same degree of responsiveness. Nevertheless a limb-specific instrument may be appropriate when the diagnosis is less certain or when more than one part of the extremity is affected. For example, a condition involving a shoulder, elbow, wrist, and hand affects, to a greater or lesser extent, the ability to use a telephone.

The Disabilities of the Arm, Shoulder and Hand (DASH) questionnaire focuses on functional limitations, symptoms, and psychosocial problems. Patient-completed limb-specific functional questionnaires such as the DASH questionnaire have been developed with careful attention to psychometric principles of instrument design. Whole-limb questionnaires can be used to assess functional outcome following the treatment of specific joint disorders in the upper extremity. The use of outcome measures that are designed to assess the function of the entire limb can help to determine the relative impact of disorders affecting various anatomic sites in the upper extremity.

It may be appropriate to use a combination of a joint-specific, a limb-specific, a disease-specific, and a generic health status instrument for detailed research studies. However, for most clinicians, the use of a generic and either a joint-specific or a limb-specific outcome instrument would be appropriate for routine assessment and follow-up.

Disease-Specific Outcome Instruments

Disease-specific outcome measures are designed to assess specific conditions in individual joints. An example of a disease-specific outcome measure is the Western Ontario Shoulder Instability Index (WOSI). As a general rule, disease-specific outcome measures are very responsive to small changes in the condition for which they were designed. The disadvantage of disease-specific outcome measures is their limited usefulness in comparing outcomes across different disorders, anatomic sites, and populations and the need for a plethora of outcome measures to assess all conditions affecting the shoulder and elbow.

Kirkley and coworkers[12] developed a disease-specific quality-of-life measurement tool for patients with shoulder instability. The steps included identification of a specific patient population, item generation, item reduction and pretesting. The final instrument had 21 items and demonstrated validity, reliability, and responsiveness. The instrument's responsiveness compared favorably to five other shoulder outcome instruments, a general health outcome measure and measurement of range of motion. The authors suggested that their instrument be used as a primary outcome measure in patients with shoulder instability. In a similar manner Watson and colleagues[12a] developed a disease-specific questionnaire to assess outcome of glenohumeral instability termed the *Melbourne Instability Shoulder Scale.*

Kirkley and coauthors[13] also developed disease-specific outcome instrument for patients with rotator cuff disorders (Western Ontario Rotator Cuff index). This instrument has been translated into Turkish, and the instrument has been shown to be valid and reliable when used in this context.[14] Kirkley's group[15] also developed an outcome measure specifically for patients with glenohumeral osteoarthritis (the Western Ontario Osteoarthritis of the Shoulder Index).

APPLICATION OF OUTCOME MEASURES

The lack of a widely accepted outcome measure can lead to confusion when one attempts to determine the severity of an impairment. Patient-completed functional questionnaires have been developed and tested by psychometric and clinometric methods. When an observer questions a patient with regard to function and then records the response, the possibility of observer bias is introduced. Patient-completed questionnaires can be answered by telephone and mail, do not require a physical examination, and can be used to derive raw scores rather than categorical rankings.

Administration of an Outcome Measure

The response methodology for outcome instruments can include yes or no answers, Likert scales, or visual analogue scales. Visual analogue scales take longer to score than other response methodologies if the value of the patients' response must be determined manually. Yes-or-no answers limit the number of possible responses and can also limit the instrument's responsiveness. Many outcome instruments use Likert scales, although the ideal number of response options for a Likert scale has not been determined.

Assessment of Pain

Some investigators question including pain and function in a total score. Because pain is an impairment, some feel that it should not be included to generate a score of functional limitations. This issue can be addressed by scoring and reporting pain and functional limitations separately. Because a clinical result is important to the clinician, the outcome of therapies designed for treating the shoulder should ideally be described on the basis of a separate patient-derived assessment of function, an assessment of pain, and a clinical examination.

Categorical Rankings Versus Aggregate Scores

A review of the literature reveals a plethora of different definitions for categorical rankings that have been used to describe the outcome after operations on the shoulder. The use of categorical ranking might lead clinicians to mistakenly assume that the categorical rankings that have been used in independently designed scoring systems describe similar levels of impairment. The variable definition of terms for categorical rankings hinders accurate communication between investigators and is an impediment to the objective comparison of the results of different studies. For example, the developers of different scoring systems have assigned different weights to each domain and different ranges of values to each categorical ranking. The outcome measures currently in general use for the shoulder are scoring systems based on the assessment domains such as range of motion, pain, and ability to perform daily activities, which are scored separately. Scores are then aggregated and assigned categorical rankings that range from excellent to poor. It is possible that the same patient can have different raw scores and different (or similar) categorical rankings, depending on which scoring system is used.

Scoring systems based on categorical rankings compartmentalize results into several categories or domains that clinicians use in decision making. Such scoring systems may be more appealing to clinicians than other outcome measures such as patient-completed functional questionnaires. However, the admixture of clinical and functional criteria can create a confusing array of variables, and questioning of a patient by an observer introduces the possibility of observer bias during the collection and interpretation of data. The differences among scoring systems are so pervasive that categorical rankings cannot be relied upon to provide meaningful comparisons either with the same cohort of patients or between cohorts. The results of studies that are based on categorical rankings of different scoring systems cannot be compared or combined. Patient-completed functional questionnaires can be valid and reliable instruments for assessing the shoulder and are not limited by observer bias.

ASSESSING OUTCOME MEASURES

A wide variety of outcome measures are available (Box 7-1). Because most clinicians use an outcome measure as an initial assessment tool and as a method of determining a patient's progress over time, the initial selection of an appropriate outcome measure is important. It is necessary to assess the measurement properties of different instruments to be certain that the outcome is being appraised accurately. Outcome measurements have varying strengths depending on the population being assessed or the reason for using the instrument. An instrument for an outcome measure must be context specific, and selection should be based on evidence that the instrument has the necessary measurement properties in the population being sampled for a study or assessment. The quality of an outcome measure can be assessed objectively, and given the plethora of outcome measures that have been developed, it is advisable to use an outcome measure for which there are data on its measurement properties. The measurement properties of an outcome measure that are important to clinicians are validity, reliability, and responsiveness.

Validity

Conceptually, an instrument is considered valid if it is measuring what it is supposed to measure. Different terms are used to describe different facets of validity. In

---

BOX 7-1 Types of Outcome Instruments to Evaluate the Shoulder

Generic
Arthritis Impact Measurement Scale
Duke Health Profile
Index of Well-Being
Nottingham Health Index
Short Form 12 (SF-12)
Short Form 36 (SF-36)
Sickness Impact Profile

Shoulder Specific
American Shoulder and Elbow Surgeons Standardized Assessment
Constant–Murley
Abbreviated Constant Score
Disability Questionnaire
L'Insalata Shoulder Rating Questionnaire
Neer Rating Sheet
Oxford Shoulder Score
Shoulder-Arm Disability Questionnaire
Shoulder Disability Questionnaire
Shoulder Function Assessment Scale
Shoulder Pain and Disability Index
Shoulder Pain Score
Shoulder Questionnaire
Shoulder Rating Scale
Shoulder Severity Index

Simple Shoulder Test
Subjective Shoulder Rating Scale
University of California at Los Angeles (UCLA) End-Result Score
University of Pennsylvania Shoulder Score
Wheelchair User's Shoulder Pain Index

Limb Specific
Disabilities of the Arm, Shoulder and Hand (DASH)
QuickDASH
Modified American Shoulder and Elbow Surgeons (M-ASES)
Musculoskeletal Functional Assessment
Toronto Extremity Salvage Score
Upper Extremity Function Scale
Upper Limb Functional Index
Functional Impairment Test: Hand and Neck/Shoulder/Arm
Gallon-Jug Shelf-Transfer Test

Disease Specific
Acromioclavicular Separation Scoring System
Melbourne Instability Shoulder Scale
Rowe's Rating for Bankart Repair
Rotator Cuff: Quality of Life
Western Ontario Rotator Cuff Index
Western Ontario Shoulder Instability Index
Western Ontario Osteoarthritis of the Shoulder Index

face validity, the items (questions) chosen appear to make sense to the subject using the instrument. Face validity is the simplest and weakest form of validity. *Content validity* is satisfied when it is proved that the scale measures all important aspects of the condition to be examined. *Construct validity* is the degree to which an outcome measure can be shown to be associated with other measures that have a specific relationship with the system being measured. Testing of construct validity builds confidence in an outcome measure. Comparison of the data generated by the outcome measure to patient-derived and physician-derived assessment of the severity of the impairment, the level of pain, the ability to perform normal activities of daily living, and the responses on other contemporary patient-completed questionnaires can be used to test validity. *Convergent validity* determines if an outcome measure correlates with similar scales or dimensions of a scale. *Divergent validity* demonstrates lack of correlation between dissimilar scales or dimensions of a scale. *Discriminant validity* is the ability of an outcome measure to discriminate across the levels of severity for a patient population. A variety of statistical measures are used in determining validity, including Pearson's product moment correlation coefficient. A detailed discussion of the methodology of determining validity is outside the scope of this chapter.

Reliability

The concept of reliability is that repeated administration of a measurement tool on stable subjects yields the same results. Shoulder outcome instruments should be sufficiently reliable that the score derived from the use of the outcome measure does not change, even if the questionnaire is completed on different occasions, providing that there has been no change in the patient's clinical problem in the intervening interval.

Reliability is assessed by recruiting a cohort of patients appropriate to the outcome measure being assessed. The outcome measure is administered and the process is completed some weeks or months hence. At the time of the second testing, patients are asked if their condition has changed. If their condition has changed, they are excluded from the analysis because, for obvious reasons, one would expect their score to change.

Reliability is determined by statistical techniques such as the one-way, random effects intraclass correlation coefficient, two-way analysis of variance to determine the intraclass correlation coefficient, Spearman rank correlation coefficients, and other measures. Clinicians can also assess the percentage of subjects having identical scores and the number of patients whose scores have changed response categories between testing sessions.

Responsiveness

Responsiveness is the ability of an instrument to detect true changes in a patient's status beyond random variability.

Some authors believe that responsiveness may be the most important property of evaluative health status instruments. Prior knowledge of an instrument's responsiveness helps the clinician to select appropriate outcome measures and allows the clinician to estimate the sample size required to ensure adequate statistical power. Responsiveness is assessed by defining a cohort of patients whose health condition has probably changed between testings. For instance, patients with advanced rotator cuff disease or glenohumeral osteoarthritis could be compared before and after rotator cuff repair or total shoulder arthroplasty.

To determine responsiveness, the difference between the preoperative and postoperative scores (change score) is determined. A statistical measure called the *standardized response mean* (mean change score divided by the standard deviation of the change scores) can be used to assess relative responsiveness of questionnaires. The standardized response mean transforms the change score into a standard unit of measurement, allowing comparison among different instruments. The standardized response mean has often been used to assess the relative responsiveness of various health status instruments used to assess the impact of musculoskeletal conditions. A higher standardized response mean indicates greater sensitivity to clinical change. Cohen's standard has been used by investigators in this field to compare responsiveness of outcome measures.

A number of other indices have been used to assess relative responsiveness of self-administered questionnaires. Other statistical measures that have been used to measure responsiveness include the effect size (mean change score divided by standard deviation of initial scores), relative efficiency (squared ratio of *t* statistic), Guyatt's responsiveness statistic (clinically important difference divided by variability in stable subjects), and correlation with external criteria. The magnitude of a responsiveness statistic can vary depending on the time that has elapsed (a 3-month score is not as high as a 6-month score) or the type of procedure that was performed (different treatments have different effects). Differences in the responsiveness statistics should not be considered by themselves to indicate the quality of a particular instrument, because such statistics must be reviewed in the context of the patient group being tested. Kirkley, Griffin and Dainty[16] noted that the responsiveness of an instrument was an important consideration in the design of research studies because it can serve to minimize the sample size required for a particular study. These authors opined that appropriate instruments exist for the "main" conditions of the shoulder.

SPECIFIC OUTCOME INSTRUMENTS

Generic Outcome Instruments

The SF-36 measures eight health concepts including physical functioning (10 items), social functioning (2 items), role limitations due to physical problems (4 items), role limitations due to emotional problems (three items), mental health (5 items), energy and fatigue (4 items), bodily pain (2 items), and general health perception (5 items). A number of studies have assessed the reliability, validity, and responsiveness of the SF-36 for conditions of the upper extremity. An abbreviated version of the SF-36 (Short Form-12 [SF-12]) has been developed, although its measurement properties have not been as well defined for musculoskeletal disorders. Concern has been expressed that the SF-36 physical functioning dimension lacks upper limb content.

Beaton and Richards[17] reported on a prospective comparison of five different shoulder questionnaires and the SF-36 in a sample of patients with shoulder pain. All the shoulder questionnaires had acceptable reliability ratings and measured responsiveness more effectively than the SF-36. These authors suggested that both types of questionnaires should be used in outcome evaluations. Crane and coworkers[18] assessed 37 shoulder items to determine if observed differences in function were due to biased test items or real differences in function. They found that the pool of shoulder function items successfully measured function across demographic groups.

Gartsman and colleagues[19] assessed 544 patients with five common shoulder conditions who completed the SF-36 health survey before undergoing treatment. Comparison with published data demonstrated that the shoulder conditions ranked in severity with five major medical conditions including hypertension, congestive heart failure, acute myocardial infarction, diabetes mellitus, and clinical depression.

McKee and Yoo[20] assessed the general health status of 71 patients who underwent open acromioplasty and subacromial bursectomy. The preoperative SF-36 scores were significantly below normative data for the domains of physical function ($P = .02$), physical role function ($P = .001$), and pain ($P = .003$). Postoperatively the scores for pain ($P = .0001$), physical role function ($P = .06$), and vitality ($P = .01$) improved. The authors concluded that surgery for chronic rotator cuff disease reliably and significantly improved general health status.

Joint-Specific Instruments for the Shoulder

The measurement properties of several joint-specific outcome measures for the shoulder have been described. The ASES Standardized Assessment Form Shoulder Score Index was developed in 1994. The instrument consists of a patient self-assessment section and a clinician assessment section. An advantage of the activities of daily living section and the pain scale is ease of administration. The patient self-assessment section of the ASES form can be completed independent of an examiner or by telephone interview. Skutek's group[21] found the ASES score to correlate with the Constant–Murley shoulder score ($r = 0.871$, $P < .01$) and to be the preferred method of outcome assessment without the patient having to return to the

clinic, at least in comparison to the Simple Shoulder Test (SST) and the DASH questionnaire (see later).

Michener and colleagues[22] validated the American Shoulder and Elbow Surgeons (ASES) standardized assessment form and found it to be a reliable, valid, and responsive outcome tool. Kocher and coworkers[23] studied the reliability, validity, and responsiveness of the ASES assessment in patients with shoulder instability, rotator cuff disease, and glenohumeral arthritis and found that the scale demonstrated overall acceptable psychometric properties for outcome assessment in these groups of patients. Chen and colleagues[24] found the ASES score to be significantly correlated with patient satisfaction following shoulder arthroplasty and emphasized the importance of patient-derived subjective assessment of symptoms and function. Lee and coauthors[25] assessed outcome after rotator cuff repair using the ASES, Constant, and pain scores. They noted significant improvement in the scores in patients with smaller rotator tears with functional improvement in patients with massive tears, although gains in strength and motion were less dramatic. Alcid and colleagues[26] used the ASES score to assess outcome following revision anterior shoulder stabilization using hamstring tendon autograft and tibialis tendon allograft. Goldhahn and coworkers[27] assessed the cross-cultural adaptation of the ASES into German and found no major problems. The German ASES showed good reliability and validity.

The Shoulder Pain and Disability Index (SPADI) was introduced in 1991. This outcome instrument uses a 100-point system incorporating visual analogue scales for all items. Williams and colleagues[28] measured shoulder function with the SPADI and found that it correlated with other measures of health outcome, was responsive, and discriminated among patients who were improved or worsened. Heald and associates[29] studied 94 patients with shoulder problems who were referred to outpatient physical therapy clinics. They found the SPADI to be more responsive than the Sickness Impact Profile (a generic outcome instrument) and determined that there was support for the construct validity of the SPADI, although it did not strongly reflect occupational and recreational disability. MacDermid and colleagues[30] assessed validity of the SPADI in a group of 129 community volunteers who identified themselves as having shoulder pain. In this study the SPADI demonstrated factor, construct, and longitudinal validity. Cross-cultural adaptation of the SPADI has been performed according to international guidelines. Angst and coworkers[31] reported in 2007 that the German SPADI was practical, reliable, and valid and that it could be recommended for self-assessment of shoulder pain and function.

The SST was developed at the University of Washington. The questionnaire consists of 12 functional items and does not directly assess pain, range of motion, or strength: 2 of the questions relate to pain, 7 to function, and 3 to range of motion. The response to each item requires either a "yes" or a "no." The dichotomous scale of the

SST provides excellent reliability but can constrain its use as an evaluative instrument. Godfrey and colleagues[32] found the SST to have acceptable test-to-retest reliability, content validity, and construct validity. Responsiveness was lower in younger patients and in patients with instability injuries to the extent that they cautioned against its use in this group of patients.

Chipcase and coauthors[33] assessed 81 patients with chronic shoulder impingement syndrome resistant to conservative treatment. The patients completed a generic (SF-36) and a shoulder-specific (SST) questionnaire. The patient scores were significantly lower on all health dimensions of the SF-36 than in the normal population. The results of the SST demonstrated that the patients were functionally very limited, particularly in being unable to work full time at their usual job and being unable to lift a weight over their head.

The UCLA end result score was first used by Ellman and colleagues in 1986.[34] It is a 35-point scale including 10 points for pain, 10 points for function, 5 points for active forward elevation, 5 points for strength and forward elevation, and 5 points for patient satisfaction. The data are reported in terms of categorical rankings. The scale has been criticized because it uses descriptive items for pain and function. The inclusion of points for patient satisfaction makes it difficult to use the scale before treatment. When using the scale, it is best to report numerical results and avoid using the categorical rankings. Roddey and colleagues[35] compared the UCLA Shoulder Scale, the SST, and the SPADI and found that the three scales demonstrated good internal consistency, although the standard errors of measurement for each of the scales were high and factor loading was inconsistent, suggesting that patients might not distinguish between pain and function.

The University of Pennsylvania Shoulder Score uses two 100% scoring systems based on patient self-assessment and objective measures of range of motion and strength. There are three pain scales, a patient satisfaction scale, and a self-assessment of function. Leggin and coworkers[36] assessed the University of Pennsylvania Shoulder Score in 40 patients in relation to the Constant shoulder score and the ASES score and found it to be a reliable and valid outcome measure for reporting patients with various shoulder disorders.

The Constant shoulder score is a 100-point scoring system in which 35 points are derived from the patient's reported pain and function and the remaining 65 points are allocated for assessment of range of motion and strength. Age- and gender-matched normative data are available for the Constant score. Grassi and Tajana[37] studied the Constant score in 563 subjects. They found that the score tended to decrease beginning at age 50 years for men and age 30 years for women. Only 4 subjects received a maximum score of 100. These investigators recommended establishing personal tables for normalizing scores, depending on the population being studied.

The Constant score has been criticized for having only one pain scale and for including a nonstandardized strength test as part of the instrument. Because a large portion of the Constant score is derived from objective measures, the patients who are unable to return for follow-up examination in person cannot be examined, which can lead to incomplete data collection. Conboy and colleagues[38] analyzed the Constant–Murley assessment for 25 patients with shoulder pathology. The score was easy to use but imprecise in repeated measurements. There was a ceiling effect (most scores high) in patients with shoulder instability that was of concern in this group of patients.

Othman and Taylor[39] compared the Constant score, the abbreviated Constant score with the strength measurement excluded, and the Oxford questionnaire. These investigators found a better correlation between the Oxford score and the Constant–Murley score when muscle strength was excluded or measured by a modified method of strength assessment with a sling over the mid-humerus. Baker and coworkers[40] compared the Constant score to the Oxford Shoulder Score and considered the Oxford score to be an alternative to longer term follow-up. These authors noted the Oxford Shoulder Score to be solely subjective and thus easier to administer.

Johansson and Adolfsson[41] found good intraobserver and interobserver reliability for the strength test in the Constant–Murley shoulder assessment, although their study only included 20 healthy young subjects and two observers. These authors concluded that a digital dynamometer could replace the conventional spring balance as originally described by Constant. Walton's group[42] found that age and sex both affected the Constant score and that methods for shoulder strength assessment (maximum strength with myometer, mean strength with myometer, and maximum strength with fixed-spring myometer) were not the same. Rocourt and colleagues[43] evaluated the intratester and intertester reliability of the Constant–Murley shoulder assessment and found that reliability could be improved by better standardization of the testing procedure. Fialka and colleagues[44] suggested that the accuracy of the Constant score could be increased by using the uninjured collateral shoulder of each patient as a reference, allowing the development of an "individual relative Constant score." This concept would be problematic for the many patients with bilateral shoulder disorders.

The Shoulder Disability Questionnaire was described in 1996. This questionnaire was found to differentiate well between high and low disability levels in patients in primary care by de Winter and coauthors.[45]

L'Insalata and colleagues[46] reported on the development of the Shoulder Rating Questionnaire. They developed this self-administered questionnaire to assess symptom severity and functionality of the shoulder. Their instrument has separate domains including global assessment, pain, daily activities, recreational and athletic activities, work, satisfaction, and areas for improvement. Each domain is graded separately and weighted to arrive at the total score. The self-administered shoulder questionnaire was found to be valid, reliable, and responsive to clinical change.

Beaton and Richards[47] reported on a prospective comparison of the validity of five questionnaires used in the assessment of shoulder function. The questionnaires (SPADI, SST, Subjective Shoulder Rating Scale [SSRS], Modified ASES Shoulder Patient Self-Evaluation Form [M-ASES], and the Shoulder Severity Index) performed similarly in describing function of the shoulder and in discriminating between levels of severity. The shoulder questionnaires performed differently than the SF-36, confirming the need to use both disease-specific and generic health status measures to assess the shoulder.

Paul and coworkers[48] assessed the SPADI, the Shoulder Rating Questionnaire (SRQ), the Dutch Shoulder Disability Questionnaire (SDQ-NL) and the United Kingdom Shoulder Disability Questionnaire (SDQ-UK) in a primary care setting. They found that all questionnaires correlated poorly with active motion, although they had similar overall validity and patient acceptability. The SPADI and SRQ were the most responsive to change.

Krepler and colleagues[49] assessed outcome following hemiarthroplasty of the shoulder using four evaluation tools. They recommended using a scoring system with emphasis on pain and patient satisfaction as opposed to strength.

Razmjou and associates[50] compared the longitudinal construct validity of two rotator cuff disease–specific outcome measures (the Rotator Cuff–Quality of Life and the Western Ontario Rotator Cuff Index) in relation to the ASES standardized assessment and the Upper Extremity Functional Index. Participants in the study received physical therapy for rotator cuff disorders treated both surgically and nonsurgically. They found that the sensitivity to change was very close among all scores and that the two disease-specific scores had similar convergent validity.

Limb-Specific Outcome Instruments

The DASH questionnaire was developed as an instrument that would measure the impact on function of a wide variety of musculoskeletal conditions affecting the upper limbs. The multidisciplinary group that developed the DASH designed the instrument to quantify disability (predominately physical function) and symptoms in persons with upper limb disorders. The DASH is a 30-item questionnaire with two optional modules to measure the impact of a disorder when playing a musical instrument or sport or when working. Respondents circle one of five responses and the score is transformed to a 0 to 100 scale. A higher score indicates greater disability. The 30-item questionnaire includes 21 physical function items, 6 symptom items, 3 social- and role-function items, plus the 4-item sports and performing arts module.

The DASH questionnaire was tested by Beaton and colleagues[51] in a group of diverse patients and compared to joint-specific questionnaires. The responsiveness of the DASH was comparable with or better than that of the joint-specific measures in the whole. This study demonstrated that the DASH had validity and responsiveness in both proximal and distal disorders, although it did not compare its responsiveness to disease-specific measures for the shoulder. The development and recommended method of use of the DASH is outlined in a detailed user's manual.

SooHoo and coworkers[52] evaluated the construct validity of the DASH questionnaire by correlating it with the SF-36. The DASH questionnaire had fewer ceiling and floor scores than most of the SF-36 subscales, supporting the use of the DASH as a valid measure of health status in patients with a wide variety of upper extremity complaints. Dowrick's group[53] has cautioned that the DASH does not exclusively assess disability in the upper extremity and that this should be taken into account when assessing upper extremity function in patients with lower extremity injuries. Jester and colleagues[54] measured levels of disability in employed adults using the DASH. These authors determined that increased disability was expressed by older workers, female workers, and manual workers.

Orfale and coauthors[55] have reported on the translation and cultural adaptation of the DASH into Brazilian Portuguese and shown it to be a reliable instrument in that context. In a similar fashion there are reports of the cross-cultural adaptation of the DASH questionnaire into Canadian French,[56] Spanish,[57] Dutch,[58] and Chinese.[59,60]

An abbreviated form of the DASH questionnaire, the QuickDASH, has been developed as a short, reliable and valid measure of physical function and symptoms related to upper limb musculoskeletal disorders. The QuickDASH was developed by Beaton and coworkers[61] using three item-reduction techniques on cross-sectional field testing data derived from a study of 407 patients with various upper limb conditions. The QuickDASH has been found to have similar discriminant ability and test-to-retest reliability to the DASH.[62] The QuickDASH has been successfully translated into Japanese.[63] Matheson and colleagues[64] report on the development of a visual analogue scale of the QuickDASH.

Medical Comorbidities

Medical comorbidities can affect the severity of disability in patients with shoulder disorders and the outcome of treatment, including operative intervention. Wolf and Green[65] studied the influence of comorbidity of self-assessment instrument scores in patients with idiopathic adhesive capsulitis. They found that patients with more comorbidities had significantly lower scores on the DASH and SF-36 questionnaires. The comfort and pain subscale of the SF-36 showed a significant correlation with increased comorbidity. Boissonnault and coworkers[66] found medical comorbidities affected outcome in patients following a physical therapy program after rotator cuff repair surgery when outcome was assessed by SF-36 scores but not with DASH function scores.

AUTHOR'S CURRENT PRACTICE

When assessing new patients, I use a 20-page survey (Fig. 7-1—see website). My practice is oriented toward assessing and treating workers with shoulder and elbow injuries. The survey is offered by way of example and would not necessarily be applicable to practices with different orientation and demographics. Nevertheless, it is my hope that the survey may be useful to the reader in terms of the type of evaluation instrument that individual practitioners can develop for their own practices.

Consent for the use of data derived from the survey for research purposes is obtained in advance of the clinic visit. The survey is configured so that the data can be read by a scanning device. The survey can also be administered by touch-screen technology. The importance of answering all of the questions is emphasized on Page 2 of the survey.

Page 3 consists of a pain diagram wherein patients are asked to localize their pain and define its severity. Page 4 of the survey asks patients to define the length of their symptoms and the nature of their onset. Pages 5 and 6 are directed toward defining the severity of the pain, its frequency, and its impact on the patient's normal daily activity and ability to take part in recreational, social, and family activity. Pages 7 and 8 are devoted to the QuickDASH questionnaire. Pages 9 to 15 are devoted to detailed questions regarding patients' ability to perform their normal occupational activity, if they can perform modified work, and their attitude toward their work. Most practices would require less emphasis on this area, and practices oriented toward patients interested in sports activity would, in contrast, have more emphasis in that area. Pages 16 to 18 are devoted to the SF-36 questionnaire. Page 19 is devoted to demographic questions and requests information regarding the patient's marital status, gender, educational background, height, weight, hand dominance, smoking history, and background language. The final page of the survey is devoted to documenting medical comorbidities, if present. As noted earlier, the presence of medical comorbidities can affect patient responses to outcome measures.

My current practice is to have this information processed by a computer and have it in a presentable format at the time I see the patient. The data are presented in a 1-page format (Fig. 7-2), which includes normative data and highlights the patient's pain profile and most prominent limitation. I find this information useful in the initial assessment of patients. Furthermore, such baseline data are very useful in assessing patients' responses to treatment, providing follow-up data are obtained in a similar fashion. It has been noted that patients' responses shift in relation to time and the effects of treatment, so the documentation of baseline data is critically important.

FUTURE DEVELOPMENTS

Various authors have called for standardization of outcome assessment because this would facilitate communication among investigators, clinicians, health care administrators, and the public. Comparison and pooling of data across studies and the conduct of multicenter trials would be encouraged by the standardization of outcome assessment.

At present, there is still much work to be done in determining the most appropriate outcome measures for various purposes. More comparative studies are needed to show one instrument is superior to another. For instance, in a study of outcomes after surgical treatment for recurrent posterior shoulder instability, we found a disease-specific measure for shoulder instability to be the most responsive, followed by a joint-specific measure and a limb-specific measure (the DASH), although the differences were not statistically significant. However, the DASH was easier to score than the other two measures and would allow comparison between studies if it were widely used. The SF-36 was not responsive to change in this patient population. Further work is needed to complete investigation of the measurement properties of a number of outcome instruments in specific patient populations.

SUMMARY

Ideally, an outcome instrument measures phenomena that are directly relevant to the patient and provides a comprehensive assessment of the impact of a condition on a patient's daily life. Although subjective complaints may be difficult to quantify, pain and disability may be the most valid outcome measures because they are directly relevant to patients. Self-administered questionnaires have been shown to be more responsive than traditional physical measures such as range of motion, strength, dexterity, and sensation. Self-administered questionnaires are not subject to observer bias. Comparisons between studies based on different scoring systems are generally not valid, and the categorical rankings of different systems are not interchangeable. When categorical rankings are used, the data should also be reported in terms of aggregate scores. In general, both generic and joint-specific measures of health status should be used when assessing function of the shoulder. The role of limb-specific and disease-specific instruments is evolving at this time. Patient-completed functional questionnaires are the optimal method of assessing the effectiveness of shoulder interventions and encourage the scientific assessment and comparison of treatment results.

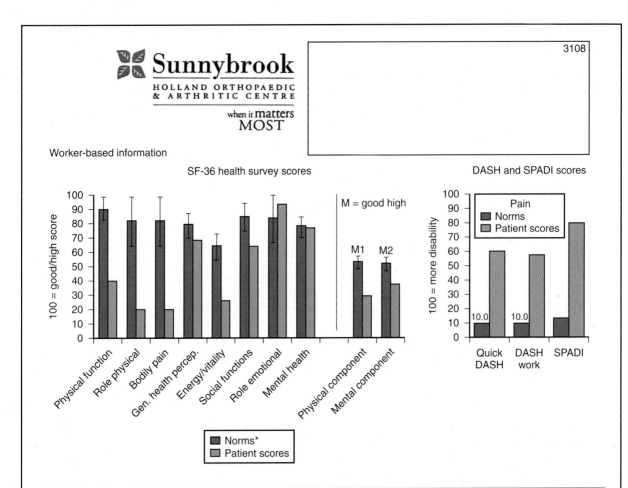

Profile

Age:	35	Sex:	F
	Current occupation:		personal support worker
	Occupation at time of injury:		

Work module

Working?	Yes
Work accomodation underway?	Yes
If 'Yes' what sort?	Modified work because of this

Other symptoms

- Arm/shoulder/hand pain
- Arm/shoulder/hand pain on activity

Pain scores (greater score = more pain)

von Korff grade (1–4):	Grade 4
Grade 4 = high disability, severely limiting	
Pain intensity scale (/100):	80.0
Days disabled (/180 days):	60
Disability score (0 low-3 high):	2

Cluster score

n/a

DASH outcome measure scores today

DASH score (0–100, 100 = more disability):	60.0
Open a tight or new jar	2
Place object on overhead shelf	4
Do heavy chores	5
Problem interferes with social activities	3
Difficulty sleeping due to pain	4

Other health problems   Total comorbidities: 1

- Low back pain

FIGURE 7-2 This 1-page summary is generated from the survey at the time the patient is assessed. The summary provides the patient's QuickDASH, SPADI, and SF-36 scores together with normative data for these scores. The summary also lists information regarding the patient's pain score, their symptoms, work profile, and comorbidities. (Redrawn from Hopman WM, Towheed T, Anastassiades T, et al: Canadian normative data for the SF-36 health survey. Canadian Multicentre Osteoporosis Study Research Group. CMAJ 163:265-271, 2000.)

REFERENCES

1. Duckworth DG, Smith KL, Campbell B, Matsen FA 3rd: Self-assessment questionnaires document substantial variability in the clinical expression of rotator cuff tears. J Shoulder Elbow Surg 8(4):330-333, 1999.
2. Codman EA: The product of a hospital. Surg Gynecol Obstet 18:491-496, 1914.
3. Hayes K, Walton JR, Szomor ZR, Murrell GA: Reliability of five methods for assessing shoulder range of motion. Aust J Physiother 47(4):289-294, 2001.
4. Ostor AJ, Richards CA, Prevost AT, et al: Interrater reproducibility of clinical tests for rotator cuff lesions. Ann Rheum Dis 63(10):1288-1292, 2004.
5. Tzannes A, Paxinos A, Callanan M, Murrell GA: An assessment of the inter-examiner reliability of tests for shoulder instability. J Shoulder Elbow Surg 13(1):18-23, 2004.
6. Terwee CB, de Winter AF, Scholten RJ, et al: Interobserver reproducibility of the visual estimation of range of motion of the shoulder. Arch Phys Med Rehabil 86(7):1356-1361, 2005.
7. Rudiger HA, Fuchs B, von Campe A, Gerber C: Measurements of shoulder mobility by patient and surgeon correlate poorly: A prospective study. J Shoulder Elbow Surg 17(2):255-260, 2008.
8. Dowrick AS, Gabbe BJ, Williamson OD, et al: A comparison of self-reported and independently observed disability in an orthopedic trauma population. J Trauma 61(6):1447-1452, 2006.
9. Hickey BW, Milosavijevic S, Bell ML, Milburn PD: Accuracy and reliability of observational motion analysis in identifying shoulder symptoms. Man Ther 12(3):263-270, 2007.
10. Cook KF, Roddey TS, Olson SL, et al: Reliability by surgical status of self-reported outcomes in patients who have shoulder pathologies. J Orthop Sports Phys Ther 32(7):336-346, 2002.
11. Beaton DE, Schemitsch E: Measures of health-related quality of life and physical function. Clin Orthop Relat Res (413):90-105, 2003.
12. Kirkley A, Griffin S, McLintock H, Ng L: The development and evaluation of a disease-specific quality of life measurement tool for shoulder instability. The Western Ontario Shoulder Instability Index (WOSI). Am J Sports Med 26:764-772, 1998.
12a. Watson L, Story I, Dalziel R, Hoy G, et al: A new clinical outcome measure of glenohumeral joint instability: the MISS questionnaire. J Shoulder Elbow Surg 14(1):22-30, 2005.
13. Kirkley A, Alvarez C, Griffin S: The development and evaluation of a disease-specific quality-of-life questionnaire for disorders of the rotator cuff: The Western Ontario Rotator Cuff Index. Clin J Sport Med 13(2):84-92, 2003.
14. El O, Bircan C, Gulbaher S, et al: The reliability and validity of the Turkish version of the Western Ontario Rotator Cuff Index. Rheumatol Int 26(12):1101-1108, 2006.
15. Lo IK, Griffin S, Kirkley: The development of a disease-specific quality of life measurement tool for osteoarthritis of the shoulder: The Western Ontario Osteoarthritis of the Shoulder Index (WOOS). Osteoarthritis Cartilage 9:8:771-778, 2001.
16. Kirkley A, Griffin S, Dainty K: Scoring systems for the functional assessment of the shoulder. Arthroscopy 19(10):1109-1120, 2003.
17. Beaton DE, Richards RR: Assessing the reliability and responsiveness of 5 shoulder questionnaires. J Shoulder Elbow Surg 7:565-572, 1998.
18. Crane PK, Hart DL, Gibbons LE, Cook KF: A 37-item shoulder functional status item pool had negligible differential item functioning. J Clin Epidemiol 59(5):478-484, 2006.
19. Gartsman GM, Brinker MR, Khan M, Karahan M: Self-assessment of general health status in patients with five common shoulder conditions. J Shoulder Elbow Surg 7:228-237, 1998.
20. McKee MD, Yoo DJ: The effect of surgery for rotator cuff disease on general health status. J Bone Joint Surg Am 82:970-979, 2000.
21. Skutek M, Fremerey RW, Zeichen J, Bosch U: Outcome analysis following open rotator cuff repair. Early effectiveness validated using four different shoulder assessment scales. Arch Orthop Trauma Surg 120(7-8):432-436, 2000.
22. Michener LA, McClure PW, Sennett BJ: American Shoulder and Elbow Surgeons Standardized Shoulder Assessment Form, patient self-report section: Reliability, validity, and responsiveness. J Shoulder Elbow Surg 11(6):587-594, 2002.
23. Kocher MS, Horan MP, Briggs KK, et al: Reliability, validity, and responsiveness of the American Shoulder and Elbow Surgeons subjective shoulder scale in patients with shoulder instability, rotator cuff disease, and glenohumeral arthritis. J Bone Joint Surg Am 87(9):2006-2011, 2005.
24. Chen AL, Bain EB, Horan MP, Hawkins RJ: Determinants of patient satisfaction with outcome after shoulder arthroplasty. J Shoulder Elbow Surg 16(1):25-30, 2007.
25. Lee E, Bishop JY, Braman JP, et al: Outcomes after arthroscopic rotator cuff repairs. J Shoulder Elbow Surg 16(1):1-5, 2007.
26. Alcid J, Powell, SE, Tibone JE: Revision anterior capsular shoulder stabilization using hamstring tendon autograft and tibialis tendon allograft reinforcement: Minimum two year follow-up. J Shoulder Elbow Surg 16:268-272, 2007.
27. Goldhahn J, Angst F, Drerup S, et al: Lessons learned during the cross-cultural adaptation of the American Shoulder and Elbow Surgeons shoulder form into German. J Shoulder Elbow Surg 17(2):248-254, 2008.
28. Williams JW, Holleman DR, Simel DL: Measuring shoulder function with the Shoulder Pain and Disability Index. J Rheumatol 22(4):727-732, 1995.
29. Heald SL, Riddle DL, Lamb RL: The shoulder pain and disability index: The construct validity and responsiveness of a region-specific disability measure. Phys Ther 77(10):1079-1089, 1997.
30. MacDermid JC, Solomon P, Prkachin K: The Shoulder Pain and Disability Index demonstrates factor, construct and longitudinal validity. BMC Musculoskelet Disord 7:12, 2006.
31. Angst F, Goldhahn J, Pap G, et al: Cross-cultural adaptation, reliability and validity of the German Shoulder Pain and Disability Index (SPADI). Rheumatology (Oxford) 46(1):87-92, 2007.
32. Godfrey J, Hamman R, Lowenstein S, et al: Reliability, validity, and responsiveness of the simple shoulder test: Psychometric properties by age and injury type. J Shoulder Elbow Surg 16(3):260-267, 2007.
33. Chipcase, LS, O'Connor DA, Costi JJ, Krishnan J: Shoulder impingement syndrome: Preoperative health status. J Shoulder Elbow Surg 9:12-15, 2000.
34. Ellman H, Hanker G, Bayer M: Repair of the rotator cuff. End-result study of factors influencing reconstruction. J Bone Joint Surg Am 68:1136-1144, 1986.
35. Roddey TS, Olson SL, Cook KF, et al: Comparison of the University of California–Los Angeles Shoulder Scale and the Simple Shoulder Test with the shoulder pain and disability index: Single-administration reliability and validity. Phys Ther 80(8):759-768, 2000.
36. Leggin BG, Michener LA, Shaffer MA, et al: The Penn shoulder score: Reliability and validity. J Orthop Sports Phys Ther 36(3):138-151, 2006.
37. Grassi FA, Tajana MS: The normalization of data in the Constant–Murley score for the shoulder. A study conducted on 563 health subjects. Chir Organi Mov 88(1):65-73, 2003.
38. Conboy VB, Morris RW, Kiss J, Carr AJ: An evaluation of the Constant–Murley shoulder assessment. J Bone Joint Surg Br 78:229-232, 1996.
39. Othman A, Taylor G: Is the Constant score reliable in assessing patients with frozen shoulder? 60 shoulders scored 3 years after manipulation under anesthesia. Acta Orthop Scand 75(1):114-116, 2004.
40. Baker P, Nanda R, Goodchild L, et al: A comparison of the Constant and Oxford shoulder scores in patients with conservatively treated proximal humeral fractures. J Shoulder Elbow Surg 17(1):37-41, 2008.
41. Johansson KM, Adolfsson LE: Intraobserver and interobserver reliability for the strength test in the Constant–Murley shoulder assessment. J Shoulder Elbow Surg 14(3):273-278, 2005.
42. Walton MJ, Walton JC, Honorez LAM, et al: A comparison of methods for shoulder strength assessment and analysis of Constant score change in patients aged over fifty years in the United Kingdom. J Shoulder Elbow Surg 16(3):285-289, 2007.
43. Rocourt MH, Radlinger L, Kalberer F, et al: Evaluation of intratester and intertester reliability of the Constant–Murley shoulder assessment. J Shoulder Elbow Surg 17(2):364-369, 2008.
44. Fialka C, Oberleitner G, Stampfl P, et al: Modification of the Constant–Murley shoulder score—introduction of the individual relative Constant score individual shoulder assessment. Injury 36(10):1159-1165, 2005.
45. deWinter AF, van der Heijden GJ, Scholten RJ, et al: The Shoulder Disability Questionnaire differentiated well between high and low disability levels in patients in primary care, in a cross-sectional study. J Clin Epidemiol 60(11):1156-1163, 2007.
46. L'Insalata JC, Warren RF, Cohen SB, et al: A self-administered questionnaire for assessment of symptoms and function of the shoulder. J Bone Joint Surg Am 79:738-748, 1997.
47. Beaton DE, Richards, RR: Measuring function of the shoulder. J Bone Joint Surg Am 78:882-890, 1996.

48. Paul A, Lewis M, Shadforth MF, et al: A comparison of four shoulder-specific questionnaires in primary care. Ann Rheum Dis 63(10):1293-1299, 2004.

49. Krepler P, Wanivenhaus AH, Wurnig C: Outcome assessment of hemiarthroplasty of the shoulder: A 5-year follow-up with 4 evaluation tools. Acta Orthop 77(5):778-784, 2006.

50. Razmjou H, Bean A, van Osnabrugge V, et al: Cross-sectional and longitudinal construct validity of two rotator cuff disease-specific outcome measures. BMC Musculoskelet Disord 7:26, 2006.

51. Beaton DE, Katz JN, Fossel AH, et al: Measuring the whole or the parts? Validity, reliability, and responsiveness of the Disabilities of the Arm, Shoulder and Hand outcome measure in different regions of the upper extremity. J Hand Ther 14(2):128-146, 2001.

52. SooHoo NF, McDonald AP, Seiler JG, McGillivary GR: Evaluation of the construct validity of the DASH questionnaire by correlation to the SF-36. J Hand Surg (Am) 27(3):537-541, 2002.

53. Dowrick AS, Gabbe BJ, Williamson OD, Cameron PA: Does the disabilities of the arm, shoulder and hand (DASH) scoring system only measure disability due to injuries to the upper limb? J Bone Joint Surg Br 88(4):524-527, 2006.

54. Jester A, Harth A, Germann G: Measuring levels of upper-extremity disability in employed adults using the DASH Questionnaire. J Hand Surg (Am) 30(5):1074.e1-1074.e10, 2005.

55. Orfale AG, Araujo PM, Ferraz MB, Natour J: Translation into Brazilian Portuguese, cultural adaptation and evaluation of the reliability of the Disabilities of the Arm, Shoulder and Hand Questionnaire. Braz J Med Biol Res 38(2):293-302, 2005.

56. Durand MJ, Vachon B, Hong QN, Loisel P: The cross-cultural adaptation of the DASH questionnaire in Canadian French. J Hand Ther 18(1):34-39, 2005.

57. Rosales RS, Delgado EB, Diez de la Lastra-Bosch I: Evaluation of the Spanish version of the DASH and carpal tunnel syndrome health-related quality-of-life instruments: Cross-cultural adaptation process and reliability. J Hand Surg (Am) 27(2):334-343, 2002.

58. Veehof MM, Sleegers EJ, van Veldhoven NH, et al: Psychometric qualities of the Dutch language version of the Disabilities of the Arm, Shoulder, and Hand questionnaire (DASH-DLV). J Hand Ther 15(4):347-354, 2002.

59. Lee EW, Lau JS, Chung MM, et al: Evaluation of the Chinese version of the Disability of the Arm, shoulder and Hand (DASH-HKPWH): cross-cultural adaptation process, internal consistency and reliability study. J Hand Ther 17(4):417-423, 2004.

60. Liang HW, Wang HK, Yao G, et al: Psychometric evaluation of the Taiwan version of the Disability of the Arm, Shoulder, and Hand (DASH) questionnaire. J Formos Med Assoc 103(10):773-779, 2004.

61. Beaton DE, Wright JG, Katz JN; Upper Extremity Collaborative Group: Development of the QuickDASH: Comparison of three item-reduction approaches. J Bone Joint Surg Am 87(5):1038-1046, 2005.

62. Gummesson C, Ward MM, Atroshi I: The shortened disabilities of the arm, shoulder and hand questionnaire (QuickDASH): Validity and reliability based on responses within the full-length DASH. BMC Musculoskelet Disord 7:44, 2006.

63. Imaeda T, Toh S, Wada T, et al; Impairment Evaluation Committee, Japanese Society for Surgery of the Hand: Validation of the Japanese Society for Surgery of the Hand Version of the Quick Disability of the Arm, Shoulder, and Hand (QuickDASH-JSSH) questionnaire. J Orthop Sci 11(3):248-253, 2006.

64. Matheson LN, Melhorn JM, Mayer TG, et al: Reliability of a visual analog version of the QuickDASH. J Bone Joint Surg Am 88(8):1782-1787, 2006.

65. Wolf JM, Green A: Influence of comorbidity on self-assessment instrument scores of patients with idiopathic adhesive capsulitis. J Bone Jone Surg Am 84(7):1167-1173, 2002.

66. Boissonnault WG, Badke MB, Wooden MJ, Ekedahl S, Fly K: Patient outcome following rehabilitation for rotator cuff repair surgery: the impact of selected medical comorbidities. J Orthop Sports Phys Ther 37(6):312-319, 2007.

Anesthesia for Shoulder Procedures

Christopher D. Kent, MD, and Laurie B. Amundsen, MD

This chapter covers unique aspects of anesthesia care as it relates specifically to shoulder surgery. The role of the interscalene brachial plexus nerve block—its indications, contraindications, benefits, and complications—in the intraoperative and postoperative care of patients undergoing shoulder procedures is central to the discussion. Developments in the use of ultrasound (US) guidance for performing interscalene brachial plexus block and advances in continuous catheter techniques are reviewed. Issues pertinent to the preoperative, intraoperative, and postoperative phases of anesthetic care for shoulder surgery are examined.

In 1884, Halsted[1] produced the first regional block of the upper extremity by injecting cocaine onto the roots of the brachial plexus under direct vision. In 1911, Hirschel[2] described the first percutaneous axillary block; this same year Kulenkampff[3] attempted a supraclavicular approach to local anesthetic block of the brachial plexus.

Etienne[4] in 1925, Burnham[5] in 1958, and Winnie and Collins in 1964[6] contributed to the development of the subclavian perivascular technique involving a single injection using a supraclavicular approach. This approach risked puncture of the subclavian artery and the lungs. Although satisfactory for the arm, the axillary, supraclavicular, and subclavian perivascular techniques did not provide good anesthesia for shoulder surgery unless dangerously large volumes of local anesthetic were used. In 1970, Winnie developed the interscalene approach, using smaller volumes of local anesthetic injected into the brachial plexus sheath at the level of the sixth cervical vertebra. This approach produced excellent anesthesia for the shoulder.[4]

ANESTHESIA

Choice of Anesthesia: Regional Versus General

The alternatives to regional anesthesia for shoulder procedures are general anesthesia or a combination of the two techniques. When compared with general anesthesia, interscalene brachial plexus block has been shown to optimize operating conditions, reduce postoperative pain, decrease postoperative nausea and vomiting, reduce postoperative anesthesia care unit stay, and, in the ambulatory setting, minimize unplanned hospital admissions.[7-18]

Each patient must be individually assessed and the final selection of the optimal anesthetic technique needs to be based on a consideration of patient preference, coexisting medical conditions, surgical procedure, surgical requirements, surgeon comfort, and the expertise of the anesthesiologist. Patients are counseled about the risks, benefits, and side effects of the anesthetic options.

Interscalene blocks can be used alone (patient awake), with sedation (light or heavy), or with a general anesthetic (laryngeal mask airway or endotracheal tube). Studies from university medical centers and community-based practices estimate the success rate of the blocks to be 81% to 100%, with the majority reporting rates around 95%.[8-10,13,17,19-27] Success in these studies has been variably defined according to the anesthetic goal for the block, that is, either as a primary anesthetic or as effective postoperative analgesia. The goals may be different for outpatient arthroscopic surgery when compared to major open inpatient procedures, such as arthroplasty.

In experienced hands, regional anesthesia can provide significant advantages to the patient having shoulder surgery, with low rates of significant long-term complications.[8,17,19,20,23,26,28-30] Advantages claimed for an interscalene brachial plexus block over a general anesthetic include decreased blood loss, decreased postoperative analgesia requirements, and avoidance of the risks and side effects of general anesthesia.[11,12,16,17,22,31] The decreased blood loss reported is postulated to be due to the dilation of capacitance vessels coupled with blood drainage away from the wound in the semi-sitting position. This mechanism is speculative,[17,32] based on the assumption that a successful interscalene brachial plexus block causes a sympathectomy, similar to the effects of spinal and epidural anesthesia in lower-extremity surgery. Interscalene block has been shown to provide adequate muscle relaxation, and some view it as superior muscle relaxation when compared with systemic muscle relaxants because it does not fluctuate like the degree of intravenous (IV) pharmacologic neuromuscular blockade.[26,32]

Initiating the interscalene block in a preoperative holding area can improve cost containment and efficiency by reducing the nonoperative time in the operating suite. Conversely, a survey of orthopaedic surgeons indicated that when regional anesthesia is not efficiently integrated into the perioperative care process, the resulting delay in the operating room schedule is one of the primary reasons for not favoring regional techniques.[33]

Postoperatively, the length of stay in the postoperative anesthesia care unit and unplanned admissions for pain, sedation, nausea, vomiting, and urinary retention can be decreased.[10-12,16,31,34] Better postoperative pain control facilitates outpatient surgery and allows earlier mobilization and physical therapy.[11,12,14] Anecdotally, in our institution interscalene blocks facilitate immediate postoperative use of continuous passive movement machines and, to a lesser extent, immediate postoperative physical therapy.

Other advantages of regional anesthesia over general anesthesia might exist in some patients with serious underlying medical conditions. Changes in physiologic function of major organ systems can often be avoided using regional anesthesia. A number of investigators have documented that a general anesthetic is unnecessary in the presence of a successful regional anesthetic block.[10-12,15,19,26,31]

Although avoiding the risk of general anesthesia is often expressed as an advantage of the interscalene block, it is common practice to use general anesthesia with the block. Patients might express the desire for the improved postoperative pain control with the block, along with concern or anxiety over recall of the sounds and other sensations associated with the intraoperative environment. Patients with a difficult airway and those who might not tolerate even light sedation without significant airway obstruction might benefit from a controlled airway at the outset of the procedure, before optimal access for airway management is relinquished for positioning and draping. Regardless of the indications for a combined technique, the general anesthetic component needs to be designed to take full advantage of a preoperatively placed block to facilitate rapid recovery by limiting the patient's exposure to longer-acting intraoperative opioids and emetogenic agents. The least desirable outcome of simultaneous regional and general anesthesia is exposure of the patient to the risks and side effects of both techniques combined with the additional time requirement for placement of the block, induction of general anesthesia, and longer postoperative recovery from a general anesthetic.

Patient refusal is an absolute contraindication to regional anesthesia. Surgical concerns can also militate against having the patient awake during surgery. Other contraindications to regional anesthesia of the shoulder include impaired coagulation and infection at the site of the block. Preexisting nerve deficits on the side of the intended nerve block could be considered relative contraindications to a block, in part because theoretically there is a potential for increased vulnerability to nerve injury. The loss of the ability to test nerve function immediately after the surgery may be considered a relative contraindication for some patients and procedures, particularly in the operative treatment of fractures at sites of nerve vulnerability. Significantly impaired pulmonary function is also a contraindication because typically the interscalene block reduces diaphragmatic excursion and vital capacity by 20% to 40%.[35,36] Patients with minimal respiratory reserve may be unable to tolerate this transient reduction in respiratory function.

Technique: Interscalene Brachial Plexus Block

The brachial plexus is formed from the ventral rami of the fifth cervical nerve to the first thoracic nerve, with variable contributions from the fourth cervical and the second thoracic nerves. These nerves travel in roots, trunks, divisions, then cords before giving rise to terminal nerves in the arm. In the neck, the nerve trunks course between the anterior and middle scalene muscles. The scalene muscles are enveloped in a fascial sheath continuing from the prevertebral fascia and the scalene fascia. This envelope provides a potential space into which local anesthetic can be deposited.

The superficial cervical plexus is composed of cervical nerves one through four and innervates parts of the anterior shoulder. The superficial cervical plexus can be blocked selectively with a field block at the posterior border of the sternocleidomastoid muscle.[37] Figure 8-1 demonstrates the distribution of cutaneous analgesia after an interscalene block and a superficial cervical plexus block.

Before a block is performed, the patient must have IV access and appropriate monitoring including electrocardiogram, noninvasive blood pressure, and continuous pulse oximetry. Interscalene blocks can be performed in a block room, a preoperative holding area, or the operating room. Specific requirements for the area include an

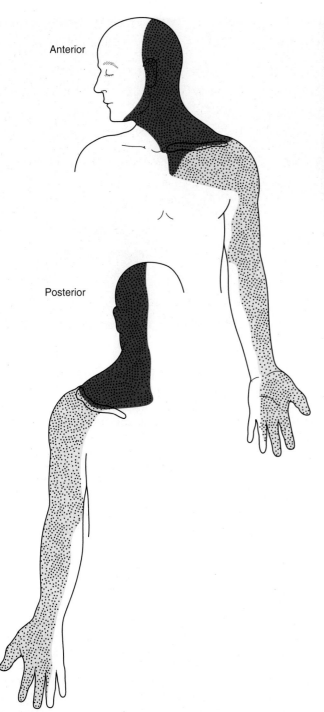

Anterior

Posterior

FIGURE 8-1 Distribution of anesthesia with an interscalene brachial plexus block *(yellow)* and a superficial cervical plexus block *(red)*.

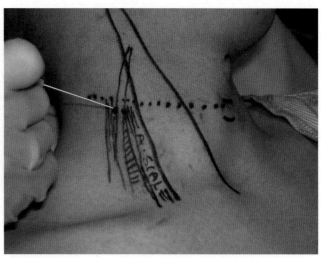

FIGURE 8-2 Winnie approach to the interscalene brachial plexus block with anatomic landmarks.

oxygen source, a bag valve mask, suction, standard airway equipment (e.g., oral airway, mask, laryngoscope, endotracheal tube), and emergency drugs immediately available (including an induction agent and a muscle relaxant).

In addition to the technique originally published by Winnie in 1970 (Fig. 8-2), Borgeat and Meier have described a modified lateral approach to the interscalene

brachial plexus,[19,38] and Boezaart has published a description of a posterior paracervical approach.[39] The authors assert that these techniques are superior to the Winnie technique for placing catheters and for avoiding injections and needle trauma to the cervical cord.

Another significant addition to the choice of techniques is US guidance for performing interscalene brachial plexus blocks. The preference for the needle insertion site and nerve localization technique (nerve stimulator, paresthesia technique, or US guidance) depends on the skills and experience of the operator. The literature consists primarily of case series reporting on a single block technique, and the very limited number of head-to-head comparisons of techniques does not conclusively demonstrate an advantage with regard to the safety and the success of one technique over the others.[17,24,30,38,40-48] Due to the relatively uncommon occurrence of significant complications with interscalene block and with published success rates in the most experienced hands of 95%, studies examining the techniques have been underpowered to adjudicate between techniques on the issues of safety and efficacy.

Even in the absence of conclusive data, there are reasons to reconsider the use of the paresthesia technique. This technique does not provide any information to the practitioner about the relative distance between the needle and the plexus, because the paresthesia either is there or it isn't. If the plexus is not encountered on the first needle pass, there is limited information on which to base a new search pattern for the nerves. The technique also involves intentionally eliciting a response that most patients would describe as uncomfortable, if not painful. The specific neurophysiologic event corresponding to the paresthesia is not known because it does not necessarily correlate with other markers of nerve-to-needle proximity, such as nerve stimulation at a current of 0.5 mA or US-visualized position of the needle tip.[40,47,48]

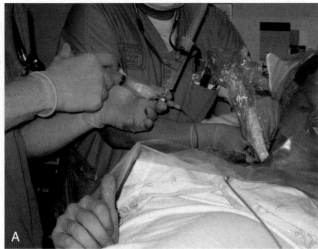
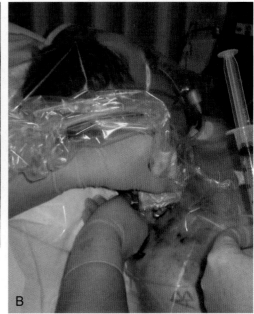

FIGURE 8-3 **A** and **B,** An interscalene block performed with US guidance. Note the sterile preparation of the site and the US transducer. The needle is inserted in line with the transducer at its posterolateral end.

Finally, it does not provide information that will guide the insertion of continuous interscalene catheters.

The peripheral nerve stimulator (PNS) provides information at a distance from the plexus and the potential for a rational redirection of the needle depending on the motor response elicited; for example, posterior shoulder muscle contraction would indicate suprascapular nerve stimulation, requiring anterior redirection of the needle. The nerve stimulator also provides an objective motor response rather than the subjective patient description of the anatomic radiation of a paresthesia.

At this early stage of its application for nerve blocks, US guidance, either added to peripheral nerve stimulation or on its own, appears to be at least comparable in efficacy to the PNS technique, with potential for further safety advantages.[49-51] For performing interscalene blocks, a linear US transducer with an upper range of 10 to 13 MHz combines good image resolution and adequate penetration depth. US guidance enables the practitioner to visualize needle and nerve proximity and monitor the spread of local anesthetic in real time, adding an extra margin of protection against problems caused by anatomic variation that might result in a failed block or intravascular injection. In both the paresthesia and nerve-stimulator techniques, the practitioner has information about the relationship between the needle and the nerve at the initiation of the injection but no information about any subsequent movement of the needle and the spread and deposition of the anesthetic, both of which are provided by US guidance (Figs. 8-3 to 8-5).[52]

The shortcomings of US guidance relate primarily to the expense of purchasing a high-resolution US machine and the possibility that practitioners experienced with other techniques might find that the time required to complete a block is increased during the early stages of learning the new technique. Because of the relative infrequency of significant complications, a very large trial would be needed to definitively determine whether the theoretical safety advantage for the use of US could be conclusively demonstrated.[52,53]

Regardless of the technique, appropriate sedation that maintains meaningful patient interaction and optimizes patient comfort is considered, and supplemental oxygen is provided.

For the Winnie technique, after locating the interscalene groove, a needle is advanced perpendicular to the skin in all planes and into the groove in a slightly caudal direction to locate the brachial plexus.[4] The modified lateral technique involves the use of the same needle insertion site, but the needle is directed toward the junction of the medial and lateral third of the clavicle at a 45- to 60-degree angle to the skin.[19,38] Boezaart's posterior cervical approach involves the use of a Tuohy needle and a loss-of-resistance technique in conjunction with peripheral nerve stimulation.[39] A variety of needles are available for performing the block. B-bevel (19-degree angle), short bevel (45-degree angle), or pencil-point needles are preferred over standard A-bevel (cutting) needles.[54]

The paresthesia technique for interscalene brachial plexus block involves directing a needle into the interscalene groove, as previously described, until a paresthesia is elicited going into the shoulder or down the arm toward the elbow.

With the PNS technique, an insulated needle with a nerve stimulator is used to determine optimal needle placement by demonstrating upper arm or forearm muscle twitching. When optimal needle placement is achieved, the needle is then held fixed by the operator while an assistant aspirates for blood. Having the needle attached

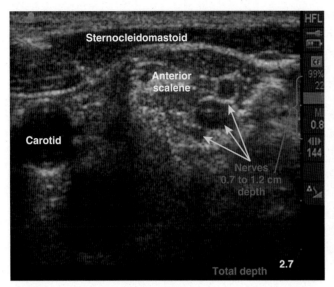

FIGURE 8-4 US image of the interscalene brachial plexus.

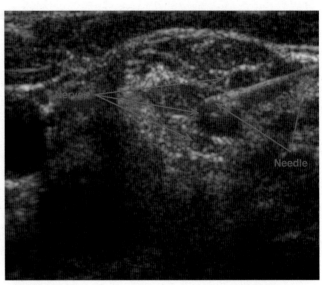

FIGURE 8-5 Needle placement for US-guided brachial plexus block.

to the syringe by extension tubing facilitates immobility of the needle during injection. If aspiration is negative, 1 mL of local anesthetic is then injected as a test dose. If there are no signs or symptoms of intra-arterial injection (transient nausea, dizziness, slurred speech, sedation, loss of consciousness, or grand mal seizures),[55-57] continued aspiration alternating with injection of 3 to 5 mL of local anesthetic solution needs to be repeated to a final volume of 20 to 40 mL total.

The US technique can be performed with the needle in line or perpendicular to the US probe and can be used simultaneously with a PNS. For the in-line technique, employed in our institution, the needle is directed from the posterolateral aspect of the neck through the middle scalene. After optimal needle placement is visualized, the injection is performed as noted with the other techniques, with the added ability of monitoring the spread of local anesthetic and the potential to carefully reposition the needle if the initial injection of anesthetic is not well distributed around the brachial plexus.

If a continuous interscalene block is desired for extended postoperative pain management, a stimulating needle or stimulating needle through a cannula can be employed to locate the brachial plexus, and a catheter can be threaded into place alongside the plexus. Needle–catheter sets specifically designed for continuous nerve block anesthesia can electrically stimulate the catheter during placement. Use of this equipment can improve the success of continuous catheter techniques. US guidance can also assist in evaluating perineural catheters because the spread of local anesthetic injected through the catheter can be monitored by scanning over the site of the catheter tip.

After the extent of the block is determined, it might have to be supplemented with a superficial cervical block.[25] From our experience and studies examining distribution of the interscalene block, it is more likely that when a block is used as the primary anesthetic for major open procedures, it will require supplementation to cover the T1-T2 dermatomes that can extend into the area of a deltoid–pectoral incision.[25,58,59] This can be accomplished through additional local anesthetic infiltration by the surgeon or through thoracic paravertebral blocks at the appropriate levels.[25,58]

The choice of local anesthetic to be used is based on the desired duration of the block, density of the block, time to onset, and the toxicity profile (Table 8-1). This decision can also be influenced by whether the interscalene block is the primary anesthetic or is used for postoperative pain control only. For single-shot analgesic blocks, concentrations of 0.125% bupivacaine or 0.2% ropivacaine appear adequate, whereas 0.375% to 0.5% bupivacaine and 0.5% to 0.75% ropivacaine may be required to provide a block appropriate for surgical anesthesia in an awake or lightly sedated patient. A perineural catheter has the advantage of allowing the use of an intermediate-acting anesthetic, such as lidocaine or mepivacaine, for denser intraoperative anesthesia, with the opportunity to transition to motor activity–sparing concentrations of bupivacaine or ropivacaine postoperatively.

Complications of Interscalene Brachial Plexus Block

Complications due to interscalene block can be separated into expected transient, associated effects (ipsilateral hemidiaphragmatic weakness, Horner's syndrome, hoarseness); shorter term, treatable complications (respiratory failure due to hemidiaphragmatic weakness,

TABLE 8-1 Characteristics of Local Anesthetics Used for Interscalene Brachial Plexus Blockade

Drug With Epinephrine 1:200,000	Usual Concentration (%)	Usual Volume (mL)	Usual Onset (min)	Usual Duration (min)
Lidocaine	2	20-40	5-20	120-240
Mepivacaine	1-1.5	20-40	5-20	180-300
Ropivacaine	0.2-0.75	20-40	10-20	360-900
Bupivacaine	0.25-0.5	20-40	15-30	360-900

Data from Casati A, Cappelleri G, Beccaria P, et al: A clinical comparison of ropivacaine 0.75%, ropivacaine 1% or bupivacaine 0.5% for interscalene brachial plexus anesthesia. European J Anesth 16:784-789, 1999; Casati G, Fanelli G, Aldegheri M, et al: Interscalene brachial plexus anaesthesia with 0.5%, 0.75% or 1% ropivacaine: A double-blind comparison with 2% mepivacaine. Br J Anaesth 83:872-875, 1999; Covino BG, Wildsmith JAW: Clinical Pharmacology of Local Anesthetic Agents. In Cousins MJ, Bridenbaugh PO (eds): Neural Blockade in Clinical Anesthesia and Management of Pain. Philadelphia: Lippincott-Raven, 1998, pp 98-109; Dagli G, Guzeldemir ME, Acar HV: The effects and side effects of interscalene brachial plexus block by posterior approach. Reg Anesth 23:87-91, 1998; Eroglu A, Uzunlar H, Sener M, et al: A clinical comparison of equal concentration and volume of ropivacaine and bupivacaine for interscalene brachial plexus anesthesia and analgesia in shoulder surgery. Reg Anesth Pain Med 29:539-543, 2004; Klein SM, Greengrass RA, Steele SM, et al: A comparison of 0.5% bupivacaine, 0.5% ropivacaine, and 0.75% ropivacaine for interscalene brachial plexus block. Anesth Analg 87:1316-1319, 1998.

pneumothorax, seizures, central nervous system local anesthetic effects); and untreatable complications (peripheral nerve injury, central nervous system injury, brachial plexitis). Figure 8-6 shows a cross section of the neck at the C6 level emphasizing the structures that are vulnerable during interscalene block.

An obvious but important consideration that applies to interscalene block anesthesia (and any other medical intervention) is that the results from centers that have the necessary case load and interest in publishing studies are in part due to the techniques used and in part due to a concentration of expertise and experience. The published results might not be readily realizable in all centers. Lenters and colleagues reported on complications associated with interscalene blocks, noting a very strong inverse association between the experience of the anesthesiologist and the frequency of complications.[60] Weber and Jain published a study in the orthopaedic literature with a lower success rate and higher rate of complications than other series, demonstrating variability in the success of the technique.[27] The exchange in the letters to the editor following the publication of this retrospective series confirmed that an anesthesiologist's and surgeon's thoughts on the risks and benefits of interscalene blocks are strongly influenced by their direct experience with or knowledge of significant complications that have occurred with their use and are not necessarily determined by the optimal published data in the literature.[22]

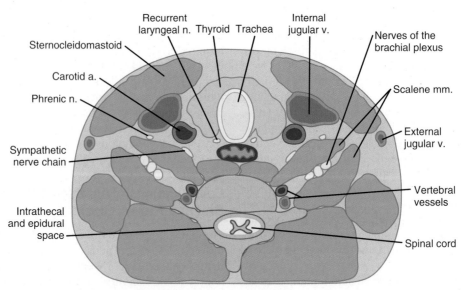

FIGURE 8-6 Cross section of the neck at the level of an interscalene block.

Transient Associated Effects

It is useful to forewarn patients of the potential for ipsilateral hemidiaphragmatic weakness, Horner's syndrome, and hoarseness to avoid undue concern. These effects usually have minimal clinical significance and are considered normal sequelae of the block.[26,59,61] The phrenic nerve, originating with the C4 nerve root and lying on the anterior surface of the anterior scalene muscle, is blocked in 100% of patients receiving an interscalene block.[35,36,62,63] Ipsilateral hemidiaphragmatic paresis has an onset of 5 to 30 minutes from the initiation of the block and lasts for the duration of the motor block. Occasionally, patients have a subjective awareness of mild shortness of breath. This is usually not a problem, but it could become so in patients with severe respiratory disease, obesity, or advanced pregnancy.

Horner's syndrome, due to blockade of the cervical sympathetic nerve, occurs in 18.5% to 75% of patients[64,65] and results in ipsilateral ptosis, miosis, anhidrosis, and nasal congestion for the duration of the block. Cases of prolonged Horner's syndrome have been reported following interscalene block.[64,66]

Recurrent laryngeal palsy is less common.[59,65] It causes ipsilateral vocal cord paralysis and hoarseness. Patients with preexisting contralateral vocal cord paresis are at risk for bilateral vocal cord paralysis and possible complete airway obstruction due to unopposed adduction of the cords.[67]

Finally, subtle and temporary auditory disturbances, possibly due to an indirect effect of blockade of the cervical sympathetic chain, have been reported in patients receiving an interscalene block.[32]

Short-Term, Treatable Complications

Interscalene blocks are not recommended in patients unable to tolerate a 25% to 30% reduction in pulmonary function,[35,43] for example, patients with contralateral diaphragm dysfunction or those dependent on intact bilateral diaphragmatic function (ankylosing spondylosis). The potential for subclinical left hemidiaphragm weakness exists after coronary artery bypass graft surgery with left internal mammary artery dissection.[62] There is a paucity of data that would enable the practitioner to predict which patients will not tolerate the hemidiaphragmatic paresis.

When an interscalene block is considered to be particularly beneficial for patients at higher risk for respiratory failure, a continuous catheter with careful induction of the block and using shorter-acting local anesthetics needs to be considered, rather than a single shot of a long-acting local anesthetic. This can shorten the period of respiratory distress and ventilator dependency if the diaphragmatic paresis from the block is not tolerated. In patients with severe pulmonary compromise, the relative risk of general anesthesia versus an interscalene block is not clear. A detailed discussion concerning the risk of respiratory failure is initiated with the patient and the surgeon regarding an immediate respiratory rescue plan including noninvasive ventilator support and sedation for intubation and ventilation. One case of persistent phrenic nerve palsy has been reported.[68]

Pneumothorax is more common with the supraclavicular approach,[63] but it can occur following interscalene block.[20,59,63,69] It is best seen on an upright chest x-ray during full expiration and is part of the differential diagnosis of dyspnea, chest pain, or persistent oxygen saturations below 95% in room air (or 5% below baseline) following interscalene block. Bronchospasm also has been reported in asthmatic and nonasthmatic patients having interscalene blocks and has been attributed to sympathetic blockade with unopposed vagal activity.[70,71]

Inadvertent intrathecal, epidural, or subdural blocks are rare but can occur during attempted interscalene block, causing apnea and hemodynamic instability and necessitating emergency intubation, ventilation, and cardiovascular support until the block resolves.[72-81] Emergency drugs and airway equipment always must be close at hand. Possible mechanisms for these problems include direct injection into the intrathecal, epidural, or subdural space secondary to incorrect needle placement, prevertebral spread of injected drug, or injection into an abnormally long dural root sleeve. There has been one reported case of inadvertent epidural catheter placement while placing a continuous interscalene block.[82] Bilateral interscalene block without evidence of central spread has also been reported.[60]

Many blood vessels are present near the injection site. Intravascular injection of a small volume of local anesthetic into the vertebral or carotid artery will cause seizures.[56,57] Negative aspirations for blood before injection and repeated several times during injection should further reduce the incidence of this uncommon complication. Theoretically, injection of local anesthetic with US guidance while monitoring the spread of local anesthetic could also reduce the incidence of misdirected injections.

Although rare, cardiac arrest and transient carotid bruit have both been reported following interscalene block.[74,83] Vasovagal episodes, manifesting with profound hypotension and bradycardia, are more common and are thought to be due to activation of the Bezold–Jarisch reflex, with patients in the sitting position.[61,84] Usually this response is transient and relatively insignificant if diagnosed and treated promptly with atropine, glycopyrrolate, or ephedrine. If it is undetected, cardiac arrest can ensue. Prophylaxis with an IV β-blocker can prevent vasovagal episodes in this setting.[85]

NEUROLOGIC INJURY AFTER SHOULDER PROCEDURES

Peripheral nerve injury following shoulder surgery usually becomes apparent once the patient is awake or the interscalene brachial plexus block has resolved. In some patients, symptoms are delayed. Many factors are consid-

---

BOX 8-1 Risk Factors Contributing to Perioperative Nerve Injury

Patient Risk Factors
Diabetes mellitus
Extremes of body habitus
Increasing age
Male gender
Preexisting neurologic disorders

Surgical Risk Factors
Hematoma
Patient positioning
Perioperative inflammation
Surgical trauma or stretch
Vascular compromise

Anesthetic Risk Factors
Ischemic injury (vasoconstrictors)
Local anesthetic neurotoxicity
Needle- or catheter-induced mechanical trauma

Adapted from Neal JM, Hebl JR, Gerancher JC, Hogan QH: Brachial plexus anesthesia: Essentials of our current understanding. Reg Anes Pain Med 27:402-428, 2002.

---

ered when trying to determine the etiology of the injury (Box 8-1). A preoperative evaluation noting and documenting preexisting neurologic deficits is crucial in differentiating preoperative and postoperative nerve deficits.

Mechanical and Surgical Causes

The suprascapular, axillary, and musculocutaneous nerves are those most commonly injured by mechanical and surgical causes during shoulder surgery, usually as a result of traction or contusion, and rarely due to direct laceration or incorporation in a suture. In contrast, nerve injury related to interscalene block is associated with a more proximal pattern involving the entire plexus, the upper trunk, or one of the cords. The incidence of nerve injuries is 1% to 2% for rotator cuff surgery, 1% to 8% for anterior instability procedures, and 1% to 4% for prosthetic arthroplasty.[86] Detailed knowledge of anatomy and careful positioning of the patient, placement of retractors and arthroscopic portals, and manipulation of the arm and joint during surgery are crucial in minimizing the occurrence of such injuries. Additional surgical risk factors include vascular compromise and postoperative swelling, hematoma, and infection.

Anesthetic Causes

In the American Society of Anesthesiologists closed claims database, anesthesia-related nerve injury accounted for 16% of total claims. Twenty percent of these involved the brachial plexus, but of the brachial plexus injuries, only 16% were due to regional anesthetic techniques[87]; the majority of nerve injuries were attributed to patient positioning during general anesthesia.

A major voluntary reporting survey and a literature review have suggested that the occurrence of postoperative nerve dysfunction after interscalene block is relatively rare,[28,29] but the incidence of short-term postoperative nerve dysfunction related to interscalene brachial plexus block is common when identified by careful follow-up in prospective studies. Borgeat and colleagues identified block-related postoperative nerve dysfunction in 7.9% of patients at 1 month and 0.4% at 9 months in their prospective study.[20] In another prospective study, Candido and colleagues noted symptoms in 3.3 % of their study patients at 1 month and 0.1% at 3 months.[23] Fanelli's prospective study described an incidence of neurologic symptoms related to interscalene block of 4%,[13] and Bishop's group reported an incidence of 2.3% in a retrospective study.[8] The majority of the injuries in these studies produced sensory symptoms only.

There are, however, case reports of disabling permanent sensory and motor injuries and chronic regional pain syndromes due to interscalene block.[72,78,87-90] The possible occurrence of these complications is described to all patients when obtaining informed consent, but with particular emphasis in patients whose livelihoods depend on manual dexterity and fine sensory discrimination.

Borgeat and colleagues performed two studies examining success rates and postoperative complications in the context of interscalene catheter insertion and did not demonstrate an increased incidence of nerve injuries associated with catheter insertion relative to single-shot techniques.[19,20] Their series pertains, however, to a specific approach (modified lateral) and a specific needle and catheter system (cannula over 20-gauge needle with a 23-gauge catheter) in the hands of an experienced group. A series reported by Capdevila[91] using the PNS and a different needle system and Bryan's series[21] of US-guided catheter placements reported similar rates of complications.

Mechanical, ischemic, or chemical injury can all be contributing factors to nerve injury. Mechanical injury can occur due to direct nerve trauma by the block needle[72,78,88] or catheter,[92] in association with paresthesia during needle insertion[23,28,47] or pain during injection,[28,88] or indirectly by nerve compression secondary to hematoma.

Selander and colleagues used a rabbit model to look at the relevance of needle type in nerve injury and found that although the overall frequency of nerve injury was significantly less with short-bevel needles compared with long-bevel needles, injury severity was greater.[54] Pencil-point needles can also reduce trauma to nerves.[93]

Assessing the comparative roles of paresthesia and the use of a PNS in nerve injury following brachial plexus block has proved extremely difficult due to the relative rarity of this complication and due to the occurrence of unintentional paresthesia in PNS study groups.[13,23,24,30,43] No statistically significant differences have been found between the techniques.[24] However, persistent nerve injuries that have been described in the literature have often been correlated with the occurrence of paresthesias during performance of the block. In some instances, paresthesias were deliberately sought; in other cases they were inadvertently elicited.

The role of epinephrine in local anesthetic solutions as a factor in anesthesia-related nerve injury has not been specifically evaluated in humans. However, peripheral nerves rely heavily on their intrinsic and extrinsic microcirculation, the latter being under adrenergic control and therefore sensitive to epinephrine-containing solutions. Rat models have shown a dramatic decrease in neural blood flow after topical application of 2% lidocaine with 1:200,000 epinephrine.[94] The risk of ischemic injury appears to be exceedingly small compared with the increased potential for local anesthetic toxicity if epinephrine is not used.

Intraneuronal injection of local anesthetic can generate extremely high pressure within the nerve sheath that compromises the intrinsic microcirculation, resulting in ischemic nerve injury.[95] Subsequent histologic changes can result in delayed presentation of symptoms some time (days or weeks) after the peripheral nerve block.[28,87] If intraneuronal injection occurs, the patient can experience severe, sharp pain on attempted injection of local anesthetic, alerting the anesthesiologist to stop injecting the local anesthetic and redirect the needle. Failure to recognize this and cease injecting can result in permanent nerve damage.[88]

Benumof reported four cases of permanent neurologic damage secondary to attempted interscalene brachial plexus block performed on patients under general anesthesia or heavy sedation.[72] Other similar cases have been reported in the literature.[78] This highlights the importance of performing these nerve blocks in awake or lightly sedated patients, who can respond appropriately. Adherence to this practice can help, but it does not guarantee good outcomes because interscalene block–related neuropathies have been reported in patients who were awake and lightly sedated and did not report any unusual symptoms or discomfort during block placement.[23]

Correspondence following the Benumof paper discussed whether interscalene block under general anesthesia should be performed.[69,96-98] No consensus on the issue of safety was reached, but at the very least it appears that the placement of interscalene blocks in patients under general anesthesia mitigates some of the advantages of the block. It requires operating room time, does not avoid the use of intraoperative opioids if placed postoperatively, and eliminates feedback from the patient.

Local anesthetic neurotoxicity can occur when inappropriately high concentrations of drug are used.[99] Continuous infusions or multiple local anesthetic injections into a perineural space appear to be safe when used at recommended concentrations.[100]

Cases of idiopathic brachial plexitis have been reported after interscalene block.[101,102] Awareness of this possibility is important to avoid misdiagnosis of nerve injury.

PREOPERATIVE CONSIDERATIONS

Preoperative Evaluation

The anesthesiologist must see all patients before surgery to assess their medical status, develop a plan of anesthesia care, and discuss the proposed plan with the patient.[103] The preoperative evaluation involves reviewing the medical record and interviewing and examining the patient. The interview needs to discuss details of medical conditions, current medications, allergies, previous anesthetic history, social history, and a review of systems. A physical examination of the airway, respiratory, cardiovascular, and neurologic systems must be conducted and documented. Good documentation of preexisting neurologic deficits, muscular deficits, and limitations in use of the operative arm is imperative. This facilitates the evaluation of any postoperative change in neuromuscular function and differentiation from a preexisting condition that would not warrant further investigation. Necessary laboratory work, electrocardiogram, radiography, and further diagnostic tests are dictated by patient history.[104]

Coexisting Medical Disease

Patients having shoulder procedures vary considerably in age and physical fitness and can present with a vast spectrum of medical conditions that can affect their anesthetic management. Many orthopaedic patients have preexisting joint problems (arthritis) leading to airway and positioning issues, notably the cervical spine and temporomandibular joint problems associated with rheumatoid arthritis.

Pulmonary disease is common and needs to be defined preoperatively, particularly if an interscalene block is considered. History, pulmonary function tests, and arterial blood gases can help to define the nature and extent of disease. Preoperative bronchodilators and minimal airway instrumentation help prevent intraoperative bronchospasm.

INTRAOPERATIVE CONSIDERATIONS

Patient Monitoring

The American Society of Anesthesiologists' "Standards for Basic Anesthesia Monitoring" dictate the minimum monitoring requirements for general, regional, and monitored anesthesia care.[46] Additional monitoring, such as a pulmonary artery catheter, arterial line, or central venous pressure catheter, is guided by the patient's medical condition.

Airway Management

There is little in the literature to guide judgment on the type of airway management to be used during shoulder surgery. The type of airway management for general anesthesia obviously is determined in part by whether or not an interscalene block has been used. In the absence of a functioning interscalene block, IV pharmacologic neuromuscular blockade may be required to optimize operating conditions.

Anesthesiologists vary in their level of comfort with using neuromuscular blockade and positive pressure ventilation with laryngeal mask airways, particularly in shoulder surgeries where access to the airway is suboptimal. Another issue to consider is the proximity of the surgeon to the airway, with the potential for displacement of a laryngeal mask airway or endotracheal tube by inadvertent pressure or traction through the surgical drapes. In spite of these considerations, there is no evidence to suggest that laryngeal mask airways are less safe than endotracheal intubation when used for airway management in shoulder surgery, and airway management should be informed by general principles.

Surgical Considerations

Antibiotics and Antithrombosis

IV antibiotics are routinely administered prior to most shoulder procedures. In the event of surgery in a patient who might require intraoperative bacterial culture, the timing of antibiotic administration needs to be discussed with the surgical team.

Sequential compression devices are placed on the patient's lower legs as an antithrombotic measure. These are started before the induction of anesthesia.

Positioning

Most surgical shoulder procedures are performed in the sitting or semi-sitting (beach chair) position, with the patient turned prone or lateral for scapular procedures. Failure to position the patient correctly can result in serious morbidity. Pressure points and vulnerable nerves must be protected and additional padding and supports used, if necessary. The most commonly injured nerves under anesthesia due to positioning are the ulnar and the common peroneal nerves. Shoulder surgery increases the risk of brachial plexus injury due to positioning or manipulation.

The sitting position has the advantage of lowering venous pressure and reducing bleeding, but it also carries the risk of postural hypotension, exacerbated by bradycardia or hypovolemia, and venous air embolism.

The prone position is used for scapular surgery. An interscalene block alone is not adequate to cover a surgical site inferior to the scapular spine; thus, a general anesthetic with or without a block is necessary. For this position, supports under the chest and pelvis are required to avoid raised intra-abdominal pressure and to facilitate

ventilation. A specially designed pillow for the face helps protect the eyes from external pressure. To avoid damage to the brachial plexus, care must be taken when positioning the patient's shoulders. In the lateral position, an axillary roll is considered and adequate peripheral pulses in the dependent arm are confirmed after final positioning. The dependent leg is padded at the knee to prevent common peroneal nerve damage.

The sitting position can require eccentric placement of the patient on the operating table for complete surgical access to the shoulder, leaving the patient at risk for intraoperative malposition of the head and neck, including loss of head and neck support due to the effects of gravity or surgical traction. With any position or head-positioning device, the patient needs to be checked frequently to ensure the airway remains unobstructed and vulnerable areas are protected from pressure and overstretching.

Specific Considerations for Arthroscopic Shoulder Surgery

In discussions over the use of interscalene block anesthesia for arthroscopic procedures, some authors maintain that the analgesic requirements for arthroscopic procedures can be met with equal success with alternative analgesic therapies alone.[22] Studies have shown that patients can require unscheduled inpatient care for analgesia after arthroscopic procedures when an interscalene block is not used,[16] suggesting that all patients require an individualized approach that takes the type of procedure and approach—open or arthroscopic—into consideration along with specific patient factors.

Arthroscopic surgery presents some concerns that are specific to the use of distending fluid for visualization. Although rare, they deserve mention to raise awareness of these problems and improve the opportunity for early detection and intervention. Significant extra-articular fluid accumulation is related to factors such as distending pressure, number of arthroscopic portals created, and surgery within the subacromial space, which does not have a containing capsule. Case reports of fluid accumulation spreading to the neck and causing airway obstruction have appeared in the literature.[105-107]

A study demonstrating an improvement in operating conditions in arthroscopic surgery, through decreased bleeding and improved optical clarity of the fluid, has encouraged the use of controlled hypotension.[108] The important factor in improving operating conditions appears to be maintaining a pressure difference between systolic blood pressure and capsular distending pressure of less than 49 mm Hg. The use of intraoperative hypotension has to be tempered by considerations of the patient's ability to tolerate this manipulation of blood pressure; case reports of postoperative cerebral ischemic deficits and visual loss have appeared in the literature with use of relatively modest intraoperative hypotension in both arthroscopic and open procedures in the sitting position.[109]

Although extremely rare and likely to be of historical interest only, venous air embolism has been described during shoulder arthroscopy, when air was injected to distend the joint.[110,111] Carbon dioxide or normal saline are safer agents for this purpose.

Posterior portals for arthroscopic surgery may be outside the anesthetized area provided by an interscalene block. They can require infiltration with local anesthetic by the surgeon, particularly when the nerve block is the primary anesthetic.

Blood Loss

Blood loss is usually only a problem in a few shoulder procedures such as revision arthroplasty and disarticulation amputations. As with any surgical procedure, the need for blood products is anticipated preoperatively and appropriate crossmatch and blood availability is confirmed. Blood loss can be minimized with regional anesthetic techniques and with positioning. Hypotensive anesthesia and blood salvaging techniques can be considered.

Methylmethacrylate

Methylmethacrylate is the acrylic cement used to secure prostheses in place in most joint replacements, including the shoulder. There is little in the literature regarding complications of methylmethacrylate in shoulder arthroplasties. One small study found no statistically significant changes in hemodynamics or pulmonary function following use of methylmethacrylate.[112] The authors suggest that the lack of evidence for microembolization with shoulder surgery is related to the fact that intramedullary pressures are lower and there is a smaller vascular surface area for absorption when compared to hip and knee arthroplasty.

POSTOPERATIVE CONSIDERATIONS

Postoperative Anesthetic Care

Following the procedure, the patient is transferred to the postoperative anesthetic care unit before being discharged to a hospital room, intensive care unit, or home. In the absence of a regional block, neurologic function may be assessed at this time. The anesthesiologist should see every patient. Any complications must be documented and further evaluation and treatment arranged as necessary.

After interscalene brachial plexus blocks, it is important to confirm return of normal neurologic function. Persistent deficits are evaluated and fully documented. The surgeon and anesthesiologist discuss such problems with the patient, offering reassurance and a plan of action. Most neurologic complications resolve over a few hours, days, or weeks. Significant or protracted injuries require

further neurologic evaluation to localize the lesion, determine the degree of injury, and coordinate further evaluation and care.[63] Baseline neurophysiologic testing can help rule out underlying pathology or preexisting conditions and needs to be performed within a week to 10 days after surgery if it is immediately important to patient care to identify lesions that preceded anesthesia and surgery. Typically, peripheral nerve injury denervation changes on EMG do not become manifest for approximately 10 days. Therefore, lesions with denervation changes evident less than 1 week postoperatively were most likely present before surgery.

Physical therapy to maintain normal range of motion of involved joints and analgesics for residual pain can contribute to the recovery process. The rare patient who suffers persistent neuropathic pain following a nerve injury might benefit from referral to a chronic pain clinic.

Postoperative Pain Management

Shoulder surgery is often associated with severe postoperative pain.[113-115] Inadequately treated postoperative pain is still a leading cause of unanticipated admission and readmission after outpatient surgery.[16,34,116] The regional anesthetic techniques for postoperative analgesia include single-shot interscalene brachial plexus block, continuous interscalene nerve block, single-shot suprascapular nerve block,[117] and intra-articular and intrabursal injections or infusions. Nonregional techniques include oral and IV opioids, oral acetaminophen, nonsteroidal anti-inflammatory agents, and cyclooxygenase-2 (COX-2) inhibitors.

Single-shot interscalene brachial plexus block, with or without general anesthesia, has been shown to reduce postoperative pain and total opioid requirements during the early postoperative period. High doses of opioids, as an alternative, can result in nausea and vomiting, sedation, and inadequate pain relief. Seltzer and colleagues[118] have suggested that decreased opioid requirements, even after the interscalene block has resolved, support the theory that regional anesthesia has a preemptive analgesic effect. Most studies, however, primarily demonstrate only a short-term benefit.[31,34,119]

Duration of the block depends largely on the local anesthetic used rather than the dose administered. One study using mepivacaine for interscalene block showed significantly lower visual analogue pain scores at 4 hours postoperatively compared with general anesthesia, but it showed no differences by 8 hours.[31] Bupivacaine has an increased duration of action. Unpublished data from our institution in patients who received 30 to 40 mL of 0.375% bupivacaine with 1:200,000 epinephrine for an interscalene brachial plexus block demonstrated a mean duration of the block of 13 ± 3 hours (range, 8-20 h). Studies directly comparing bupivacaine 0.5% with ropivacaine 0.5% and 0.75% show similar mean durations of 10 to 15 hours with all concentrations sand agents.[120-122]

Prolonging the duration of an interscalene block has many benefits, but it must be weighed against the possible hazard of a totally anesthetized extremity, particularly in the outpatient setting, and the possibility for serious injury.[55] Outpatients are sent home with a properly fitted sling for the arm, and the sling should not be removed until the interscalene block has completely resolved. Patients are instructed about protecting the anesthetized extremity. Interscalene blocks with low-dose local anesthetics, combined with general anesthesia, have been shown to provide good duration of postoperative analgesia for arthroscopic shoulder surgery, with minimal somatic block.[7,121] Although 12.5 mg of bupivacaine (10 mL 0.125% bupivacaine) produced excellent immediate postoperative analgesia, compared with placebo, it only lasted 2 to 3 hours.[7] However, 12.5 mg, 25 mg, and 50 mg of ropivacaine all provided approximately 10 hours of postoperative analgesia. Complete analgesia was achieved more consistently with 25 and 50 mg of ropivacaine, but recovery of hand and arm function was still more rapid in comparison to conventional longer-acting local anesthetic doses.[123] The goal is to provide the best analgesia with the least motor impairment.

Continuous interscalene nerve blocks are increasingly being used by experienced teams in both the inpatient or outpatient setting to provide prolonged postoperative analgesia after shoulder surgery.[19,39,113,114,124,130] The challenges of accurate catheter placement and fixation have resulted in reports of catheter failure up to 25%.[125,126,130] Boezaart and Borgeat have reported that the use of subcutaneous tunneling of the catheter to prevent dislodgement improve the reliability of the technique.[19,39,113]

For inpatients, patient-controlled interscalene analgesia with local anesthetics has been compared to IV patient-controlled analgesia (PCA). The former provides better pain relief, less nausea and pruritus, and greater patient satisfaction than IV PCA after major shoulder surgery.[113,114]

The development of sophisticated disposable infusion pumps with larger reservoirs that can be programmed to vary the infusion rate and bolus dose has improved the flexibility of outpatient interscalene catheter analgesia.[125-127,131-133] In the outpatient setting the use of catheters places greater responsibility on patients, emphasizing the importance of careful patient selection and the provision of an education program regarding the perineural catheter and pump. The pain-management team should be available by phone to troubleshoot any problems with catheter analgesia and an immediately available back-up analgesic plan needs to be in place to deal with the possibility of a displaced catheter or pump malfunction.

The prolonged use of local anesthetic infusions generates concerns regarding toxicity, but the most commonly used infusions for continuous interscalene nerve block (0.25% bupivacaine or 0.2% ropivacaine) do not raise plasma levels near the threshold for toxicity.[129,134,135]

A significant concern, particularly in patients undergoing total shoulder arthroplasty, is the possibility that perineural interscalene catheters can add to the risk of infection. In the single largest published series evaluating complication rates of interscalene catheters (700 patients) signs of infection (local pain, redness, and induration) were noted in one patient after 3 days and in four patients after 4 days.[19] Two of the culture tips were positive—one for coagulase-negative staphylococcus, one for *Staphylococcus aureus*—and two were culture negative. All patients were successfully treated with antibiotics. In one diabetic patient, a collection was demonstrated by US after 5 days. The catheter tip was positive for coagulase-negative staphylococcus, but blood cultures were negative. Surgical drainage was performed, followed by administration of antibiotics, with complete recovery after 10 days of treatment.

In a specific practice setting, the decision to offer patients continuous catheter analgesia needs to be considered in light of the resources available to meet the added technical and time demands that will be required of practitioners placing and maintaining the catheters.

Alternative analgesic methods include intra-articular or subacromial bursa injection or infusion of local anesthetic, with or without opioids. The techniques are simple[136] and catheters can be placed under direct vision or arthroscopic guidance. Subacromial block with plain bupivacaine has not been shown to significantly reduce postoperative pain compared with placebo.[137] A cautionary note regarding the use of intra-articular catheters was raised by investigators studying a rabbit model that indicated that intra-articular bupivacaine may be associated with chondrolysis.[138] The addition of opioids to bupivacaine placed in intra-articular and subacromial bursae appears to be effective.[44,102,139] Action on peripheral opioid receptors has been postulated as the mechanism. As with continuous interscalene nerve blocks, intra-articular infusion pumps have been developed to optimize outpatient analgesia following shoulder surgery.[127,140,141]

After upper extremity amputation, placement of a catheter in the amputated nerve sheath before closure of the incision, and infusion of local anesthetic, can provide excellent postoperative analgesia, but it does not decrease the incidence of phantom limb pain.[142] Horn's group has successfully used wound infiltration with drain lavage with a local anesthetic after shoulder surgery.[143]

In situations in which regional anesthesia is contraindicated or where patients refuse it, IV PCA is the postoperative analgesia of choice. A meta-analysis and review of postoperative PCA versus intramuscular analgesia showed a strong patient preference for PCA, as well as better pain relief without an increase in side effects.[144,145]

Despite all the available techniques and drugs, postoperative pain control can be inadequate after resolution of the regional block. A study of 50 outpatients who received analgesia with single-shot interscalene blocks followed by oral analgesics for open rotator cuff repairs found that 20% had maximal pain on a visual analogue pain score after resolution of the block.[119] The patients in this study often did not take their medications as prescribed, a finding that highlights the importance of detailed written instructions for analgesia, an analgesic rescue plan for the time of resolution of the block, and the continuous availability of a competent adult care giver for the first 24 hours for outpatients after interscalene block.

Inpatients after major open shoulder surgery might require transition to IV opioid PCA, but a combination of extended and immediate-release oral opioids is sufficient for others. The unpredictability of the duration of single-shot block often results in a period of increased pain if the patient has to wait for medications to be prescribed and delivered. Preempting this problem by preoperatively prescribing an extended release opioid could bridge this gap. In our experience, the mean block duration was 13 hours, with a range of 8 to 20 hours. Therefore, an extended release opioid given orally about 8 hours after placement of the block would establish analgesia in 95% of subjects before the block resolves. This can then be continued twice a day for several days postoperatively.

IV medications for breakthrough and rescue analgesia need to be available for the possibility of an analgesic gap inadequately bridged with oral analgesics. In conjunction with an extended release opioid, oxycodone 5 to 20 mg every 3 to 4 hours can be used to control breakthrough pain. If not contraindicated, NSAIDs throughout the postoperative period will provide additional postoperative analgesia and reduce opioid requirements. COX-2 inhibitors, such as celecoxib, avoid some of the side effects of traditional NSAIDs while providing effective analgesia. In particular, COX-2 inhibitors do not alter platelet function and therefore do not predispose to bleeding postoperatively, as has been observed with non-specific COX-1 and COX-2 inhibitors such as ibuprofen or aspirin.

Although there are no specific studies addressing the treatment of postoperative shoulder pain in patients with preexisting chronic pain syndromes, general principles from the pain management literature would favor a multimodal approach. Regardless of the use of a regional technique, the patient's preoperative opioid needs must be met intravenously, orally, or transdermally. If an interscalene catheter is not an option and a single-shot block is placed, then special consideration has to be given to the resources available to the patient at the time of resolution of the interscalene block. If the patient requires rapid titration of IV opioids, then skilled nursing care and pulse oximetry monitoring need to be available.

SUMMARY

Shoulder procedures, as with most orthopaedic procedures, lend themselves to regional anesthetic techniques. The emphasis has been on the techniques, benefits, risks, and complications of the interscalene brachial plexus block. The literature reviewed supports the role of both single-shot and continuous regional anesthetic techniques, by experienced personnel in providing good intraoperative anesthesia, postoperative pain control, and facilitating the transition from inpatient to outpatient care.

REFERENCES

1. Halstead WS: Practical comments on the use and abuse of cocaine, suggested by its invariably successful employment in more than a thousand minor surgical operations. N Y State J Med 42:294-295, 1885.
2. Hirschel G: Anesthesia of the brachial plexus for operations on the upper extremity. München Med Wochenschr 58:1555-1556, 1911.
3. Kulenkampff D: Anesthesia of the brachial plexus. Zentralbl Chir 38:1337-1350, 1911.
4. Winnie AP: Interscalene brachial plexus block. Anesth Analg 49:455-466, 1970.
5. Burnham PJ: Regional block of the great nerves of the upper arm. Anesthesiology 19:281-284, 1958.
6. Winnie AP, Collins VJ: The subclavian perivascular technique of brachial plexus anesthesia. Anesthesiology 25:353-363, 1964.
7. Al-Kaisy A, McGuire G, Chan VWS, et al: Analgesic effect of interscalene block using low-dose bupivacaine for outpatient arthroscopic shoulder surgery. Reg Anesth Pain Med 23(5):469-473, 1998.
8. Bishop JY, Sprague M, Gelber J, et al: Interscalene regional anesthesia for shoulder surgery. J Bone Joint Surg Am 87:974-979, 2005.
9. Brown AR: Regional anesthesia for shoulder surgery. Tech Reg Anesth Pain Manag 3:64-78, 1999.
10. Brown AR, Weiss R, Greenberg C, et al: Interscalene block for shoulder arthroscopy: Comparison with general anesthesia. Arthroscopy 9(3):295-300, 1993.
11. D'Allessio JG, Freitas DG, Rosenblum M, et al: Is general anesthesia superior to interscalene block for shoulder surgery? Anesth Analg 76(suppl):S67, 1993.
12. D'Allessio JG, Rosenblum M, Shea KP, et al: A retrospective comparison of interscalene block and general anesthesia for ambulatory surgery shoulder arthroscopy. Reg Anesth 20:62-68, 1995.
13. Fanelli G, Casati A, Garancini P, et al: Nerve stimulator and multiple injection technique for upper and lower limb blockade: Failure rate, patient acceptance, and neurological complications. Anesth Analg 88:847-852, 1999.
14. Gohl MR, Moeller RK, Olson RL, et al: The addition of interscalene block to general anesthesia for patients undergoing open shoulder procedures. AANA 69(2):105-109, 2001.
15. Greek R, Maurer P, Torjman M, et al: Effect of general anesthesia vs interscalene block for shoulder surgery: Postoperative pain and neuroendocrine responses. Reg Anesth 18(2s):68, 1993.
16. Hadzic A, Williams B, Karaca P, et al: For outpatient rotator cuff surgery, nerve block anesthesia provides superior same-day recovery over general anesthesia. Anesthesiology 102:1001-1007, 2005.
17. Tetzlaff JE, Dilger J, Yap E, et al: Idiopathic brachial plexitis after total shoulder replacement with interscalene brachial plexus block. Anesth Analg 85:644-646, 1997.
18. Tetzlaff JE, Yoon HJ, Brems J: Interscalene brachial plexus block for shoulder surgery. Reg Anesth 19:339-343, 1994.
19. Borgeat A, Dullenkopf A, Ekatodramis G, et al: Evaluation of the lateral modified approach for continuous interscalene block after shoulder surgery. Anesthesiology 99:436-442, 2003.
20. Borgeat A, Ekatodramis G, Kalberer F, et al: Acute and nonacute complications associated with interscalene block and shoulder surgery. Anesthesiology 95:875-880, 2001.
21. Bryan NA, Swenson JD, Greis PE, et al: Indwelling interscalene catheter use in an outpatient setting for shoulder surgery: Technique, efficacy, and complications. J Shoulder Elbow Surg 16:388-395, 2007.
22. Brown AR, Levine WN, et al: Complication rates of scalene regional anesthesia. J Bone Joint Surg Am 84:1891-1893, 2002.
23. Candido KD, Sukhani R, Doty R, et al: Neurologic sequelae after interscalene brachial plexus block for shoulder/upper arm surgery: The association of patient, anesthetic, and surgical factors to the incidence and clinical course. Anesth Analg 100:1489-1495, 2005.
24. Liguori GA, Zayas VM, YaDeau JT, et al: Nerve localization techniques for interscalene brachial plexus blockade: A prospective, randomized comparison of mechanical paresthesia versus electrical stimulation. Anesth Analg 103:761-767, 2006.
25. Peterson DO: Shoulder block anesthesia for shoulder reconstruction surgery. Anesth Analg 64:373-375, 1985.
26. Sandin R, Stan H, Sternlo JE: Interscalene plexus block for arthroscopy of the humero-scapular joint. Acta Anaesthesiol Scand 36:493-494, 1992.
27. Weber SC, Jain R: Scalene regional anesthesia for shoulder surgery in a community setting: An assessment of risk. J Bone Joint Surg Am 84(5):775-779, 2002.

28. Auroy Y, Narchi P, Messiah A, et al: Serious complications related to regional anesthesia. Anesthesiology 87(3):479-486, 1997.
29. Brull R, McCartney CJ, Chan VW, et al: Neurological complications after regional anesthesia: Contemporary estimates of risk. Anesth Analg 104:965-974, 2007.
30. Urban MK, Urquhart B: Evaluation of brachial plexus anesthesia for upper extremity surgery. Reg Anesth 19(3):175-182, 1994.
31. Wu CL, Rouse LM, Chen JM, et al: Comparison of postoperative pain in patients receiving interscalene block or general anesthesia for shoulder surgery. Orthopedics 25(1):45-48, 2002.
32. Rosenberg PH, Lamberg TS, Tarkila P, et al: Auditory disturbance with interscalene brachial plexus block. Br J Anaesth 74:89-91, 1995.
33. Oldman M, McCartney CJ, Leung A, et al: A survey of orthopedic surgeons' attitudes and knowledge regarding regional anesthesia. Anesth Analg 98:1486-1490, 2004.
34. Gold BS, Kitz DS, Lecky JH, et al: Unanticipated admission to the hospital following ambulatory surgery. JAMA 262(21):3008-3010, 1989.
35. Urmey WF, McDonald M: Hemidiaphragmatic paresis during interscalene brachial plexus block: Effects on pulmonary function and chest wall mechanics. Anesth Analg 74:352-357, 1992.
36. Urmey WF, Talts KH, Sharrock NE: One hundred percent incidence of hemidiaphragmatic paresis associated with interscalene brachial plexus anesthesia as diagnosed by ultrasonography. Anesth Analg 72:498-503, 1991.
37. Masters RD, Castresana EJ, Castresana MR: Superficial and deep cervical plexus block: Technical considerations. AANA J 63:235-243, 1995.
38. Meier G, Bauereis C, Heinrich C: Interscalene brachial plexus catheter for anesthesia and postoperative pain therapy: Experience with a modified technique. Anaesthesist 46:715-719, 1997.
39. Boezaart AP, de Beer JF, du Toit C, et al: A new technique of continuous interscalene nerve block. Can J Anesth 46:275-281, 1999.
40. Choyce A, Chan VWS, Middleton WJ, et al: What is the relationship between paresthesia and nerve stimulation for axillary brachial plexus block. Reg Anesth Pain Med 26:100-104, 2001.
41. Dagli G, Guzeldemir ME, Acar HV: The effects and side effects of interscalene brachial plexus block by posterior approach. Reg Anesth 23:87-91, 1998.
42. Gologorsky E, Tenicella RA: Does the interscalene block require paresthesia? Reg Anesth 22:387-388, 1997.
43. Moore DC: "No paresthesias—No anesthesia," the nerve stimulator or neither? Reg Anesth 22:388-390, 1997.
44. Muittari P, Kirvela O: The safety and efficacy of intrabursal oxycodone and bupivacaine in analgesia after shoulder surgery. Reg Anesth Pain Med 23:474-478, 1998.
45. Roch JJ, Sharrock NE, Neudachin L: Interscalene brachial plexus block for shoulder surgery: A proximal paresthesia is effective. Anesth Analg 75:386-388, 1992.
46. Standards of the American Society of Anesthesiologists: Standards for Basic Anesthetic Monitoring. Available at http://www.asahq.org/publicationsAndServices/standards/02.pdf (accessed March 1, 2008).
47. Urmey WF: Interscalene block: The truth about twitches. Reg Anesth 25:340-342, 2000.
48. Urmey WF, Stanton J: Inability to consistently elicit a motor response following sensory paresthesia during inter-scalene block administration. Anesthesiology 96:552-554, 2002.
49. Standards of the American Society of Anesthesiologists: Standards for Basic Anesthetic Monitoring. Available at http://www.asahq.org/publicationsAndServices/standards/02.pdf (accessed March 1, 2008).
50. Sites B, Spence BC, Gallagher JD, et al: Characterizing novice behavior associated with learning ultrasound-guided peripheral regional anesthesia. Reg Anesth Pain Med 32:107-115, 2007.
51. Soeding PE, Sha S, Royse CE, et al: A randomized trial of ultrasound-guided brachial plexus anaesthesia in upper limb surgery. Anaesth Intensive Care 33:719-725, 2005.
52. Hopkins PM: Ultrasound guidance as a gold standard in regional anaesthesia. Br J Anaesth 98:299-301, 2007.
53. Borgeat A, Capdevila X: Neurostimulation/ultrasonography: The Trojan War will not take place. Anesthesiology 106:896-898, 2007.
54. Selander D, Ghuner K-G, Lundborg G: Peripheral nerve injury due to injection needles used for regional anesthesia. An experimental study of the acute effects of needle point trauma. Acta Anaesthesiol Scand 21:182-188, 1977.
55. Hume MA, Stevenson J: Unusual complication of brachial plexus anaesthesia. Anaesthesia 49:837-838, 1994.
56. Korman B, Riley RH: Convulsions induced by ropivacaine during interscalene brachial plexus block. Anesth Analg 85:1128-1129, 1997.
57. Kozody R, Ready LB, Barsa JE, et al: Dose requirement of local anesthetic to produce grand mal seizure during stellate ganglion block. Can Anaesth Soc J 29:489-491, 1982.
58. Moore DC: Regional Block, 4th ed. Springfield Ill: Charles C Thomas, 1965, pp 200-204.
59. Vester-Andersen T, Christiansen C, Hansen A, et al: Interscalene brachial plexus block: Area of analgesia, complications and blood concentrations of local anesthetics. Acta Anaesthesiol Scand 25:81-84, 1981.
60. Cobcroft MD: Bilateral spread of analgesia with interscalene brachial plexus block [letter]. Anaesth Intensive Care 4:73, 1976.
61. Ayad S, Tetzlaff JE: Interscalene brachial plexus anesthesia for shoulder surgery: Report of a complicated intraoperative course. J Clin Anesth 13:514-516, 2001.
62. Hashim MS, Shevde K: Dyspnea during interscalene block after recent coronary bypass surgery. Anesth Analg 89:55-56, 1999.
63. Neal JM, Hebl JR, Gerancher JC, et al: Brachial plexus anesthesia: Essentials of our current understanding. Reg Anesth Pain Med 27:402-428, 2002.
64. Al-Khafaji JM, Ellias MA: Incidence of Horner syndrome with interscalene brachial plexus block and its importance in the management of head injury. Anesthesiology 64:127, 1986.
65. Seltzer JL: Hoarseness and Horner's syndrome after interscalene brachial plexus block. Anesth Analg 56:585-586, 1977.
66. Sukhani R, Barclay J, Aasen M: Prolonged Horner's syndrome after interscalene block: A management dilemma. Anesth Analg 79:601-603, 1994.
67. Kempen PM, O'Donnell J, Lawler R, et al: Acute respiratory insufficiency during interscalene plexus block. Anesth Analg 90:1415-1416, 2000.
68. Bashein G, Robertson HT, Kennedy WF: Persistent phrenic nerve paresis following interscalene brachial plexus block. Anesthesiology 63:102-104, 1985.
69. White JL: Catastrophic complications of interscalene nerve block. Anesthesiology 95:1301, 2001.
70. Lim E: Interscalene brachial plexus block in the asthmatic patient. Anaesthesia 34:370, 1979.
71. Thiagarajah S, Lear E, Azar I, et al: Bronchospasm following interscalene brachial plexus block. Anesthesiology 61:759-761, 1984.
72. Benumof JL: Permanent loss of cervical spinal cord function associated with interscalene block performed under general anesthesia. Anesthesiology 93:1541-1544, 2000.
73. Dutton R, Eckhardt W, Sunder N: Total spinal anesthesia after interscalene blockade of the brachial plexus. Anesthesiology 80:939-941, 1994.
74. Edde RR, Deutsch S: Cardiac arrest after interscalene brachial plexus block. Anesth Analg 56:446-447, 1977.
75. Huang KC, Fitzgerald MR, Tsueda K: Bilateral block of cervical and brachial plexuses following interscalene block. Anaesth Intensive Care 14:87-88, 1986.
76. Kumar A, Battit GE, Froese AB, et al: Bilateral cervical and thoracic epidural blockade complicating interscalene brachial plexus block: Report of two cases. Anesthesiology 35:650-652, 1971.
77. Norris D, Klahsen A, Milne B: Delayed bilateral spinal anesthesia following interscalene brachial plexus block. Can J Anaesth 43:303-305, 1996.
78. Passannante AN: Spinal anesthesia and permanent neurological deficit after interscalene block. Anesth Analg 82:873-874, 1996.
79. Ross S, Scarborough CD: Total spinal anesthesia following brachial plexus block. Anesthesiology 39:458, 1973.
80. Scammell SJ: Inadvertent epidural anaesthesia as a complication of interscalene brachial plexus block. Anaesth Intensive Care 7:56-57, 1979.
81. Tetzlaff JE, Yoon HJ, Dilger J, et al: Subdural anesthesia as a complication of an interscalene brachial plexus block. Reg Anesth 19:357-359, 1994.
82. Cook L: Unsuspected extradural catheterization in an interscalene block. Br J Anaesth 67:473-475, 1991.
83. Siler JN, Lief PL, Davis JF: A new complication of interscalene brachial plexus block. Anesthesiology 38:590-591, 1973.
84. D'Alessio JG, Weller RS, Rosenblum M: Activation of the Bezold–Jarisch reflex in the sitting position for shoulder arthroscopy using interscalene block. Anesth Analg 80:1158-1162, 1995.
85. Liguori GA, Kahn RL, Gordon J, et al: The use of metoprolol and glycopyrrolate to prevent hypotensive/bradycardic events during shoulder arthroscopy in the sitting position under interscalene block. Anesth Analg 87:1320-1325, 1998.
86. Boardman ND, Cofield RH: Neurologic complications of shoulder surgery. Clin Orthop Relat Res (368):44-53, 1999.
87. Cheney FW, Domino KB, Caplan RA, et al: Nerve injury associated with anesthesia: A closed claims analysis. Anesthesiology 90:1062-1069, 1999.
88. Barutell C, Vidal F, Raich M, et al: A neurological complication following interscalene brachial plexus block. Anaesthesia 35:365-367, 1980.
89. Dullenkopf A, Zingg P, Curt A, et al: Persistent neurological deficit of the upper extremity after a shoulder operation under general anesthesia combined with a preoperatively placed interscalene catheter. Anaesthesist 51:547-551, 2002.
90. Lenters TR, Davies J, Matsen FA 3rd: The types and severity of complications associated with interscalene brachial plexus block anesthesia: Local and national evidence. J Shoulder Elbow Surg 16:379-387, 2007.
91. Capdevila X, Pirat P, Bringuier S, et al: Continuous peripheral nerve blocks in hospital wards after orthopedic surgery: A multicenter prospective analysis of the quality of postoperative analgesia and complications in 1,416 patients. Anesthesiology 103:1035-1045, 2005.
92. Ribeiro FC, Georgousis H, Bertram R, et al: Plexus irritation caused by interscalene brachial plexus catheter for shoulder surgery. Anesth Analg 82:870-872, 1996.
93. Galindo A, Galindo A: Special needle for nerve blocks. Reg Anesth 5:12-13, 1980.

94. Myers RR, Heckman HM: Effect of local anesthesia on nerve blood flow: Studied using lidocaine with and without epinephrine. Anesthesiology 71:757-762, 1989.

95. Selander D, Sjöstrand J: Longitudinal spread of intraneurally injected local anesthetics. Acta Anaesthesiol Scand 22:622-634, 1978.

96. Bittar D: Attempted interscalene block procedures. Anesthesiology 5:1303-1304, 2001.

97. Borgeat A, Ekatodramis G, Gaertner E: Performing an interscalene block during general anesthesia must be the exception. Anesthesiology 5:1302-1303, 2001.

98. Chelly JE, Greger J, Gebhard R, et al: How to prevent catastrophic complications when performing interscalene blocks. Anesthesiology 5:1302, 2001.

99. Selander D, Brattsand R, Lundborg G, et al: Local anesthetics: Importance of mode of application, concentration and adrenaline for the appearance of nerve lesions. Acta Anaesthesiol Scand 23:127-136, 1979.

100. Kroin JS, Penn RD, Levy FE, et al: Effect of repetitive lidocaine infusion on peripheral nerve. Exp Neurology 94:166-173, 1986.

101. Fibuch EE, Mertz J, Geller B: Postoperative onset of idiopathic brachial plexitis. Anesthesiology 84:455-458, 1996.

102. Tetzlaff JE, Brems J, Dilger J: Intraarticular morphine and bupivacaine reduces postoperative pain after rotator cuff repair. Reg Anesth Pain Med 25:611-614, 2000.

103. American Society of Anesthesiologists: Basic standards for preanesthesia care, 2005. Available at http://www.asahq.org/publicationsAndServices/standards/03.pdf (accessed March 1, 2008).

104. Barash PG, Cullen BF, Stoelting RK (eds): Clinical Anesthesia. Philadelphia: Lippincott Williams & Wilkins, 2001.

105. Blumenthal S, Nadig M, Gerber C, et al: Severe airway obstruction during arthroscopic shoulder surgery. Anesthesiology 99:1455-1456, 2003.

106. Hynson JM, Tung A, Guevara JE, et al: Complete airway obstruction during arthroscopic shoulder surgery Anesth Analg 76:875-878, 1993.

107. Yoshimura E, Yano T, Ichinose K, Ushijima K: Airway obstruction involving a laryngeal mask airway during arthroscopic shoulder surgery. J Anesth 19:325-327, 2005.

108. Morrison DS, Schaefer RK, Friedman RL: The relationship between subacromial space pressure, blood pressure, and visual clarity during arthroscopic subacromial decompression. Arthroscopy 11:557-560 1995.

109. Pohl A, Cullen D: Cerebral ischemia during shoulder surgery in the upright position: A case series. J Clin Anesth 17:463-469, 2005.

110. Faure EAM: Air embolism during anesthesia for shoulder arthroscopy. Anesthesiology 89:805-806, 1998.

111. Hegde RT, Avatgere RN: Air embolism during anaesthesia for shoulder arthroscopy. Br J Anaesth 85(6):926-927, 2000.

112. Huffnagle S, Seltzer JL, Torjman M, et al: Does the use of methylmethacrylate cement in total shoulder replacement induce hemodynamic or pulmonary instability? J Clin Anesth 5:404-407, 1993.

113. Borgeat A, Schappi B, Biasca N, et al: Patient-controlled analgesia after major shoulder surgery. Anesthesiology 87:1343-1346, 1997.

114. Borgeat A, Tewes E, Biasca N, et al: Patient-controlled interscalene analgesia with ropivacaine after major shoulder surgery: PCIA vs PCA. Br J Anaesth 81:603-605, 1998.

115. Sriwatanakul K, Weis OF, Alloza JL, et al: Analysis of narcotic analgesic usage in the treatment of postoperative pain. JAMA 250:926-929, 1983.

116. Twersky R, Fishman D, Homel P: What happens after discharge? Return hospital visits after ambulatory surgery. Anesth Analg 84:319-324, 1997.

117. Ritchie ED, Tong D, Chung F, et al: Suprascapular nerve block for postoperative pain relief in arthroscopic shoulder surgery: A new modality? Anesth Analg 84:1306-1312, 1997.

118. Seltzer J, Greek R, Maurer P, et al: The preemptive analgesic effect of regional anesthesia for shoulder surgery. Anesthesiology 79(3A):A815, 1993.

119. Wilson AT, Nicholson E, Burton L, Wild C: Analgesia for day-case shoulder surgery. Br J Anaesth 92:414-415, 2004.

120. Casati A, Cappelleri G, Beccaria P, et al: A clinical comparison of ropivacaine 0.75%, ropivacaine 1% or bupivacaine 0.5% for interscalene brachial plexus anesthesia. European J Anesth 16:784-789, 1999.

121. Casati G, Fanelli G, Aldegheri M, et al: Interscalene brachial plexus anaesthesia with 0.5%, 0.75% or 1% ropivacaine: A double-blind comparison with 2% mepivacaine. Br J Anaesth 83:872-875, 1999.

122. Klein SM, Greengrass RA, Steele SM, et al: A comparison of 0.5% bupivacaine, 0.5% ropivacaine, and 0.75% ropivacaine for interscalene brachial plexus block. Anesth Analg 87:1316-1319, 1998.

123. Krone SC, Chan VWS, Regan J, et al: Analgesic effects of low-dose ropivacaine for interscalene brachial plexus block for outpatient shoulder surgery: A dose-finding study. Reg Anesth Pain Med 26(5):439-443, 2001.

124. Bauer GS, Bauereis C, Heinrich C: Interscalene brachial plexus catheter for anaesthesia and postoperative pain therapy. Experience with a modified technique. Anaesthetist 46:715-719, 1997.

125. Ilfeld BM, Morey TE, Wright TW, et al: Continuous interscalene brachial plexus block for postoperative pain control at home: A randomized, double-blinded, placebo-controlled study. Anesth Analg 96:1089-1095, 2003.

126. Ilfeld BM, Morey TE, Wright TW, et al: Interscalene perineural ropivacaine infusion: A comparison of two dosing regimens for postoperative analgesia. Reg Anesth Pain Med 29:9-16, 2004.

127. Klein SM, Nielsen KC, Martin A, et al: Interscalene brachial plexus block with continuous intraarticular infusion of ropivacaine. Anesth Analg 93:601-605, 2001.

128. Singelyn FJ, Seguy S, Gouverneur JM: Interscalene brachial plexus analgesia after open shoulder surgery: Continuous versus patient-controlled infusion. Anesth Analg 89:1216-1220, 1999.

129. Tuominen M, Haasio J, Hekali R, et al: Continuous interscalene brachial plexus block: Clinical efficacy, technical problems and bupivacaine plasma concentrations. Acta Anaesthesiol Scand 33:84-88, 1989.

130. Tuominen M, Pitkanen M, Rosenberg PH: Postoperative pain relief and bupivacaine plasma levels during continuous interscalene brachial plexus block. Acta Anaesthesiol Scand 31:276-278, 1987.

131. Ilfeld BM, Enneking FK: A portable mechanical pump providing over four days of patient-controlled analgesia by perineural infusion at home. Reg Anesth Pain Med 27(1):100-104, 2002.

132. Ilfeld BM, Morey TE, Enneking FK: Continuous infraclavicular brachial plexus block for post-operative pain control at home: A randomized double blind placebo controlled study. Anesthesiology 96:1297-1304, 2002.

133. Rawal N, Allvin R, Axelsson K, et al: Patient-controlled regional analgesia (PCRA) at home. Anesthesiology 96:1290-1296, 2002.

134. Kirkpatrick AF, Bednarcyzk LR, Hime GW, et al: Bupivacaine blood levels during continuous interscalene block. Anesthesiology 62:65-67, 1985.

135. Rosenberg PH, Pere P, Hekali R, et al: Plasma concentrations of bupivacaine and two of its metabolites during continuous interscalene brachial plexus block. Br J Anaesth 66:25-30, 1991.

136. Laurila PA, Lopponen A, Kangas-Saarela T, et al: Interscalene brachial plexus block is superior to subacromial bursa block after arthroscopic shoulder surgery. Acta Anaesthesiol Scand 46:1031-1036, 2002.

137. de Nadal M, Agreda G, Massenet S, et al: Efficacy of bupivacaine infiltration upon postoperative pain after ambulatory shoulder arthroscopy under general anaesthesia. Br J Anaesth 80(Suppl 1):A595, 1998.

138. Gomoll AH, Kang RW, Williams JM, et al: Chondrolysis after continuous intra-articular bupivacaine infusion: An experimental model investigating chondrotoxicity in the rabbit shoulder. Arthroscopy 22:813-819, 2006.

139. Park J-Y, Lee G-W, Kim Y, et al: The efficacy of continuous intrabursal infusion with morphine and bupivacaine for postoperative analgesia after subacromial arthroscopy. Reg Anesth Pain Med 27:145-149, 2002.

140. Barber FA, Herbert MA: The effectiveness of an anesthetic continuous-infusion device on postoperative pain control. Arthroscopy 18(1):76-81, 2002.

141. Savoie FH, Field LD, Jenkins RN, et al: The pain control infusion pump for postoperative pain control in shoulder surgery. Arthroscopy 16:339-342, 2000.

142. Enneking FK, Scarborough MT, Radson EA: Local anesthetic infusion through nerve sheath catheters for analgesia following upper extremity amputation. Reg Anesth 22:351-356, 1997.

143. Horn EP, Schroeder F, Wilhelm S, et al: Wound infiltration and drain lavage with ropivacaine after major shoulder surgery. Anesth Analg 89:1461-1466, 1999.

144. Ballantyne JC, Carr DB, Chalmers TC, et al: Postoperative patient-controlled analgesia: Meta-analyses of initial randomised control trials. J Clin Anesth 5:182-190, 1993.

145. Walder B, Schafer M, Henzi I, et al: Efficacy and safety of patient-controlled opioid analgesia for acute postoperative pain. A quantitative systematic review. Acta Anaesthesiol Scand 45:795-804, 2001.

Fractures of the Proximal Humerus

Kamal I. Bohsali, MD, and Michael A. Wirth, MD

With regard to shoulder girdle injuries, proximal humerus fractures remain challenging in both their initial diagnosis and treatment. Proximal humerus fractures account for nearly 5% of all fractures,[1,2] and incidence increases secondary to an aging population and associated osteoporosis.[3-6] Nonoperative versus operative management of these injuries depends upon the mechanism of injury, the patient's physiologic age including activity level, and fracture pattern.[7] In general, proximal humerus fractures occur more in female patients than male patients (3:1 ratio), and the overall incidence increases with age.

Nearly three fourths of all proximal humerus fractures occur in patients older than 60 years, and they generally occur as a result of low-energy trauma such as a fall from standing height.[7,8] A majority of these injuries are nondisplaced or minimally displaced and have a good overall prognosis with nonsurgical management.[2,7] Specific risk factors associated with the development of proximal humerus fractures in the elderly include low bone density, impaired vision and balance, lack of hormone replacement therapy, previous fracture, three or more chronic illnesses, and smoking.[7-9]

In contradistinction to the elderly, younger patients generally sustain proximal humerus fractures during high-energy situations such as motor vehicle collisions, seizures, or electrical shock. These injuries tend to be more severe regarding soft tissue compromise and fracture displacement requiring operative intervention.[2,7]

ANATOMY

To appropriately manage proximal humerus fractures, it is crucial to understand the complex anatomy of the shoulder girdle. Stability and function of the glenohu-meral joint is provided by an interaction of mechanisms that promote near global range of motion and purposeful function. Loads of increasing severity are initially offset by joint surface anatomy, joint volume, atmospheric pressure, and joint fluid cohesion and adhesion. Moderate loads are counteracted by the deltoid and rotator cuff, and larger loads are counterbalanced by capsulolabral structures and bone structure. Proximal humerus fractures alter these complex interactions, resulting in pain, decreased range of motion, and disability.[10]

The proximal humerus consists of the humeral head, greater tuberosity, lesser tuberosity, and humeral shaft. Fractures of the proximal humerus occur in predictable patterns based upon the muscular insertions of the pectoralis major, subscapularis, supraspinatus, and infraspinatus (Fig. 9-1).[10] The articular head is spherical and has a diameter of 37 to 57 mm.[11,12] The most superior portion of the articular surface of the humeral head averages 8 mm above the greater tuberosity,[11] and humeral version averages 29.8 degrees (range, 10-55 degrees).[13] The head is inclined approximately 130 degrees with respect to the humeral shaft.[12]

The bicipital groove lies between the greater and lesser tuberosities and serves as a pathway for the long head of the biceps as it traverses from its intra-articular origin from the superior glenoid-labrum complex into the proximal arm.[10] The distal aspect of the groove is internally rotated with respect to the proximal portion.[14]

The anatomic neck of the proximal humerus is located at the junction of the articular surface and the tuberosities. The surgical neck represents an indistinct region (metaphysis) below the tuberosities but above the humeral shaft. There are direct implications regarding injuries to these separate locations, because injury to the former (anatomic neck) portends a poor prognosis with

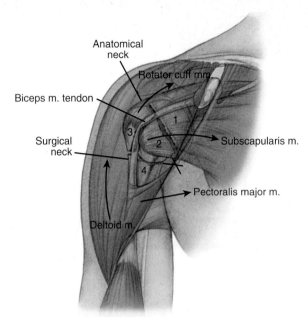

Anatomical neck

Rotator cuff mm.

Biceps m. tendon

Surgical neck

Subscapularis m.

Pectoralis major m.

Deltoid m.

FIGURE 9-1 The anatomy of the shoulder is complex, and shoulder function depends on proper alignment and interaction of anatomic structures. Displacement of fracture fragments is due to the pull of muscles attaching to the various bony components. The four anatomic components of the proximal part of the humerus are the head (*1*), lesser tuberosity (*2*), greater tuberosity (*3*), and shaft (*4*). The anatomic neck is at the junction of the head and tuberosities, and the surgical neck is below the greater and lesser tuberosities. The subscapularis inserts on the lesser tuberosity and causes medial displacement, whereas the supraspinatus and infraspinatus insert on the greater tuberosity and cause superior and posterior displacement. The pectoralis major inserts on the humeral shaft and displaces it medially.

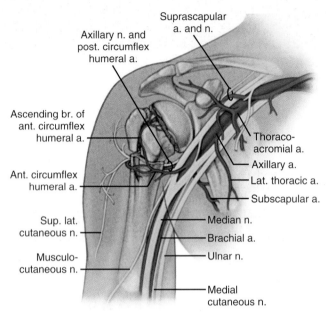

Suprascapular a. and n.

Axillary n. and post. circumflex humeral a.

Ascending br. of ant. circumflex humeral a.

Ant. circumflex humeral a.

Sup. lat. cutaneous n.

Musculo-cutaneous n.

Thoraco-acromial a.

Axillary a.

Lat. thoracic a.

Subscapular a.

Median n.

Brachial a.

Ulnar n.

Medial cutaneous n.

FIGURE 9-2 The brachial plexus and axillary artery lie adjacent to the coracoid process and can be injured with fractures of the proximal end of the humerus. The major blood supply to the humeral head is through the ascending branch of the anterior humeral circumflex artery, which penetrates the head at the superior aspect of the bicipital groove and becomes the arcuate artery. Three important nerves are located about the shoulder: the axillary, suprascapular, and musculocutaneous. ant., anterior; br., branch; lat., lateral; post., posterior; sup., superior.

complete disruption of the vascular supply to the humeral head (Fig. 9-2).[10]

The greater tuberosity, which is located in a posterior-superior location with respect to the humeral shaft, serves as the attachment site for the supraspinatus, infraspinatus, and teres minor. The subscapularis, which lies on the anterior aspect of the humerus, inserts on the lesser tuberosity.

The glenoid is a convex structure of shallow depth shaped like an inverted comma. It articulates with the humeral head and serves as the attachment for the labrum and joint capsule.[15]

The acromion, the coracoacromial ligament, and the coracoid process form the coracoacromial arch, a rigid bony-ligamentous structure that imparts stability to the shoulder girdle (see Fig. 9-2). The rotator cuff, subacromial bursa, and subdeltoid bursa (synovial membranes) pass underneath the coracoacromial arch. Displaced proximal humerus fractures can impede normal movement of these structures, causing impingement and dis-

ruption of normal glenohumeral motion.[10] In proximal humerus fractures, the subdeltoid bursa can thicken and become fibrotic. These adhesions can limit normal glenohumeral motion. Early range-of-motion exercises after a fracture have been hypothesized to decrease the formation of these adhesions.[10]

The proximal humerus receives its blood supply from the anterior and posterior humeral circumflex branches from the third division of the axillary artery. The posterior humeral circumflex artery travels with the axillary nerve, enters the quadrilateral space posteriorly, and anastomoses with the anterior circumflex branch, supplying the posterior cuff. The anterior humeral circumflex artery arises from the axillary artery at the inferior border of the subscapularis and provides the majority of vascular inflow to the humeral head by way of its terminal anterolateral branch known as the *artery of Laing*.[10,16,17] This vessel courses parallel to the lateral aspect of the long head of the biceps and enters the humeral head at interface of the intertubercular groove and the greater tuberosity.

Additional extraosseous collateral branches can permit humeral head perfusion despite complete ligation of the arcuate artery.[18] Injury to the arcuate artery can result in osteonecrosis of the humeral head.[16,17]

Vascular injuries with proximal humerus fractures are uncommon (5%-6%). Most axillary artery injuries occur in patients older than 50 years, suggesting that comorbid conditions (e.g., arteriosclerosis) play a role in this increased incidence.[19,20] Most axillary artery injuries occur at the level of the surgical neck, just proximal to the trifurcation of the anterior and posterior circumflex and subscapular branches.[19,20] A careful neurologic examination must be performed in addition to the vascular assessment secondary to a high correlation between axillary artery injury and brachial plexus traction injuries.[19,20]

The brachial plexus (nerve roots C5-T1, with small contributions from C3 and C4 nerve roots) provides innervation to the shoulder. The most commonly injured nerve in proximal humerus fractures is the axillary nerve and it is most susceptible to injury during anterior fracture dislocations of the proximal humerus.[21] The axillary nerve arises from the posterior cord of the brachial plexus (C5 and C6 nerve roots) and travels posterior to the surgical neck through the quadrilateral space with the posterior humeral circumflex artery, lying on the deep surface of the deltoid.

Previous anatomic studies documenting the course of the axillary nerve have demonstrated that the average distance from the proximal end of the humerus to the nerve is 6.1 cm (range, 4.5-6.9 cm), and the distance from the surgical neck of the humerus to the nerve is 1.7 cm (range, 0.7-4.0 cm).[22] The nerve sends three distinct branches (including an articular branch) that provide innervation to the deltoid and teres minor. The lateral brachial (cutaneous branch) provides sensation to the overlying deltoid region (see Fig. 9-2).

The suprascapular nerve, the second most commonly injured nerve, originates form the upper trunk and supplies input to the supraspinatus and infraspinatus muscles. It is most susceptible to traction injury at two locations: the origin from the upper trunk and the suprascapular notch where the nerve passes underneath the transverse scapular ligament.[21,23]

The musculocutaneous nerve obtains neural input from C5, C6, and C7. It originates from the lateral cord of the plexus, passes through the conjoint tendon at a variable distance from the coracoid process (3.1-8.2 cm), and terminates into the lateral antebrachial cutaneous nerve, supplying sensation to the anterolateral forearm. Injury to the musculocutaneous nerve is a rare event, but it can occur with blunt trauma and traction injuries to the shoulder.[24,25]

Electromyographic studies should be completed at 3 weeks if clinical recovery is not apparent by physical examination. Documentation of motor denervation without improvement on additional studies might warrant surgical exploration for complete injuries at 3 months.[7,21,23]

MECHANISM OF INJURY

The most common cause of proximal humerus fractures is a fall on an outstretched hand from standing height (or less), particularly in patients older than 60 years.[4,5,6-30] Less commonly, high-energy trauma such as motor vehicle accidents, falls from height, seizures, and electrical shock can occur in younger patients. These injuries tend to be more severe with regard to fracture pattern and soft tissue compromise.[31-33] In the setting of metastatic bone disease or primary malignancy, a pathologic fracture can occur with minimal trauma.[7]

CLINICAL EVALUATION

Regardless of the age of the patient, a thorough history and physical examination should be performed. The history should include assessment of mechanism of action, velocity of the injury (associated injuries to ribs, cervical spine, and scapula), premorbid level of function, occupation, hand dominance, history of malignancy, and the ability to participate in a structured rehabilitation program.[34] A review of systems should include queries regarding paresthesias, loss of consciousness, and ipsilateral elbow or wrist pain. On physical examination, the surgeon should look for swelling, soft tissue injuries, ecchymosis, and gross deformity. Most patients present with guarding, with the arm in internal rotation. Any attempts at active or passive movement elicit significant pain. Palpation of the shoulder reveals crepitus.[7] A careful neurovascular assessment should include evaluation of the axillary nerve, brachial plexus, and axillary artery. Posterior fracture-dislocations can demonstrate flattening of the anterior aspect of the shoulder, with an associated prominence; anterior fracture-dislocations manifest with opposite findings.[35] The surgeon should assume a vascular injury (even in the presence of a benign examination) with four-part proximal humerus fractures with axillary dislocation of the humeral head.[7,18,19]

IMAGING

Radiographic evaluation of the shoulder is often difficult but crucial during surgical decision making. The shoulder trauma series includes a true anteroposterior (AP) scapular view, an axillary lateral view, and a scapular Y lateral view.

The true AP view may be taken with the patient's arm in the sling and with the patient standing, seated, or prone. The glenohumeral joint does not lie in either the coronal or sagittal plane, and the glenoid is angled 35 to 40 degrees anteriorly. To obtain the true AP view, the unaffected shoulder must be rotated away 40 degrees, thus allowing the injured side to rest upon the x-ray plate (Fig. 9-3A).

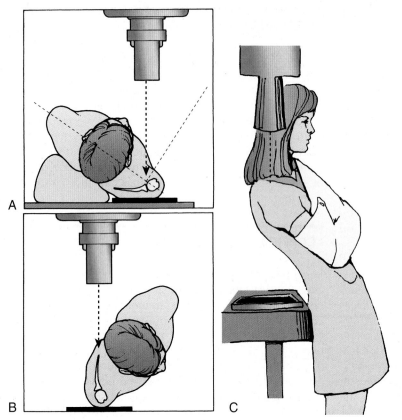

FIGURE 9-3 The trauma series consists of anteroposterior and lateral radiographs in the scapular plane, as well as an axillary view. These views may be taken with the patient sitting, standing, or prone. The scapula sits obliquely on the chest wall, and the glenoid surface is tilted approximately 35-40 degrees anteriorly. **A,** For the anteroposterior radiograph in the scapular plane, the posterior aspect of the affected shoulder is placed up against the x-ray plate and the opposite shoulder is tilted forward approximately 40 degrees. **B,** For the lateral radiograph in the scapular plane, the anterior aspect of the affected shoulder is placed against the x-ray plate, and the other shoulder is tilted forward approximately 40 degrees. The x-ray tube is then placed posteriorly along the scapular spine. **C,** The Velpeau axillary view is preferred after trauma when the patient can be positioned for this view because it allows the shoulder to remain immobilized and avoids further displacement of the fracture fragments. (Modified from Rockwood CA Jr, Green DP, Bucholz RW, Heckman JD: Fractures in Adults, 4th ed. Philadelphia: Lippincott-Raven, 1996, p 1065.)

The scapular Y lateral view is obtained by placing the anterior aspect of the affected shoulder against the x-ray plate with the unaffected side rotated out 40 degrees (see Fig. 9-3B). The axillary view is essential in evaluating the relationship of the humeral head to the glenoid, the displacement of the greater tuberosity, and the glenoid articular surface.[36-38] This view can be obtained in the seated, standing, or prone position. The arm is gently held in 30 degrees of abduction with an x-ray plate placed on the posterosuperior aspect of the shoulder. The x-ray tube is directed cephalad from a level slightly below the plane of the patient.

Because of the nature of the injury, the patient may be unable or unwilling to participate in the abducted axillary view. The Velpeau axillary view is an excellent alterative and the preferred view in the trauma series (see Fig. 9-3C). The view is obtained by directing the x-ray beam from superior to inferior as the patient leans back over the x-ray cassette with the arm in a sling. Internal-rotation and external-rotation AP views can portray lesser or greater tuberosity fractures, respectively.[7,20]

Magnetic resonance imaging (MRI) is rarely indicated in the setting of an acute injury. If primary or metastatic disease from malignancy is a possibility, then MRI may be useful for staging of the disease. Computed tomography (CT) analysis may be helpful in evaluating tuberosity displacement, degree of comminution, and glenoid articular surface involvement.[7,20,35]

CLASSIFICATION

A functional classification scheme should be easy to use and easy to reproduce (good inter- and intraobserver reliability), and it should direct appropriate management. The system must be comprehensive enough to include all variables but at the same time be specific enough to allow accurate diagnosis and treatment.

The most commonly used system is Neer's four-part fracture classification, initially reported in 1970.[39] Prior to Neer's system, several persons attempted to classify these injuries according to fracture location (Kocher [Fig. 9-4]),[40] fracture pattern (Codman [Fig. 9-5], De Anquin and De Anquin, and De Palma and Cautilli),[41-43] and mechanism of injury (Watson-Jones, Dehne).[44,45]

Jakob and Ganz from the AO (Arbeitsgemeinschaft für Osteosynthesefragen) group proposed a classification scheme involving 27 subgroups based upon articular involvement, location, and degree of comminution and dislocation, with special emphasis on the integrity of vascular supply. This system helped distinguish valgus impacted four-part proximal humerus fractures from other four-part injuries with partial preservation of vascular inflow to the articular segment through the medial capsule.[46-48] The complexity of this system has generally precluded its routine use, despite similar intra- and interobserver reliability when compared to Neer's classification.[49]

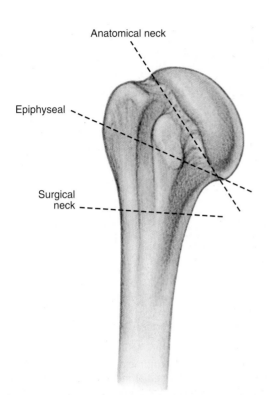

FIGURE 9-4 The Kocher classification is based on three anatomic levels of fractures: anatomic neck, epiphyseal region, and surgical neck. This classification does not allow differentiation of multiple fractures at two different sites, nor does it differentiate between displaced and nondisplaced fractures. (Modified from Kocher T: Beitrage zur Kenntnis einiger praktisch wichtiger Fracturenformen. Basel: Carl Sallman Verlag, 1896.)

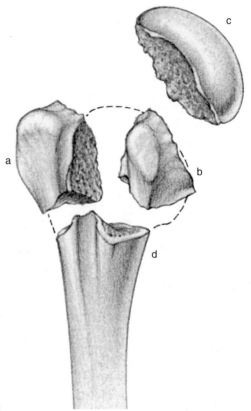

FIGURE 9-5 Codman divided the proximal end of the humerus into four distinct fragments that occur along anatomic lines of epiphyseal union. He differentiated the four major fragments as *a*, greater tuberosity; *b*, lesser tuberosity; *c*, head; and *d*, shaft. (Modified from Codman EA: The Shoulder: Rupture of the Supraspinatus Tendon and Other Lesions in or About the Subacromial Bursa. Boston: Thomas Todd, 1934.)

The intra- and interobserver reliability of the Neer classification system has been previously challenged, but it still remains the most reliable and commonly used system for assessment of proximal humerus fractures.[50-55] The classification scheme is based upon four segments: the humeral shaft, articular surface, greater tuberosity, and lesser tuberosity, with emphasis on identifying fracture patterns associated with vascular injury to the humeral head (Fig. 9-6). Displacement of a segment occurs when the part (articular segment, greater or lesser tuberosity, shaft) has separated more than 1 cm or angulated more than 45 degrees. If this criterion is not met, the fracture is considered minimally displaced, even if multiple segments are involved.[39]

Neer additionally focused on fracture-dislocations of the proximal humerus, head-splitting fractures, and impression fractures of the humeral head. Fracture-dislocations are classified according to direction of head dislocation (anterior or posterior) in conjunction with additional displaced fracture segments. Head-splitting and impression fractures have specific features of articular surface involvement and have been subdivided according to percentage involvement in order to direct treatment (<20%, 25%-40%, and >45%). Classification of these injuries depends on proper radiographs (AP, scapular Y lateral, and axillary lateral views) and adequate knowledge of the proximal humerus anatomy, including the rotator cuff insertions.

Some authors have attempted to improve the reliability of the Neer classification with CT scan augmentation, but they have demonstrated no evidence of decreased variability with this modality. The same authors have concluded that classification of proximal humerus fractures remains a difficult task, with reproducibility depending on the surgeon's experience and level of expertise.[50-58] Shrader and colleagues assert that the problem lies not with an understanding of the classification scheme but with the comprehension of the complex images.[59]

Hertel and colleagues have modified Codman's original classification in order to evaluate the predictors of humeral

DISPLACED FRACTURES

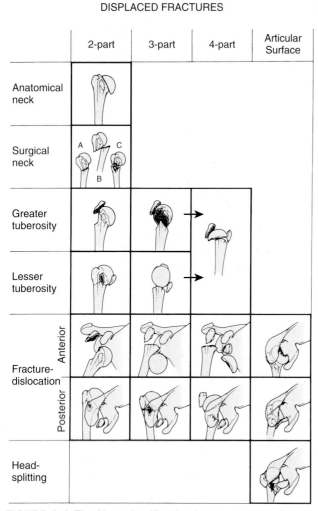

FIGURE 9-6 The Neer classification is a comprehensive system that encompasses anatomy and biomechanical forces that result in the displacement of fracture fragments. It is based on accurate identification of the four major fragments and their relationship to each other. A displaced fracture is either two part, three part, or four part. In addition, fracture-dislocations can be either two part, three part, or four part. A fragment is considered displaced when it has more than 1 cm of separation or is angulated more than 45 degrees from the other fragments. Impression fractures of the articular surface also occur and are usually associated with an anterior or posterior dislocation. Head-splitting fractures are generally associated with fractures of the tuberosities or surgical neck. (Adapted from Neer CS: Displaced proximal humeral fractures. Part I. Classification and evaluation. J Bone Joint Surg Am 52:1077-1089, 1970.)

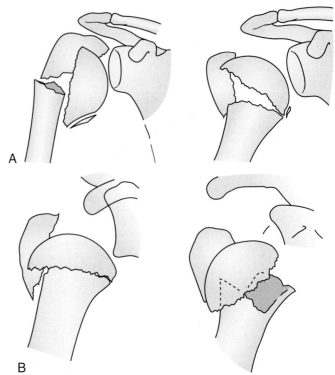

FIGURE 9-7 Predictors of humeral head ischemia. **A,** The longer the length of the medial metaphyseal extension (>8 mm), the more likely the humeral head is perfused. **B,** Integrity of the medial hinge at the pivot point of the dorsomedial fracture line predicts vascular perfusion and feasibility of reduction. (Redrawn from Hertel R, Hempfing A, Stiehler M, Leunig M: Predictors of humeral head ischemia after intracapsular fracture of the proximal humerus. J Shoulder Elbow Surg 13:427-433, 2004.)

head ischemia after intracapsular fractures of the proximal humerus. According to the authors, the most relevant predictors of ischemia were the length of the dorsomedial metaphyseal extension, the integrity of the medial hinge, and basic fracture pattern (Fig. 9-7).[60] The combination of an anatomic neck fracture, short calcar (<8 mm of metaphyseal extension), and disrupted medial hinge demonstrated a positive predictive value of 97% when determining humeral head ischemia. Fracture displacement proved less important with regard to humeral head viability.

Despite these newer findings, the Neer classification remains the most commonly used system by orthopaedic surgeons for the treatment of proximal humerus fractures.

METHODS OF TREATMENT

The vast majority of proximal humerus fractures are minimally displaced or angulated and do not require surgical intervention.[7,41,61-65] Early protection with gradual mobilization is the guiding principle with nondisplaced injuries. The patient generally wears a sling for 7 to 10 days with or without an axillary pad for comfort. The patient is encouraged to perform active finger, hand, wrist, and

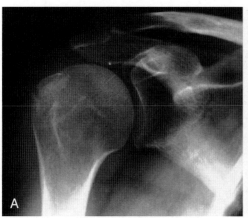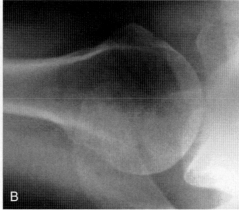

FIGURE 9-8 A, True anteroposterior radiograph showing a nondisplaced to minimally displaced greater tuberosity fracture in a 68-year-old, right hand–dominant woman after a fall onto her outstretched hand. **B,** Axillary radiograph showing no significant displacement of the fracture.

elbow exercises. By 2 weeks, active assisted range-of-motion and pendulum exercises may be initiated under the supervision of a physical therapist. Delay of motion beyond 2 weeks has deleterious effects on shoulder range of motion, pain, and function.[66-69] Intermittent biplanar radiographs should be obtained to monitor interval fracture displacement or angulation. By 6 weeks, light-resistance shoulder exercises may be performed. Range-of-motion gains are generally noted between weeks 3 and 8.[69]

Approximately 20% of proximal humerus fractures are comminuted or displaced and can require surgical intervention by means of closed reduction with splinting, percutaneous fixation, open reduction with internal fixation, or humeral head replacement.[7,43] In addition to the severity of the fracture, bone quality, rotator cuff status, patient's physiologic age, activity level, and premorbid health status should be considered when deciding to pursue operative treatment. Patients with low demands and significant medical comorbidities (e.g., dementia) should be managed nonsurgically.[68] The ideal goal of treatment, whether surgical or nonsurgical, is to reestablish functional pain-free range of motion.

Greater Tuberosity Fractures

Epidemiology
Isolated displaced fractures of the greater tuberosity account for a small percentage of proximal humerus fractures.[70] Chun and colleagues, in their review of two-part proximal humerus fractures, recorded 26 out of 141 (18%) displaced greater tuberosity fractures.[71] As an uncommon event, these injuries may be overlooked or trivialized by orthopaedic surgeons and other health care providers (Fig. 9-8).

Nature of the Injury
The amount of tuberosity displacement guides decision making regarding surgical intervention. In view of Neer's

criteria regarding displacement, most authors agree that the shoulder has little tolerance for greater tuberosity displacement. McLaughlin suggested that displacement of 5 mm or more can cause impingement and rotator cuff dysfunction.[72] Park and colleagues have suggested that fractures in manual laborers or athletes with 3 mm of displacement should be reduced.[73]

The direction of displacement of the tuberosity is just as important as the degree of displacement. Posterior displacement can affect external rotation, but it is generally more tolerated than superior displacement, which results in subacromial impingement.

Different mechanisms of injury have been proposed for greater tuberosity fractures, including impaction (fall onto shoulder in hyperabduction) or avulsion and shearing (anterior glenohumeral dislocation), though the pathomechanics have not been clearly elucidated.[74]

Peripheral nerve injury is the most commonly associated injury, occurring in nearly 33% of patients.[75-77] Nearly 50% of patients older than 50 years who have an anterior proximal humerus fracture-dislocation demonstrate a peripheral nerve injury, and the axillary nerve is most commonly affected (Fig. 9-9).[78,79]

Evaluation
The initial evaluation of a patient with an injured shoulder includes a detailed history with a careful neurovascular examination. Radiographic evaluation should include the trauma series: true anteroposterior, scapular Y lateral, and axillary view. CT and MRI are not routinely used, though three-dimensional CT may be used to better delineate greater tuberosity displacement.[70]

Treatment
Nonsurgical
Nonsurgical treatment of nondisplaced and minimally displaced greater tuberosity fractures should be limited to low-demand patients. This treatment includes a brief period of sling immobilization for 1 to 2 weeks followed

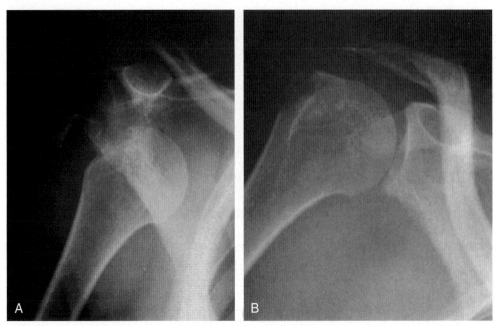

FIGURE 9-9 A, Anteroposterior radiograph of a two-part anterior fracture-dislocation with a displaced greater tuberosity fracture. **B,** After closed reduction, the greater tuberosity fracture reduced and healed without further displacement. The patient achieved normal range of motion without any further anterior dislocations. (From Rockwood CA Jr, Green DP, Bucholz RW, Heckman JD: Fractures in Adults, 4th ed. Philadelphia: Lippincott-Raven, 1996, p 1069.)

by passive motion. By 6 weeks, active range-of-motion and progressive strengthening exercises may be initiated.[70]

Surgical

Operative intervention is deemed appropriate for greater tuberosity fractures with more than 5 mm of displacement.[72] Patients are placed in the semi-sitting (beach chair) position under general anesthesia augmented by an interscalene nerve block for postoperative pain control. An articulated headrest and arm positioning device (McConnell, Greenville, Tex) is used with a standard operating table, with the patient's affected shoulder placed over the edge of the table. A C-arm image intensifier may be used to obtain anteroposterior and axillary views (Fig. 9-10).

Surgical exposure for open reduction and internal fixation can proceed by way of a superior deltoid-splitting or deltopectoral approach. Some authors have advocated the use of the deltoid-splitting approach due to the relative ease in visualization of the greater tuberosity fragment. If necessary, an acromioplasty can also be performed with this technique.[80] The deltopectoral approach avoids detachment of the deltoid and allows exposure of the surgical neck when there is a concomitant proximal humeral shaft fracture.

Screw and heavy suture fixation are two techniques used for internal fixation of greater tuberosity fractures. Isolated screw fixation is not recommended because the tuberosity can fragment or displace around the screw.[70] Screws may be used as a post when placed distal to the fracture site, using sutures for tension band fixation. We recommend fixation with multiple sutures (e.g., No. 5 nonabsorbable) placed at the interface of the rotator cuff tendon and the tuberosity, with cortical approximation through distal bone tunnels through a figure-of-eight technique (Fig. 9-11). If there is an additional rotator cuff tear, this should also be repaired at the time of surgery.

Some authors have advocated percutaneous reduction with fixation to minimize soft tissue dissection, though fixation with a single screw or pin remains a disadvantage.[81]

Recovery

Postoperative rehabilitation begins the day after surgery with pendulum and passive forward-flexion and external-rotation exercises. Internal-rotation and adduction maneuvers are prohibited until 6 weeks. After 6 weeks, active range-of-motion exercises are initiated, with concurrent passive stretching exercises tolerated in all planes. Rotator cuff strengthening exercises are postponed until 10 to 12 weeks after surgery. All patients need to be informed that clinical improvement might not be maximized until 1 year.[70]

Stiffness, malunion, and nonunion remain the most common complications that can occur after nonoperative or operative treatment of greater tuberosity fractures. Shoulder stiffness may be treated early with aggressive passive stretching exercises, but it can require arthroscopic capsular release with acromioplasty to address posttraumatic impingement.

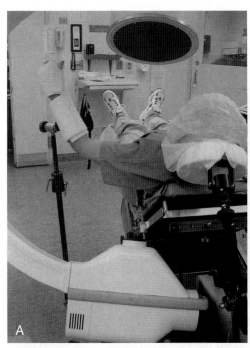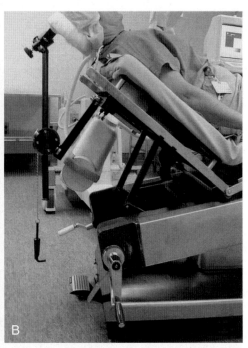

FIGURE 9-10 Intraoperative beach chair positioning for concomitant use of C-arm during open reduction and internal fixation of greater tuberosity fracture. **A,** Posterior view. **B,** Lateral view. (From Green A, Izzi J Jr: Isolated fractures of the greater tuberosity of the proximal humerus. J Shoulder Elbow Surg 12:641-649, 2003.)

Osteotomy and mobilization of a malunited greater tuberosity fragment has unpredictable results, often requiring rotator cuff interval slides to reduce the fragment and the rotator cuff. Fixation of the mobilized tuberosity can prove tenuous due to significant osteopenia.

In the setting of nonunion, the tuberosity may be markedly displaced, making mobilization and repair difficult secondary to scarring.[72,82,83]

Follow-up

There are limited published follow-up data regarding surgical treatment of displaced greater tuberosity fractures. Jakob and colleagues[84] treated 17 displaced greater tuberosity fractures but did not report the results of their treatment. Paavolainen and colleagues reported good results in the surgical treatment of six displaced fractures with screw fixation.[85] Chun and colleagues treated 10 greater tuberosity fractures with open reduction and internal fixation (8 with screws). At a mean follow-up of 5.1 years, results were graded as (according to Neer's criteria) excellent in 1 patient, good in 7, and fair in 3. The average active forward flexion and external rotation were 118 and 35 degrees, respectively.[71] Flatow and colleagues reported their experience with surgical fixation of 16 displaced greater tuberosity fractures using heavy nonabsorbable suture. At 4.5 years of follow-up, the authors reported 6 excellent and 6 good results according to Neer's criteria.[80]

Lesser Tuberosity Fractures

Isolated lesser tuberosity fractures without an associated posterior shoulder dislocation or surgical neck fracture is a rare event.[86] Because of the subscapularis insertion, the lesser tuberosity fragment can displace medially in the event of an injury. If the fragment is small, minimally displaced, and does not block internal rotation, a short period of immobilization in slight external rotation is appropriate (Fig. 9-12).[71,84,86,87]

In the more common situation involving a posterior dislocation and lesser tuberosity fracture, closed reduction and immobilization is also appropriate if the fracture is addressed within 2 weeks of the event. Surgical intervention is warranted for displaced large tuberosity fragments and lesser tuberosity injuries with articular surface involvement.[84,86,87] The tuberosity may be fixed either anatomically or into the base of the humeral head defect (reverse Hill–Sachs lesion) if the shoulder is unstable after open reduction.[87]

Surgical Neck Fractures

Epidemiology

Surgical neck fractures account for the majority (60%-65%) of proximal humerus fractures. Nearly 80% of these fractures are minimally displaced and warrant nonoperative management. Surgical indications include displacement, polytrauma, ipsilateral upper extremity injuries,

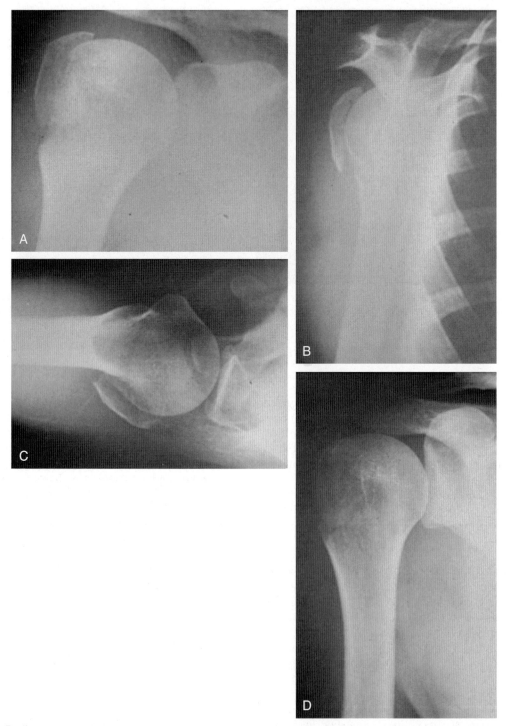

FIGURE 9-11 Radiographs depicting a displaced greater tuberosity fracture. **A,** Anteroposterior view. **B** and **C,** Lateral and axillary views. Note the posterior-superior displacement of the large greater tuberosity fragment on the lateral and axillary views. The anteroposterior view shows superior displacement. **D,** Postoperative radiograph after open reduction and internal fixation with multiple nonabsorbable sutures.

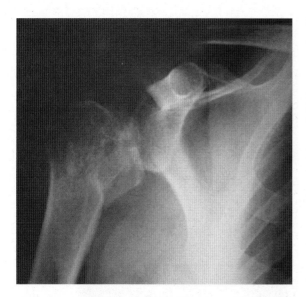

FIGURE 9-12 Anteroposterior radiograph of a two-part posterior fracture-dislocation after reduction. The lesser tuberosity fragment was minimally displaced and did not block medial rotation. This injury was treated in closed fashion, with excellent return of function. (From Rockwood CA Jr, Green DP, Bucholz RW, Heckman JD: Fractures in Adults, 4th ed. Philadelphia: Lippincott-Raven, 1996, p 1070.)

vascular compromise, open fractures, and patient compliance with a postoperative therapy regimen.[88] Malunion can be tolerated fairly well if the tuberosity and articular surface relationships are not distorted.

As Iannotti and colleagues have suggested, there are two distinct patient populations: young, male patients with high-energy trauma and elderly, female patients with low-energy trauma. These should be treated differently even with the same fracture pattern.[88] The young patient typically has good bone quality and can generally comply with postoperative therapy, allowing the surgeon to employ surgical methods such as open reduction and internal fixation. The elderly patient might not fully understand or appreciate her role in the postoperative rehabilitation process. Bone quality in elderly patients tends to be poor, with evidence of comminution after minor trauma. Fixation options may be limited, and in some cases, hemiarthroplasty may be a more viable option.[88]

Evaluation

The amount of displacement is critical when assessing nonoperative versus operative treatment for surgical neck fractures (Fig. 9-13). In the elderly patient, bony contact of fracture segments may be all that is necessary for a functional result. In active patients, less than 50% shaft diameter displacement and less than 45 degrees of angulation may be tolerated.[20] Varus deformity, valgus deformity, comminution, and 100% displaced surgical neck fractures are unstable and require surgical intervention.

Treatment

If the initial evaluation reveals a displaced fracture (<50%) without impaction, a closed reduction maneuver may be performed under conscious sedation or hematoma block. Because of the deforming force of the pectoralis major muscle, the arm should be adducted and flexed to 90 degrees. While in this position, a posterolateral translation force is applied in conjunction with longitudinal traction to promote impaction of the shaft and humeral head–tuberosity segments. If the maneuver is not successful, the surgeon should suspect that interposed soft tissues such as muscle, capsule, or the long head of the biceps are preventing the reduction.[20] If manipulation is successful, sling immobilization is performed, with weekly examination and radiographs. Two-part surgical neck fracture-dislocations may similarly be treated with immobilization if the fragments are minimally displaced following reduction of the glenohumeral joint.

Management of surgical neck fractures depends on fracture displacement, bone quality, functional demands of the patient, and mental status of the patient. Closed reduction with immobilization is generally reserved for patients with minimally displaced or less than 50% displaced surgical neck fractures who can participate in a rehabilitation program. Not all of these patients do well; Chun and colleagues reported 55% good or excellent results in 56 surgical neck fractures treated nonoperatively with a mean forward flexion arc of 104 degrees.[71] Displaced fractures in active patients should undergo open reduction with internal fixation. An alternative option, though tedious and technically difficult, may be percutaneous fixation after closed reduction. The main advantage to this technique is the lack of soft tissue dissection, which can theoretically minimize the risk of iatrogenic injury to the vascular supply of the articular segment.[88]

Three-Part Fractures

In three-part fractures, cleavage lines occur through the surgical neck and the greater or lesser tuberosity. Degree of displacement of the segments depends largely on the deforming forces of the rotator cuff muscles. The greater tuberosity is more commonly involved than the lesser tuberosity and is usually displaced into a posterior and superior position by the pull of the attached supraspinatus, infraspinatus, and teres minor.[88,89] The humeral head is pulled into internal rotation secondary to the subscapularis, while the humeral shaft is displaced anteromedially due to the insertion of the pectoralis major. If the fracture involves the lesser tuberosity, the subscapularis pulls the segment medially. The intact greater tuberosity and articular surface segment are pulled into adduction and external rotation, and the humeral shaft is similarly pulled in an anteromedial direction. Surgical treatment options include closed reduction, closed reduction and percutaneous fixation, open reduction with internal fixation, intramedullary fixation with suture supplementation, and hemiarthroplasty.

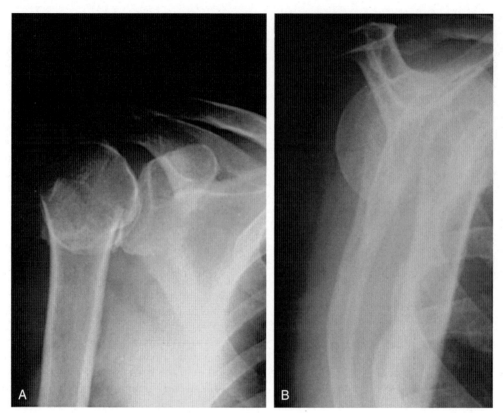

FIGURE 9-13 Anteroposterior (**A**) and scapular Y lateral (**B**) radiographs of a displaced surgical neck fracture.

Nonoperative management of three-part fractures should follow the same principles that guide treatment of minimally displaced fractures. Closed reduction may be attempted in the medically unfit patient, but it is often unsuccessful secondary to rotatory instability and degree of displacement. Multiple attempts at closed reduction should be avoided to prevent further displacement, fragmentation, and soft tissue injury.[20,88-90] If the reduction is successful, the patient should be placed in a sling for 7 to 10 days followed by physical therapy when the patient can tolerate motion.

Neer in 1970 initially reported his experience in 39 patients with three-part proximal humerus fractures treated by closed reduction. Only 3 patients demonstrated a satisfactory result by his criteria. Poor results were due to malreduction, nonunion, humeral head resorption, and osteonecrosis. He concluded that nonoperative intervention for these injuries was inadequate in active patients.[39] More recent studies by Lill and colleagues[91] and Zyto and colleagues[92,93] suggest that good functional outcomes after nonsurgical management of these injuries may be achieved. Zyto prospectively evaluated 40 patients with displaced three- and four-part proximal humerus fractures randomized to nonoperative management or tension band fixation. At 3 to 5 years of follow-up, he found no differences in functional outcome between the two methods, despite radiographic evidence revealing improved position of the humeral head in the surgical patient.[93]

The majority of three-part proximal humerus fractures require operative fixation or hemiarthroplasty due to the residual humeral deformity and functional deficits that can prevent the patient from returning to premorbid level of activity (Fig. 9-14).

Four-Part Fractures

Nonsurgical management of four-part proximal humerus fractures should only be employed in the medically unfit patient. Because of the poor outcomes and high incidence of complications (osteonecrosis, malunion, nonunion, and post-traumatic arthritis) associated with nonoperative treatment, most fractures are treated surgically.[91,94] Options include closed reduction, open reduction with internal fixation, and hemiarthroplasty.

The impacted valgus four-part fracture is an uncommon but important subtype to identify.[47,84,95-98] This injury has a more favorable prognosis when compared to other multipart proximal humerus fractures secondary to the integrity of the medial capsular blood supply.[97,98] The fracture pattern is characterized by impaction of the lateral aspect of the humeral articular surface due to a fracture of the anatomic neck (Fig. 9-15).[95-98] The articular surface faces superiorly toward the acromion rather than the glenoid. The tuberosities typically displace secondary to impaction of the articular surface on the humeral metaphysis. The prevalence of osteonecrosis approaches

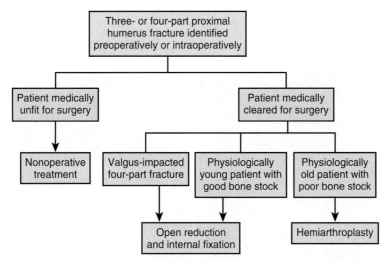

FIGURE 9-14 Treatment algorithm for three- and four-part proximal humerus fractures. (Adapted from Naranja RJ Jr, Iannotti JP: Displaced three- and four-part proximal humerus fractures: Evaluation and management. J Am Acad Orthop Surg 8:373-382, 2000.)

5% to 10%, much less than the corresponding standard four-part proximal humerus fractures.[47,95,96,98,99]

Surgical treatment options include early mobilization, percutaneous reduction with internal fixation, and hemiarthroplasty.[88] Nonoperative management is reserved for elderly and sedentary patients with medical comorbidities that prevent intervention. Percutaneous reduction with internal fixation is a viable option for acute injuries (<7-10 days old) with good bone stock and minimal comminution. Open reduction is generally performed for fractures not amenable to reduction by closed means, for fractures with comminution, and for injuries that are 10 days to 4 months old.

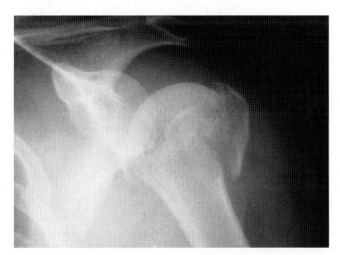

FIGURE 9-15 Anteroposterior radiograph of a valgus-impacted four-part proximal humerus fracture. The medial periosteal hinge remains intact, preserving partial vascular inflow into the articular surface. (From Iannotti JP, Ramsey ML, Williams GR, Warner JJP: Nonprosthetic management of proximal humeral fractures. J Bone Joint Surg Am 85:1578-1593, 2003.)

Jakob and colleagues achieved a satisfactory outcome in 74% of the patients in his study who underwent closed reduction or limited open reduction with internal fixation. The major reason for failure was avascular necrosis, which occurred in five cases (26%).[47] Resch and colleagues performed limited open reduction and internal fixation on 22 patients with four-part valgus-impacted fractures, demonstrating no evidence of osteonecrosis at a mean follow-up of 36 months (minimum, 18 months). Results were graded as excellent, particularly in cases in which anatomic reduction was maintained (12 of 22).[98]

Hemiarthroplasty is reserved for the elderly and sedentary patient with poor bone stock.[88]

Proximal Humerus Fracture-Dislocations

Two-part fracture dislocations are amenable to open reduction and internal fixation due to the integrity of the vascular supply that is maintained by the soft tissue attachments to the intact tuberosities.[20] Three-part and four-part fracture-dislocations with articular surface involvement similarly require operative intervention. Repeated attempts at closed reduction or delayed open reduction and internal fixation can result in an increased incidence of myositis ossificans.[7] Results of internal fixation for four-part proximal humerus fracture-dislocations are poor, and hemiarthroplasty serves as the appropriate treatment method for these injuries (Fig. 9-16). Closed management should only be considered in the medically moribund patient.

AUTHORS' PREFERRED METHOD OF TREATMENT

There are two basic surgical approaches that can be used to treat proximal humerus fractures. The superior

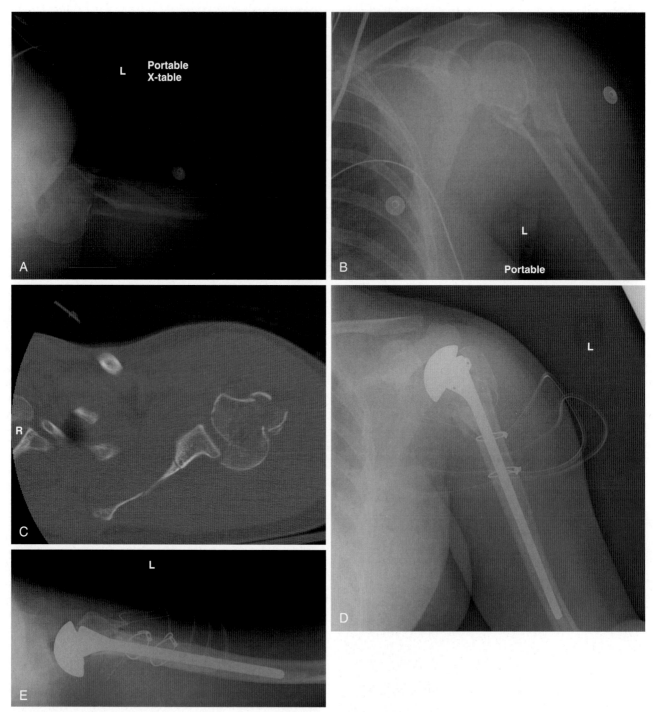

FIGURE 9-16 A, Axillary lateral radiograph of a four-part proximal humerus fracture. **B,** Anteroposterior radiograph of the same fracture with diaphyseal involvement. **C,** Axial computed tomography image demonstrating articular surface involvement. **D,** Postoperative anteroposterior view demonstrating a modular hemiarthroplasty. **E,** Axillary view of modular implant with reapproximation of lesser tuberosity. L, left; R, right.

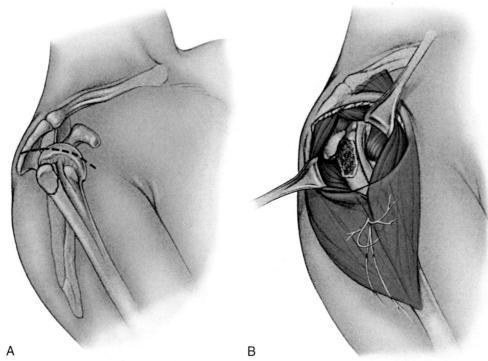

FIGURE 9-17 Superior approach to the shoulder. **A,** The skin incision for the superior approach to the shoulder consists of an oblique incision along Langer's lines beginning on the anterolateral aspect of the acromion and extending down obliquely for approximately 8-9 cm. **B,** Two Richardson retractors are placed in the deltoid as it is split approximately 4-5 cm from the tip of the acromion. This technique generally provides adequate exposure for fractures of the greater tuberosity. Great care is taken to not extend the split below 5 cm to avoid injury to the axillary nerve.

approach to the shoulder involves a skin incision made in Langer's lines just lateral to the anterolateral aspect of the acromion (Fig. 9-17A). The deltoid can be split from the edge of the acromion distally for approximately 4 to 5 cm, but, to protect the axillary nerve, the split should not be extended (see Fig. 9-17B).[7,20,88] The deltoid origin is not removed during exposure of the superior aspect of the proximal end of the humerus. This approach is useful for internal fixation of greater tuberosity fractures and is helpful for intramedullary fixation of two-part proximal humerus fractures. Rotation, flexion, or extension of the humerus can allow exposure of the underlying structures for appropriate reduction and internal fixation.[7,20,88]

The workhorse approach is the deltopectoral approach (Fig. 9-18A). In this technique, both the deltoid origin and insertion are preserved. The skin incision begins just inferior to the clavicle and extends across the coracoid process and down to the region of insertion of the deltoid. The cephalic vein should be preserved and retracted laterally with the deltoid. The deltopectoral interval is dissected proximally and distally (see Fig. 9-18B). If more exposure is needed, the superior 50% of the pectoralis major tendon insertion can be divided. This approach is useful for internal fixation of two-part surgical neck fractures and for hemiarthroplasty of three-part and four-part fractures.[7,20,88]

These approaches are useful because they preserve deltoid function, which allows more rapid rehabilitation in the postoperative period. Detachment of the deltoid origin is unnecessary because it deleteriously affects the function of this important muscle and can prohibit progression during the postoperative rehabilitation program.

Nondisplaced or Minimally Displaced Proximal Humerus Fractures

Nondisplaced and minimally displaced fractures are treated with a sling for comfort. Elbow, wrist, and hand exercises are encouraged during the initial immobilization period. If the fracture is stable, range-of-motion exercises may be started within 10 days, if the pain is tolerable. The physician can evaluate the fracture for gross stability by manipulating the elbow and forearm with gentle rotation while palpating the proximal humerus with the other hand. If the entire humerus appears to move as a unit, then the fracture is stable, and gentle passive range-of-motion exercises may be started. It is important to have the patient begin exercises within 14 days of the date of injury to avoid late sequelae such as stiffness, limited activities of daily living, and a poor functional outcome.[67] Weekly radiographic evaluation is needed to check for displacement of fracture fragments.[67]

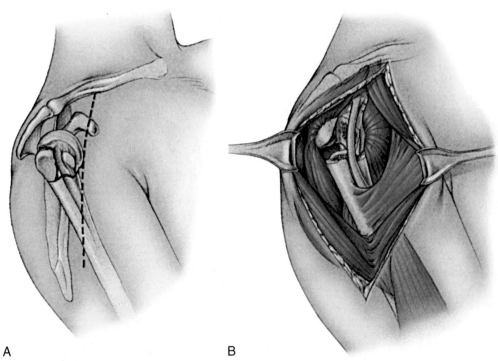

A   B

FIGURE 9-18 The extended deltopectoral approach is a utilitarian approach for two-, three-, and four-part fractures. **A,** The incision is made from the clavicle, passes over the coracoid, and extends down to the shaft of the humerus near the deltoid insertion. **B,** The insertion of the pectoralis major can also be released to improve exposure. Care is taken to never remove the deltoid origin from the clavicle. If more exposure is needed, the deltoid insertion can be elevated, although such elevation is rarely necessary.

Percutaneous Treatment of Proximal Humerus Fractures

The purpose of surgical fixation of proximal humerus fractures is twofold: to restore the anatomic relationship between the articular surface and the tuberosities and to preserve the vascularity of the articular fragment. Closed reduction with percutaneous fixation minimizes soft tissue dissection and can preserve vascular inflow for anatomic healing. The caveat to this technique is that it involves an increased level of technical skill and ancillary support (cooperation among surgeon, anesthesiologist, nursing staff, surgical assistant, and radiology).[100,101] Percutaneous fixation of proximal humerus fractures was initially used by Bohler to treat pediatric injuries,[102] but it was subsequently applied to adult surgical neck fractures.[103] Because of the growing emphasis on biological fixation, some authors have advocated percutaneous treatment of three- and four-part fractures.[95,99,103,104] The learning curve is substantial, but proponents of this method cite a decreased incidence of osteonecrosis because the region of the ascending branch of the anterior humeral circumflex artery is left undisturbed (Fig. 9-19).[105-109]

The indications for closed reduction and percutaneous pinning include proximal humerus fractures (ideally, two-part surgical neck) without comminution in compliant patients with good bone stock. Frequent (weekly) radiographic evaluation and shoulder immobilization for a duration of 4 to 6 weeks are required. Severe comminution and osteopenia are absolute contraindications to this technique. Additionally, numerous attempts to reduce fracture fragments should be avoided. In this situation, the surgeon might need to convert to an open procedure to achieve the goal of anatomic or near-anatomic reduction. Fracture-dislocations can prove extremely difficult to manage with this method as well, so it is generally not recommended.[88,101,103-109]

Surgical Technique

The most important decision occurs before surgery: selecting the appropriate patient. The ideal indication for this procedure is a displaced two-part surgical neck fracture without comminution. Specific technical steps are required to assure a positive outcome from this intervention. Adequate nursing, anesthesia, and radiologic staff (C-arm fluoroscopic operator) are necessary for this procedure. Biplanar images should be obtained with the patient positioned before draping. A surgical assistant who can maintain reduction during the fixation process is also recommended.

Two-Part Fracture

The patient is placed in the beach chair position that allows access to the entire shoulder. Commercially available beach chair positioners (alternative: bean bag) and mechanical arm holders can help significantly. Reduction

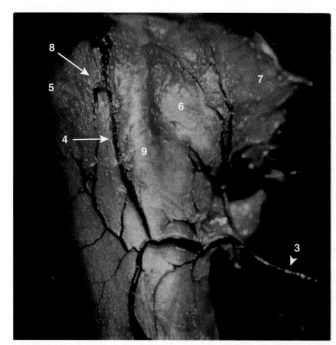

FIGURE 9-19 Vascular supply of the humeral head. *3,* Anterior humeral circumflex artery; *4,* anterolateral branch of anterior humeral circumflex artery (arcuate artery); *5,* greater tuberosity; *6,* lesser tuberosity; *7,* insertion of the subscapularis; *8,* site of terminal entry of arcuate artery into bone; *9,* intertubercular groove. (From Gerber C, Schneeberger AG, Vinh TS: The arterial vascularization of the humeral head: An anatomical study. J Bone Joint Surg Am 72:1486-1494, 1990.)

instruments should include bone elevators and hooks to manipulate fragments into position. Terminally threaded 2.5-mm pins and 4.0-mm cannulated screws are commonly used as fixation implants with this technique. The C-arm image intensifier is placed parallel to the table to allow anteroposterior and axillary views (Fig. 9-20). The image receiver is placed at the foot of the table for evaluation of reduction adequacy and pin placement. Anesthesia should provide neuromuscular relaxation in the form of general anesthesia and muscle relaxants (or an interscalene block) to facilitate the reduction maneuver.[101]

A provisional reduction maneuver should be performed to determine the feasibility of a closed reduction. With two-part surgical neck fractures, there is apex anterior angulation at the fracture site. The arm should first be placed in 20 to 30 degrees of abduction. Longitudinal traction is then applied to the arm, while the humeral shaft is directed lateral to the humeral head. Concomitant pressure against the anterior surface of the shoulder will help reduce the apex anterior angulation (Fig. 9-21).[88,103] A single pin is placed anterior to the shoulder in a distal-to-proximal direction from the lateral humeral cortex to the humeral head. An anteroposterior image confirms the inclination, and a skin marker is used to document pin positioning.

A 1-cm incision is placed on the lateral aspect of the shoulder at the level determined by the C-arm image. Blunt dissection is performed down to bone with a hemostat. The hemostat is then used to palpate the anterior and posterior cortices of the humerus. The initial pin is then guided under power at the previously determined angle. Initial horizontal pin placement can prevent the pin from skating across the cortex.

While the assistant maintains the reduction, the pin is advanced under C-arm fluoroscopy to engage the humeral head. Because of the approximate 30 degrees of retroversion of the humeral shaft, C-arm fluoroscopy must be used to confirm appropriate pin placement. A second pin is then advanced in parallel to the first with approximately 1.5 to 2 cm of separation. Jiang and colleagues have shown that parallel pin placement increases torsional stability in biomechanical testing when compared to converging pins.[110] A third pin is then placed from the anterior humeral shaft into the humeral head. A fourth pin from anterior to posterior may be necessary to augment the fixation (Fig. 9-22).[88,103] The axillary nerve, radial nerve, biceps tendon, and anterior humeral circumflex vessels are all at risk with this method. Soft tissue dissection should proceed carefully down to bone before pin placement. It is critical to obtain biplanar radiographic views before completing the procedure to confirm correct pin placement.[88,103]

Three-Part and Four-Part Fractures

Three- and four-part proximal humerus fractures add a level of complexity that proves difficult to manage with this technique even in the most experienced hands.[111]

With a three-part valgus-impacted fracture, the humeral head is tilted into valgus while the greater tuberosity remains at the correct height. After positioning the humeral shaft under the humeral head, a small incision is made laterally to allow placement of an elevator into the fracture site under the humeral head. Under C-arm fluoroscopy, the humeral head is then levered upward and into varus alignment. As the humeral head is reduced, the greater tuberosity will be pulled below the articular surface due to the integrity of the rotator cuff insertion. A 2.5-mm threaded pin or 4.0-mm cannulated screw guidewire is then advanced through a separate superior incision to capture the greater tuberosity and the humeral head. Cannulated screws are usually placed to hold the tuberosity and articular surface reduction while additional pins or screws are inserted in an antegrade fashion to stabilize the tuberosity to the humeral shaft.[88,103,111] Resch and colleagues reported good to very good functional results (Constant score, 91% in three-part and 87% in four-part fractures) in 27 patients (9 three-part, 18 four-part) with percutaneous treatment of three- and four-part proximal humerus fractures at 24 months of follow-up without evidence of humeral head necrosis.[95]

Four-part fractures, except for the valgus-impacted subtype (Fig. 9-23), generally require open reduction with internal fixation rather than hemiarthroplasty. On the

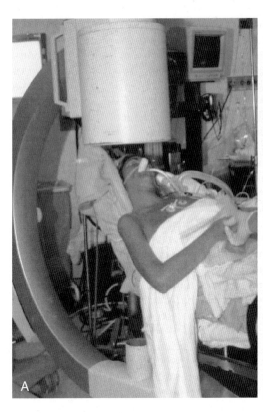
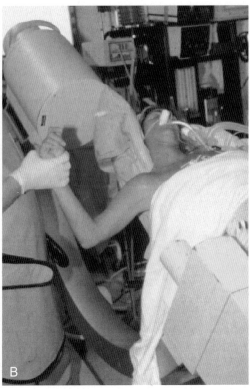

FIGURE 9-20 A, The patient is positioned in the beach chair position and the body is held in place with a large bean bag. The image intensifier is placed at the head of the table. **B,** The image intensifier can be positioned for both anteroposterior and axillary views of the proximal part of the humerus. (From Iannotti JP, Ramsey ML, Williams GR, Warner JJP: Nonprosthetic management of proximal humeral fractures. J Bone Joint Surg Am 85:1578-1593, 2003.)

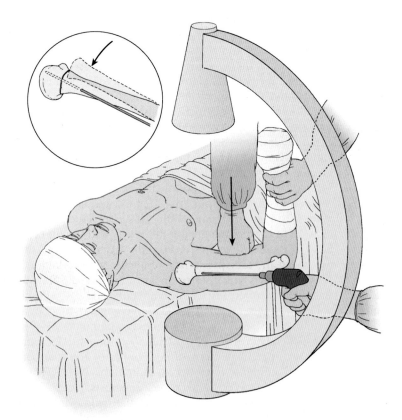

FIGURE 9-21 The reduction maneuver involves slight shoulder abduction, longitudinal traction of the arm, and posterior pressure on the humeral shaft. Anteroposterior and axillary views using C-arm fluoroscopy confirm the reduction. (Redrawn from Jaberg H, Warner JJ, Jakob RP: Percutaneous stabilization of unstable fractures of the humerus. J Bone Joint Surg Am 74:508-515, 1992.)

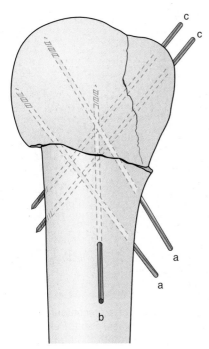

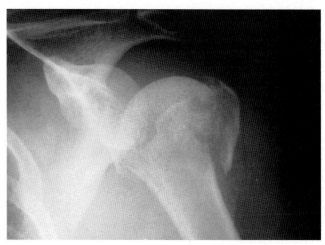

FIGURE 9-23 Anteroposterior view of a four-part valgus-impacted proximal humerus fracture. (From Iannotti JP, Ramsey ML, Williams GR, Warner JJP: Nonprosthetic management of proximal humeral fractures. J Bone Joint Surg Am 85:1578-1593, 2003.)

FIGURE 9-22 Two 2.5 mm AO terminally threaded pins are inserted from the lateral shaft, just above the deltoid insertion (*a*). A third pin (*b*) is placed through the anterior cortex and directed posteriorly toward the humeral head. If there is an associated greater tuberosity fracture, it is reduced and held in place with two additional pins (*c*). (Redrawn from Jaberg H, Warner JJ, Jakob RP: Percutaneous stabilization of unstable fractures of the humerus. J Bone Joint Surg Am 74:508-515, 1992.)

infrequent occasion that percutaneous fixation is attempted, the same steps to reduce the greater tuberosity, articular surface, and humeral shaft are employed. The lesser tuberosity may be reduced by internally rotating the arm and by placing a hook on the fragment through a laterally based incision. Once reduced, the fragment is held in place with a 4.0-mm cannulated screw (Fig. 9-24). A follow-up study by Resch and colleagues in the treatment of four-part fractures indicated good to very good results, with a Constant score of 87% and an osteonecrosis rate of 11% in 18 patients.[99]

Keener and colleagues reported their positive results after percutaneous reduction and fixation of two-, three-, and four-part proximal humerus fractures in 35 patients from three institutions. The mean follow-up was 35 months, with mean visual analogue pain, American Shoulder and Elbow Surgeons (ASES), and Constant scores of 1.4, 83.4, and 73.9, respectively. Fracture type, age at presentation, malunion, or osteoarthritis had no significant influence on measured outcomes. The authors concluded that this technique remained a viable and predictable option in the treatment of proximal humerus fractures.[112]

The threaded pins are trimmed below the skin, which is closed with suture. Tenting of the skin due to the pin can occur as the shoulder swelling diminishes. In some cases, the pin needs to be trimmed on an outpatient basis. Most patients are admitted postoperatively for 24-hour observation and continued parenteral antibiotics.

The shoulder is placed in a shoulder immobilizer for comfort, and pendulum, hand, wrist, and elbow exercises are encouraged. Passive forward flexion and external rotation exercises are initiated during the third postoperative week. Weekly physical examination and radiographs are obtained. The pins are generally removed at 4 weeks, and active assisted shoulder exercises are performed under the supervision of a physical therapist. Radiographic union should be apparent by 2 or 3 months. Shoulder strengthening may be initiated by 3 months postoperatively.[88,95,99,101,103]

Open Reduction and Internal Fixation of Proximal Humerus Fractures

Numerous techniques of internal fixation for two-, three-, and four-part proximal humerus fractures have been delineated in the literature. These methods include plate and screw fixation, blade plates, tension banding, antegrade or retrograde nailing, or a combination of internal fixation with sutures and metallic implant fixation.[88,89,111,113-121] Though the ideal fixation for these injuries has not been defined, current advances in locking plate technology have provided surgeons another viable option in the treatment of multipart proximal humerus fractures.[113,121]

The osseus architecture of the humeral head is variable with respect to the density of cancellous bone stock.[122] Particularly in elderly patients, this proves problematic when the goal is to achieve rigid internal fixation capable of withstanding a progressive rehabilitation program. Attempts at rigid fixation with prior implants have indicated high risk of failure due to osteonecrosis, nonunion, malunion, screw cutout, and screw loosening.[115,123-125]

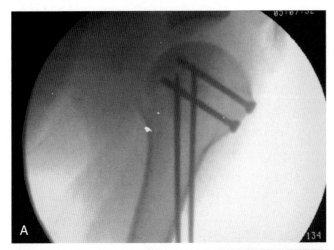

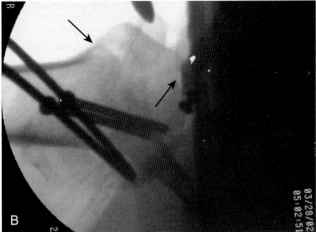

FIGURE 9-24 A, Anteroposterior C-arm view of the same four-part fracture as in Figure 9-23 after reduction and fixation of the articular surface and greater tuberosity fragments. **B,** Axillary view of the fracture with mild displacement of the lesser tuberosity fragment (*arrows*). (From Iannotti JP, Ramsey ML, Williams GR, Warner JJP: Nonprosthetic management of proximal humeral fractures. J Bone Joint Surg Am 85:1578-1593, 2003.)

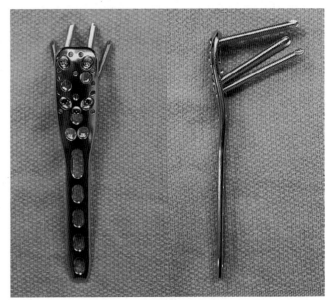

FIGURE 9-25 Photograph of a precontoured proximal humeral locking plate (Synthes, Paoli, Penn). The proximal screws allow locking fixation into the humeral head. The diaphyseal screws may be conventional or locking. Peripheral holes allow suture or wire augmentation to tuberosity fragments. (From Rose PS, Adams CR, Torchia ME, et al: Locking plate fixation for proximal humerus fractures: Initial results with a new implant. J Shoulder Elbow Surg 16:202-207, 2007.)

Blade plate fixation was used to overcome concerns regarding early hardware failure, but this challenging technique only allows a single point of proximal fixation in the humeral head.[88,126] In addition to the soft tissue dissection required with this technique, some authors have reported unacceptable complication rates related to blade plate protrusion into the glenohumeral joint (8 of 36 patients, 22%).[117] Weinstein and colleagues demonstrated in a three-part cadaveric model significantly increased torsional stiffness of the locking plate when compared to the blade plate.[127] Percutaneous pinning and intramedullary fixation can preserve the soft tissue envelope and decrease the risk of osteonecrosis, but the indirect reduction techniques can make anatomic alignment of the fracture fragments difficult to achieve. At this point, there is no consensus regarding the optimal form of fixation for these injuries.[128]

The indications for plate and screw fixation include comminuted two-, three-, and some four-part proximal humerus fractures. The ideal patient is compliant, physiologically young with good bone stock, and capable of undergoing surgery (see Fig. 9-14).[88,111] Based upon a current review of the literature, Nho and colleagues recommended buttress plate fixation in young patients with diaphyseal cortices greater than 3.5 mm. Metaphyseal comminution, however, prevented the use of the nonlocking device.[111]

The proximal humeral locking plate has been developed to overcome some of the limitations of conventional plating and to address issues specifically related to osteoporotic bone and metaphyseal comminution. Stability of this implant is based upon the fixed-angle relationship between the screws and the plate. The threaded screw heads lock into the corresponding threaded plate holes, preventing toggle, pullout, and sliding. The stability of the fracture-and-plate construct does not depend on any single screw because of the fixed-angle contruct.[129] As a single unit, the plate is better able to withstand bending and torsional forces.[121] Precontoured proximal humeral locking plates provide a mechanical advantage in fractures with metaphyseal comminution (Fig. 9-25).

Nonlocking and Locking Plate Surgical Technique
The patient may be positioned in the beach chair, lateral decubitus, or supine position on a radiolucent table. We

generally prefer the beach chair position and use an extended deltopectoral approach. The anterior third of the deltoid might need to be partially elevated from its insertion on the deltoid tubercle. If necessary, the displaced greater and lesser tuberosity fragments are tagged with No. 5 braided nonabsorbable suture for later repair through the peripheral plate holes.

For three-part and four-part fractures, the tuberosity fragments are initially reduced to the lateral humeral shaft cortex. The medial calcar may be re-established by using an elevator to disimpact the humeral head. Threaded or smooth 1.6-mm pins may be used to provisionally hold the fracture fragments reduced. The plate should then be positioned on the anterolateral aspect of the greater tuberosity. Previously placed sutures from the tuberosity fragment may be delivered through the peripheral holes at this time. On the anteroposterior view, the plate should be placed approximately 8 mm below the superior tip of the greater tuberosity to avoid impingement. Adequate spacing is necessary between the plate and the biceps tendon to prevent injury to the arcuate artery.

After anteroposterior and axillary (or scapular Y lateral) views document a satisfactory reduction, an initial screw is placed in the elongated hole of the plate. Locked screws are then inserted into the humeral head using the insertion guide. Tingart and colleagues investigated the appropriate positioning of these screws by evaluating the bone mineral density of 18 unpaired cadaveric humeri. They concluded that the pullout strength was least in the anterosuperior portion of the humeral head, and suggested screws be placed in regions of highest bone mineral density (central, posteroinferior, posterosuperior, inferoposterior, and inferoanterior).[122] At least three distal shaft screws (locking or nonlocking) are inserted. In the event that there is a residual metaphyseal defect, bone graft or bone graft substitute may be used as an adjuvant to fracture healing (Fig. 9-26).[111] The stability of the fixation is evaluated intraoperatively to allow specific tailoring of the postoperative physician-directed rehabilitation regimen.

With rigid fixation, patients should begin pendulum and passive range-of-motion exercises on postoperative day 1 as allowed by intraoperative stability assessment. Radiographic union should be apparent by 6 to 8 weeks postoperatively, and active and active assisted range of motion may be performed under the supervision of a physical therapist. By 3 months, strengthening exercises should be added, and the patient is made aware that maximal improvement may not be achieved for up to 1 year.

Saudan and colleagues,[130] Frankauser and colleagues,[131] and Bjorkenheim and colleagues[132] have reported early favorable results with a similar titanium implant. All authors reported excellent results, with union rates greater than 90%. Rose and colleagues reported their 1-year experience with a stainless steel proximal humeral locking plate of similar design. They followed 16 patients (9 with three-part fractures, 5 with two-part fractures, and 2 four-part fractures) until union or revision at a mean follow-up

of 12 months. Of the 4 nonunions, 3 were three-part fractures with extensive metaphyseal comminution in smokers. Patients with united fractures demonstrated mean forward elevation and external rotation of 132 degrees and 43 degrees, respectively. The authors were encouraged by the early positive findings, but they emphasized that there are limitations with this method based upon degree of comminution and patient factors (e.g., smoking).[113] Longer term follow-up will be necessary with this surgical technique to better elucidate long-term outcomes and negative sequelae.

Intramedullary Fixation Surgical Technique

There are two distinct types of intramedullary fixation for two- and three-part proximal humerus fractures. One is intramedullary fixation with a nail alone, and the other is fixation with modified Ender rods supplemented by tension band.[88] Both of these methods can be technically demanding, particularly with three-part fractures. In three-part proximal humerus fractures with involvement of the greater tuberosity, the entry point for commercially available nails (e.g., Polarus nail, Acumed, Beaverton, Oregon) is compromised.[88,133-135] If the lesser tuberosity is involved, the insertion point at the junction of the articular surface and the greater tuberosity is left intact.

Nail Fixation. The patient is placed in the beach chair position on a radiolucent table. A 3-cm longitudinal incision is made in line with the greater tuberosity of the humerus. The deltoid is then split in line with its fibers.[133] Under C-arm fluoroscopy, the entry hole of the nail is made with a curved awl or guide pin just medial to the greater tuberosity and approximately 1.5 cm posterior to the bicipital groove.[134] Adduction of the arm and extension of the shoulder provide adequate clearance from the acromion for the awl and subsequent nail insertion. If closed reduction can be performed (acute cases), it is generally accomplished with longitudinal traction on an adducted arm in neutral forearm rotation.[133] If closed reduction is not possible secondary to soft tissue interposition or adhesions (chronic cases), open reduction may be performed before the nail is inserted.[133,134]

A 2-mm guidewire is passed across the fracture and down the intramedullary canal. The nail is inserted and locked proximally and distally. Care must be taken when placing the distal locking screws to avoid injury to the neurovascular structures, including the radial nerve, brachial artery, and median nerve (depending on lateral or anterior screw placement). Gentle blunt soft tissue dissection (nick-and-spread method) and screw placement under C-arm guidance are a must to avoid iatrogenic injury to these structures.[133]

The arm is placed in sling or shoulder immobilizer. Gentle pendulum and elbow range-of-motion exercises are initiated on postoperative day 1. Patients are seen at 2 and 6 weeks with biplanar radiographs. With radiographic union, active range-of-motion exercises may be initiated. By 3 months, strengthening may begin.[133-135]

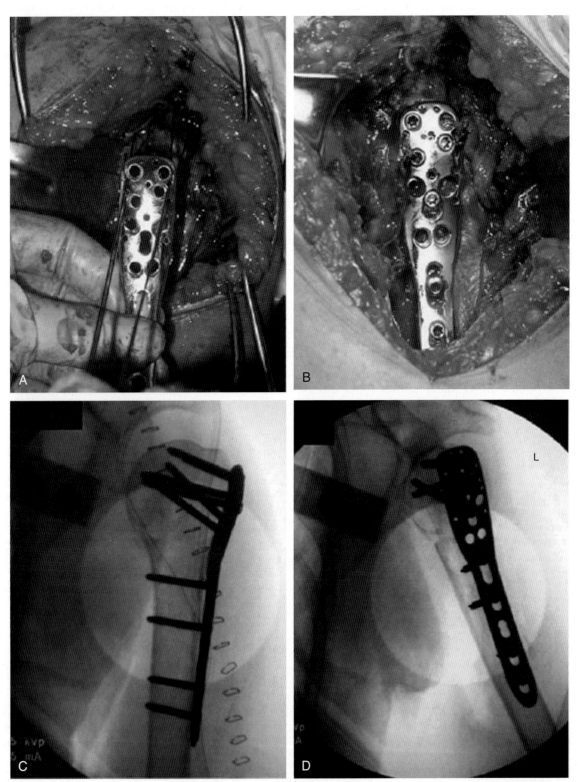

FIGURE 9-26 A, Tagged sutures from the greater tuberosity are placed through the plate. **B,** Locking plate placed in the anterolateral aspect of the greater tuberosity and humeral shaft. Anteroposterior (**C**) and internal rotation (**D**) views of the proximal humerus after locking plate fixation. (© 2007 American Academy of Orthopaedic Surgeons. Reprinted from the *Journal of the American Academy of Orthopaedic Surgeons*, Volume 15(1), pp 12-26 with permission.)

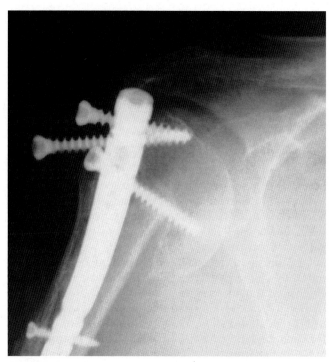

FIGURE 9-27 Intramedullary fixation for a surgical neck nonunion resulting in malunion and hardware prominence in the subacromial space. (From Iannotti JP, Ramsey ML, Warner JJP: Nonprosthetic management of proximal humeral fractures. J Bone Joint Surg Am 85:1578-1593, 2003.)

This technique has limitations, particularly when there is significant metaphyseal comminution or humeral head involvement. Nonunions associated with intramedullary nailing appear to be unique to proximal humerus (and humeral shaft) fractures and tend to be more refractory to secondary intervention (Fig. 9-27).[133] Infection remains a rare event after nailing, occurring in 1% to 2% of cases. More commonly, intramedullary nails are associated with shoulder pain and loss of motion. Subacromial impingement, bursitis, and rotator cuff irritation can occur if the nail is prominent proximally. Iatrogenic fractures can also occur with vigorous attempts at nail insertion.[133]

Early reports on intramedullary fixation of two- and three-part fractures by Lin and colleagues,[136] Adedapo and colleagues,[137] and Rajasekhar and colleagues[134] suggested that this is a reliable technique of fixation, with union rates of 100% (21 patients), 97% (29 patients), and 100% (23 patients), respectively. A more recent evaluation by Agel and colleagues[135] placed emphasis on the location of the appropriate nail insertion site medial to the greater tuberosity and suggested that lateral metaphyseal comminution can contribute to implant failure. Of the 20 fractures treated by the authors, only 65% achieved union; 6 of the 7 nonunions had not healed at the latest follow-up reported by the investigators (range, 4-9 months). Only 3 of the 20 nails placed (15%) demonstrated proximal screw loosening. Agel and colleagues concluded that the intramedullary implant is not effective for fixation

of proximal humerus fractures if the insertion site is incorrect, if the insertion site is violated by fracture, or if the fracture contains extensive lateral metaphyseal comminution.[135]

Park and colleagues performed intramedullary fixation augmented with a tension band and locking suture technique and noted fracture union in 25 of 26 patients at an average of 8.7 weeks (range, 7-12 weeks).[120] At a mean follow-up of 39 months (range, 24-59 months), ASES scores averaged 85 (range, 40-100), with no statistical difference evident when comparing patients younger or older than 65 years of age (range, 27-79 years old).[120] The authors concluded that open intramedullary nailing remained a viable technique for proximal humerus fractures in elderly patients, and, more importantly, good functional outcomes could be expected at mid-term follow-up.

Ender Rod and Tension Band. The combination of tension band sutures with Ender rod fixation serves as an alternative form of fixation for two- and three-part proximal humerus fractures. Intraoperative management of the rods and sutures can be tedious, even in two-part fractures. Additional complexity is encountered when an additional fracture plane involves the lesser or the greater tuberosity.[88]

A deltopectoral approach is used as the approach for surgical exposure in both two- and three-part fractures. The fracture sites are cleared of hematoma and debris. The humeral head can be mobilized with traction sutures at the bone–tendon interface. Small stab incisions are made in line with the rotator cuff fibers lateral to the articular surface at the greater or lesser tuberosity. Modified Ender nails contain proximal eyelets that allow suture management and deeper insertion of the implant, thus reducing the incidence of rotator cuff irritation (Fig. 9-28A).

While the reduction is maintained, an initial nail is placed in the posterior portion of the entry point created by a supplied awl. A second nail is advanced 1 to 1.5 cm anterior to the first.[114] The combination of two different length nails can reduce the risk of a distal stress riser.[138] Before fully seating the nails, drill holes are made in the humeral shaft to accept tension band sutures or wires. The sutures or wires are initially placed through the nail eyelets deep to the rotator cuff and are then crossed in a figure-of-eight fashion through the shaft holes (see Fig. 9-28B). The nails are then impacted below the cuff tissue. With three-part fractures, the tuberosity fragment is reduced first and secured to the articular segment with heavy nonabsorbable sutures through drill holes. Ender nails are then inserted into the unaffected tuberosity (two for the greater tuberosity, one rod for the lesser tuberosity). Two drill holes are placed medial and lateral to the bicipital groove for figure-of-eight fixation of both the tuberosity and articular surface segments. The surgical neck fracture is then repaired, as previously outlined, with an intramedullary nail–tension band construct.[138,139]

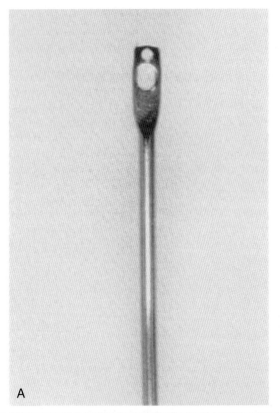

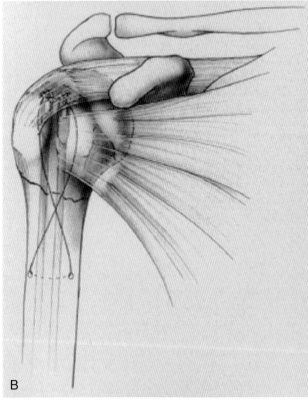

FIGURE 9-28 A, Modified Ender rod with proximal eyelet that allows suture or wire passage. **B,** Ender rod fixation with figure-of-eight tension band technique. (From Iannotti JP, Ramsey ML, Warner JJP: Nonprosthetic management of proximal humeral fractures. J Bone Joint Surg Am. 85:1578-1593, 2003.)

The stability of the fixation is assessed intraoperatively and to help guide the postoperative rehabilitation regimen.

Pendulum and passive range-of-motion exercises are started after surgery within the defined intraoperative limits. At 6 to 8 weeks, active assisted and active exercises may begin, followed by strengthening at 3 months.[88,114,138]

Intramedullary Fixation Versus Locking Plate Fixation

Kitson and colleagues investigated the biomechanical behavior of a locking plate versus a locking intramedullary nail for the treatment of three-part proximal humerus fractures. Paired cadaveric specimens were tested with four directional loads: flexion, extension, varus, and valgus. When cantilever bending loads were below the failure threshold, the nail construct demonstrated a significantly higher stiffness value in valgus, flexion, and extension. Valgus load to failure was also significantly higher for the locking intramedullary nail (157 versus 84 N). The authors also noted different modes of failure for each implant. In all samples, the nail construct failed at the bone–screw interface, whereas the plates all failed due to bending of the implant at the surgical neck fracture site. Kitson and colleagues cautioned the extrapolation of this data to clinical scenarios encountered by surgeons in which the results of controlled osteotomies cannot be equated with the setting of proximal humerus fractures with cortical and metaphyseal comminution.[140]

Sanders and colleagues performed a similar evaluation with paired cadaveric specimens and reported opposite results with the locking plate, demonstrating greater stiffness in valgus loading compared to the nail construct (420 versus 166 N/mm). All other loading vectors showed no statistical differences between the two constructs. If failure occurred in the plate fixation, it occurred in a similar manner through the osteotomy site as described by Kitson and colleagues.[140,141]

Both studies used similar biomechanical testing techniques. Kitson and colleagues used a locking humeral nail. It is unclear whether Sanders and colleagues performed their study with a locking version of the humeral nail tested (Polarus humeral nail, Acumed, Portland, Oregon).[140,141] Both studies were limited by sample size, and conclusions must be applied with caution to clinical practice.

Shoulder Arthroplasty for Three- and Four-Part Proximal Humerus Fractures

In the 1950s, Neer initially developed the technique of humeral head arthroplasty for treating proximal humerus fractures.[142] Before this method was developed, these injuries were treated with benign neglect or humeral head resection. By 1970, Neer reported uniformly poor results of open reduction and internal fixation of four-part fractures and fracture-dislocations and again suggested humeral head replacement for these fractures.[38] Because of the high risk of humeral head osteonecrosis with three-part and four-part proximal humerus fractures, Neer believed that even with anatomic reconstruction with internal fixation, post-traumatic osteoarthritis would develop, resulting in poor outcomes for the patients. Neer reiterated that humeral head replacement and stable fixation of the tuberosities could provide a reasonable result for the patient.

Similar principles are applied to three- and four-part fractures in the present. Advances have been made in metallurgy, implant modularity, surgical technique, rehabilitation, and validated outcome tools (Constant score,[143] ASES score[144]). The current indications for primary hemiarthroplasty include most four-part fractures, three-part fractures and dislocations in elderly patients with osteoporotic bone, head-splitting articular segment fractures, and chronic anterior or posterior humeral head dislocations with more than 40% of the articular surface involved.[38,145]

Iannotti and colleagues outlined specific anatomic parameters in their cadaveric study that are vital to consider when performing a primary hemiarthroplasty, including humeral head height (8 mm from greater tuberosity to top of articular surface), radius of curvature (22-25 mm), and humeral version (average, 29.8 degrees; range, 10-55 degrees).[146]

Initial implant designs were monoblock and did not offer variations in humeral head sizes. Second- and third-generation implants have added modularity and stem body size reduction to match the patient's anatomy while accommodating for tuberosity reduction.[147,148] Several studies have indicated that outcomes following primary hemiarthroplasty for acute proximal humerus fractures are superior to results from late reconstruction.[149,150]

Though some studies have recommended urgent intervention (<48 hours), most authors suggest preoperative planning with a careful neurovascular assessment of the injured shoulder, medical optimization of the patient, and preoperative templating with standard radiographs of the contralateral uninjured shoulder.[151] Nerve injuries (up to 67%) tend to be more common with proximal humerus fractures and fracture-dislocations than usually reported in studies involving hemiarthroplasty.[152-154]

Surgical Technique

The goal of surgery is to anatomically reconstruct the glenohumeral joint with restoration of humeral length, placement of appropriate prosthetic retroversion, and secure tuberosity fixation. An interscalene block (regional anesthesia) may be used to augment general anesthesia. Endotracheal intubation is generally recommended to allow intraoperative muscle relaxation, although laryngeal mask intubation may be used.[20,151,155]

The patient is placed on an operative table in the beach chair position with the arm positioned in a sterile articulating arm holder or draped free if an appropriate number of assistants are available (Fig. 9-29).[20,151,155] The surgical preparation site should include the entire upper extremity and shoulder region, including the scapular and pectoral

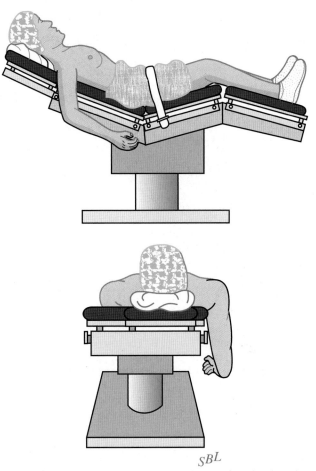

SBL

FIGURE 9-29 Beach chair position. The patient is placed with the thorax at the end of the table. A kidney post and a McConnell head holder are used to allow free and unencumbered access to the medullary canal of the humerus. (Modified from Matsen FA III, Lippitt SB: Shoulder Surgery: Principles and Procedures. Philadelphia: WB Saunders, 2004, p 628.)

region. Appropriate prophylactic intravenous antibiotics are given to the patient within 30 minutes of skin incision.

A standard deltopectoral incision is used. The incision begins superior and lateral to the coracoid process and extends toward the anterior aspect of the deltoid insertion. The cephalic vein is identified, preserved, and retracted laterally with the deltoid muscle. The pectoralis major is retracted medially. If additional exposure is necessary, the proximal 1 cm of the pectoralis major insertion is released (Fig. 9-30). Fracture hematoma is usually encountered once the clavipectoral fascia is incised. Fracture fragments and the rotator cuff musculature become evident.[151,155] The axillary and musculocutaneous nerves may be identified through digital palpation of the anteroinferior aspect of the subscapularis muscle and the posterior aspect of the coracoid muscles, respectively.

External rotation of the humerus results in reduced tension on the axillary nerve.[20,151,155] The tendon of the

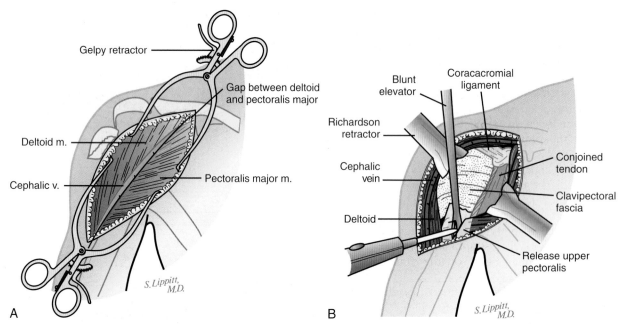

FIGURE 9-30 A, The skin incision is centered over the anterior deltoid. The deltopectoral interval is developed with lateral retraction of the cephalic vein. **B,** For more exposure, the superior 1 cm of the pectoralis major tendon may be incised. (**A** Modified from Matsen FA III, Lippitt SB: Shoulder Surgery: Principles and Procedures, Philadelphia: WB Saunders, 2004, p 629. **B** modified from DePuy Orthopaedics: Global Fx Shoulder Fracture System Surgical Technique. DePuy Orthopaedics, 1999, p 8.)

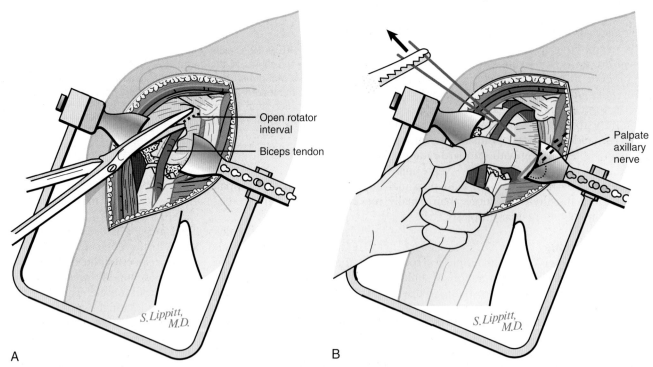

FIGURE 9-31 A, The long head of the biceps is identified and traced superiorly to the rotator interval. The tendon serves as a key landmark when re-establishing the anatomic relationship between the greater and lesser tuberosities. **B,** The axillary nerve is identified at the anteroinferior border of the subscapularis. (Modified from DePuy Orthopaedics: Global Fx Shoulder Fracture System Surgical Technique, DePuy Orthopaedics, 1999, pp 9, 10.)

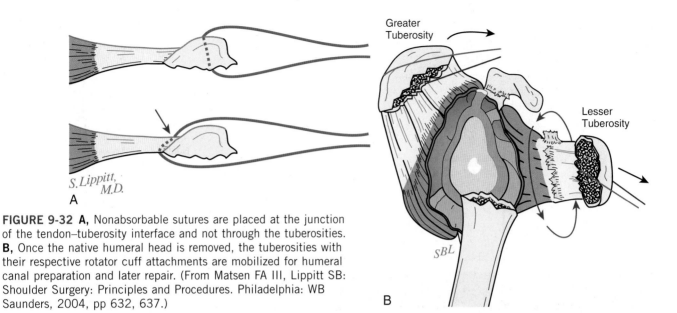

FIGURE 9-32 A, Nonabsorbable sutures are placed at the junction of the tendon–tuberosity interface and not through the tuberosities. **B,** Once the native humeral head is removed, the tuberosities with their respective rotator cuff attachments are mobilized for humeral canal preparation and later repair. (From Matsen FA III, Lippitt SB: Shoulder Surgery: Principles and Procedures. Philadelphia: WB Saunders, 2004, pp 632, 637.)

long head of the biceps is identified as it courses in the bicipital groove toward the rotator interval. The tendon serves as a key landmark when re-establishing the anatomic relationship between the greater and lesser tuberosities. The rotator interval and coracohumeral ligament are both released to allow mobilization of the tuberosities (Fig. 9-31).[20,151,155] An osteotome or saw may be used to create a cleavage plane for mobilizing the lesser or greater tuberosity, if the fracture does not involve the bicipital groove. Preservation of the coracoacromial ligament is advisable to maintain the coracoacromial arch and prevent upward migration of the humeral head.

Heavy, nonabsorbable traction sutures (e.g., 1-mm Cottony Dacron, Deknatel, Mansfield, Mass) are placed through the rotator cuff insertions on the tuberosities. Two or three should be placed through the subscapularis tendon and three or four through the supraspinatus. Tuberosity fragments vary in size and might require trimming for reduction and repair (Fig. 9-32). With the tuberosities retracted on their muscular insertions, the humeral head and shaft fragments are removed.[20,151,155] The native articular surface is removed and sized with a template for trial humeral head replacement (Fig. 9-33).The glenoid must be examined for concomitant pathology. Hematoma, cartilaginous fragments, and bone fragments are removed with sterile saline irrigation. Glenoid fractures should be stabilized with internal fixation. If the glenoid exhibits significant degenerative wear or irreparable damage, a glenoid component must be used.[20,151,155]

The proximal end of the humeral shaft is delivered into the incisional wound. Loose bone fragments and hematoma are removed from the canal of the humeral shaft. Axial reamers, preferably without power, are used to prepare the humeral shaft for trial implantation. The trial humeral implant is placed with the lateral fin slightly posterior to the bicipital groove and with the medial

aspect of the trial head at least at the height of the medial calcar. We previously used a sponge to anchor the trial stem within the intramedullary canal of the humerus. We currently use a commercially available fracture jig that can maintain the height and retroversion of the trial component through a functional range of motion (Fig. 9-34).[151]

Correct humeral retroversion is critical when recreating the glenohumeral articulation. Most techniques suggest 30 degrees as a guide during reconstruction, although

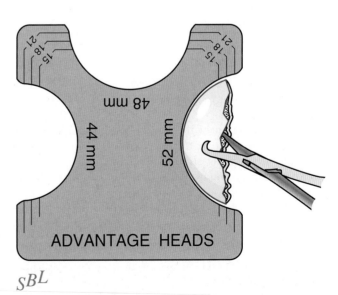

FIGURE 9-33 The extracted native humeral head is sized with the use of a commercially available template guide. (Modified from Matsen FA III, Lippitt SB: Shoulder Surgery: Principles and Procedures. Philadelphia: WB Saunders, 2004, p 634.)

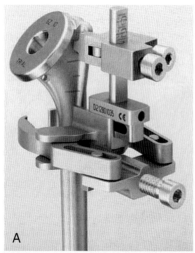

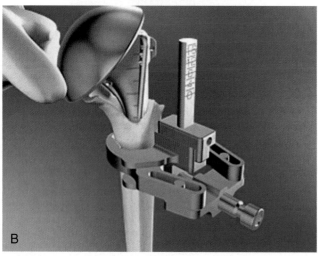

FIGURE 9-34 A, Commercially available fracture jig (Depuy Orthopaedics, Warsaw, Ind). **B,** The jig stably situates implant at appropriate height and retroversion.

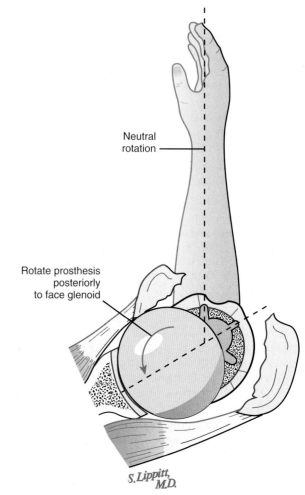

FIGURE 9-35 The anterior fin of the prosthesis is aligned with the forearm in neutral rotation, and the lateral fin is positioned approximately 8 mm posterior to the biceps groove, establishing a retroversion angle of approximately 30 degrees. (Modified from Matsen FA III, Lippitt SB: Shoulder Surgery: Principles and Procedures. Philadelphia: WB Saunders, 2004, p 638.)

native retroversion varies from 10 to 50 degrees.[146] Several methods are used to gauge this angle:

1. External rotation of the humerus to 30 degrees from the sagittal plane of the body with the humeral head component facing straight medially
2. An imaginary line from the distal humeral epicondylar axis that bisects the axis of the prosthesis
3. Positioning of the lateral fin of the prosthesis approximately 8 mm posterior to the bicipital groove (Fig. 9-35)[151,156]

The prosthetic height is also critical in re-establishing appropriate muscle tension and shoulder mechanics. Preoperative templating may be helpful. Intraoperative examination of soft tissue tension including the deltoid, the rotator cuff, and the long head of the biceps combined with fluoroscopic imaging aids in prosthetic height placement.[151,155] Common errors involve placing the pros-

thesis too low, resulting in poor deltoid muscle tension and lack of space for the tuberosities (Fig. 9-36). In the event of significant proximal humerus comminution, Murachovsky and colleagues have suggested that the pectoralis major insertion (if intact) may be a useful landmark in restoring humeral length. According to their cadaveric study, the distance from the top of the pectoralis major tendon to the articular surface averaged 5.6 cm (±0.5 cm).[157] Drill holes are placed in the proximal humerus medial and lateral to the bicipital groove, with 1-mm Cottony Dacron sutures subsequently passed for tuberosity-to-shaft fixation (Fig. 9-37). A trial reduction is then performed with the mobilized tuberosities fitted below the head of the modular prosthesis. A towel clip may be used to hold the tuberosities for fluoroscopic examination and assessment of glenohumeral stability

FIGURE 9-36 A, A commercially available fracture jig allows intraoperative height adjustment. (Similarly, a sponge may be placed to hold the trial stem at a determined level and allow intraoperative assessment). **B,** Placing the prosthesis too low results in poor deltoid muscle tension and lack of space for the tuberosities. (Modified from Global Fx Shoulder Fracture System Surgical Technique, DePuy Orthopaedics, Inc, 1999, pp 18, 15.)

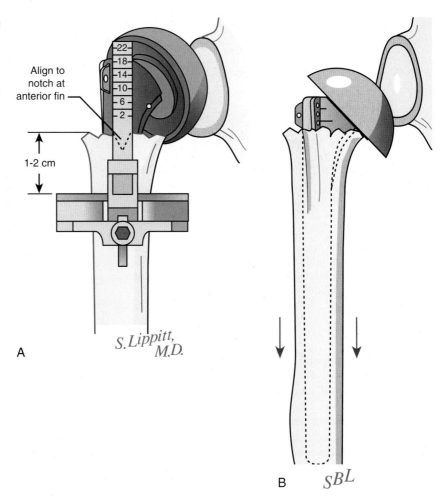

FIGURE 9-37 Drill holes are placed in the proximal humerus medial and lateral to the bicipital groove with 1-mm Cottony polyethylene (Dacron) sutures. (Modified from Global Fx Shoulder Fracture System Surgical Technique, DePuy Orthopaedics, 1999, p 24.)

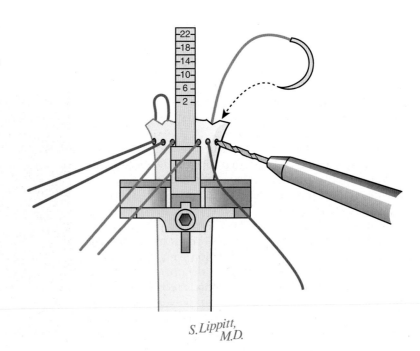

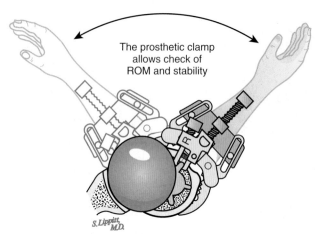

FIGURE 9-38 A trial reduction may be performed with the fracture jig in place, allowing assessment of the functional range of motion (ROM). (Modified from Global Fx Shoulder Fracture System Surgical Technique, DePuy Orthopaedics, 1999, p 21.)

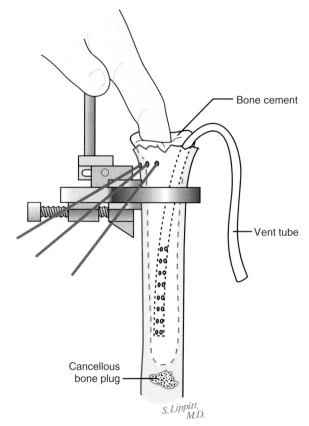

FIGURE 9-39 A cement restrictor is placed to prevent cement extravasation distally. Pulsatile lavage and retrograde injection of cement with suction pressurization is also used. (Modified from Global Fx Shoulder Fracture System Surgical Technique, DePuy Orthopaedics, 1999, p 24.)

(Fig. 9-38). The humeral head should not subluxate more than 25% to 30% of the glenoid height inferiorly.[151,155]

The final humeral component should be cemented in all fracture patients. A cement restrictor is placed to prevent extravasation into the distal humerus. Pulsatile lavage and retrograde injection of cement with suction pressurization is also used (Fig. 9-39).[151,155] Excess cement is removed during the curing phase. Spaces between the tuberosities, prosthesis, and shaft are packed with autogenous cancellous bone graft from the resected humeral head (Fig. 9-40). A second trial reduction may be performed with a trial head after cement fixation of the humeral stem. The final head may be impacted before the stem is implanted or after the repeat trial reduction.[151,155] A cerclage suture is placed circumferentially around the greater tuberosity and through the supraspinatus insertion and then medial to the prosthesis and through the subscapularis insertion (lesser tuberosity). Several authors have indicated superior fixation with the cerclage suture when compared to tuberosity–tuberosity and tuberosity–fin fixation alone.[158-160]

Over-reduction of the tuberosities should be avoided to prevent limitations in external rotation (lesser tuberosity) and internal rotation (greater tuberosity).[158-160] Sutures are then tied beginning with tuberosity to shaft, followed by tuberosity-to-tuberosity closure using the previously placed suture limbs (Fig. 9-41). The lateral portion of the rotator interval is then closed with the arm in approximately 30 degrees of external rotation with a No. 2 nonabsorbable suture (Fig. 9-42). The deltopectoral interval is generally not closed. Drain suction is recommended in both acute and chronic injuries to prevent hematoma formation. A commercially available pain pump may be used to augment postoperative analgesia and to reduce narcotic medication use. The subcutaneous tissues are reapproximated with 2-0 absorbable suture. Subcuticular

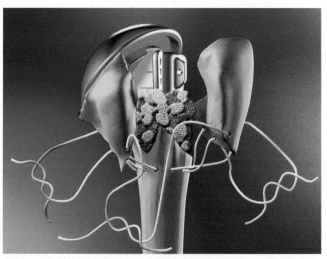

FIGURE 9-40 Morselized cancellous bone graft is placed between the tuberosities and shaft.

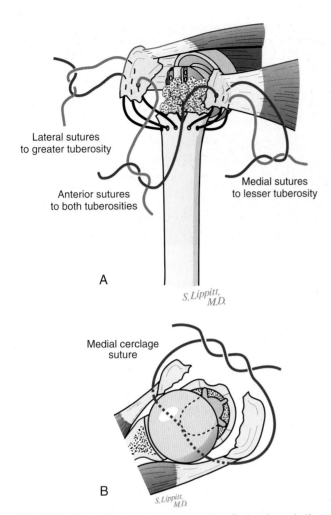

Lateral sutures
to greater tuberosity

Anterior sutures
to both tuberosities

Medial sutures
to lesser tuberosity

A

Medial cerclage
suture

B

FIGURE 9-41 A, Previously placed suture limbs through the tuberosities and shaft are reapproximated. **B,** Medial cerclage suture is placed circumferentially around the greater tuberosity and through the supraspinatus insertion, and then medial to the prosthesis and through the subscapularis insertion (lesser tuberosity), and tied. (Modified from Global Fx Shoulder Fracture System Surgical Technique, DePuy Orthopaedics, 1999, p 27.)

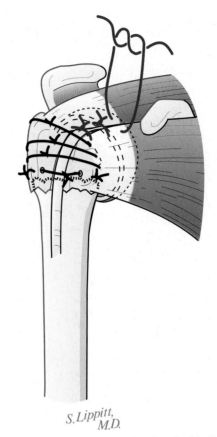

FIGURE 9-42 The rotator interval is closed with No. 2 nonabsorbable suture, with the arm in approximately 30 degrees of external rotation. (Modified from Global Fx Shoulder Fracture System Surgical Technique, DePuy Orthopaedics, 1999, p 28.)

closure is performed with 2-0 monofilament suture. The patient is then placed in a sling or shoulder immobilizer with 30 to 45 degrees of abduction for comfort (Fig. 9-43).[151,155]

Rehabilitation

Physician-directed therapy is initiated on postoperative day 1 with gentle, gravity-assisted pendulum exercises and with passive pulley-and-stick exercises to maintain forward flexion and external rotation. Motion limits are placed by the surgeon based on intraoperative stability. After discharge, the patient's wound is reexamined and sutures are removed at 10 to 14 days. Gentle range-of-motion exercises are continued. At 6 weeks, repeat radiographs are obtained to evaluate tuberosity healing. When

tuberosity healing is evident, phase-two exercises are initiated with isometric rotator cuff exercises and active assisted elevation with the pulley. At 3 months, strength training (phase three) with graduated rubber bands is implemented. Patients should be aware that maximal motion and function can take approximately 12 months from the date of surgery to achieve.[151,155]

COMPLICATIONS AFTER ARTHROPLASTY

Complications include delays in wound healing, infection, nerve injury, humeral fracture, component malposition, instability, nonunion of the tuberosities, rotator cuff tearing, regional pain syndrome, periarticular fibrosis, heterotopic bone formation, component loosening, and glenoid arthritis.[161-163] The most common problems in acute fracture treatment involve stiffness, nonunion, malunion, or resorption of the tuberosities.[161,162] In patients with chronic fractures treated with hemiarthroplasty, the most common problems encountered were instability, heterotopic ossification, tuberosity malunion or nonunion, and rotator cuff tears.[162]

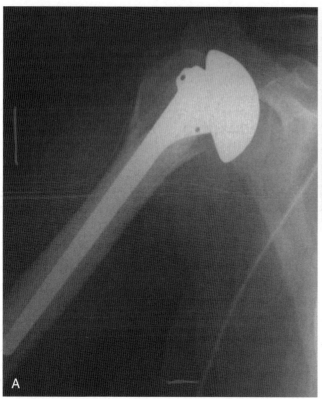

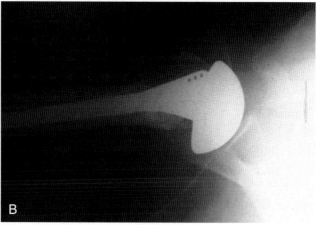

FIGURE 9-43 Anteroposterior (**A**) and axillary (**B**) radiographs demonstrate a cemented hemiarthroplasty of a four-part proximal humerus fracture, with anatomic reconstruction of the greater and lesser tuberosities.

RESULTS AFTER ARTHROPLASTY

Approximately 90% of patients treated with hemiarthroplasty demonstrate minimal pain, despite a wide range of function, motion, and strength. Factors that predict a poor outcome after hemiarthroplasty for fractures include tuberosity malposition, superior migration of the humeral prosthesis, stiffness, persistent pain, and poor initial positioning of the implant (excessive retroversion, decreased height); women older than 75 years also are at risk for poor outcome.[164] When comparing acute intervention versus late reconstruction, most authors report poorer outcomes with surgical intervention delayed longer than 2 weeks, particularly with respect to functional results.[82,149,162,165] Robinson and colleagues reported satisfactory results in patients treated with primary hemiarthroplasty at an average prosthetic survival of 6.3 years. In this study, a majority of the shoulders were pain free at last follow-up, despite a wide variation in motion, function, and power. Poorer results were noted in elderly patients, especially in the settings of a neurologic deficit, postoperative complication, or instability with retracted tuberosities. Good functional outcomes at 1 year could be anticipated in younger (nonsmoking) patients who have no postoperative complications or neurologic deficits and who have satisfactory radiographs at 6 weeks.[166]

At present, there are investigations regarding the feasibility of computer-assisted hemiarthroplasty in the treatment of proximal humerus fractures. Bicknell and colleagues have initiated a pilot study with cadaveric specimens to develop a computer-assisted system in the treatment of four-part fractures. Seven pairs of specimens underwent surgery by way of computer-assisted and traditional methods to anatomically reconstruct the following seven characteristics: humeral head version, humeral head inclination, humeral head offset, humeral length, medial articulation point, greater tuberosity position, and lesser tuberosity position. The differences between the intact and reconstructed proximal humeral anatomic values were improved in five of seven characteristics, but only humeral head offset demonstrated statistically significant improvement with the computer-assisted method. Though computer-assisted hemiarthroplasty is promising, the authors emphasized the need for further investigation and refinement of this technique to allow reproducibility and facile use in the patient setting.[167]

REVERSE SHOULDER ARTHROPLASTY FOR PRIMARY AND SECONDARY MANAGEMENT OF PROXIMAL HUMERUS FRACTURES

Overview

The North American literature is limited with regard to results of primary reverse shoulder arthroplasty for three- and four-part proximal humerus fractures. Boulahia and colleagues reported their initial results (average follow-up, 35 months) of a mixed patient population (16 patients) with cuff tear arthropathy and fracture sequelae who underwent reverse shoulder arthroplasty. The average preoperative-to-postoperative forward elevation increased from 70 to 139 degrees, with a corresponding Constant score of 31 to 59. The authors did note a revision rate of 12.5%.[168]

Boileau and colleagues reviewed their results with the Delta III (Depuy, Warsaw, Ind) prosthesis in the management of three distinct patient groups: cuff tear arthropathy (21 patients), implant revision (19 patients), and fracture sequelae with arthritis (5 patients). Although all groups demonstrated significant increases in forward elevation (55 to 121 degrees) and Constant score (17 to 58), the authors noted no improvement in external rotation. More importantly, they reported a 20% (1 of 5 cases) complication rate with the fracture-sequelae group (one implant revised to hemiarthroplasty due to glenoid fracture). Boileau and colleagues emphasized that functional results are less predictable and complication rates are higher when comparing revision and fracture cases to cuff tear arthropathy alone.[169]

Cazenueve and Cristofari retrospectively analyzed 23 patients who underwent primary reverse arthroplasty with the Delta III prosthesis for acute three- and four-part proximal humerus fractures (18 patients) and fracture-dislocations (5 patients). Tuberosity reduction was amenable in only 5 patients. There were 16 patients available for follow-up at last review secondary to patient death (7 patients). The average Constant score was 60 (83 for the uninjured side) at a mean follow-up of 86 months. Significant gains in forward elevation, abduction, and pain relief were reported. Complications included regional pain syndrome (2 patients), infection (1 patient, requiring revision), and anterior dislocation (1 patient, requiring revision). Because of their results, they recommended reverse shoulder arthroplasty as a suitable technique for elderly patients with unmanageable tuberosities (resorption, rotator cuff atrophy, and scarring) to attain gains in pain relief and forward elevation.[170]

Reverse Arthroplasty for Revision of Hemiarthroplasty

Revision of a failed hemiarthroplasty is extremely difficult to accomplish, even in experienced hands. Failures might have resulted from excessive glenoid wear, tuberosity malunion, tuberosity nonunion, tuberosity resorption, humeral-stem loosening, or infection. Associated soft-tissue deficits and contractures, bone loss, and instability all play a role in the loss of glenohumeral function. Nerve paralysis may be present and can complicate revision surgery. An electromyogram is helpful in the evaluation before any surgery is attempted.

Expectations and goals of revision surgery should be realistic and frankly understood by both the patient and the surgeon. Revision of a prosthesis is generally indicated for pain relief, because it can be difficult to significantly improve function as a result of long-standing nerve and muscle damage.

Levy and colleagues have suggested that until recently, surgeons have not had a viable option for this clinical scenario. The authors have offered the reverse shoulder prosthesis as a salvage procedure to address the issue of failed hemiarthroplasty for proximal humerus fractures. They operated on 29 patients of mean age 69 years (range, 42-80 years) to remove a hemiarthroplasty and subsequently to convert to a reverse shoulder prosthesis (with or without proximal humeral allograft). Mean follow-up was 35 months, with an overall complication rate of 28% (8 of 29 patients). The average ASES score improved from 22.3 to 52.1 postoperatively. Active forward flexion and abduction improved from 38.1 and 34.1 degrees to 72.7 and 70.4 degrees, respectively. Six patients reported dissatisfaction with the procedure; 4 of the 6 dissatisfied patients were treated with the prosthesis alone. The authors found the early results to be encouraging and recommended this implant as a salvage solution for failed hemiarthroplasty with rotator cuff deficiency or tuberosity failure.[171]

LATE COMPLICATIONS OF PROXIMAL HUMERUS FRACTURES

Minimally displaced and displaced proximal humerus fractures remain difficult to diagnose and appropriately manage. Negative consequences can occur as a result of the initial injury or from the surgical treatment itself. Some of these complications include shoulder stiffness, osteonecrosis, malunion, nonunion, and heterotopic bone formation.[20,172]

Shoulder Stiffness

Shoulder stiffness remains one of the most common complications after a proximal humerus fracture. Contributing factors include the severity of the initial injury, the duration of the immobilization, articular surface malunion, and patient noncompliance with rehabilitation.[172]

Koval and colleagues assessed the functional outcome of 104 patients with minimally displaced proximal humerus fractures treated with a standardized therapy program. At a mean follow-up of 41 months (range, 12-117 months), patients who began a therapy program fewer than 2 weeks from the date of injury demonstrated significantly better results (forward elevation, external rotation, pain level) than did the patients who began therapy more than 2 weeks after injury.[173]

Hodgson and colleagues have reaffirmed the necessity for early physical therapy with two-part proximal humerus fractures, noting prolonged recovery (2 years vs. 1 year) in patients immobilized longer than 3 weeks. With regard to hemiarthroplasty, numerous studies have indicated more-favorable outcomes with early intervention due to the presence of soft tissue contractures with chronic injuries.[174-176] The consensus is that an early physician-directed rehabilitation program for both surgically and nonsurgically managed fractures should be performed to minimize stiffness.

Osteonecrosis

The incidence of avascular necrosis depends on the severity of the initial injury and surgical technique (soft tissue stripping, hardware placement). Avascular necrosis is not uncommon after three- and four-part fractures and fracture-dislocations.

Hagg and colleagues reported an avascular necrosis rate of 3% to 14% after closed reduction of displaced three-part fractures and a rate of 13% to 34% after four-part fractures. In addition to the severity of the fracture, exuberant soft tissue dissection has been identified as a major contributing factor.[177] Sturzenegger and colleagues reported a nearly 34% incidence of avascular necrosis in a series of 17 patients treated with open reduction and internal fixation with a T plate.[178]

Osteonecrosis may be initially detected by MRI. Conventional radiographs might later demonstrate humeral head collapse with secondary degenerative changes on the glenoid side. The treatment of choice for avascular necrosis in the setting of severe pain and functional loss is a hemiarthroplasty or total shoulder replacement, if the glenoid is involved.[172]

Malunion

Malunion can occur after inadequate closed reduction or failed open reduction and internal fixation. Greater tuberosity malunion (superior, posterior, or both) can lead to impingement against the acromion, resulting in pain, weakness, and diminished forward elevation.[20,172] If displacement of the malunited greater tuberosity is greater than 5 mm with functional limitations and pain, this problem is best managed with fragment mobilization and reduction.[172] For greater tuberosity malunions that are symptomatic but have lesser degrees of displacement, partial removal of the tuberosity along with anterior acromioplasty and lysis of adhesions can provide an alternative treatment option.[20] Care should be taken to avoid greater tuberosity osteotomy when possible because of reported failure rates and poor outcomes.[164]

Two-part surgical neck malunions infrequently cause pain or functional limitations. The occasional varus malunion can result in impingement and require surgical management with arthroscopic acromioplasty or tuberoplasty, or both.[172] Osteotomy and open reduction with internal fixation is reserved for severe angulation that prohibits forward flexion.[179] Prosthetic replacement is generally required for three- and four-part malunions

with joint incongruity. Tuberosity osteotomies are usually performed to allow adequate placement of the humeral head prosthesis. Anatomic restoration of the glenohumeral joint must be performed; particular attention must be paid to humeral head retroversion and humeral head height, otherwise function will be impaired.[20,172] Secondary prosthetic arthroplasty for proximal humeral malunions has demonstrated less-favorable outcomes secondary to soft tissue scarring and retraction of the tuberosities.[20,163,172] Pain relief is usually satisfactory, but it is less predictable than primary arthroplasty.[20,172]

Nonunion

Nonunion of proximal humeral fractures is uncommon and is usually associated with displaced fractures.[38,180-183] Nonunion often occurs in elderly, debilitated patients with osteoporotic bone.[34,39] The incidence of nonunion in this patient population is estimated to be 23%.[184] Factors that predispose to nonunion include soft tissue interposition, hanging arm casts, inadequate open reduction with internal fixation, alcohol abuse, and medical comorbidities such as diabetes mellitus.[180,182,185-187]

Indications for surgical treatment are significant pain, deformity, and functional loss. Open reduction and internal fixation (proximal humeral locking plate) with the addition of autogenous iliac crest bone graft is the preferred method of treatment if adequate bone stock remains. In the setting of humeral head resorption and cavitation, a prosthesis may be necessary to reconstruct the glenohumeral joint.[172] Outside of this situation, humeral head excision and arthrodesis should be avoided.[20]

The surgical reconstruction for nonunion of surgical neck fractures results in pain relief for a majority of patients, but the overall results with regard to motion and strength are less than satisfactory.[188-190] Reconstruction is often difficult and associated with a significant risk of postoperative complications with limited results. The risks and benefits of surgical intervention should be discussed in detail with the patient. Nonoperative treatment may be an option in elderly patients who have minimal symptoms in the nondominant extremity.[20]

Heterotopic Bone Formation

Formation of ectopic bone is a common and often incidental finding noted on radiographs in patients with proximal humerus fractures and fracture-dislocations.[20,38,191-193] Neer's report in 1970 on 117 patients treated for three-part and four-part fractures and fracture-dislocations indicated an overall rate of 12% of heterotopic bone formation. Factors that increased the likelihood of ectopic bone included degree of soft tissue injury, repetitive manipulations, and delayed reduction beyond 7 days from injury.[38] In the rare situation that ankylosis occurs from heterotopic bone formation, surgical resection is indicated to restore functional range of motion.[172]

REFERENCES

1. DeFranco MJ, Brems JJ, Williams GR Jr, et al: Evaluation and management of valgus impacted four-part proximal humerus fractures. Clin Orthop Relat Res (442):109-114, 2006.

2. Green A, Norris T: Proximal humerus fractures and fracture-dislocations. In Jupiter J (ed): Skeletal Trauma, 3rd ed. Philadelphia: Saunders, 2003, pp 1532-1624.

3. Hagino H, Yamamoto K, Ohshiro H, et al: Changing incidence of hip, distal radius, and proximal humerus fractures in Tottori Prefecture, Japan. Bone 24:265-270, 1999.

4. Kannus P, Palvanen M, Niemi S, et al: Osteoporotic fractures of the proximal humerus in elderly Finnish persons: Sharp increase in 1970-1998 and alarming projections for the new millennium. Acta Orthop Scand 71:465-470, 2000.

5. Palvanen M, Kannus P, Parkkari J, et al: The injury mechanisms of osteoporotic upper extremity fractures among older adults: A controlled study of 287 consecutive patients and their 108 controls. Osteoporos Int 1:822-831, 2000.

6. Court-Brown CM, Caesar B: Epidemiology of adult fractures: A review. Injury 37(8):691-697, 2006.

7. Lobo MJ, Levine WN: Classification and closed treatment of proximal humerus fractures. In Wirth MA (ed): Proximal Humerus Fractures. Chicago: American Academy of Orthopaedic Surgeons, 2005, pp 1-13.

8. Court-Brown C, Garg A, McQueen M: The epidemiology of proximal humerus fractures. Acta Orthop Scand 72:365-371, 2001.

9. Huopio J, Kroger H, Honkanen R, et al: Risk factors for perimenopausal fractures: A prospective study. Osteoporos Int 11:219-227, 2000.

10. Matsen FA 3rd, Rockwood CA Jr, Wirth MA, et al: Glenohumeral arthritis and its management. In Rockwood CA Jr, Matsen FA 3rd, Wirth MA, Lippitt SB (eds): The Shoulder, 3rd ed. Philadelphia: WB Saunders, 2004, pp 879-1008.

11. Boileau P, Walch G: The three-dimensional geometry of the proximal humerus: Implications for surgical technique and prosthetic design. J Bone Joint Surg Br 79:857-865, 1997.

12. Iannotti JP, Gabriel JP, Schneck SL, et al: The normal glenohumeral relationships: An anatomical study of one hundred and forty shoulders. J Bone Joint Surg Am 74:491-500, 1992.

13. Pearl ML, Volk AG: Retroversion of the proximal humerus in relationship to the prosthetic replacement arthroplasty. J Shoulder Elbow Surg 4:286-289, 1995.

14. Itamura J, Dietrick T, Roidis N, et al: Analysis of the bicipital groove as a landmark for humeral head replacement. J Shoulder Elbow Surg 11:322-326, 2002.

15. DePalma AF: Fractures and fracture-dislocations of the shoulder girdle. Surgery of the Shoulder, 3rd ed. Philadelphia: JB Lippincott, 1983, pp 372-403.

16. Gerber C, Schneeberger A, Vinh T: The arterial vascularization of the humeral head: An anatomical study. J Bone Joint Surg Am 72:1486-1494, 1990.

17. Laing P: The arterial supply of the adult humerus. J Bone Joint Surg Am 38:1105-1116, 1956.

18. Brooks CH, Revell WJ, Heatley FW: Vascularity of the humeral head after proximal humerus fractures: An anatomical cadaver study. J Bone Joint Surg Br 75:132-136, 1993.

19. McLaughlin JA, Light R, Lustrin I: Axillary artery injury as a complication of proximal humerus fractures. J Shoulder Elbow Surg 7:292-294, 1998.

20. Blaine TA, Bigliani LU, Levine WN: Fractures of the proximal humerus. In Rockwood CA Jr, Matsen FA 3rd, Wirth MA, Lippitt SB (eds): The Shoulder, 3rd ed. Philadelphia: WB Saunders, 2004, pp 355-412.

21. Visser CP, Coene LN, Brand R, et al: Nerve lesions in the proximal humerus. J Shoulder Elbow Surg 10:421-427, 2001.

22. Bono CM, Grossman MG, Hochwald N, Tometta P 3rd: Radial and axillary nerves. Anatomic considerations for humeral fixation. Clin Orthop Relat Res (373):259-264, 2000.

23. Visser CP, Tavy DL, Coene LN, Brand R: Electromyographic findings in shoulder dislocations and fractures of the proximal humerus: Comparison with clinical neurological examination. Clin Neurol Neurosurg 101:86-91, 1999.

24. Flatow EL, Bigliani LU, April EW: An anatomic study of the musculocutaneous nerve and its relationship to the coracoid process. Clin Orthop Relat Res (244):166-171, 1989.

25. Flatow EL, Cuomo F, Maday MG, et al: Open reduction and internal fixation of two-part displaced fractures of the greater tuberosity of the proximal part of the humerus. J Bone Joint Surg Am 73:1213-1218, 1991.

26. Lind T, Kroner TK, Jensen J: The epidemiology of fractures of the proximal humerus. Arch Orthop Trauma Surg 108:285-287, 1989.

27. Baron JA, Karagas M, Barrett J, et al: Basic epidemiology of fractures of the upper and lower limb among Americans over 65 years of age. Epidemiology 7:612-618, 1996.

28. Ivers RQ, Cumming RG, Mitchell P, Peduto AJ: Risk factors for fractures of the wrist, shoulder and ankle: The Blue Mountains Eye Study. Osteoporos Int 13:513-518, 2002.

29. Nguyen TV, Center JR, Sambrook PN, Eisman JA: Risk factors for proximal humerus, forearm, and wrist fractures in elderly men and women: The Dubbo Osteoporosis Epidemiology Study. Am J Epidemiol 153:587-595, 2001.

30. Sporer SM, Weinstein JN, Koval KJ: The geographic incidence and treatment variation of common fractures of elderly patients. J Am Acad Orthop Surg 14(4):246-255, 2006.

31. Salem MI: Bilateral anterior fracture-dislocation of the shoulder joints due to severe electric shock. Injury 14:361-363, 1983.

32. Desai KB, Ribbans WJ, Taylor GJ: Incidence of five common fracture types of the greater tuberosity of the proximal humerus. Injury 27:97-100, 1996.

33. Green A, Izzi J Jr: Isolated fractures of the greater tuberosity of the proximal humerus. J Shoulder Elbow Surg 12:641-649, 2003.

34. Rose SH, Melton LJ III, Morrey BF, et al: Epidemiologic features of humeral fractures. Clin Orthop Relat Res (168):24-30, 1982.

35. Hartsock LA, Estes WJ, Murray CA, Friedman RJ: Shoulder hemiarthroplasty for proximal humeral fractures. Orthop Clin North Am 29(3):467-475, 1998.

36. Funsten RV, Kinser P: Fractures and dislocations about the shoulder. J Bone Joint Surg 18:191-198, 1936.

37. Meyerding HW: Fracture-dislocation of the shoulder. Minn Med 20:717-726, 1937.

38. Neer CS 2nd: Displaced proximal humeral fractures. II. Treatment of three-part and four-part displacement. J Bone Joint Surg Am 52:1090-1103, 1970.

39. Neer CS 2nd: Displaced proximal humeral fractures. I. Classification and evaluation. J Bone Joint Surg Am 52:1077-1089, 1970.

40. Kocher T: Beitrage zur Kenntnis einiger praktisch wichtigen Fracturenformen. Basel: Carl Sallman Verlag, 1896.

41. Codman E: Rupture of the supraspinatus tendon and other lesions in or about the subacromial bursa. In Codman E (ed): The Shoulder. Boston, Thomas Todd, 1934.

42. De Anquin C, De Anquin C: Prosthetic replacement in the treatment of serious fractures of the proximal humerus. In Bayley I, Kessel L (eds): Shoulder Surgery. Berlin: Springer-Verlag, 1982, pp 207-217.

43. De Palma A, Cautilli R: Fractures of the upper end of the humerus. Clin Orthop 20:73-93, 1961.

44. Watson-Jones R: Fracture of the neck of the humerus. In Watson-Jones R: Fractures and Other Bone and Joint Injuries. Baltimore: Williams and Wilkins, pp 289-297, 1940.

45. Dehne E: Fractures of the upper end of the humerus. Surg Clin N Am 25:28-47, 1945.

46. Green A: Proximal humerus fractures. In Norris T (ed): Orthopaedic Knowledge Update: Shoulder and Elbow 2. Rosemont, Ill: American Academy of Orthopaedic Surgeons, 2002, pp 209-217.

47. Jakob R, Miniaci A, Anson P, et al: Four-part valgus impacted fractures of the proximal humerus. J Bone Joint Surg Br 73:295-298, 1991.

48. Orthopaedic Trauma Association Committee for Coding and Classification: Fracture and Dislocation Compendium. J Orthop Trauma 10(suppl):1-155, 1996.

49. Siebenrock KA, Gerber C: The reproducibility of classification of fractures of the proximal end of the humerus. J Bone Joint Surg Am 75:1751-1755, 1993.

50. Brorson S, Bagger J, Sylvest A, et al: Improved interobserver variation after training of doctors in the Neer system. A randomised trial. J Bone Joint Surg Br 84:950-954, 2002.

51. Sallay PI, Pedowitz RA, Mallon WJ, et al: Reliability and reproducibility of radiographic interpretation of proximal humeral fracture pathoanatomy. J Shoulder Elbow Surg 6:60-69, 1997.

52. Sjoden GO, Movin T, Guntner P, et al: Poor reproducibility of classification of proximal humeral fractures. Additional CT of minor value. Acta Orthop Scand 68:239-242, 1997.

53. Bigliani LV, Flatow EL, Pollock RG: Fracture classification systems: Do they work and are they useful? [comment]. J Bone Joint Surg Am 76:790-792, 1994.

54. Neer CS 2nd: Fracture classification systems: Do they work and are they useful? [comment]. J Bone Joint Surg Am 76:789-790, 1994.

55. Rockwood CA Jr: Fracture classification systems: Do they work and are they useful? [comment]. J Bone Joint Surg Am 76:790, 1994.

56. Sjoden GO, Movin T, Aspelin P, et al: 3D-radiographic analysis does not improve the Neer and AO classifications of proximal humeral fractures. Acta Orthop Scand 70:325-328, 1999.

57. Sjoden GO, Movin T, Guntner P, et al: Poor reproducibility of classification of proximal humeral fractures. Additional CT of minor value. Acta Orthop Scand 68:239-242, 1997.

58. Bernstein J, Adler LM, Blank JE, et al: Evaluation of the Neer system of classification of proximal humeral fractures with computerized tomographic scans and plain radiographs. J Bone Joint Surg Am 78:1371-1375, 1996.

59. Shrader MW, Sanchez-Sotelo J, Sperling JW, et al: Understanding proximal humerus fractures: Image analysis, classification, and treatment. J Shoulder Elbow Surg 14:497-505, 2005.

60. Hertel R, Hempfing A, Stiehler A, et al: Predictors of humeral head ischemia after intracapsular fracture of the proximal humerus. J Shoulder Elbow Surg 13:427-433, 2004.

61. Einarsson F: Fracture of the upper end of the humerus. Acta Orthop Scand Suppl 32:1-215, 1958.

62. Moriber LA, Patterson RL: Fractures of the proximal end of the humerus. J Bone Joint Surg Am 49:1018, 1967.

63. Rasmussen S, Hvass I, Dalsgaard J, et al: Displaced proximal humeral fractures: Results of conservative treatment. Injury 23:41-43, 1992.

64. Roberts SM: Fractures of the upper end of the humerus. An end-result study which shows the advantage of early active motion. JAMA 98:367-373, 1932.

65. Rowe CR, Colville M: The glenohumeral joint. In Rowe CR (ed): The Shoulder. New York: Churchill Livingstone, 1988, pp 331-358.

66. Koval KJ, Gallagher MA, Marsciano JG, et al: Functional outcome after minimally displaced fractures of the proximal part of the humerus. J Bone Joint Surg Am 79:203-207, 1997.

67. Koval KJ, Zuckerman JD: Orthopaedic challenges in the aging population: Trauma treatment and related clinical issues. Instr Course Lect 46:423-430, 1997.

68. Hodgson S: Proximal humerus fracture rehabilitation. Clin Orthop Relat Res (442):131-138, 2006.

69. Bertoft ES, Lundh I, Ringqvist I: Physiotherapy after fracture of the proximal end of the humerus. Comparison between two methods. Scand J Rehabil Med 16:11-16, 1984.

70. Green A, Izzi J Jr: Isolated fractures of the greater tuberosity of the proximal humerus. J Shoulder Elbow Surg 12:641-649, 2003.

71. Chun JM, Groh GI, Rockwood CA Jr: Two-part fractures of the proximal humerus. J Shoulder Elbow Surg 3:273-287, 1994.

72. McLaughlin HL: Dislocation of the shoulder with tuberosity fracture. Surg Clin North Am 43:1615-1620, 1963.

73. Park TS, Choi IY, Kim YH, et al: A new suggestion for the treatment of minimally displaced fractures of the greater tuberosity of the proximal humerus. Bull Hosp Jt Dis 56:171-176, 1997.

74. Bahrs C, Lingenfelter E, Fischer F, et al: Mechanism of injury and morphology of the greater tuberosity fracture. J Shoulder Elbow Surg 15:140-147, 2006.

75. Garg A, McQueen MM, Court-Brown CM: Nerve injury after greater tuberosity fracture dislocation. J Orthop Trauma 14(2):117-118, 2000.

76. Leffert RD, Seddon H: Infraclavicular brachial plexus injuries. J Bone Joint Surg Br 47:9-22, 1965.

77. Toolanen G, Hildingsson C, Hedlund T, et al: Early complications after anterior dislocation of the shoulder in patients over 40 years. Acta Orthop Scand 64:549-552, 1993.

78. De Laat EA, Visser CP, Coene LN, et al: The lesions in primary shoulder dislocations and humeral neck fractures. J Bone Joint Surg Br 3:273-287, 1994.

79. Pasila M, Jeroma H, Kivilnoto O, et al: Early complications of primary shoulder dislocations. Acta Orthop Scand 49:260-263, 1978.

80. Flatow EL, Cuomo F, Maday MG, et al: Open reduction and internal fixation of two-part displaced fractures of the greater tuberosity of the proximal humerus. J Bone Joint Surg Am 73:1213-1218, 1991.

81. Gartsman GM, Taverna E, Hammerman SM, et al: Arthroscopic treatment of acute traumatic anterior glenohumeral dislocation and greater tuberosity fracture. Arthroscopy 15:648-650, 1999.

82. Beredjiklian PK, Iannotti JP, Norris TR: Operative treatment of malunion of a fracture of the proximal aspect of the humerus. J Bone Joint Surg Am 80:1484-1494, 1998.

83. Norris TR, Turner JA, Bovill D: Nonunion of the upper humerus: An analysis of the etiology and treatment in 28 cases. In Post M, Hawkins RJ, Morrey BF (eds): Surgery of the Shoulder. St Louis: Mosby, 1990, pp 63-67.

84. Jakob RP, Kristiansen T, Mayo K, et al: Classification and aspects of treatment of fractures of the proximal humerus. In Bateman JE, Welsh JP (eds): Surgery of the Shoulder. St Louis: Mosby, 1984, pp 330-343.

85. Paavolainen P, Bjorkenheim JM, Slatis P, et al: Operative treatment of severe proximal humeral fracture. Acta Orthop Scand 54:374-379, 1983.

86. Robinson CM, Aderinto J: Current concepts review: Posterior shoulder dislocations and fracture-dislocations. J Bone Joint Surg Am 87:639-650, 2005.

87. Ross J, Lov JB: Islolated evulsion fracture of the lesser tuberosity of the humerus: Report of two cases. Radiology 172:833-834, 1989.

88. Iannotti JP, Ramsey ML, Williams GR, et al: Nonprosthetic management of proximal humerus fractures. J Bone Joint Surg Am 85:1578-1593, 2003.

89. Naranja RJ Jr, Iannotti JP: Displaced three- and four-part proximal humerus fractures: Evaluation and management. J Am Acad Orthop Surg 8:373-382, 2000.

90. Schlegel TF, Hawkins RJ: Displaced proximal humerus fractures: Evaluation and treatment. J Am Acad Orthop Surg 2:54-66, 1994.

91. Lill H, Brewer A, Korner J: Conservative treatment of dislocated proximal humerus fractures. Zentralbl Chir 126:205-210, 2001.

92. Zyto K: Non-operative treatment of comminuted fractures of the proximal humerus in elderly patients. Injury 29:349-352, 1998.

93. Zyto K, Ahrengart L, Sperber A, et al: Treatment of displaced proximal humeral fractures in elderly patients. J Bone Joint Surg Br 79:412-417, 1997.

94. Stableforth PG: Four-part fractures of the neck of the humerus. J Bone Joint Surg Br 66:104-108, 1984.

95. Resch H, Povacz F, Frohlich R, et al: Percutaneous fixation of three- and four-part fractures of the proximal humerus. J Bone Joint Surg Br 79:295-300, 1997.

96. Robinson CM, Page RS: Severely impacted valgus proximal humeral fractures. J Bone Joint Surg Am 85:1647-1655, 2003.

97. Brooks CH, Revell WJ, Heatley FW: Vascularity of the humeral head after proximal humeral fractures. An anatomical cadaver study. J Bone Joint Surg Br 75:132-136, 1993.

98. Resch H, Beck E, Bayley I: Reconstruction of the valgus-impacted humeral head fracture. J Shoulder Elbow Surg 4:73-80, 1995.

99. Resch H, Hubner C, Schwaiger R: Minimally invasive reduction and osteosynthesis of articular fractures of the humeral head. Injury 32(suppl 1): SA25-SA32, 2001.

100. Gerber C, Warner JJP: Alternatives to hemiarthroplasty for complex proximal humeral fractures. In Warner JJP, Iannotti JP, Gerber C (eds): Complex and Revision Problems in Shoulder Surgery. Philadelphia, Lippincott Williams & Wilkins, 1997, pp 215-243.

101. Millet PJ, Warner JJP: Percutaneous treatment of proximal humerus fractures. In Wirth MA (ed): Proximal Humerus Fractures. Chicago: American Academy of Orthopaedic Surgeons, 2005, pp 15-26.

102. Bohler J: Les fractures recentes de l'epaule. Acta Orthop Belg 30:235-242, 1964.

103. Jaberg H, Warner JJ, Jakob RP: Percutaneous stabilization of unstable fractures of the humerus. J Bone Joint Surg Am 74:508-515, 1992.

104. Herscovici D Jr, Saunders DT, Johnson MP, et al: Percutaneous fixation of proximal humeral fractures. Clin Orthop Relat Res (375):97-104, 2000.

105. Chen CY, Chao EK, Tu YK, et al: Closed management and percutaneous fixation of unstable proximal humerus fractures. J Trauma 45:1039-1045, 1998.

106. Ebraheim N, Wong FY, Biyani A: Percutaneous pinning of the proximal humerus. Am J Orthop 25:500-506, 1996.

107. Kocialkowski A, Wallace WA: Closed percutaneous K-wire stabilization for displaced fractures of the surgical neck of the humerus. Injury 21:209-212, 1990.

108. Soete PJ, Clayson PE, Costenoble VH: Transitory percutaneous pinning in fractures of proximal humerus. J Shoulder Elbow Surg 8:569-573, 1999.

109. Williams GR Jr, Wong KL: Two-part and three-part fractures. Open reduction and internal fixation versus closed reduction and percutaneous pinning. Orthop Clin North Am 31:1-21, 2000.

110. Jiang C, Zhu Y, Wang M, et al: Biomechanical comparison of different pin configurations during percutaneous pinning for the treatment of proximal humeral fractures. J Shoulder Elbow Surg 16:235-239, 2007.

111. Nho SJ, Brophy RH, Barker JU, et al: Innovations in the management of displaced proximal humerus fractures. J Am Acad Orthop Surg 15:12-26, 2007.

112. Keener JD, Parsons BO, Flatow EL, et al: Outcomes after percutaneous reduction and fixation of proximal humeral fractures. J Shoulder Elbow Surg 16(3):330-338, 2007.

113. Rose PS, Adams CR, Torchia ME, et al: Locking plate fixation for proximal humerus fractures: Initial results with a new implant. J Shoulder Elbow Surg 16:202-207, 2007.

114. Boes MT, Moutoussis M, Cuomo F: Open reduction and internal fixation of two- and three-part fractures. In Wirth MA (ed): Proximal Humerus Fractures. Chicago: American Academy of Orthopaedic Surgeons, 2005, pp 27-38.

115. Gerber C, Werner CM, Vienne P: Internal fixation of complex fractures of the proximal humerus. J Bone Joint Surg Br 86:848-855, 2004.

116. Koukakis A, Apostolou CD, Taneja T, et al: Fixation of proximal humerus fractures with the PHILOS plate: Early experience. Clin Orthop Relat Res (442):115-120, 2006.

117. Meier RA, Messmer P, Regazzoni P, et al: Unexpected high complication rate following internal fixation of unstable proximal humerus fractures with an angled blade plate. J Orthop Trauma 20:253-260, 2006.

118. Agel J, Jones CB, Sanzone AG, et al: Treatment of proximal humerus fractures with Polarus nail fixation. J Shoulder Elbow Surg 13:191-195, 2004.

119. Wijgman AJ, Rookler W, Patt TW, et al: Open reduction and internal fixation of three- and four-part fractures of the proximal part of the humerus. J Bone Joint Surg Am 84:1919-1925, 2002.

120. Park JY, An JW, Oh JH: Open intramedullary nailing with tension band and locking sutures for proximal humeral fracture: Hot air balloon technique. J Shoulder Elbow Surg 15:594-601, 2006.

121. Haidukewych GJ: Perspectives on modern orthopaedics: Innovations in locking plate technology. J Am Acad Orthop Surg 12:205-212, 2004.

122. Tingart MJ, Lehtinen J, Zurakowski D, et al: Proximal humeral fractures: Regional differences in bone mineral density of the humeral head affect the fixation strength of cancellous screws. J Shoulder Elbow Surg 15:620-624, 2006.

123. Hall MC, Rosser M: The structure of the upper end of the humerus with reference to osteoporotic changes in senescence leading to fractures. Can Med Assoc J 88:290-294, 1963.

124. Hawkins RJ, Bell RH, Gurr K: The three-part fracture of the proximal part of the humerus. Operative treatment. J Bone Joint Surg Am 68:1410-1414, 1986.

125. Kristiansen B, Christensen SW: Plate fixation of proximal humeral fractures. Acta Orthop Scand 57:320-323, 1986.
126. Instrum K, Fennell C, Shrive N, et al: Semitubular blade plate fixation in proximal humeral fractures: A biomechanical study in a cadaver model. J Shoulder Elbow Surg 17:462-466, 1998.
127. Weinstein DM, Bratton DR, Ciccone WJ, et al: Locking plates improve torsional resistance in the stabilization of three part proximal humerus fractures. J Shoulder Elbow Surg 15:239-243, 2006.
128. Handoll HHG, Gibson JNA, Madhok R: Interventions for treating proximal humeral fractures in adults. Cochrane Database Syst Rev (4):CD000434, 2003.
129. Wagner M: General principles for the clinical use of the LCP. Injury 34(suppl 2):B31-B42, 2003.
130. Saudan M, Strern RE, Lubbeke A, et al: Fixation of fractures of the proximal humerus: Experience with a new locking plate. Presented at the 2003 Annual Meeting of the Orthopedic Trauma Association, Salt Lake City, Utah, October 9-11, 2003.
131. Frankhauser F, Boldin C, Schippinger G, et al: A new locking plate for unstable fractures of the proximal humerus. Clin Orthop Relat Res (430):176-181, 2005.
132. Bjorkenheim JM, Pajarinen J, Savolainen V: Internal fixation of proximal humeral fractures with a locking compression plate: A retrospective evaluation of 72 patients followed for a minimum of 1 year. Acta Orthop Scand 72:741-745, 2004.
133. Roberts CS, Walz BM, Yerasimides J: Humeral shaft fractures: Intramedullary nailing. In Wiss D (ed): Fractures. Master Techniques in Orthopaedic Surgery, 2nd ed. Philadelphia: Lippincott Williams & Wilkins, 2006, pp 81-96.
134. Rajasekhar C, Ray PS, Bhamra MS: Fixation of proximal humeral fractures with the Polarus nail. J Shoulder Elbow Surg 10:7-10, 2001.
135. Agel J, Jones CB, Sanzone AG, et al: Treatment of proximal humeral fractures with Polarus nail fixation. J Shoulder Elbow Surg 13:191-195, 2004.
136. Lin J, Hou SM, Hang YS: Locked nailing for displaced surgical neck fractures of the humerus. J Trauma 45:1051-1057, 1998.
137. Adedapo AO, Ikempe JO: The results of internal fixation of three and four-part proximal humeral fractures with the Polarus nail. Injury 32:115-121, 2001.
138. Cuomo F, Flatow EL, Maday MG, et al: Open reduction and internal fixation of two- and three-part displaced surgical neck fractures of the proximal humerus. J Shoulder Elbow Surg 1:287-295, 1992.
139. Williams GR, Copley LA, Iannotti JP, et al: The influence of intramedullary fixation on figure-of-eight wiring for surgical neck fractures of the proximal humerus: A biomechanical comparison. J Shoulder Elbow Surg 6:423-428, 1997.
140. Kitson J, Booth G, Day R: A biomechanical comparison of locking plate and locking nail implants used for fractures of the proximal humerus. J Shoulder Elbow Surg 16(3):362-366, 2007.
141. Sanders BS, Bullington AB, McGillivary GR, et al: Biomechanical evaluation of locked plating in proximal humeral fractures. J Shoulder Elbow Surg 16:229-234, 2007.
142. Neer CS II: Articular replacement for the humeral head. J Bone Joint Surg Am 37:215-228, 1955.
143. Constant C, Murley A: A clinical method of functional assessment of the shoulder. Clin Orthop Relat Res (214):160-164, 1987.
144. Richards RR, An KN, Bigliani LU, et al: A standardized method for the assessment of shoulder function. J Shoulder Elbow Surg 3:347-352, 1994.
145. Zuckerman JD, Cuomo F, Koval KJ: Proximal humeral replacement for complex fractures: Indications and surgical technique. Instr Course Lect 46:7-14, 1997.
146. Iannotti JP, Gabriel JP, Schneck SL, et al: The normal glenohumeral relationships: An anatomical study of one hundred and forty shoulders. J Bone Joint Surg Am 74:491-500, 1992.
147. Dines DM, Warren RF: Modular shoulder hemiarthroplasty for acute fractures: Surgical considerations. Clin Orthop Relat Res (307):18-26, 1994.
148. Moeckel BH, Dines DM, Warren RF, et al: Modular hemiarthroplasty for fractures of the proximal part of the humerus. J Bone Joint Surg Am 74:884-889, 1992.
149. Norris TR, Green A, McGuigan FX: Late prosthetic shoulder arthroplasty for displaced proximal humerus fractures. J Shoulder Elbow Surg 4:271-280, 1995.
150. Bosch U, Skutek M, Fremery RW, Tscherne H: Outcome after primary and secondary hemiarthroplasty in elderly patients with fractures of the proximal humerus. J Shoulder Elbow Surg 7:479-484, 1998.
151. Green A, Lippitt SB, Wirth MA: Humeral head replacement arthroplasty. In Wirth MA (ed): Proximal Humerus Fractures. Rosemont, Ill: American Academy of Orthopaedic Surgeons, 2005, pp 39-48.
152. de Laat EA, Visser CP, Coene LN, et al: Nerve lesions in primary shoulder dislocations and humeral neck fractures: A prospective clinical and EMG study. J Bone Joint Surg Br 76:381-383, 1994.
153. Visser CP, Tavy DL, Coene LN, et al: Electromyographic findings in shoulder dislocations and fractures of the proximal humerus: Comparison with clinical neurological examination. Clin Neurol Neurosurg 101:86-91, 1999.
154. Visser CP, Coene LN, Brand R, et al: Nerve lesions in proximal humerus fractures. J Shoulder Elbow Surg 10:421-427, 2001.
155. Hartsock LA, Estes WJ, Murray CA, Friedman RJ: Shoulder hemiarthroplasty for proximal humeral fractures. Orthop Clin North Am 29(3):467-475, 1998.
156. Itamura J, Dietrick T, Roidis N, et al: Analysis of the bicipital groove as a landmark for humeral head replacement. J Shoulder Elbow Surg 11:322-326, 2002.
157. Murachovksy J, Ikemoto RY, Nascimento LGP, et al: Pectoralis major tendon reference (PMT): A new method for accurate restoration of humeral length with hemiarthroplasty for fracture. J Shoulder Elbow Surg 15:675-678, 2006.
158. Frankle MA, Ondrovic LE, Markee BA, et al: Stability of tuberosity attachment in proximal humeral arthroplasty. J Shoulder Elbow Surg 11:413-420, 2002.
159. Frankle MA, Greenwald DP, Markee BA, et al: Biomechanical effects of malposition of tuberosity fragments on the humeral prosthetic reconstruction for four-part proximal humerus fractures. J Shoulder Elbow Surg 10:321-326, 2001.
160. Frankle MA, Mighell MA: Techniques and principles of tuberosity fixation for proximal humeral fractures treated with hemiarthroplasty. J Shoulder Elbow Surg 13:239-247, 2004.
161. Compito CA, Self EB, Bigliani LU: Arthroplasty and acute shoulder trauma. Clin Orthop Relat Res (307):27-36, 1994.
162. Muldoon MP, Cofield RH: Complications of humeral head replacement for proximal humerus fractures. Instr Course Lect 46:15-24, 1997.
163. Bohsali KI, Wirth MA, Rockwood Jr CA: Current concepts review: Complications of total shoulder arthroplasty. J Bone Joint Surgery Am 88:2279-2292, 2006.
164. Boileau P, Krishnan SG, Tinsi L, et al: Tuberosity malposition and migration: Reason for poor outcomes after hemiarthroplasty for displaced fractures of the proximal humerus. J Shoulder Elbow Surg 11:401-412, 2002.
165. Boileau P, Walch G, Trojani C, et al: Surgical classification and limits of shoulder arthroplasty. In Walch G, Boileau P (eds): Shoulder Arthroplasty. Berlin, Springer-Verlag, 1999, pp 349-358.
166. Robinson CM, Page RS, Hill RMF, et al: Primary hemiarthroplasty for treatment of proximal humeral fractures. J Bone Joint Surg Am 85:1215-1223, 2003.
167. Bicknell RT, Delude JA, Kedgley AE, et al: Early experience with computer-assisted shoulder hemiarthroplasty for fractures of the proximal humerus: Development of a novel technique and an in vitro comparison with traditional methods. J Shoulder Elbow Surg 16(3 suppl):S117-S125, 2007.
168. Boulahia A, Edwards TB, Walch G, et al: Early results of a reverse design prosthesis in the treatment of arthritis of the shoulder in elderly patients with a large rotator cuff tear. Orthopedics 25:129-133, 2002.
169. Boileau P, Watkinson D, Hatzidakis AM, et al: Neer Award 2005: The Grammont reverse shoulder prosthesis: Results in cuff tear arthritis, fracture sequelae, and revision arthroplasty. J Shoulder Elbow Surg 15:527-540, 2006.
170. Cazeneuve JF, Cristofari DJ: Grammont reversed prosthesis for acute complex fracture of the proximal humerus in an elderly population with 5 to 12 years follow-up. Rev Chir Orthop Reparatrice Appar Mot 6:534-548, 2006.
171. Levy J, Frankle M, Mighell M, et al: The Use of the reverse shoulder prosthesis for the treatment of failed hemiarthroplasty for proximal humeral fracture. J Bone Joint Surg Am 89:292-300, 2007.
172. Wirth MA: Late sequelae of proximal humerus fractures. In Wirth MA (ed): Proximal Humerus Fractures. Chicago: American Academy of Orthopaedic Surgeons, 2005, pp 49-55.
173. Koval KJ, Gallagher MA, Marsicano JG, et al: Functional outcome after minimally displaced fractures of the proximal part of the humerus. J Bone Joint Surg Am 79:203-207, 1997.
174. Frich LH, Sojbjerg JO, Sneppen O: Shoulder arthroplasty in complex acute and chronic proximal humeral fractures. Orthopedics 14:949-954, 1991.
175. Neer CS II: Glenohumeral arthroplasty. In Neer CS II (ed): Shoulder Reconstruction. Philadelphia: WB Saunders, 1990, pp 143-269.
176. Tanner MW, Cofield RH: Prosthetic arthroplasty for fractures and fracture-dislocations of the proximal humerus. Clin Orthop Relat Res (179):116-128, 1983.
177. Hagg O, Lundberg B: Aspects of prognostic factors in comminuted and dislocated proximal humeral fractures. In Bateman JE, Welsh RP (eds): Surgery of the Shoulder. Philadelphia: BC Decker, 1984, pp 51-59.
178. Sturzenegger M, Fornaro E, Jakob RP: Results of surgical treatment of multifragmented fractures of the humeral head. Arch Orthop Trauma Surg 100:249-259, 1982.
179. Benegas E, Filho AZ, Filho AA, et al: Surgical treatment of varus malunion of the proximal humerus with valgus osteotomy. J Shoulder Elbow Surg 16:55-59, 2007.
180. Coventry MB, Laurnen EL: Ununited fractures of the middle and upper humerus: Special problems in treatment. Clin Orthop Relat Res 69:192-198, 1970.
181. Leach RE, Premer RF: Nonunion of the surgical neck of the humerus. Method of internal fixation. Minn Med 48:318-322, 1965.
182. Rooney PJ, Cockshott WP: Pseudarthrosis following proximal humeral fractures: A possible mechanism. Skeletal Radiol 15:21-24, 1986.
183. Speck M, Lang FJ, Regazzoni P. Proximal humeral multiple fragment fractures—failures after T-plate osteosynthesis. Swiss Surg 2:51-56, 1996.

184. Neer CS II: Non-union of the surgical neck of the humerus. Orthop Trans 7:389, 1983.
185. Ray RD, Sankaran B, Fetrow KO: Delayed union and nonunion of fractures. J Bone Joint Surg Am 46:627-643, 1964.
186. Mayer PJ, Evarts CM: Nonunion, delayed union, malunion, and avascular necrosis. In Epps CH Jr (ed): Complications in Orthopaedic Surgery, 2nd ed. Philadelphia, JB Lippincott, 1986, pp 207-230.
187. Muller ME, Thomas RJ: Treatment of non-union in fractures of long bones. Clin Orthop Relat Res 138:141-153, 1979.
188. Duralde XA, Flatow EL, Pollock RG, et al: Operative treatment of nonunions of the surgical neck of the humerus. J Shoulder Elbow Surg 5:169-180, 1996.
189. Healy WL, Jupiter JB, Kristiansen TK, et al: Nonunion of the proximal humerus. J Orthop Trauma 4:424-431, 1990.
190. Rosen H: The treatment of nonunions and pseudoarthroses of the humeral shaft. Orthop Clin North Am 21:725-742, 1990.
191. Wirth MA, Rockwood CA Jr: Complications of shoulder arthroplasty. Clin Orthop Relat Res (307):47-69, 1993.
192. Wirth MA, Rockwood CA Jr: Complications of total shoulder replacement arthroplasty. J Bone Joint Surg Am 78:603-616, 1996.
193. Post M: Fractures of the upper humerus. Orthop Clin North Am 11:239-252, 1980.

Fractures of the Scapula

Thomas P. Goss, MD, and Brett D. Owens, MD

The scapula is quite important to upper extremity function. Lying over the posterior chest wall, it is an integral part of the connection between the upper extremity and the axial skeleton via the glenohumeral and acromioclavicular joints, as well as the sternoclavicular articulation. It functions as a semi-stable, fairly mobile platform for the humeral head and upper extremity to work against. Finally, it serves as a point of attachment for a variety of soft tissue structures (musculotendinous and ligamentous) (Fig. 10-1).

Scapular fractures are usually the result of high-energy trauma (most often direct, but occasionally indirect). Avulsion, stress, and even fatigue fractures can also occur. Quite a number of fracture patterns have been described.

Fractures of the scapula account for 1% of all fractures, 5% of shoulder fractures, and 3% of injuries to the shoulder girdle (Box 10-1). This relative infrequency occurs for two reasons: (1) the scapula lies over the posterior chest wall and is protected by the rib cage and the thoracic cavity anteriorly and a thick layer of soft tissues posteriorly, and (2) the relative mobility of the scapula allows considerable dissipation of traumatic forces. The vast majority of scapula fractures (>90%) are insignificantly displaced, primarily because of the strong support provided by the surrounding soft tissues, thus making nonoperative management the treatment of choice.[1] As a result, these injuries have received little attention in the literature. However, scapula fractures involve a major articulation, occur in patients with a mean age of 35 to 45 years, and, when significantly displaced, can cause considerable morbidity. Consequently, these injuries deserve more respect and recently have received more consideration in major texts,[2-17] general and review articles, and papers dealing with specific issues.[18-39]

Because of the significant trauma often involved, patients sustaining a scapula fracture have an 80% to 95% incidence of associated osseous and soft tissue injuries (local and distant) that may be major, multiple, and even life threatening. These patients need to be carefully evaluated when they arrive in the emergency department, and appropriate supportive care must be rendered. As a result, scapula fractures are often diagnosed late or definitive treatment is delayed, or both. Such delay can compromise the patient's final functional result. In addition, if the associated injuries involve the shoulder complex, the patient's scapula fracture recovery may be even further compromised.

ANATOMY

A thorough knowledge of the local bony, soft tissue, and neurovascular anatomy is necessary when evaluating and treating scapula fractures, especially if operative management is required. The subscapularis muscle lies over the anterior (ventral) scapular surface, and the serratus anterior inserts along the anteromedial (vertebral) border. Posteriorly, the supraspinatus and infraspinatus muscles lie within the supraspinatus and infraspinatus fossae, respectively. More superficially, the trapezius muscle inserts along the scapular spine and clavicle, whereas the deltoid muscle originates along the scapular spine, acromial process, and distal end of the clavicle. The levator scapulae and rhomboids attach along the medial scapular border, and the teres minor and teres major muscles attach along its lateral border. Tendons of the pectoralis minor, short head of the biceps, and coracobrachialis attach to the coracoid process and form the conjoined tendon. The long head of the biceps originates at the superior glenoid margin, and the long head of the triceps attaches along the inferior glenoid margin.

Arising from the superior border of the scapula, the coracoid process curves superiorly, anteriorly, and later-

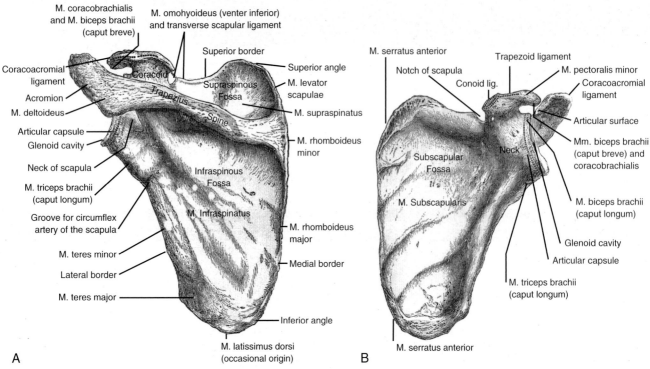

FIGURE 10-1 Illustrations showing the many musculotendinous and ligamentous attachment sites on the scapula.
A, Posterior or dorsal surface of the scapula. **B,** Anterior or costal surface of the scapula. (From Anson B: Morris' Human Anatomy. New York: McGraw-Hill, 1966, pp 247-248.)

ally. The brachial plexus and axillary vessels pass medial to the coracoid process and deep to the pectoralis minor tendon. The suprascapular notch is found along the superior scapular border, just medial to the base of the coracoid process, and is bridged by the transverse scapular ligament. The suprascapular nerve courses through the notch beneath the ligament, and the suprascapular artery passes above the ligament. The acromion projects laterally and then anteriorly from the scapular spine. Its junction with the glenoid neck constitutes the spinoglenoid notch, through which the suprascapular nerve and vessels pass from the supraspinatus fossa into the infraspinatus fossa. The dorsal scapular and accessory nerves accompany the deep and superficial branches of the transverse cervical artery, respectively, medial to the vertebral border of the scapula.

Most shoulder functions involve complex glenohumeral and scapulothoracic movements that occur in a precise sequence. The scapula is capable of six basic movements over the posterior chest wall: elevation, depression, upward rotation, downward rotation, protraction, and retraction. Combinations of these movements allow positioning of the upper extremity optimally in space. Trauma to the scapular region resulting in fracture nonunion, fracture malunion, soft tissue scarring, muscle damage, and nerve injury can have adverse mechanical and functional consequences.

CLASSIFICATION OF FRACTURES OF THE SCAPULA

Quite a number of scapula fracture patterns occur. Typically, they are classified by anatomic area: body and spine, glenoid neck, glenoid cavity, acromial process, and coracoid process. Most scapula fractures involve the body and spine (~50%).[27] The remaining 50% involve its three processes (Fig. 10-2).

BOX 10-1 Fractures of the Scapula

1% of all fractures
≥90% insignificantly displaced
Incidence

- Body and spine: 50%
- Glenoid process: 35% (glenoid cavity, 10%; glenoid neck, 25%)
- Acromial process: 8%
- Coracoid process: 7%

Incidence of associated injuries is 80%-90%, including major, multiple, and life-threatening injuries

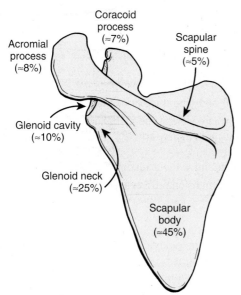

FIGURE 10-2 Incidence of scapular fractures according to region: the scapular body, approximately 45%; the scapular spine, approximately 5%; the glenoid neck, approximately 25%; the glenoid cavity, approximately 10%; the acromial process, approximately 8%; and the coracoid process, approximately 7%.

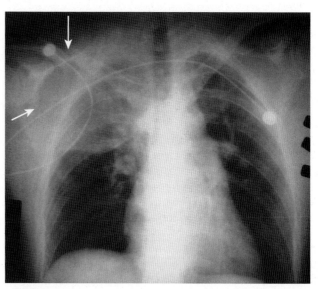

FIGURE 10-3 AP chest radiograph of a patient who sustained multiple trauma. The fractured clavicle and scapula (*arrows*) were incidental findings. (From Goss TP: Fractures of the scapula: Diagnosis and treatment. In Iannotti JP, Williams GR Jr [eds]: Disorders of the Shoulder: Diagnosis and Management. Philadelphia: Lippincott Williams & Wilkins, 1999, p 600.)

Fractures of the glenoid neck constitute approximately 25% of the total, and fractures of the glenoid cavity (the glenoid rim and glenoid fossa) make up approximately 10%. Fractures of the glenoid process therefore account for approximately 35% of all scapula fractures. Approximately 8% of these injuries involve the acromial process and approximately 7% involve the coracoid process.[27] An acromial fracture is defined as any fracture that runs from the posterior margin of the scapular spine or acromion to the undersurface of the acromial process all the way to the deepest point of the spinoglenoid interval.

A group of injuries termed *double disruptions* of the superior shoulder suspensory complex (SSSC) also have been described and often involve fractures of the coracoid, acromial, or glenoid processes.[40] Avulsion, stress, and fatigue fractures can also occur.

CLINICAL FEATURES

The physician's attention is initially drawn to the scapular region by the patient's complaints of pain. Characteristically, the arm is held adducted and all movement is resisted, particularly abduction, which is especially painful. Local tenderness is typical. Abnormal physical findings in the area include swelling and crepitus. Ecchymosis is less than what might be expected given the degree of bony injury. The specific diagnosis of a scapula fracture, however, is ultimately radiographic. These injuries are often initially missed[41] or detected incidentally on the patient's admission chest radiograph (Fig. 10-3). It

cannot be overemphasized that scapula fractures are typically accompanied by associated injuries that often require more urgent management.

ASSOCIATED INJURIES AND COMPLICATIONS

The most significant complications associated with scapula fractures are those that result from accompanying injuries to adjacent and distant osseous and soft tissue structures.[1,42] Because of the severe traumatic forces involved, these patients have an average of 3.9 additional injuries, with the most common sites being the ipsilateral shoulder girdle,[43] upper extremity, lung, and chest wall.[44] Twenty-five percent to 45% of patients have accompanying rib fractures, 15% to 40% have fractures of the clavicle, 15% to 55% have pulmonary injuries[45] (e.g., hemopneumothorax, pulmonary contusion), 12% have humeral fractures, and 5% to 10% sustain injuries to the brachial plexus and peripheral nerves.[46-48] Fractures of the skull are found in approximately 25% of patients, cerebral contusions in 10% to 40%, central neurologic deficits in 5%, tibia and fibula fractures in 11%,[48-50] major vascular injuries in 11%, and injuries that result in splenectomy in 8%. Two percent of these patients die. Landi and colleagues have described a compartment syndrome associated with a scapula fracture.[51] A variety of other cardiothoracic, genitourinary, and gastrointestinal injuries have also been reported. Interestingly, Stephens and associates reviewed 173 blunt trauma patients (92 with scapula fractures and 81 controls) and concluded that scapula fractures are not a significant marker for greater mortality or neurovascular morbidity.[52] Veysi and colleagues also showed no increase in mortality, but they did confirm significantly greater severity scores in trauma patients sustaining scapula fractures.[53]

Complications related to scapula fractures themselves are relatively uncommon. Nonunion, although possible, is quite rare. Malunion can occur in a variety of forms, depending on the particular fracture type. Malunion of a scapular body fracture is generally well tolerated; however, painful scapulothoracic crepitus has been described on occasion. Fractures of the glenoid cavity can result in symptomatic glenohumeral degenerative joint disease. Shoulder instability can occur after significantly displaced fractures of the glenoid neck (angular displacement) and fractures of the glenoid rim. Fractures of the glenoid neck with significant translational displacement can give rise to glenohumeral pain and dysfunction related to altered mechanics of the surrounding tissues.

Complications associated with surgical management are possible and include infection (both superficial and deep), intraoperative neurovascular injury, loss of fixation because of poor surgical technique, and others. A poorly supervised postoperative physical therapy and rehabilitation program can lead to unnecessary postoperative shoulder stiffness.

Finally, complications related to poor patient compliance can occur. Examples include suboptimal shoulder range of motion caused by unwillingness to follow the postoperative physical therapy program and hardware failure associated with reluctance to observe postoperative instructions.

RADIOGRAPHIC EVALUATION

A fracture of the scapula is an x-ray diagnosis, but precisely defining the injury can be difficult. If a scapula fracture is suspected or noted on other radiographs, a scapula trauma series is indicated, including true anteroposterior (AP) and lateral views of the scapula, as well as a true axillary projection of the glenohumeral joint (Fig. 10-4 and Box 10-2).

The scapula is a complex bony structure. One must be able to visualize and evaluate the scapular body and spine, as well as its three processes: the glenoid process, the acromial process, and the coracoid process. The glenoid process is composed of the glenoid neck and the glenoid cavity; the glenoid cavity is made up of the glenoid fossa and the glenoid rim. The scapula takes part in three articulations (the acromioclavicular joint, the glenohumeral joint, and the scapulothoracic articulation), each of which must be carefully evaluated. One also needs to look for associated shoulder girdle injuries, including those involving the clavicle, proximal part of the humerus, and sternoclavicular joint.

If an injury to the SSSC (the linkage system between the clavicle and the scapula) is suspected (e.g., a disrup-

---

BOX 10-2 Radiographic Evaluation of the Scapula

Often detected incidentally on chest radiograph
Scapula trauma series

- AP and lateral views of the scapula
- Axillary view of the glenohumeral joint
- Weight-bearing AP view of the shoulder

CT with and without reconstructions
Three-dimensional CT scan

---

tion of the coracoclavicular and/or acromioclavicular ligaments), a weight-bearing AP film is obtained (see Fig. 10-4). In some situations, transthoracic lateral and oblique projections of the region may be of value. The scapula trauma series should suffice for most injuries.

If the fracture pattern appears to be complex (multiple fracture lines and significant displacement), computed tomography (CT) scanning is necessary. Images in the superior plane allow evaluation of the acromioclavicular joint and acromial process, whereas the inferior images allow visualization of the scapular body and spine and the scapulothoracic articulation (Fig. 10-5). The middle images allow one to see the glenoid neck, the glenoid cavity (glenoid rim and glenoid fossa), the coracoid process, and the glenohumeral articulation (Fig. 10-6). In certain clinical situations, reconstructed views can be of great value. The proximal part of the humerus can be eliminated for optimal visualization of the glenoid cavity, and other reconstructed images are also possible (Fig. 10-7). Three-dimensional (3D) scanning can be extremely helpful to an orthopaedist trying to evaluate the most complex fracture patterns (Fig. 10-8). Images rotated at 15-degree increments in the horizontal, vertical, and oblique planes can be examined and the most useful printed for later reference. McAdams and colleagues found that CT scanning did not improve the evaluation of glenoid fractures over plain films but did help in identifying associated injuries to the SSSC.[54]

The exact role, if any, of arthroscopy (both diagnostic and therapeutic) is yet to be defined.

One must be careful to avoid mistaking nontraumatic radiographic findings (epiphyseal lines, os acromiale, glenoid dysplasia, and normal scapular foramina) for true traumatic changes.

TYPES OF FRACTURES AND METHODS OF TREATMENT

Glenoid Neck (Extra-articular) Fractures

Fractures of the glenoid neck make up 25% of all scapula fractures (Box 10-3). It is somewhat surprising that these injuries are not more common because this portion of

FIGURE 10-4 The scapula trauma series. **A,** True AP projection of the scapula. **B,** True axillary projection of the glenohumeral joint and scapula. **C,** True lateral projection of the scapula. **D,** Weight-bearing AP projection of the shoulder complex designed to evaluate the integrity of the clavicular–scapular linkage (optional and depending on the clinical situation). (**A to C,** from Goss TP: Fractures of the scapula: Diagnosis and treatment. In Iannotti JP, Williams GR Jr [eds]: Disorders of the Shoulder: Diagnosis and Management. Philadelphia: Lippincott Williams & Wilkins, 1999, p 600. **D,** Modified from Rockwood CA: Fractures. Philadelphia: JB Lippincott, 1975, p 733.)

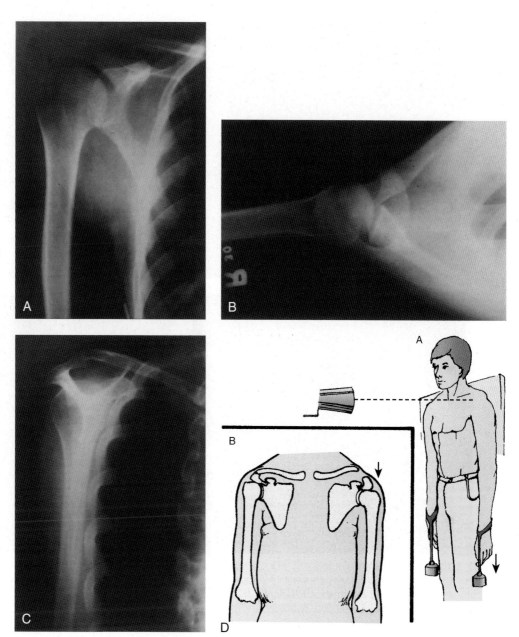

the glenoid process is quite narrow. These fractures may be caused by the following:

1. Direct blow over the anterior or posterior aspect of the shoulder
2. Fall on the outstretched arm with impaction of the humeral head against the glenoid process
3. In rare cases, a force applied over the superior aspect of the shoulder complex

The glenoid neck is that portion of the glenoid process which lies between the scapular body and the glenoid cavity. The coracoid process arises from its superior aspect. Its stability is primarily osseous—specifically, its junction medially with the scapular body. Secondary support is provided by its attachments superiorly to the clavicular–acromioclavicular joint–acromial strut via the clavicular–coracoclavicular ligamentous–coracoid (C-4) linkage and the coracoacromial ligament (Fig. 10-9). Tertiary soft tissue support is provided anteriorly by the subscapularis muscle, superiorly by the supraspinatus muscle, and posteriorly by the infraspinatus and teres minor muscles.

To be a glenoid neck fracture, the disruption must be complete: exiting along the lateral scapular border and the superior scapular margin, either just lateral or just

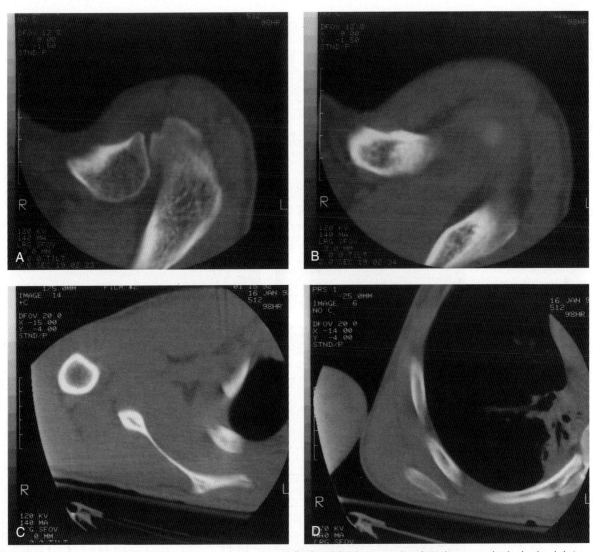

FIGURE 10-5 Multiple axial CT images of the scapula. **A** and **B,** Superior images showing the acromioclavicular joint and the acromion. **C** and **D,** Inferior images showing the scapular body and scapulothoracic articulation. (From Goss TP: Fractures of the scapula: Diagnosis and treatment. In Iannotti JP, Williams GR Jr [eds]: Disorders of the Shoulder: Diagnosis and Management. Philadelphia: Lippincott Williams & Wilkins, 1999, p 601.)

medial to the coracoid process (Fig. 10-10). Displacement can then occur. If, in addition, its secondary support is compromised (a coracoid process fracture, a coracoclavicular ligament disruption with or without a coracoacromial ligament injury, a clavicle fracture, an acromioclavicular joint disruption, or an acromial fracture; i.e., a double disruption of the SSSC), the fracture has the potential for severe displacement.[55] Hardegger and coauthors[56] described a rare case in which the fracture line exited the superior scapular border lateral to the coracoid process (the anatomic neck) (see Fig. 10-10), thereby allowing the glenoid fragment to be displaced laterally and distally by the pull of the long head of the triceps muscle. Arts and Louette[57] described a similar injury. They saw these fractures as inherently unstable (the primary support is completely disrupted and the fracture is lateral to the

secondary support system) and in need of open reduction and internal fixation (ORIF), as opposed to fractures of the surgical neck, which require associated injuries to their secondary support system to be rendered unstable and in need of surgical management.

Type I fractures include all insignificantly displaced injuries and constitute more than 90% of the total. Management is nonoperative, and a good to excellent functional result can be expected. Type II fractures include all significantly displaced injuries; *significant displacement* is defined as translational displacement of the glenoid fragment of 1 cm or more or angular displacement of the fragment of at least 40 degrees (Fig. 10-11).[58] Limb and McMurray described the case of a patient with a glenoid neck fracture so severely displaced and inferiorly angulated that the humeral head was articulating

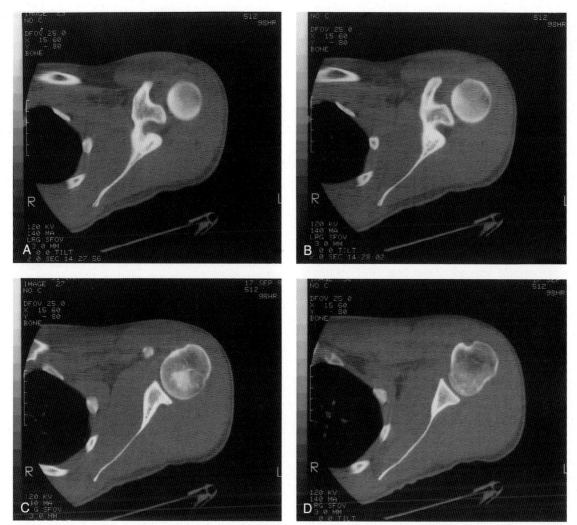

FIGURE 10-6 Multiple axial CT images through the glenohumeral region of the scapula. **A** and **B,** Most superior. **C** and **D,** Most inferior. (From Goss TP: Fractures of the scapula: Diagnosis and treatment. In Iannotti JP, Williams GR Jr [eds]: Disorders of the Shoulder: Diagnosis and Management. Philadelphia: Lippincott Williams & Wilkins, 1999, p 601.)

FIGURE 10-7 Reconstructed CT image showing the glenoid cavity en face with the humeral head eliminated. Note the large anteroinferior glenoid rim fragment with severe separation of the articular surface. (From Goss TP: Fractures of the scapula: Diagnosis and treatment. In Iannotti JP, Williams GR Jr [eds]: Disorders of the Shoulder: Diagnosis and Management. Philadelphia: Lippincott Williams & Wilkins, 1999, p 602.)

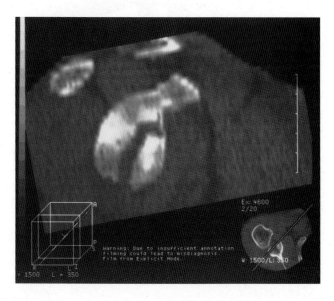

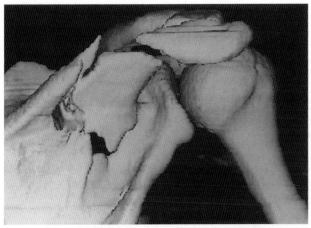

FIGURE 10-8 3D CT image of a patient who sustained a segmental fracture of the acromion. Note the severely displaced intermediate segment. (From Goss TP: Fractures of the scapula: Diagnosis and treatment. In Iannotti JP, Williams GR Jr [eds]: Disorders of the Shoulder: Diagnosis and Management. Philadelphia: Lippincott Willims & Wilkins, 1999, p 602.)

with the medial fracture surface and lateral margin of the scapular body rather than the glenoid fragment.[59] Translational displacement of 1 cm was chosen by Zdravkovic and Damholt,[60] Nordqvist and Petersson,[61] and Miller and Ada[62,63] as separating major from minor injuries. Bateman[2] stated that this degree of displacement could interfere with abduction.

Hardegger and coworkers[56] pointed out that significant translational displacement changes the normal relationships between the glenohumeral articulation and the

undersurface of the distal end of the clavicle, the acromioclavicular joint, and the acromial process. This alters the mechanics of nearby musculotendinous units, resulting in a functional imbalance of the shoulder complex as a whole (a disorganization of the coracoacromial arch). Miller and Ada[62,63] stated that the resultant weakness (especially abductor weakness), decreased range of motion, and pain (particularly subacromial pain) were largely due to rotator cuff dysfunction. The premise that significant translational displacement of the glenoid process can lead to shoulder discomfort and dysfunction certainly makes sense intuitively. The complex bony relationships in the glenohumeral region are clearly altered, as are the mechanics of the musculotendinous structures that pass from the scapula to the proximal part of the humerus (the deltoid muscle and rotator cuff, in particular). The fracture line usually exits the superior scapular margin medial to the coracoid process (the surgical neck region). The glenoid fragment is then drawn inferiorly by the weight of the arm and either anteromedially or posteromedially by the adjacent muscle forces (Fig. 10-12).

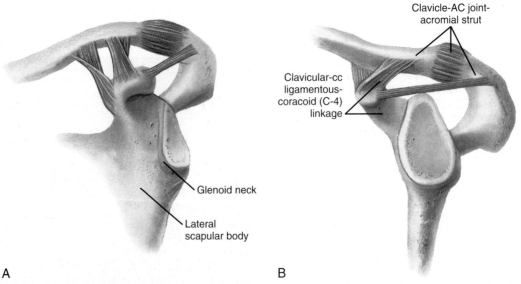

A   B

FIGURE 10-9 Illustrations depicting structures providing stability to the glenoid process in the region of the glenoid neck. **A,** Lateral aspect of the scapular body. **B,** Clavicle–acromioclavicular (AC) joint–acromial strut via the clavicular–coracoclavicular (cc) ligamentous–coracoid [C-4] linkage and the coracoacromial ligament.

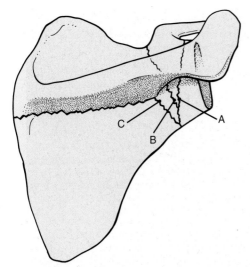

FIGURE 10-10 Illustration depicting three basic fracture patterns involving the glenoid neck: *A*, fracture through the anatomic neck; *B*, fracture through the surgical neck; and *C*, fracture involving the inferior glenoid neck, which then courses medially to exit through the scapular body (this type is managed as a scapular body fracture). (From Goss TP: Fractures of the glenoid neck. J Shoulder Elbow Surg 3[1]:42-52, 1994.)

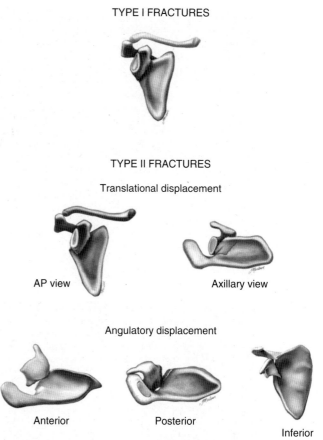

TYPE I FRACTURES

TYPE II FRACTURES

Translational displacement

AP view   Axillary view

Angulatory displacement

Anterior   Posterior

Inferior

FIGURE 10-11 Classification scheme for fractures of the glenoid neck.

(Van Noort and van der Werken think that the scapular body is displaced laterally rather than the glenoid fragment displaced medially).[64]

Bateman[2] and DePalma[65] stated that excessive angulation of the glenoid fragment could result in glenohumeral instability (anterior, posterior, or inferior). Normally, the glenoid cavity faces 15 degrees superiorly and is retroverted 6 degrees relative to the plane of the scapular body. With increasing angulation, the humeral head loses the normal bony support provided by the glenoid cavity (bony instability), which translates into glenohumeral discomfort and dysfunction.[2,5,62,63] Miller and Ada[62,63] stated that angular displacement of 40 degrees or more in either the coronal or sagittal plane was unacceptable. They saw this degree of displacement as adversely altering not only glenohumeral but also other bony relationships, as well as musculotendinous dynamics, particularly those of the rotator cuff, with resultant pain and overall shoulder dysfunction (diminished range of motion and loss of strength) (Fig. 10-13). Van Noort and van Kampen recommended surgical management for glenoid neck fractures with inferior angulation greater than 20 degrees (4 degrees of superior angulation being the mean in normal persons).[66]

Imatani,[24] McGahan and associates,[27] and Lindholm and Leven[67] recommended nonsurgical treatment of all glenoid neck fractures, but their studies give few details to justify this conclusion. Although somewhat ambivalent in their recommendations, two studies do mention surgical management as an option in selected cases. Armstrong and Vanderspuy[68] said that although most of these injuries

do well, more aggressive treatment, including ORIF, may be indicated in patients who are young and fit. Wilbur and Evans[36] stated that ORIF might be indicated if the glenoid fragment is markedly displaced or angulated but did not think that they had enough information or experience to warrant definitive surgical indications. Judet,[69] Magerl,[70] Ganz and Noesberger,[71] and Tscherne and Christ[72] said that operative management of displaced glenoid neck fractures prevents late disability and yields better results. Neer,[9] as well as Rockwood[10] and Butters,[3] presented the recommendations of other investigators, as did a review article by Guttentag and Rechtine.[22] Boerger and Limb[73] reported the case of a patient with a fracture of the glenoid neck, acromial and coracoid fractures, a dislocated acromioclavicular joint, and incomplete paralysis of the infraspinatus muscle treated with ORIF of the acromial and glenoid neck fractures. DeBeer and colleagues described the operative treatment of a professional cyclist who was able to return to competition after 6 weeks and urged more aggressive management in high-demand patients.[74]

Bozkurt and colleagues reported on 18 patients treated nonoperatively and found that decreased functional outcome correlated significantly with increased inferior angulation of the fracture and the presence of associated

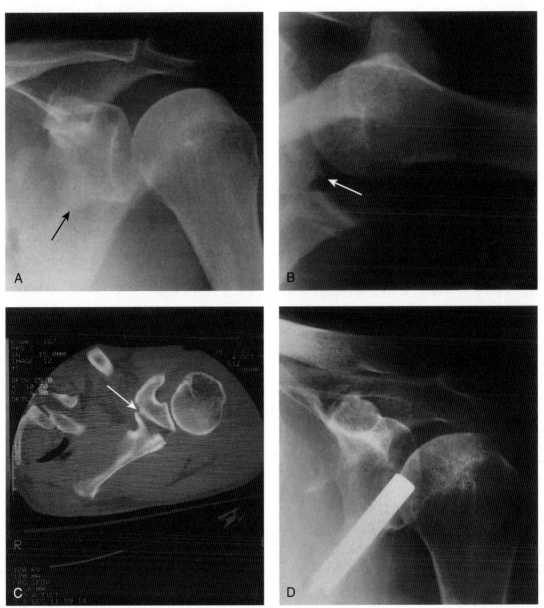

FIGURE 10-12 Radiographs of a patient who sustained a type II fracture of the glenoid neck with significant translational displacement of the glenoid fragment. **A,** Preoperative AP radiograph showing the glenoid neck fracture (*arrow*) and medial translation of the glenoid fragment. **B,** Preoperative axillary radiograph revealing that the unstable glenoid fragment is severely displaced anteromedially (*arrow*) (the glenohumeral joint is medial to the most lateral aspect of the scapular body), probably as a result of an associated disruption of the coracoclavicular ligament (a violation of the C-4 linkage and, therefore, a double disruption of the superior shoulder suspensory complex) and possibly the coracoacromial ligament. **C,** Preoperative axial CT image revealing the glenoid neck fracture to be complete and exiting the superior scapular border medial to the intact coracoid process (*arrow*) (a surgical neck fracture). **D,** Postoperative AP radiograph showing anatomic reduction and stabilization of the glenoid neck fracture and glenoid process fragment. (From Goss TP: Fractures of the scapula: Diagnosis and treatment. In Iannotti JP, Williams GR Jr [eds]: Disorders of the Shoulder: Diagnosis and Management. Philadelphia: Lippincott Williams & Wilkins, 1999, p 618.)

injuries.[75] Van Noort and van Kampen managed 13 patients without significant angular displacement, neurologic injury, and associated ipsilateral shoulder injuries, all of whom had a good to excellent outcome regardless of the degree of translational displacement when treated nonoperatively.[66]

Miller and Ada[62,63] retrospectively reviewed 16 displaced glenoid neck fractures (≥1 cm of translational displacement or ≥40 degrees of angulation) managed nonoperatively (36-month average follow-up). They found that 20% had decreased range of motion, 50% had pain (75% of which was night pain), 40% had weakness

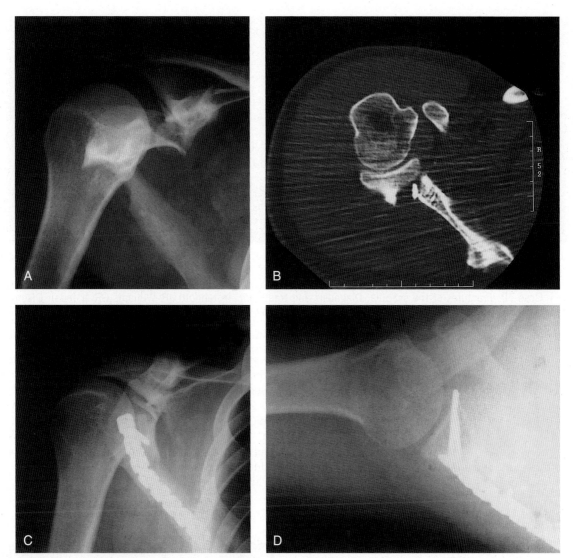

FIGURE 10-13 Type II fracture of the glenoid neck with significant angular displacement of the glenoid fragment. **A,** Preoperative AP radiograph showing the glenoid neck fracture with severe angulation of the glenoid fragment and a fractured coracoid process. Also note the fracture of the scapular body with displacement of the lateral scapular border. **B,** Preoperative axial CT projection showing the coracoid process fracture (a violation of the clavicular–coracoclavicular ligamentous–coracoid [C-4] linkage), which further destabilized the glenoid fragment and allowed severe angulatory displacement to occur (a double disruption of the superior shoulder suspensory complex). Postoperative AP (**C**) and axillary (**D**) radiographs show the glenoid fragment is reduced and stabilized with a contoured reconstruction plate (the coracoid process was allowed to heal spontaneously).

with exertion, and 25% noted popping. In particular, these patients often had shoulder abductor weakness and subacromial pain that was due at least in part to rotator cuff dysfunction. They recommended ORIF of glenoid neck fractures with this degree of displacement. Chadwick and colleagues agreed.[77]

Pace and colleagues reviewed 9 patients with insignificantly displaced fractures and found the majority had some activity-related pain that was believed to be due to impingement and cuff arthropathy despite 90% good to excellent results.[78] A long-term follow-up study by Zdravkovic and Damholt[60] included 20 to 30 patients (it

is difficult to determine the exact number from the text) with displaced glenoid neck fractures and noted that nonoperative treatment yielded satisfactory results. Nordqvist and Petersson[61] evaluated 37 glenoid neck fractures treated without surgery (10- to 20-year follow-up) and found the functional result to be either fair or poor in 32%. They said that for some fractures, early ORIF might have improved the result. Hardegger and coauthors[56] reported 80% good to excellent results in five displaced glenoid neck fractures treated surgically (6.5-year follow-up). They said that operative management of such injuries prevented late disability and yielded better

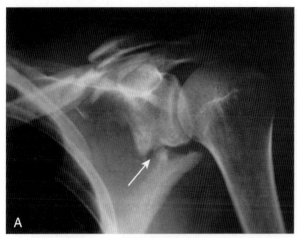
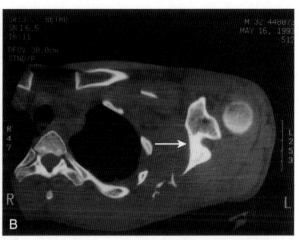

FIGURE 10-14 Radiographs showing what initially, but erroneously, appeared to be a complete fracture of the glenoid neck. **A,** AP radiograph of the shoulder showing a fracture (*arrow*) involving the inferior aspect of the glenoid neck. **B,** Axial CT image showing the superior portion of the glenoid neck to be uninvolved (*arrow*) (the fracture exited through the scapular body). (From Goss TP: Fractures of the scapula: Diagnosis and treatment. In Iannotti JP, Williams GR Jr [eds]: Disorders of the Shoulder: Diagnosis and Management. Philadelphia: Lippincott Williams & Wilkins, 1999, p 619.)

results. Gagey and colleagues[79] found a good result in only 1 of 12 displaced fractures treated nonoperatively. They stated that such injuries could "disorganize the coracoacromial arch" and recommended ORIF.

Clearly, these investigators agree that the vast majority of glenoid neck fractures can and should be treated without surgery. However, most authors think that more aggressive treatment, including ORIF, is at least a consideration if not clearly indicated when the glenoid fragment is severely displaced (i.e., type II injuries).

The diagnosis is ultimately radiographic. Plain radiographs are helpful, but because of the complex bony anatomy in the area, CT scanning is generally necessary to decide whether a glenoid neck fracture is indeed complete, to determine the degree of displacement, if any, and to identify injuries to adjacent bony structures and articulations.[54] One must not confuse these injuries with the more common fractures that course through the inferior glenoid neck and the scapular body (see Fig. 10-10). CT scanning readily reveals that the latter are not complete disruptions of the glenoid process because the superior aspect of the glenoid neck is intact. These injuries are essentially fractures of the scapular body and do quite well with nonoperative care because the normal relationships between the glenohumeral articulation and the distal end of the clavicle acromion are unaltered (Fig. 10-14).[80] Finally, if an injury to the SSSC (the clavicular–scapular linkage) is suspected, a weight-bearing AP view of the shoulder is obtained.

Glenoid Cavity (Intra-articular) Fractures

Fractures of the glenoid cavity make up 10% of scapula fractures. The majority (>90%) are insignificantly displaced and are managed nonoperatively (Fig. 10-15 and Box 10-4). Significantly displaced fractures require surgi-

cal treatment or at least merit surgical consideration. Ideberg reviewed more than 300 such injuries and proposed the first detailed classification scheme,[43,81,82] which was subsequently expanded by Goss (Fig. 10-16).[83] Type I fractures involve the glenoid rim: type Ia, the anterior rim; and type Ib, the posterior rim. Fractures of the glenoid fossa make up types II to V. Type VI fractures include all comminuted injuries (more than two glenoid cavity fragments).

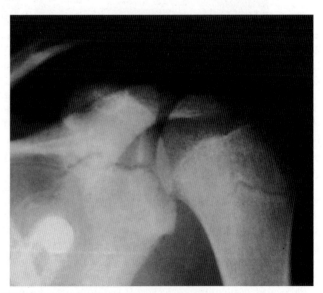

FIGURE 10-15 AP radiograph showing an undisplaced fracture of the scapula involving the glenoid process. (From Goss TP: Fractures of the scapula: Diagnosis and treatment. In Iannotti JP, Williams GR Jr [eds]: Disorders of the Shoulder: Diagnosis and Management. Philadelphia: Lippincott Williams & Wilkins, 1999, p 603.)

BOX 10-4 Significantly Displaced
Glenoid Cavity Fractures

Glenoid Rim Fractures

Displacement of a fragment ≥10 mm *and*

Involvement of one quarter or more of the glenoid cavity anteriorly or one third or more of the glenoid cavity posteriorly

Glenoid Fossa Fractures

Articular step-off of ≥5 mm

Failure of the humeral head to lie within the center of the glenoid concavity

Severe separation of the glenoid fragments

Fractures of the glenoid rim occur when the humeral head strikes the periphery of the glenoid cavity with considerable violence (Fig. 10-17).[84] These injuries are true fractures, distinct from the small avulsion injuries that occur when a dislocating humeral head applies a tensile force to the periarticular soft tissues.[65] A true axillary view of the glenohumeral joint, CT imaging (routine and reconstructive), and, if necessary, 3D scanning allow one to determine the size and displacement of the rim fragment, whether persistent subluxation of the humeral head is present, and therefore whether stability of the glenohumeral articulation is significantly compromised (Figs. 10-18 and 10-19).

Fractures of the glenoid fossa occur when the humeral head is driven with significant force into the center of the concavity. The fracture generally begins as a transverse disruption (or slightly oblique) for several possible reasons:

GLENOID RIM FRACTURES

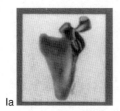
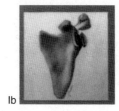

GLENOID FOSSA FRACTURES

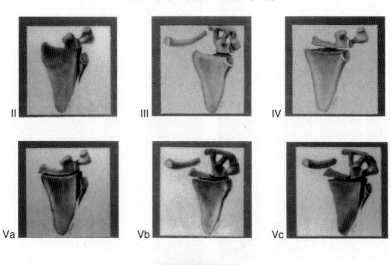

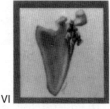

FIGURE 10-16 Goss–Ideberg classification scheme for fractures of the glenoid cavity. (From Goss TP: Fractures of the glenoid cavity [Current Concepts Review]. J Bone Joint Surg Am 74[2]:299-305, 1992.)

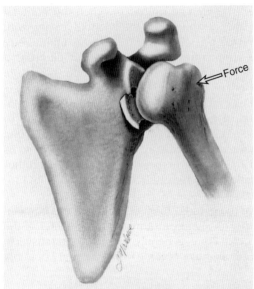

FIGURE 10-17 Illustration depicting one mechanism of injury responsible for fractures of the glenoid rim: a force applied over the lateral aspect of the proximal end of the humerus. A fall on an outstretched arm driving the humeral head against the periphery of the glenoid cavity with considerable violence could also cause this injury. (From Goss TP: Fractures of the shoulder complex. In Pappas AM [ed]: Upper Extremity Injuries in the Athlete. New York: Churchill Livingstone, 1995, p 267.)

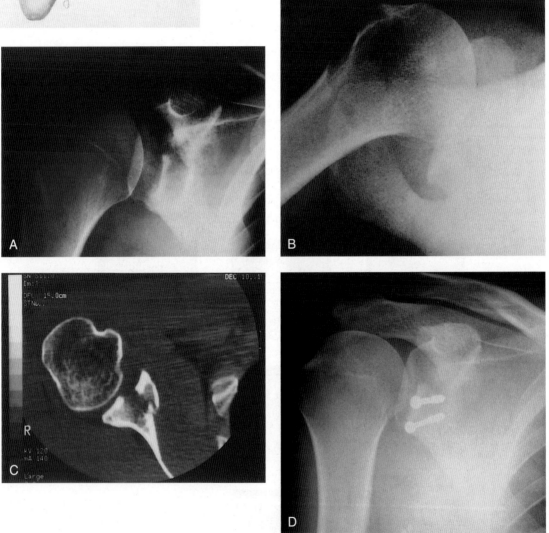

FIGURE 10-18 Radiographs of a patient who sustained a type Ia fracture of the glenoid cavity. **A,** Preoperative AP radiograph showing what appears to be a fracture of the anteroinferior glenoid rim. **B,** Preoperative axillary radiograph showing what appears to be a fracture of the anterior glenoid rim with anterior subluxation of the humeral head. **C,** Axial CT image showing a severely displaced fracture of the anterior glenoid rim. **D,** Postoperative AP radiograph showing reduction and stabilization of the anteroinferior glenoid rim fragment with two cannulated interfragmentary screws. (**A** to **C,** From Goss TP: Fractures of the scapula: Diagnosis and treatment. In Iannotti JP, Williams GR Jr [eds]: Disorders of the Shoulder: Diagnosis and Management. Philadelphia: Lippincott Williams & Wilkins, 1999, p 610.)

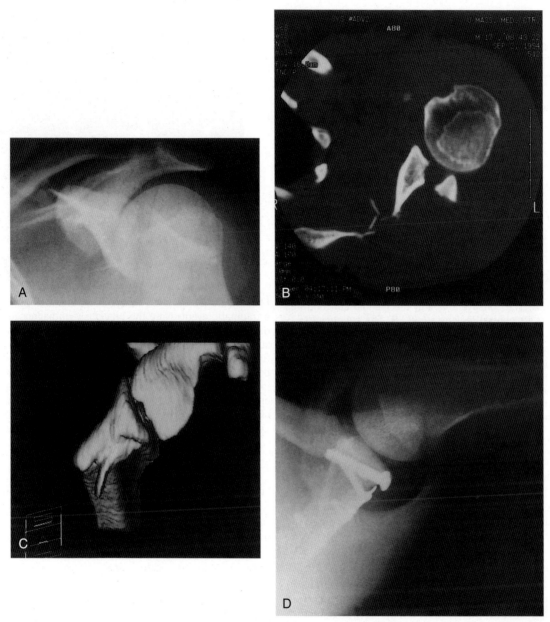

FIGURE 10-19 Radiographs of a patient who sustained a type Ib fracture of the glenoid cavity. **A,** Preoperative lateral scapula radiograph showing what appears to be a fracture of the glenoid cavity with significant posterior involvement. **B,** Axial CT image showing a severely displaced fracture of the posterior glenoid rim with posterior subluxation of the humeral head. **C,** 3D CT image of the glenoid cavity with the humeral head subtracted showing the severely displaced and rotated posteroinferior glenoid rim fragment. **D,** Postoperative axillary radiograph showing anatomic reduction and stabilization of the posterior glenoid rim fragment with restoration of articular congruity. (From Goss TP: Fractures of the scapula: Diagnosis and treatment. In Iannotti JP, Williams GR Jr [eds]: Disorders of the Shoulder: Diagnosis and Management. Philadelphia: Lippincott Williams & Wilkins, 1999, p 611.)

1. The glenoid cavity is concave; therefore, forces tend to be concentrated over its central region.
2. The subchondral trabeculae are transversely oriented; therefore, fractures tend to occur in this plane.
3. The glenoid cavity is formed from two ossification centers; therefore, the central region can remain a persistently weak area.
4. The glenoid cavity is narrow superiorly and wide inferiorly, with an indentation along its anterior rim.

This anatomy constitutes a stress riser where fractures are particularly prone to originate before coursing over to the posterior rim (Fig. 10-20).

Once a transverse disruption occurs, the fracture can propagate in a variety of directions, depending on the exact direction of the humeral head force. An AP projection of the glenohumeral joint, reconstructed CT images in the coronal plane, and even 3D CT scanning

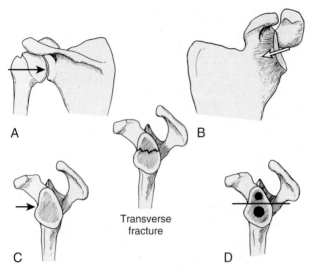

FIGURE 10-20 Illustrations depicting a transverse disruption of the glenoid cavity and the factors responsible for this orientation. **A,** The concave shape of the glenoid concentrates forces across its central region (*arrow*). **B,** The subchondral trabeculae are oriented in the transverse plane. **C,** A crook along the anterior rim (*arrow*) is a stress riser where fractures tend to originate. **D,** Formed from a superior and an inferior ossification center, the glenoid cavity may have a persistently weak central zone. (From Goss TP: Fractures of the shoulder complex. In Pappas AM [ed]: Upper Extremity Injuries in the Athlete. New York: Churchill Livingstone, 1995, p 268.)

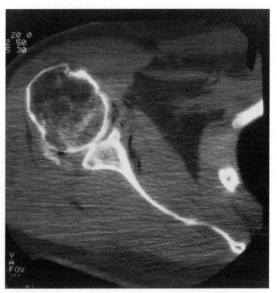

FIGURE 10-21 Axial CT image of a patient 8 months after a traumatic event. Note the previously undiagnosed displaced type Ia fracture of the glenoid cavity with anterior subluxation of the humeral head and bone-on-bone contact (intraoperatively the patient was found to have significant post-traumatic degenerative disease of the glenohumeral joint). (From Goss TP: Fractures of the scapula: Diagnosis and treatment. In Iannotti JP, Williams GR Jr [eds]: Disorders of the Shoulder: Diagnosis and Management. Philadelphia: Lippincott Williams & Wilkins, 1999, p 610.)

may be necessary to accurately determine whether and to what degree articular incongruity, separation, or both are present. If an injury to the SSSC (the scapular–clavicular linkage) is suspected, a weight-bearing AP view of the shoulder is obtained.

Type I

Surgical management of fractures of the glenoid rim is indicated if the fracture results in persistent subluxation of the humeral head (failure of the humeral head to lie concentrically within the glenoid cavity) or if the fracture or humeral head is unstable after reduction. DePalma[65] stated that instability could be expected if the fracture is displaced 10 mm or more and if a quarter or more of the glenoid cavity anteriorly or a third or more of the glenoid cavity posteriorly is involved. Hardegger and coworkers[56] concurred and stated that operative reduction plus fixation of the fragment is indicated to prevent recurrent or permanent dislocation of the shoulder. Guttentag and Rechtine[22] and Butters[3] agreed with these recommendations. Several papers describing operative management of glenoid rim fractures have also appeared in the literature.[85-89] Surgery, if necessary, is designed to restore articular stability and prevent post-traumatic degenerative joint disease (Fig. 10-21).

Type II

With type II glenoid fossa fractures, the humeral head is driven inferiorly and an inferior glenoid fragment is

created. Surgery is indicated if an articular step-off of 5 mm or more is present or if the fragment is displaced inferiorly and carries the humeral head with it such that the humeral head fails to lie in the center of the glenoid cavity (Fig. 10-22). These injuries can result in post-traumatic degenerative joint disease or glenohumeral instability, or both.[90]

Type III

Type III (glenoid fossa) fractures occur when the force of the humeral head is directed superiorly and causes the transverse disruption to propagate upward, generally exiting through the superior scapular margin in the vicinity of the suprascapular notch.[91,92] One might question whether this is a fracture of the glenoid cavity or a fracture of the coracoid process because the superior third of the glenoid cavity and the base of the coracoid process are formed from the same ossification center. Displacement is usually minimal, with the fragment lying medially. Consequently, as with base of the coracoid fractures, these injuries are generally treated nonoperatively and heal uneventfully.

Any glenoid cavity fracture may be associated with neurovascular injury due to the proximity of the brachial plexus and axillary vessels, as well as the considerable violence involved. Type III injuries, as well as Type Vb, Vc, and VI injuries, however, are particularly prone to

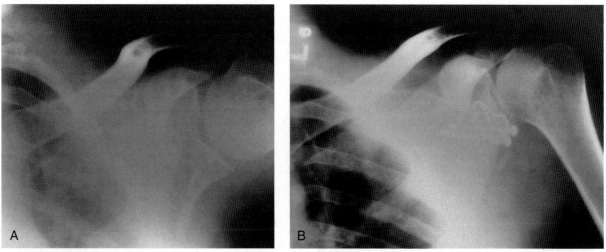

FIGURE 10-22 Radiographs of a patient who has sustained a type II fracture of the glenoid cavity. **A,** Preoperative AP radiograph showing significant displacement of the inferior glenoid fragment and a severe articular step-off. **B,** Postoperative AP radiograph showing anatomic reduction and stabilization of the inferior glenoid fragment with restoration of articular congruity. (From Goss TP: Fractures of the scapula: Diagnosis and treatment. In Iannotti JP, Williams GR Jr [eds]: Disorders of the Shoulder: Diagnosis and Management. Philadelphia: Lippincott Williams & Wilkins, 1999, p 613.)

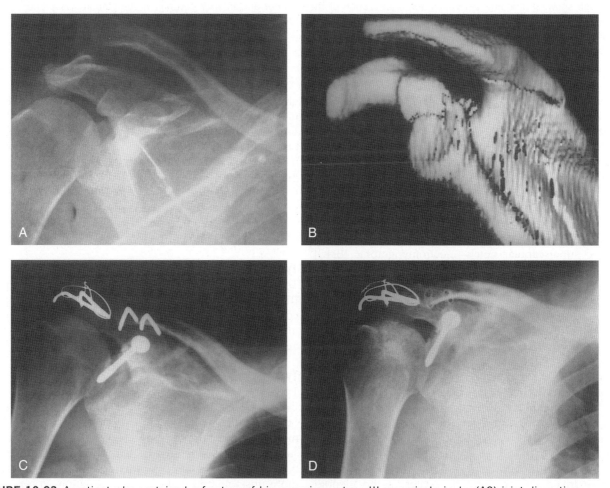

FIGURE 10-23 A patient who sustained a fracture of his acromion, a type III acromioclavicular (AC) joint disruption, and a type III glenoid cavity fracture. **A,** Preoperative AP radiograph. **B,** Preoperative 3D CT radiograph. **C,** Postoperative AP radiograph showing the acromial fracture reduced and stabilized with a tension band construct, the type III glenoid cavity fracture reduced and stabilized with a compression screw, and the AC joint disruption reduced and stabilized with Kirschner wires passed through the clavicle and into the acromial process. **D,** Postoperative AP radiograph showing maintenance of the normal clavicle–scapula relationships after removal of the clavicular–acromial Kirschner wires.

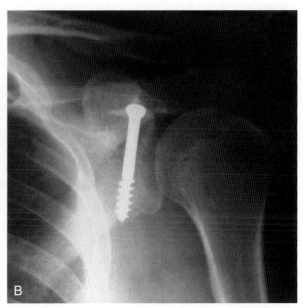

FIGURE 10-24 Radiographs of a patient who sustained a type IV fracture of the glenoid cavity. **A,** Preoperative AP radiograph showing severe separation of the superior and inferior portions of the glenoid fossa and scapular body. **B,** Postoperative AP radiograph showing anatomic reduction and stabilization of the superior and inferior portions of the glenoid fossa and scapular body with restoration of articular congruity. (From Goss TP: Fractures of the scapula: Diagnosis and treatment. In Iannotti JP, Williams GR Jr [eds]: Disorders of the Shoulder: Diagnosis and Management. Philadelphia: Lippincott Williams & Wilkins, 1999, p 614.)

such neurovascular involvement, especially if the superiorly directed force continues further upward and damages the SSSC—that is, if there is an associated disruption of the C-4 linkage or the clavicular–acromioclavicular joint–acromial strut. Neer and Rockwood considered compression of the adjacent neurovascular structures by these and fractures of the coracoid process indications for surgery.[10] They and others also described the occurrence of suprascapular nerve paralysis associated with fractures involving the coracoid process and the glenoid neck that extend into the suprascapular notch (electromyographic [EMG] testing was essential to make the diagnosis, and early exploration was recommended).[4,93-94]

Surgical management of type III fractures is indicated if the fracture has an articular step-off of 5 mm or more with lateral displacement of the superior fragment or if a significantly displaced additional disruption of the SSSC is present (a double disruption injury) (Fig. 10-23). Examples include an associated disruption of the C-4 linkage or of the clavicular–acromioclavicular joint–acromial strut.[55] These injuries can result in post-traumatic degenerative joint disease and severe functional impairment.

Type IV

Type IV (glenoid fossa) injuries occur when the humeral head is driven directly into the center of the glenoid cavity.[95] The fracture courses transversely across the entire scapula and exits along its vertebral border. If there is an unacceptable articular step-off (≥5 mm) with the superior fragment displaced laterally, or if the superior and inferior

glenoscapular segments are severely separated, ORIF is indicated to prevent symptomatic degenerative joint disease, nonunion at the fracture site (an extremely rare occurrence but a definite concern in the case shown [Fig. 10-24]), and instability of the glenohumeral joint. Ferraz and colleagues described a Type IV glenoid fossa fracture that progressed to a nonunion. When explored surgically less than 2 years after injury, a 7 mm articular step-off was noted as well as grade III cartilaginous erosion of the humeral head.[96]

Type V

These glenoid fossa injuries are combinations of type II, III, and IV injuries and are caused by more violent and complex forces. The same clinical concerns and operative indications detailed for the type II, III, and IV fractures apply to type V fractures (Fig. 10-25).

Type VI

Type VI glenoid cavity fractures are caused by the most violent forces and include all disruptions in which two or more articular fragments are present. Operative treatment is contraindicated because exposing these injuries surgically does little more than disrupt whatever soft tissue support remains, rendering the fragments even more unstable and making a bad situation worse.

Reports by Aulicino and coauthors[97] and Aston and Gregory[85] lend support to the role of surgery in managing significantly displaced glenoid fossa fractures. Lee and colleagues[98] reported the case of a child who sustained

FIGURE 10-25
Radiographs of a patient involved in a motor vehicle accident who sustained a type Vc fracture of the glenoid cavity. **A,** AP radiograph of the glenoid cavity fracture. **B,** Axial CT image showing a large anterosuperior glenoid fragment including the coracoid process. **C,** Axial CT image showing the lateral aspect of the scapular body lying between the two glenoid fragments, abutting the humeral head. **D,** Axial CT image showing a large posteroinferior cavity fragment. **E,** Postoperative AP, and **F,** axillary radiographs, showing the glenoid cavity fragments secured together with cannulated screws and the glenoid unit secured to the scapular body with a malleable reconstruction plate (the acromial fracture was reduced and stabilized with a tension band construct.) (From Goss TP, Owens BD: Fractures of the scapula: Diagnosis and treatment. In Iannotti JP, Williams GR Jr [eds]: Disorders of the Shoulder: Diagnosis and Management, 2nd ed. Philadelphia: Lippincott Williams & Wilkins, 2007, p 814.)

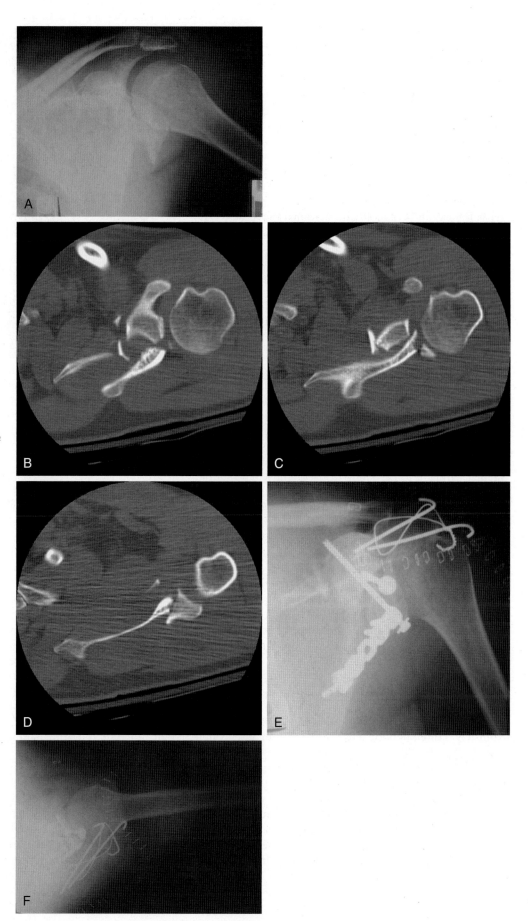

a type II fracture that required ORIF. Ruedi and Chapman[15] stated that "grossly displaced intra-articular fractures of the glenoid that render the joint incongruent and unstable profit from operative reconstruction and internal fixation as incongruities result in osteoarthritic changes." Rowe[14] advocated surgical management of severely displaced injuries. Bauer and coworkers[99] reviewed 20 patients treated surgically for significantly displaced fractures of the scapula (6.1-year average follow-up) and reported greater than 70% good or very good results based on the Constant score. They recommended early ORIF for grossly displaced fractures of the glenoid fossa, glenoid rim, glenoid neck, and coracoid and acromial processes. Hardegger and associates[56] reported that if "there is significant displacement, conservative treatment alone cannot restore congruency," and stiffness and pain can result— "for this reason open reduction and stabilization are indicated."

Kavanagh and colleagues[100] presented their experience at the Mayo Clinic in which 10 displaced intra-articular fractures of the glenoid cavity were treated with ORIF. They found ORIF to be "a useful and safe technique" that "can restore excellent function of the shoulder." In their series, the major articular fragments were displaced 4 to 8 mm. The authors emphasized that they remained uncertain how much incongruity of the glenoid articular surface can be accepted without risking the long-term sequelae of pain, stiffness, and traumatic osteoarthritis. Soslowsky and coworkers[101] found the maximal depth of the glenoid articular cartilage to be 5 mm. Consequently, if a glenoid fossa fracture is associated with an articular step-off of 5 mm or more, subchondral bone is exposed. Schandelmaier and coauthors[102] reported a series of 22 fractures of the glenoid fossa treated with ORIF. They stated that "if the postoperative courses are uneventful, excellent to good results can be expected." Leung and colleagues[103] reviewed 14 displaced intra-articular fractures of the glenoid treated with ORIF (30.5-year average follow-up) and reported nine excellent and five good results.

On the basis of these reports, it seems reasonable to conclude that there is a definite role for surgery in the treatment of glenoid fossa fractures.

Fractures of the Scapular Body

These injuries are often rather alarming radiographically: Extensive comminution and displacement are often present (Fig. 10-26). However, there is very little enthusiasm in the literature for operative treatment[104] because bone stock for fixation is at a premium and these injuries seem to heal quite nicely with nonoperative or symptomatic care,[105] and a good to excellent functional result can be expected. The vast majority of fractures of the scapular body and insignificantly displaced fractures (>90% of glenoid, coracoid, acromial, and avulsion fractures) are managed nonoperatively.

This prognosis is positive probably because the scapulothoracic interval is cushioned by a thick layer of soft

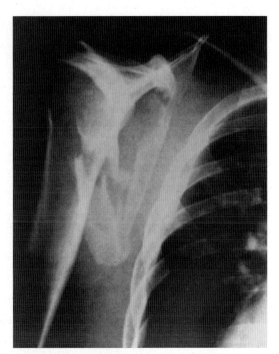

FIGURE 10-26 AP radiograph showing a severely comminuted fracture of the scapular body. (From Neer CS II: Less frequent procedures. In Neer CS II [ed]: Shoulder Reconstruction. Philadelphia: WB Saunders, 1990, pp 421-485.)

tissues and the mobility of the scapulothoracic articulation compensates for most residual deformities of the scapular body. The literature does mention a fracture of the scapular body with a lateral spike entering the glenohumeral joint as an indication (albeit extremely uncommon) for surgical management,[56] and a similar recommendation was made in two cases involving patients with fractures of the scapular body and intrathoracic penetration by one of the fragments.[106,107] Bowen and colleagues reported a case of a significantly angulated greenstick fracture of the scapular body that required a closed reduction.[108] On rare occasions, malunion of a scapular body fracture can result in scapulothoracic pain and crepitus requiring surgical exposure of its ventral surface and removal of the responsible bony prominence or prominences.[109] Nonunion of a scapular body fracture requiring surgical management has been described.[96,110-112]

Fractures of the scapular body and spine, as well as insignificantly displaced fractures of the glenoid, acromial, and coracoid processes, are managed nonoperatively. These patients are initially placed in a sling and swathe immobilizer for comfort. Local ice packs to the affected area are helpful during the first 48 hours, followed by moist heat thereafter. Analgesic medications are prescribed as needed. Absolute immobilization is generally short (48 hours), but it can continue for up to 14 days, depending on the clinical situation. The patient is then permitted to gradually increase the functional use of the upper extremity as symptoms allow, and sling and swathe protection is gradually decreased until the 6-week point.

Physical therapy is prescribed during this period and focuses on maintaining and regaining shoulder range of motion. The program begins with dependent circular and pendulum movements, as well as external rotation to but not past neutral, gradually moving on to progressive stretching techniques in all ranges. Close follow-up is necessary to monitor and guide the patient's recovery, and radiographs are obtained at 2-week intervals to ensure that unacceptable displacement does not occur at the fracture site or sites.

At 6 weeks, osseous union is usually sufficient to discontinue all external protection and encourage functional use of the upper extremity. The rehabilitation program continues until range of motion, strength, and overall function are maximized. Six months to 1 year may be required for full recovery, but a good to excellent result should be readily obtainable.

Isolated Acromial Fractures

The acromial process is formed from two ossification centers: one for its most anterior end and one for its posterolateral tip (its base is actually an extension of the scapular body and spine). The acromial process has four basic functions:

1. It provides one side of the acromioclavicular articulation.
2. It serves as a point of attachment for various musculotendinous and ligamentous structures.
3. It lends posterosuperior stability to the glenohumeral joint.
4. It is an important component of the SSSC (the scapular–clavicular linkage).

Acromial fractures may be caused by a direct blow from the outside or a force transmitted via the humeral head. Avulsion fractures are the result of purely indirect forces occurring where musculotendinous or ligamentous structures (the deltoid and trapezius muscles as well as the coracoacromial and acromioclavicular ligaments) attach to the acromion. Even stress and fatigue fractures have been reported.[113,114] These injuries may be minimally or significantly displaced.[115] Kuhn and colleagues proposed a classification scheme that drew some discussion.[116-119] They emphasized the need for ORIF if an acromial fragment is displaced inferiorly by the pull of the deltoid muscle and is compromising the subacromial space, thereby resulting in impingement symptoms and interfering with rotator cuff function.[120]

The diagnosis is radiographic. True AP and lateral views of the scapula and a true axillary projection of the glenohumeral joint detect most acromial fractures. An os acromiale can complicate the evaluation. On occasion, however, CT scanning may be needed to precisely define the injury and disclose involvement of adjacent bony and articular structures. A weight-bearing AP projection is obtained if disruption of the scapular–clavicular linkage (SSSC) is suspected. Arthrography to evaluate the rotator cuff is considered if an acromial fracture is the result of traumatic superior displacement of the humeral head or chronic superior migration of the proximal humerus as seen in long-standing rotator cuff disease (e.g., cuff tear arthropathy with a stress fracture of the acromion). Madhavan and coauthors[121] described a case in which an acromial fracture was associated with an avulsed subscapularis tendon.

Although significantly displaced, isolated, nonavulsion acromial fractures have been described,[122,123] the vast majority are nondisplaced or minimally displaced. Symptomatic nonoperative care reliably led to union and a good to excellent functional result. Significantly displaced injuries, however, require surgical management. Symptomatic acromial nonunion, although uncommon, has been reported in the literature.[124-126] No more than a small fragment should ever be excised.[127] The presence of a large fragment requires surgical stabilization and bone grafting (Fig. 10-27).

Isolated Coracoid Fractures

The coracoid process develops from two constant ossification centers: one at its base, which also forms the upper third of the glenoid process, and one that becomes its main body. In addition, it has at least two inconstant centers: one at its angle where the coracoclavicular ligament attaches and one at its tip where the conjoined tendon is located. The regions at which the centers finally unite are relatively weak, especially in young adults, thus making fractures more likely to occur when direct or indirect forces are applied.[128,129]

The coracoid process, which has been called the *lighthouse of the anterior shoulder*, has three basic functions:

1. It serves as a point of attachment for a number of musculotendinous and ligamentous structures (Fig. 10-28).
2. It provides the glenohumeral joint with some anterosuperior stability.
3. It is an integral part of the SSSC (the scapular–clavicular linkage).

Coracoid fractures may be caused by a blow from the outside[130] or contact by a dislocating humeral head or by indirect forces applied through the musculotendinous and ligamentous structures at their attachment sites (avulsion fractures fall into this category).[131-134] Fatigue fractures have also been described.[135,136] Other causes include fractures associated with coracoclavicular tape fixation used in acromioclavicular joint reconstructions[137] and fractures associated with massive rotator cuff tears. Despite

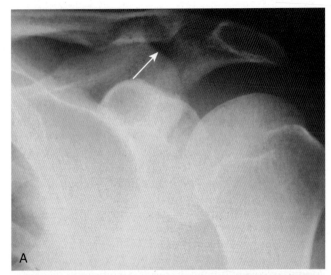

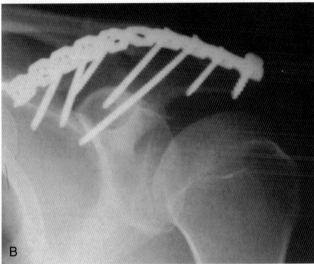

FIGURE 10-27 Radiographs of a patient who sustained a significantly displaced fracture of his acromial process, which went on to a nonunion. **A,** Preoperative AP radiograph showing significant displacement (*arrow*) at the acromial fracture site and minimal healing. **B,** Postoperative AP radiograph showing anatomic reduction at the fracture site and stabilization using a plate-and-screw construct (the site was also bone grafted).

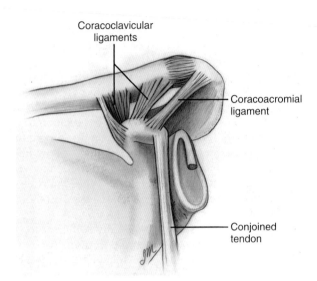

FIGURE 10-28 Illustration showing the coracoid process as the point of attachment for the conjoined tendon, the coracoacromial ligament, and the coracoclavicular ligament.

the relative scarcity of isolated coracoid fractures, several types have been described.[91,127] These injuries can be anatomically divided into the following categories:

1. Fractures of the tip of the coracoid
2. Fractures of the coracoid between the coracoclavicular and coracoacromial ligaments
3. Fractures at the base of the coracoid process

The diagnosis is ultimately radiographic. True AP and axillary projections of the glenohumeral joint disclose, or at least suggest, the presence of most coracoid fractures. Because of the complex bony anatomy in the area,

oblique views[138,139] or even CT scanning[140] may be necessary to detect and accurately define some fractures, as well as injuries to adjacent bony and articular structures. Accessory ossification centers and epiphyseal lines can complicate the evaluation. A weight-bearing AP view of the shoulder is obtained if the integrity of the scapular–clavicular (SSSC) linkage is a concern.

Fractures of the coracoid tip are avulsion injuries—the result of an indirect force applied through the conjoined tendon and concentrated over its attachment to the coracoid process (see Fig. 10-38D). Displacement may be quite marked, but nonsurgical treatment is usually in order.[141,142] Open surgical reduction plus internal fixation has been advocated in athletes, especially those participating in sports that require optimal upper extremity function, and in persons who perform heavy manual labor. Wong-Chung and Quinlan described a case in which a fractured coracoid tip prevented closed reduction of an anterior glenohumeral dislocation.[143] Late surgical treatment may be necessary if the displaced bone fragment causes irritation of the surrounding soft tissues.

Fractures between the coracoclavicular and the coracoacromial ligaments may be the result of either a direct or an indirect force.[144] The distal coracoid fragment is usually significantly displaced, drawn distally by the pull of the conjoined tendon and rotated laterally by the tethering effect of the coracoacromial ligament (Fig. 10-29). Treatment may be nonsurgical or surgical, following the same reasoning described for significantly displaced avulsion fractures of the coracoid tip. Because the fragment is larger, however, symptomatic irritation of the local soft tissues is more common and late surgical management is more likely.

Fractures at the base of the coracoid process are the most common coracoid fractures. They may be caused

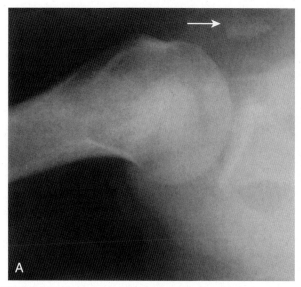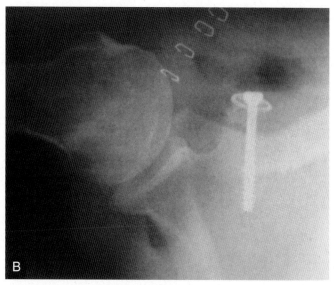

FIGURE 10-29 A patient who sustained a fracture of the distal coracoid process between the coracoclavicular ligament and the coracoacromial ligament. **A,** Preoperative axillary radiograph showing the significantly displaced distal portion of the coracoid process (*arrow*). **B,** Postoperative axillary radiograph showing the bony fragment reduced and stabilized with an interfragmentary screw and a ligament washer. (From Goss TP: Fractures of the scapula: Diagnosis and treatment. In Iannotti JP, Williams GR Jr [eds]: Disorders of the Shoulder: Diagnosis and Management. Philadelphia: Lippincott Williams & Wilkins, 1999, p 628.)

by a direct blow from the outside or by a dislocating humeral head.[145] Avulsion fractures caused by strong traction forces are also possible.[146-149] These injuries are generally minimally displaced due to the stabilizing effect of the surrounding soft tissues, in particular the coracoclavicular ligament (Fig. 10-30). Symptomatic nonsurgical care is usually sufficient, and union occurs within 6 weeks.[141,142,150] McLaughlin said that fibrous union is not uncommon but is rarely associated with discomfort.[29] If a fibrous union is symptomatic, however, bone grafting and compression screw fixation must be considered.

Double Disruptions of the Superior Shoulder Suspensory Complex

The SSSC is a ring of bony and soft tissue at the end of a superior and an inferior bony strut (Fig. 10-31). The ring is composed of the glenoid process, the coracoid process, the coracoclavicular ligament, the distal end of the clavicle, the acromioclavicular joint, the coracoacromial ligament, and the acromial process. The superior strut is the middle third of the clavicle, and the inferior strut is the junction of the most lateral portion of the scapular body and the most medial portion of the glenoid neck. The complex can be divided into three units: the clavicular–acromioclavicular joint–acromial strut, the three-process–scapular body junction, and the C-4 linkage, with additional support provided by the coracoacromial ligament (Fig. 10-32).

The SSSC is an extremely important structure with regard to the biomechanics of the shoulder complex: Each of its components has its own individual function(s),

it serves as a point of attachment for a variety of musculotendinous and ligamentous structures, it allows limited but very important motion to occur through the coracoclavicular ligament and the acromioclavicular articulation, and it maintains a normal stable relationship between the upper extremity and the axial skeleton. The clavicle is the only bony connection between the upper extremity and the axial skeleton, and the scapula is hung or suspended from the clavicle by the coracoclavicular ligament

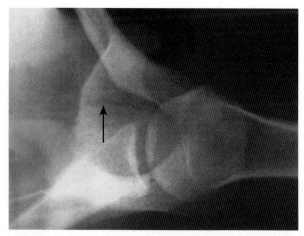

FIGURE 10-30 Axillary radiograph showing an undisplaced fracture of the base of the coracoid process (*arrow*). (From Goss TP: Fractures of the scapula: Diagnosis and treatment. In Iannotti JP, Williams GR Jr [eds]: Disorders of the Shoulder: Diagnosis and Management. Philadelphia: Lippincott Williams & Wilkins, 1999, p 630.)

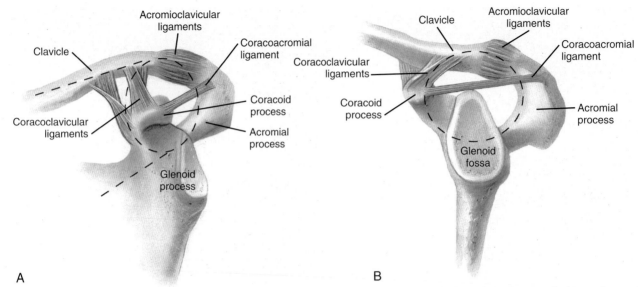

FIGURE 10-31 Illustrations depicting the superior shoulder suspensory complex. **A,** AP view of the bone–soft tissue ring and the superior and inferior bony struts. **B,** Lateral view of the bone–soft tissue ring.

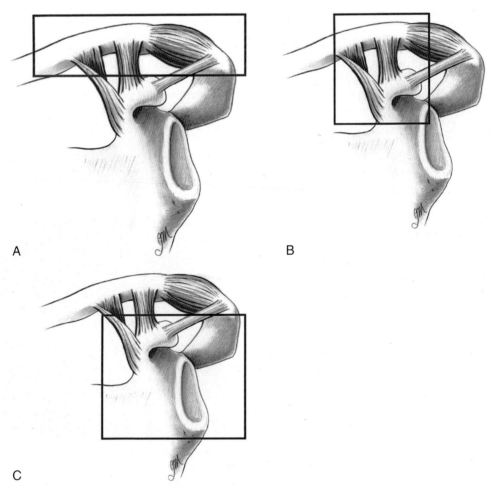

FIGURE 10-32 The three components of the superior shoulder suspensory complex: **A,** the clavicular–acromioclavicular joint–acromial strut; **B,** the clavicular–coracoclavicular ligamentous–coracoid (C-4) linkage; **C,** the three-process–scapular body junction.

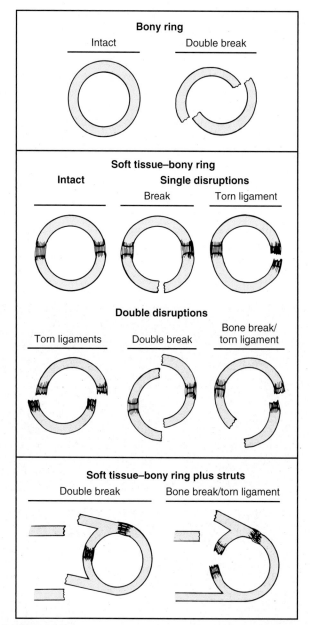

FIGURE 10-33 Illustrations depicting the many possible traumatic ring–strut disruptions. (From Goss TP: Double disruptions of the superior shoulder suspensory complex. J Orthop Trauma 7[2]:99-106, 1993. © Raven Press, Ltd., New York.)

and the acromioclavicular articulation. It is, in fact, the linkage system between the scapula and the clavicle.

The *double-disruption* concept (Box 10-5) is a principle that underlies and allows one to understand a variety of difficult-to-treat injuries of the shoulder complex that have previously been described in isolation but are actually united by a single biomechanical theme. This double-disruption concept also has a certain predictive value regarding injuries that have been encountered only rarely.[40]

Single traumatic disruptions of the SSSC are common (e.g., a type I fracture of the distal end of the clavicle). These are anatomically stable situations because the overall integrity of the complex is not significantly violated, and nonoperative management generally yields a good to excellent result. When the complex is disrupted in two (or more) places (a double disruption), however, the integrity of the SSSC is compromised and a *potentially* unstable anatomic situation is created. Significant displacement can occur at either or both sites and result in bony healing problems (delayed union, malunion, and nonunion[151]), as well as adverse long-term functional difficulties (subacromial impingement, decreased strength, muscle fatigue discomfort, neurovascular compromise from a drooping shoulder, and degenerative joint disease), depending upon the particular injury. Double disruptions can take a variety of forms: two fractures of the bone–soft tissue ring, two ligamentous disruptions of the ring, a fracture and a ligamentous disruption of the ring, fractures of both bony struts, or a fracture of one strut combined with ring disruption (either a fracture or a ligamentous disruption) (Fig. 10-33). When particularly severe forces are involved, there is the potential for complex injury patterns due to multiple ring and strut disruptions. Because the glenoid, acromial, and coracoid processes are all components of the SSSC, many double-disruption injuries involve the scapula. In addition, many, if not most, significantly displaced coracoid and acromial fractures are part of a double disruption.

The coracoid process is a vital part of the SSSC, serving as one of the bony components of the C-4 linkage that joins the scapula to the clavicular–acromioclavicular joint–acromial strut and part of the three-process–scapular body junction. Consequently, if a coracoid process fracture is present and associated with another SSSC injury, the potential adverse consequences of a double disruption must be considered and treatment tailored accordingly.[55] Ogawa and coworkers[152] stated that such fractures were usually deep to the coracoclavicular ligament. They classified them as type I fractures and said that they represented dissociation between the scapula and the clavicle and as such often required ORIF.

The acromial process is one of the components of the clavicular–acromioclavicular joint–acromial strut and part of the three-process–scapular body junction. Acromial fractures that are significantly displaced are usually the result of instability created when other fractures or ligamentous disruptions of the SSSC are present.[55] These injuries are generally the result of high-energy trauma and often require surgical intervention. Ogawa and Naniwa[153] divided acromial fractures into two types: type I (lateral to the spinoglenoid notch) and type II (descending into the spinoglenoid notch). They said that the mechanism of each was different and that type I injuries were more likely to be associated with other injuries to the SSSC (i.e., a double disruption), more likely to be significantly displaced, and more likely to require ORIF.

If a single disruption is noted on routine radiographs (a true AP view of the shoulder, a true axillary view of the glenohumeral joint, and a weight-bearing AP view of the shoulder to evaluate the integrity of the clavicular–scapular linkage [SSSC]), one needs to look carefully for other disruptions (CT scanning is often necessary because

of the complex bony anatomy in the area). If two or more disruptions are present, one must decide whether the displacement at one or both sites is unacceptable ("acceptable" being a relative term, dependent upon the particular clinical situation). If so, surgical management is generally necessary.

The Floating Shoulder (Ipsilateral Fractures of the Midshaft Clavicle and the Glenoid Neck)

The floating shoulder represents a double disruption of the SSSC. In isolation, each fracture is generally minimally displaced and managed nonoperatively. In combination, however, each disruption has the potential to make the other unstable (the glenoid neck fracture allowing severe displacement to occur at the clavicular site, and vice versa) (Fig. 10-34). The situation is rendered even more unstable if an additional disruption of the clavicular–

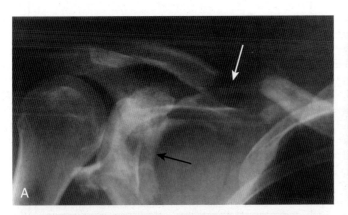
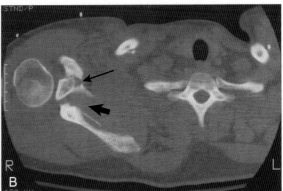
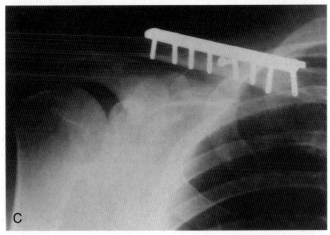

FIGURE 10-34 Radiographs of a patient who sustained a double disruption of the superior shoulder suspensory complex, resulting in a floating shoulder. **A,** Preoperative AP radiograph showing a fracture of the glenoid neck with medial translation (*black arrow*) and a severely displaced fracture of the middle third of the clavicle (*white arrow*). **B,** Preoperative axial CT image showing the glenoid neck fracture to be complete (*thick black arrow*), with the glenoid fragment and the entire superior shoulder suspensory complex rendered particularly unstable by the associated fracture of the coracoid process (*thin black arrow*). **C,** Postoperative AP radiograph showing anatomic reduction and stabilization of the clavicle fracture. The glenoid neck fracture was managed nonoperatively, although a strong case could be made for open reduction and internal fixation in light of its persistent medial translational displacement (the glenoid fragment remained unstable because of the fractured coracoid process, i.e., a double disruption of the superior shoulder suspensory complex was still present). (From Goss TP: Fractures of the scapula: Diagnosis and treatment. In Iannotti JP, Williams GR Jr [eds]: Disorders of the Shoulder: Diagnosis and Management. Philadelphia: Lippincott Williams & Wilkins, 1999, p 624.)

acromioclavicular joint–acromial strut is present or if the C-4 linkage is violated with or without involvement of the coracoacromial ligament. Hardegger and colleagues[56] stated that these injuries represented a "functional imbalance" as a result of "altered glenohumeral–acromial relationships." Both they and Butters[3] recommended surgery to reduce and stabilize the injury.

Surgical reduction plus stabilization of the clavicular fracture site (most commonly with plate fixation) is advisable if displacement is unacceptable in order to avoid nonunion, alleviate tensile forces on the brachial plexus, restore normal anatomic relationships, and ensure restoration of normal shoulder function.[154,155] The glenoid neck fracture can reduce satisfactorily with stabilization of the clavicle. However, if significant displacement persists, it can also require surgical management[156,157] (see "Glenoid Neck [Extra-articular] Fractures"). Additional injuries to the clavicular–acromioclavicular joint–acromial strut can require operative treatment, whereas associated injuries involving the C-4 linkage usually heal satisfactorily if the glenoid neck and other disruption sites are treated appropriately.

Leung and Lam[158] reported on 15 patients treated surgically (average follow-up, 25 months). In 14 of the 15 patients, the fractures healed with a good to excellent functional result. Herscovici and coauthors[159] reported the results of nine patients with ipsilateral clavicular and glenoid neck fractures (average follow-up, 48.5 months). Seven patients were treated surgically with plate fixation of the clavicular fracture site and achieved excellent results. Two patients were treated without surgery and had decreased range of motion and drooping of the involved shoulder. The authors strongly recommended ORIF of the clavicle to prevent glenoid neck malunion. Simpson and Jupiter[160] in a review article indicated that these injuries often require operative treatment. Rikli and associates expanded this concept somewhat, saying that a fracture of the glenoid neck combined with either a fracture of the clavicle or a disruption of the acromioclavicular or sternoclavicular joint results in an unstable shoulder girdle. They reviewed 13 cases (12 in which the clavicular injury was surgically stabilized) and reported excellent results in nearly all.[161]

There has been considerable interest recently in floating shoulders, including both clinical and basic science studies. Edwards and colleagues reported excellent results with conservative treatment of consecutive patients with ipsilateral clavicle and scapula fractures; however, in 5 of the 20 patients the scapula fracture did not involve the glenoid neck.[162] Hashiguchi and Ito reported excellent results in five patients with ipsilateral clavicle and glenoid neck fractures in whom fixation of the clavicle alone was performed.[163] Egol and colleagues reviewed their results in 19 patients (some treated surgically based upon surgeon preference and some treated nonoperatively) and reported good results with each approach.[164] Ramos and coworkers published a series of patients treated nonoperatively who did quite well.[165]

Williams and coworkers conducted a cadaveric study to determine the stability afforded by specific structures. Using a model with ipsilateral glenoid neck and clavicular fractures, they found that instability of the glenoid segment occurred only with subsequent coracoacromial and acromioclavicular ligamentous sectioning. They concluded that floating shoulders only become unstable when there is an associated disruption of those structures.[166]

Van Noort and van der Werken reported on 46 patients with floating shoulder injuries treated operatively or nonoperatively, with mixed results in both groups. They agreed that additional ligamentous disruptions (the coracoacromial, coracoclavicular, or acromioclavicular ligaments) are necessary for significant displacement to occur. They said that significantly displaced clavicular fractures required ORIF and that glenoid neck fractures with significant persistent inferior angulation also needed to be addressed surgically.[64]

Pasapula and colleagues in a review article stated that in the presence of a glenoid neck and a clavicle fracture, various combinations of bony and ligamentous injuries must be present for a true floating shoulder to occur. These were injuries affecting the attachment of the glenoid fragment to the proximal fragment (the acromion, the scapular spine, and the scapular body) via the coracoacromial and acromioclavicular ligaments and the attachment of the glenoid fragment to the axial skeleton through the clavicular shaft via the coracoclavicular ligament. They also said that due to these associated injuries, ORIF of the clavicular fracture alone might not satisfactorily reduce the glenoid neck fracture.[167] Labler and colleagues reviewed 17 patients with such injuries and echoed these sentiments.[168] This would help explain the nature of the injury shown in Figure 10-34. This patient had an associated coracoid process fracture that effectively detached the coracoacromial and coracoclavicular ligaments from the glenoid fragment. These ideas are similar to those expressed for isolated glenoid neck fractures that may require damage to their secondary support system to displace significantly.

Other articles by Van Noort and van der Werken[64] and by DeFranco and Patterson[169] concluded that most floating shoulder injuries do well with nonoperative management and that the criterion for operative treatment is not well established, namely, how much displacement at the fracture site(s) is unacceptable. Current experience seems to indicate that the mere presence of a clavicular and a glenoid neck fracture does not demand operative treatment, and many or most do well nonoperatively. However, the more displacement at one or both sites, the greater the need for ORIF, and another disruption of the SSSC may be necessary for significant displacement to occur.[170]

Fracture of the Coracoid Process and a Grade III Disruption of the Acromioclavicular Joint

On occasion, especially in young adults, a force that would otherwise cause a grade III sprain of the acromioclavicular joint results in an avulsion fracture of the base of the coracoid process or the bony attachment of the coracoclavicular ligament to the angle of the coracoid process instead of a disruption of the coracoclavicular ligament (see Fig. 10-38C). A weight-bearing AP projection of the shoulder complex shows displacement of the distal end of the clavicle above the superior border of the acromion, but the coracoclavicular interval remains normal. Treatment of injuries associated with a small bony avulsion fracture of the angle of the coracoid process follows the principles developed for grade III acromioclavicular joint disruptions—specifically, surgical repair of the acromioclavicular joint needs to be considered in young people engaged in athletics or heavy manual labor. Disruptions associated with a fracture of the base

of the coracoid process (especially if the fracture is significantly displaced) are considered for surgical ORIF of both sites to avoid the adverse long-term effects of a grade III acromioclavicular separation and a nonunion of the coracoid process. Reports in the literature have described both operative and nonoperative management of these injuries.[91,92,128,129,155,171-178]

Fractures of the Ipsilateral Coracoid and Acromial Processes

Isolated fractures of the coracoid and acromial processes (Fig. 10-35) are usually minimally displaced and therefore managed nonoperatively. When they occur together, however, they constitute a double disruption of the SSSC,

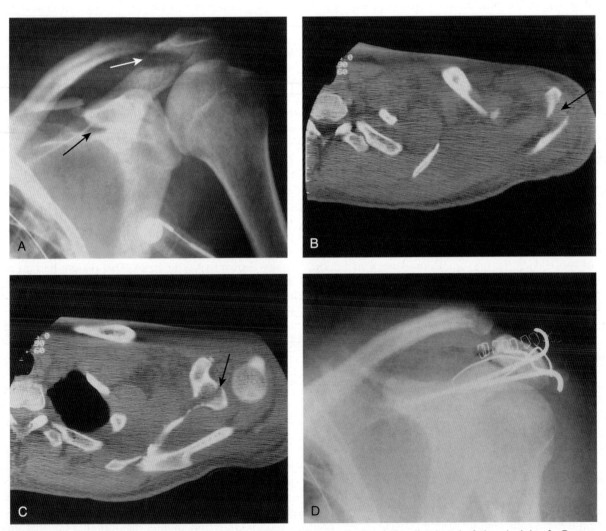

FIGURE 10-35 Ipsilateral fractures of the coracoid and acromial processes and the distal end of the clavicle. **A,** Preoperative AP radiograph of the involved area. The *white arrow* indicates the acromial fracture; the *black arrow* indicates the coracoid fracture. **B,** Preoperative axial CT image showing wide separation at the acromial fracture site (*arrow*) as a result of the associated coracoid process fracture. **C,** Preoperative axial CT image showing the fractured coracoid process (*arrow*). **D,** Postoperative AP radiograph of the shoulder showing reduction and stabilization of the acromial fracture with a tension band construct. The coracoid process fracture and distal clavicle fracture were not addressed surgically and healed spontaneously. (From Goss TP: Fractures of the scapula: Diagnosis and treatment. In Iannotti JP, Williams GR Jr [eds]: Disorders of the Shoulder: Diagnosis and Management. Philadelphia: Lippincott Williams & Wilkins, 1999, p 625.)

a *potentially* unstable anatomic situation.[142] If displacement at either or both sites is unacceptable, surgical management is indicated. ORIF of the acromial fracture may be all that is required. It often indirectly reduces and stabilizes the coracoid fracture satisfactorily and is technically less difficult than addressing the coracoid injury. If ORIF of the acromial fracture does not improve the coracoid fracture, however, the coracoid fracture may need to be reduced and stabilized as well. Lim and coworkers described such an injury managed with ORIF of both sites.[179]

Fracture of the Base of the Coracoid Process and a Fracture of the Glenoid Neck

A fracture of the glenoid neck can become displaced only if it is complete (i.e., if the fracture line exits the lateral scapular border and the superior scapular margin adjacent to the coracoid process). Even so, if continuity of the glenoid fragment with the clavicular–acromioclavicular joint–acromial strut via the C-4 linkage is intact, the displacement is usually minimal. If, however, this secondary support system is disrupted with or without involvement of the coracoacromial ligament (e.g., a fracture of the base of the coracoid process), significant displacement of the glenoid fragment is particularly likely (translational displacement of ≥ 1 cm, or angular displacement of ≥ 40 degrees, or both), and surgical management must be considered (see Fig. 10-13).[58] Operative treatment consists of ORIF of the glenoid neck fracture via either a posterior or a posterosuperior approach (see "Glenoid Neck [Extra-articular] Fractures"). The coracoid fracture usually heals without direct intervention.

Fracture of the Coracoid Process and a Type I Fracture of the Distal Third of the Clavicle

Fractures of the distal third of the clavicle can become unacceptably displaced if the continuity of the coracoclavicular ligament between the coracoid process and the proximal clavicular segment is disrupted (type II and type V fractures).[9,180-183] The same situation can occur with type I fractures if the coracoid process is fractured (Fig. 10-36). It would probably make most sense to call all of these injuries type II fractures—that is, situations in which the distal third of the clavicle is fractured and the linkage between the proximal segment and the scapula (the C-4 linkage) is disrupted (Box 10-6).

If displacement at the clavicular fracture site is of such a degree that delayed union or nonunion is likely, treatment consists of surgical reduction and stabilization of the injury (usually by means of tension band fixation). The coracoid fracture can reduce secondarily and heal uneventfully. If it does not, the coracoid fracture may need to be addressed surgically as well.

Acromial Fracture and a Grade III Disruption of the Acromioclavicular Joint

The combination of acromial fracture and a grade III disruption of the acromioclavicular joint creates a free-

---

BOX 10-6 Type II Distal Clavicular Fractures

Features
Fracture of the distal third of the clavicle plus a disruption of the linkage between the proximal clavicular segment and the scapula

Treatment
Open reduction and internal fixation for significant displacement

---

floating acromial fragment and can lead to a nonunion as well as the well-described adverse long-term functional consequences associated with an acromioclavicular joint disruption. A case report by McGahan and Rab described a patient with an associated axillary nerve deficit.[184] Acutely, isolated grade III acromioclavicular joint disruptions are usually managed nonoperatively.

However, in this situation, if displacement at the acromial fracture site is unacceptable, surgical reduction and stabilization of both injuries is indicated. Kurdy and Shah[86] described a patient treated nonoperatively who had "a satisfactory outcome; however, he was 74 years old and an acromial non-union occurred." Gorczyca and coauthors[185] described an injury that gradually displaced over time and eventually required surgical ORIF. Torrens and colleagues described a combined type VI acromioclavicular joint disruption and an acromial fracture requiring ORIF of both injury sites.[186]

Segmental Fracture of the Acromion

As with segmental fractures of other bones, two acromial disruptions create an unstable intermediate segment (Fig. 10-37). If the displacement at one or both sites is unacceptable and nonunion is likely, ORIF with plate fixation or a tension band construct, or both, is performed via a posterolateral approach.

Other Combinations

Type III, Vb, and Vc glenoid cavity fractures and another disruption of the superior shoulder suspensory complex are discussed in the section "Glenoid Cavity (Intra-articular) Fractures" (see Fig. 10-23).

Avulsion Fractures of the Scapula

Most of the scapula is formed by intramembranous ossification, but it also has at least six or seven secondary ossification centers. As with other scapula fractures, avulsion injuries are uncommon. By definition, they are caused by indirect forces applied to the surrounding musculotendinous and ligamentous tissues and concentrated at their scapular attachment sites. Three mechanisms are possible: a severe, uncontrolled muscular contraction caused by electroconvulsive treatment, an electric shock, or an epileptic seizure[42,76,174,187-195]; a strong

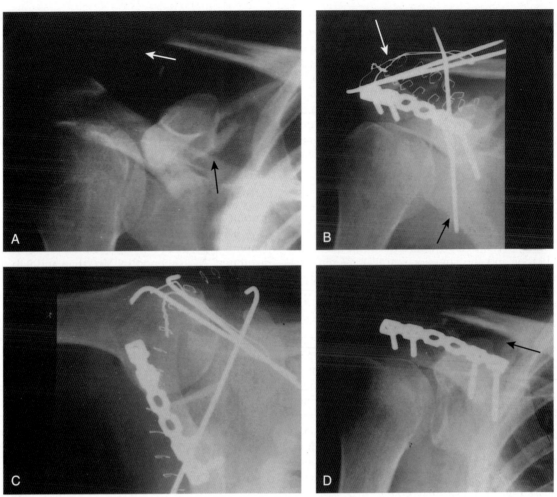

FIGURE 10-36 A patient who sustained a fracture at the base of the coracoid process, a type I fracture of the distal end of the clavicle, and a nondisplaced fracture of the acromion. **A,** Preoperative AP radiograph showing severe displacement at the distal clavicular fracture site (*white arrow*) and the coracoid fracture site (*black arrow*). Postoperative AP (**B**) and axillary (**C**) radiographs show reduction and stabilization of the clavicular fracture with a tension band construct (*white arrow*) and reduction and stabilization of the coracoid process fracture by means of a transfixing Kirschner wire passed into the glenoid process (a cannulated interfragmentary screw would now be used). The acromial fracture was plated (*black arrow*). **D,** An AP radiograph taken 3 months postoperatively after removal of hardware shows the distal clavicle and coracoid fractures to be healed and the superior shoulder suspensory relationships re-established (*arrow*). (From Goss TP: Fractures of the scapula: Diagnosis and treatment. In Iannotti JP, Williams GR Jr [eds]: Disorders of the Shoulder: Diagnosis and Management. Philadelphia: Lippincott Williams & Wilkins, 1999, p 626.)

indirect force associated with a single traumatic event[78,178,196,197]; and a gradual bony failure caused by lesser but repetitive traumatic events (stress[198] or fatigue[114] fractures). The potential varieties are numerous, and many have been described.

Diagnosis and Treatment

True AP and lateral projections of the scapula and a true axillary view of the glenohumeral joint constitute the diagnostic trauma series. It may be supplemented as needed by CT scanning and a weight-bearing view of the shoulder complex. Treatment is, by and large, symptom-atic and nonoperative. However, if the fracture is significantly displaced and of functional importance, ORIF must be considered.[127]

Nonoperative Treatment

Some injuries are managed quite successfully nonoperatively.[97] These include avulsion fracture of the superior angle of the scapula (insertion of the levator scapulae) (Fig. 10-38A)[125]; avulsion fracture through the body of the scapula caused by an accidental electrical shock[174,195,200,201]; avulsion fracture of the infraglenoid tubercle (origin of the long head of the triceps) and the lateral border of the

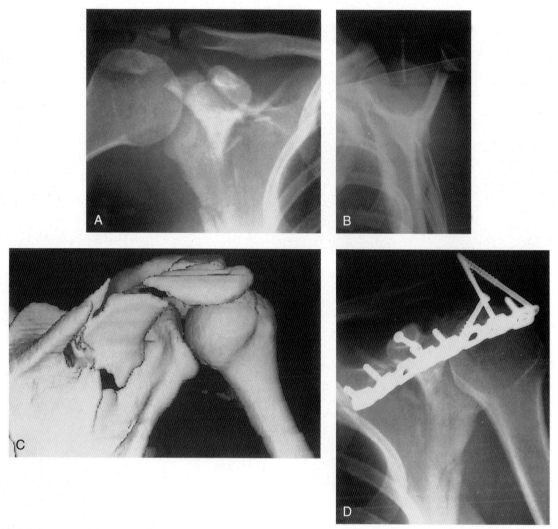

FIGURE 10-37 Segmental fracture of the acromial process and a comminuted fracture of the scapular body. **A,** Preoperative AP radiograph. **B,** Preoperative lateral scapula radiograph. **C,** Preoperative 3D CT radiograph. **D,** Postoperative AP radiograph showing the acromial fractures reduced and stabilized with a malleable reconstruction plate. (From Goss TP: The scapula: Coracoid, acromial, and avulsion fractures. Am J Orthop 25[2]:106-115, 1996.)

scapula (origin of the teres major and minor muscles)[174]; and avulsion fracture of the infraspinatus fossa (origin of the infraspinatus muscle[202]), which must be differentiated from a developmental anomaly.[165]

Avulsion fracture of the superior border of the scapula can also be managed nonoperatively.[199] This injury is often associated with a fracture of the base of the coracoid process and an acromioclavicular joint disruption.[85,202] Some have attributed it to indirect stress applied via the omohyoid muscle,[203-205] and others have considered it an extension of a coracoid fracture.[206]

Operative Treatment

Some avulsion fractures deserve, at the very least, operative consideration, such as avulsion fracture of the lateral margin of the acromial process (see Fig. 10-38B) (origin of the deltoid muscle).[174]

The deltoid muscle is the most important dynamic structure about the glenohumeral joint. Consequently, if this fracture is significantly displaced, surgical reattachment is indicated. Reattachment is rather simply accomplished with multiple nonabsorbable sutures passed in a horizontal mattress fashion through the deltoid and drill holes made along the periphery of the acromial process.

Two cases of an avulsion fracture through the body of the acromion have been described.[207,208] Both were caused by a significant force transmitted through the surrounding musculature, especially the deltoid. One was treated nonsurgically, and the second was managed surgically. Bony union and satisfactory return of function were realized in both.

Isolated avulsion fractures of the coracoid process may benefit from surgery (see Fig. 10-29) (see "Isolated Coracoid Fractures").

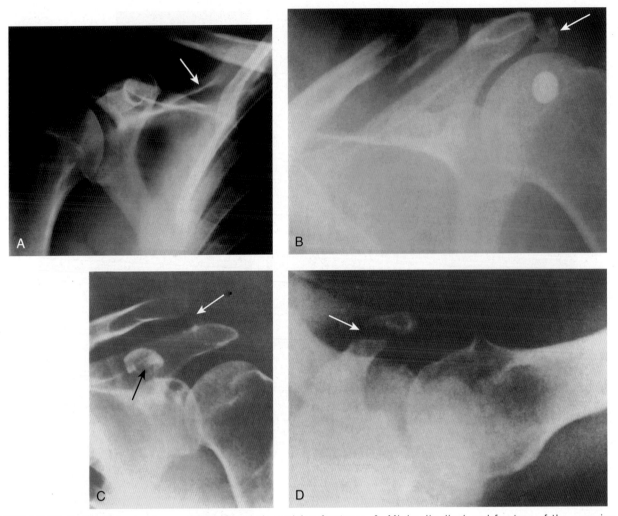

FIGURE 10-38 Radiograph showing a variety of scapula avulsion fractures. **A,** Minimally displaced fracture of the superior angle of the scapula (attachment of the levator scapulae [*arrow*]). **B,** Displaced fracture of the lateral margin of the acromial process (origin of the deltoid muscle [*arrow*]). **C,** Type III disruption of the acromioclavicular joint (*white arrow*) with an associated avulsion fracture at the base of the coracoid process (*black arrow*). **D,** Displaced fracture of the tip of the coracoid process (attachment of the conjoined tendon [*arrow*]). (From Goss TP: Fractures of the scapula: Diagnosis and treatment. In Iannotti JP, Williams GR Jr [eds]: Disorders of the Shoulder: Diagnosis and Management. Philadelphia: Lippincott Williams & Wilkins, 1999, p 632.)

Avulsion fracture of the superior angle of the coracoid process (attachment of the coracoclavicular ligament)[128] or the base of the coracoid process can occur in association with a disruption of the acromioclavicular joint (see Fig. 10-38C) (see "Fracture of the Coracoid Process and a Grade III Disruption of the Acromioclavicular Joint").

Avulsion fracture of the inferior angle of the scapula (Fig. 10-39) (insertion of the serratus anterior muscle) is a rare injury.[209] If significantly displaced, this injury causes winging of the scapula and can compromise shoulder function considerably, in which case, ORIF is indicated.[210] (This might be the fracture Longabaugh described in 1924.[211]) Franco and colleagues described an avulsion fracture of the inferior angle of the scapula presumably caused by prolonged coughing.[212]

Avulsion fracture of the supraglenoid tubercle (origin of the long head of the biceps muscle) indicates a dis-

placed, possibly symptomatic SLAP (superior labral anterior to posterior) lesion.[213]

OTHER DISORDERS

Lateral Dislocation of the Scapula (Scapulothoracic Dissociation)

Scapulothoracic dissociation is a rare traumatic disruption of the scapulothoracic articulation caused by a severe direct force applied over the shoulder accompanied by traction applied to the upper extremity (Box 10-7).[14,20,46,214-222] Although the skin remains intact, the scapula is torn away from the posterior chest wall, prompting some to call this injury a *closed traumatic forequarter amputation*.

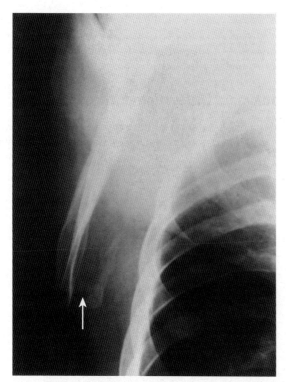

FIGURE 10-39 Lateral radiograph of the scapula showing a severely displaced avulsion fracture of the inferior angle (insertion of the serratus anterior muscle [*arrow*]). (From Goss TP: Fractures of the scapula: Diagnosis and treatment. In Iannotti JP, Williams GR Jr [eds]: Disorders of the Shoulder: Diagnosis and Management. Philadelphia: Lippincott Williams & Wilkins, 1999, p 633.)

Because of the violent forces involved, any of the three bones in the shoulder complex (the clavicle, the scapula, and the proximal end of the humerus) may be fractured, and any of the remaining three articulations (the glenohumeral, acromioclavicular, and sternoclavicular joints) may be disrupted. Neurovascular injury is common. Disruption of the subclavian or axillary artery (more commonly the former) and complete or partial disruption of the brachial plexus are well described. In addition, the

---

BOX 10-7 Scapulothoracic Dissociation

Features
Violent trauma

Massive swelling

Neurovascular compromise

Lateral displacement on chest radiograph

Awareness of entity

Treatment
Reduce and stabilize the sternal–clavicular–acromial linkage

---

soft tissue supporting structures can suffer severe damage, especially those that run from the chest wall to the scapula or from the chest wall to the humerus. Complete or partial tears of the trapezius, levator scapulae, rhomboids, pectoralis minor, and latissimus dorsi have all been reported.

A presumptive diagnosis is based on a history of violent trauma and the presence of massive soft tissue swelling over the shoulder girdle. A pulseless upper extremity, indicating a complete vascular disruption, and a complete or partial neurologic deficit, indicating an injury to the brachial plexus, are quite suggestive. Significant lateral displacement of the scapula seen on a nonrotated chest radiograph confirms the diagnosis. As with all rare injuries, awareness of the clinical entity is critical to making the diagnosis.

Treatment recommendations have focused on care of the accompanying neurovascular injury. If the vascular integrity of the extremity is in question, an emergency arteriogram is performed, followed by surgical repair, if necessary. The brachial plexus is explored at the same time. If a neurologic deficit is present, EMG testing is performed 3 weeks after injury to determine the extent of damage and assess the degree of recovery, if any. Cervical myelography can be performed at 6 weeks. If nerve root avulsion or a complete neurologic deficit is present, the prognosis for functional recovery is poor.[223,224] Partial plexus injuries, however, have a good prognosis, and most patients achieve complete recovery or regain functional use of the extremity. If some portions of the plexus are intact and others are disrupted, neurologic repair is a possibility. Late reconstructive efforts are guided by the degree of neurologic return, and musculotendinous transfers are performed as needed.

Care of the surrounding soft tissue supportive structures (musculotendinous and ligamentous) has been nonoperative and consists of protection of the shoulder complex for 6 weeks to allow healing, combined with a closely monitored progressive physical therapy program designed to restore range of motion initially and then restore strength. Magnetic resonance imaging (MRI) of the involved area now offers the ability to visualize important disruptions that may be amenable to surgical repair.

Injury to the sternal–clavicular–acromial linkage (a disruption of the sternoclavicular or acromioclavicular joint or a fracture of the clavicle) is usually, if not invariably, present for posterolateral displacement of the scapula to occur. This component of scapulothoracic dissociation has been largely ignored in terms of diagnosis and treatment. Of the three possible disruptions, a fracture of the clavicle seems to be the most common. This anatomic situation is very unstable—the clavicular injury allows maximal displacement of the scapula, and the unstable scapulothoracic articulation often leads to significant displacement at the clavicular fracture site. Consequently, ORIF of the clavicle (screw-and-plate fixation for fractures of the middle third, and tension band fixation for fractures of the distal third) is considered in order to avoid delayed union or nonunion, restore as much stability as possible to the shoulder complex to avoid adverse long-term functional consequences, and protect the brachial plexus as well as the subclavian and axillary vessels from further injury caused by tensile forces (Fig. 10-40).[225]

Uhl and Hospeder[226] described a lesser injury characterized by progressive subluxation of the scapulothoracic articulation and a clavicle fracture (no neurovascular involvement) requiring ORIF of the clavicle. Similar thera-peutic reasoning would apply to scapulothoracic dissociations accompanied by a disruption of the acro-mioclavicular or the sternoclavicular joint, although with the latter, metallic fixation devices must be avoided.

Intrathoracic Dislocation of the Scapula

Intrathoracic dislocation of the scapula is extremely rare. Cases associated with minimal violence and a preexisting factor (generalized laxity or a locking osteochondroma)

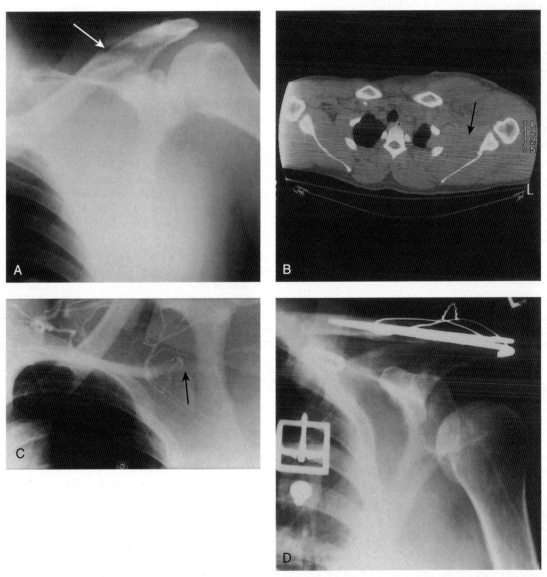

FIGURE 10-40 Patient who sustained a left scapulothoracic dissociation. **A,** Preoperative AP radiograph showing significant lateral displacement of the scapula (*arrow*) and a significantly displaced fracture of the distal end of the clavicle. **B,** CT image showing significantly increased distance between the left scapula and the rib cage (*arrow*) as compared to the opposite (uninjured) side. **C,** Arteriogram showing disruption of the subclavian artery (*arrow*). **D,** Postoperative AP radiograph showing reduction and stabilization of the distal clavicle fracture (and secondarily the scapulothoracic articulation) by means of a tension band construct. (From Goss TP: Fractures of the scapula: Diagnosis and treatment. In Iannotti JP, Williams GR Jr [eds]: Disorders of the Shoulder: Diagnosis and Management. Philadelphia: Lippincott Williams & Wilkins, 1999, p 634.)

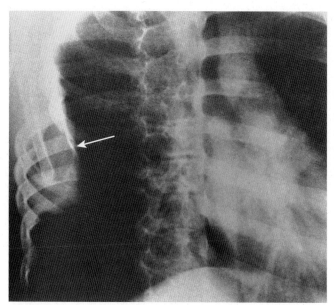

FIGURE 10-41 An anterior oblique radiograph taken of a patient who sustained an intrathoracic dislocation of his right scapula (*arrow*). (From Nettrour LF, Krufky EL, Mueller RE, Raycroft JF: Locked scapula: Intrathoracic dislocation of the inferior angle. J Bone Joint Surg Am 54:413-416, 1972.)

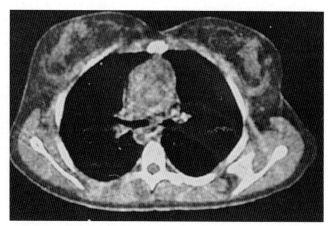

FIGURE 10-42 CT scan of the scapular body showing a large osteochondroma on the costal surface, which caused a snapping scapula.

have been described.[227] The scapula becomes locked within the posterior aspect of one of the upper intercostal spaces.[228] A second type is caused by more violent trauma, either a direct blow over the posterior aspect of the scapula or a violent outward distractive force applied to the arm. The scapular body is displaced anterolaterally, and its inferior angle becomes lodged between the ribs (Fig. 10-41). The severity of the event usually causes a fracture of the scapula and ribs and a marked disruption of the periscapular soft tissues.[229] Pell and Whipple described a patient who sustained a fracture of the scapular body with the inferior angle locked within the fourth intercostal space that was managed successfully by closed reduction.[230]

The diagnosis may be missed initially because of associated injuries, inadequate radiographic projections, or both.[228] Displacement of the scapula might not be readily apparent on routine AP chest radiographs. Tangential views (anterior oblique or lateral scapular projections) or a chest CT may be necessary to establish the diagnosis.

Acute injuries are reduced in a closed fashion under anesthesia by hyperabducting the arm and manually manipulating the scapula (rotating the scapula forward and pushing it backward)[5] while steady traction is applied to the arm. The reduction is usually stable, but securing the scapula to the chest wall with adhesive tape or immobilizing the arm in a sling and swathe binder is advisable for comfort and soft tissue healing.[229] The dressing and immobilizer are changed at 7 to 10 days and discontinued 2 weeks thereafter. Unprotected, progressive functional use of the shoulder and arm is then encouraged. In long-standing cases, open reduction with soft tissue detachment may be necessary, followed by reconstruction of the periscapular tissues to re-establish stability.[228]

Scapulothoracic Crepitus

Scapulothoracic crepitus (described under various terms but most often called *snapping scapula*)[8,9,231-234] was first described by Boinet[235] in 1867. Mauclaire[236] noted three varieties: *froissemant* (an asymptomatic gentle sound thought to be physiologic); *froittemant* (a louder sound, possibly symptomatic and, if so, more likely to be due to soft tissue pathology); and *craquemont* (a loud sound, often symptomatic and, if so, more likely to result from bony pathology). These sounds were believed to have two general etiologies: abnormalities within the tissues between the scapula and the chest wall and abnormalities of scapulothoracic congruence.

Etiology

Pathologic conditions affecting the musculature lying within the scapulothoracic interval that can cause crepitus include atrophy,[33,233,237] tears, fibrosis and scarring,[233,238,239] and anomalous muscle insertions.[237,240] Representative cases have been described by Milch,[233,238,241] Bateman,[2] Strizak and Cowen,[242] and Rockwood.[33]

Bony abnormalities within the scapulothoracic interval that can cause crepitus include osteochondromas over the ventral surface of the scapula (Fig. 10-42),[128,238,241,243-245] rib exostoses,[65] Luschka's tubercle[233,246] (a bony prominence at the superomedial angle of the scapula), a hooked superomedial angle of the scapula,[233,247] malunited fractures of the ribs or scapula,[17,233,238] and reactive bony spurs secondary to repeated microtrauma at soft tissue attachment sites (Fig. 10-43).[2,242,248]

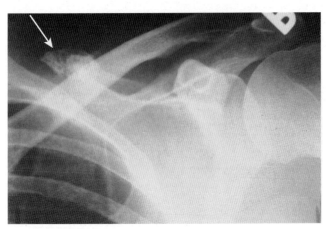

FIGURE 10-43 Radiograph of a patient with pain and crepitus over the superomedial aspect of her scapula (*arrow*). Note the significant exostosis, which was subsequently surgically removed, alleviating the patient's discomfort and dysfunction.

Scapulothoracic bursitis can also be accompanied by scapulothoracic crepitus.[232,249-255] The most common sites are at the superomedial angle of the scapula between the serratus anterior and subscapularis muscles, between the serratus anterior and the lateral chest wall, and at the inferior angle of the scapula.[256-258]

Other rather rare causes have been described, including Sprengel's deformity (possibly related to the omohyoid bone or the abnormal scapular shape), tuberculous lesions[233] in the region, and syphilitic lues.[233] Finally, scoliosis[259,260] and thoracic kyphosis[231] can cause scapulothoracic incongruence leading to localized crepitus.

Diagnosis

When evaluating such patients, the history, physical examination, and radiologic evaluation can provide a number of clues to the diagnosis. Does the patient have a history of acute trauma involving the scapular body, the ribs, or the scapulothoracic articulation? Does the patient have a history of forceful or repetitive use of the scapulothoracic articulation? Can the patient identify the location of the crepitus or can the physician do the same by palpation or auscultation as the shoulder girdle is put through a range of motion? Visual inspection can disclose fullness or pseudowinging of the scapula, suggesting a deep surface mass. EMG testing may be indicated to evaluate the neuromuscular status of the shoulder girdle. AP and especially lateral views of the scapula are obtained to visualize the scapulothoracic interval, and CT or MRI scanning may be indicated in an effort to identify bony or soft tissue pathology (or both) in the region. One must always bear in mind that the presence of scapulothoracic crepitus may be clinically insignificant, in which case other sources of posterior shoulder discomfort must be considered, including local pathology and referred pain from nearby or distant sources.

Treatment

When considering treatment, one must ultimately decide whether the scapulothoracic crepitus is truly associated with pain and therefore reflects localized scapulothoracic pathology. In this regard it is important to remember that scapulothoracic crepitus has been noted in 35% of asymptomatic persons[261] and that those with hidden agendas or psychiatric conditions can misrepresent its importance. Patients with a well-defined bony prominence within the scapulothoracic interval usually respond quite nicely to surgical removal (see Fig. 10-43).[3,245,262]

With most persons, however, the etiology of the painful crepitus is not obvious, making nonoperative care the treatment of choice, at least initially. Such management can include a number of modalities: local application of ice, heat, or both; exercises to strengthen the shoulder girdle musculature[233,254,256]; postural training (a figure-of-eight dressing may be used to remind patients to maintain an upright posture)[256,263]; local injections of lidocaine (Xylocaine) and a steroid into particularly symptomatic areas for diagnostic and therapeutic purposes[3,231,253,254,264]; rest or avoidance of aggravating positions and activities; analgesics; nonsteroidal antiinflammatory medications; massage; phonophoresis; ultrasound; and application of ethyl chloride to trigger points. Most patients respond satisfactorily to these measures.

For those who fail nonoperative therapy, surgery may be an option if the physician thinks that a definable pathologic lesion is present—the procedure depends the nature of the presumed pathology. Procedures have been described wherein a local muscle flap is sutured over the undersurface of the scapula.[236] Rockwood[33] described excision of an avulsed flap of rhomboid muscle with satisfactory relief of pain and crepitus. Partial scapulectomy, including resection of the medial border of the scapula[265] or the superomedial angle,[231,233,237,242,247,249,266] has been fairly popular when symptoms can be localized to these areas. For symptomatic bursitis associated with crepitus, procedures described have included open bursectomy[252,253,267] and arthroscopic bursectomy.[79,256,257,268,269]

AUTHORS' PREFERRED METHOD OF TREATMENT

Scapular Body and Spine Fractures

Patients with fractures of the body and spine of the scapula are examined carefully for associated injuries, which are quite common and may be life threatening. Symptomatic and nonoperative care is almost always indicated and consists of immobilization initially, followed by a progressive rehabilitation program focusing on regaining range of motion at first and then strength. Six weeks is usually necessary for healing, although continued therapy is generally required to achieve an optimal result. A good to excellent outcome can be expected.[20,21]

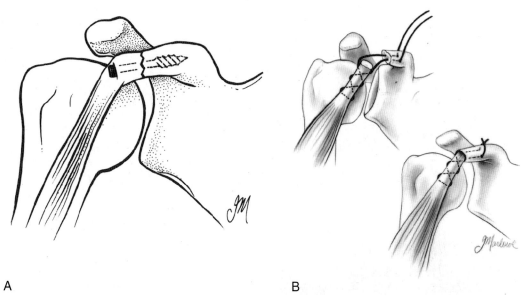

A   B

FIGURE 10-44 Illustrations showing two surgical techniques for managing coracoid process fractures. **A,** Interfragmentary screw fixation may be used if the fragment is sufficiently large and not comminuted. **B,** Excision of the distal fragment for small or comminuted fractures and suture fixation of the conjoined tendon to the remaining coracoid process. (Redrawn from Goss TP: Fractures of the scapula: Diagnosis and treatment. In Iannotti JP, Williams GR Jr [eds]: Disorders of the Shoulder: Diagnosis and Management. Philadelphia: Lippincott Williams & Wilkins, 1999, p 628.)

Isolated Coracoid Process Fractures[20]

Fractures of the coracoid tip are generally managed nonoperatively initially. However, late surgical management may be necessary if the displaced bony fragment causes irritation of the surrounding soft tissues.[270] Surgical management (either acute or late) takes two forms[271]: ORIF of the bony fragment if it is sufficiently large and not comminuted and excision of the fragment if comminuted with suture fixation of the conjoined tendon to the remaining coracoid process (Fig. 10-44). With fractures occurring between the coracoclavicular and coracoacromial ligaments, the fragment is larger and symptomatic irritation of local soft tissues is more likely. Consequently, surgical management (acute or late) is more likely. The size of the fragment generally makes it amenable to interfragmentary screw fixation. Cannulated 3.5- and 4.0-mm compression screws are particularly useful. With fractures of the base of the coracoid process, nonoperative care is usually sufficient. However, in the event of symptomatic nonunion, bone grafting and compression screw fixation must be considered. As with all coracoid process fractures managed surgically, an anterior deltoid–splitting approach is used, and the rotator interval is opened as need be for optimal exposure of the fracture site (Fig. 10-45).

Isolated Acromial Process Fractures[20]

Symptomatic, nonoperative care generally leads to union and a good to excellent functional result. If unacceptable displacement is present, however, surgical reduction and stabilization must be considered. A tension band construct is usually chosen for distal disruptions where the acromial process is quite thin, whereas 3.5-mm malleable reconstruction plates are generally chosen for more proximal injuries (Fig. 10-46).[19]

Double Disruptions of the Superior Shoulder Suspensory Complex

If two (or more) disruptions of the SSSC are present, one must decide whether displacement at one or both sites is unacceptable (unacceptable being a relative term that depends upon the particular clinical situation), and if so, surgical management is generally necessary. Reducing and stabilizing one of the disruptions often indirectly reduces and stabilizes the other disruption satisfactorily (whichever injury is easier to manage is chosen). If unsuccessful, both disruptions might need to be addressed. The results, as always, depend on the adequacy of the reduction, the quality of the fixation, and the rigor of the postoperative rehabilitation program.

Avulsion Fractures of the Scapula

The majority of these injuries are managed nonoperatively; however, ORIF is indicated if the fracture is significantly displaced and functionally significant.

Glenoid Process Fractures (General Considerations)

The glenoid process includes the glenoid neck and the glenoid cavity. Each of these areas may be fractured in

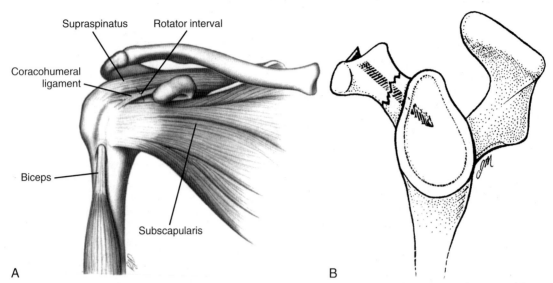

FIGURE 10-45 A, The rotator interval incised and the surrounding soft tissues retracted to expose the coracoid process, including its junction with the glenoid process. **B,** A coracoid process fracture reduced and stabilized with an interfragmentary compression screw.

a variety of ways. The vast majority (>90%) of these injuries are managed satisfactorily nonoperatively, and a good to excellent result can be expected. Most investigators, however, agree that if displacement is significant, surgical management is indicated or should at least be considered.

Principles of Surgery

Several operative principles apply (Box 10-8). The glenoid process may be approached from three directions or combinations thereof, depending on the clinical situation.[272] The anterior approach is used for fractures of the anterior glenoid rim and at least in part for some fractures involving the superior aspect of the glenoid fossa (Fig. 10-47). Some injuries require only opening the rotator interval (see Fig. 10-45) without detaching the subscapularis tendon. The posterior approach is used for fractures of the posterior rim, most fractures of the glenoid fossa, and fractures of the glenoid neck (Figs. 10-48 and 10-49). The superior approach may be used for fractures of the

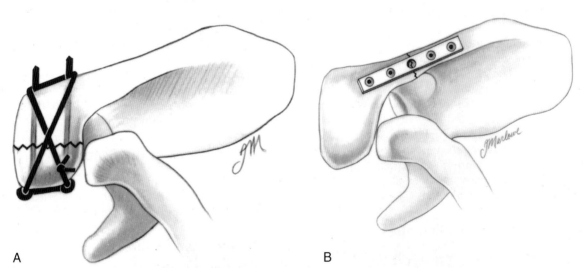

FIGURE 10-46 Two surgical techniques for managing fractures of the acromial process. **A,** A tension band construct (most appropriate for fractures of the distal portion of the acromion). **B,** Plate and screw fixation (most appropriate for proximal fractures). (From Goss TP: The scapula: Coracoid, acromial, and avulsion fractures. Am J Orthop 25[2]:106-115, 1996.)

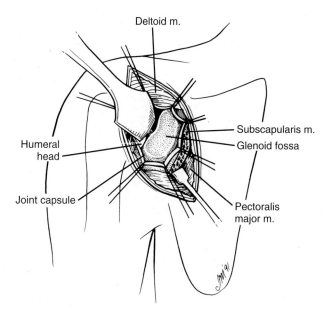

FIGURE 10-47 Anterior surgical approach to the glenoid cavity. (From Goss TP: Fractures of the glenoid cavity: Operative principles and techniques. Techniques in Orthopaedics 8[3]:199-204, 1993. © Raven Press, Ltd., New York.)

glenoid fossa that have a difficult-to-control superior fragment (in conjunction with a posterior exposure) and fractures of the glenoid neck that have a difficult-to-control glenoid fragment (in conjunction with a posterior exposure) (Figs. 10-50 and 10-51). Klingman and Roffman described a variation of the posterior approach which they stated allowed ORIF of anterior as well as posterior glenoid fragments.[257] Van Noort and colleagues described

a limited posterior approach,[273] and Ombremsky and Lyman described a modified Judet (posterior) approach for ORIF of glenoid process fractures.[274]

Thick, solid bone for fixation is at a premium because much of the scapula is paper thin. Four areas, however,

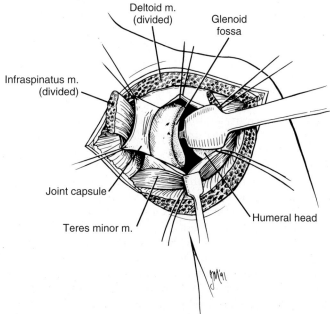

FIGURE 10-48 Posterior surgical approach to the glenoid cavity: standard exposure. (From Goss TP: Fractures of the glenoid cavity: Operative principles and techniques. Techniques in Orthopaedics 8[3]:199-204, 1993. © Raven Press, Ltd., New York.)

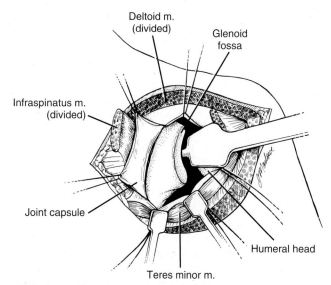

FIGURE 10-49 Posterior surgical approach to the glenoid cavity with development of the infraspinatus–teres minor interval to expose the posteroinferior glenoid cavity and the lateral scapular border. (From Goss TP: Fractures of the glenoid cavity: Operative principles and techniques. Techniques in Orthopaedics 8[3]:199-204, 1993. © Raven Press, Ltd., New York.)

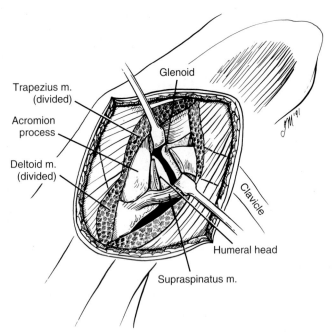

FIGURE 10-50 Superior surgical approach to the glenoid cavity: soft tissue and bony anatomy. (From Goss TP: Fractures of the glenoid cavity: Operative principles and techniques. Techniques in Orthopaedics 8[3]:199-204, 1993. © Raven Press, Ltd., New York.)

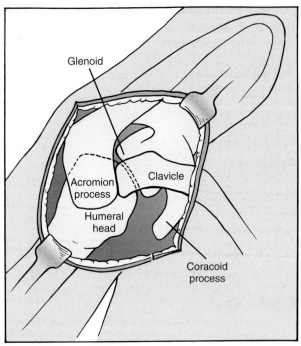

FIGURE 10-51 Superior surgical approach to the glenoid cavity: bony anatomy. (From Goss TP: Fractures of the glenoid cavity: Operative principles and techniques. Techniques in Orthopaedics 8[3]:199-204, 1993. © Raven Press, Ltd., New York.)

are satisfactory: the glenoid neck, the lateral scapular border, the acromial process and scapular spine, and the coracoid process (Fig. 10-52).[275] A variety of fixation devices are available (Fig. 10-53). The most useful, however, are Kirschner wires, malleable reconstruction plates, and cannulated interfragmentary compression screws (Figs. 10-54 and 10-55).[80,276,277] Kirschner wires can be used for temporary or permanent fixation. They are used for permanent fixation when significantly displaced fracture fragments are too small to allow more substantial fixation, but one must be sure to bend the Kirschner wire at its point of entry to prevent migration. For managing glenoid neck fractures, 3.5-mm malleable reconstruction plates are particularly helpful, and 3.5- and 4.0-mm cannulated compression screws are especially useful in stabilizing fractures of the glenoid rim and the glenoid fossa. These devices may be used alone or in combination, depending on the clinical situation and the available bone stock, as well as the surgeon's preference and experience. Rigid fixation is desirable, but inability to achieve this goal does not preclude an excellent anatomic and functional result.

Bauer and colleagues reported on five patients with intra-articular fractures of the glenoid cavity who were treated with arthroscopic reduction and fixation.[278] Sugaya and colleagues described eight patients with significantly displaced type Ia fractures managed arthroscopically.[267]

Postoperative Management

Postoperative management of glenoid process fractures depends on the fixation and stability achieved. Immobilization in a sling and swathe bandage is prescribed for the first 24 to 48 hours after surgery. If fixation is rigid, dependent circular and pendulum movements are then initiated, as well as external rotation of the shoulder to but not past neutral. During postoperative weeks 3 to 6, progressive range-of-motion exercises in all directions (especially forward flexion, internal rotation up the back, and external rotation) are prescribed with the goal of achieving full range of motion by the end of the 6-week period. The patient is allowed to use the arm actively in a progressive manner within clearly defined limits (moving the weight of the extremity alone when sitting in a protected setting during weeks 3 and 4 and when up and about indoors during weeks 5 and 6).

The patient is evaluated clinically and radiographically every 2 weeks to make sure that displacement does not occur at the fracture site and to monitor and update the rehabilitation program. At 6 weeks, healing is sufficient to discontinue all external protection and encourage progressive functional use of the extremity. Kirschner wires spanning bones that move relative to each other are removed at this time, as are those passing through soft tissues (Kirschner wires embedded within a single osseous structure and bent at their entry site to prevent migration

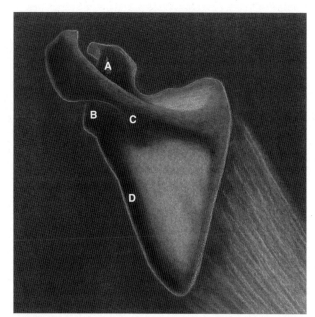

FIGURE 10-52 Illustration depicting the scapula and areas of sufficient bone stock for internal fixation. *A*, the coracoid process; *B*, the glenoid process; *C*, the scapular spine and acromial process; and *D*, the lateral scapular border. (From Goss TP: Fractures of the glenoid cavity: Operative principles and techniques. Techniques in Orthopaedics 8[3]:199-204, 1993. © Raven Press, Ltd., New York.)

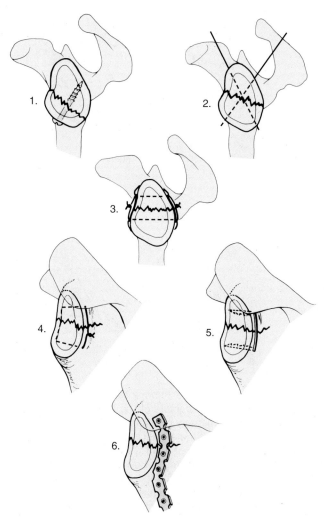

FIGURE 10-53 Illustrations depicting fixation techniques available for stabilization of fractures of the glenoid cavity. *1*, An interfragmentary compression screw; *2*, Kirschner wires; *3*, a construct using Kirschner wires and cerclage wires or Kirschner wires and cerclage sutures; *4*, a cerclage wire or suture; *5*, a staple; *6*, a 3.5-mm malleable reconstruction plate. (From Goss TP: Fractures of the glenoid cavity [Current Concepts Review]. J Bone Joint Surg Am 74[2]:299-305, 1992.)

may be left in place). Physical therapy continues to focus on regaining range of motion as progressive strengthening exercises are added.

The patient's rehabilitation program continues until range of motion, strength, and overall function are maximized. Light use of the shoulder is emphasized through postoperative week 12, but heavy physical use of the shoulder, including athletic activities, is prohibited until the 4- to 6-month point. If surgical fixation is less than rigid, the shoulder may need to be protected in a sling and swathe binder, in an abduction brace, or even in overhead olecranon pin traction for 7, 10, or 14 days (depending on the clinical situation) before the physical therapy program is prescribed. The patient must be encouraged to work diligently on the rehabilitation program because range of motion and strength can improve and the end result is often not achieved for approximately 6 months to 1 year after injury. Hard work, perseverance, and dedication on the part of the patient, the physician, and the physical therapist are critical to an optimal functional result.

Although the literature remains somewhat deficient because of the rarity of these injuries, an increase in interest in recent years has resulted in a growing number of case reports and personal series. Although more data are needed, it is reasonable to anticipate a good to excellent functional result if surgical management restores normal or near-normal glenoid anatomy, articular congruity, and glenohumeral stability; the fixation is secure; and

a well-structured, closely monitored postoperative rehabilitation program is prescribed.

Glenoid Cavity Fractures[55,58,83,90]

Type I (glenoid rim) fractures are managed surgically if the fracture results in persistent subluxation of the humeral head or if the fracture or the humeral head is unstable after reduction. Instability can be expected if the fracture is displaced 10 mm or more and if a quarter or more of the glenoid cavity anteriorly or a third or more of the glenoid cavity posteriorly is involved. Type Ia (anterior rim) fractures are approached anteriorly. The displaced fragment is mobilized, reduced anatomically, and fixed in

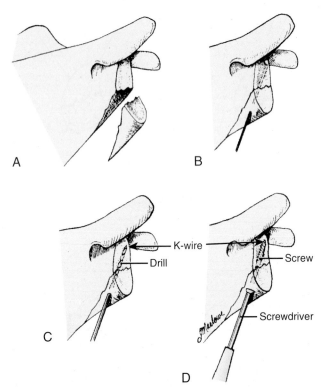

A

B

K-wire

Drill

C

Screw

Screwdriver

D

FIGURE 10-54 Illustrations showing reduction and stabilization of a type II fracture of the glenoid cavity with a cannulated interfragmentary compression screw. **A,** Fracture of the glenoid cavity with a significantly displaced inferior glenoid fragment. **B,** Reduction of the glenoid fragment and stabilization with a guidewire. **C,** Use of the guidewire (K-wire) to pass a cannulated drill and eventually a cannulated tap. **D,** Use of the guidewire to place a cannulated interfragmentary compression screw to securely fix the glenoid fragment in position. (From Goss TP: Fractures of the glenoid cavity: Operative principles and techniques. Techniques in Orthopaedics 8[3]:199-204, 1993. © Raven Press, Ltd., New York.)

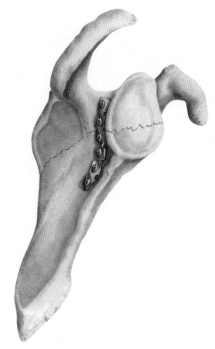

FIGURE 10-55 Illustration showing reduction and stabilization of a glenoid cavity fracture with a 3.5-mm malleable reconstruction plate. (From Goss TP: Glenoid fractures: Open reduction internal fixation. In Wiss DA [ed]: Master Techniques in Orthopaedic Surgery. Fractures. Philadelphia: Lippincott-Raven, 1998, p 10.)

position with cannulated interfragmentary compression screws (ideally, two screws are used to provide rotational stability) (see Fig. 10-18). Type Ib (posterior fractures) are approached posteriorly and reduced and stabilized in the same manner (see Fig. 10-19). If the fracture is comminuted, the fragments are excised. A tricortical graft harvested from the iliac crest is then placed intra-articularly to fill the defect (Fig. 10-56). A simple repair of the periarticular soft tissues to the intact glenoid cavity is an option if the bone defect is less than 20% of the AP dimension, but restoration of the rim contour is preferable.

On the basis of available reports, it seems reasonable to conclude that surgery has a definite role in the treatment of glenoid fossa fractures (types II-V). An injury with an articular step-off of 5 mm or more should be considered for surgical intervention to restore articular congruity, and displacement of 10 mm or more is an absolute indication for surgery to avoid post-traumatic osteoarthritis. Another indication is such severe separa-

tion of the fracture fragments that nonunion at the injury site, chronic instability of the glenohumeral joint, or both, are likely.

Type II fractures are approached posteriorly. The infraspinatus–teres minor interval is developed to expose the displaced inferior glenoid process fragment and the lateral scapular border. The fragment is reduced as anatomically as possible and stabilized, generally with two cannulated interfragmentary compression screws passed posteroinferiorly to anterosuperiorly (see Fig. 10-22) or with a contoured reconstruction plate placed along the posterior aspect of the glenoid process and the lateral scapular border. Excision of the fracture fragment and placement of a bone graft from the iliac crest is an option in a severely comminuted fracture. Associated tears of the labral–capsular–ligamentous complex are repaired if possible, as they are with all fractures of the glenoid cavity. Detachments are corrected with nonabsorbable sutures passed through drill holes or with suture anchors. Intrasubstance tears are reapproximated with nonabsorbable sutures passed in a figure-of-eight fashion.

Type III fractures are approached either via a posterosuperior exposure or anteriorly through the rotator interval. A Kirschner wire can be placed into the superior glenoid fragment and used to manipulate it into satisfactory position relative to the remainder of the glenoid process, thereby restoring articular congruity. The Kirschner wire is then driven across the fracture site and used

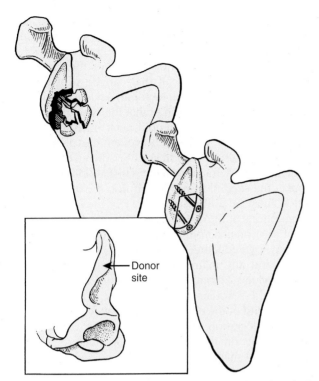

FIGURE 10-56 Illustration depicting the use of a tricortical graft harvested from the iliac crest to re-establish bony stability in a patient with a severely comminuted type Ia fracture of the glenoid cavity.

to place a cannulated interfragmentary compression screw. In patients with a significantly displaced additional disruption of the SSSC, reduction and stabilization of the superior glenoid fragment can restore the integrity of the complex satisfactorily. If not, that injury might need to be addressed as well (see Fig. 10-23). Conversely, if the superior glenoid fragment is severely comminuted and difficult to fix, operative restoration of the additional SSSC disruption can improve glenoid articular congruity indirectly and satisfactorily.

Type IV fractures are approached posterosuperiorly or with a combined posterior-anterior (through the rotator interval) exposure. A Kirschner wire is placed into the superior glenoscapular segment and used to manipulate the fragment into position relative to the inferior segment while directly visualizing the reduction via the posterior exposure. The Kirschner wire is then driven across the fracture site and used to place a cannulated interfragmentary compression screw (see Fig. 10-24). A cerclage wire or cerclage suture passed around the glenoid neck may also be used for fixation, as well as a malleable reconstruction plate. As always, one must take care to avoid injury to adjacent neurovascular structures, in particular the suprascapular nerve and vessels that pass through the spinoglenoid interval.

Type Va fractures are approached, reduced, and stabilized according to the principles described for significantly displaced type II fractures, although a superior approach might need to be added to gain control over the superior glenoscapular fragment. Type Vb injuries are approached, reduced, and stabilized according to the principles described for significantly displaced type III fractures. If an additional disruption of the SSSC is present, it can require operative reduction and stabilization. Type Vc fractures are exposed via a posterosuperior or a combined posterior–anterior (via the rotator interval) approach. The superior and inferior glenoid fragments are reduced anatomically and rigidly fixed to each other, ideally with a lag screw passed superiorly to inferiorly. Other alternatives are cerclage wires or sutures passed through drill holes or suture anchors placed in the superior and inferior fragments. The glenoid fragment is then reduced and stabilized relative to the inferomedial portion of the scapular body using the principles described for ORIF of glenoid neck fractures (see Fig. 10-25). Additional disruptions of the SSSC can require attention as well.

Type VI fractures are managed nonoperatively. However, an associated disruption of the SSSC might warrant surgical correction and indirectly improve glenoid articular congruity. The upper extremity is initially protected in a sling and swathe bandage, an abduction brace, or even overhead olecranon pin traction—whichever maximizes articular congruity as determined radiographically. Gentle passive circular and rotatory range-of-motion exercises performed by a therapist and the patient are initiated immediately, hoping that movement of the humeral head molds the articular fragments into a maximally congruous position. By 2 weeks, healing is sufficient to allow protection of such injuries in a sling and swathe binder. Exercises designed to gradually increase range of motion and progressive functional use of the shoulder out of the sling (within clearly defined limits) are prescribed during the subsequent 4 weeks. At 6 weeks, these fractures are sufficiently healed to allow discontinuation of all external protection. Functional use of the shoulder is encouraged and physical therapy continues until range of motion and strength are maximized. These injuries obviously have the highest potential for post-traumatic degenerative joint disease and glenohumeral instability.

Glenoid Neck Fractures[80]

Clearly, the vast majority of glenoid neck fractures can and should be treated nonoperatively; however, more-aggressive management, including ORIF, is indicated when the glenoid fragment is severely displaced (type II injuries). Some might quarrel with 1 cm of translational displacement being an indication for surgery; however, the decision to proceed operatively becomes easier with increasing degrees of displacement, especially if the glenoid rim lies medial to the lateral margin of the scapular body (see Fig. 10-12). Forty degrees (or certainly more) of angular displacement of the glenoid fragment also seems to be a reasonable indication for surgical management (see Fig. 10-13).

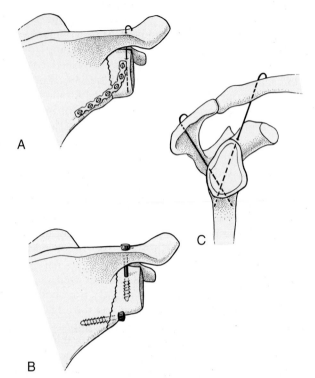

FIGURE 10-57 Illustrations depicting fixation techniques available for stabilization of glenoid neck fractures. **A,** Stabilization with a 3.5-mm malleable reconstruction plate (note the Kirschner wire running from the acromial process into the glenoid process, which can be used for temporary or permanent fixation). **B,** Stabilization with 3.5-mm cannulated interfragmentary screws. **C,** Stabilization with Kirschner wires (in this case, Kirschner wires passed from the acromion and clavicle into the glenoid process). (From Goss TP: Fractures of the glenoid neck. J Shoulder Elbow Surg 3[1]:42-52, 1994.)

The glenoid process and fracture site are approached posteriorly. The interval between the infraspinatus and teres minor is developed to expose the posteroinferior glenoid neck and lateral scapular border. A superior approach can be added to gain control over the free glenoid fragment. Once satisfactory reduction has been achieved, temporary fixation can be provided by placing Kirschner wires between the glenoid fragment and the adjacent bony structures (e.g., through the glenoid fragment and into the scapular body or through the acromial process and into the glenoid fragment). Firm fixation is generally achieved by means of a contoured 3.5-mm malleable reconstruction plate applied along the lateral border of the scapula and the posterior aspect of the glenoid process. Supplemental fixation can be provided by Kirschner wires or lag screws. Kirschner wires providing temporary fixation can be retained or used for placing 3.5-mm cannulated lag screws (Fig. 10-57).

Conceivably, comminution of the scapular body and spine can be so severe or the size of the glenoid fragment so small that plate fixation is precluded. In these cases, Kirschner-wire or lag-screw fixation of the reduced glenoid fragment to adjacent intact bony structures (e.g., the acromial process, the distal end of the clavicle, or other structures) may be all that can be provided. If a disruption of the clavicular–acromioclavicular joint–acromial strut is present, fixation of that injury might indirectly reduce and stabilize the glenoid neck fracture. If significant displacement persists, however, the glenoid neck fracture must also be addressed.[80] Conversely, ORIF of the glenoid neck fracture might satisfactorily reduce and stabilize the second disruption. If not, the associated disruption must be addressed.

Disruptions of the C-4 linkage with or without a disruption of the coracoacromial ligament are usually managed indirectly by reducing and stabilizing the glenoid neck fracture and any injuries compromising the integrity of the clavicular–acromioclavicular joint–acromial strut. Rarely, if the scapular body and spine, acromial process, and distal end of the clavicle are all severely comminuted, overhead olecranon pin traction must be considered or displacement of the glenoid neck fracture must be accepted and managed nonoperatively.

Scapulothoracic Dissociation

One of us (TPG) has treated five such cases. The key to diagnosis is awareness of the clinical entity; these injuries, though rare, may be more common than previously thought. All the injuries seen have included a disruption of the sternal–clavicular–acromial linkage, most commonly a fracture of the distal part of the clavicle. Every effort is made to reduce and stabilize this component of the injury for the reasons noted earlier.[20] The upper extremity is protected for 6 weeks while a progressive rehabilitation program is instituted. Late reconstructive efforts are dictated by the degree of neurologic return.

Intrathoracic Dislocation

We have not encountered this rare injury. Therapeutic principles presented in the literature and detailed earlier would be followed.

Scapulothoracic Crepitus

Active management is indicated if scapulothoracic crepitus is truly painful and therefore represents an underlying pathologic condition. Clearly defined bony prominences within the scapulothoracic interval refractory to nonoperative treatment are resected, but they are rare. Other presumed etiologies are best managed nonoperatively, and the majority respond satisfactorily. Surgery is a consideration in those that do not, especially if symptoms are relatively localized. Exploration of the symptomatic area with judicious bony resection and removal of questionable soft tissue is generally performed, but the results are quite mixed.

REFERENCES

1. Brown CV, Velmahos G, Wang D, et al: Association of scapular fractures and blunt thoracic aortic injury: Fact or fiction? Am Surg 71:54-57, 2005.
2. Bateman JE: The Shoulder and Neck, 2nd ed. Philadelphia: WB Saunders, 1978.
3. Butters KP: The scapula. In Rockwood CA, Matsen FA (eds): The Shoulder. Philadelphia: WB Saunders, 1990, pp 335-366.
4. Crenshaw AH: Fractures. In Crenshaw AH (ed): Campbell's Operative Orthopaedics, 8th ed. St Louis: CV Mosby, 1992.
5. DeRosa GP, Kettelkamp DB: Fracture of the coracoid process of the scapula: A case report. J Bone Joint Surg Am 59:696-697, 1977.
6. Goss TP, Owens BD: Fractures of the scapula: Diagnosis and treatment. In Iannotti JP, Williams GR (eds): Disorders of the Shoulder: Diagnosis and Management, 2nd ed. Philadelphia, Lippincott, 2007, pp 793-840.
7. McKoy BE, Bensen CV, Hartsock LA: Fractures about the shoulder. Orthop Clin North Am 31:205-216, 2000.
8. Moseley HF: Shoulder Lesions, 2nd ed. New York: Paul Hoeber, 1953.
9. Neer CS II: Less frequent procedures. In Neer CS II (ed): Shoulder Reconstruction. Philadelphia: WB Saunders, 1990, pp 421-485.
10. Neer CS, Rockwood CA: Fractures and dislocations of the shoulder. In Rockwood CA, Green DP (eds): Fractures in Adults, 2nd ed. Philadelphia: JB Lippincott, 1984.
11. Norris TR: Fractures and dislocations of the glenohumeral complex. In Chapman M (ed): Operative Orthopedics. Philadelphia: JB Lippincott, 1988.
12. Post M: The Shoulder: Surgical and Non-surgical Management, 2nd ed. Philadelphia: Lea & Febiger, 1988.
13. Rockwood CA Jr, Matsen FA III: The Shoulder. Philadelphia: WB Saunders, 1990.
14. Rowe CR (ed): The Shoulder. New York: Churchill Livingstone, 1988.
15. Ruedi T, Chapman MW: Fractures of the scapula and clavicle. In Chapman M (ed): Operative Orthopedics. Philadelphia: JB Lippincott, 1988.
16. Scudder CL (ed): The Treatment of Fractures, 4th ed. Philadelphia: WB Saunders, 1904.
17. Steindler A: Traumatic Deformities and Disabilities of the Upper Extremity. Springfield, Ill: Charles C Thomas, 1946, pp 112-118.
18. Findlay RT: Fractures of the scapula and ribs. Am J Surg 38:489-494, 1937.
19. Gleich JJ: The fractured scapula: Significance and prognosis. Mo Med 77:24-26, 1980.
20. Goss TP: The scapula: Coracoid, acromial and avulsion fractures. Am J Orthop 25:106-115, 1996.
21. Cuomo F, Goss TP: Shoulder trauma: Bone. In Kasser JR (ed): Orthopaedic Knowledge Update 5. Rosemont Ill: American. Academy of Orthopaedic Surgeons, 1996, pp 217-232.
22. Guttentag IJ, Rechtine GR: Fractures of the scapula. A review of the literature. Orthop Rev 17:147-158, 1988.
23. Herscovici D, Sanders R, DiPasquale T, Gregory P: Injuries of the shoulder girdle. Clin Orthop Relat Res (318):54-60, 1995.
24. Imatani RJ: Fractures of the scapula: A review of 53 fractures. J Trauma 15:473-478, 1975.
25. Laing R Dee R: Fracture symposium. Orthop Rev 13:717, 1984.
26. McCally WC, Kelly DA: Treatment of fractures of the clavicle, ribs and scapula. Am J Surg 50:558-562, 1940.
27. McGahan JP, Rab GT, Dublin A: Fractures of the scapula. J Trauma 20:880-883, 1980.
28. McGinnis M, Denton JR: Fractures of the scapula: A retrospective study of 40 fractured scapulae. J Trauma 29:1488-1493, 1989.
29. McLaughlin HL: Trauma. Philadelphia: WB Saunders, 1959.
30. Neviaser J: Traumatic lesions: Injuries in and about the shoulder joint. Instr Course Lect 13:187-216, 1956.
31. Newell ED: Review of over 2,000 fractures in the past seven years. South Med J 20:644-648, 1927.
32. Papagelopoulos PJ, Koundis GL, Kateros KT, et al: Fractures of the glenoid cavity: Assessment and management. Orthopedics 22:956-961, 1999.
33. Rockwood CA: Management of fractures of the scapula. J Bone Joint Surg 10:219, 1986.
34. Rowe CR: Fractures of the scapula. Surg Clin North Am 43:1565-1571, 1963.
35. Thompson DA, Flynn TC, Miller PW, et al: The significance of scapular fractures. J Trauma 25:974-977, 1985.
36. Wilber MC, Evans EB: Fractures of the scapula. An analysis of forty cases and a review of the literature. J Bone Joint Surg Am 59:358-362, 1977.
37. Wilson PD: Experience in the Management of Fractures and Dislocations (Based on an Analysis of 4390 Cases) by the Staff of the Fracture Service MGH, Boston. Philadelphia: JB Lippincott, 1938.
38. Zlowodzki M, Bhandari M, Zelle BA, et al: Treatment of scapula fractures: Systematic review of 520 fractures in 22 case series. J Orthop Trauma 20:230-233, 2006.
39. Zuckerman JD, Koval KJ, Cuomo F: Fractures of the scapula. Instr Course Lect 42:271-281, 1993.
40. Goss TP: Double disruptions of the superior shoulder complex. J Orthop Trauma 7:99-106, 1993.
41. Harris RD, Harris JH: The prevalence and significance of missed scapular fractures in blunt chest trauma. AJR Am J Roentgenol 151:747-750, 1988.
42. Weening B, Walton C, Cole PA, et al: Lower mortality in patients with scapular fractures. J Trauma 59:1477-1481, 2005.
43. Ideberg R, Grevsten S, Larsson S: Epidemiology of scapular fractures. Acta Orthop Scand 66:395-397, 1995.
44. Fischer RP, Flynn TC, Miller PW, et al: Scapular fractures and associated major ipsilateral upper-torso injuries. Curr Concepts Trauma Care 1:14-16, 1985.
45. McLennan JG, Ungersma J: Pneumothorax complicating fractures of the scapula. J Bone Joint Surg Am 64:598-599, 1982.
46. Ebraheim NA, An HS, Jackson WT, et al: Scapulothoracic dissociation. J Bone Joint Surg Am 70:428-432, 1988.
47. Nunley RL, Bedini SJ: Paralysis of the shoulder subsequent to comminuted fracture of the scapula: Rationale and treatment methods. Phys Ter Rev 40:442-447, 1960.
48. Tomaszek DE: Combined subclavian artery and brachial plexus injuries from blunt upper-extremity trauma. J Trauma 24:161-153, 1984.
49. Halpern AA, Joseph R, Page J, Nagel DA: Subclavian artery injury and fracture of the scapula. JACEP 8:19-20, 1979.
50. Stein RE, Bono J, Korn J, Wolff WI: Axillary artery injury in closed fracture of the neck of the scapula: A case report. J Trauma 11:528-531, 1971.
51. Landi A, Schoenhuber R, Funicello R, et al: Compartment syndrome of the scapula. Ann Chir Main Memb Super 11:383-388, 1992.
52. Stephens NG, Morgan AS, Corvo P, Bernstein BA: Significance of scapular fracture in the blunt trauma patient. Ann Emerg Med 26:439-442, 1995.
53. Veysi VT, Mittal R, Agarwal S, et al: Multiple trauma and scapula fractures: So what? J Trauma 55:1145-1147, 2003.
54. McAdams TR, Blevins FT, Martin TP, DeCoster TA: The role of plain films and computed tomography in the evaluation of scapular neck fractures. J Trauma 16:7-11, 2002.
55. Goss TP: Fractures of the Glenoid Cavity. Video J Orthopedics VII(6), 1992, and AAOS Physician Videotape Library.
56. Hardegger FH, Simpson LA, Weber BG: The operative treatment of scapular fractures. J Bone Joint Surg Br 66:725-731, 1984.
57. Arts V, Louette L: Scapula neck fracture: An update of the concept of floating shoulder. Injury 30:146-148, 1999.
58. Goss TP: Fractures of the glenoid cavity (operative principles and techniques). Tech Orthop 8:199-204, 1994.
59. Limb D, McMurray D: Dislocation of the glenoid fossa. J Shoulder Elbow Surg 14:338-339, 2005.
60. Zdravkovic D, Damholt VV: Comminuted and severely displaced fractures of the scapula. Acta Orthop Scand 45:60-65, 1974.
61. Nordqvist A, Petersson C: Fracture of the body, neck or spine of the scapula. Clin Orthop Relat Res (283):139-144, 1992.
62. Ada JR, Miller ME: Scapular fractures. Analysis of 113 cases. Clin Orthop Relat Res (269):174-180, 1991.
63. Miller ME, Ada JR: Injuries to the shoulder girdle. In Browner BD, Jupiter JB, Levine AM, Trafton PY (eds): Skeletal Trauma, 2nd ed. Philadelphia: WB Saunders, 1992, pp 1291.
64. Van Noort A, van der Werken C: The floating shoulder. Injury 37:218-227, 2006.
65. DePalma AF: Surgery of the Shoulder, 3rd ed. Philadelphia: JB Lippincott, 1983.
66. Van Noort A, van Kampen A: Fractures of the scapula surgical neck: Outcome after conservative treatment in 13 cases. Arch Orthop Trauma Surg 125:696-700, 2005.
67. Lindholm A, Leven H: Prognosis and fractures of the body and neck of the scapula. Acta Surg Chir Scand 140:33-36, 1994.
68. Armstrong CP, Van der Spuy J: The fractured scapula: Importance in management based on a series of 62 patients. Injury 15:324-529, 1984.
69. Judet R: Traitement chirurgical des fractures de l'omoplate. Acta Orthop Belg 30:673, 1954.
70. Magerl F: Osteosynthesen in Bereich der Schulter: Pertuberkulare Humerusfracturen. Scapulahalsfrakturen. Helv Chir Acta 41:225-232, 1974.
71. Ganz R, Noesberger B: Die Behandlung der Scapula-Frakturen. Hefte Unfallheilkd 126:59-62, 1975.
72. Tscherne H, Christ M: Konservative und operative Therapie der Schulterblattbruche. Hefte Unfallheilkd 126:52-59, 1975.
73. Boerger TO, Limb D: Suprascapular nerve injury at the spinoglenoid notch after glenoid neck fracture. J Shoulder Elbow Surg 9:236-237, 2000.
74. DeBeer JF, Berghs BM, van Rooyen KS, du Toit DF: Displaced scapular neck fracture: A case report. J Shoulder Elbow Surg 13:123-125, 2004.
75. Bozkurt M, Can F, Kirdemir V, et al: Conservative treatment of scapular neck fracture: The effect of stability and glenopolar angle on clinical outcome. Injury 36:1176-1181, 2005.
76. Mathews RE, Cocke TB, D'Ambrosia RD: Scapular fractures secondary to seizures in patients with osteodystrophy. J Bone Joint Surg Am 65:850-853, 1983.
77. Chadwick EK, van Noort A, van der Helm FC: Biomechanical analysis of scapular neck malunion—a simulation study. Clin Biomech 19:906-912, 2004.

78. Binazzi R, Assiso JR, Vaccari V, Felli L: Avulsion fractures of the scapula: Report of 8 cases. J Trauma 33:785-789, 1992.

79. Gagey O, Curey JP, Mazas F: Les fractures récentes de l'omoplate à propos de 43 cas. Rev Chir Orthop 70:443-447, 1984.

80. Goss TP: Fractures of the glenoid neck. J Shoulder Elbow Surg 3:42-52, 1994.

81. Ideberg R: Fractures of the scapula involving the glenoid fossa. In Bateman JE, Welsh RP (eds): Surgery of the Shoulder. Philadelphia: BC Decker, 1984, pp 63-66.

82. Ideberg R: Unusual glenoid fractures. A report on 92 cases [abstract]. Acta Orthop Scand 58:191, 1987.

83. Goss TP: Fractures of the glenoid cavity: Current concepts review. J Bone Joint Surg Am 74:299-305, 1992.

84. Heggland EJH, Parker RD: Simultaneous bilateral glenoid fractures associated with glenohumeral subluxation/dislocation in a weightlifter. Orthopedics 20:1180-1183, 1997.

85. Aston JW Jr, Gregory CF: Dislocation of the shoulder with significant fracture of the glenoid. J Bone Joint Surg Am 55:1531-1533, 1973.

86. Kurdy NM, Shah SV: Fracture of the acromion associated with acromioclavicular dislocation. Injury 26:636-637, 1995.

87. Niggebrugge AHP, van Heusden HA, Bode PJ, van Vugt AB: Dislocated intra-articular fracture of the anterior rim of glenoid treated by open reduction and internal fixation. Injury 24:130-131, 1993.

88. Sinha J, Miller AJ: Fixation of fractures of the glenoid rim. Injury 23:418-419, 1992.

89. Varriale PL, Adler ML: Occult fracture of the glenoid without dislocation. J Bone Joint Surg Am 65:688-689, 1983.

90. Goss TP: Fractures of the glenoid cavity. J Bone Joint Surg Am 74:299-305, 1992.

91. Eyres KS, Brooks A, Stanley D: Fractures of the coracoid process. J Bone Joint Surg Br 77:425-428, 1995.

92. Martín-Herrero T, Rodriquez-Merchán C, Munuera-Martínez L: Fractures of the coracoid process: Presentation of seven cases and review of the literature. J Trauma 30:1597-1599, 1990.

93. Edeland HG, Zachrisson BE: Fracture of the scapular notch associated with lesion of the suprascapular nerve. Acta Orthop Scand 46:758-763, 1975.

94. Solheim LF, Roaas A: Compression of the suprascapular nerve after fracture of the scapular notch. Acta Orthop Scand 49:338-340, 1978.

95. Fischer WR: Fracture of the scapula requiring open reduction: Report of a case. J Bone Joint Surg 21:459-461, 1939.

96. Ferraz IC, Papadimitriou NG, Sotereanos DG: Scapular body nonunion: A case report. J Shoulder Elbow Surg 11:98-100, 2002.

97. Aulicino PL, Reinert C, Kornberg M, et al: Displaced intraarticular glenoid fractures treated by open reduction and internal fixation. J Trauma 26:1137-1141, 1986.

98. Lee SJ, Meinhard BP, Schultz E, Toledano B: Open reduction and internal fixation of a glenoid fossa fracture in a child: A case report and review of the literature. J Orthop Trauma 11:452-454, 1997.

99. Bauer G, Fleischmann W, DuBler E: Displaced scapular fractures: Indication and long term results of open reduction and internal fixation. Arch Orthop Trauma Surg 114:215-219, 1995.

100. Kavanagh BF, Bradway JK, Cofield RH: Open reduction of displaced intra-articular fractures of the glenoid fossa. J Bone Joint Surg Am 75:479-484, 1993.

101. Soslowsky LJ, Flatow EL, Bigliani LU, Mow DC: Articular geometry of the glenohumeral joint. Clin Orthop Relat Res (285):181-190, 1992.

102. Schandelmaier P, Blauth M, Schneider C, Krethek C: Fractures of the glenoid treated by operation. A 5- to 23-year follow-up of 22 cases. J Bone Joint Surg Br 84:173-177, 2002.

103. Leung KS, Lam TP, Poon KM: Operative treatment of displaced intra-articular glenoid fractures. Injury 24:324-328, 1993.

104. Harmon PH, Baker DR: Fracture of the scapula with displacement. J Bone Joint Surg 25:834-838, 1943.

105. Heatly MD, Breck LW, Higinbotham NL: Bilateral fracture of the scapula. Am J Surg 71:256-259, 1946.

106. Blue JM, Anglen JO, Helikson MA: Fracture of scapula with intrathoracic penetration. J Bone Joint Surg Am 79:1076-1078, 1997.

107. Schwartzbach CC, Seuodi H, Ross AE, et al: Fracture of a scapula with intrathoracic penetration in a skeletally mature patient: A case report. J Bone Joint Surg Am 88:2735-2738, 2006.

108. Bowen TR, Miller F: Greenstick fracture of the scapula: A cause of scapular winging. J Orthop Trauma 20:147-149, 2006.

109. Martin SD, Weiland AJ: Missed scapular fracture after trauma. A case report and a 23-year follow-up report. Clin Orthop Relat Res (299):259-262, 1994.

110. Gupta R, Sher J, Williams GR, Iannotti JP: Non-union of the scapular body: A case report. J Bone Joint Surg Am 80:428-430, 1998.

111. Kaminsky SB, Pierce VD: Nonunion of a scapula body fracture in a high school football player. Am J Orthop 31:456-457, 2002.

112. Michael D, Fazal MA, Cohen B: Nonunion of a fracture of the body of the scapula: Case report and literature review. J Shoulder Elbow Surg 10:385-386, 2001.

113. Hall RJ, Calvert PT: Stress fracture of the acromion: An unusual mechanism and review of the literature. J Bone Joint Surg Br 77:153-154, 1994.

114. Warner J, Port I: Stress fracture of the acromion. J Shoulder Elbow Surg 3:262-265, 1994.

115. Mencke JB: The frequency and significance of injuries to the acromion process. Ann Surg 59:233-238, 1914.

116. Kuhn JE, Blasier RB, Carpenter JE: Letter to the editor. J Orthop Trauma 8:14, 1994.

117. Kuhn JE, Blasier RB, Carpenter JE: Letter to the Editor. J Orthop Trauma 8:359, 1994.

118. Miller ME: Letter to the editor. J Orthop Trauma 8:14, 1994.

119. Taylor J: Letter to the editor. J Orthop Trauma 8:359, 1994.

120. Kuhn JE, Blasier RB, Carpenter JE: Fractures of the acromion process: A proposed classification system. J Orthop Trauma 8:6-13, 1994.

121. Madhavan P, Buckingham R, Stableforth PG: Avulsion injury of the subscapularis tendon associated with fracture of the acromion. Injury 25:271-272, 1994.

122. Goodrich JA, Grosland E, Pye J: Acromion fracture associated with posterior shoulder dislocation. J Orthop Trauma 12:521-523, 1998.

123. Weber D, Sadri H, Hoffmeyer P: Isolated fracture of the posterior angle of the acromion: A case report. J Shoulder Elbow Surg 9:534-535, 2002.

124. Dounchis JS, Pedowtiz RA, Garfin SR: Symptomatic pseudoarthrosis of the acromion: Report of a case and review of the literature. J Orthop Trauma 13:63-66, 1999.

125. Gordes W, Hessert GR: Seltene Verletzungsfolgen an der Spina Scapulae. Arch Orthop Unfall Chir 68:315-324, 1970.

126. Mick CA, Weiland AJ: Pseudarthrosis of a fracture of the acromion. J Trauma 23:248-249, 1983.

127. Goss TP: Glenoid fractures—open reduction and internal fixation. In Wiss DA (ed): Master Techniques in Orthopaedic Surgery: Fractures. Philadelphia: Lippincott-Raven, 1998, pp 3-17.

128. Montgomery SP, Loyd RD: Avulsion fracture of the coracoid epiphysis with acromioclavicular separation. Report of 2 cases in adolescents and review of the literature. J Bone Joint Surg Am 59:963-965, 1977.

129. Protass JJ, Stampfli FB, Osmer JC: Coracoid process fracture diagnosis in acromioclavicular separation. Radiology 116:61-64, 1975.

130. Cottalorda J, Allard D, Dutour N, Chavrier Y: Fracture of the coracoid process in an adolescent. Injury 27:436-437, 1996.

131. Cottias P, le Bellec Y, Jeanrot C, et al: Fractured coracoid with anterior shoulder dislocation and greater tuberosity fracture—report of a bilateral case. Acta Orthop Scand 71:95-97, 2000.

132. Coues WP: Fracture of the coracoid process of the scapula. N Engl J Med 212:727-728, 1935.

133. Fery A, Sommelet J: Fractures de l'apophyse coracoide. Rev Chir Orthop 65:403-407, 1979.

134. Rush LV: Fracture of the coracoid process of the scapula. Ann Surg 90:1113, 1929.

135. Borges JLP, Shah A, Torres BC, Bowen JR: Modified Woodward procedure for Sprengel deformity of the shoulder: Long-term results. J Pediatr Orthop 16:508-513, 1996.

136. Sandrock AR: Another sports fatigue fracture. Stress fracture of the coracoid process of the scapula. Radiology 117:274, 1975.

137. Moneim MS, Balduini FC: Coracoid fracture as a com-plication of surgical treatment by coracoclavicular tape fixation. A case report. Clin Orthop Relat Res (168):133-135, 1982.

138. Froimson AI: Fracture of the coracoid process of the scapula. J Bone Joint Surg Am 60:710-711, 1978.

139. Goldberg RP, Vicks B: Oblique angle view for coracoid process fractures. Skeletal Radiol 9:195-197, 1983.

140. Kopecky KK, Bies JR, Ellis JH: CT diagnosis of fracture of the coracoid process of the scapula. Comput Radiol 8:325-327, 1984.

141. Wood VE, Marchinski L: Congenital anomalies of the shoulder. In Rockwood CA, Matsen FA (eds): The Shoulder. Philadelphia: WB Saunders, 1990, pp 98-148.

142. Zilberman Z, Rejovitzky R: Fracture of the coracoid process of the scapula. Injury 13:203-206, 1982.

143. Wong-Chung J, Quinlan W: Fractured coracoid process preventing closed reduction of anterior dislocation of the shoulder. Injury 20:296-297, 1989.

144. Deltoff MN, Bressler HB: Atypical scapular fracture. A case report. Am J Sports Med 17:292-295, 1989.

145. Benchetrit E, Friedman B: Fracture of the coracoid process associated with subglenoid dislocation of the shoulder. A case report. J Bone Joint Surg Am 61:295-296, 1979.

146. Asbury S, Tennent TD: Avulsion fracture of the coracoid process: A case report. Injury 36:567-568, 2005.

147. Mariani PP: Isolated fracture of the coracoid process in an athlete. Am J Sports Med 8:129-130, 1980.

148. Ramin JE, Veit H: Fracture of the scapula during electroshock therapy. Am J Psychiatry 110:153-154, 1953.

149. Rounds RC: Isolated fracture of the coracoid process. J Bone Joint Surg Am 31:662, 1949.

150. Gil JF, Haydar A: Isolated injury of the coracoid process: Case report. J Trauma 31:1696-1697, 1991.

151. Charlton WP, Kharrazi D, Alpert S, et al: Unstable nonunion of the scapula: A case report. J Shoulder Elbow Surg 12:517-519, 2003.

152. Ogawa K, Yoshida A, Takahashi M, Ui M: Fractures of the coracoid process. J Bone Joint Surg Br 79:17-19, 1997.

153. Ogawa K, Naniwa T: Fractures of the acromion and the lateral scapular spine. J Shoulder Elbow Surg 6:544-548, 1997.

154. Herscovici D: Correspondence. J Bone Joint Surg Am 76:1112, 1994.

155. Kumar VP, Satku K: Fractures of the clavicle and scapular neck. Correspondence. J Bone Joint Surg Br 75:509, 1993.

156. Herscovici D: Fractures of the clavicle and scapular neck. Correspondence. J Bone Joint Surg Br 75:509, 1993.

157. Leung KS, Lam TP: Open reduction and internal fixation of ipsilateral fractures of the scapular neck and clavicle. J Bone Joint Surg Am 75:1015-1018, 1993.

158. Leung K, Lam T: Correspondence. J Bone Joint Surg Am 76:1112, 1994.

159. Herscovici D Jr, Fiennes AG, Allgöwer M, Ruëdi TP: The floating shoulder: Ipsilateral clavicle and scapular neck fractures. J Bone Joint Surg Br 74:362-364, 1992.

160. Simpson NS, Jupiter JB: Complex fracture patterns of the upper extremity. Clin Orthop Relat Res (318):43-53, 1995.

161. Rikli D, Regazzoni P, Renner N: The unstable shoulder girdle: Early functional treatment utilizing open reduction and internal fixation. J Orthop Trauma 9:93-97, 1995.

162. Edwards SG, Whittle AP, Wood GW 2nd: Nonoperative treatment of ipsilateral fractures of scapula and clavicle. J Bone Joint Surg Am 82:774-780, 2000.

163. Hashiguchi H, Ito H: Clinical outcome of the treatment of floating shoulder by osteosynthesis for clavicle fracture alone. J Shoulder Elbow Surg 12:589-591, 2003.

164. Egol KA, Connor PM, Karunakar MA, et al: The floating shoulder: Clinical and functional results. J Bone Joint Surg Am 83:1188-1194, 2001.

165. Ramos L, Mencia R, Alonso A, Ferrandez L: Conservative treatment of ipsilateral fractures of the scapula and clavicle. J Trauma 42:239-242, 1997.

166. Williams GR Jr, Naranja J, Klimkiewicz J, et al: The floating shoulder: A biomechanical basis for classification and management. J Bone Joint Surg Am 83:1182-1187, 2001.

167. Pasapula C, Mandalia V, Aslam N: The floating shoulder. Acta Orthop Belg 70:393-400, 2004.

168. Labler L, Platz A, Weishaupt D, Trentz O: Clinical and functional results after floating shoulder injuries. J Trauma 57:595-602, 2004.

169. DeFranco MJ, Patterson BM: The floating shoulder. J Am Acad Orthop Surg 14:499-509, 2006.

170. Owens BD, Goss TP: The floating shoulder. J Bone Joint Surg Br 88:1419-1424, 2006.

171. Bernard TN, Brunet ME, Haddad RJ Jr: Fractured coracoid process in acromioclavicular dislocations. Report of four cases and review of the literature. Clin Orthop Relat Res (175):227-232, 1983.

172. Combalía A, Arandes JM, Alemany X, Ramón R: Acromioclavicular dislocation with epiphyseal separation of the coracoid process: Report of a case and review of the literature. J Trauma 38:812-815, 1995.

173. Hak DJ, Johnson EE: Avulsion fracture of the coracoid associated with acromioclavicular dissociation. J Orthop Trauma 7:381-383, 1993.

174. Heyse-Moore GH, Stoker DJ: Avulsion fractures of the scapula. Skeletal Radiol 9:27-32, 1982.

175. Lasda NA, Murray DG: Fracture separation of the coracoid process associated with acromioclavicular dislocation: Conservative treatment—A case report and review of the literature. Clin Orthop Relat Res (134):222-224, 1978.

176. Smith DM: Coracoid fracture associated with acromioclavicular dislocation. A case report. Clin Orthop Relat Res (108):165-167, 1975.

177. Wang K, Hsu K, Shih C: Coracoid process fracture combined with acromioclavicular dislocation and coracoclavicular ligament rupture. A case report and review of the literature. Clin Orthop Relat Res (300):120-122, 1994.

178. Zettas JP, Muchnic PD: Fracture of the coracoid process base and acute acromioclavicular separation. Orthop Rev 5:77-79, 1976.

179. Lim KE, Wang CR, Chin KC, et al: Concomitant fractures of the coracoid and acromion after direct shoulder trauma. J Orthop Trauma 10:437-439, 1996.

180. Baccarani G, Porcellini G, Brunetti E: Fracture of the coracoid process associated with fracture of the clavicle: Description of a rare case. Chir Organi Mov 78:49-51, 1993.

181. Bezer M, Aydin N, Guven O: The treatment of distal clavicle fractures with coracoclavicular ligament disruption: A report of 10 cases. J Orthop Trauma 19:524-528, 2005.

182. Neer CS: Fractures of the distal third of the clavicle. Clin Orthop Relat Res 58:43-50, 1968.

183. Parkes JC, Deland JT: A three-part distal clavicle fracture. J Trauma 23:437-438, 1983.

184. McGahan JP, Rab GT: Fracture of the acromion associated with axillary nerve deficit: A case report and review of the literature. Clin Orthop Relat Res (147):216-218, 1980.

185. Gorczyca JT, Davis RT, Hartford JM, Brindle TJ: Open reduction internal fixation after displacement of a previously nondisplaced acromial fracture in a multiply injured patient: Case report and review of literature. J Orthop Trauma 15:369-373, 2001.

186. Torrens C, Mestre C, Perez P, Marin M: Subacromial dislocation of the distal end of the clavicle. Clin Orthop Relat Res (348):121-123, 1998.

187. Beswick DR, Morse SD, Barnes AU: Bilateral scapular fractures from low voltage electrical injury. Ann Emerg Med 11:676-677, 1982.

188. Dumas JL, Walker N: Bilateral scapular fractures secondary to electric shock. Arch Orthop Trauma Surg 111:287-288, 1992.

189. Henneking K, Hofmann D, Kunze K: Skapulafrakturen nach Electrounfall. Unfallchirurgie 10:149-151, 1984.

190. Kam ACA, Kam PCA: Scapular and proximal humeral head fractures. An unusual complication of cardiopulmonary resuscitation. Anaesthesia 49:1055-1057, 1994.

191. Kelly JP: Fractures complicating electro-convulsive therapy in chronic epilepsy. J Bone Joint Surg Br 36:70-79, 1954.

192. Kotak BP, Haddo O, Iqbal M, Chissell H: Bilateral scapula fracture after electrocution. J R Soc Med 93:143-144, 2000.

193. Peraino RA, Weinman EJ, Schloeder FX: Unusual fractures during convulsions in two patients with renal osteodystrophy. South Med J 70:595-596, 1977.

194. Simon JP, Van Delm I, Fabry G: Comminuted fracture of the scapula following electric shock. A case report. Acta Orthop Belg 57:459-460, 1991.

195. Tarquinio T, Weinstein ME, Virgilio RW: Bilateral scapular fractures from accidental electric shock. J Trauma 19:132-133, 1979.

196. DeMarquay J: Exostosis of rib. In Jaccoud S (ed): Dictionnaire de Médicine et de Chirurgie Pratiques. Paris: Balliere, 1868.

197. Wyrsch RB, Spindler KP, Stricker BR: Scapular fracture in a professional boxer. J Shoulder Elbow Surg 4:395-398, 1995.

198. Boyer DW: Trapshooter's shoulder: Stress fracture of the coracoid process. Case report. J Bone Joint Surg Am 57:862, 1975.

199. Houghton GR: Avulsion of the cranial margin of the scapula: A report of two cases. Injury 11:45-46, 1980.

200. De Villiers RV, Pritchard M, de Beer J, Koenig J: Scapular stress fracture in a professional cricketer and a review of the literature. S Afr Med J 95:312-317, 2005.

201. Rana M, Banerjee R: Scapular fracture after electric shock. Ann R Coll Surg Engl 88:3-4, 2006.

202. Banerjee AK, Field S: An unusual scapular fracture caused by a water skiing accident. Br J Radiol 58:465-467, 1985.

203. Arenas AJ, Pampligea T: An unusual kind of fracture. Acta Orthop Belg 59:398-400, 1993.

204. Ishizuki M, Yamaura I, Isobe Y, et al: Avulsion fracture of the superior border of the scapula. Report of five cases. J Bone Joint Surg Am 63:820-822, 1981.

205. Williamson DM, Wilson-MacDonald J: Bilateral avulsion fractures of the cranial margin of the scapula. J Trauma 28:713-714, 1988.

206. Wolf AW, Shoji H, Chuinard RG: Unusual fracture of the coracoid process. Case report and review of the literature. J Bone Joint Surg Am 58:423-424, 1976.

207. Mugikura S, Hirayama T, Tada H, et al: Avulsion fracture of the scapular spine: A case report. J Shoulder Elbow Surg 2:39-42, 1993.

208. Rask MR, Steinberg LH: Fracture of the acromion caused by muscle forces. J Bone Joint Surg Am 60:1146-1147, 1978.

209. Cain TE, Hamilton WP: Scapular fractures in professional football players. Am J Sports Med 20:363-365, 1992.

210. Hayes J, Zehr D: Traumatic muscle avulsion causing winging of the scapula. J Bone Joint Surg Am 68:495-497, 1981.

211. Longabaugh RI: Fracture simple, right scapula. US Naval Med Bull 27:341-342, 1924.

212. Franco M, Albano L, Blaimont A, et al: Spontaneous fracture of the lower angle of scapula. Possible role of cough. Joint Bone Spine 71:580-582, 2004.

213. Iannotti JP, Wang ED: Avulsion fracture of the supraglenoid tubercle: A variation of the SLAP lesion. J Shoulder Elbow Surg 1:26-30, 1992.

214. An HS, Vonderbrink JP, Ebraheim NA, et al: Open scapulothoracic dissociation with intact neurovascular status in a child. J Orthop Trauma 2:36-38, 1988.

215. Ebraheim NA, Pearlstein SR, Savolaine ER, et al: Scapulothoracic dissociation (avulsion of the scapula, subclavian artery, and brachial plexus): An early recognized variant, a new classification, and a review of the literature and treatment options. J Orthop Trauma 1:18-23, 1987.

216. Hollinshead R, James KW: Scapulothoracic dislocation (locked scapula). A case report. J Bone Joint Surg Am 61:1102-1103, 1979.

217. Johansen K, Sangeorzan B, Copass MK: Traumatic scapulothoracic dissociation: Case report. J Trauma 31:147-149, 1991.

218. Kelbel JM, Hardon OM, Huurman WV: Scapulothoracic dissociation: A case report. Clin Orthop Relat Res (209):210-214, 1986.

219. Lange RH, Noel SH: Traumatic lateral scapular displacement: An expanded spectrum of associated neurovascular injury. J Orthop Trauma 7:361-366, 1993.

220. Nagi ON, Dhillon MS: Traumatic scapulothoracic dissociation. A case report. Arch Orthop Trauma Surg 111:348-349, 1992.

221. Oreck SL, Burgess A, Levine AM: Traumatic lateral displacement of the scapula: A radiologic sign of neurovascular disruption. J Bone Joint Surg Am 66:758-763, 1984.

222. Tuzuner S, Yanat AN, Urguden MD, Ozkaynak C: Scapulothoracic dissociation: A case report. Isr J Med Sci 32:70-74, 1996.
223. Brucker PU, Gruen GS, Kaufmann RA: Scapulothoracic dissociation: Evaluation and management. Injury 36:1147-1155, 2005.
224. Zelle BA, Pape HC, Gerich TG, et al: Functional outcome following scapulothoracic dissociation. J Bone Joint Surg Am 86:2-8, 2004.
225. Clark ML, Jomha NM: Musculoskeletal. Scapulothoracic dissociation. J Can Chir 47:456-457, 2004.
226. Uhl RL, Hospodar PP: Progressive scapulothoracic subluxation after fracture of the clavicle. Am J Orthop 25:637-638, 1996.
227. Ainscow DA: Dislocation of the scapula. J Coll Surg Edinb 27:56-57, 1982.
228. Nettrour LF, Krufky LE, Mueller RE, Raycroft JF: Locked scapula: Intrathoracic dislocation of the inferior angle. A case report. J Bone Joint Surg Am 54:413-416, 1972.
229. Kolodychuk LB, Regan WD: Visualization of the scapulothoracic articulation using an arthroscope: A proposed technique. Orthop Trans 17:1142, 1993-1994.
230. Pell RF 4th, Whipple RR: Fracture-dislocation of the scapula. Orthopedics 24:595-597, 2001.
231. Cobey MC: The rolling scapula. Clin Orthop Relat Res 60:193-194, 1968.
232. Cohen JA: Multiple congenital anomalies. The association of seven defects including multiple exostoses, von Willebrand's disease, and bilateral winged scapula. Arch Intern Med 129:972-974, 1972.
233. Milch H: Partial scapulectomy for snapping in the scapula. J Bone Joint Surg Am 32:561-566, 1950.
234. Shull JR: Scapulocostal syndrome: Clinical aspects. South Med J 62:956-959, 1969.
235. Boinet W: Societe Imperiale de Chiruge, 2nd series. 8:458, 1867.
236. Mauclaire M: Craquments sous-scapulaires pathologiques traités par l'interposition musculaire interscapulo-thoracique. Bull Mem Soc Chir Paris 30:164-168, 1904.
237. Kouvalchouk JF: Subscapular crepitus. Orthop Trans 9:587-588, 1985.
238. Milch H: Snapping scapula. Clin Orthop 20:139-150, 1961.
239. Von Gruber W: Kie bursae musocae der inneren aschselwand. Arch Anat Physiol Wiss Med 358-366, 1864.
240. Ssoson-Jaroschewitsch JA: Über Skapularkrache. Arch Klin Chir 123:378, 1923.
241. Milch H, Burma MS: Snapping scapula and humerus varus. Arch Surg 26:570-588, 1933.
242. Strizak AM, Cowen MH: The snapping scapula syndrome. J Bone Joint Surg Am 64:941-942, 1982.
243. Cooley LH, Torg JS: "Pseudo-winging" of the scapula secondary to subscapular osteochondroma. Clin Orthop Relat Res (162):119-124, 1982.
244. McWilliams CA: Subscapular exostosis with adventitious bursa. JAMA 63:1473-1474, 1914.
245. Parsons TA: The snapping scapula and subscapularis exostosis. J Bone Joint Surg Br 55:345-349, 1973.
246. Von Luschka H: Über ein Costo-scapular-gelenk des Menschen. Wierteljahrasschr Prakt Heilkd 107:51-57, 1870.
247. Richards RR, McKee MD: Treatment of painful scapulothoracic crepitus by resection of the superomedial angle of the scapula. Clin Orthop Relat Res (247):111-116, 1989.
248. Roldan R, Warren D: Abduction deformity of the shoulder secondary to fibrosis of the central portion of the deltoid muscle. J Bone Joint Surg Am 54:1332-1336, 1972.
249. Arntz CT, Matsen FA III: Partial scapulectomy for disabling scapulothoracic snapping. Orthop Trans 14:252, 1990.
250. Codman EA: The anatomy of the human shoulder. In Codman EA (ed): The Shoulder, suppl ed. Malabar, Fla: Kreiger, 1984, pp 1-31.
251. Cuomo F, Blank K, Zuckerman JD, Present DA: Scapular osteochondroma presenting with exostosis bursata. Bull Hosp Jt Dis 52:55-58, 1993.
252. McCluskey GM III, Bigliani LU: Surgical management of refractory scapulothoracic bursitis. Orthop Trans 15:801, 1991.
253. McCluskey GM III, Bigliani LU: Scapulothoracic disorders. In Andres JR, Wilk KE (eds): The Athlete's Shoulder. New York: Churchill Livingstone, 1994, pp 305-316.
254. Percy EL, Birbrager D, Pitt MJ: Snapping scapula: A review of the literature and presentation of 14 patients. Can J Surg 31:248-250, 1988.
255. Shogry ME, Armstrong P: Case report 630: Reactive bursa formation surrounding an osteochondroma. Skeletal Radiol 19:465-467, 1990.
256. Ciullo JV, Jones E: Subscapular bursitis: Conservative and endoscopic treatment of "snapping scapula" or "washboard syndrome." Orthop Trans 16:740, 1992-1993.
257. Klingman M, Roffman M: Posterior approach for glenoid fracture. J Trauma 42:733-735, 1997.
258. Sisto DJ, Jobe FW: The operative treatment of scapulothoracic bursitis in professional pitchers. Am J Sports Med 14:192-194, 1986.
259. Gorres H: Ein Fall von schmerzhaften Skapularkrachen durch operation Geheilt.
260. Volkmann J: Über sogenannte Skapularkrachen. Klin Wochenschr 37:1838-1839, 1922.
261. Grunfeld G: Beitrag zur Genese des Skapularkrachens und der Skapulargerausche. Arch Orthop J Unfall Chir 24:610-615, 1927.
262. Morse JB, Ebraheim NA, Jackson WT: Partial scapulectomy for snapping scapula syndrome. Orthop Rev 22:1141-1144, 1993.
263. Michele A, Davies JJ, Krueger FJ, Lichtor JM: Scapulocostal syndrome (fatigue-postural paradox). N Y J Med 50:1352-1356, 1950.
264. Brower AC, Neff JR, Tillema DA: An unusual scapular stress fracture. AJR Am J Roentgenol 129:519-520, 1977.
265. Cameron HU: Snapping scapulae. A report of three cases. Eur J Rheumatol Inflamm 7:66-67, 1984.
266. Wong-Pack WK, Bobechko PE, Becker EJ: Fractured coracoid with anterior shoulder dislocation. J Can Assoc Radiol 31:278-279, 1980.
267. Sugaya H, Kon Y, Tsuchiya A: Arthroscopic repair of glenoid fractures using suture anchors. Arthroscopy 21:635, 2005.
268. Bizousky DT, Gillogly SD: Evaluation of the scapulothoracic articulation with arthroscopy. Orthop Trans 16:822, 1992-1993.
269. Matthews LS, Poehling CG, Hunter DM: Scapulothoracic endoscopy: Anatomical and clinical considerations. In McGinty JB, Caspari RB, Jackson RW, Poehling GG (eds): Operative Arthroscopy, 2nd ed. Philadelphia: Lippincott-Raven, 1996, pp 813-820.
270. Benton J, Nelson C: Avulsion of the coracoid process in an athlete. Report of a case. J Bone Joint Surg Am 53:356-358, 1971.
271. Garcia-Elias M, Salo JM: Non-union of a fractured coracoid process after dislocation of the shoulder. A case report. J Bone Joint Surg Br 67:722-723, 1985.
272. Owens BD, Goss TP: Surgical approaches for glenoid fractures. Tech Shoulder Elbow Surg 5:103-115, 2004.
273. Van Noort A, van Loon CJ, Rijnberg WJ: Limited posterior approach for internal fixation of a glenoid fracture. Arch Orthop Trauma Surg 124:140-144, 2004.
274. Obremskey W, Lyman JR: A modified Judet approach to the scapula. J Orthop Trauma 18:696-699, 2004.
275. Burke CS, Roberts CS, Nyland JA, et al: Scapular thickness—implications for fracture fixation. J Shoulder Elbow Surg 15:645-648, 2006.
276. Goss TP: Scapular fractures and dislocation: Diagnosis and treatment. J Am Acad Orthop Surg 3:22-33, 1995.
277. Goss TP, Busconi BD: Scapula fractures: Surgical principles and treatment. In Fu FH, Ticker JB, Imhoff AB (eds): An Atlas of Shoulder Surgery. London: Martin Funitz, 1998, pp 259-273.
278. Bauer T, Abadie O, Hardy P: Arthroscopic treatment of glenoid fractures. Arthroscopy 22:569.e1-e6, 2006.

BIBLIOGRAPHY

Borens O, Kloen P, Richmond J, et al: Complex open trauma of the shoulder: A case report. Am J Orthop 33:149-152, 2004.
Brown MA, Sikka RS, Guanche CA, Fischer DA: Bilateral fractures of the scapula in a professional football player: A case report. Am J Sports Med 32:237-242, 2004.
Fukuda H, Mikasa M, Ogawa K: Ring retractor. J Bone Joint Surg Am 64:289, 1982.
Gillogly SD, Bizouski DT: Arthroscopic evaluation of the scapulothoracic articulation. Orthop Trans 16:196, 1992-1993.
Gramstad GD, Marra G: Treatment of glenoid fractures. Tech Shoulder Elbow Surg 3:102-110, 2002.
Key JA and Conwell HE: The Management of Fractures, Dislocations and Sprains. St Louis: CV Mosby, 1964.
Kumar A: Management of coracoid process fracture with acromioclavicular joint dislocation. Orthopedics 13:770-771, 1990.
Pace AM, Stuart R, Brownlow H: Outcome of glenoid neck fractures. J Shoulder Elbow Surg 14:585-590, 2005.
Rao KG: Correspondence. Br J Radiol 58:1057, 1985.
Van Noort, A te Slaa RL, Marti RK, van der Werken C: The floating shoulder—a multi centre study. J Bone Joint Surg Br 83:795-798, 2001.
Wertheimer C, Mogan J: Bilateral scapular fractures during a seizure in a patient following subtotal parathyroidectomy. Orthopedics 13:656-659, 1990.

Fractures of the Clavicle

Carl J. Basamania, MD, and Charles A. Rockwood, Jr, MD

A fracture of the clavicle has been greatly underrated in respect to pain and disability. . . . The "usual or routine treatment" is perhaps far short of satisfying, relieving therapy.

CARTER R. ROWE, 1968

Although fractures of the clavicle typically do not pose a significant diagnostic dilemma, there have been few injuries with as much controversy in regard to treatment as this fracture. This clinical relevance is underscored when one considers that the clavicle is the most common fracture site in children,[1,2] that an estimated 1 in 20 fractures involves the clavicle,[3] and that fractures of the clavicle constitute as much as 44% of shoulder girdle injuries.[4] Furthermore, it appears that the pattern of these fractures is changing, with fractures of much higher energy now being seen. Possibly as a consequence of this changing pattern, recent studies have shown poorer results with nonoperative treatment than with surgical intervention. There also seems to be a trend to recommend operative treatment for these more-displaced fractures.

HISTORICAL REVIEW

The clavicle is entirely subcutaneous and thus is easily accessible to inspection and palpation. This fact may account for its inclusion in some of the earliest descriptions of injuries of the human skeleton and their treatment. As early as 400 BC, Hippocrates recorded several observations about clavicle fractures. With a fractured clavicle, the distal fragment and the arm sag, whereas the proximal fragment, held securely by the attachments of the sternoclavicular joint, points upward. It is difficult to reduce the fracture and maintain the reduction:

They act imprudently who think to depress the projecting end of the bone. But it is clear that the underpart ought to be brought to the upper, for the former is the movable part, and that which has been displaced from its natural position.[5]

Union is usual and rapid and produces a prominent callus, and despite the deformity, healing usually proceeds uneventfully.

A fractured clavicle, like all other spongy bone, gets speedily united; for all such bone forms callus in a short time. When, then, a fracture has recently taken place, the patients attach much importance to it, as supposing the mischief greater than it really is; but, in a little time, the patients having no pain, nor finding any impediment to their walking or eating, become negligent, and the physician, finding they cannot make the parts look well, take themselves off, and are not sorry at the neglect of the patients, and in the mean time the callus is quickly formed.[5]

The Edwin Smith papyrus provides what is probably the earliest description of the accepted method of fracture reduction; an unknown Egyptian surgeon in 3550 BC recommended the following treatment of fractures of the clavicle:

Thou shouldst place him prostrate on his back with something folded between his shoulder blades, thou shouldst spread out with his two shoulders in order to stretch apart his collar bone until that break falls into place.[1,3,6]

Paul of Aegina, a 17th century Byzantine, reported that all that could ever be written about fractures of the clavicle had been written and that treatment included the supine position and the application of potions of olive oil, pigeon dung, snake oil, and other essences.[3]

Some of the earliest documented cases resulted from reports of riding accidents. William III in 1702 died of a fracture of the clavicle 3 days after falling when his horse shied at a molehill. Sir Benjamin Brodie described a "diffuse false venous aneurysm" that complicated a fracture of the clavicle in the case of Sir Robert Peel, who fell from his horse in 1850 on the way to Parliament. As Peel lapsed into unconsciousness, a pulsatile swelling rapidly developed behind the fracture, and his arm was paralyzed. *The Lancet* defended the physician's handling of the case even though many skeptics doubted that death could occur from a clavicle fracture.[7-9]

In 1839, Dupuytren, a keen, though controversial anatomist and observer, noted that the cumbersome devices of his day used to hold the reduction were often unnecessary; he advocated simply placing the arm on a pillow until union occurred. Several devices at that time often appeared to aggravate the difficulty created by the fracture or seemed to engender new problems. Dupuytren described a case in which bleeding could not be arrested: "When I was summoned I merely removed the apparatus (the pressure of which was the cause of the mischief) and placed the arm on a pillow. The bleeding immediately ceased."[9,10] He railed against cumbersome and painful treatment methods.

In the late 1860s, the current ambulatory treatment (early mobilization of the patient) was described by Lucas Championniere, who advocated a figure-of-eight dressing and suggested that recumbency, a popular treatment method of his day, be abandoned.[11] In 1871, Sayre, recognizing the difficulty in maintaining the reduction, advocated a method of ambulatory treatment involving a rigid dressing to maintain the reduction and support the extremity, a method that was echoed and taught in the textbooks of his time and still has many advocates.[12]

In 1859, Malgaigne concluded:

> But while for a century and a half we see the most celebrated surgeons striving to prefer, or perhaps more strictly to complicate, the contrivances for treating fractured clavicle we may follow parallel to them another series of no less estimable surgeons, who disbelieving in these so-called improvements, return to the simplest means, as to Hippocrates before them. If now we seek to judge of all these contrivances by their results we see that most of them are extolled as producing cures without deformity; but we see also that subsequent experience has always falsified these promises. I therefore regard the thing (absence of deformity) as not impossible, although for my own part I have never seen such an instance.[13]

This quotation well summarizes the results of most conservative methods of treatment of the fractured clavicle—that is, most fractures unite by various treatment methods. However, many patients are left with residual deformity, some shortening, and a lump. Interference with function, cosmesis, activity level, and satisfaction used to be considered minimal, but more-recent studies have suggested that the satisfaction patients achieve after treatment of fractures of the clavicle might not be as high as we previously thought.[14-16] In fact, Jesse Jupiter probably best summarized these shortcomings when he noted that "we are not meeting our patient expectations with current non-operative treatment."[17]

Although ambulatory treatment of fractures of the clavicle with support of the arm remains the mainstay of care today, there are few other fractures in humans where as much deformity, angulation, and shortening are accepted as the standard of care. Recent studies have shown that nonoperative treatment of clavicle fractures has been associated with chronic pain, weakness, and overall dissatisfaction on the part of the patients.[18,19] In a multicenter, prospective study, patients who were treated nonoperatively did significantly worse in terms of DASH (disabilities of the arm, shoulder, and hand) and Constant scores than those treated operatively.[20] Moreover, the patients treated nonoperatively had a more than threefold increase in the rate of nonunion than the operative patients, and the nonoperative patients had a significant risk of malunion and significantly longer time to radiographic healing.[20] Another study showed significant functional deficits in terms of DASH and Constant scores, with a strength deficit of 20% to 30% at an average follow-up of 55 months after conservative treatment of a clavicle shaft fracture.[18] Although some of these deficits in patients with malunions and nonunions improved with delayed treatment, there were still significant deficits as compared to patients who were treated acutely.[21] Other studies showed that displacement of more than one bone width was the most significant predictor of poor outcome in nonoperatively treated clavicle fractures,[22] and less than half of the patients returned to their previous recreational and professional activities after a clavicle fracture.[23]

ANATOMY

Development

The embryology of the clavicle is unique in that it is the first bone in the body to ossify (fifth week of fetal life) and is the only long bone to ossify by intramembranous ossification without going through a cartilaginous stage.[24-27] The ossification center begins in the central portion of the clavicle; this area is responsible for growth of the clavicle up to about 5 years of age.[1,28] Epiphyseal growth plates develop at both the medial and lateral ends of the clavicle, but only the sternal ossification center is present radiographically.[1,29] This medial growth plate of the clavicle is responsible for the majority of its longitudinal growth and probably contributes as much as 80% of the length of the clavicle.[30] The sternal ossification center appears and fuses relatively late in life, with ossification occurring between the ages of 12 and 19 years and fusion to the clavicle occurring at 22 to 25 years of age.[31,32] Thus, many of the so-called sternoclavicular dislocations in young adults are, in fact, epiphyseal fractures and are a potential source of confusion unless the late sternoclavicular epiphyseal closure is remembered.

MORPHOLOGY AND FUNCTION

The superior surface of the clavicle is essentially subcutaneous over its course, with only the thin platysma providing any muscular coverage and then only to the inner two thirds of the bone. The supraclavicular nerves, which provide sensation to the overlying skin, are consistently found just deep to the platysma muscle layer. These nerves have been known to cause painful neuromas when damaged by fracture shards or iatrogenic injury (Fig. 11-1).[33] The clavicle is the sole bone strut connecting the trunk to the shoulder girdle and arm, and it is the only bone of the shoulder girdle that forms a synovial joint with the trunk.[34] Its name is derived from the Latin word *clavis* (key), the diminutive of which is *clavicula,* a reference to the musical symbol of similar shape.[26]

The shape and configuration of the clavicle are not only important for its function but also provide an explanation for the pattern of fractures encountered in this bone. In 1993, Harrington and colleagues[35] described an image-processing system that was used to evaluate the histomorphometric properties of 15 adult male and female human clavicles. Variations in porosity, cross-sectional area, and anatomic and principal moments of inertia were assessed at 2.5% to 5% increments along the length of the bones. The clavicle's biomechanical behavior (axial, flexural, and proportional rigidity and the critical forceful buckling) was modeled from these data by using beam theory. More than threefold variations in porosity and moments of inertia were found along the length of the S-shaped clavicle, with the greatest porosity and moments of inertia being located in the variably shaped sternal and acromial thirds of the bone as opposed to the denser, smaller, and more circular central third of the bone.

Clavicle orientation, as indicated by the direction of greatest resistance to bending (maximal principal moment of inertia), was found to rotate from a primarily craniocaudal orientation at the sternum to a primarily anteroposterior (AP) orientation at the acromion. Based on cross-sectional geometry, sectional moduli, and estimates of flexural and proportional rigidity, the clavicle was found to be weakest in the central third of its length. These data concur with the fracture location most commonly reported clinically.

An analysis by Euler predicted a minimal critical force for buckling during axial loading of about two to three body weights for an average adult. Thus, buckling, or a combination of axial loading and bending or proportional loading, must be considered as a possible failure mechanism for this commonly injured bone.[35] Although it appears almost straight when viewed from the front, when viewed from above, the clavicle appears as an S-shaped double curve that is concave ventrally on its outer half and convex ventrally on its medial half (Fig. 11-2). Even though some reports have noted differences in the shape and size of the clavicle in male and female subjects and in the dominant and nondominant arm, others have not found such to be the case or have discounted their clinical significance.[30,34,36,37]

DePalma found that the outer third of the clavicle exhibited varying degrees of anterior torsion and suggested that changes in torsion might be responsible for the altered stresses that lead to primary degenerative changes in the acromioclavicular joint.[36] The cross section

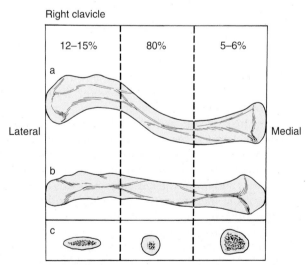

Right clavicle

12–15%   80%   5–6%

Lateral   Medial

a. Superior view
b. Frontal view
c. Cross sections

FIGURE 11-2 The clavicle appears as an S-shaped double curve when viewed from above *(a)*. It appears nearly straight when viewed from in front *(b)*. The outer end of the clavicle is flat in cross section but becomes more tubular in its medial aspect *(c)*.

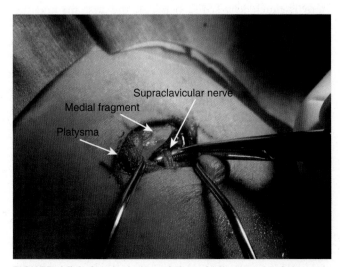

FIGURE 11-1 Surgical view of the middle branch of the supraclavicular nerve entrapped in the fracture site.

of the clavicle differs in shape along its length: It varies from flat along its outer third to prismatic along its inner third. The exact curvature of the clavicle and its thickness, to a high degree, vary according to the attachments of muscles and ligaments.[34] The flat outer third is most compatible with pull from muscles and ligaments, whereas the tubular medial third is a shape consistent with axial pressure or pull. The junction between the two cross sections varies with regard to its precise location in the middle third of the clavicle. This junction is a weak spot, particularly with axial loading,[34] which may be one of several reasons why fractures occur so commonly at the middle third. Another reason may be that it is an area not reinforced by muscles and ligaments and that it is just distal to the subclavius insertion.[3,38,39] It is curious that nature has strengthened, through ligaments or muscular reinforcement, every part of the clavicle except the end of the outer part of the middle third, which is the thinnest part of the bone.[40]

The clavicle articulates with the sternum through the sternoclavicular joint, which has little actual articular contact but surprisingly strong ligamentous attachments. The medial end of the clavicle is moored firmly against the first rib by the intra-articular sternoclavicular joint cartilage (which functions as a ligament), the oblique fibers of the costoclavicular ligaments, and to a lesser degree, the subclavius muscle.[36] The scapula and clavicle are bound securely by both the acromioclavicular and coracoclavicular ligaments, the mechanism and function of which have been reported extensively, and these ligaments contribute significantly to movement and stability of the entire upper extremity (Fig. 11-3).[41] The tubular third of the clavicle, which is thicker in cross section, offers protection for the important neurovascular structures that pass beneath the medial third of the clavicle. The intimate relationship between these structures and the clavicle assumes great importance both in acute fractures, in which direct injury can occur, and in the unusual fracture sequelae of malunion, nonunion, or production of excessive callus, in which compression of these structures can lead to late symptoms.

The brachial plexus, at the level at which it crosses beneath the clavicle, consists of three main branches (see Fig. 11-3). Of these branches, two are anterior. One (lateral) branch originates from the fifth, sixth, and seventh cervical roots and forms the musculocutaneous nerve and a branch of the median nerve; the other (medial) originates from the eighth cervical and first thoracic roots and forms another branch of the median nerve, the entire ulnar nerve, and the medial cutaneous nerve. The posterior branch of the plexus forms the axillary and radial nerves. The cord of the brachial plexus, which contains the first components of the ulnar nerve, crosses the first rib directly under the medial third of the clavicle. The other two cords are farther to the lateral side and posterior. Therefore, the ulnar nerve is more often involved in complications arising from fractures of the medial third of the clavicle.

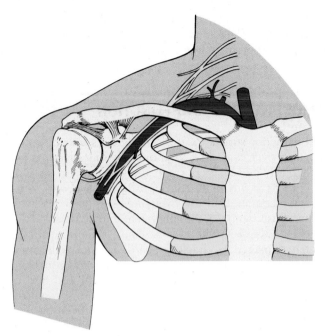

FIGURE 11-3 The clavicle is bound securely by ligaments at both the sternoclavicular and acromioclavicular joints. It is the only bony strut from the torso to the extremity. The brachial plexus and greater vessels are seen posterior to the medial third of the clavicle between the clavicle and the first rib.

The space between the clavicle and the first rib has been called the *costoclavicular space*. This space has been measured in gross anatomic studies and often appears to be quite adequate. However, it is not as large in a living subject as in a cadaver, possibly because in a living subject the vessels are distended and the dimensions of the cords of the brachial plexus are larger than in a cadaver. In addition, in a living subject the space is diminished as the first rib elevates because of contraction of the scalenus anticus. Hence, when the inner end of the outer fragment of the fractured clavicle is depressed, there is much less space between the first rib and the clavicle; the result is that the vessels (especially the subclavian and axillary vessels) and nerves (especially the ulnar nerve) are potentially subject to injury, pressure, or irritation.[40] The internal jugular, which is adjacent to the sternoclavicular joint (see Fig. 11-3), is not usually injured with middle third fractures but has the potential for injury in more medial trauma involving the sternum and sternoclavicular joint. The subclavian vessels, because of their relative proximity to the medial third of the clavicle, can also be injured during operative treatment of clavicle fractures.[42]

The clavicle also appears to be unique as a long bone in that it has only a periosteal blood supply and little, if any, intramedullary or nutrient arterial blood supply. More importantly, the periosteal blood supply has been found to be primarily on the anterior and superior surface of the clavicle. This blood supply, coupled with the poor soft tissue coverage of the clavicle, may be an important consideration in fixation of the clavicle, particularly when significant soft tissue stripping is necessary.[35,43]

Surgical Anatomy

The surgical anatomy relative to the fascial arrangements about the clavicle has been extensively described by Abbott and Lucas.[44] Such knowledge will reduce the risk of damage to neurovascular structures during surgical dissection.[45] It is useful to divide these structures into areas above, below, and behind the clavicle.

Above the Clavicle

At the sternal notch, a layer of cervical fascia splits into two layers, a superficial layer attached to the front and a deep layer attached to the back of the manubrium. The space between these layers contains lymphatics and a communicating vessel between the two anterior jugular veins. The two layers of fascia proceed laterally to enclose the sternocleidomastoid muscle before passing down to the clavicle. For 2.5 cm above the clavicle, they are separated by loose fat. The superficial layer is ill defined and is continuous with the fascia covering the undersurface of the trapezius muscle. A prolongation from the deep layer forms an inverted sling for the posterior belly of the omohyoid muscle, and it continues below to blend with the fascia enclosing the subclavius muscle. Medially, the omohyoid fascia covers the sternohyoid muscle.

Below the Clavicle

Two layers consisting of muscle and fascia form the anterior wall of the axilla. The pectoralis major and pectoral fascia form the superficial layer; the pectoralis minor and clavipectoral fascia form the deep layer. The pectoral fascia closely envelops the pectoralis major. Above, it is attached to the clavicle, and laterally, it forms the roof of the superficial infraclavicular triangle (formed by the pectoralis major, a portion of the anterior deltoid, and the clavicle). The deep layer—the clavipectoral fascia—extends from the clavicle above to the axillary fascia below. At the point where it attaches to the clavicle, it consists of two layers that enclose the subclavius muscle. The subclavius muscle arises from the manubrium and first rib and inserts into the inferior surface of the clavicle.

At the lower border of the subclavius, the two fascial layers join to form the costocoracoid membrane. This membrane fills a space between the subclavius above and the pectoralis minor below and is attached medially to the first costal cartilage and laterally to the coracoid process. Below, it splits into two layers that ensheathe the pectoralis minor. The costocoracoid membrane is pierced by the cephalic vein, the lateral pectoral nerve, and the thoracoacromial artery and vein.[44]

Behind the Clavicle

A continuous myofascial layer, which has not been commonly appreciated in surgical anatomy, lies in front of the large vessels and nerves as they pass from the root of the neck to the axilla. From above to below, this layer consists of the omohyoid fascia enclosing the omohyoid muscle and the clavipectoral fascia enclosing the pectoralis minor and subclavius muscles.[44] Behind the medial part of the clavicle and the sternoclavicular joint, the internal jugular and subclavian veins join to form the innominate vein. These veins are covered by the omohyoid fascia and by its extension medially over the sternohyoid and sternothyroid muscles. Behind the clavicle, at the junction between the middle and medial thirds, the junction of the subclavian and axillary veins lies very close to the clavicle and is also protected by this myofascial layer.

Between the omohyoid fascia posteriorly and the investing layer of cervical fascia anteriorly is a space, described by Grant, in which the external jugular vein usually joins the subclavian vein at its confluence with the internal jugular vein.[46] Before this junction, the external jugular is joined on its lateral aspect by the transverse cervical and scapular veins and on its medial aspect by the anterior jugular vein. This anastomosis usually lies just behind the fascial envelope and the angle formed by the posterior border of the sternocleidomastoid muscle and clavicle.[2]

FUNCTION

The function of the clavicle may be inferred, in part, by some study of comparative anatomy. Codman has stated:

> [W]e are proud that our brains are more developed than the animals: we might also boast of our clavicles. It seems to me that the clavicle is one of man's greatest skeletal inheritances, for he depends to a greater extent than most animals, except the apes and monkeys, on the use of his hands and arms.[47]

Mammals that depend on swimming, running, or grazing have no clavicles, whereas species with clavicles appear to be predominantly fliers or climbers. Codman theorized that animals with strong clavicles needed to use their arms more in adduction and abduction. The long clavicle may facilitate placement of the shoulder in a more lateral position so that the hand can be positioned more effectively to deal with the three-dimensional environment.[48]

The teleologic role of the clavicle has been disputed, however, because of reports of entirely normal function of the upper limb after complete excision of the clavicle.[49-51] These reports, combined with observations in patients with congenital absence of the clavicle (cleidocranial dysostosis) who do not appear to have any impairment in limb function, are probably responsible for the often-stated belief that this bone is a surplus part that can be excised without any disturbance in function. However, others have noted drooping of the shoulder, weakness, and loss of motion after excision of the clavicle and have

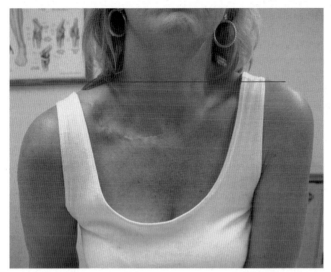

FIGURE 11-4 Appearance of a patient who has had a complete clavulectomy. Note the significant drooping of the right shoulder. The patient complained of chronic pain, hand numbness, and an inability to keep her bra strap on her shoulder.

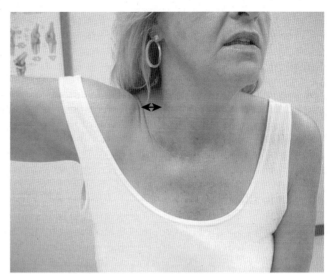

FIGURE 11-5 Note the medial collapse of the shoulder during attempted abduction.

used these observations to attribute to the clavicle its important role in normal function of the extremity (Figs. 11-4 and 11-5).[52,53]

The clavicle does have several important functions, each of which would be expected to be altered not only by excision of the bone but also by fracture, nonunion, or malunion.

Power and Stability of the Arm

The clavicle, by serving as a bony link from the thorax to the shoulder girdle, provides a stable linkage of the arm–trunk mechanism and contributes significantly to the power and stability of the arm and shoulder girdle, especially in movement above shoulder level.[27] It transmits the support and force of the trapezius muscle to the scapula and arm via the coracoclavicular ligaments.

Although patients with cleidocranial dysostosis and absence of the clavicle do not appear to have significantly decreased range of motion and can, in fact, have an increase in protraction and retraction of the scapula (because of absence of the clavicle), they can exhibit some weakness in supporting a load overhead. This limitation further suggests that the clavicle adds stability to the extremity under load in extreme ranges of motion.[51]

The clavicle is predominantly supported and stabilized by passive structures,[34] particularly the sternoclavicular ligaments.[54,55] Although evidence of trapezius muscle activity at rest has been demonstrated electromyographically, thus suggesting a role for that muscle in support of the clavicle,[54] other authors have not been able to demonstrate that muscle activity plays any role in supporting the clavicle.

Motion of the Shoulder Girdle

When the arm is elevated 180 degrees, the clavicle angles upward 30 degrees and backward 35 degrees at the sternoclavicular joint. It also rotates upward on its longitudinal axis approximately 50 degrees. During combined glenohumeral, acromioclavicular, and sternoclavicular movement, the humerus moves approximately 120 degrees at the glenohumeral joint and the scapula moves along the chest wall approximately 60 degrees. These complex and combined simultaneous movements of the joints and their articulating bony structures (scapula, humerus, and clavicle) seem to imply an important role for the clavicle in range of motion of the arm. This role is debatable, however, because it has been observed by some that loss of the clavicle does not in fact impair abduction of the arm at all[44,56] and that excision of the clavicle can permit range of motion just as well. However, Rockwood has observed loss of the clavicle to result in disabling loss of function, weakness, drooping of the arm, and pain secondary to irritation of the brachial plexus (see Figs. 11-4 and 11-5).[52]

It has been stated that its contribution to motion may be the most important function of the clavicle and that this role is related to its curvature, especially its lateral curvature. The 50-degree rotation of the clavicle on its axis appears to be important for free elevation of the extremity. In fact, a direct relationship has been found among the line of attachment of the coracoclavicular ligaments, the amount of clavicular rotation, the extent and relative lengthening of the ligaments, and scapula rotation itself. Of the total 60 degrees of scapular rotation, the first 30 degrees is due to elevation of the clavicle as a whole by movement of the sternoclavicular joint, and the second 30 degrees is permitted through the acromioclavicular joint by clavicular rotation and elongation of the coracoclavicular ligaments. Thus, the lateral curvature of the

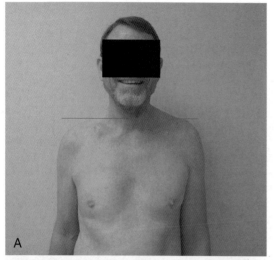

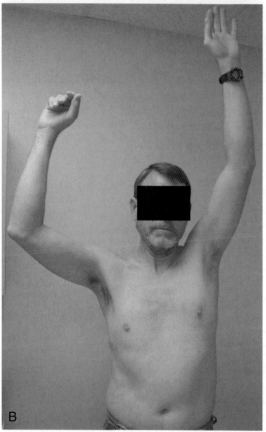

FIGURE 11-6 A, Clinical appearance of a patient with clavicle malunion. **B,** Note the drooping of the right shoulder and loss of forward flexion.

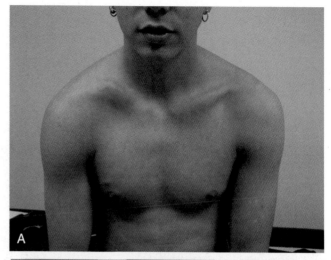

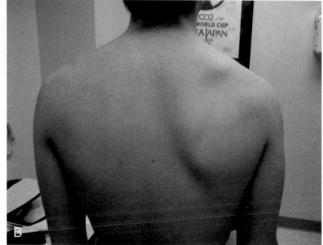

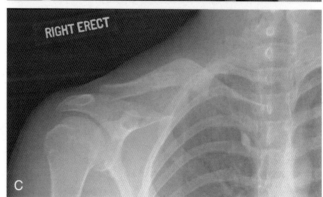

FIGURE 11-7 Clinical appearance and radiograph of a patient with a clavicle malunion. **A,** Anterior view. **B,** Posterior view. Note the scapular pseudowinging. **C,** AP radiograph.

clavicle permits it to act as a crankshaft, effectively allowing half of scapular movement.[57]

The smooth, rhythmic movement of the shoulder girdle is a complex interaction of muscle groups acting on joints and both the subacromial and scapulothoracic spaces. Although it is difficult to break down all the contributions of the clavicle to total motion of the shoulder, it appears that its geometric and kinematic design, by permitting

rotation, maximizes the stability of the upper limb against the trunk while permitting mobility, particularly of the scapula along the chest wall. The practical result is that the glenoid fossa continually moves, facing and contacting the humeral head as the arm is used overhead.[51]

Nonunion and malunion can cause significant alterations in orientation of the scapula and glenohumeral joint[58,59] (Figs. 11-6 and 11-7). This altered orientation is typically

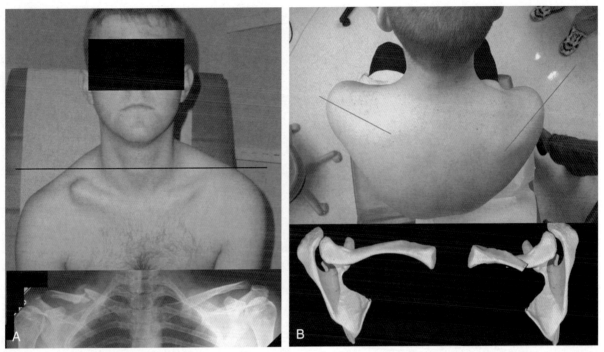

FIGURE 11-8 A, Clinical appearance and AP radiograph of an acute fracture. Note the inferior displacement of the involved shoulder relative to the normal shoulder. **B,** Same patient viewed from above. Note the anterior rotation of the right shoulder relative to the coronal plane of the body. The changes in orientation of the scapula are shown in the schematic drawing.

an anteromedial and inferior rotatory deformity. Malunion represents a fixed or static change in orientation of the scapula, whereas nonunion is a dynamic deformity, much as one would see in a significant acromioclavicular separation (Figs. 11-8 and 11-9). This change in orientation of the scapula results in a change in the resting length of the muscles about the shoulder. Basamania[60] and McKee[16] found significant weakness in the affected limbs of patients with clavicle malunion, regardless of the time since their injury. This weakness corrected with return of the clavicle to its normal length in spite of no formal physical therapy.

Muscle Attachments

The clavicle also acts as a bony framework for muscle origin and insertion. The upper third of the trapezius inserts on the superior surface of the outer third of the clavicle, opposite the site of origin of the clavicular head of the deltoid along its anterior edge. The clavicular head of the sternocleidomastoid muscle arises from the posterior edge of the inner third of the clavicle. The clavicular head of the pectoralis major muscle arises from the anterior edge of the clavicle. During active elevation of the arm, these muscles contract simultaneously. It has been suggested that in theory, the muscles above the clavicle could be directly attached to the muscles below the clavicle as a continuous muscular layer without an interposed bony attachment,[44] but the stable bony framework

clearly provides the advantage of a solid foundation for muscle attachment.

The other muscle that inserts on the clavicle is the subclavius muscle. After it arises from the first rib anteriorly at the costochondral junction, it proceeds obliquely and posteriorly into a groove on the undersurface of the clavicle. This muscle appears to aid in depressing the middle third of the clavicle. Fractures of the clavicle often occur at the distal portion of its insertion. In midclavicle fractures, this muscle can offer some protection to the neurovascular structures beneath; however, it can also become entrapped within the fracture site and delay or inhibit healing.

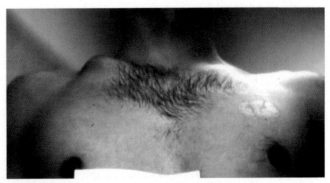

FIGURE 11-9 Significant right clavicle malunion.

Protection of Neurovascular Structures

The clavicle also provides skeletal protection for adjacent neurovascular structures and the superior aspect of the lung. The subclavian and axillary vessels, the brachial plexus, and the lung are directly behind the medial third of the clavicle. The tubular cross section of the medial third of the clavicle increases its strength and adds to its protective function at this level. The anterior curve of the medial two thirds of the clavicle provides a rigid arch beneath which the great vessels pass as they move from the mediastinum and thoracic outlet to the axilla. It has been shown that during elevation of the arm, the clavicle, as it rotates upward, also moves backward, with the curvature providing increased clearance for the vessels.[61] Loss of the clavicle eliminates this bony barrier against external trauma.[62] In addition, loss of the clavicle can cause exacerbation of thoracic outlet symptoms because of drooping of the shoulder and resultant draping of the brachial plexus over the first rib (see Figs. 11-3 and 11-4).

Respiratory Function

Elevation of the lateral part of the clavicle results in increased pull on the costoclavicular ligament and subclavius muscle. Because of the connection between the clavicle and the first rib and between the first rib and the sternum, elevation of the shoulder girdle brings about a cephalad motion of the thorax corresponding to an inspiration. This relationship is used in some breathing exercises and in some forms of artificial respiration.[44]

Cosmesis

By providing a graceful curve to the base of the neck, the smooth, subcutaneous bony clavicle serves a cosmetic function. After surgical excision of the clavicle, the upper limb in some patients falls downward and forward and gives a foreshortened appearance to this area. Female patients have complained of difficulty keeping their bra strap on their affected shoulder because of this drooping (see Figs. 11-4 and 11-5). The cosmetic function of the clavicle is noted by many patients who are concerned by excessive formation of callus after a clavicle fracture or by deformity after clavicular malunion (see Fig. 11-9).[62]

CLASSIFICATION OF CLAVICLE FRACTURES

To be effective, a classification system should be accurate in terms of identifying the pathologic anatomy, and it should be able to predict outcome, thereby serving as a basis for deciding on proper treatment. Ideally, a classification system should also be sufficiently straightforward that it is easily reproducible with good intraobserver and interobserver reliability. Unfortunately, most clavicle fracture classification systems are merely descriptive and give no guidance in terms of prognosis. Although clavicle fractures have been classified by fracture configuration (e.g., greenstick, oblique, transverse, comminuted),[63] the usual classification is by location of the fracture because location appears to better compartmentalize our understanding of fracture anatomy, mechanism of injury, clinical findings, and alternative methods of treatment.[64-68] One of the early classifications of clavicle fractures was Allman's classification. He divided these fractures into three groups[64]:

Group I: Fractures of the middle third
Group II: Fractures of the distal third
Group III: Fractures of the medial third

Neer[3,67,69,70] and Jager and Breitner[71] devised a specific classification for fractures of the distal third of the clavicle.

Craig's Classification

In 1990, Craig[72] introduced a more detailed classification of clavicle fractures that was based on the variable fracture patterns seen within the three broad groups of Allman's clavicle fracture classification (Box 11-1).

Group I Fractures

Group I fractures, or fractures of the middle third, are the most common fractures seen in adults and children. They occur at the point at which the clavicle changes to a flat-

---

BOX 11-1 Craig's Classification of Clavicle Fractures

Group I: Fracture of the Middle Third

Group II: Fracture of the Distal Third
Type I: Minimal displacement (interligamentous)
Type II: Displaced secondary to a fracture medial to the coracoclavicular ligaments
   A. Conoid and trapezoid attached
   B. Conoid torn, trapezoid attached
Type III: Fractures of the articular surface
Type IV: Ligaments intact to the periosteum (children), with displacement of the proximal fragment
Type V: Comminuted, with ligaments attached neither proximally nor distally, but to an inferior, comminuted fragment

Group III: Fracture of the Proximal Third
Type I: Minimal displacement
Type II: Displaced (ligaments ruptured)
Type III: Intra-articular
Type IV: Epiphyseal separation (children and young adults)
Type V: Comminuted

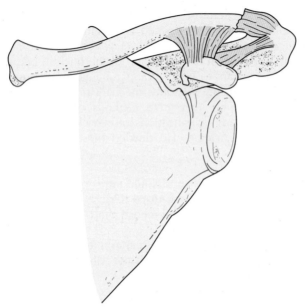

FIGURE 11-10 Type I fracture of the distal end of the clavicle (group II). The intact ligaments hold the fragments in place. (From Rockwood CA, Green DP [eds]: Fractures [3 vols], 2nd ed. Philadelphia: JB Lippincott, 1984.)

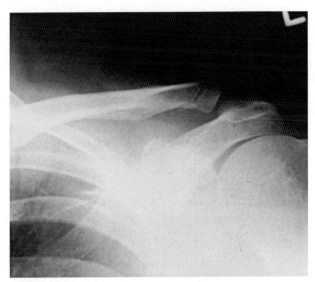

FIGURE 11-11 A type I fracture of the distal end of the clavicle seen radiographically. The fragments are held in place securely by the intact coracoclavicular and acromioclavicular ligaments.

tened cross section from a prismatic cross section. The force of the traumatic impact follows the curve of the clavicle and disperses on reaching the lateral curve.[73-76] In addition, the proximal and distal segments of the clavicle are mechanically secured by ligamentous structures and muscular attachments, whereas the central segment is relatively free. This fracture accounts for 80% of clavicle fractures.[3,4]

Group II Fractures

Group II fractures account for 12% to 15% of all clavicle fractures and are subclassified according to the location of the coracoclavicular ligaments relative to the fracture fragments.[77] Neer first pointed out the importance of this fracture while subdividing it into four types.

Type I fractures are the most common by a ratio of 4:1. In this fracture, the ligaments remain intact to hold the fragments together and prevent rotation, tilting, or significant displacement. This fracture is an interligamentous fracture that occurs between the conoid and the trapezoid or between the coracoclavicular and acromioclavicular ligaments (Figs. 11-10 and 11-11).[70]

In type II distal clavicle fractures, the coracoclavicular ligaments are detached from the medial segment. Both the conoid and trapezoid may be on the distal fragment (IIA) (Fig. 11-12), or the conoid ligament may be ruptured while the trapezoid ligament remains attached to the distal segment (IIB) (Fig. 11-13).[1] There is really no functional difference between these two fractures. The high rate of nonunion in these fractures may be secondary to excessive motion at the fracture site. These fractures are equivalent to a serious acromioclavicular separation in

which the normal constraints to anteromedial rotation of the scapula relative to the clavicle are lost.

Four forces that may impair healing and may be contributing factors to the reported high incidence of nonunion act on this fracture: When the patient is erect, the outer fragment, which retains the attachment of the trapezoid ligament to the scapula through the intact acromioclavicular ligaments, is pulled downward and forward by the weight of the arm; the pectoralis major, pectoralis minor, and latissimus dorsi draw the distal segment downward and medially, thereby causing overriding; the scapula might rotate the distal segment as the arm is moved; and the trapezius muscle attaches to the entire outer two thirds of the clavicle, whereas the sternocleidomastoid muscle attaches to the medial third, and these muscles act to draw

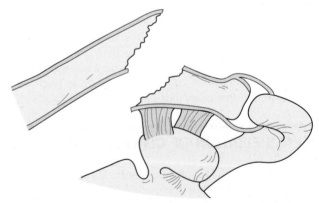

FIGURE 11-12 Type II distal clavicle fracture. In type IIA, both the conoid and trapezoid ligaments are on the distal segment, and the proximal segment, without ligamentous attachments, is displaced. (From Rockwood CA, Green DP [eds]: Fractures [3 vols], 2nd ed. Philadelphia: JB Lippincott, 1984.)

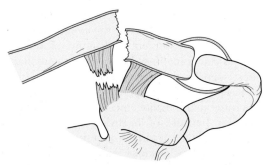

FIGURE 11-13 Type IIB fracture of the distal part of the clavicle. The conoid ligament is ruptured, and the trapezoid ligament remains attached to the distal segment. The proximal fragment is displaced. (From Rockwood CA, Green DP [eds]: Fractures [3 vols], 2nd ed. Philadelphia: JB Lippincott, 1984.)

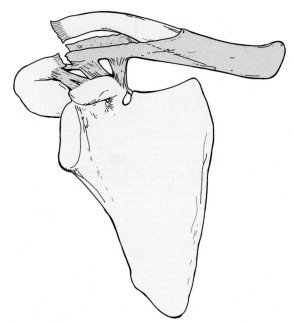

FIGURE 11-14 A type IV fracture occurring in children that has been called a *pseudodislocation of the acromioclavicular joint.* The coracoclavicular ligaments remain attached to the bone or the periosteum, and the proximal fragment ruptures through the thin superior periosteum and may be displaced upward by muscle forces. (From Rockwood CA, Green DP [eds]: Fractures [3 vols], 2nd ed. Philadelphia: JB Lippincott, 1984.)

the clavicular segment superiorly and posteriorly, often into the substance of the trapezius muscle.[67]

Type III distal clavicle fractures involve the articular surface of the acromioclavicular joint alone. Although type II fractures can have intra-articular extension, type III fractures are characterized by a break in the articular surface without a ligamentous injury. A type III injury may be subtle, may be confused with a first-degree acromioclavicular separation, and can require special views to visualize. In fact, it may be manifested as late degenerative joint arthrosis of the acromioclavicular joint. In addition, it has been suggested that weightlifter's clavicle, or resorption of the distal end of the clavicle, might occur from increased vascularity secondary to the microtrauma or microfractures that lead to such resorption.[3,78-80]

It appears logical to add a fourth and fifth type of distal clavicle fracture because in a certain series of fractures, bone displacement occurs as a result of deforming muscle forces, but the coracoclavicular ligaments remain attached to bone or periosteum.

Type IV fractures occur in children and may be confused with complete acromioclavicular separation (Fig. 11-14). Called *pseudodislocation* of the acromioclavicular joint, these fractures typically occur in children younger than 16 years.[81] The distal end of the clavicle is fractured, and the acromioclavicular joint remains intact. In children and young adults, the attachment between bone and the periosteum is relatively loose. The proximal fragment ruptures through the thin periosteum and may be displaced upward by muscular forces. The coracoclavicular ligaments remain attached to the periosteum or may be avulsed with a small piece of bone.[65,66,81]

Group III Fractures

Group III fractures, or fractures of the inner third of the clavicle, constitute 5% to 6% of clavicle fractures. As with distal clavicle fractures, they can be subdivided according to the integrity of the ligamentous structures. If the costoclavicular ligaments remain intact and attached to the outer fragment, little or no displacement develops.[64,82]

When these lesions occur in children, they are usually epiphyseal fractures.[83] In adults, articular surface injuries can also lead to degenerative changes.[3,84]

Panclavicular dislocation, or a traumatic floating clavicle, is neither a clavicle fracture nor an isolated sternoclavicular or acromioclavicular separation.[85-89] In this injury, both sternoclavicular ligaments and the coracoclavicular and the acromioclavicular ligamentous structures are disrupted.

Rockwood's Classification

Clinically and radiographically, it may be impossible to distinguish between grade III acromioclavicular separations, type II fractures of the distal end of the clavicle, and type IV fractures involving rupture of the periosteum.[3,67,70] Rockwood has classified these fractures in a manner that is roughly analogous to his classification system for acromioclavicular joint injuries in adults (Fig 11-15) (see Chapter 12). This system is based on the amount of energy imparted to the distal part of the clavicle, which determines the degree of displacement, and the direction of the applied force, which determines the direction of the displacement. The subtypes are based on the position of the distal end of the clavicle relative to the periosteal tube.[81]

Type I is a minor strain of the acromioclavicular ligaments without disruption of the periosteal sleeve of the

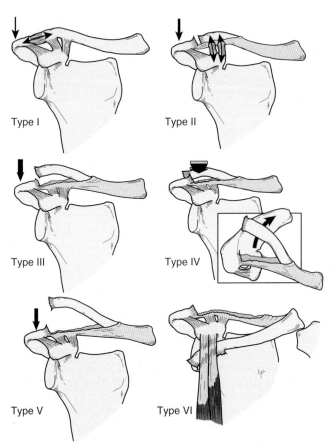

Type I

Type II

Type III

Type IV

Type V

Type VI

FIGURE 11-15 The Rockwood classification of distal clavicle injuries in children. Refer to the text for a complete description of this classification system. (From Rockwood CA Jr and Green DP [eds]: Fractures [3 vols], 2nd ed., Philadelphia: JB Lippincott, 1984.)

clavicle. A patient with this injury might have tenderness to palpation of the acromioclavicular joint but no significant side-to-side radiographic changes.

In a *type II* fracture, some disruption of the periosteal sleeve with a minimal increase in the coracoclavicular interval is noted on radiographs when compared with the uninjured side. The acromioclavicular interval might appear to be slightly widened.

Type III fracture is a gross disruption of the dorsal aspect of the periosteal sleeve, with the clavicle appearing to be displaced upward relative to the scapula. On plain radiographs taken with both shoulders on the same cassette, the clavicles actually appear to be of the same relative height, with the scapula on the injured side drooping downward. This finding is usually confirmed clinically. The coracoclavicular interval can appear to be increased 50% to 100% more than on the uninjured side. Swelling and ecchymosis may be present over the dorsal aspect of the acromioclavicular joint and the distal end of the clavicle in addition to ecchymosis over the posterolateral aspect of the acromion. If the coracoclavicular interval is not widened but the acromioclavicular space is significantly widened, the physician should be suspi-

cious of a coracoid base fracture. With these injuries, the force is dissipated in fracturing the coracoid before the periosteal tube is disrupted. A fracture of the base of the coracoid can sometimes be seen on the axillary view but is best seen on the Stryker notch view.

Type IV is posterior displacement of the clavicle relative to the acromion. In reality, the clavicle remains in the same position because of its strong medial attachments; however, the scapula is driven anteriorly relative to the clavicle. The coracoclavicular interval might not appear to be significantly increased, thereby leading the physician to conclude that it is a less-significant injury. Key to examination of the patient is palpating the distal part of the clavicle relative to the acromion and obtaining a good axillary view to look for the relative posterior displacement of the clavicle. In our experience, these injuries are the most problematic in children and adolescents, just as type IV injuries in adults are so disabling, because the distal end of the clavicle can be buttonholed out of the trapezius muscle. Such buttonholing not only prevents reduction but also causes considerable pain for the patient.

Type V is essentially a severe type III injury with complete disruption of the dorsal periosteal tube and significant superior displacement of the distal part of the clavicle relative to the acromion. This injury is presumably due to the additional disruption of the deltotrapezial fascia. Again, the distal end of the clavicle really stays in its anatomic position but the scapula drops away. The coracoclavicular interval is typically increased more than 100%. In type V fractures in adults, neither of the main fracture fragments has a functional coracoclavicular ligament. These fracture fragments are displaced by the deforming muscles as in type I distal clavicle fractures, but the coracoclavicular ligaments are intact and remain attached to a small, third comminuted intermediary segment.[68] This fracture is thought to be more unstable than type II distal clavicle fractures.

Type VI injuries are extremely rare and are associated with displacement of the clavicle under the coracoid process.

Robinson's Classification

The classification proposed by Robinson (Fig. 11-16) is perhaps the only validated classification system in terms of correlating the type of fracture with the typical outcome.[45] His system was based on the observation of 1000 adult clavicle fractures and takes into account the anatomic site, extent of displacement, comminution, and articular extension and stability of the fracture.

Much like Allman's classification, the primary anatomic sites are medial (*type 1*), middle (*type 2*), and lateral (*type 3*). Displacement further subdivides these primary groups if they are displaced less than 100% (subgroup A) or more than 100% (subgroup B). Type 1 and 3 fractures are subdivided with regard to their articular involvement, with subgroup 1 being no intra-articular involvement and

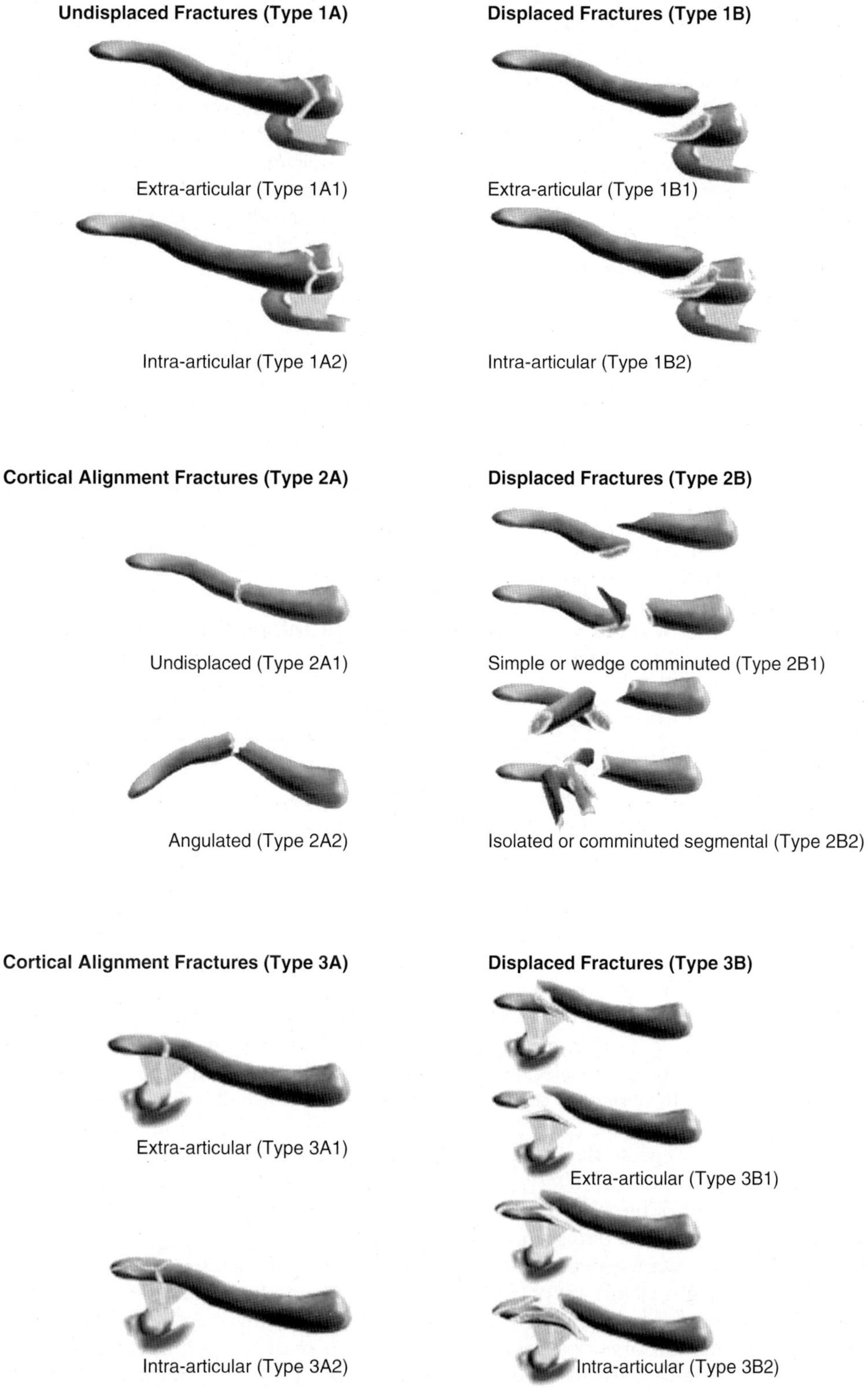

Undisplaced Fractures (Type 1A)

Extra-articular (Type 1A1)

Intra-articular (Type 1A2)

Displaced Fractures (Type 1B)

Extra-articular (Type 1B1)

Intra-articular (Type 1B2)

Cortical Alignment Fractures (Type 2A)

Undisplaced (Type 2A1)

Angulated (Type 2A2)

Displaced Fractures (Type 2B)

Simple or wedge comminuted (Type 2B1)

Isolated or comminuted segmental (Type 2B2)

Cortical Alignment Fractures (Type 3A)

Extra-articular (Type 3A1)

Intra-articular (Type 3A2)

Displaced Fractures (Type 3B)

Extra-articular (Type 3B1)

Intra-articular (Type 3B2)

FIGURE 11-16 Robinson classification of clavicle fractures. (From Robinson CM: Fractures of the clavicle in the adult. Epidemiology and classification. J Bone Joint Surg Br 80:476-484, 1998.)

subgroup 2 having intra-articular extension. Type 2 fractures are subdivided with regard to their comminution. Simple or wedge comminution is subgroup 1, and segmental or comminuted fractures are subgroup 2.

By combining these groups and subgroups, virtually all fractures can be described. For example, a comminuted, displaced midshaft fracture is described as a *type 2B2* fracture, and a nondisplaced intra-articular lateral clavicle fracture is a *type 3A2*. Robinson found that both displacement and comminution were associated with an increased risk of delayed union or nonunion.[45]

MECHANISM OF INJURY

Because the clavicle is the bone that is most often fractured, numerous causes of fracture of the clavicle, both traumatic and nontraumatic, have been reported.[90]

Trauma in Children

Fractures of the clavicle in children share many of the same mechanisms of injury as in adults and can result from a direct blow to the clavicle or the point of the shoulder or from an indirect blow such as a fall on the outstretched hand. However, other features are unusual and unique to children, including obstetric fracture of the clavicle and plastic bowing injury.

Birth Fractures

In 15,000 deliveries from 1954 to 1959, Rubin found that fractures of the clavicle were the most common injury at birth.[91] Although it has been stated that intrapartum traumatic injuries are decreasing as a result of improvements in obstetric care,[41,92-95] the incidence of clavicle fracture remains quite high, and in infants it might actually be increasing.[96] Moir and Myerscough found an incidence of clavicle fractures of 5 per 1000 vertex births, which increased to 160 per 1000 with a breech presentation.[97] The mechanism of injury in a full-term newborn infant delivered vaginally, when the baby is in a cephalic presentation, is compression of the leading clavicle against the maternal symphysis pubis.[98,99] In a breech delivery, direct traction can occur and produce the same bone injury as the obstetrician tries to depress the shoulders and free the arm during delivery of the head.[100,101]

The overall incidence of fracture of the clavicle during birth is approximately 0.5 to 7.2 per 1000 births. In addition to the presentation of the infant, several factors appear to be involved. Birth weight clearly plays a role because the incidence of fractures of the clavicle increases with increasing birth weight and in larger babies.[102,103] Babies who weigh 3800 to 4000 g or measure 52 cm or longer seem to be at higher risk for fracture. Increased maternal age has likewise been shown to be a risk factor for birth fracture.[104] The experience of the physician is probably also related. Cohen and Otto reported an increased incidence of fractures of the clavicle when babies were delivered by less-experienced residents, and a decrease in incidence was noted for each year of obstetrics experience.[105] This statistic certainly merits consideration in obstetrics house staff training. The method of delivery is also important because of an increase in the risk of fracture with midforceps deliveries, which calls into question the wisdom of this obstetric maneuver. On the other hand, Balata and coworkers noted no fractures in babies delivered by cesarean section.[96]

Fracture of the clavicle does not seem to be related to the type of anesthesia, length of active labor, length of second-stage labor, Apgar score, or parity of the mother. The exact anatomy of fractures that occur during delivery varies, and incomplete, greenstick, and bicortical disruptions with or without displacement have all been reported.[2] In one study, boys were more commonly affected than girls, and the right clavicle was fractured more often than the left clavicle.[96] In 1992, a study suggested a relationship between fractures of the clavicle and mothers with a second childbirth.[106]

All the literature suggests that more frequent and systematic clinical examination might reduce the incidence or make the diagnosis of clavicle fractures more timely because of what we now know to be risk factors.

Injuries in Infancy and Childhood

Fractures of the clavicle are particularly common in childhood, and almost half occur in children younger than 7 years.[107] Fractures commonly result from a fall on the point of the shoulder or on an outstretched hand. In younger children, such a fall is not uncommonly from a highchair, bed, or changing table. The fracture is occasionally caused by a direct violent force applied from the front of the clavicle; like other fractures of long bones, fractures of the clavicle may be one of several signs of trauma in a physically abused child.

Unlike the situation in adults, direct and indirect trauma to a child's clavicle can result in incomplete or greenstick fractures rather than displaced fractures.[75] In addition, trauma to a child's clavicle can result in plastic bowing alone without evident cortical disruption. Despite an initial appearance of only bowing, on later examination these fractures usually show evidence of gross healing of complete fractures, with obvious callus visible on radiographs.[108,109]

Trauma in Adults

The incidence of fractures of the clavicle in adults appears to be increasing because of several factors, including the occurrence of many more high-velocity vehicular injuries and the increase in popularity of contact sports.[36] The mechanism of injury of fractures of the clavicle in adults has been widely reported to consist of either direct or indirect force. It has generally been assumed that the most common mechanism of fractures in adults is a fall onto the outstretched hand.[36] Allman, in dividing fractures of the clavicle into three groups, proposed different mechanisms of injury for each group.[64] He thought that in group I (fractures of the middle third), the most common mechanism of injury is a fall onto an outstretched hand, with the force being transmitted up the arm and across the glenohumeral joint and dispersing along the clavicle. Group II fractures, those distal to the coracoclavicular ligaments, occur from a fall on the lateral aspect of the shoulder that drives the shoulder and scapula downward. Group III fractures, or proximal clavicle fractures, are usually due to direct violence caused by a force applied from the lateral side.

In 1994, Nordqvist and Petersson investigated the incidence of fractures of the clavicle. They reviewed 2035 fractures that occurred between 1952 and 1987.[110] The fractures were classified into three groups according to the Allman system.[64] Each group was further divided into nondisplaced fracture subgroups, with an extra subgroup of comminuted midclavicle fractures in group I. Of the fractures, 76% were classified as Allman group I. The median age of patients in this group was 13 years. Significant differences in age- and gender-specific incidence were noted between the nondisplaced, displaced, and comminuted fracture subgroups. Allman group II accounted for 21% of fractures. The median age of these patients was 47 years, and no difference in age was found between the subgroups with nondisplaced and displaced fractures. Three percent of the fractures were classified as Allman group III, and the median age of patients in this group was 59 years. All three groups were characterized by a significant preponderance of male patients.

A study by Nowak in 2000 showed that the incidence of clavicle fractures in Uppsala, Sweden, was 50 per 100,000 population; however, the incidence in male patients was 71 per 100,000, and the incidence in female patients was 30 per 100,000.[111,112] Bicycle accidents were the most common cause of injury, and male patients tended to be younger and to have more comminuted, high-energy injuries. Most (75%) of the injuries were midshaft fractures, and the nonunion rate was 5%.

In 1962, Fowler[113] pointed out that all clavicular injuries almost always follow a fall or a blow on the point of the shoulder, whereas a blow on the bone itself is rarely a cause (although a direct blow has certainly been recognized in sports, particularly in stick sports such as lacrosse and hockey[114]). In a large series of fractures of the clavicle (342 patients) studied by Sankarankutty and Turner, 91% sustained a fall or blow to the point of the shoulder, whereas only 1% had a fall onto the outstretched hand.[115]

More recently, Stanley and colleagues studied a consecutive series of 150 patients with fractures of the clavicle; 81% of the patients described information about the mechanism of injury.[116] The researchers found that 94% had fractured the clavicle from a direct blow on the shoulder, whereas only 6% had fallen onto an outstretched hand. Further biomechanical analysis of the force involved in fracture of the clavicle by this group revealed that direct injury produces a critical buckling load that is exceeded at a compression force equivalent to body weight and thereby results in fracture of the bone. When force is applied along the axis of the arm, the buckling force is rarely reached in the clavicle. These investigators recorded fractures at every site along the clavicle with a direct injury to the point of the shoulder and found little support for Allman's concept that fractures at different anatomic sites have different mechanisms of injury. In addition, they theorized that a direct blow to the shoulder might even be the mechanism of injury in those who described a fall on the outstretched hand: as the hand makes contact with the ground, the patient's body weight and falling velocity are such that the fall continues, with the shoulder becoming the upper limb's next point of contact with the ground.

Harnroongroj and coworkers found that when clavicles were axially loaded, they tended to fracture at the middle third of the clavicle in the region where the curve of the lateral aspect of the clavicle changes to the curve of the medial aspect of the clavicle.[117] The force required to fracture the clavicle was 1526.19 N. The ratio of the lateral fragment to the total length of the clavicle was 0.49.

Another indirect mechanism of fracture of the clavicle is a direct force applied to the top of the shoulder; the clavicle is forced against the first rib, and a spiral fracture of the middle third is often produced.[36] Another variation of this mechanism is what we refer to as *seat-belt fractures*. The shoulder strap from the seat belt acts as a fulcrum, typically at the midpoint of the clavicle, and the forward force of the clavicle against this fulcrum causes the clavicle to fracture in a transverse or oblique pattern with little or no comminution. Although we cannot explain why, it appears that this fracture is more prone to nonunion than a more typical fracture is (Fig 11-17). It may be because the amount of energy required to cause a transverse fracture is more than that required to cause a fracture as one sees with an axial load.

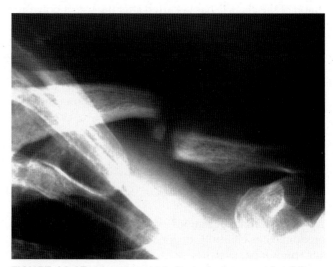

FIGURE 11-17 Atrophic midshaft clavicular nonunion 18 months after a seat-belt injury.

Stress Fractures

Stress fractures of the clavicle have been reported in athletes. They have been seen in a variety of sports, including baseball, diving, gymnastics, and cheerleading.[44,118-121] It appears that the mechanism of injury is repeated axial loading of the clavicle in all the activities except cheerleading. These fractures tend to be more medial and should be suspected in patients with chronic clavicular pain associated with overuse. Although plain radiographs can appear normal, bone scintigraphy usually reveals endosteal thickening; however, magnetic resonance imaging (MRI) can easily detect these injuries and also help rule out pathologic fractures. Most of these fractures occur after changes or an increase in the athlete's training routine and typically heal uneventfully with rest and activity modification. Stress fractures have also been reported in conjunction with coracoclavicular cerclage fixation of acromioclavicular joint separation.[122]

Nontraumatic Fractures

It is well recognized that the clavicle can be the site of neoplastic or infectious destruction of bone, and a fracture can occur after relatively minor trauma. Certainly, lack of a traumatic episode should lead the clinician to focus on the possibility that a long bone fracture has occurred in pathologic bone. In addition to both malignant and benign lesions producing pathologic fractures of the clavicle,[53,123] pathologic fracture has also been described in association with arteriovenous malformation, an entity that can mimic a neoplasm.[124]

Atraumatic stress fracture has also been reported in the clavicle.[83] In addition, spontaneous fracture of the medial end of the clavicle has been reported as a pseudotumor after radical neck dissection (Fig. 11-18).[125-128]

The synthetic material used to treat coracoclavicular disruption has also been reported to produce stress fractures in the clavicle, with subsequent nonunion. Nonunion of the clavicle has occurred after the use of polyester mesh (Mersilene) tape and polyethylene (Dacron) to repair a grade III dislocation of the acromioclavicular joint.[129] Such nonunion is probably the result of the differential motion between the clavicle and the scapula with normal arm motion. When the tape or suture is passed over the clavicle, the differential motion can result in the tape's sawing through the clavicle.

CLINICAL FINDINGS

Birth Fractures

Two clinical manifestations of birth fractures appear to predominate: clinically unapparent and clinically apparent (pseudoparalysis).

Diagnosis of clinically unapparent fracture may be very difficult because of the presence of few clinical

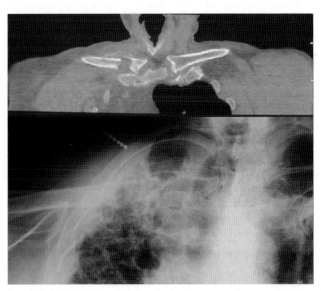

FIGURE 11-18 Medial right clavicular stress fracture 1 year after radical neck dissection for squamous cell carcinoma. Biopsy showed only evidence of a healing fracture with no evidence of tumor.

symptoms. A crack heard during the delivery may be the only clue to fracture of the clavicle.[130] Whether the lesion in this group of fractures is truly asymptomatic and is overlooked in the neonatal examination is uncertain, but Farkas and Levine emphasized that many of these fractures are not initially diagnosed. Of the five cases of fracture of the clavicle in 355 newborns in their series, none were suspected after routine physical examination in the delivery room and newborn nursery.[131] On reexamination, however, crepitus could usually be demonstrated at the fracture site. Thus, it appears that fractures can easily be overlooked. However, because they are generally unilateral, close examination can reveal asymmetry of clavicular contour or shortening of the neck line. The fracture is often first recognized by the mother after noticing the swelling, which is caused by fracture callus, and typically appears 7 to 11 days after the fracture.[132]

The infant with a clinically apparent fracture is disinclined or unwilling to use the extremity, and clinicians note a unilateral lack of movement of the whole upper limb either spontaneously or during elicitation of Moro's reflex.[133,134] Because these fractures are often complete, local swelling, tenderness, and crepitus can suggest the diagnosis. This injury must be distinguished from other conditions that can make the infant disinclined or unable to use the extremity, such as birth brachial plexus injury, separation of the proximal humeral epiphysis, and acute osteomyelitis of the clavicle or proximal end of the humerus. It is important to remember that a fractured clavicle and a brachial plexus injury can coexist.[2]

FIGURE 11-19 Clavicle fracture in a 2-year-old child. Prominent callus formation is evident and is manifested clinically as a bump.

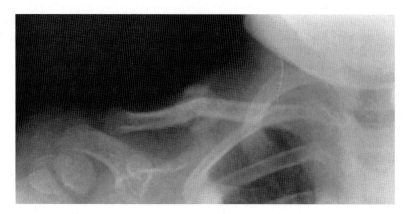

Fractures in Children

Almost half of fractures of the clavicle in children occur in those younger than 7 years. Because clavicle fractures in these young children may be incomplete or of the greenstick variety, they might not be obvious and thus may be overlooked. The mother of the infant might notice that the baby cries after being picked up and appears to be hurt.[107] The baby does not seem to use the arm naturally and cries when the arm is used for any activities or is moved during dressing. On palpation, a tender, uneven upper border of the clavicle may be felt that is asymmetric when compared with the contralateral side. As with a newborn, the mother may take the baby to the pediatrician because of the "sudden" appearance of a lump (Fig. 11-19).[1]

However, if the fracture is complete in children who are ambulatory and verbal, the diagnosis is usually obvious. In addition to the child's complaints of pain localized to the clavicle, when these fractures are displaced, a typical deformity caused by muscle displacement of the fracture fragments is apparent. The shoulder on the affected side can appear lower and droop forward and inward. The child splints the involved extremity against the body and supports the affected elbow with the contralateral hand. Because of the pull of the sternocleidomastoid muscle on the proximal fragment, the child tilts the head toward and the chin away from the side of the fracture in an effort to relax the pull of this muscle (Fig. 11-20).[2] Physical examination reveals tenderness, crepitus, and swelling, which are typical for this fracture at any age.

Complete acromioclavicular separations are very unusual in children younger than 16 years. What may be evident clinically as a high-riding clavicle above the acromioclavicular joint and an apparent acromioclavicular separation is often either a transperiosteal distal clavicle fracture or, more commonly, a rupture through the periosteum plus a distal clavicle fracture, with the coracoclavicular ligaments remaining behind attached to the periosteum. This lesion is not often recognized in children younger than 16 years.[65]

Similarly, because the sternal epiphysis is the last epiphysis of the long bones to fuse with the metaphysis (fusion usually occurs from ages 22-25 years), the joint may be subject to the usual types of epiphyseal injury. Many misdiagnosed sternoclavicular dislocations are, in fact, separations through the medial clavicular epiphysis. Occasionally, sternoclavicular separations occur with adjacent clavicle fractures in children.[135,136]

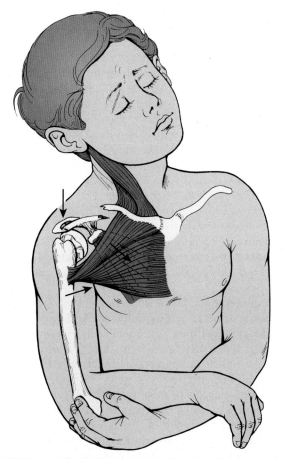

FIGURE 11-20 Clinical manifestation of a displaced clavicle fracture in a child. The shoulder on the affected side appears lower and droops forward and inward. The child splints the involved extremity against the body, supports the affected elbow with the contralateral hand, and tilts the head toward and the chin away from the site of the fracture to relax the pull of the sternocleidomastoid muscle.

Fractures in Adults

Because of the characteristic clinical features in adults, displaced fractures of the clavicle present little difficulty with diagnosis if the patient is seen soon after injury. The patient usually provides a clear history of some form of either direct or indirect injury to the shoulder. The clinical deformity is obvious and may be out of proportion to the amount of discomfort that the patient experiences.[107] The proximal fragment is displaced upward and backward and may be tenting the skin. Compounding of this fracture is unusual but can occur.[137] The patient is usually splinting the involved extremity at the side because any movement elicits pain. The involved arm droops forward and down because of the weight of the arm and pull of the pectoralis minor muscle. This drooping further accentuates the posterosuperior angulation seen in most clavicle fractures. Although the initial deformity may be obvious later, it may be obscured by acute swelling of soft tissue and hemorrhage. In a fracture near the ligamentous structures (acromioclavicular and sternoclavicular joints), the deformity can mimic a purely ligamentous injury.

Examination of the patient reveals tenderness directly over the fracture site, and any movement of the arm is painful. Ecchymosis may be noted over the fracture site, especially if severe displacement of the bone fragments has produced associated tearing of soft tissue. Patients might angle their head toward the injury in an attempt to relax the pull of the trapezius muscle on the fragment. As in children, the patient may be more comfortable with the chin tilted to the opposite side. Gentle palpation and manipulation usually produces crepitus and motion, and the site of the fracture is easily palpable because of the subcutaneous position of the bone. The skin over the clavicle, the scapula, or the chest wall might give a clue to the mechanism of injury and might indicate other areas to be evaluated for associated injuries. The lungs must be examined for the presence of symmetrical breath sounds, and the whole extremity must be examined carefully.

Nondisplaced fractures or isolated fractures of the articular surfaces might not cause deformity and thus may be overlooked unless they are specifically sought radiographically. If the diagnosis is in doubt, special radiographs or a repeat radiograph of the clavicle in 7 to 10 days may be indicated.

A panclavicular dislocation is typically produced by extreme and forceful protraction of the shoulder. This injury is usually the result of a major traumatic episode such as a high-speed motor vehicle accident, a fall from a height, or a very heavy object falling on the shoulder,[86] although it has been reported after a minor fall at home.[87] Clinically, patients usually have bruising over the spine of the scapula, and swelling and tenderness at both ends of the clavicle. This injury is associated with anterosuperior sternoclavicular dislocation and either posterosuperior or subjacent displacement of the clavicle. The whole clavicle may be freely mobile and may feel as though it is floating. Radiographs usually confirm this injury.

Associated Injuries

In 1830 Gross reported that "fractures of the clavicle usually assume a mild aspect, being seldom accompanied by any serious accident."[138] Although statistically most clavicle fractures are relatively innocuous injuries, serious associated injuries can occur, and a delay in treatment may be potentially life threatening.[8,139] Therefore, in a patient with a clavicle fracture, it is critical that a careful examination of the entire upper extremity be performed, with particular emphasis on neurovascular status, in addition to careful examination of the lungs.[140]

Associated injuries accompanying acute fractures of the clavicle may be divided into associated skeletal injuries, injuries to the lung and pleura, vascular injuries, and brachial plexus injuries.

Associated skeletal injuries can include sternoclavicular or acromioclavicular separations or fracture-dislocations through these joints (Fig. 11-21).[136,141-143] As might be anticipated with ipsilateral sternoclavicular or acromioclavicular joint injuries, closed reduction of the ligamentous injury is usually impossible because of the accompanying clavicle fracture.[142] Baccarani and colleagues reported a fracture of the coracoid process associated with a fracture of the clavicle that they treated by open reduction and internal fixation of the coracoid.[144]

Head and neck injuries may be present,[145] especially with displaced distal clavicle fractures. In one series, 10% of patients were comatose.[70]

Fractures of the first rib are not infrequent and are easily overlooked (Fig. 11-22).[146,147] These rib fractures may be directly responsible for accompanying lung, brachial plexus, or subclavian vein injury. First-rib fractures may be under-recognized because they are not easily seen on standard chest radiographs. Weiner and O'Dell recommended either an AP view of the cervical spine or an AP view of the thoracic spine associated with a lateral view of the thoracic spine to decrease the likelihood that

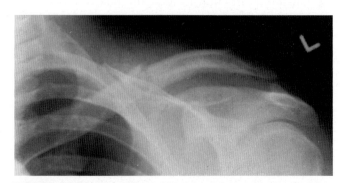

FIGURE 11-21 An unusual case of a fracture of the clavicle associated with complete acromioclavicular separation. The associated clavicle fracture makes treatment of the ligamentous injury very difficult.

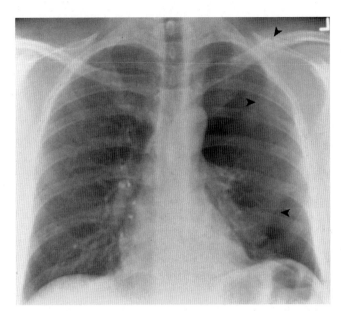

FIGURE 11-22 Fracture of the left clavicle (*top arrowhead*) associated with a left pneumothorax (*bottom arrowhead*). The lung markings are absent on the left side. This patient also has a fracture of the second rib (*middle arrowhead*).

this injury would be overlooked.[147] The location of a first-rib fracture may be either the ipsilateral or contralateral rib to the clavicle fracture.

Weiner and O'Dell have outlined how several of these rib fractures occur. The scalenus anticus muscle attaches on a tubercle of the first rib. On either side of this tubercle lies a groove for the subclavian vein anteriorly and the subclavian artery posteriorly. Posterior to the groove for the subclavian artery lies a roughened area for attachment of the scalene medius muscle. These two muscles elevate the rib during inspiration. The serratus anterior muscle arises from the outer surfaces of the upper eight ribs and fixes the rib posteriorly during inspiration. These structures can interact to contribute to the occurrence of fractures of the first rib as the clavicle is fractured.

Three basic mechanisms have been theorized to be responsible for this combination of injuries: indirect force transmitted via the manubrium, avulsion fracture at the weakest portion of the rib by the scalenus anticus, and injury to the lateral portion of the clavicle, causing an acromioclavicular separation that leads to indirect force from the subclavius muscle to the costal cartilage and the anterior aspect of the first rib.[147,148] Because of loss of the suspensory function of the clavicle and splinting secondary to pain from the clavicle and rib fractures, care should be taken to monitor respiratory function, especially in those with already compromised function, such as patients with chronic obstructive pulmonary disease. These patients can easily decompensate unless given appropriate respiratory and analgesic support.

Fractures of the clavicle may also be associated with dissociation-disruption of the scapulothoracic articulation

manifested as swelling of the shoulder, lateral displacement of the clavicle, severe neurovascular injury, and fracture of the clavicle or the acromioclavicular or sternoclavicular joint.[149]

In a combination injury, the floating shoulder consists of fractures of both the clavicle and the scapula and is associated with an extremely unstable shoulder girdle. In this injury, sequelae such as a drooping shoulder and limited range of motion can develop if this fracture is treated conservatively. Rockwood surveyed members of the American Shoulder and Elbow Surgeons and concluded that treatment should be directed primarily at stabilization of the clavicle. The primary indication for internal fixation of the scapula is to reduce and internally stabilize a grossly displaced intra-articular fracture of the glenoid fossa.[150,151] Stabilization of the clavicle alone has been shown to produce good and excellent functional results.[152,153] In a case of multiple trauma, Herscovici and coworkers recommended internal fixation of only the clavicle fracture.[154,155]

Other authors have suggested that although operative fixation does give good results, most cases of floating shoulder are not really unstable and can be managed with nonoperative treatment.[156-158] Williams and colleagues studied double disruptions of the superior suspensory mechanism and did not find any significant loss of stability unless the coracoacromial and acromioclavicular ligaments were disrupted in addition to fractures of the clavicle and glenoid neck.[158]

A number of authors have commented on the potentially serious complication of associated pneumothorax or hemothorax with fractures of the clavicle because the apical pleura and upper lung lobes lie adjacent to this bone[159] (see Fig. 11-22). Rowe reported a 3% incidence of pneumothorax in a series of 690 clavicle fractures, but he did not comment on how many had associated rib or scapular fractures.[4,160] Although it is easy to see how a severely displaced fracture can puncture the pleura with a sharp shard of bone to produce this lesion, the x-ray appearance may be misleadingly benign, with little evidence to suggest what might have been significant fragment displacement at the time of injury.[140] It is essential that a careful physical examination of the lung be undertaken at the initial evaluation and that the presence and symmetry of breath sounds be identified. In addition, an upright chest film appears to be important in the assessing all patients with fractures of the clavicle who have decreased breath sounds or other physical findings that suggest pneumothorax, with particularly close attention paid to the outline of the lung.[161] Such assessment is especially necessary in multiply traumatized or unconscious patients who have neither obvious blunt chest trauma nor any external signs of trauma to the chest that might yield a clue to potential lung or pleural complications.[9,140,161-164]

Although nerve injuries are rare with clavicle fractures, acute injuries to the brachial plexus do occur.[8] The neurovascular bundle emerges from the thoracic outlet under

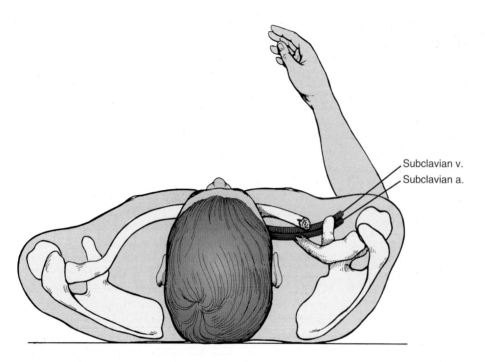

FIGURE 11-23 As the clavicle fractures and displaces, the subclavian vessels immediately posterior to the clavicle may be injured by sharp shards of bone.

Subclavian v.
Subclavian a.

the clavicle on top of the first rib.[165] As it passes under the clavicle, it is protected to a certain extent by the thick medial clavicular bone; considerable trauma is usually necessary to damage the brachial plexus and break the clavicle at the same time. When the force is severe enough to break the clavicle and injure the brachial plexus, a subclavian vascular injury often occurs concomitantly (Fig. 11-23). The force resulting in nerve injury usually comes in a direction from above downward or from in front downward. As the force is applied, the nerves may be stretched, with the fulcrum of maximal tension being the transverse process of the cervical vertebra. The roots can also be torn above the clavicle, or they may be avulsed from their attachment to the spinal cord.[166] Although the posterior periosteum, subclavius muscles, and bone offer some protection to the underlying plexus, the plexus may be injured directly by the fragments of bone. Such injury is especially worthy of emphasis: Clavicle fragments should not be manipulated without adequate x-ray studies of the position of these fracture fragments.[167]

Direct injury to the brachial plexus usually involves the ulnar nerve because this portion of the plexus lies adjacent to the middle third of the clavicle.

Acute vascular injuries are unusual because of many of the same local anatomic factors that protect the nerves from direct injury. The subclavius muscle and the thick, deep cervical fascia also act as barriers against direct injury to the vessels. If the initial displacement of the fracture fragment has not injured the adjacent vessels, they are unlikely to be injured further, because the distal fragment is pulled downward and forward by the weight of the limb and the proximal fragment is pulled upward and backward by the trapezius muscle. Thus, as with

acute nerve injury, a major injury is usually required to produce an acute vascular insult.[168] Nevertheless, injury has been reported even with a greenstick fracture.[169] In addition, acute vascular compression resulting from fracture angulation has been described (Fig. 11-24).[170]

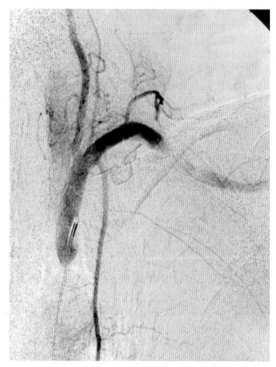

FIGURE 11-24 Subtraction arteriogram showing nearly complete cutoff of the left subclavian artery after a clavicle malunion.

When they occur, vascular injuries include laceration, occlusion, spasm, or acute compression; the vessels most commonly injured are the subclavian artery, subclavian vein, and internal jugular vein.[171-174] The subclavian vein is particularly vulnerable to tearing because it is fixed to the clavicle by a fascial aponeurosis.[175,176] Injuries to the suprascapular and axillary arteries have also been reported.[177,178] Laceration can result in life-threatening hemorrhage, whereas arterial thrombus and occlusion can lead to distal ischemia. Damage to the arterial wall can, in addition, lead to aneurysm formation and late embolic phenomena. Venous thrombosis may be problematic as well; although it does not typically threaten life or limb, it has the potential for pulmonary embolism, which can constitute a threat.[179]

Clinical recognition of an acute vascular injury may be difficult, particularly in an unconscious patient or one in shock. Although a complete laceration can cause life-threatening hemorrhage or result in an extremity that is cold, pulseless, and pale, a partial laceration is more likely to be manifested as uncontrolled bleeding and life-threatening blood loss. The color and temperature of the extremity may be normal, but the absence of a pulse, the presence of a bruit, or a pulsatile hematoma (as the hematoma is walled off or produces a false aneurysm) should make the clinician strongly suspect a major vascular injury.[178] If blood flow is significantly obstructed, the injured limb is usually colder than the uninjured limb, but there might also be a difference in blood pressure between the two.[9] Vascular contusion or spasm can result in thrombotic and, later, thromboembolic phenomena.[180] It is sometimes difficult to recognize the difference between arterial spasm and interruption or occlusion, and it may be reasonable to consider a sympathetic block to help distinguish a spasm from a more serious injury.

If major injury to a vessel is suspected, an arteriogram should be performed.[9] In the rare event of a tear of a large vessel, surgical exploration is mandatory. To gain adequate exposure, as much of the clavicle should be excised as needed to isolate and repair the injured major vessel. Although the vessel may be ligated in some cases, ligation of a major vessel in an elderly patient might well be dangerous because of inadequate remaining circulation to the extremity. In any event, a surgeon skilled in decision making and in the techniques of vascular repair is essential if a major injury has occurred.

Of particular importance is the association of medial clavicle fractures with occurrence of almost all of these injuries. Medial clavicle fractures are relatively uncommon in comparison to midshaft and lateral fractures, but they have been associated with a very high incidence of pulmonary problems such as pneumothorax, hemothorax, or hemopneumothorax and pulmonary contusion as well as head, face, and cervical injuries.[181] Most impressive is the very high mortality rate found in association with medial clavicle injuries. Throckmorton and Kuhn found that 20% of patients with medial clavicle fractures die as a result of their associated injuries.[181]

RADIOGRAPHIC EVALUATION

Fractures of the Shaft

With most clavicular shaft fractures, the diagnosis is not in doubt because of the clinical deformity and confirmatory radiographs. Unfortunately, many physicians obtain only an AP radiograph of the shoulder to image clavicle fractures. Because of the multiplanar nature of the clavicle, it is almost impossible to determine displacement and angulation on a single AP radiograph. The primary problem is that the plane of the fracture is oblique to the plane of the x-ray beam. Therefore, what is measured as displacement or shortening on an AP radiograph is really equivalent to the base of a triangle, but the true amount of shortening is really the hypotenuse of the triangle (Fig. 11-25). If one takes into account that the clavicle not only shortens but also becomes angulated inferiorly and rotated medially, the deformity is truly in three planes. Aside from using a three-dimensional Cartesian coordinate system, it is really difficult, if not impossible, to characterize the true deformity on plane radiographs.

To obtain as accurate an evaluation of fragment position as possible, at least two projections of the clavicle

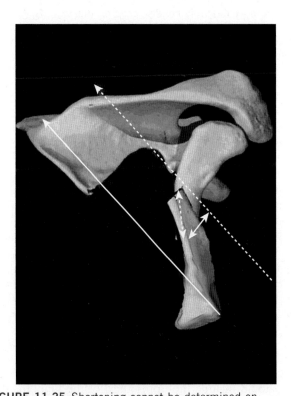

FIGURE 11-25 Shortening cannot be determined on standard radiographs because the deformity is not orthogonal to the beam of the x-ray. The x-ray beam is represented by the *dashed line* and the apparent shortening by the *short solid line*. The true shortening *(short, dotted line)* is really the hypotenuse of the triangle and is longer than the apparent shortening.

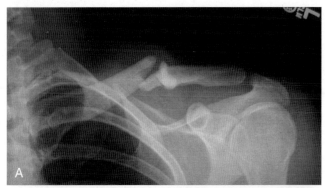

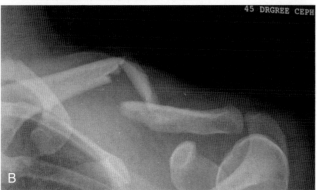

FIGURE 11-26 A, AP radiograph of an acute midshaft left clavicle fracture sustained in a mountain bike accident. It appears to be relatively nondisplaced on this view. **B,** Forty-five-degree cephalic tilt radiograph of the clavicle showing marked displacement and a transversely oriented butterfly fragment.

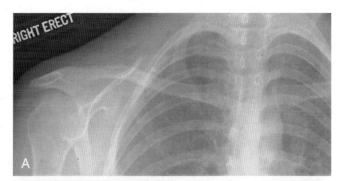

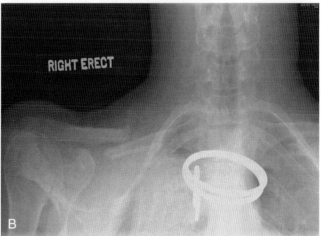

FIGURE 11-27 A, Benign-looking AP radiograph of a fracture sustained while playing Frisbee. **B,** Significant deformity unseen on the AP radiograph. The hint on the AP view of significant deformity is the markedly oblique orientation of scapula.

should always be obtained: an AP view and a 45-degree cephalic tilt view. In the former, the proximal fragment is typically displaced upward and the distal fragment is displaced downward (Figs. 11-26A and 11-27A). In the latter, the tube is directed from below upward and more accurately assesses the AP relationship of the two fragments (see Figs. 11-26B and 11-27B).[182] Displacement of the fracture is best assessed on the 45-degree cephalic tilt projection. An axillary view with the beam angled slightly cephalad can also help determine fracture displacement and can be useful in assessing possible nonunion (Figs. 11-28 and 11-29). Quesana recommended two views at right angles to each other, a 45-degree angle superiorly and a 45-degree angle inferiorly, to assess the extent and displacement of fractures of the clavicle.[183] In our practice, we have not really found the 45-degree caudal tilt view to be of benefit.

Rowe has suggested that with an AP radiograph, the film should include the upper third of the humerus, the shoulder girdle, and the upper lung fields so that other shoulder girdle fractures and pneumothorax can be identified more speedily.[4] The configuration of the fracture is also important to assess because it can give a clue to the presence of associated injuries. The usual clavicular shaft fracture in adults is slightly oblique; a fracture that is more comminuted, and especially if the middle spike is projecting in a superior-to-inferior direction, has generally resulted from a greater force and can alert the surgeon to the potential for associated neurovascular or pulmonary injuries.

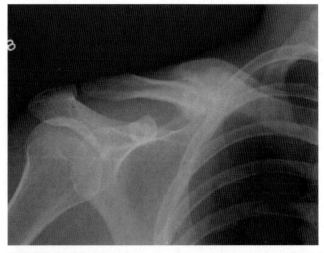

FIGURE 11-28 AP radiograph of a clavicle nonunion. On this view, the fracture appears to be healed in acceptable alignment and has adequate callus.

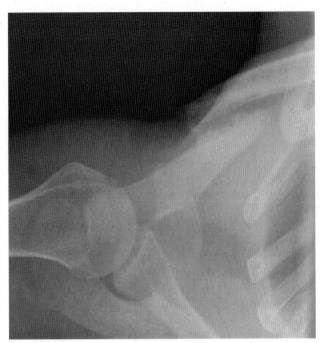

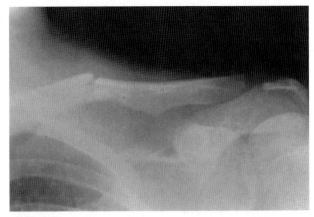

FIGURE 11-30 Greenstick fracture of the left clavicle in a 14-year-old patient. In such a patient, the diagnosis may be more difficult to make.

FIGURE 11-29 Axillary radiograph of the clavicle in Figure 11-28. The nonunion is obvious, with significant shortening at the fracture site.

Children's fractures may be greenstick or nondisplaced, or they can appear only as bony bowing, and thus the diagnosis of shaft fractures may be more difficult to make (Fig. 11-30), especially in newborns or infants, in whom the clinical findings may be difficult to assess. Movement by the child or bone overlap can obscure radiographic detail, and an incomplete fracture might not be recognized. However, the surrounding soft tissues of the clavicle are normally displayed as parallel shadows above the body of the clavicle. Although this accompanying shadow might not be seen along the proximal third of the clavicle medial to the crossing of the first rib, it is invariably present on most radiographs. Suspicion of fractures of the clavicle should be aroused by loss of the accompanying shadow unilaterally.[109] If one has any doubt about the presence of a fracture in a child, a repeat radiograph taken 5 to 10 days after the injury will usually reveal callus formation.

In 1988, the technique of ultrasonography was described for evaluation of clavicular birth fractures.[100] These birth fractures can easily be overlooked and may be confused clinically with birth palsy. In their study, Katz and associates noted no difference in diagnostic accuracy between ultrasonography and plain radiography.[100] In addition, a medial clavicle fracture not seen on plain film was picked up by ultrasonography. In fact, the authors noted that the individual fracture fragments were seen to move up and down with respiration.

With either plain radiography or ultrasonography, it may be difficult to differentiate congenital pseudarthrosis from an acute fracture. However, the radiographic features, the lack of trauma, and the absence of callus usually help distinguish an atraumatic condition such as congenital pseudarthrosis from a birth fracture.

Fractures of the Distal Third

In both children and adults, the usual radiographic views obtained for shaft fractures are inadequate to completely assess distal clavicle fractures. The standard exposure for evaluation of shoulder or shaft fractures overexposes the distal end of the clavicle. The usual exposure for the distal part of the clavicle should be approximately one third that used for the shoulder joint, especially if it is important to determine articular surface involvement.

Type II distal clavicle fractures can be particularly difficult to diagnose because the usual AP and 40-degree cephalic tilt views typically do not reveal the extent of the injury.[70] If the exposure is appropriate, this distal clavicle fracture may be identified on the AP and lateral views of the trauma series, but to accurately assess the extent of the injury and the presence or absence of associated ligamentous damage, Neer has recommended three views: the AP view, an anterior 45-degree oblique view, and a posterior 45-degree oblique view.

The AP view includes both shoulders on one plate with the patient erect and with 10 lb of weight strapped to each wrist (Figs. 11-31 and 11-32). If the distance between the coracoid and the medial fragment is increased in comparison to the normal side, ligamentous detachment from the medial fragment can be assumed to be present. However, because much of the displacement of the fracture is in the AP plane, two additional views were suggested. An anterior 45-degree oblique view, with the patient erect and the injured shoulder against the plate, gives a lateral view of the scapula and shows the medial fragment posteriorly with the outer fragment displaced anteriorly. A posterior 45-degree oblique view, with the patient erect and the injured shoulder against the plate, also demonstrates the extent of separation of the two fragments. Alternatively, a cross-body adduction AP radio-

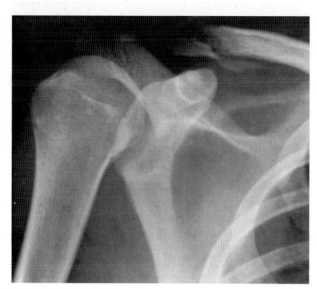

FIGURE 11-31 Fracture of the distal end of the right clavicle. In an AP view, the location of the fracture suggests ligamentous involvement, with the ligaments attached to the distal fragment.

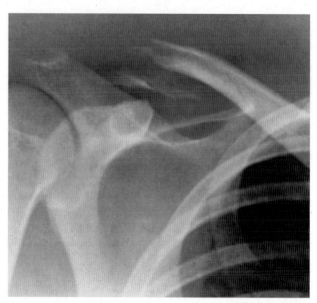

FIGURE 11-32 The extent of ligamentous involvement is confirmed on a weighted view in which separation of the coracoclavicular distance is apparent. The coracoclavicular ligaments are attached to the distal clavicular segment.

graph can be obtained to assess for ligamentous injury. An AP radiograph is taken with the patient pulling the elbow of the affected shoulder to the midline. If significant ligamentous injury is present, there will be no restraint to anteromedial subluxation of the shoulder relative to the clavicle, and it will appear on the radiograph that the distal fragment is subluxating under the medial fragment.

In a type II distal clavicle fracture, if x-ray views at right angles to a cephalic tilt view show good bone overlap and proximity of the fragments and if the presence of crepitation confirms contact between the fragments, stress radiographic views with weights are probably not necessary; in fact, the use of weights can further displace otherwise minimally displaced fracture fragments (Fig. 11-33). Posterior displacement of type II distal clavicle fractures is best assessed with an axillary radiograph.

Articular surface fractures of the distal end of the clavicle are easily overlooked unless high-quality radiographs are obtained. A Zanca view with a 15-degree cephalic tilt and soft tissue technique can detect intra-articular fractures much better than standard radiographs can. If the fracture is not seen on a plain x-ray view and clinical suspicion is strong, tomography or a computed tomography (CT) scan can reveal the presence and extent of the articular surface injury (Fig. 11-34).

Fractures of the Medial Third

These fractures may be particularly difficult to detect by routine radiographs because of the overlap of ribs, vertebrae, and mediastinal shadows. However, a cephalic tilt

view of 40 to 45 degrees or a serendipity view often reveals the fracture, whether in a child or an adult. In children particularly, fractures of the medial end of the clavicle are often misdiagnosed as sternoclavicular dislocations when in fact they are usually epiphyseal injuries. As with distal clavicular injuries, tomography or a CT scan may be useful in demonstrating the intra-articular or epiphyseal nature of the injury in this location.

DIFFERENTIAL DIAGNOSIS

In adults, fractures of the shaft of the clavicle are not usually confused with any other diagnosis, although pathologic fractures are occasionally difficult to recognize as such. However, fractures of the distal or medial end of the clavicle can clinically appear to be complete acromioclavicular or sternoclavicular separations, although these injuries rarely cause confusion once proper radiographic studies are performed.

In children, it can be easy to confuse injuries to the clavicle with other entities, including congenital disorders and other traumatic conditions.

Congenital Pseudarthrosis

When recognized at birth or shortly thereafter, congenital pseudarthrosis may be confused with either cleidocranial dysostosis or a birth fracture, especially if some trauma has been associated with the delivery. However, birth fractures unite rapidly and leave no disability. The deformity of congenital pseudarthrosis can become more conspicuous as the child grows.[184] Clinically, the lump is

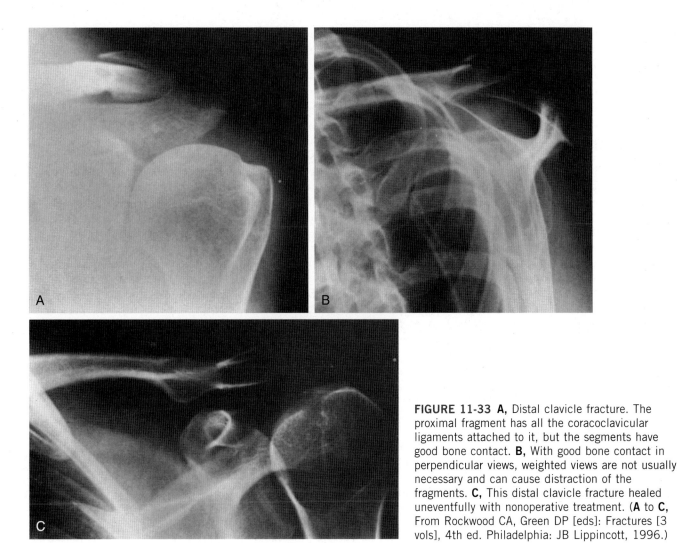

FIGURE 11-33 A, Distal clavicle fracture. The proximal fragment has all the coracoclavicular ligaments attached to it, but the segments have good bone contact. **B,** With good bone contact in perpendicular views, weighted views are not usually necessary and can cause distraction of the fragments. **C,** This distal clavicle fracture healed uneventfully with nonoperative treatment. (**A** to **C,** From Rockwood CA, Green DP [eds]: Fractures [3 vols], 4th ed. Philadelphia: JB Lippincott, 1996.)

painless; the child usually has no history of injury, pain, or disability with this lesion.[185,186] It is invariably in the lateral portion of the middle third of the clavicle and usually affects the right clavicle except in children with dextrocardia, in which case it can occur on the left side.[187,188] Bilateral congenital pseudarthrosis has been

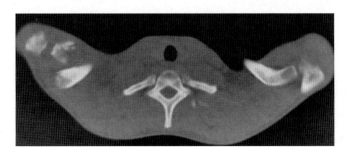

FIGURE 11-34 CT scan of a right clavicle fracture. The CT scan confirms the site of fracture at the distal end of the clavicle and it identifies a previously unsuspected intra-articular extension of the distal clavicle fracture.

reported, particularly in the presence of bilateral cervical ribs.[1]

The cause of this entity is unclear. Although a family history is not typical, some reports have noted a familial incidence, thus raising the question of genetic transmission.[184]

Although there may be a history of trauma with the birth, it is probably incidental; most investigators now agree that congenital pseudarthrosis is not a nonunion of normal bone after trauma.[189] It is probable that abnormal intrauterine development plays the primary role in its appearance, and it has been suggested that pressure from the subclavian artery as it arches over the first rib and under the clavicle may be a primary factor in its development.[187,190] The cervical ribs can also displace the subclavian artery and cause pressure in the same area of the clavicle.[1]

Radiographically, characteristic changes can be noted in congenital pseudarthrosis. The sternal fragment, which consists of the medial third of the clavicle, is larger and protrudes forward and upward, whereas the lateral half is situated below, points upward and backward, and ends in a bulbous mass at the pseudarthrosis site. Other identifying features are an increase in the deformity with age, the proximity of the bone ends to one another, and a large lump palpable clinically. These findings contrast quite markedly with cleidocranial dysostosis.

Cleidocranial Dysostosis

Cleidocranial dysostosis is a hereditary abnormality of membranous bone, such as the skull, and the clavicle is the most commonly involved. The abnormality varies from a central defect in the clavicle to complete absence of the clavicle; the most common manifestation is absence of the distal portion of the clavicle.[1,191] Radiographically, it is distinguished from congenital pseudarthrosis by the larger gap between the bone ends and by the tapered ends of the clavicle rather than the larger bulbous ends.[184] It is more clearly aplastic bone. In addition, multiple membranous bones are involved, and they can each have their own clinical manifestations. Some children have bossing or other skull defects, smallness of the facial bones, scoliosis, abnormal epiphyses of the hands or feet, and deficiencies of the pelvic ring. Usually, a familial history of bone disorders can be elicited.[192,193]

Sternoclavicular Dislocation

Epiphyseal fractures of the medial end of the clavicle can mimic sternoclavicular separations in children because of the late closure of the sternal epiphysis. If it is important to distinguish between these two entities, tomography or CT scanning may be indicated.

Acromioclavicular Separation

Fracture of the lateral aspect of the clavicle in children can also be identical with a complete acromioclavicular separation, clinically and radiographically. If plain radiography does not identify the small fracture fragment, tomography or CT scanning can. However, because the coracoclavicular ligaments remain attached to the periosteal tube in children and healing is uneventful, it is difficult to justify these more-elaborate diagnostic modalities in children with this injury.[81]

COMPLICATIONS

Nonunion

One of the greatest fallacies of orthopaedics is that "all clavicles heal well." Although many clavicles do heal with nonoperative treatment, the incidence of nonunion is probably much higher than previously thought. Nonunion of nonoperated shaft fractures was thought to be rare, with a reported incidence of 0.9% to 4%.[4,69,144,194-200] However, more recent research suggests that the actual

nonunion rate may be much higher than previously thought, with an incidence of 15% to 25%.[14,15] A review at one of our institutions showed a 10% nonunion rate of fractures that were treated nonoperatively. However, 40% of the fractures in this series were treated acutely with surgery, which means that it could be assumed that the more serious fractures were treated operatively and that this 10% nonunion rate was seen in less-severe injuries.

Despite some debate in the literature about the definition, most authors consider clavicular nonunion to be defined as failure to show clinical or radiographic progression of healing at 4 to 6 months,[57,201-203] although there is some temporal difference between atrophic and hypertrophic nonunion. Manske and Szabo reported that bone ends that were tapered, sclerotic, and atrophic at 16 weeks were unlikely to unite, whereas they classified other fractures as delayed union at the 16-week period as long as some potential for healing was present.[204] Bilateral post-traumatic pseudarthrosis has been reported in an adult.[205]

Although nonunion of the clavicle is predominantly a problem after fracture in adults, it has been described in children.[206] However, apparent nonunion in a child is likely to be congenital pseudarthrosis. Several factors appear to predispose to nonunion of the clavicle: inadequate immobilization, severity of the trauma, refracture, location of the fracture (outer third), degree of displacement (marked displacement), and primary open reduction.

Predisposing Factors
Inadequate Immobilization
It has long been recognized that the clavicle is one of the most difficult bones to immobilize properly and completely after fracture while providing the patient with the simplicity and comfort that is ideal and practical in fracture treatment. Immobilization, by whatever means, should be continued until union is complete, although it may be difficult to determine this time with certainty. Rowe has provided some guidelines for the usual healing period of fractures of the middle third of the clavicle[4]:

Infants: 2 weeks
Children: 3 weeks
Young adults: 4 to 6 weeks
Adults: 6 weeks or longer

It has been recognized, moreover, that radiographic union can progress more slowly than clinical union, with x-ray evidence of union not appearing for 12 weeks or longer.[207] When in doubt, immobilization should probably be continued. It has been suggested that once clinical union has occurred along with absence of motion or tenderness at the fracture site, a gradual increase in activity can safely be permitted, even if radiographic union is incomplete.[207]

Severity of Trauma

Up to half of fractures resulting in nonunion follow severe trauma.[208] In their series, Wilkins and Johnston reviewed 33 ununited clavicle fractures.[203] Many of their patients had severe trauma that was manifested by the degree of displacement of the fracture fragments, the amount of soft tissue damage, and associated injuries such as multiple long bone, spine, pelvic, and rib fractures. They pointed out the similarities between the clavicle and another subcutaneous long bone, the tibia, which is also susceptible to nonunion, and emphasized that the subcutaneous position of the clavicle predisposes it to more severe trauma, more severe soft tissue damage, and thus, nonunion. As with other bones, open fractures have been implicated as a factor in nonunion of the clavicle.[57] Late perforation of the skin with a free compounding fragment has also been reported.[137]

In a severely traumatic situation, although actual skin defects overlying a clavicle fracture are uncommon, soft tissue coverage appears to be essential to avoid the potential complication of osteomyelitis and nonunion. It may be that most factors associated in some series with clavicular nonunion, such as the degree of displacement, compounding, operative management, poor immobilization, and soft tissue interposition, can simply reflect the cases that have been associated with more severe trauma to the clavicle. The independent statistical importance of some of these associations with nonunion may be questioned.

The increased incidence of nonunion seen in more-recent series can reflect more-accurate follow-up or the fact that we are seeing more high-energy fractures. If one looks at the patients in the 1968 Rowe study,[4] most were either children or older adults who experienced falls from a standing height. It has been our experience that the fractures we see now are often in bicyclists, particularly mountain bikers.[112,209] In fact, two recent studies showed that the most common injury in bicycle racers is a clavicle fracture. Most of these bikers report flipping over their handlebars at fairly high speeds. Because of the forward momentum in these bikers, they transmit far higher energy to the clavicle when they land on the outer aspect of their shoulders.

We have also seen an increase in what we refer to as *seat-belt fractures* (see Fig. 11-17). These injuries are typically right-sided fractures in passengers and left-sided fractures in drivers. They are generally simple, transverse fractures; however, as a group, they tend to heal very slowly and have a greater propensity for nonunion than lateral impact–type fractures do.

Refracture

A number of studies have identified refracture of a previously healed clavicle fracture as a factor contributing to the development of nonunion.[197,210] In Wilkins and Johnston's series, 7 of 31 nonunions occurred in such patients.[203] There appears to be no relationship among the length of time between injuries, the age of the patient,

the duration of immobilization of the original fracture, or the severity of the initial or subsequent traumatic injuries and the complication of nonunion after refracture. It has been theorized that because the vascular anatomy of a fractured bone remains altered for a long period even after fracture union,[211] reinjury might in some way prevent this altered blood supply from reacting to the new fracture.[203]

Location of Fracture

Approximately 85% of nonunions of the clavicle occur in the middle third of the bone.[212] Nonetheless, it appears that fractures of the distal third of the clavicle are much more susceptible to nonunion than shaft fractures are. In his series of clavicular nonunions, Neer noted that distal clavicle fractures accounted for more than half of the ununited clavicles after closed treatment.[69] He found the reasons for this increased incidence of nonunion to be multifactorial: the fracture is very unstable, and the muscle forces and weight of the arm tend to displace the fracture fragments[213]; because these distal clavicular injuries are often the result of severe trauma, local soft tissue injury is extensive, and associated injuries may be present and affect generalized biological and specific fracture healing[70]; and it may be difficult to secure adequate external immobilization.

Even in fractures in which union can occur with closed methods, the union time for distal clavicle fractures is often delayed. This long healing time, combined with the associated degree of soft tissue trauma, can lead to stiffness and prolonged disability from disuse. For these reasons, Neer advocated early open reduction and internal fixation for this injury.[67,70]

Degree of Displacement

In a large series reported by Jupiter and Leffert, the degree of displacement was the most significant factor in nonunion.[210] Wick found that 91% of delayed unions and nonunions had initial shortening of at least 2 cm.[214] However, in many clavicle fractures, marked displacement is often associated with other factors that delay fracture healing, such as severe trauma, soft tissue damage, open fractures, and soft tissue interposition. Manske and Szabo thought that soft tissue interposition alone was a major contributing factor in fractures that failed to heal, and at surgery they often found a fracture fragment impaled in the trapezius muscle.[204] They particularly implicated soft tissue interposition in the development of atrophic nonunion. However, others have reported that muscle interposition is uncommon.[210]

Primary Open Reduction

A number of authors have associated primary open reduction of acute clavicular shaft fractures with an increased incidence of nonunion.[215] Rowe reported an incidence of nonunion of 0.8% in fractures treated nonoperatively, which rose to 3.7% in those treated operatively.[4] Neer had a similar experience, with a nonunion rate of 0.1%

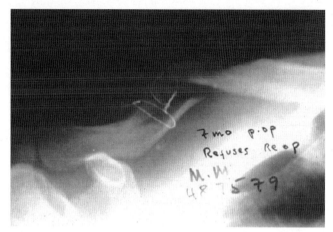

FIGURE 11-35 Failure of fixation in a midshaft clavicle fracture.

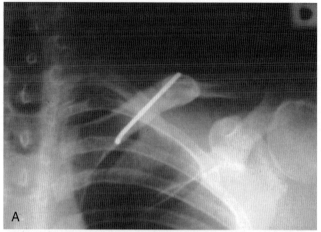

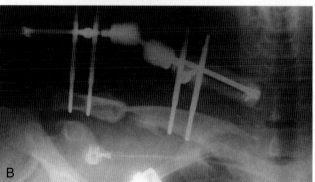

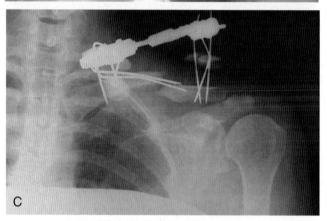

FIGURE 11-36 A, Failure of fixation in a midshaft clavicle fracture treated with a single smooth Steinmann pin. **B,** Nonunion and malalignment of a midshaft clavicle fracture treated with an external fixator. **C,** Nonunion and malalignment of a midshaft clavicular malunion that was treated with a fine-wire external fixator.

in fractures treated nonoperatively and 4.6% when the initial fracture was treated surgically.[69] Schwartz and Leixnering reported a nonunion rate of 13% in patients with clavicle fractures treated by primary open reduction, although they suggested that inadequate internal fixation might have played a prominent role in this high incidence.[215] Poigenfurst and coworkers reported a complication rate of 10%, with four nonunions in 60 fresh clavicle fractures that were plated.[216]

Poor internal fixation rather than the surgery itself can play the primary role in the increased incidence of nonunion in patients treated by primary surgery. Zenni and associates reported a series of 25 acute clavicle fractures treated by primary open reduction with intramedullary pins or cerclage suture and bone grafting, all of which healed without complication.[217] In some series reporting an increased incidence of nonunion after open reduction, it is probable that the operative fractures also included many of the more difficult fractures, such as those with more severe trauma, soft tissue damage, and associated injuries, thus contributing to the poor results.

One cannot overlook the fact that most of the surgical complications are related to poor fixation techniques, and it is not the concept of surgical treatment that is the problem but, rather, the choice of fixation (Figs. 11-35 and 11-36), possibly because of the tenuous soft tissue coverage about the clavicle and its marginal blood supply. As Wilkins and Johnston have pointed out, the clavicle is very much like the tibia[203] in that it has poor soft tissue coverage. However, very few surgeons, who would never even consider plating a midshaft tibia fracture, see any problem with plating a midshaft clavicle fracture. It may be that the soft tissue injury, combined with the soft tissue stripping that is required for plate fixation, is what contributes to the higher rate of nonunion seen with this popular form of operative fixation.

Diagnosis
Radiographic Evaluation
Although nonunion is often demonstrated clinically by motion at the fracture site, radiographic confirmation is obtained by AP and 45-degree cephalic tilt views. The radiographic signs of nonunion might not always be clear. In patients with minimal displacement of the fracture fragments and no gross motion, tomography or even

a bone scan may be useful to demonstrate the presence of nonunion in a symptomatic patient. As with other fractures, nonunion of the clavicle may be manifested as hypertrophic or atrophic bone ends. Patients can have real or apparent bone loss, particularly with comminuted fractures.

Obtaining an AP view of both clavicles on a single large cassette is particularly helpful in evaluating nonunion. In this way the distance from the sternum to the acromion can be measured on the normal side and compared with the symptomatic side. Such comparison can help when deciding whether primary osteosynthesis with bone grafting will be adequate or whether an intercalary segment of bone will be needed to span the area of segmental bone loss. It is very difficult to appreciate the true shortening or deformity of a clavicle on plain radiographs alone.

Symptoms

Approximately 75% of patients with an ununited fracture of the clavicle are symptomatic with moderate to severe pain.[204,210] However, some evidence indicates that patients with atrophic nonunion, though symptomatic initially, may become less so with time.[203] Pain from nonunion can radiate to the neck, down into the forearm, or even into the hand, especially if nerve irritation is present.[202] The patient might complain of grating or crepitation, which is often palpable. The shoulder can appear to sag forward, inward, and medially, and the apex of the medial fragment may be observed angling upward underneath the trapezius. The rotation of the scapula can also contribute to the posterior medial scapular border pain that can be seen in these patients. Twenty-five percent or more of patients are also affected by neurologic symptoms, which are often caused by compromise of the brachial plexus by overabundant callus.[202,210,218,219] Similarly, chronic vascular symptoms may be present as a result of pressure on the subclavian vein, producing symptoms of thoracic outlet syndrome.[210,220-224]

When considering nonunion as the cause of a patient's painful symptoms, it must be emphasized that nonunion may be an incidental finding. A careful history and physical examination must be obtained because many soft tissue and bone abnormalities around the shoulder, including post-traumatic arthrosis of either the sternoclavicular or acromioclavicular joint, can mimic the symptoms of nonunion. These degenerative changes in the joint can appear several years after the injury.[203]

Physical Examination

Physical examination can reveal motion as the clavicle is manipulated or pain on pressure at a nonunion site. The prominent bone of comminuted fragments may be palpable. Occasionally, patients have limited range of motion at the shoulder joint, but this finding is often associated with soft tissue, subacromial, or glenohumeral joint disease rather than being a direct result of the clavicular

nonunion. Loss of motion can occur secondary to malposition of the scapula in the case of significant shortening. If neurologic symptoms are noted, they are often referred to the ulnar nerve distribution, and intrinsic weakness can occur.[202,225]

Malunion

In children with clavicle fractures, foreshortening is common but has not been reported to be a problem, and the angular deformity often remodels. Adults, however, have no remodeling potential, and shortening or angulation can occur. This defect has been described by some authors as a purely cosmetic deformity with little interference with function.[107] However, Eskola and associates reported that patients with shortening of the clavicular segments of more than 15 mm at follow-up examination had significantly more pain than did those without these findings, and they recommended taking care to avoid acceptance of a shortened clavicle.[14]

Patients can present with pseudowinging of the scapula secondary to the fixated anteromedial rotation of the scapula caused by a malunion of the clavicle (see Fig. 11-7B). Although this is not true winging, it represents a static, fixed condition similar to the dynamic dysfunction seen with long thoracic nerve injuries. Ledger and colleagues found that a malunion with shortening of at least 15 mm caused increased upward angulation of the clavicle at the sternoclavicular joint and increased anterior scapular version, and it also caused significant loss of strength in adduction, extension, and internal rotation of the humerus as well as a reduced peak abduction velocity.[226]

If a malunited fracture is a significant cosmetic or functional problem, simply shaving down the bone may be inadequate.[3] This procedure does not correct the primary deformity, which is shortening and angulation, and it can significantly weaken the clavicle. Because of overlapping of the fracture ends, removing the prominence of the deformity can create a unicortical clavicle that is not capable of remodeling. This outcome can predispose the clavicle to refracture and can cause chronic pain. Several authors have recommended osteotomy, internal fixation, and bone grafting.[107,227] The patient must, however, be made aware that nonunion may be a sequela and that the cosmetic appearance of the surgical scar required for plate fixation may be more troublesome than the bump from the malunited bone (Fig. 11-37 and see Fig. 11-52). Furthermore, it must be kept in mind that the deformity is multiplanar and a single osteotomy can correct only one plane of the deformity.

Another approach to this problem is to remove the callus about the fracture site to get down to the original fracture fragments.[228] We have found that even years after the original injury, there is a qualitative difference between the normal cortical bone and the callus. Removal of the callus can be aided through the use of image intensification at the time of surgery to make sure that all of the

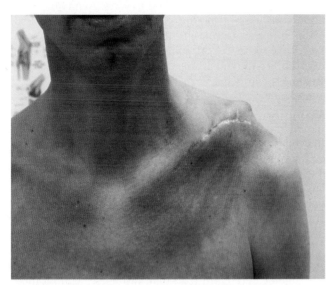

FIGURE 11-37 Clinical appearance of a patient who had undergone plate fixation of a clavicle malunion with an intercalary graft. Loss of distal fixation had occurred.

callus is removed. The fracture fragments are then fixed with an intramedullary pin, which is removed at a later date. The callus is morselized and placed around the fracture site. This procedure can be accomplished through a small cosmetic incision in Langer's lines.

Neurovascular Sequelae

Despite the large amount of callus that follows healing of a fracture in children, the callus mass rarely causes any compression of the costoclavicular space and usually decreases with time.[1] In adults, however, late neurovascular sequelae can follow both united and ununited fractures.[229-234]

Normally, the sternoclavicular angle and anterior bow of the clavicle provide abundant room for the brachial plexus and subclavian vessels in the costoclavicular space. Despite some normal variability in the width and space between the clavicle and the first rib, this room is usually adequate.[235] Occasionally, a congenital anomaly such as a bifid clavicle or a straight clavicle with no medial or anterior angulation can narrow the costoclavicular space and cause neurovascular compression.[236] Thus, it is not surprising that abundant callus or significant fracture deformity in some patients can narrow this space sufficiently to cause symptoms that most often involve the subclavian vessels, the carotid artery, or the brachial plexus.[237] These compression phenomena, though uncommon, are important because their clinical manifestation may be confusing to the clinician and problematic for the patient until definitive treatment is instituted. Vascular structures that have been reported to be involved in compression syndromes include the carotid artery, the subclavian vein, and the subclavian artery. Aneurysms and pseudoaneurysms producing brachial plexus compression are also seen.

Vascular Compression Syndromes

Obstruction of the carotid artery can lead to syncope. Such obstruction is associated with fracture deformity or callus at the medial end of the clavicle.

Compression of the subclavian vein between the clavicle and the first rib, with subsequent obstruction, is probably the most common late vascular complication and may be accompanied by plexus and subclavian artery involvement. The point of this obstruction has been shown by Lusskin and coworkers to be the site where the vein crosses the first rib and passes beneath the subclavius muscle and costoclavicular ligament.[238] A number of authors have emphasized the role of the subclavius muscle and the condensation of the clavipectoral fascia known as the *costocoracoid ligament* in producing venous obstruction and subsequent thrombosis.[239] The syndrome is characterized by dilatation of the veins of the upper extremity and the anterior aspect of the chest on the affected side as a result of congestion of the collateral venous network. This compression is relieved by a downward thrust of the shoulder.[219,239-241]

Lusskin and associates[238] reported that this costoclavicular syndrome could be distinguished from the typical anterior scalene, cervical rib, and thoracic outlet compression syndromes, which can also produce arterial and neurologic symptoms but are typically reproduced by Adson's maneuver. The other syndromes are not generally accentuated by shoulder girdle extension.[235,242-244] The treatment described by a number of authors has depended on the offending structure. If overabundant callus is causing the problem, addressing the surgery to the clavicle may be indicated. If the clavicle is more normal, however, it might make more sense to resect the first rib. Under no circumstance should the clavicle be removed.[245]

Subclavian artery compression was reported by Guilfoil and Christiansen, who described a case of thrombosis secondary to clavicular nonunion.[243] Although injury to this artery is recognized to occur with acute clavicular injuries,[246,247] it is unusual as a late complication secondary to overabundance of clavicular callus or nonunion (see Fig. 11-24). However, Yates and Guest reported a patient who died as a result of an embolus to the basilar artery that originated from a thrombosis in the subclavian artery after an ununited clavicle fracture.[248]

Traumatic aneurysm[249-251] and pseudoaneurysm[252] have been reported after fractures of the clavicle. They may be manifested as pulsatile masses or soft tissue densities in the area of the clavicle fracture or nonunion, and they may be the source of thrombi as well. We have also seen a late vascular injury secondary to a nonunion. Figures 11-38 and 11-39 show an orthopaedic surgeon who underwent emergency surgery because of an aneurysm of his subclavian artery that extended into his carotid artery. The aneurysm developed after failed plating of a fracture that progressed to nonunion. Hansky and associates reported a case of aneurysm of the subclavian artery that produced compression of the brachial plexus.[253]

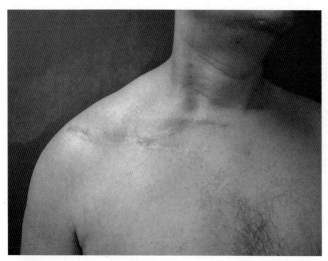

FIGURE 11-38 Clinical appearance of a patient in whom a subclavian artery aneurysm developed and extended into his carotid artery after nonunion of a midshaft clavicle fracture.

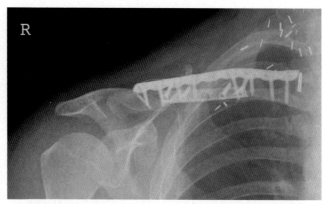

FIGURE 11-39 AP radiograph of the patient in Figure 11-38 after successful double plating of the midshaft nonunion.

Neurologic Syndromes

A number of neurologic symptoms have been described as late complications of fractures of the clavicle.[40,74,202,235,238,254-257] Symptoms can involve the entire brachial plexus or a single nerve. Suso and coworkers reported an injury to the anterior interosseous nerve secondary to fracture of the distal end of the clavicle.[258] Bartosh and associates reported an injury to the musculocutaneous nerve after a refracture of the midshaft of the clavicle that occurred 3 weeks after the original injury.[259] Because the onset of symptoms may be variable between the occurrence of a fracture and the establishment of nonunion, the late sequelae can be confused with nerve injuries that occurred at the time of the acute injury. Thus, it is particularly important to perform a careful neurologic examination of patients with an acute fracture. Rumball and colleagues suggest that a patient with a displaced fracture of the medial part of the clavicle be advised to immediately report the development of any new symptoms.[260]

An early nerve injury is usually a traction neurapraxia, involves the lateral cord, and has a guarded prognosis, but late compression neuropathies typically affect the medial cord, produce ulnar nerve symptoms, and have a more benign prognosis. In this complication, which is typically associated with middle-third fractures, the proximal tip of the distal nonunion fragment is pulled downward and posterior, thereby bringing it into contact with the neurovascular bundle, which is squeezed by the nonunion site above and the first and second ribs below. As one would expect, compression neuropathy is more commonly a problem with hypertrophic rather than atrophic nonunion (Figs. 11-40 and 11-41). Ivey and associates reported a case of reflex sympathetic dystrophy of the anterior chest wall after an injury to the supraclavicular nerve that was associated with a midshaft clavicle fracture.[261]

Ring and Holovacs also reported transient postoperative plexopathies in three patients who had undergone intramedullary fixation of their clavicle fractures. They thought that this might have been due to the force applied to the fragments as they were delivered into the surgical incision and subsequent traction on the plexus.[262]

In addition to compression syndromes, Eilanberger and coworkers described a patient in whom cardiac arrest occurred after a medial clavicle fracture. They explained the complication as vagus nerve irritation secondary to hematoma of the fracture.[263]

Though seemingly minor in comparison to a brachial plexus injury, we have seen five cases in which the middle branch of the supraclavicular nerve has either formed a neuroma over the fracture site or has become entrapped within the fracture callus itself. This complication may be the source of the chronic superficial pain that can be seen after clavicle fractures (see Fig. 11-1). With midshaft clavicle fractures, the middle branch of the supraclavicular nerve is at highest risk for damage either at the fracture site from the original injury or during an internal fixation procedure, whether an open or closed reduction is carried out.

Diagnosis

The diagnosis of late compression syndrome is usually made by a careful history, physical examination, and electrical studies such as electromyography and nerve conduction velocities.[28,107,132,154,185,225,264,265] MRI may be helpful to outline the relationship between the brachial plexus and hypertrophic callus or clavicular fragments. Dela Santo reported that in 16 cases of clavicle fracture, two patients had early neurovascular complications and 14 had late symptoms of costoclavicular syndrome.[266]

Post-Traumatic Arthritis

Post-traumatic arthritis of the joint can follow intra-articular injuries to both the sternoclavicular and acromioclavicular joints, although degenerative disease of the

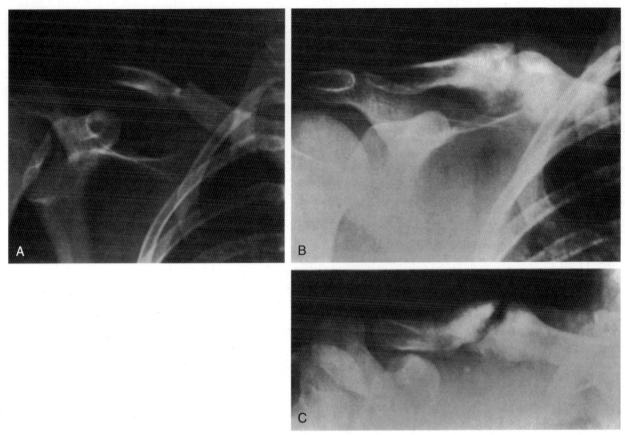

FIGURE 11-40 A, Midclavicle fracture with a mild degree of displacement in an adult. This fracture was treated with a figure-of-eight splint, which was discontinued early so that motion could be started. **B,** AP view showing abundant callus formation. It is unclear whether the fracture has united. **C,** A cephalic tilt view confirms the nonunion with hypertrophic callus. The patient is symptomatic with paresthesias, which suggests irritation of the brachial plexus. (From Rockwood CA, Green DP [eds]: Fractures [3 vols], 4th ed. Philadelphia: Lippincott-Raven, 1996.)

distal end of the clavicle is much more common. Often, this arthritis is a result of the trauma transmitted to these joints at the time of the original injury. It can also be the result of an intra-articular fracture that has gone unrecognized (type III distal clavicle fracture). The patient can have symptoms specifically related to pain at the acromioclavicular joint or symptoms of impingement as a result of extrinsic pressure on the subacromial bursa and rotator cuff by an inferiorly protruding osteophyte of the acromioclavicular joint.[267] Radiographically, cystic changes, spur formation, or narrowing of the acromioclavicular joint may be noted, or resorption of the distal part of the

clavicle may be found. Further radiologic studies may be needed to define the lesion, especially in the area of the sternoclavicular joint, and additional tomograms or a CT scan may be indicated. The patient often symptomatically improves after a diagnostic injection of 1% lidocaine (Xylocaine) into the affected joint.

If appropriate nonoperative treatment, including the administration of nonsteroidal medications or a steroid injection, does not provide lasting relief, surgical excision of the joint may be indicated. If the outer portion of the clavicle is to be resected, no more than the distal 10 mm of bone should be removed to prevent injury to the cora-

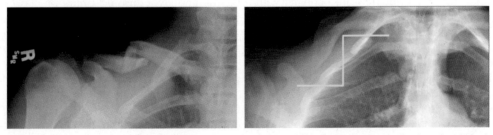

FIGURE 11-41 AP radiograph of a 20-year-old woman in whom a left midshaft clavicular malunion developed.

coclavicular ligaments, and the deltoid is repaired to the trapezius fascia. If resection of the sternoclavicular joint is indicated, the intra-articular disk can be sutured into the end of the clavicle to help stabilize the medial end, and the clavicular head of the sternocleidomastoid muscle may be used to fill in the area of resection.[16]

TREATMENT

As early as the late 1920s, more than 200 different treatment methods had already been described for fractures of the clavicle.[268,269] In general, excellent results have been reported with nonoperative treatment of these fractures.[270]

The exact method of treatment of a fractured clavicle depends on several factors, including the age and medical condition of the patient, the location of the fracture, and associated injuries. Often overlooked are the functional demands of the patient and the patient's expectations in terms of cosmesis.

Children

Because of their excellent healing potential and the tremendous remodeling that accompanies growth, there is little role for any form of treatment other than nonoperative in children; in fact, it has been stated that operative treatment is contraindicated in children.[2] Occasionally, however—such as for débridement of an open fracture, for neurovascular compromise that does not resolve with closed reduction, or for severe irreducible displacement of the fragments—operative management may be indicated.[39,169,271,272] Although it is generally agreed that closed treatment methods are usually successful, the exact method can vary because children can differ in their comprehension or ability to cooperate with nonoperative treatment regimens.

In a newborn with a birth fracture, little treatment is needed other than measures to keep the baby comfortable. Healing is usually rapid and occurs within the first 2 weeks with no untoward effects. However, both the nurse and the mother must be instructed in methods of careful, safe, and gentle turning of the infant to minimize discomfort. The arm may be gently bound to the child for a few days to increase the comfort level.[1] Direct pressure over the clavicle while dressing the child is avoided.

In children with a greenstick or nondisplaced fracture, treatment often consists of the use of a sling until the symptoms have subsided.[273] In displaced fractures or those requiring reduction, most treatment methods have entailed the use of some form of a figure-of-eight bandage or splint, either alone or reinforced with plaster, to hold the shoulder upward and backward in an attempt to reduce the degree of displacement. Fortunately, in children these fractures heal rapidly without much morbidity.[274] Treatment of older children and teenagers may be

more troublesome and more often requires plaster reinforcement because of their high level of activity.

Frequent adjustment is often needed by the physician or parent when attempting to treat these young patients with figure-of-eight methods, which can prove frustrating for both patients and surgeons. It has been questioned whether any significant long-term advantage is gained by aggressive attempts at maintaining reduction with these treatment methods.

Adults

In adults with clavicle fractures, the goal of treatment (as with other fractures) is to achieve healing of bone with minimal morbidity, loss of function, and residual deformity. If this objective is kept in mind, re-evaluation of some of the traditional, cumbersome methods of immobilization of clavicle fractures might be considered. The main principles of nonoperative treatment historically have included bracing of the shoulder girdle to raise the outer fragment upward, outward, and backward; depression of the inner fragment; maintenance of reduction; and use of the ipsilateral elbow and hand so that associated problems with immobilization can be avoided.

An extensive review of the literature generally leads one to conclude that immobilization is almost impossible to achieve and that deformity and shortening are usual. Although this shortening was previously not seen as a problem, more recent studies have suggested that shortening alone is probably one of the most significant predictors of dissatisfaction with the outcome of clavicle fractures (see Figs. 11-29 and 11-41).[15,16] The literature is replete with methods of various complexity to immobilize the clavicle, and treatment has ranged from long-term recumbency alone[107,275] to various forms of ambulatory treatment,[276] and various internal fixation methods.[39,217,275,277-285]

In general, methods of treatment of fractures of the clavicle can be broadly grouped into simple support of the arm, reduction, open or closed reduction with fixation, and primary excision.

Support

With simple support of the arm (Fig. 11-42) whether by sling alone, a sling and swathe, a Sayre bandage, or a Velpeau bandage,[269] no attempt is made to maintain a clavicular reduction, provided that the bone appears to be positioned satisfactorily so that union is anticipated.[286] Although sling treatment is certainly the simplest way to treat a fractured clavicular shaft, it is often unsettling to an orthopaedic surgeon who wishes to realign the fracture fragments; this mindset probably explains the popularity of the numerous methods of effecting and maintaining a closed reduction. Placing the arm in a sling with the forearm across the abdomen can exaggerate the shortening of the fracture and the anterior medial rotation of the scapula.

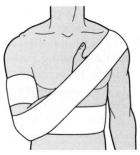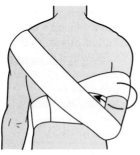

FIGURE 11-42 Modification of a Sayre bandage, which is not intended to reduce the fracture but to simply support the arm. (From Rockwood CA, Green DP [eds]: Fractures [3 vols], 2nd ed. Philadelphia: JB Lippincott, 1984.)

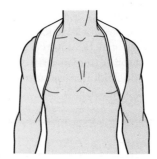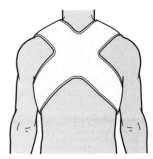

FIGURE 11-43 A Billington yoke: a method of attempting to maintain reduction by plaster reinforcement of a figure-of-eight type of immobilization. (From Rockwood CA, Green DP [eds]: Fractures [3 vols], 2nd ed. Philadelphia: JB Lippincott, 1984.)

Reduction

After reduction, an attempt is made to maintain and hold the reduction by bringing the distal fragment up and back, which may be achieved by a bandage alone (including a figure-of-eight dressing),[275,287] by plaster reinforcement,[288,289] or by full immobilization of the shoulder in various forms of spica casts (Figs. 11-43 and 11-44).[3,4,32,290,291] A variety of materials have been used to maintain a closed reduction, including metal, leather, plastic, plaster, and muslin.[3] The position required to reduce the fracture and maintain the reduction (upward, lateral, and backward) is difficult to achieve, is virtually

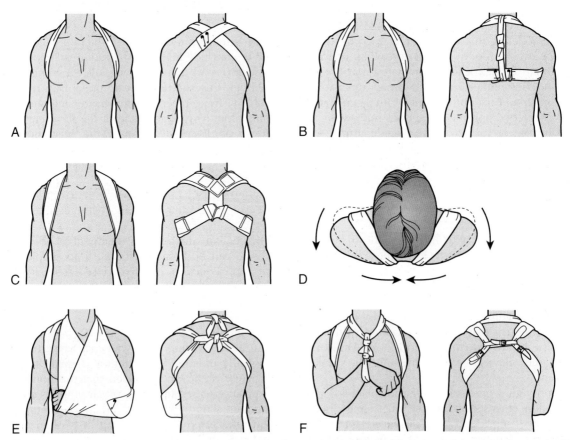

FIGURE 11-44 Various types of figure-of-eight bandages. The figure-of-eight method is intended to maintain a reduction that has been achieved by closed means. **A,** Stockinette that has been padded with three layers of sheet wadding and held in place with safety pins. **B,** Padded stockinette that is not crossed in the back. The upper and lower borders are tied to each other and tightened daily to increase tension to maintain the reduction. **C,** Commercial figure-of-eight support. **D,** Superior view of the patient showing how the figure-of-eight support pulls the shoulder up and backward. **E,** Modified figure-of-eight bandage with a sling. **F,** Figure-of-eight support used with a collar and cuff. (From Rockwood CA, Green DP [eds]: Fractures [3 vols], 2nd ed. Philadelphia: JB Lippincott, 1984.)

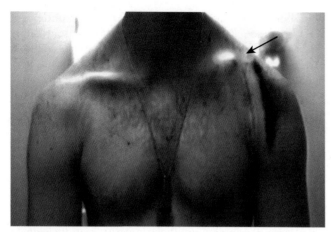

FIGURE 11-45 Clinical appearance of a patient treated with a figure-of-eight harness after a midshaft fracture of the left clavicle. Note that the striations caused by the harness pass directly over the fracture site *(arrow)*.

impossible to maintain, may often be uncomfortable for the patient, and has occasionally been reported to cause symptoms of either neurovascular compression or displacement of the fragment[4] if careful attention is not paid to placing the external immobilization precisely. The figure-of-eight dressing can also lie over the apex of the fracture and cause the patient considerable pain and possibly compromise the skin over the fracture (Fig. 11-45).

Few studies have tried to evaluate in controlled fashion whether a vigorous attempt to effect and maintain a reduction provides a greater chance for a better outcome than does simple arm support for comfort. In two studies directly comparing a figure-of-eight dressing with sling support, it was noted that figure-of-eight dressings were time consuming, required frequent adjustment, might contribute to other problems, and had more complications than simple sling treatment did. The authors concluded that the functional and cosmetic sequelae of the two methods of treatment were identical and that alignment of the healed fracture was unchanged from the initial displacement.[292,293]

Another group studied the recovery time after conservation treatment of fractures of the clavicle in 155 patients. No difference was found in the speed of recovery in those treated with a sling and those treated with a figure-of-eight bandage, although the patient's age at the time of fracture did affect the recovery, with 33% of patients older than 20 years still having symptoms 3 months after injury.

Reduction With Fixation

A number of techniques have been described for the treatment of clavicle fractures with open or closed reduction with internal fixation.[294-296] These techniques have included cerclage sutures,[32] intramedullary devices (Stein-

mann pins, Kirschner wires, Knowles pins, Perry pins, modified Hagie pins, Kuntscher nails, or Rush pins[297]), or plate fixation.[217,277,280-285,298-301]

Reduction With External Fixation

In some cases, such as open fractures or septic nonunion, open or closed reduction with external fixation can be considered.[302] In one study using the Hoffmann device, the average time for the external fixator to be left on was 51 days; no pleural or vascular complications occurred, and all fractures united.[303] However, this technique is not one with which orthopaedists have extensive experience, and this procedure is associated with the potential for serious complications. Xiao reported on a new external fixation device that produced nearly anatomic reduction in 87.4% of his patients.[304] In another report, a small AO (Arbeitsgemeinschaft für Osteosynthesefragen) fixator was used in treatment of fractures of the clavicle.[303] Although Nowak and associates found no difference in the rate of healing in comparing a reconstruction plate to an external fixator, most patients with an external fixator found the device cumbersome.[305]

In rare instances, primary excision of both ends of the fracture with skin closure and intentional formation of a pseudarthrosis has been advocated.[306]

Open Reduction With Internal Fixation

Although distal clavicle fractures can heal without surgical treatment,[81,307] because of the deforming forces, loss of the stabilizing ligaments, and the high incidence of nonunion, many authors continue to recommend primary open reduction and internal fixation,[308,309] either with an intramedullary pin[67,70] or with some method of dynamic fixation to bring the proximal clavicular segment to the distal segment.[278,310]

Winkler and associates[311] described treating lateral clavicle fractures by suturing the acromioclavicular and coracoclavicular ligaments with tension band wiring. However, they noted a 14% complication rate because of the implant.

Poigenfurst and associates reported on 25 fractures of the distal end of the clavicle.[312] Only two patients who were treated without surgery had a successful result. These authors recommended using a coracoclavicular lag screw for simple fractures associated with rupture of the coracoclavicular ligament and plating for fragmented fractures.

Brunner and coworkers reported 283 clavicle fractures, 75 of which (32%) involved the lateral third of the bone.[313] At a 5-year follow-up after extensive conservative treatment, good results were found in Neer type I and type III fractures, but a 31% rate of pseudarthrosis was reported for Neer type II (Jager–Breitner type IIA) fractures. These authors described a new bandage to prevent posterior and upward displacement of the proximal fragment. However, they recommended open reduction and internal fixation for Neer type II and Jager–Breitner fractures and the use of extra-articular implants.

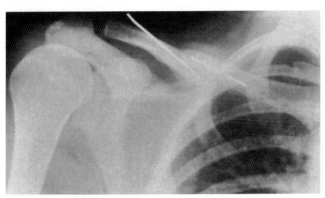

FIGURE 11-46 Complication of intramedullary fixation with a Kirschner wire or Steinmann pin. Insufficient bone purchase combined with motion can lead to hardware failure and migration of pins, with potentially catastrophic results. (From Rockwood CA, Green DP [eds]: Fractures [3 vols], 4th ed. Philadelphia: JB Lippincott, 1996.)

Nordqvist and Petersson described 110 patients with fractures of the lateral end of the clavicle who were treated without surgery.[110] After an average follow-up of 15 years, they reported on 73 nondislocated Neer type I fractures, 23 dislocated type II fractures, and 14 intra-articular type III fractures.[314] The average age of the patients at the time of injury was 36 years (range, 2-71 years). At follow-up, 95 shoulders were asymptomatic. Fifteen shoulders had moderate pain and dysfunction and were rated as fair. No patient had severe residual shoulder disability. Of the 10 cases of nonunion, 8 were asymptomatic. These authors concluded that a fractured end of the clavicle does not require an operation.

Complications have been reported with each of these methods, including the well-known migration of intramedullary wires[315] (Fig. 11-46). In addition, musculocutaneous nerve injuries have been reported with transfer of the coracoid process to the proximal clavicular segment in this fracture.[249] Plate fixation is often impractical because of the small distal segment and the weakness of fixation in this metaphyseal-type bone. One alternative is to extend the fixation onto the acromion. There are a number of problems with this:

1. The bone of the acromion can be thin and not lend itself well to screw fixation.[316]
2. Screws through the acromion can abrade the tissue of the rotator cuff.
3. The normal differential motion been the clavicle and acromion necessitates removing the plate before the patient can start normal motion.

To get around these limitations, a number of studies have examined the use of a hook plate to treat both lateral clavicle fractures and acromioclavicular joint separations.[317] A variety of plates have been marketed by different companies; however, they all have the same common feature of a hook or finger-like extension that goes behind the acromioclavicular joint and under the acromion (see Fig. 11-82). Some versions use locking screws, and others use traditional nonlocking fixation. The supposed advantage of these plates is that they enhance the fixation by incorporating the acromion without limiting the motion at the acromioclavicular joint. The primary problems associated with the use of these plates have been instability, due to dislocation of the hook from under the acromion, wearing of the hook into the underside of the acromion, fracture of the acromion, and impingement. Because of these limitations, the plate typically has to be removed 2 to 3 months after placement, requiring a second operative procedure and, because the incision to place these plates is somewhat large, it requires another similarly large incision to remove it.

In 1994, Voight and associates reported on use of the Rahmanzadeh plate, which permits rotation and tilting, in acute treatment of distal clavicle fractures as well as high-degree acromioclavicular separations.[318] However, these authors also noted a higher rate of infection than with other types of osteosynthesis because of the limited tissue covering for the implant in this area. Haidar and associates reported a union rate of 95% and a satisfaction rate of 85% with a nonlocking hook plate.[319] Unfortunately, they also found a very high rate of complication (80% major complication rate) in patients older than 60 years. Muramatsu and associates reported migration of the hook plate into the acromion in 87% of patients treated for unstable distal clavicle fractures.[320] In a comparison of hook plate fixation to coracoclavicular screw fixation, McKee found that a single coracoclavicular screw was significantly stronger than a hook plate (744 ± 184 N vs. 459 ± 188 N), although the hook plate had less stiffness than the coracoclavicular screw.[321] A number of authors have reported on the use of coracoclavicular screw fixation of distal clavicle fractures and acromioclavicular joint separations.[303,322-326]

For fracture of the medial end of the clavicle, treatment is indeed difficult. The problems encountered here are similar to those seen with lateral factures: The medial fragment is often small and more cancellous-type metaphyseal bone. It is further complicated by the important structures that lie very close to the medial clavicle. Although internal fixation of these fractures has been described, the type of fixation has been under some discussion. The medial fragment is often too small to be effectively stabilized by a plate. Internal fixation with Kirschner wires has led in some instances to severe problems as the pins migrate. One study suggested that these medial para-articular fractures of the clavicle could be treated effectively with a resorbable 2-mm polydioxanone cord.[327]

Nonunion

Asymptomatic clavicular nonunion need not be treated. In addition, nonoperative treatment should probably be considered for nonunion in the elderly. Although nonoperative methods to obtain union have been reported—particularly the use of electrical stimulation and ultrasound—only a few cases of healing of clavicular nonunion by pulsed electromagnetic fields have been documented.[58,192,328,329] Most authors share the view that electrical stimulation has little role in the treatment of clavicular nonunion, especially because operative methods have shown such a high degree of success.[208,330]

Indications for surgical treatment include pain or aching clearly attributable to the nonunion; shoulder girdle dysfunction, weakness, or fatigue; and neurovascular compromise.[284,331] Although bone drilling has been suggested as a means of stimulating a delayed union to progress,[332] such drilling has little role in established nonunion. Alternatively, some authors have advocated resection of the nonunion. Lateral-third nonunions can occasionally be treated with excision of the distal fragment. Because excision does not address the instability of the remaining medial fragment, some type of ligament reconstruction has to be carried out, such as a Weaver–Dunn type of reconstruction.[333,334]

Partial claviculectomy, with excision of the nonunion site, has been reported by some as a means of treating ununited clavicle fractures. Certainly, in the short term this procedure can alleviate the crepitus and often eliminates the pain.[204] However, many patients treated in this manner remain mildly to moderately symptomatic,[203,210,245] the stabilizing function of the clavicle is lost, and neurogenic symptoms can be a problem.[57,203] Nonetheless, resection of the nonunion and filling of the defect with cancellous bone chips can stimulate regeneration of the clavicle and, in addition, can decompress the neurovascular structures if the nonunion is accompanied by symptoms of thoracic outlet syndrome.[221,222,335,336] Surgical treatment most commonly consists of an attempt to gain union through some means of internal fixation with bone grafting. The techniques for surgical treatment of nonunion have evolved, as have internal fixation techniques for other long bone fractures and nonunion.

A number of open treatment methods have been detailed. Some authors have used wire sutures through the ends of either clavicular fragment and through an iliac crest graft.[69,107,225] Sutures consisting of other materials, including catgut, braided suture, and even loops of kangaroo tendon, have been used in the past.[3] Simple intrafragmentary screw fixation has been advocated, with fixation of the iliac bone as an onlay graft and cancellous bone grafting at either junction.[202,337] However, because of the amount of movement in multiple planes that the clavicle exhibits and because these methods control rotation poorly, neither suture nor screw fixation is secure enough to be reliable when used independently of additional protection. An external cast or brace support is necessary to prevent screw or wire breakage and potential wire fragment migration, which can produce disastrous results.[315,338-341]

Open reduction plus internal intramedullary fixation with the use of Kirschner wires (with or without screws),[3,29,197,207,217,342,343] Steinmann pins,[4,67,298] Knowles pins,[283] or modified Hagie pins[344] has been a popular method of internal fixation. Although reports have been encouraging with these methods (and they can be successful), rotation is poorly controlled under most circumstances, and the intramedullary fixation can be difficult to insert if the bone ends are atrophic (especially with a flat, curved clavicle). In addition, distraction of the fracture at the nonunion site can occur with the use of threaded pins.[298] If an improper form of intramedullary fixation is chosen, the device can bend or break. Several complications have been reported with pin migration.[315,339-341]

However, in 1991 Rockwood and associates[345] described a series of 21 patients with nonunion of the clavicle who were treated successfully with an intramedullary pin that was specifically designed for clavicle fixation. It had threads with a differential pitch on either end and a blunt medial tip to prevent penetration of the medial cortex. Furthermore, it had a nut that was secured over the lateral portion of the pin that virtually ensured that the pin would not migrate. The lateral nut and the differential pitch threads also allowed compression of the fragments. These patients underwent open reduction, internal fixation with a modified Hagie intramedullary pin, and autogenous bone grafting. The average duration of follow-up was 35 months (range, 5 months-11 years). Healing occurred in 20 (95%) of the 21 patients. When compared with other treatment methods, such as fixation with a plate and screws, intramedullary fixation has several advantages. The intramedullary pin can be inserted through a cosmetically acceptable incision in Langer's lines. The pin requires less soft tissue dissection, and after healing, it can be removed through a small incision under local anesthesia (see "Surgical Technique for Intramedullary Fixation" later).

The application of rigid internal fixation for acute fractures has aided the management of many traditionally difficult fractures, and this concept of rigidly immobilizing fragment ends has had its natural application in the treatment of nonunion as well. Although rigid internal fixation techniques using AO plates without bone grafting have been reported to be just as successful for clavicular nonunion as for nonunion of other long bones,[346,347] the addition of supplemental bone graft to rigid plating has been the most popular treatment of clavicular nonunion. With this method of treatment, reports in the literature have approached a union rate of 100%.[347-353] Manske and Szabo reported a 100% incidence of union by 10 weeks postoperatively without complications when using open reduction and internal fixation with compression plating and bone grafting.[204] Jupiter and Leffert reported on 23 clavicular nonunions, including two resulting from clavicular osteotomies for surgical access, with an overall success rate of 89% in achieving union. However, 93.7% of those treated with grafting and dynamic compression plating achieved union.[210]

A number of series using an AO reconstruction plate for clavicular nonunion and delayed union have been reported, with results equal to those achieved with the larger dynamic compression plates and semitubular plates.[354] Advantages of the reconstruction plate include its lower profile and its relative ease of contouring to the available clavicular bone. The primary disadvantage of these plates is that they are weaker and do not allow compression at the fracture site.

Eskola and colleagues reported that 20 of 22 clavicular nonunions healed with rigid plate fixation and bone grafting, but they warned against shortening the clavicle to achieve union.[194] For this reason, if resection of the sclerotic edges of the atrophic margin to achieve primary osteosynthesis would result in significant clavicular shortening, many authors recommend intercalary bone grafting along with plate fixation[40,57] (see Fig. 11-80). The reconstruction ratio has been used as an adjunctive means of assessing restoration of clavicular length. A reconstruction ratio of 1 means that the restored length of the clavicle is equal to the length of the contralateral uninjured clavicle. In one series, 16 midclavicular nonunions were treated with a 3.5-mm plate, and 15 of 16 achieved union with a reconstruction ratio of 0.96.[7] Plate fixation with bone grafting is reliable and safe and has few complications; it has the additional benefit that the rigid internal fixation is usually secure enough that no postoperative external cast immobilization is needed; use of a sling alone is usually adequate. The plate does have the disadvantage of requiring a second operation to remove the hardware if its prominent position irritates the skin. In addition, the screw holes weaken the bone, and protection is thus needed after hardware removal. Some have used this argument to advocate the use of intramedullary fixation if previous plate fixation has failed; they contend that removal of previous hardware and the presence of screw holes from plate fixation make the use of a new plate for rigid internal fixation more difficult.[355]

The advent of low-contact dynamic compression plates has enabled further refinement of well-established principles of plating.[356] The structured undersurface of the plate allows the blood supply to plated bone segments to be preserved, and avoidance of the stress risers produced at plate removal reduces the possibility of refracture after removal of the plate.[357] The excellent biocompatibility of titanium ensures superb tissue tolerance and increases the possibility of leaving plates in situ, thus obviating a second procedure (see Fig. 11-49).

Despite apparent success in treating nonunion with rigid internal fixation, a report by Pedersen and associates suggested that care must be taken when choosing the correct plate size.[358] These authors reported 12 patients with clavicular nonunion treated by plate fixation and bone grafting. Although 9 of 12 patients achieved a good end result, the primary treatment failed in half the cases. The authors theorized that a short (four-holed) semitubular plate and insufficient postoperative immobilization were two factors that were significant in the failure of treatment in these patients.

Medial clavicular nonunion, though rare, is particularly troublesome to treat. The proximity to the sternoclavicular joint and vital structures makes intramedullary fixation worrisome, and often little proximal bone is available to secure a standard dynamic compression plate. Center plates are often prone to breakage. A postoperative spica cast may be required.

Rehabilitation After Clavicle Fracture

Rehabilitation after a clavicle fracture is started almost immediately, regardless of the treatment modality used. Assuming that no associated injuries have occurred, the patient is allowed to continue lower-body strengthening exercises as before the injury. Aerobic conditioning on an exercise bike or other stationary apparatus is encouraged. The patient is allowed to perform wrist and elbow range-of-motion exercises and grip-strength maintenance exercises immediately. Running is discouraged until the acute pain has resolved. As soon as the acute pain resolves, gentle pendulum exercises and isometric strengthening of the rotator cuff, deltoid, biceps, and triceps are initiated. Normal use of the ipsilateral hand for activities of daily living is also encouraged.

Generally, active range of motion is limited to less than 90 degrees of forward flexion or abduction if any operative fixation has been performed. Such restriction helps limit the initial stress on the hardware. In the absence of hardware, the patient is allowed to advance to active range of motion within the arc of pain tolerance. If no operative fixation is performed, full active range of motion is allowed when the patient is completely pain free, usually after 4 to 6 weeks of healing. When the patient has achieved full pain-free range of motion with radiographic evidence of callus, resistive exercises may be instituted. When the patient has near-normal strength in the injured upper extremity, a plyometrics program may be started.

Return-to-Play Criteria in Athletes

The criteria for return to sport activity are always controversial and essentially come down to a judgment call by the treating orthopaedist. This decision is affected by several factors, including the athlete, the specific fracture, the sport, the position played, the level of sports competition, the level of compensation, and the needs of the team. Occasionally, these factors are in direct opposition to common sense. The treating surgeon must realize that this decision is ultimately a compromise and that all compromises come with inherent risks. The athlete, coaches, and team may be willing to take risks that the orthopaedist is unwilling to shoulder. It is our job to protect the athlete from these competing forces just long enough to allow adequate healing of the clavicle fracture. The key word here is *adequate*. We know that fracture remodeling is a long and ongoing process that takes 9 months to 1 year or longer. In theory, the risk of refracture is increased until the bone remodels completely. Stopping sports participation for a year is obviously overkill. We have to make the athlete understand that returning to sports earlier is a compromise and that by doing so, we increase the risk of reinjury. The goal is caution to allow adequate healing without overprotection.

For noncontact athletes, return to sports may be allowed when painless full active range of motion and nearly normal strength have been achieved, as well as evidence of bridging callus, which usually occurs about 6 weeks after fracture. Contact athletes and, in particular, those involved in collision sports are obviously at greater risk for refracture. The position played and the type of fracture also affect this risk. Even if we cannot authorize a return to full participation, we can often permit the athlete to return to practice with the team on a noncontact basis, which allows the athlete to remain at least mentally in sync with the team. We generally permit such participation when the athlete meets the same criteria as those for noncontact athletes. The team trainer can be extremely valuable in keeping the athlete from doing too much, too soon because the trainer is with the team every day at practice. Generally, between 2 and 3 months would be the earliest return to contact sports. In football, extra protection can at times be afforded by the use of donut pads or, sometimes, fabrication of a fiberglass shoulder shell to dissipate impact forces to the clavicle. If the fracture required operative fixation of any type, the season is generally over for the athlete.

Neurovascular Complications

In general, treatment of late neurovascular lesions has depended on the cause of the compromised structure.

If neurovascular compromise is present and due to massive callus formation and callus debulking is risky, if internal fixation of pseudarthrosis with bone grafting is impractical because of comminution, or if malunion with a severe deformity has occurred and realignment osteotomy cannot be achieved, *resection* of the middle third of the clavicle may be the best choice if the lesion is in this portion. Abbott and Lucas outlined the various areas of the clavicle that can be resected without untoward sequelae and areas that do less well with resection.[44] Although some authors have advocated total claviculectomy, it is probably wiser to perform careful subtotal resections when possible.

If excessive callus buildup or malunion of the clavicle has occurred and the lesion is amenable to bone grafting and plate fixation, removal of the hypertrophic callus and realignment osteotomy with or without segmental interposition of bone graft and cancellous bone grafting often relieves the neurovascular symptoms.

If the clavicle has a satisfactory appearance and is stable, enlargement of the costoclavicular space—and thus neurovascular decompression—can be accomplished by resecting the first rib, with partial excision of the scalene or subclavius muscle.[232,359]

POSTOPERATIVE CARE

After operative treatment of a nonunion or an acute fracture, patients are placed in a sling and swathe in the operating room; however, they are told to remove this sling and start simple activities of daily living, such as eating, washing, and writing, as soon as possible. A postoperative radiograph is reviewed. It should include not only the fracture site and the internal fixation, to determine fracture alignment and hardware placement, but also enough of the lung to ensure that no injury has occurred during the surgical procedure. When the patient is comfortable, he or she is discharged, and wound care is the same as for any surgical procedure on the shoulder.

If the glenohumeral joint and the subacromial bursa have not been surgically violated and are not otherwise diseased, there appears to be no need for instituting early range-of-motion exercises because shoulder range of motion, if normal preoperatively, usually remains normal. Thus, the patient may be kept safely supported in a sling or immobilizer until radiographic signs of union occur without fear of producing a frozen shoulder.

Early in the postoperative period, isometric exercises for the rotator cuff may be initiated, although isometric strengthening of the trapezius and deltoid is delayed until their suture junction is healed securely (3-4 weeks). Range of motion after surgery is not permitted past 90 degrees of flexion in the plane of the scapula until clinical signs of union are apparent, usually at 4 to 6 weeks.

When clinical or radiographic union is present, the patient may begin full range of motion, particularly in forward elevation (using an overhead pulley); external rotation (with the use of a cane or stick) and hyperextension–internal rotation are then added. Resistive exercises of the deltoid, trapezius, cuff, and scapula muscles are also added. When radiographic union is evident, full active use of the arm is permitted.

The patient is not permitted to return to full, strenuous work or athletic activities until nearly full range of motion of the shoulder has been achieved, strength has returned to nearly normal, and bone healing is presumed to be solid. In adults, 4 to 6 months is usually required to achieve these goals.

AUTHORS' PREFERRED METHOD OF TREATMENT

Newborns and Infants

Despite some information that fracture of the clavicle in newborns may be asymptomatic, we prefer to ensure comfort by treating clavicle birth fractures for a few days.

The newborn is supine for many hours in the day; one who is not particularly active may be treated simply by avoiding pressure on the clavicle when dressing the infant and taking care to handle the infant gently and avoid movement of the affected arm during feeding, diapering, and dressing changes. When the newborn is prone, soft padding may be placed under the anterior aspect of the shoulder, with the weight of the body used to help keep the lateral portion of the clavicle back. Avoiding handling of a newborn is neither practical nor desirable.

If pseudoparalysis is present and the infant avoids using the arm because of pain, we prefer to place a cotton abdominal pad under the infant's arm, flex the elbow fully to 90 degrees, and gently strap the arm to the chest with a padded elastic, Kling, or Kerlix bandage. A sling is difficult to apply and maintain and is not necessary. Parents may be taught to reapply the bandage for skin care and after bathing. Usually within 7 to 10 days the patient is asymptomatic, and healing is generally complete by 2 weeks.

The infant will use the arm normally once symptoms subside. Unrestricted use of the arm is permitted once the wrap is off, and parents may be reassured that the deformity and exuberant callus will remodel in time. After adequate healing, the infant is retested with Moro's reflex to ensure that the disinclination to move the arm was, in fact, pseudoparalysis rather than an inability to move the arm secondary to an injury to the brachial plexus.[2]

Children

Ages 2 to 12 Years
Young children are treated symptomatically. In children younger than 6 years, no attempt is made to reduce the fracture because the fracture will remodel and the large lump will be gone in 6 to 9 months.[2] The child is made more comfortable with some type of applied figure-of-eight bandage.

Commercial figure-of-eight bandages are usually too large; the simplest way to construct one is to fill a 2-inch stockinette with cotton wadding, cast padding, or felt. The child is seated and the dressing is applied as follows: the surgeon, standing behind the patient, passes the stockinette across the front of the uninjured clavicle, through the uninjured axilla and across the back, through the axilla on the fracture side, across the front of the anterior of the shoulder and the clavicle on the fracture side, and across the back behind the neck. To help keep the shoulder up and back, tension is placed on the stockinette, and a safety pin binds both ends of the stockinette together as the tension is maintained. An elastic bandage or 2-inch tape securing the bandage can be placed from one posterior strap to the other to maintain tension and secure the position. Alternatively, the figure-of-eight stockinette may be crisscrossed behind the patient before being applied to the fracture side and subsequently pinned and tightened. If the 2-inch stockinette appears

to irritate the skin, an abdominal cotton pad can be placed beneath the anterior straps.

Parents should be instructed on how to tighten the figure-of-eight bandage to maintain tension by reapplying the anchoring safety pin. Such adjustments should be done in situ without taking the stockinette off. The stockinette can have a tendency to loosen quickly; it should be retightened 2 or 3 days after the initial application and then weekly thereafter. We prefer to see the child weekly to ensure that the bandage is secure and that no skin problems, neurovascular irritation, or any other problems with treatment are occurring. Parents should be made aware of potential circulatory difficulties or skin problems if the bandage is too tight, and we ask them to practice tightening the bandage under our supervision to minimize the anxiety of having to bear the responsibility for handling the bandage adjustment themselves.

In young children, 3 weeks is usually adequate immobilization, but in an older ambulatory child, clinical signs of union, such as absence of tenderness to pressure over the fracture site or movement of the arm, are good signs that can help the physician decide when immobilization may be discontinued. Although union typically occurs in 3 to 6 weeks, symptoms are often dramatically diminished within the first 2 to 3 weeks.

Nondisplaced fractures, incomplete fractures, or plastic bone bowing need not be treated with a figure-of-eight bandage because the position is unlikely to change with ambulatory treatment if activity can be curtailed and reinjury avoided. A simple sling for comfort until clinical union takes place is sufficient. The child should avoid unusually vigorous activity such as gym class until the bone is solid, typically at about 3 months.

Repeat radiographic evaluation is not necessary at each return visit. We typically order a radiograph of the involved shoulder with the immobilization in place, another radiograph to check the progress of healing and the amount of callus, and one final radiograph when union is definite (between 6 and 12 weeks). An additional radiograph showing healing is helpful; in the event of reinjury, radiographic interpretation can be confusing if no radiograph is available that shows union after the first injury.

Ages 12 to 16 Years
This group may be difficult to treat because their activity level often frustrates the most aggressive attempts to maintain reduction and immobilization. Whereas in very young children little or no attempt is made to reduce the fracture, the teenage population has limited remodeling potential, and an attempt can be made to reduce the fracture before applying the immobilization. However, most, if not all, fractures return to their final length within a week after injury.

In cooperative older children, a commercial figure-of-eight clavicular splint—usually an elastic bandage with well-padded areas for the axilla—may be applied. A commercial splint has several advantages, including easy removal for bathing and more resistance to stretching out over time than is the case with a fashioned stockinette. This figure-of-eight bandage does not reduce or rigidly immobilize the fracture, but it may be a reminder to hold the shoulders back when the child wants to slump forward.[1]

Despite reports that there might not be any long-term difference between the use of a sling and a figure-of-eight bandage, we still prefer the latter after an attempt is made to reduce the fracture while maintaining alignment of the clavicle. A figure-of-eight bandage has one advantage that a sling lacks—it leaves both hands and elbows free for use in activities of daily living. In addition, a sling in its usual position holds the arm forward and inward, and the distal clavicular segment is not in position to be lined up with the proximal segment.

In older children, fractures usually heal within 6 weeks. However, we generally maintain the clavicular immobilizer for another 4 weeks after healing to remind the patient to restrict activities. Vigorous athletic activity

should be avoided until union is solid, which in a teenager should be after 12 to 16 weeks.[1,360]

In a multiply traumatized child, the clavicle fracture may be treated by recumbency if a small pillow is placed between the scapulae to allow the weight of the arm to reduce the fracture. If recumbent treatment is to be instituted, a sling might make the arm more comfortable.

Medial and Distal Fractures in Children

We prefer to treat both medial and distal clavicle fractures in children with a sling for support and an elastic (Ace) wrap for comfort. Medial clavicle fractures are rare problems and seldom produce significant displacement. Lateral clavicle fractures, though clinically dramatic (appearing to be a high-grade acromioclavicular separation), are stable because the coracoclavicular ligaments and acromioclavicular ligaments remain attached to the periosteal tube and both sides of the joint, respectively. Despite the degree of displacement, the bone will remodel in time (Fig. 11-47). For lateral clavicle fractures, we find that a

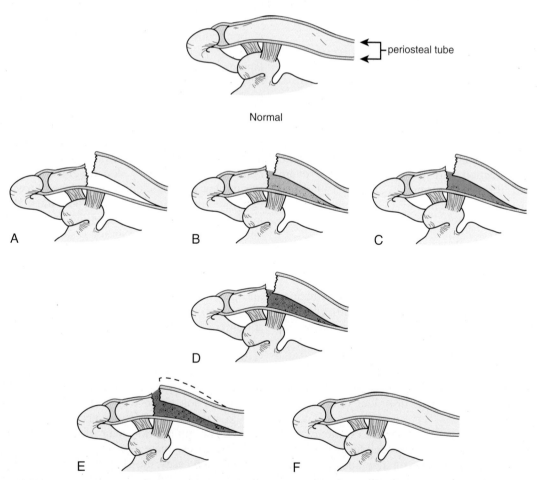

FIGURE 11-47 Sequence of events in a typical type IV distal clavicle fracture in children. **A,** The ligaments have remained attached to the periosteal tube as the medial clavicular fragment ruptures through the superior thin periosteum. This injury can mimic an acromioclavicular separation. **B,** Early filling of the area between the periosteum and the bone is seen. **C,** Further filling in of the bone is apparent. **D,** Bridging callus is seen to reach the top of the medial clavicular segment. **E,** Early remodeling has begun to occur with further consolidation of the fracture. **F,** Remodeling has occurred with complete union. This fracture is best treated nonoperatively, and excellent results can be expected. (From Rockwood CA, Green DP [eds]: Fractures [3 vols], 2nd ed. Philadelphia: JB Lippincott, 1984.)

figure-of-eight bandage is difficult to maintain over the most lateral aspect of the shoulder; the sling and swathe is more practical and quite comfortable, and the healing potential in children negates the need for precise maintenance of reduction.

Adults

Fractures of the Shaft

Fractures of the clavicle in adults are much more difficult to treat because the quality of the bone and periosteum is different from that in children, and associated soft tissue or bone injury is often greater. In addition, the potential for healing is less in adults. In the past, it was thought that all clavicle fractures heal and the patient is left with little discomfort or disability. From more-recent studies, we now know that displaced midshaft clavicle fractures have a far higher nonunion rate than previously thought and that up to half of all patients are still symptomatic as long as 10 years after injury.[15,360] Consequently, it is probably justified to consider operative intervention on displaced and shortened midshaft clavicle fractures, particularly in high-demand patients.

Indications for Primary Open Fixation

Our indications for operative treatment of acute clavicle fractures include the following:

- Neurovascular injury or compromise that is progressive or that fails to reverse with closed reduction of the fracture
- Severe displacement caused by comminution, with resultant angulation and tenting of the skin severe enough to threaten its integrity and that fails to respond to closed reduction
- An open fracture that requires operative débridement
- Multiple trauma, when mobility of the patient is desirable and closed methods of immobilization are impractical or impossible
- A floating shoulder with a displaced clavicle fracture and an unstable scapula fracture or with compromise of the acromioclavicular and coracoacromial ligaments[154,155]
- Type II distal clavicle fractures (see later)
- Factors that render the patient unable to tolerate closed immobilization, such as the neurologic problems of parkinsonism, seizure disorders, or other neurovascular disorders[217]
- The occasional patient for whom the cosmetic lump over the healed clavicle is intolerable and who is willing to exchange this bump for a potentially equally noncosmetic surgical scar and the possibility of nonunion

Relative indications include shortening of more than 15 to 20 mm and displacement more than the width of the clavicle.

Medial-Third Fractures

Medial-third fractures are rare and account for about 5% of all clavicle fractures in adults. The medial clavicular physis is the last in the body to close, and closure occurs between the ages of 22 and 25 years.[85,361] Many medial clavicle fractures are therefore physeal injuries, which inherently have great healing potential. Physeal arrest is not a concern. Even in cases in which the medial physis has already fused, these fractures heal well. Anterior displacement, even if complete, is not a concern. The great majority of these fractures are best treated nonoperatively with a figure-of-eight bandages or a sling. Healing can be expected to be rapid with a very low risk of nonunion. This being said, we must emphasize that accurate diagnosis is important for several reasons. These injuries can be misdiagnosed as sternoclavicular joint injuries, which can confound treatment. Medial clavicle fractures that include extension into the sternoclavicular articulation carry some risk of post-traumatic arthrosis, which is something to consider when counseling the patient about the injury.

A medial clavicle fracture that can be very problematic is one with posterior displacement severe enough to impinge on the vital structures at the root of the neck. Patients with complaints of difficulty swallowing or breathing or with any neurovascular compromise require operative reduction of the fracture. Patients without symptoms but with documented CT evidence of impingement of the fragments on vital structures should be considered for operative reduction. Reduction maneuvers or a towel-clip reduction should not be performed in the clinic or the emergency department unless the posterior position of the fragment is causing an airway or hemodynamic emergency. This reduction must be performed in the operating room under general anesthesia. The chest must be prepared as for a sternotomy, and a thoracic surgeon must be available in case a vascular problem occurs.

A towel clip can be used to grasp the distal fragment and pull it forward to the proximal fragment. Traction on the upper extremity, or a towel placed between the shoulder blades, might assist in unlocking the fragments and allowing reduction. The reduction is generally stable.

In cases in which the reduction is unstable or cannot be achieved, open reduction is necessary. Removing interposed soft tissue will probably allow reduction and should stabilize the fracture. Fixation may be obtainable with heavy suture and repair of the soft tissue envelope. In some cases, plate-and-screw fixation may be necessary. In such cases, the vital structure beneath the clavicle must be protected with a curved Crego or other such retractor to prevent plunging with the drill. You must use all available willpower to resist pinning across the fracture and into the sternum. The literature has many reports of broken hardware that migrated to the mediastinum and neck and even into the great vessels and heart.

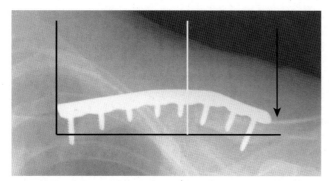

FIGURE 11-48 Cantilever effect when using plate fixation. In the ideal situation, the primary fixation point is at the medial aspect of the plate. With a superiorly placed plate, compression occurs at the fracture site. *Arrow* points to compression on distal fragment of clavicle. However, with comminution, the cantilever point is moved laterally to the fracture site, thereby increasing the force on the distal fixation. This model would predict loss of distal fixation as the primary mode of failure in comminuted fractures.

Middle-Third Fractures

Many middle-third fractures or shaft fractures of the clavicle can be managed best by closed means either with a figure-of-eight splint or a sling. Keep in mind, however, that what you see clinically and on the original injury films is likely to foretell the ultimate result after healing has occurred. Reduction maneuvers and figure-of-eight bandages have not been conclusively shown to hold a reduction or improve cosmesis in these fractures. A fracture that is completely displaced or severely shortened, or both, is likely to stay in this position or revert to this position despite one's best efforts at reduction and the tightest figure-of-eight bandage.

An attempt at reduction can be useful in several circumstances. In extremities with acute neurovascular compromise as a result of a clavicle fracture, an attempt at reduction may be helpful. These cases are rare, but when they occur, a reduction maneuver can turn an emergency into just an urgency and might provide the necessary time for planning or to call in appropriate equipment. Another case in which a reduction maneuver may be useful is in a completely displaced middle-third fracture. This fracture is at greater risk for nonunion according to Thompson and Batten.[352] Crepitus felt with a reduction maneuver suggests that the fracture fragments are less likely to have interposed muscle or other soft tissues. If crepitus is felt and the fracture has no other indications for operative intervention, you might wish to attempt nonoperative treatment of this fracture with the realization that there might still be an increased risk of nonunion. If no crepitus is felt, we must assume that something is interposed between the fracture fragments. Such interposition of tissue raises concern for the development of nonunion.

Problematic fractures of the midshaft of the clavicle are generally those that have absorbed greater energy. In our

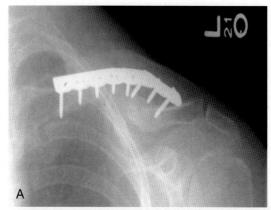

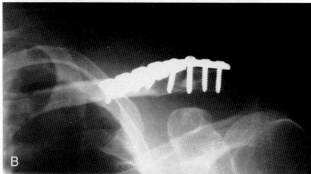

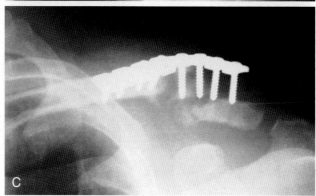

FIGURE 11-49 Loss of distal fixation. **A,** Bending of plate. **B,** Plate on distal clavicle fracture. **C,** Nonunion of distal clavicle previously treated with plate.

experience, these higher-energy fractures tend to have a remarkably consistent pattern. They are generally shortened and comminuted and have a butterfly fragment that is consistently inferior. Soft tissue injury and stripping are usually significant, and therefore greater instability is commonly present. All of these problems raise the risk of nonunion in any fractured bone.

We believe that these fractures are best treated by open reduction and internal fixation, for which we have essentially two options: plate-and-screw fixation and intramedullary fixation.

Fixation

In terms of fixation, the two primary choices are plate-and-screw fixation and intramedullary fixation. The former

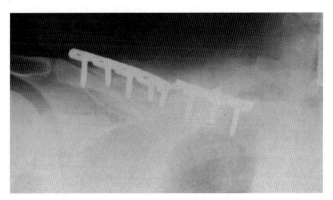

FIGURE 11-50 Loss of distal fixation and plate failure with a locking 3.5-mm reconstruction plate.

has the advantage of being a familiar operation to most surgeons. The primary disadvantage is that plate fixation requires a large skin incision and significant soft tissue stripping. In a study by Bostman, the complication rate with plating was 43%, with major complications noted in 15%, and the reoperation rate was 14%.[362]

Plate Fixation

Because the clavicle has a rather marginal blood supply that is entirely periosteal, plate fixation might not be a wise choice. Although plate fixation provides excellent rotational control, which intramedullary fixation does not, its strength as a tension band is dramatically weakened in cases of comminution. Plate fixation is akin to a cantilever effect in that a dorsally placed plate acts as a tension band. In the case of a perfect transverse fracture, the point of fixation of the cantilever is the sternoclavicu-

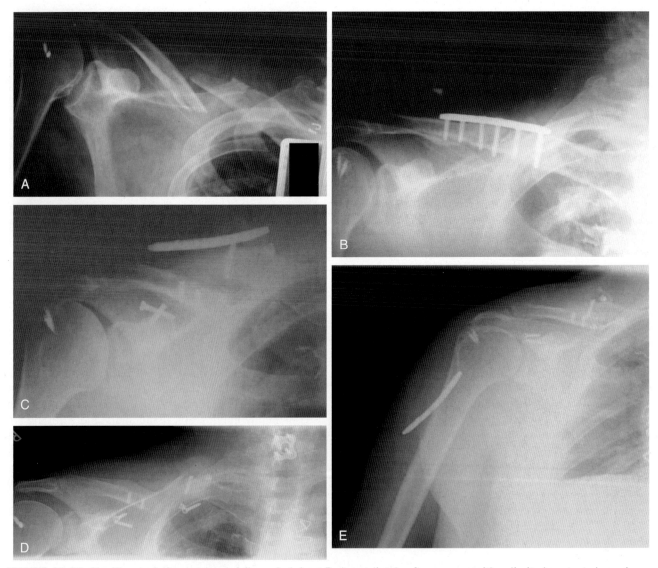

FIGURE 11-51 Significant plating hardware failure. **A,** Injury. **B,** Immediately after surgery with a limited-contact dynamic compression plate. **C,** Six months after surgery **D** and **E,** One year after surgery.

lar joint, and the plate acts to compress the fracture with bending. Unfortunately, most high-energy clavicle fractures are comminuted, and in this setting, the fixation point of the cantilever moves laterally to the fracture site itself, thereby negating the compression effect at the fracture site and putting significant force on the lateral-most screws (Fig. 11-48). In fact, it has been our experience that when plates fail, they typically do so by pullout of the lateral-most screws (Figs. 11-49 to 11-52). Another problem with plate fixation is that the plate itself sits subcutaneously and can be the source of irritation and poor cosmesis. If the plate needs to be removed, another involved procedure is required, and the patient is left with multiple stress risers in the clavicle.

If a plate is chosen, it should be a dynamic compression plate, preferably a low-contact dynamic compression type of plate such as the AO limited-contact dynamic compression plate (LC-DCP). The other choice is a reconstruction plate. The advantage of a reconstruction plate is that it can be easily contoured; however, it provides no compression and is weaker than a dynamic compression plate in terms of bending (see Fig. 11-50). A one-third tubular plate is not recommended because it does not provide strong enough fixation.

Pertinent Anatomy. Plate fixation of the clavicle is complicated because it is an S-shaped bone that is flattened on its lateral end and pyramid-shaped on its medial end. There is considerable variation of the length and curvature of the clavicle; however, the medial arch of curvature always matches the lateral arch. In addition to its S-shaped curve, the clavicle also has a superior bow that has its apex in a variable position on the clavicle.[363] The superior surface tends to be flat medially and laterally; however, the mid portion tends to have a convex shape due to the tubular middle clavicle. The anterior medial portion of the clavicle tends to be flat, and the lateral portion tends to be convex and almost angular, making plate fixation laterally more difficult.

Choice of Plate. There are a number of choices in terms of plate fixation. The traditional choices are the 2.7-mm dynamic compression plate, the 3.5-mm reconstruction plate, and the 3.5-mm LC-DCP. A number of new clavicle-specific plates have been introduced, such as the Acumed clavicle plate and the Smith & Nephew Peri-Loc Upper Extremity plate, both of which are precontoured for the clavicle and have locked screw capabilities. However, the Smith & Nephew plate is more of a precontoured 3.5-mm locking reconstruction plate. One of the primary advantages of using precontoured plates versus traditional straight plates is that there is a significant risk of losing the locking screw capabilities of the locking plates when they are contoured. The one-third tubular plate is far too weak to be used in fixation of clavicle fractures.

There is great variability in the curvature of the clavicle and in the caudal-to-cephalic bow of the clavicle. Huang noted that precontoured plates could fit well on the majority of male clavicles but not female clavicles because of the superior bow, with a poor fit being seen in 38% of specimens from white female donors.[363] Huang also found that precontoured Acumed plates tended to work best with fixation of fractures occurring in the medial three fifths of the clavicle. Unfortunately, most fractures occur at the junction of the middle and lateral third of the clavicle.

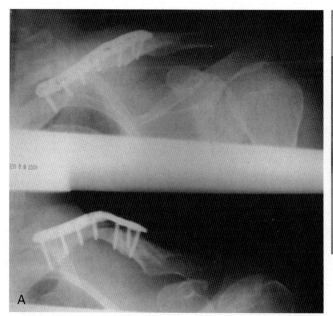

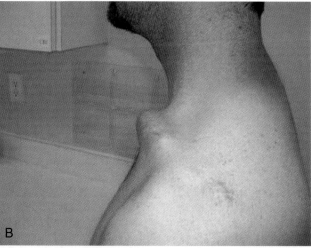

FIGURE 11-52 Loss of distal fixation and plate failure with resultant nonunion of a midshaft clavicle fracture treated with a locking precontoured plate. **A,** Plate fixation that developed failure with angulation of fracture. **B,** Clinical appearance of angulated clavicle secondary to nonunion of left clavicle.

Innanoti and Crosby[364] found that the LC-DCP provided the most biomechanical stability in terms of fracture rigidity, construct stiffness, and strength. In terms of clinical results, Shahid[365] found that the time to union was faster using a 3.5-mm dynamic compression plate (DCP) compared to a 3.5-mm reconstruction plate; however, hardware had to be removed in half of the patients treated with a DCP because prominence of the plate caused discomfort.

Although gross motion of fracture fragments can lead to nonunion, a certain amount of micromotion may be a stimulus to bone healing. Because of the considerable forces acting on the clavicle, fracture fixation must be very strong. The paradox in choosing plate fixation for clavicle fractures is that the stiffer the plate, the better able it is to resist these forces but the more likely it is to inhibit healing and allow weakening of the underlying bone due to excessive stress shielding. The stripping of soft tissue about the clavicle to allow placement of a plate can also contribute to osteopenia under the plate, further weakening the bone.

Placement of the Plate. There has been debate about the best position for application of plate fixation, the primary choices being anterior or superior placement. The advantage of superior placement is that is can be accomplished with minimal soft tissue stripping and there is a broad surface medially for fixation of the plate; however, there is the inherent problem of plate prominence and the risk of injury to the underlying neurovascular structures when drilling in a superior-to-inferior direction, especially medially.[42,366] The primary advantage of anterior placement is decreased incidence of plate-prominence problems and less risk of damage to the underlying neurovascular structures. However, anterior placement has the problem of more soft tissue stripping for placement of the plate. Furthermore, the anterior surface of the clavicle tends to be more angular compared to the flatter superior surface, making fixation more difficult.

There have been no clinical studies directly correlating clinical outcome with placement of the plate; however, there have been biomechanical studies comparing plate placement. Iannoti and Crosby found that constructs plated on the superior aspect of the clavicle exhibited significantly greater fracture rigidity and stiffness than the anterior location.[364] It should be noted, however, that the model used in this study was a straight, transverse osteotomy that would have favored a tension-band construct offered by the superior plate position. Unfortunately, this is not the pattern typically seen in real clavicle fractures. In our experience, the vast majority of midshaft clavicle fractures have some element of comminution, usually with an anterior-to-inferior butterfly fragment.

Harnroongroj and associates found that superior plating of a clavicle fracture without an inferior cortical defect provided more stability against the bending moment than the anterior plating; however, anterior plating of a fracture with an inferior cortical defect provided more stability than a superior plate.[367]

Intramedullary Fixation

The primary advantage of intramedullary fixation is that it can be performed through a small skin incision in Langer's lines. It requires minimal soft tissue stripping and can be removed under local anesthesia. Furthermore, in the setting of comminution, the cantilever effect for a pin extends to the medial-most portion of the pin, thereby providing better fixation in bending loads. It also allows axial compression, which should enhance healing.

The concept of intramedullary fixation of the clavicle is certainly not new. One of the earliest, and more interesting, methods of intramedullary fixation was described in 1930 by Brockway.[368] He described using beef bone inserted into the intramedullary canal for fixation of displaced clavicle fractures. Gerhard Kuntscher beautifully described the anatomy of the clavicle and suggested that intramedullary fixation should be used in the fixation of clavicle fractures.[369]

Murray also thought that the tubular structure of the clavicle lent itself well to intramedullary fixation.[282] He noted that most clavicle fractures were comminuted and many had a transversely oriented butterfly fragment that made closed reduction difficult. He used a smooth pin to accomplish reduction, and the pin was passed through the intramedullary canal in a medial-to-lateral direction after drilling a pilot hole through the anterior medial cortex (see Fig. 11-58). He also described the technique similar to the one we prefer for open intramedullary fixation. He made a small incision over the fracture site, passed a pin in an antegrade direction out through the lateral fragment, and then passed the pin in a retrograde fashion into the medial fragment after the fracture was held reduced. Zenni described a similar technique in 1981.[217] Unfortunately, it was not long after this period that Mazet[340] described migration of smooth wires from the shoulder into the lung.

There are basically three types of intramedullary fixation devices (not including beef bone):

1. Smooth
2. Threaded
3. Partially threaded

These can be rigid or flexible and can be described as nails, pins, or screws.

Pertinent Anatomy. It has been said that intramedullary fixation cannot be used in the clavicle because of its complex shape. Although the clavicle has an S-shape with a superior bow, most clavicle fractures occur in its mid-section, where it tends to be relatively straight. If one simply draws a tangent to the straightest portion of the clavicle (Fig. 11-53), it is easy to see that a fixation device inserted either medially or laterally can traverse this area without difficulty.

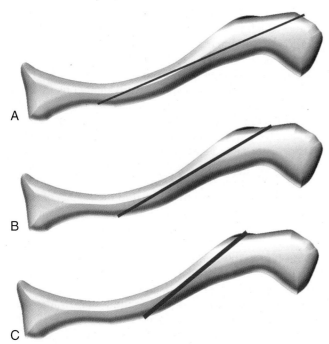

FIGURE 11-53 The length of fixation is determined by the length, diameter, and curvature of the clavicle in addition to the diameter of the pin. As the diameter of the pin increases, it has less fixation because the length of fixation decreases. The larger pin is also forced to exit the lateral fragment more medially than a smaller pin. **A,** Use of small diameter pin in clavicle. **B,** Medium diameter pin. **C,** Larger diameter pin.

Two important determinants of intramedullary fixation are the diameter of the intramedullary canal and the length of fixation. The intramedullary canal determines the maximum size of the device. The average size of the intramedullary canal at its narrowest point is approximately 6 mm. Although this sounds like a fairly large caliber, one has to keep in mind that curve of the clavicle makes the effective diameter of the canal much smaller because to span the area of the fracture, the pin has to travel through the isthmus of the clavicle obliquely as shown in Figure 11-53. For the pin to travel the most effective length, it actually makes three-point contact with the walls of the canal: anterolaterally, then posteriorly at the apex of the posterior curve, and then again anteromedially when it makes contact with the anterior medial curve.

The diameter of the device also determines the length of fixation that is possible. Harnroongroj and associates found that there was a significant increase in the length of fixation using a 3.2-mm pin as compared to a 4.0-mm pin.[370] Although this seems like a small difference in pin size, they found that the ratio of engagement length to total length of the clavicle was 0.59 with a 3.2-mm pin and 0.47 with a 4-mm pin, with the smaller pin having almost 2 cm greater fixation length. They also found that the engagement of the 4-mm pin was equivalent to a

six-hole reconstruction plate, whereas that of the 3.2-mm pin was equivalent to an eight-hole reconstruction plate. The larger pin had significantly less fixation in the lateral fragment.

Another consideration in the diameter of pin fixation is that the stiffness of the pin is directly proportional to the fourth power of the radius of the pin ($I = \pi r^4/4$); in other words, as the pin becomes larger, its stiffness increases considerably. Just as with plate fixation, one would prefer to have some micromotion to enhance healing. If the pin is too large, it will be excessively stiff, and this may actually inhibit healing.

We can now see an important relationship here in that a larger diameter form in intramedullary fixation, whether it be a screw, pin or smooth wire, will be stiffer and will have potentially less fixation length. Healing can be compromised and there will also be greater stresses on the short fixation, which could lead to greater risk of loosening, failure of the fixation, and healing. The conclusion from all of this is that the surgeon should pick the smallest pin that has stable fixation within the bone. In our experience, most midshaft clavicle fractures in female patients can be stabilized with a 2.5-mm pin, and most male patients should receive a 3-mm pin. Seldom do we use a larger pin except in very large patients or in older patients who have age-related increases in their canal diameters.

Because the clavicle has very little soft tissue coverage about it, any type of intramedullary fixation that protrudes from the bone can cause soft tissue problems. This was one of the primary factors in the complications in Grassi's study.[371] Although he had a good union rate, he found significant problems with the pin causing irritation to the skin. This was also seen in a study by Zuckerman and associates.[372] It is imperative that the portion of any intramedullary device outside of the bone have the lowest profile possible. The quandary here is that the lower the profile of the device, the harder it is to remove, but the more prominent the hardware, the easier the removal will be.

Choice of Intramedullary Fixation. The primary choices of intramedullary fixation are smooth, threaded, and partially threaded devices. Fully threaded devices are seldom used in the treatment of clavicle fractures because of the risk of gapping at the fracture site. These have far less risk of migration than smooth devices; however, they can prevent compression of the fracture fragments and thereby impede healing.[371]

There are numerous reports of migration of smooth devices used in clavicle fixation.[315] If these devices are to be used, they need to followed closely for any radiographic signs of migration. Although smooth pin fixation has declined in popularity, there seems to be new interest in the use of smooth titanium elastic nails (TENs) in treating clavicle factures.[17,82,373-376] One of the primary advantages in using a flexible nail is that is allows considerable length of fixation as compared to a rigid device.

The fixation of these devices is said to be facilitated by jamming the end of the device into the lateral fragment. In spite of this, there still remains the risk of implant migration, and some studies show a rate of loosening or migration of 5% to 25%.[375,377]

Kettler and associates examined the use of a TEN in 95 midshaft clavicle fractures. They found that an open fracture reduction was required in 53 patients (56%) and they had a nonunion rate of 2%, a malunion rate of 8%, and pin migration in 4%; 5% of patients required a revision surgery.[82] Mueller and associates used a TEN in 32 cases and they reported a union rate of 100%[377]; however, they also noted that an open reduction was necessary in 50%. They also had shortening greater than 5 mm in 38% and nail migration in 8 patients (25%) that required revision shortening of the nail in 5 of those 8. They also reported breakage of the nail in 2 patients after the clavicle was healed.[377] It is somewhat difficult to understand how this could have happened after healing unless there were some repetitive micromotion from a subtle nonunion.

One additional problem with the TEN fixation is that most studies have relied on insertion of the pin through an anterior medial approach. The dilemma of intramedullary fixation is that unlike plate fixation, the device is intended to be removed once the fracture has healed. The quandary with this is that the device needs to have a low profile so it does not cause skin and soft tissue irritation, but it must be prominent enough to be easily retrieved. In the case of the TEN fixation, or any other pin relying on medial insertion, there is very little tissue overlying the medial clavicle, and any prominence can cause significant soft tissue irritation.

Another limitation with intramedullary fixation is that the device length is quite variable, and the surgeon has limited choice of device sizes in terms of length and diameter. There is the risk of compromising fracture fixation. This is particularly true is the case of intramedullary screw fixation, especially cannulated screws where the length of the device is limited by the mechanical properties of the metal used to make the screw. In other words, it is difficult to make a screw of small enough diameter and sufficient length to achieve adequate fixation. For example, studies have suggested using a Herbert cannulated bone screw for midshaft clavicle fractures.[378-380] However, the smallest diameter is 4.5 mm and the longest screw is 100 mm. Low-profile devices do not need to be removed, which is considered an advantage, except in competitive athletes who are at high risk for clavicle refracture.

For most of these fractures, we prefer intramedullary fixation with a modified Hagie pin (Depuy Orthopaedics). We believe this method to be superior for several reasons. The exposure needed to place an intramedullary pin is significantly smaller than that needed for a formal open reduction and internal fixation with plates and screws. This restricted exposure limits further damage to the already injured soft tissue envelope. The intramedul-

lary pin allows compression at the fracture site and load sharing, which have been advantageous in the healing of other long-bone fractures. The intramedullary pin can be removed easily under local anesthesia. Intramedullary pins come in different sizes to allow filling of the canal, which again has been shown to be advantageous in other fractures treated with intramedullary devices. Unlike plate-and-screw fixation, placement of an intramedullary pin does not require drilling perpendicularly through the clavicle. This fact decreases the risk to neurovascular structures and obviates the need to strip the soft tissues to allow protection of these structures.

Few studies have directly compared the results of intramedullary pinning to plate fixation; however, in a randomized prospective study of 51 acute midshaft fractures, Thyagarajan found that patients who had undergone pinning had a 100% union within 2 to 4 months with a shorter hospital stay. Plate patients also had a 100% healing rate, but 23.5% also had scar-related pain and 17.5% had discomfort from prominent hardware. The nonoperative group had a 23.5% nonunion rate, 29.4% had cosmetic complaints, and 6% had malunion.[381] Wu examined patients with middle-third clavicular aseptic nonunions treated by plating in 11 patients and intramedullary nailing in 18 patients with supplementary cancellous bone grafting. The time to union was not significantly different, but the union rate of 81.8% (9 of 11) for plating was significantly lower than the 88.9% (16 of 18) for intramedullary nailing, and the complication rate was 27.3% (3 of 11) for plating and only 11.1% (2 of 18) for intramedullary nailing.[382]

Surgical Technique for Intramedullary Fixation
Patient Positioning

Place the patient in a beach chair position on the operating table. Clavicle and shoulder access is facilitated by using a radiolucent shoulder-positioning device. An image-intensification device or C-arm greatly facilitates pin placement. Bring the C-arm base in from the head of the bed, with the C-arm gantry rotated slightly away from the operative shoulder and oriented in a cephalic tilt. Drape the C-arm with standard split sheets (Fig. 11-54).

The procedure may also be performed without C-arm equipment. However, great care must be taken when passing the drill and pin, particularly into the medial fragment, because the subclavian vessels are in very close approximation to the junction of the medial and middle third of the clavicle. If a C-arm is not available, an x-ray cassette can be placed posterior to the shoulder before preparation and draping. Radiographs can then be taken during the procedure to verify pin position. Unfortunately, they only tell you after the fact where the pin is.

Incision

Make a 3-cm incision in Langer's lines over the distal end of the medial fragment (Fig. 11-55). This technique is used because the clavicle skin is more easily moved

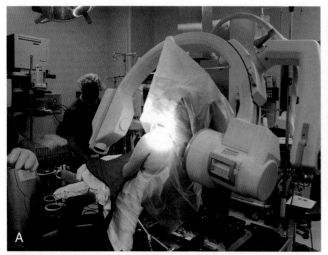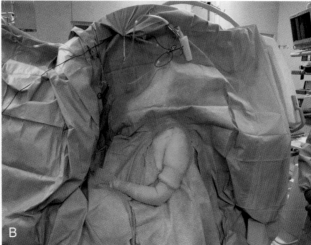

FIGURE 11-54 A, The patient is placed in the beach chair position on the operating table with the use of a radiolucent positioner. **B,** The image intensifier is then brought over the top of the patient and draped into the surgical field.

medially than laterally. Most patients have a deep skin crease in the same area where the incision is made. Placing the incision in this crease results in a more cosmetically pleasing scar.

Because there is little subcutaneous fat in this region, take care to prevent injury to the underlying platysma muscle. Use scissors to free the platysma muscle from the overlying skin. Once the platysma muscle has been identified, divide its fibers longitudinally (Fig. 11-56). Take care to prevent injury to the middle branch of the supraclavicular nerve, which is usually found directly beneath the platysma muscle near the midportion of the clavicle.

Identify and retract the nerve to prevent injury. With acute fractures, the periosteum over the fracture site is disrupted and usually requires no further division. In most cases, muscle and soft tissue are interposed in the fracture. Carefully remove them with an elevator or curette. Leave small butterfly fragments, usually found anteriorly, attached to their soft tissue envelope.

Drilling and Tapping the Intramedullary Canal
Elevate the proximal end of the medial part of the clavicle through the incision with a towel clip, elevator, or bone-holding forceps (Figs. 11-57 and 11-58). Because the drill bits, taps, and intramedullary pins are in sets, use either

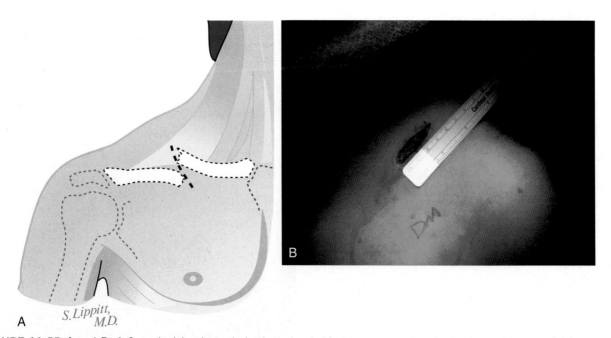

S. Lippitt, M.D.

FIGURE 11-55 A and **B,** A 3-cm incision is made in the natural skin creases over the distal aspect of the medial fragment. Because of tethering of the skin by the platysma muscle, it is easier to move the skin medially than laterally.

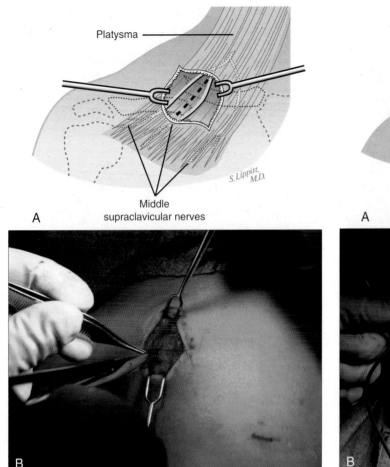

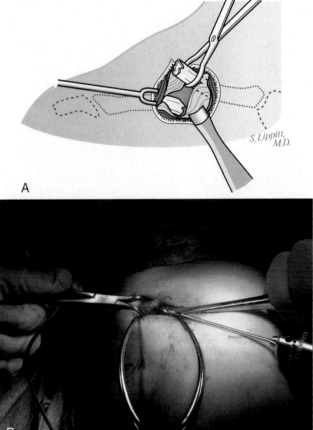

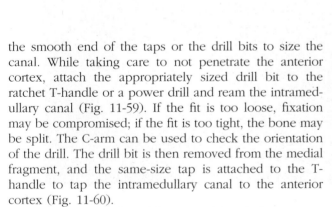

FIGURE 11-56 A and **B,** The platysma muscle is typically directly under the skin because of the usually little subcutaneous fat in this region. The middle branches of the supraclavicular nerve are generally found directly under the platysma muscle, and care must be taken to protect them during the surgical exposure, regardless of whether intramedullary or plate fixation is used.

FIGURE 11-57 A and **B,** The medial fragment is grasped with a towel clip or bone reduction forceps.

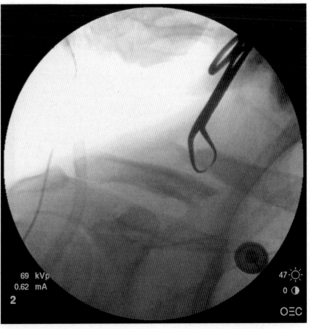

FIGURE 11-58 Image intensifier view of Figure 11-57.

the smooth end of the taps or the drill bits to size the canal. While taking care to not penetrate the anterior cortex, attach the appropriately sized drill bit to the ratchet T-handle or a power drill and ream the intramedullary canal (Fig. 11-59). If the fit is too loose, fixation may be compromised; if the fit is too tight, the bone may be split. The C-arm can be used to check the orientation of the drill. The drill bit is then removed from the medial fragment, and the same-size tap is attached to the T-handle to tap the intramedullary canal to the anterior cortex (Fig. 11-60).

Next, elevate the lateral fragment through the incision. If the arm is left in a neutral or internally rotated position, it can be difficult to drill the lateral fragment because of interference from the drapes and the patient's head and chin. The ability to work with the distal fragment is

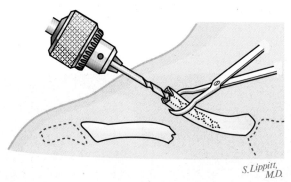

FIGURE 11-59 Drilling of the intramedullary canal of the medial fragment. The drill is advanced until it contacts the anteromedial cortex. The cortex is not typically penetrated.

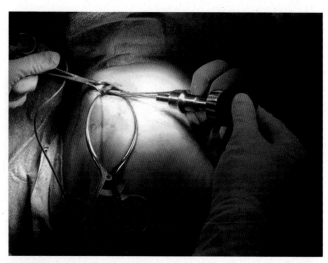

FIGURE 11-60 Tapping of the medial fragment.

greatly facilitated by externally rotating the patient's arm (Fig. 11-61). Because the scapula is no longer tethered by the clavicle, the patient's arm can be externally rotated much more than with an intact clavicle. By externally rotating the arm, the fragment is in more of an anterior-to-posterior orientation. This greatly facilitates passing the drill, tap, and pin into the distal fragment. It also seems to lessen the traction and amount of force needed to deliver the distal fragment into the incision.

Connect the same-size drill bit used in the medial fragment to the drill and drill the intramedullary canal (Fig. 11-62). Under C-arm guidance, pass the drill out through the posterolateral cortex of the clavicle, which will be posterior to the acromioclavicular joint. When viewed under fluoroscopy, the drill bit should appear to be just lateral to the coracoid when it makes contact with the posterolateral cortex. It should also be at the equator or midpoint of the posterolateral acromion to prevent irritation by the pin and securing nuts to the overlying soft tissue (Fig. 11-63). Then remove the drill bit from the lateral fragment, attach the same-size tap to the T-handle, and tap the intramedullary canal so that the large threads are fully advanced into the canal (Fig. 11-64).

Insertion of the Clavicle Pin

While holding the distal fragment with a bone clamp, remove the nuts from the pin assembly and pass the trocar end of the DePuy clavicle pin into the medullary canal of the distal fragment. The pin should exit through the previously drilled hole in the posterolateral cortex. Once the pin exits the clavicle, its tip can be felt subcutaneously.

Make a small incision over the palpable tip and spread the subcutaneous tissue with a hemostat (Fig. 11-65). Place the tip of the hemostat under the tip of the clavicle pin to facilitate passage through the incision. Alternatively, the medial or lateral wrench from the clavicle pin set can be placed over the lateral pin as it exits the clavicle to protect the surrounding soft tissue. Then drill the pin out laterally until the large medial threads start to engage the cortex. Attach the Jacobs chuck to the end of the pin protruding laterally, and carefully advance the

medial end of the clavicle pin into the lateral fragment until only the smooth tip is protruding from the lateral fragment (Fig. 11-66).

Reduce the fracture and pass the pin into the medial fragment. The weight of the patient's arm usually pulls the arm downward; therefore, the shoulder needs to be lifted up to facilitate passage of the pin into the medial fragment. Place the medial nut on the pin, followed by the smaller lateral nut. Cold-weld the two nuts together by grasping the medial nut with a needle driver or needle-nosed pliers and tightening the lateral nut against the medial nut with the lateral nut wrench (Fig. 11-67). Then use the T-handle and wrench on the lateral nut to medially advance the pin down into the medial fragment until it comes into contact with the anterior cortex (Fig. 11-68). This position can be verified by the C-arm or a radiograph.

Securing the Pin

Break the cold weld between the nuts by grasping the medial nut with a needle driver or pliers and quickly turning the lateral nut counterclockwise with the insertion wrench. Advance the medial nut until it is against the lateral cortex of the clavicle. Tighten the lateral nut until it engages the medial nut. This technique cold-welds the two nuts together again. Cut the excess pin by backing the pin out of the clavicle with the medial wrench until the lateral nut can be seen near the skin surface; take care to not back the pin completely out of the medial fragment. Use a double-action pin cutter to cut the pin near the lateral nut (Fig. 11-69). Any remaining burrs or sharp edges on the cut surface can be removed by turning the pin 90 degrees and recutting any remaining pin by placing one jaw of the pin cutter on the lateral nut and the other on the far surface of the pin (Fig. 11-70). This maneuver both crimps the lateral nut on to the pin and rivets the end of the pin so it is smooth and is flush with the lateral nut. Advance the pin back into the medial fragment. The

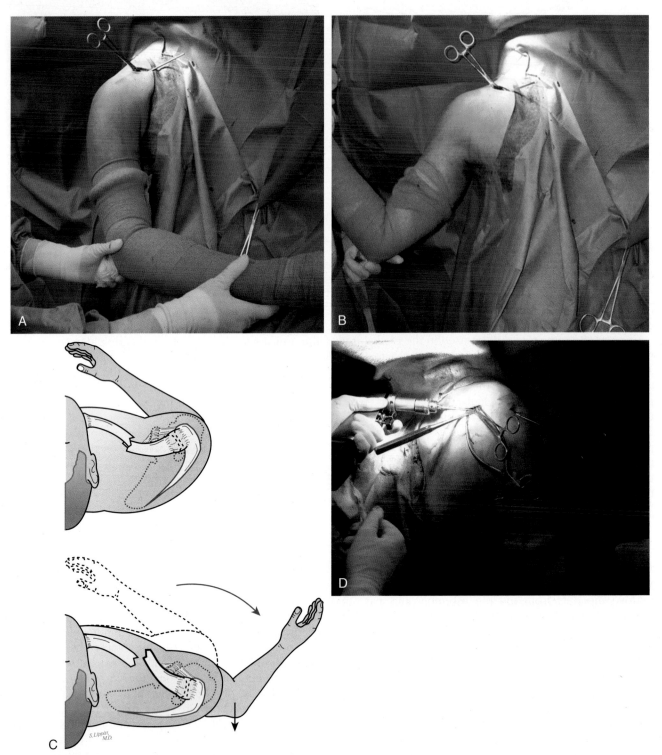

FIGURE 11-61 A and **C** (*top*), When the arm is internally rotated, access to the lateral fragment can be difficult. **B** and **C** (*bottom*), By externally rotating the arm, the lateral fragment is in more of an AP orientation, facilitating passage of the drill bit into the distal fragment (**D**).

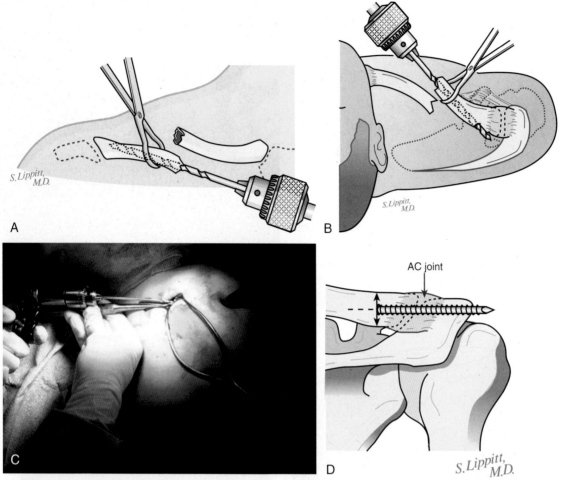

FIGURE 11-62 Drilling of the distal fragment. **A** to **C,** The drill is passed along the posterior cortex of the distal fragment until it contacts the posterolateral cortex. **D,** At this point, the drill tip should appear to be lateral to the coracoid when viewed under the image intensifier. Note that the arm is externally rotated. AC, acromioclavicular.

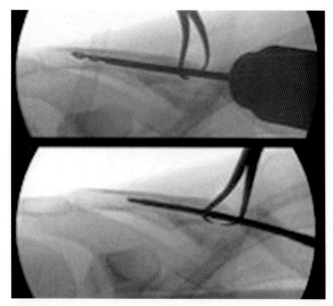

FIGURE 11-63 Fluoroscopic view of the ideal position of the drill and pin in the lateral fragment. Note how they both exit the posterolateral clavicle at its equator.

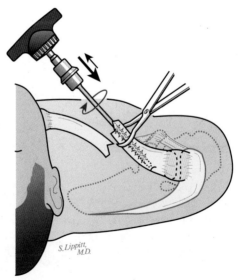

FIGURE 11-64 The lateral fragment is tapped. The tap first drills the lateral fragment and then is withdrawn.

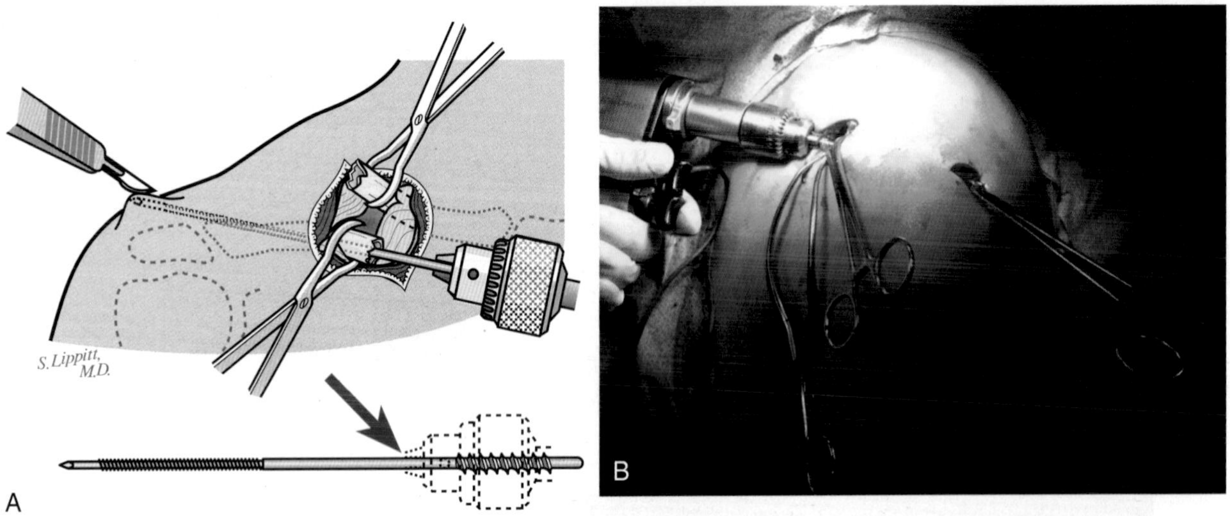

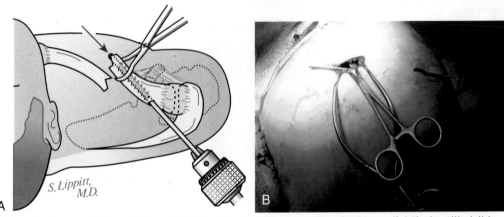

FIGURE 11-65 A and **B,** The clavicle pin is directed in antegrade fashion out the distal fragment. Once the tip is felt under the lateral skin, a small, 1.5-cm is incision made over the pin tip and the subcutaneous tissue is spread with a small hemostat. *Arrow* points to the chuck of the drill placement on the pin.

FIGURE 11-66 The pin is completely withdrawn into the lateral fragment until only the medial tip is still visible. *Arrow,* The tip of the pin is withdrawn to the medial end of the distal fragment.

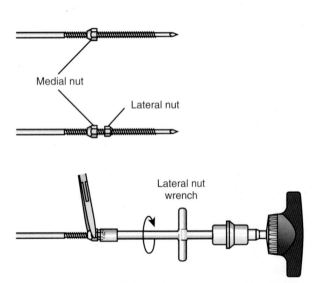

FIGURE 11-67 The medial and lateral nuts are placed on the lateral aspect of the pin and cold-welded together by grasping the medial nut with pliers or a needle driver.

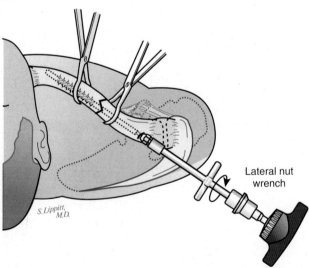

FIGURE 11-68 The fracture is reduced and the pin inserted in a retrograde manner into the medial fragment. Once the pin has passed to the anteromedial cortex of the medial fragment, the cold weld between the two nuts is broken and the medial nut is tightened against the lateral cortex. The lateral nut is tightened against the medial nut, thereby cold-welding them together again.

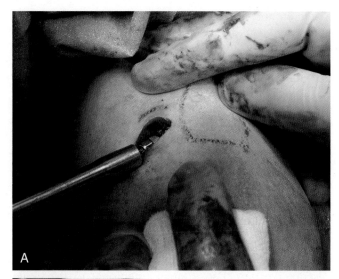

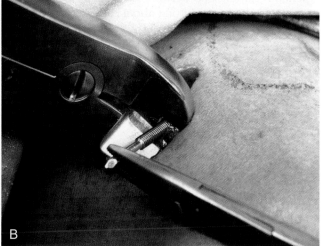

FIGURE 11-69 A, Excess pin is cut by backing the pin out with the medial wrench until the lateral nut is just visible at the lateral incision. **B,** Any pin cutter can be used to cut the excess pin right at the level of the lateral nut. The pin is passed back into the medial fragment until the medial nut makes contact with the lateral cortex.

pin can generate considerable compression force, so care must be taken to not over-reduce the fracture.

Soft Tissue Closure

To reapproximate the anterior butterfly fragments, pass the Crego elevator beneath the clavicle in an anterior-to-posterior direction to protect the underlying structures. Use absorbable Ethicon No. 0 or No. 1 PDS or Panacryl suture loaded on a CTX or CT1 needle and pass it through the periosteum attached to the butterfly fragment. Then pass it around and beneath the clavicle (Fig. 11-71). Carefully direct the needle toward the Crego elevator so that it will be deflected by the elevator. Retrieve the needle posteriorly. Pass the suture in a figure-of-eight manner or use multiple simple sutures to cerclage the butterfly fragment to the main fracture fragments. Close the periosteum overlying the fracture with multiple figure-of-eight

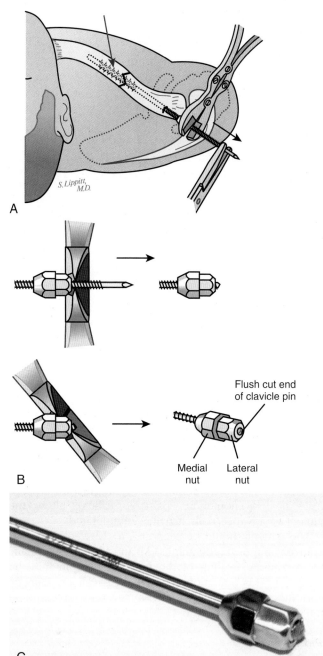

FIGURE 11-70 A, *Red arrow* points to the location of the threads into the medial fragment. **B,** The pin should be cut as flush as possible by turning the pin 90 degrees and recutting any remaining pin by placing one jaw of the pin cutter on the lateral nut and the other on the far surface of the pin. **C,** Image of properly cut pin.

sutures of No. 0 absorbable suture. Reapproximate the platysma muscle with simple nonabsorbable Ethicon 2-0 Vicryl sutures. Close both incisions with a running subcuticular suture.

Postoperative Care of Acute Fractures

The patient may resume activities of daily living as soon as tolerated but should avoid strenuous activities such as

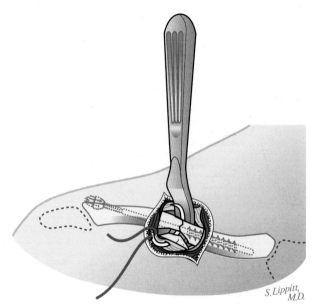

S. Lippitt, M.D.

FIGURE 11-71 If a butterfly fragment is present, a Crego elevator can be passed under the clavicle and the fragments bound in cerclage fashion with an absorbable suture.

pulling, lifting, or pushing and arm elevation higher than face level for 4 to 6 weeks. Excessive arm motion, particularly forward flexion, can result in rotation of the fracture fragments and irritation of the soft tissue by the lateral pin and nuts. Remove the sutures at 7 to 10 days. Postoperative radiographs should be taken at the 4- to 6-week postoperative clinic visit. If the fracture is clinically healed (nontender, palpable callus), allow the patient to advance daily activities as tolerated.

The patient should be seen at 8 to 12 weeks postoperatively. If repeat radiographs (AP and 45-degree cephalic tilt AP) show healing of the fracture, the pin may be removed. This operation can give an excellent cosmetic and functional result even with severely comminuted fractures (Figs. 11-72 and 11-73).

Pin Removal

The pin can be removed in the office or in an ambulatory surgery setting. We typically use local anesthesia, which may be supplemented with intravenous sedation. The patient is placed in a lateral decubitus or beach chair position. The skin about the lateral incision is infiltrated with a local anesthetic. A hemostat is used to spread the soft tissue from around the nuts, and the lateral wrench is placed on the lateral nut. The nut is turned about one-half turn to make sure that the cold weld is re-established. The medial wrench is placed on the medial nut, and the pin is removed (Fig. 11-74).

Middle-Third Malunion and Nonunion

Symptomatic nonunion and malunion are treated with the same intramedullary technique as acute fractures. Clavicle malunion and nonunion represent cases in which a pin may also be used. These fractures require only minor modifications to the technique noted earlier.

Surgical Techniques

For clavicle malunion, incise the periosteum overlying the deformity longitudinally as described earlier. Once the periosteum is circumferentially elevated from the deformity, use a small osteotome to remove the callus from the fracture site. This procedure is best performed under C-arm guidance to ensure adequate removal of the fracture callus (Fig. 11-75).

Use a rongeur to remove the callus from the ends of the medial and lateral fracture fragments. Then find the canal by using the smallest size drill bit, verify its position with a C-arm or a radiograph, and drill the canal with the appropriate-size drill. Pass the DePuy clavicle pin as described earlier. Use a small osteotome to fish scale (rose petal) the cortical bone about the fracture site (Fig. 11-76). Morselize the previously removed callus, and pack it about the fracture site (Fig. 11-77). Autogenous bone graft from the patient should be used when indicated. The periosteum is then carefully closed over the fracture site. Because of the relative loss of mass with débridement of the callus, the periosteum is easily closed. An excellent radiographic and clinical result can be obtained (Fig. 11-78).

Hypertrophic nonunion can be treated the same as a clavicle malunion. In the case of atrophic nonunion, remove any tapered ends of the clavicle fragments. Carefully remove the scar tissue with a rongeur. Proceed with treatment as described for clavicle malunion, with the exception of using autologous or autograft bone.

In the case of an atrophic nonunion, the bone ends might have resorbed. It is important to return the clavicle to its normal length (Fig. 11-79), but this can be difficult to do with intramedullary fixation. In this situation, we remove any nonviable bone from the ends of the fragments. If there is significant loss of clavicular length, a tricortical graft of appropriate length is placed into the defect.[199,383] Because of the difficulty in controlling the intercalary fragment, we prefer to use an LC-DCP. If there is loss of soft tissue coverage in this area, a portion of the clavicular head of the pectoralis major muscle can be swung over the fracture site without difficulty (Fig. 11-80). In the case of severe bone and soft tissue loss, a free vascularized fibular graft can be used in conjunction with an LC-DCP plate as shown in Figure 11-80.[384]

Postoperative Care

Postoperative care for malunion and nonunion needs to be modified as required because these fractures typically take longer to heal. On average, the pin is removed in malunion cases at between 12 and 16 weeks, whereas nonunion can take up to 6 months to adequately heal.

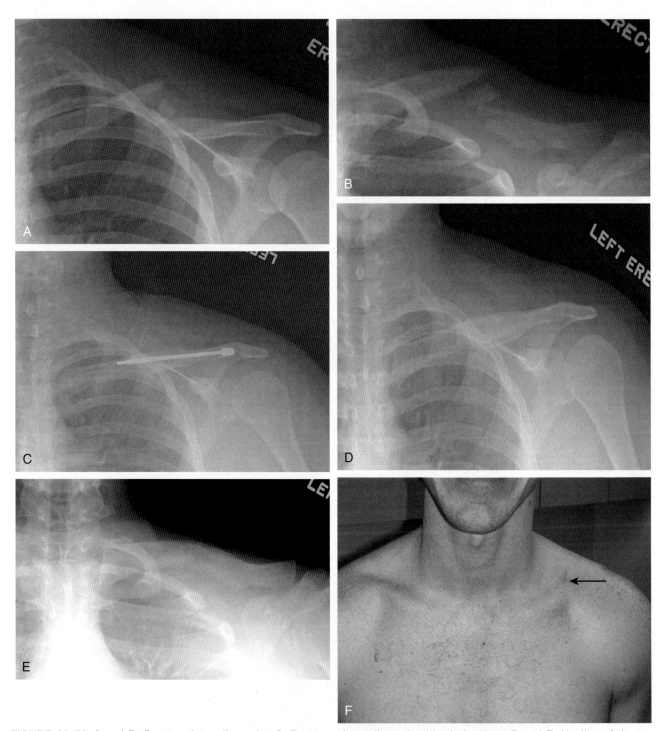

FIGURE 11-72 A and **B,** Preoperative radiographs. **C,** Postoperative radiograph with pin in place. **D** and **E,** Healing of the fracture. **F,** Clinical view of healed left fractured clavicle (*arrow*) showing cosmetic appearance.

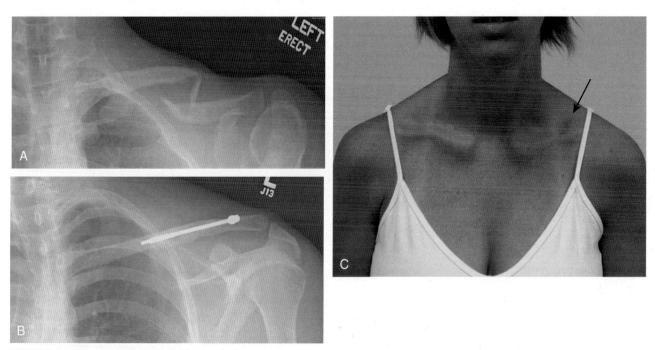

FIGURE 11-73 A, Preoperative radiograph. **B,** Postoperative radiograph with pin in place. **C,** Cosmetic appearance of healed left fractured clavicle.

FIGURE 11-74 Pin removal with the medial wrench. *Red arrow* indicates direction of pin movement; *black arrow* indicates direction of wrench rotation.

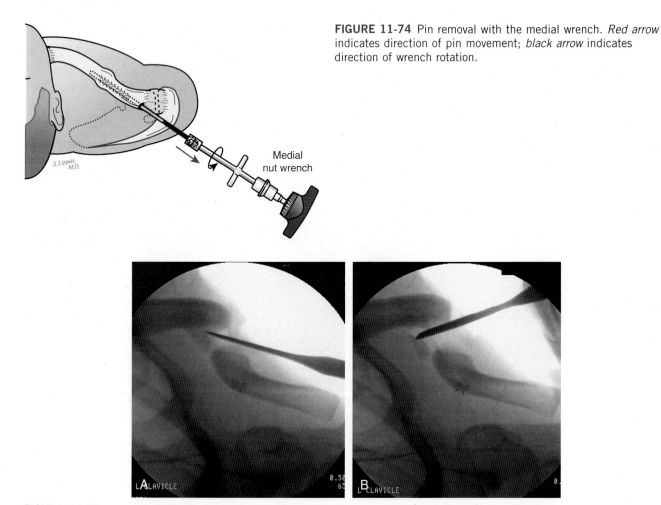

FIGURE 11-75 Resection of callus in a clavicle malunion under image intensifier guidance. **A,** Osteotome identifying callus on distal end of medial fragment. **B,** Osteophyte removed and will be used for bone graft.

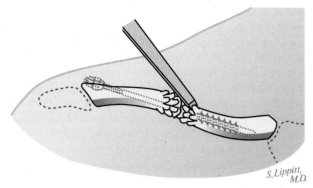

FIGURE 11-76 Fish scaling of the clavicle on both sides of the fracture site.

FIGURE 11-77 Bone graft is placed about the fracture site with care taken to not place too much graft on the inferior surface.

Distal Clavicle Fractures

Distal clavicle fractures include fractures with differing treatments and prognoses that depend on the location and displacement of the fracture. In this section we consider fractures that involve or are distal to the conoid tubercle of the clavicle. The reason for this distinction is that fractures that are medial to the conoid tubercle can generally be treated like middle-third fractures, but those lateral to the conoid present different concerns and treatment requirements because of the presence of the coracoclavicular ligaments and their effects on fracture stability.

Nondisplaced fractures of the distal end of the clavicle are best treated with a sling. As symptoms allow, the patient is weaned from the sling and started on a shoulder rehabilitation program. The earliest return to sports activity is generally around 2 months after injury. In collision sports, extra padding or a fiberglass shell may be necessary to protect the distal end of the clavicle. The patient must be advised that even though he or she feels well, early return to sports is a compromise that involves some risk of refracture or displacement.

Nondisplaced fractures that involve the acromioclavicular joint deserve special note. The treatment is the same,

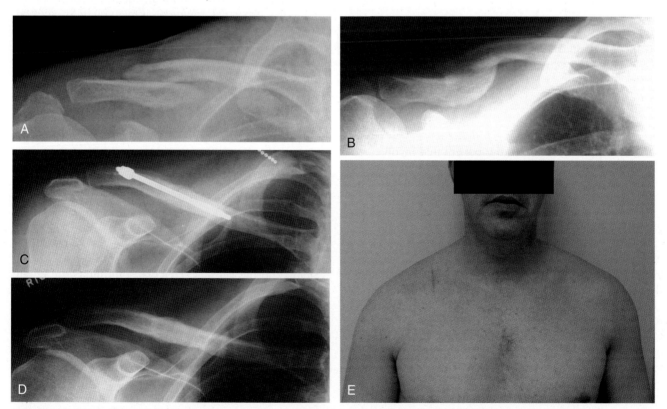

FIGURE 11-78 A, Preoperative radiograph of fracture of the right clavicle. **B,** Nonunion of fracture. **C,** Postoperative radiograph with pin in place. **D,** Postoperative radiograph with pin removed. **E,** Clinical appearance of patient with a very small skin incision.

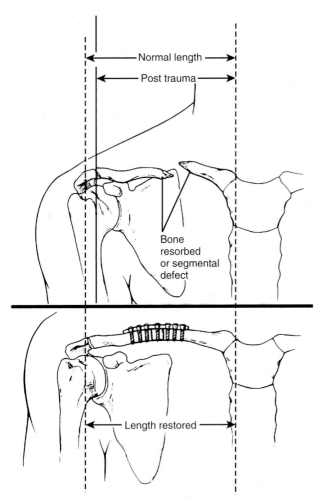

FIGURE 11-79 In cases of nonunion, care must be taken to return the clavicle to its normal length after removal of nonviable bone.

but it is important to inform the patient that involvement of the joint increases the likelihood of chronic pain and post-traumatic arthrosis of the acromioclavicular joint. If this complication occurs, a subsequent surgical procedure may be required to alleviate these symptoms, and the patient needs to be aware of this fact.

Treatment of a displaced distal clavicle fracture hinges on the integrity of the coracoclavicular and acromioclavicular ligaments. More precisely, treatment generally depends on whether the conoid portion of the coracoclavicular ligaments is still attached to the medial fragment of the clavicle. If the conoid continues to be attached to the medial fragment, this strong ligament will maintain the coracoclavicular interval and thereby help prevent large displacement at the fracture site. In fact, it is rare to have a markedly displaced distal clavicle fracture if the conoid ligament remains intact and attached to the medial fragment of the clavicle. The ligamentous stability does not easily allow displacement to occur.

If the conoid ligament is intact, the coracoclavicular interval will be maintained, and the ligamentous and bony anatomy will help prevent the distal clavicular fragment from becoming markedly displaced. The fracture fragments should remain relatively close to one another, and this fracture can be expected to heal with sling treatment. If the conoid ligament is disrupted, the distal clavicular fragment with the attached scapula (through the acromioclavicular and coracoclavicular ligaments) will droop inferiorly and medially under the weight of the attached upper extremity. The medial clavicular fragment, now unencumbered, will elevate away from the distal fragment. Such elevation raises the risk of nonunion and chronic medial rotational instability of the shoulder through the fracture site.

Several clues can be used to ascertain the integrity of the conoid ligament. Often, rupture of the conoid ligament is obvious on radiographs because the fracture is lateral to the conoid tubercle, the coracoclavicular interval is markedly increased, and the fracture is markedly displaced. With fractures occurring at or very near the conoid tubercle, this call sometimes becomes more difficult. When both coracoclavicular ligaments are attached to the distal fragment, the fracture line is usually oblique, and the coracoclavicular interval is maintained with the lateral fragment. The fracture is typically widely displaced. In equivocal cases, medial rotational instability at the fracture site can be demonstrated by performing a cross-body adduction view of the shoulder (Fig. 11-81). This stress radiograph accentuates conoid ligament detachment from the medial clavicular fragment. One generally sees an increase in fracture displacement, an increase in the coracoclavicular interval, and marked underriding of the distal fragment beneath the proximal fragment. These findings represent medial rotational instability occurring through the fracture site. Failure of these findings to occur suggests that the conoid ligament is still attached to the medial fragment of the clavicle. MRI also demonstrates the coracoclavicular ligaments.

Lateral Clavicle Fractures

Treatment options for lateral clavicle fractures include coracoclavicular fixation, plate fixation, and (some advocate) Kirschner-wire fixation.

Plate fixation of this fracture can be problematic. The exposure required is relatively large. The distal fragment is small, and the acromioclavicular joint limits the length of plate that can be used. A small T-plate sometimes allows enough screws in the distal fragment for adequate fixation. Newer specialized plates allow better fit of the plate onto the distal clavicle.

One significant problem with plate fixation of distal fractures is that there are significant forces on the distal fixation. The distal fragment is softer metaphyseal bone and can be quite small, which makes it hard to get even 2 or 3 screws into the distal fragment. Because of this problem, some authors have advocated the use of a hook

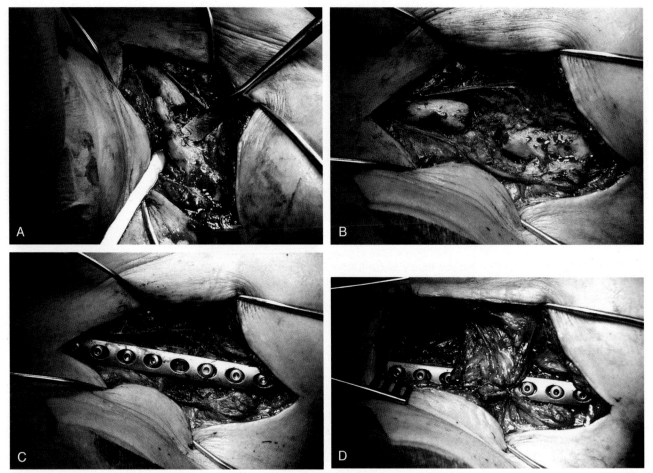

FIGURE 11-80 A, Initial appearance of a clavicle nonunion. **B,** After resection of nonviable bone with resultant bone loss. **C,** Limited contact dynamic compression plate incorporating an intercalary tricortical graft. **D,** The lateral position of the clavicular head of the pectoralis major is swung over the fracture site to provide soft tissue coverage.

plate that relies on a finger-like projection that goes under the acromion to give added stability while still allowing some rotational movement at the acromioclavicular joint.[294,319,320,385-389] Although in concept this may be better than carrying the fixation out onto the acromion, a number of authors have reported complications such as dislocation of and mechanical failure of the plate, acromial erosion or osteolysis, and impingement (Fig. 11-82).[319,387,390] Muramatsu and associates found evidence of hook migration into the acromion in 87% of patients.[320] This necessitates early removal of the plate, which must be carried out through the same large incision.

Kirschner-wire fixation down the intramedullary canal of the distal end of the clavicle can create problems as well. The force on this area is large, and hardware breakage is quite possible. Migration of broken hardware in this region is well documented,[315] and we prefer to avoid this possibility.

For the unstable variety of this fracture we generally prefer placement of a coracoclavicular screw, which reduces the coracoclavicular interval and brings the fragments into close proximity to allow healing. Use of the

coracoclavicular screw is limited by comminution extending medial to the conoid tubercle. Comminution distal to the conoid tubercle is not a factor. The coracoclavicular screw offers several advantages. The exposure required is small, and sometimes we do not even have to open

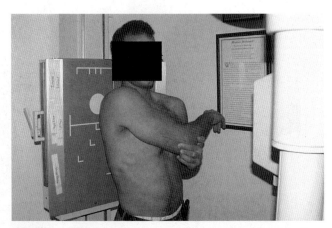

FIGURE 11-81 Method for obtaining a cross-body adduction AP radiograph. The patient pulls the elbow to the midline while keeping the arm against the chest.

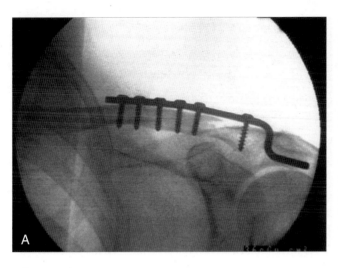
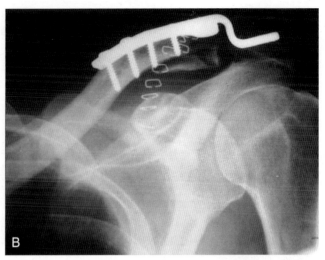

FIGURE 11-82 A, Hook plate for a distal-third clavicle fracture. **B,** Dislocation of the acromial portion of the plate. (From Haidar SG, Krishnan KM, Deshmukh SC: Hook plate fixation for type II fractures of the lateral end of the clavicle. J Shoulder Elbow Surg 15[4]:419-423, 2006.)

the fracture site. The fixation is solid, with true bicortical fixation in the coracoid giving nearly 750 to 1000 N of strength to failure, which nearly approximates the strength of the native acromioclavicular and coracoclavicular ligament complex,[391] whereas a hook plate has only 460 N load to failure.[295,321] In comparison to a hook plate, a coracoclavicular screw is can be inserted with minimal exposure and minimal soft tissue stripping. Under C-arm guidance, this procedure can be performed almost percutaneously. After fracture healing, the screw can be removed easily under local anesthesia, thereby avoiding breakage of the hardware, whereas a hook plate requires significantly greater exposure for removal.

Coracoclavicular Screw Technique

The patient is positioned much the same as for intramedullary pinning. The primary difference is that the C-arm is oriented in a posteromedial-to-anterolateral direction (Fig. 11-83). This gives what we refer to as a *cortical ring sign* of the coracoid. We have found that when the cora-

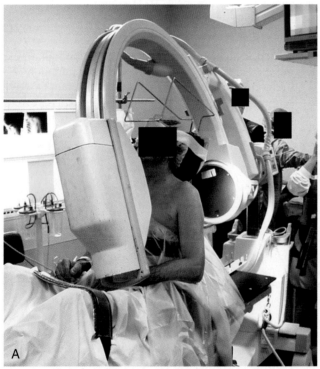
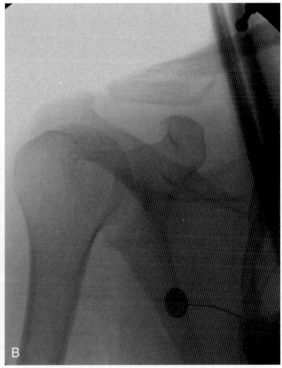

FIGURE 11-83 A, Position of the C-arm for coracoclavicular screw placement. **B,** Radiograph of clavicle superior to the corocoid and ready for screw placement.

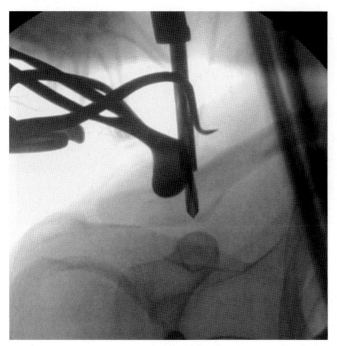

FIGURE 11-84 Fracture is held reduced and a 4.5-mm drill is used to produce the hole through both cortices of the clavicle directly above the ring of the coracoid.

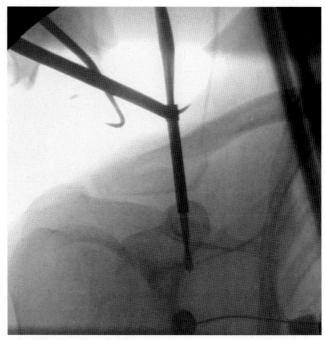

FIGURE 11-85 The drill hole in the coracoid is made by passing the drill guide for a 3.2-mm drill through the hole in the clavicle.

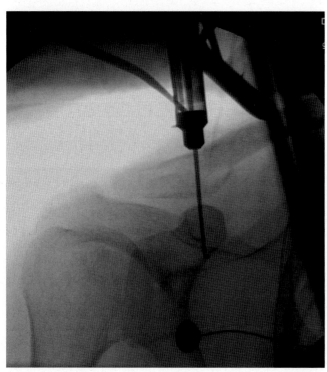

FIGURE 11-86 Position and length of the screw is checked with a depth gauge.

coid is viewed in this position, placement of the coracoclavicular screw into the superior apex of this ring virtually guarantees placement in the center of the coracoid.

A skin incision that allows exposure of the fracture site is then made in line with the clavicle. The fracture is held reduced with a reduction forceps, and the clavicle is drilled by placing a 4.5-mm drill bit directly above the coracoid in the midportion of the clavicle (Fig. 11-84). A 3.2-mm drill guide is passed through this hole until it makes contact with the coracoid. This allows a collinear placement of the screw holes, which facilitates passage of the screw. This position is verified under C-arm guidance (Fig. 11-85).

Both cortices of the coracoid are drilled with a 3.2-mm drill bit. It is very important to drill both the superior and deep cortex of the coracoid because bicortical fixation has significantly greater resistance to pullout than a unicortical screw. A depth gauge is used to measure for the length of the screw, and an appropriate-sized screw with a washer is passed through the clavicle and into the coracoid (Figs. 11-86 and 11-87).

If there is significant comminution, the coracoclavicular screw can be used in conjunction with a small T-plate for what we call *hybrid fixation*. This combination is still significantly stronger than a hook plate and prevents compromise of the acromion (Fig. 11-88).

Postoperative Care

The patient is placed in a sling for the first 4 weeks. The patient is allowed out of the sling for hand, wrist, and elbow range of motion. Repeat x-rays are taken at 4

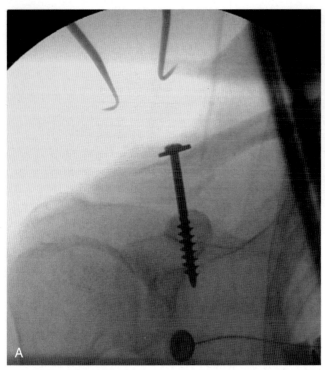

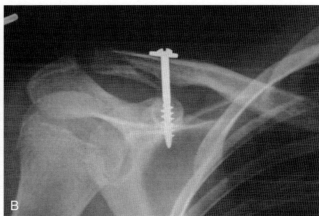

FIGURE 11-87 Fluoroscopic view (**A**) and radiographic view (**B**) showing placement of the appropriate length screw and washer.

weeks. If there has been no change in position of the screw fixation, the sling is discontinued and the patient is allowed to perform activities of daily living with a lifting restriction of 5 lb and no repeated use of the operative-side hand above shoulder level. Once healing has been confirmed on follow-up radiographs, the screw is removed under local anesthesia approximately 8 to 12 weeks post-operatively. The patient is instructed to avoid contact sports for 6 weeks and advance activities as tolerated. If a hybrid-type fixation is used, only the coracoclavicular screw needs to be removed, and this can still be done under local anesthesia. There is no need to remove the rest of the plate and screws unless the patient so desires (Fig. 11-89).

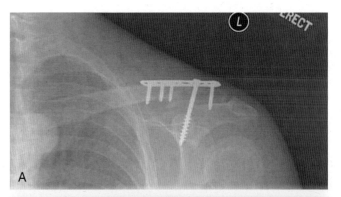

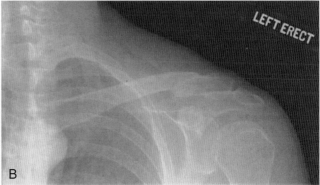

FIGURE 11-89 A, Postoperative radiograph of a hybrid fixation technique. **B,** After removal of both the plate and screws.

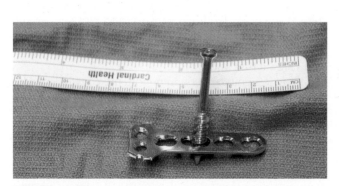

FIGURE 11-88 A hybrid plate and coracoclavicular screw combination may be used when the fracture is significantly comminuted.

REFERENCES

1. Dameron TB Jr, Rockwood CA Jr: Fractures of the shaft of the clavicle. In Rockwood CA, Wilkins KE, King RE (eds): Fractures in Children. Philadelphia: JB Lippincott, 1984, pp 608-624.
2. Tachdjian MO: Pediatric Orthopaedics. Philadelphia: WB Saunders, 1972.
3. Neer CS II: Fractures of the clavicle. In Rockwood CA, Green DP (eds): Fractures in Adults. Philadelphia: JB Lippincott, 1984, pp 707-713.
4. Rowe CR: An atlas of anatomy and treatment of mid-clavicular fractures. Clin Orthop 58:29-42, 1968.
5. Adams CF: The Genuine Works of Hippocrates. Baltimore: Williams & Wilkins, 1939.
6. Fry J: Photo of the "Edwin Smith Surgical Papyrus." In Rockwood CA, Wilkins KE, King RE (eds): Fractures in Children. Philadelphia: JB Lippincott, 1984, p 679.
7. Davids PH, Luitese JS, Strating RP, van der Hart CP: Operative treatment for delayed union and nonunion of midshaft clavicle fractures: AO reconstruction plate, fixation plate, and early mobilization. J Trauma 40:985-986, 1996.
8. Lancet editorial: Sir Robert Peel's death. Lancet 2:19, 1850.
9. Yates DW: Complications of fractures of the clavicle. Injury 7:189-193, 1976.
10. Dupuytren LB: On the Injuries and Diseases of Bone (trans L Clark.) London: Sydenham Society, 1847.
11. Gibbon JH: Lucas-Championniere and mobilization in the treatment of fractures. Surg Gynecol Obstet 43:271-278, 1926.
12. Sayre L: A simple dressing for fractures of the clavicle. Am Practitioner 4:1, 1871.
13. Malgaigne JF: A Treatise on Fractures, trans JH Packard. Philadelphia: JB Lippincott, 1859, pp 374-401.
14. Eskola A, Vainionpaa S, Myllynen P, et al: Outcome of clavicular fracture in 89 patients. Arch Orthop Trauma Surg 105:337-338, 1986.
15. Hill JM, McGuire MH, Crosby LA: Closed treatment of displaced middle-third fractures of the clavicle gives poor results. J Bone Joint Surg Br 79:537-539, 1997.
16. McKee MD, Wild LM, Schemitsch EH: Midshaft malunions of the clavicle. J Bone Joint Surg Am 85:790-797, 2003.
17. Jupiter JB: Paper presented at the First Open Meeting of the American Shoulder and Elbow Surgeons, Miami, 2000.
18. McKee MD, Pedersen EM, Jones C, et al: Deficits following nonoperative treatment of displaced midshaft clavicular fractures. J Bone Joint Surg Am 88(1):35-40, 2006.
19. Nowak J, Holgersson M, Larsson S: Sequelae from clavicular fractures are common: A prospective study of 222 patients. Acta Orthop 76(4):496-502, 2005.
20. Nonoperative treatment compared with plate fixation of displaced midshaft clavicular fractures. A multicenter, randomized clinical trial. J Bone Joint Surg Am 89(1):1-10, 2007.
21. Potter JM, Jones C, Wild LM, Schemitsch EH, McKee MD. Does delay matter? The restoration of objectively measured shoulder strength and patient-oriented outcome after immediate fixation versus delayed reconstruction of displaced midshaft fractures of the clavicle. J Shoulder Elbow Surg 16(5):514-518, 2007.
22. Nowak J, Holgersson M, Larsson S. Can we predict long-term sequelae after fractures of the clavicle based on initial findings? A prospective study with nine to ten years of follow-up. J Shoulder Elbow Surg 13(5):479-486, 2004.
23. Rosenberg N, Neumann L, Wallace AW: Functional outcome of surgical treatment of symptomatic nonunion and malunion of midshaft clavicle fractures. J Shoulder Elbow Surg 16(5):510-513, 2007.
24. Gardner E: The embryology of the clavicle. Clin Orthop 58:9-16, 1968.
25. Gardner ED, Grey DJ, O'Rahilly R: Anatomy. Philadelphia: WB Saunders, 1960.
26. Moseley HF: The clavicle: Its anatomy and function. Clin Orthop Relat Res 58:17-27, 1968.
27. Moseley HF: Shoulder Lesions. Edinburgh: Churchill Livingstone, 1972, pp 207-235.
28. Fawcett J: The development and ossification of the human clavicle. J Anat 47:225-234, 1913.
29. Tregonning G, Macnab I: Post-traumatic pseudoarthrosis of the clavicle. Proceedings of the New Zealand Orthopaedic Association. J Bone Joint Surg Br 58:264, 1976.
30. Ogden JA, Conologue GJ, Bronson NL: Radiology of postnatal skeletal development, vol 3. The clavicle. Skeletal Radiol 4:196-203, 1979.
31. Jit I, Kulkrani M: Times of appearance and fusion of epiphysis at the medial end of the clavicle. Indian J Med Res 64:773-792, 1976.
32. Tyrnin AH: The Bohler clavicular splint in the treatment of clavicular injuries. J Bone Joint Surg 19:417-424, 1937.
33. Mehta A, Birch R: Supraclavicular nerve injury: The neglected nerve? Injury 28:491-492, 1997.
34. Ljunggren AE: Clavicular function. Acta Orthop Scand 50:261-268, 1979.
35. Harrington MA Jr, Keller TS, Seiler JG III, et al: Geometric properties and the predicted mechanical behavior of adult human clavicles. J Biomech 26:417-426, 1993.
36. DePalma A: Surgery of the Shoulder, 3rd ed. Philadelphia: JB Lippincott, 1983.
37. Fich R: Handbuch der Anatomie und Mechanic der Galanke. In Bvdeleben V (ed): Handbuch der Anatomie des Menschen, vol 2, Section 1. Jena, Germany: Gustava Discher, 1910, pp 163-187.
38. Hoyer HE, Kindt R, Lippert H: Zur Biomechanik der menschlichen Clavicula. Z Orthop 118:915-922, 1980.
39. Jablon M, Sutker A, Post M: Irreducible fractures of the middle third of the clavicle. J Bone Joint Surg Am 61:296-298, 1979.
40. Berkheiser EJ: Old ununited clavicular fractures in the adult. Surg Gynecol Obstet 64:1064-1072, 1937.
41. Fukuda K, Craig EV, An KN, et al: Biomechanical study of the ligamentous system of the acromioclavicular joint. J Bone Joint Surg Am 68:434-440, 1986.
42. Johnson B, Thursby P: Subclavian artery injury caused by a screw in a clavicular compression plate. Cardiovasc Surg 4:414-415, 1996.
43. Knudsen FW, Andersen M, Krag C: The arterial supply of the clavicle. Surg Radiol Anat 11:211-214, 1989.
44. Abbott LC, Lucas DB: The function of the clavicle: Its surgical significance. Ann Surg 140:583-599, 1954.
45. Robinson CM: Fractures of the clavicle in the adult. Epidemiology and classification. J Bone Joint Surg Br 80:476-484, 1998.
46. Grant JCB: A Method of Anatomy, 5th ed. Baltimore: Williams & Wilkins, 1952.
47. Codman EA: The Shoulder: Rupture of the Supraspinatus Tendon and Other Lesions in or about the Subacromial Bursa. Boston: Thomas Todd, 1934.
48. Oxnard CE: The architecture of the shoulder in some mammals. J Morphol 126:249-290, 1968.
49. Copeland SM: Total resection of the clavicle. Am J Surg 72:280-281, 1946.
50. Gurd FB: The treatment of complete dislocation of the outer end of clavicle: A hitherto undescribed operation. Ann Surg 113:1094-1097, 1941.
51. Inman VT, Saunders JB: Observation in the function of the clavicle. Calif Med 65:158-165, 1946.
52. Rockwood CA: Personal communication, 1989.
53. Spar I: Total claviculectomy for pathological fractures. Clin Orthop Relat Res (129):236-237, 1977.
54. Bearn JG: An electromyographic study of the trapezius, deltoid, pectoralis major, biceps, and triceps muscles during static loading of the upper limb. J Anat 140:103-108, 1961.
55. Bearn JG: Direct observation in the function of the capsule to the sterno-clavicular joint in clavicular support. J Anat 10:159-170, 1967.
56. Wood VE: The results of total claviculectomy. Clin Orthop Relat Res (207):186-190, 1986.
57. Lipton HA, Jupiter JB: Nonunion of clavicular fractures: Characteristics and surgical management. Surg Rounds Orthop 1c:344, 1988.
58. Andermahr J, Jubel A, Elsner A, et al: Malunion of the clavicle causes significant glenoid malposition: A quantitative anatomic investigation. Surg Radiol Anat 28(5):447-456, 2006.
59. Edelson JG: The bony anatomy of clavicular malunions. J Shoulder Elbow Surg 12:173-178, 2003.
60. Basamania CJ: Medial instability of the shoulder: A new concept of the pathomechanics of acromioclavicular separations. Paper presented at a day meeting of the American Orthopaedic Society for Sports Medicine Specialty, Orlando, Fla, 2000.
61. Thomas CB Jr, Freidman RJ: Ipsilateral sternoclavicular dislocation and clavicular fracture. J Orthop Trauma 3:355-357, 1989.
62. Abbot AE, Hannafin JA: Stress fracture of the clavicle in a female lightweight rower. A case report and review of the literature. Am J Sports Med 29:370-372, 2001.
63. Taylor AR: Nonunion of fractures of the clavicle: A review of 31 cases. Proceedings of the British Orthopaedic Association. J Bone Joint Surg Br 51:568-569, 1969.
64. Allman FL: Fractures and ligamentous injuries of the clavicle and its articulation. J Bone Joint Surg Am 49:774-784, 1967.
65. Eidman DK, Siff SJ, Tullos HS: Acromioclavicular lesions in children. Am J Sports Med 9:150-154, 1981.
66. Falstie-Jensen S: Pseudodislocation of the acromioclavicular joint. J Bone Joint Surg Br 64:368-369, 1982.
67. Neer CS II: Fractures of the distal third of the clavicle. Clin Orthop Relat Res 58:43-50, 1968.
68. Parkes JC, Deland JD: A three-part distal clavicle fracture. J Trauma 23:437-438, 1983.
69. Neer CS II: Nonunion of the clavicle. JAMA 172:1006-1011, 1960.
70. Neer CS II: Fracture of the distal clavicle with detachment of coracoclavicular ligaments in adults. J Trauma 3:99-110, 1963.
71. Jager N, Breitner S: [Therapy related classification of lateral clavicular fracture.] Unfallheilkund 87:467-473, 1984.
72. Craig EV: Fractures of the clavicle. In Rockwood CA Jr, Matsen FA III (eds): The Shoulder. Philadelphia, WB Saunders, 1990, pp 367-412.
73. Neviaser JS: Injuries in and about the shoulder joint. Instr Course Lect 13:187-216, 1956.
74. Neviaser JS: The treatment of fractures of the clavicle. Surg Clin North Am 43:1555-1563, 1963.

75. Neviaser JS: Injuries of the clavicle and its articulations. Orthop Clin North Am 11:233-237, 1980.
76. Sorrells RB: Fracture of the clavicle. J Ark Med Soc 71:253-256, 1975.
77. Heppenstall RB: Fractures and dislocations of the distal clavicle. Orthop Clin North Am 6:477-486, 1975.
78. Cahill BR: Osteolysis of the distal part of the clavicle in male athletes. J Bone Joint Surg Am 64:1053-1058, 1982.
79. Jacobs P: Posttraumatic osteologies of the outer end of the clavicle. J Bone Joint Surg Br 46:705-707, 1964.
80. Quinn SF, Glass TA: Post-traumatic osteolysis of the clavicle. South Med J 76:307-308, 1983.
81. Rockwood CA: Treatment of the outer clavicle in children and adults. Orthop Trans 6:472, 1982.
82. Kettler M, Schieker M, Braunstein V, et al: Flexible intramedullary nailing for stabilization of displaced midshaft clavicle fractures: Technique and results in 87 patients. Acta Orthop 78(3):424-429, 2007.
83. Kaye JJ, Nance EP Jr, Green NE: Fatigue fracture of the medial aspect of the clavicle: An academic rather than athletic injury. Radiology 144:89-90, 1982.
84. Worcester JN, Green DP: Osteoarthritis of the acromioclavicular joint. Clin Orthop Relat Res 58:69-73, 1968.
85. Beckman T: A case of simultaneous luxation of both ends of the clavicle. Acta Chir Scand 56:156-163, 1923.
86. Gearen PF, Petty W: Panclavicular dislocation: Report of a case. J Bone Joint Surg Am 64:454-455, 1982.
87. Jain AS: Traumatic floating clavicle: A case report. J Bone Joint Surg Br 66:560-561, 1984.
88. Lukin AV, Grishkin VA: Two cases of successful treatment of fracture dislocation of the clavicle. Ortop Travmatol Protez 11:35, 1987.
89. Porral A: Observation d'une double luxation de la clavicule droite. Juniva Hibd Med Chir 2:78-82, 1931.
90. Elliott AC: Tripartite injury of the clavicle: A case report. S Afr Med J 70:115-119, 1986.
91. Rubin A: Birth injuries: Incidents, mechanisms and end result. Obstet Gynecol 23:218-221, 1964.
92. Gilbert WM Tshabo JG: Fractured clavicle in newborns. Int Surg 73:123-125, 1988.
93. Gresham EL: Birth trauma. Pediatr Clin North Am 22:317-328, 1975.
94. Joseph PR, Rosenfeld W: Clavicular fractures in neonates. Am J Dis Child 144:165-167, 1990.
95. Valdes-Dapena MA, Arey JB: The causes of neonatal mortality: An analysis of 501 autopsies on new born infants. J Pediatr 77:366-375, 1970.
96. Balata A, Olzai MG, Porcu A, et al: Fractures of the clavicle in the newborn. Riv Ital Pediatr 6:125-129, 1984.
97. Moir JC, Myerscough PR: Operative Obstetrics, 7th ed. Baltimore: Williams & Wilkins, 1964.
98. Madsen ET: Fractures of the extremities in the newborn. Acta Obstet Gynecol Scand 34:41-74, 1955.
99. Tanchev S, Kolishev K, Tanches P, et al: Etiology of a clavicle fracture due to the birth process. Akush Ginekol (Mosk) 24:39-43, 1985.
100. Katz R, Landman J, Dulitzky F, et al: Fracture of the clavicle in the newborn: An ultrasound diagnosis. J Ultrasound Med 7:21-23, 1988.
101. Swischuk LE: Radiology of Newborn and Young Infants, 2nd ed. Baltimore: Williams & Wilkins, 1981, p 630.
102. Cayford EH, Tees FJ: Traumatic aneurysm of the subclavian artery as a late complication of fractured clavicle. Can Med Assoc J 25:450-452, 1931.
103. Gitsch VG, Schatten C: Frequenz und potentielle Faktoren in der Genese der geburtstraumatisch bedingten Klavicula fraktur. Zentralbl Gynakol 109:909-912, 1987.
104. Beall MH, Ross MG: Clavicle fracture in labor: Risk factors and associated morbidities. J Perinatol 21(8):513-515, 2001.
105. Cohen AW, Otto SR: Obstetric clavicular fractures. J Reprod Med 25:119-122, 1980.
106. Jelic A, Marin L, Pracny M, Jelic N: Fractures in neonates. Litjec Vjesn 114:1-4, 32-35, 1992.
107. Bateman JE: The Shoulder and Neck. Philadelphia: WB Saunders, 1978.
108. Bowen AD: Plastic bowing of the clavicle in children: A report of two cases. J Bone Joint Surg Am 65:403-405, 1983.
109. Snyder LA: Loss of the accompanying soft tissue shadow of clavicle with occult fracture. South Med J 72:243, 1979.
110. Nordqvist A, Petersson C: The incidence of fractures of the clavicle. Clin Orthop Relat Res (300):127-132, 1994.
111. Nowak J: Clavicular Fractures: Epidemiology, Union, Malunion, Nonunion. Uppsala, Sweden: Acta Universitatis Upsalaiensis, 2002.
112. Nowak J, Mallmin H, Larsson S: The aetiology and epidemiology of clavicle fractures: A prospective study during a two-week period in Uppsala, Sweden. Injury 31:5, 353-358, 2000.
113. Fowler AW: Fractures of the clavicle. J Bone Joint Surg Br 44:440, 1962.
114. Silloway KA, Mclaughlin RE, Edlichy RC, et al: Clavicular fractures and acromioclavicular joint injuries in lacrosse: Preventable injuries. J Emerg Med 3:117-121, 1985.
115. Sankarankutty M, Turner BW: Fractures of the clavicle. Injury 7:101-106, 1975.
116. Stanley D, Trowbridge EA, Norris SH: The mechanism of clavicular fracture. J Bone Joint Surg Br 70:461-464, 1988.
117. Harnroongroj T, Tantikul C, Keatkor S: The clavicular fracture: A biomechanical study of the mechanism of clavicular fracture and modes of the fracture. J Med Assoc Thai 83:663-667, 2000.
118. Fallon KE, Fricker PA: Stress fracture of the clavicle in a young female gymnast. Br J Sports Med 35:448-449, 2001.
119. Roset-Llobet J, Salo-Orfila JM: Sports-related stress fracture of the clavicle: A case report. Int Orthop 22:266-268, 1998.
120. Waninger KN: Stress fracture of the clavicle in a collegiate diver. Clin J Sport Med 7:66-68, 1997.
121. Wu CD, Chen YC: Stress fracture of the clavicle in a professional baseball player. J Shoulder Elbow Surg 7:164-167, 1998.
122. Dust WN, Lenczner AN: Stress fracture of the clavicle leading to nonunion secondary to coracoclavicular reconstruction with Dacron. Am J Sports Med 17:128-129, 1989.
123. Bernard TN, Haddad RJ: Enchondroma of the proximal clavicle: An unusual cause of pathologic fracture dislocation of the sternoclavicular joint. Clin Orthop Relat Res (167):239-241, 1982.
124. Mnaymneh W, Vargas A, Kaplan J: Fractures of the clavicle caused by arteriovenous malformation. Clin Orthop Relat Res (148):256-258, 1980.
125. Cummings CW, First R: Stress fracture of the clavicle after a radical neck dissection: Case report. Plast Reconstr Surg 55:366-367, 1975.
126. Fini-Storchi O, LoRusso D, Agostini V: "Pseudotumors" of the clavicle subsequent to radical neck dissection. J Laryngol Otol 99:73-83, 1985.
127. Ord RA, Langon JD: Stress fracture of the clavicle: A rare late complication of radical neck dissection. J Maxillofac Surg 14:281-284, 1986.
128. Strauss M, Bushey MJ, Chung C, Baum S: Fractures of the clavicle following radical neck dissection or postoperative radiotherapy: A case report and review of the literature. Laryngoscope 92:1304-1307, 1982.
129. Martell JR: Clavicular nonunion: Complication with the use of Mersilene tape. Am J Sports Med 20:360-362, 1992.
130. Schrocksnadel H, Hein K, Dapunt O: The clavicular fracture—a questionable achievement in modern obstetrics. Geburtshilfe Frauenheilkd 49:481-484, 1989.
131. Farkas R, Levine S: X-ray incidence of fractured clavicle in vertex presentation. Am J Obstet Gynecol 59:204-206, 1950.
132. Cumming WA: Neonatal skeletal fractures: Birth trauma, or child abuse? J Can Assoc Radiol 30:30-33, 1979.
133. Freedman M, Gamble J, Lewis C: Intrauterine fracture simulating a unilateral clavicular pseudoarthrosis. J Assoc Radiol 33:37-38, 1982.
134. Sandford HN: The Moro reflex as a diagnostic aid in fracture of the clavicle in the newborn infant. Am J Dis Child 41:1304-1306, 1931.
135. Brooks AL, Henning GD: Injuries to the proximal clavicular epiphysis. J Bone Joint Surg Am 54:1347-1348, 1972.
136. Lemire L, Rosman M: Sternoclavicular epiphyseal separation with adjacent clavicular fracture. J Pediatr Orthop 4:118-120, 1984.
137. Redmond AD: A complication of fracture of the clavicle [letter]. Injury 13:352, 1982.
138. Gross SD: The Anatomy, Physiology, and Diseases of the Bones and Joints. Philadelphia: John Grigg, 1830.
139. Dickson JW: Death following fractured clavicle. BMJ 2:666-667, 1952.
140. Dugdale TW, Fulkerson JB: Pneumothorax complicating a closed fracture of the clavicle: A case report. Clin Orthop Relat Res (221):212-214, 1987.
141. Butterworth RD, Kirk AA: Fracture dislocation sternoclavicular joint: Case report. Virginia Med Month 79:98-100, 1952.
142. Kanoksikarin S, Wearne WN: Fracture and retrosternal dislocation of the clavicle. Aust N Z J Surg 48:95-96, 1978.
143. Wurtz LD, Lyons FA, Rockwood CA Jr: Fracture of the middle third of the clavicle and dislocation of the acromioclavicular joint. J Bone Joint Surg Am 74:133-137, 1992.
144. Apeli L, Burch HB: Study on the pseudoarthrosis of the clavicle. In Chapchal G (ed): Pseudoarthroses and Their Treatment. Eighth International Symposium on Topical Problems in Orthopaedic Surgery. Stuttgart, Germany: Thieme, 1979, pp 188-189.
145. Wilkes J, Hoffer M: Clavicle fractures in head-injured children. J Orthop Trauma 1:55-58, 1987.
146. Aitken AD, Lincoln RE: Fractures of the first rib due to muscle pull: Report of a case. N Engl J Med 220:1063-1064, 1939.
147. Weiner DS, O'Dell HW: Fractures of the first rib associated with injuries to the clavicle. J Trauma 9:412-422, 1969.
148. Post M: Injury to the shoulder girdle. In Post M (ed): The Shoulder: Surgical and Non-surgical Management. Philadelphia: Lea & Febiger, 1988.
149. Ebraheim NA, An HS, Jackson WT, et al: Scapulothoracic dissociation. J Bone Joint Surg Am 70:428-432, 1988.
150. Leung KS, Lin TP: Open reduction and internal fixation of ipsilateral fractures of the scapular neck and clavicle. J Bone Joint Surg Am 75:1015-1018, 1993.
151. Rockwood CA: Personal communication, 1995.
152. Low CK, Lam AW: Results of fixation of clavicle alone in managing floating shoulder. Singapore Med J 41:452-453, 2000.
153. Tseng RC, Shu RJ, Chen RJ, Shih CH: Floating shoulder (ipsilateral scapula, neck and clavicle fracture)—two case reports [Chinese]. Chang Keng I Hsueh-Chang Gung Med J 17:403-406, 1994.

154. Herscovici D Jr, Fiennes AGT, Allgower N, Ruedi TP: The floating shoulder: Ipsilateral clavicle and scapular neck fractures. J Bone Joint Surg Br 74:362-364, 1992.

155. Herscovici D Jr, Fiennes AGT, Ruedi TP: The floating shoulder: Ipsilateral clavicle and scapular neck fractures [abstract]. J Orthop Trauma 6:499, 1992.

156. Egol KA, Connor PM, Karunakar MA, et al: The floating shoulder: Clinical and functional results. J Bone Joint Surg Am 83:1188-1194, 2001.

157. Van Noort A, te Slaa RL, Marti RK, van der Werken C: The floating shoulder. A multicentre study. J Bone Joint Surg Br 83:795-798, 2001.

158. Williams GR Jr, Naranja J, Klimkiewicz J, et al: The floating shoulder: A biomechanical basis for classification and management. J Bone Joint Surg Am 83:1182-1187, 2001.

159. Meeks RJ, Riebel GD: Isolated clavicle fracture with associated pneumothorax: A case report. Am J Emerg Med 9:555-556, 1991.

160. Rowe CR (ed): The Shoulder. New York: Churchill Livingstone, 1988.

161. Malcolm BW, Ameli FM, Simmons EH: Pneumothorax complicating a fracture of the clavicle. Can J Surg 22:84, 1979.

162. Jackson WJ: Clavicle fractures: Therapy is dictated by the patient's age. Consultant p 177, 1982.

163. Steenburg RW, Ravitch MM: Cervico-thoracic approach for subclavian vessel injury from compound fracture of the clavicle: Considerations of subclavian axillary exposures. Ann Surg 1:839-846, 1963.

164. Stimson LA: A Treatise on Fractures. Philadelphia: Henry A Lea's Son & Co, 1883, p 332.

165. Reid J, Kenned J: Direct fracture of the clavicle with symptoms simulating a cervical rib. BMJ 2:608-609, 1925.

166. Bateman JE: Nerve injuries about the shoulder in sports. J Bone Joint Surg Am 49:785-792, 1967.

167. Van Vlack HG: Comminuted fracture of the clavicle with pressure on brachial plexus: Report of case. J Bone Joint Surg Am 22:446-447, 1940.

168. Penn I: The vascular complications of fractures of the clavicle. J Trauma 4:819-831, 1964.

169. Mital MA, Aufranc OE: Venous occlusion following greenstick fracture of clavicle. JAMA 206:1301-1302, 1968.

170. Curtis RJ Jr: Operative treatment of children's fractures of the shoulder region. Orthop Clin North Am 21:315-324, 1990.

171. Javid H: Vascular injuries of the neck. Clin Orthop 28:70-78, 1963.

172. Klier I, Mayor PB: Laceration of the innominate internal jugular venous junction: Rare complication of fracture of the clavicle. Orthop Rev 10:81-82, 1981.

173. Lim E, Day LJ: Subclavian vein thrombosis following fracture of the clavicle: A case report. Orthopedics 10:349-351, 1987.

174. Matry C: Fracture de la clavicule gauche au tiers interne. Blessure de la vein sous-clavière. Osteosynthese Bull Mem Soc Nat Chir 58:75-78, 1932.

175. Guillemin A: Dechirure de la veine sous-clavière par fracture fermée de la clavicule. Bull Mem Soc Nat Chir 56:302-304, 1930.

176. Steinberg I: Subclavian vein thrombosis associated with fractures of the clavicle: Report of two cases. N Engl J Med 264:686-688, 1961.

177. Iqbal O: Axillary artery thrombosis associated with fracture of the clavicle. Med J Malaysia 26:68-70, 1971.

178. Tse DHW, Slabaugh PB, Carlson PA: Injury to the axillary artery by a closed fracture of the clavicle. J Bone Joint Surg Am 62:1372-1373, 1980.

179. Scarpa FJ, Levy RM: Pulmonary embolism complicating clavicle fracture. Conn Med 43:771-773, 1979.

180. Weh L, Torklus DZ: Fracture of the clavicle with consecutive costoclavicular compression syndrome. Z Orthop 118:140-142, 1980.

181. Throckmorton T, Kuhn JE: Fractures of the medial end of the clavicle. J Shoulder Elbow Surg 16(1):49-54, 2007.

182. Widner LA, Riddewold HO: The value of the lordotic view in diagnosis of fractured clavicle. Rev Int Radiol 5:69-70, 1980.

183. Quesana F: Technique for the roentgen: Diagnosis of fractures of the clavicle. Surg Gynecol Obstet 42:4261-4281, 1926.

184. Gibson DA, Carroll N: Congenital pseudoarthrosis of the clavicle. J Bone Joint Surg Br 52:629-643, 1970.

185. Kite JH: Congenital pseudarthrosis of the clavicle. South Med J 61:703-710, 1968.

186. Quinlan WR, Brady PG, Regan BF: Congenital pseudoarthrosis of the clavicle. Acta Orthop Scand 51:489-492, 1980.

187. Lloyd-Roberts GC, Apley AG, Owen R: Reflections upon the etiology of congenital pseudoarthrosis of the clavicle. J Bone Joint Surg Br 57:24-29, 1975.

188. Wall JJ: Congenital pseudoarthrosis of the clavicle. J Bone Joint Surg Am 52:1003-1009, 1970.

189. Owen R: Congenital pseudoarthrosis of the clavicle. J Bone Joint Surg Br 52:642-652, 1970.

190. Lombard JJ: Pseudoarthrosis of the clavicle: A case report. S Afr Med J 66:151-153, 1984.

191. Marie P, Sainton P: On hereditary cleidocranial dysostosis. Clin Orthop Relat Res 58:5-7, 1968.

192. Alldred AJ: Congenital pseudoarthrosis of the clavicle. J Bone Joint Surg Br 45:312-319, 1963.

193. Fairbank H: Cranio-cleido-dysostosis. J Bone Joint Surg Br 31: 608-617, 1949.

194. Eskola A, Vainionpaa S, Myllynen P: Surgery for ununited clavicular fracture. Acta Orthop Scand 57:366-367, 1986.

195. Johnson EW Jr, Collins HR: Nonunion of the clavicle. Arch Surg 87:963-966, 1963.

196. Koch F, Papadimitriou G, Groher W: [Clavicular pseudarthrosis, its development and treatment]. Unfallheilkunde 74:330-337, 1971.

197. Marsh HO, Hazarian E: Pseudoarthrosis of the clavicle. In Proceedings of the American, British, Canadian, Australia, New Zealand, and South African Orthopaedic Associations. J Bone Joint Surg Br 52:793-970, 1970.

198. Schewior T: Die Durckpallenostesynthese bei Schlusselpein pseudarthrosen. Acta Traumatol 4:113-125, 1974.

199. Simpson NS, Jupiter JB: Clavicular nonunion and malunion: Evaluation and surgical management. J Am Acad Orthop Surg 4:1-8, 1996.

200. Wachsmudh W: Allgemiene und Specielle Operationslettie. Berlin: Martin Kirschner, Springer-Verlag, 1956, p 375.

201. Joukainen J, Karaharju E: Pseudoarthrosis of the clavicle. Acta Orthop Scand 48:550, 1977.

202. Sakellarides H: Pseudoarthrosis of the clavicle. J Bone Joint Surg Am 43:130-138, 1961.

203. Wilkins RM, Johnston RM: Ununited fractures of the clavicle. J Bone Joint Surg Am 65:773-778, 1983.

204. Manske DJ, Szabo RM: The operative treatment of mid-shaft clavicular nonunions. J Bone Joint Surg Am 67:1367-1371, 1985.

205. Hargan B, Macafee AL: Bilateral pseudoarthrosis of the clavicles. Injury 12:316-318, 1981.

206. Nogi J, Heckman JD, Hakula M, Sweet DE: Non-union of the clavicle in the child: A case report. Clin Orthop Relat Res (110):19-21, 1975.

207. Neviaser RJ: Injuries to the clavicle and acromioclavicular joint. Orthop Clin North Am 18:433-438, 1987.

208. Basom WC, Breck LW, and Herz JR: Dual grafts for nonunion of the clavicle. South Med J 40:898-899, 1987.

209. Frobenius H, Betzel A: Injuries and their causes in bicycle accidents. Unfallchirurgie 13:135-141, 1987.

210. Jupiter JB, Leffert RD: Nonunion of the clavicle. J Bone Joint Surg Am 69:753-760, 1987.

211. Rhinelander FW: Tibial blood supply in relation to fracture healing. Clin Orthop Relat Res (105):34-81, 1974.

212. Rabenseifner L: Zur Ätiologie und Therapie bei Schlusselbeinpseudarthosen. Aktuelle Traumatol 11:130-132, 1981.

213. Smith RW: A Treatise on Fractures in the Vicinity of Joints. Dublin: Hodges & Smith, 1847, pp 209-224.

214. Wick M, Muller EJ, Kollig E, Muhr G: Midshaft fractures of the clavicle with a shortening of more than 2 cm predispose to nonunion. Arch Orthop Trauma Surg 121:207-211, 2001.

215. Schwartz N, Leixnering M: Technik und Ergebienisse der Klavikula-markdrahtung. Zentralbl Chir 111:640-647, 1986.

216. Poigenfurst J, Reiler T, Fischer W: Plating of fresh clavicular fractures: Experience with 60 operations. Unfallchirurg 14:26-37, 1988.

217. Zenni EJ Jr, Krieg JK, Rosen MJ: Open reduction and internal fixation of clavicular fractures. J Bone Joint Surg Am 63:147-151, 1981.

218. Chen CE, Liu HC: Delayed brachial plexus neurapraxia complicating malunion of the clavicle. Am J Orthop 29:321-322, 2000.

219. Lord JW, Rosati JM: Neurovascular Compression Syndromes of the Upper Extremity. Ciba Clinical Symposia, vol 10. Basel: Ciba, 1958, pp 35-62.

220. Bargar WL, Marcus RE, Ittleman FP: Late thoracic outlet syndrome secondary to pseudoarthrosis of the clavicle. J Trauma 24:857-859, 1984.

221. Connolly JF, Dehne R: Delayed thoracic outlet syndrome from clavicular non-union: Management by morseling. Nebr Med J 71:303-306, 1986.

222. Hughes AW, Sherlock DA: Bilateral thoracic outlet syndrome following nonunion of clavicles, associated with radio-osteodystrophy injury. Injury 19:40-41, 1988.

223. Koss SD, Giotz HT, Redler NR, et al: Nonunion of a midshaft clavicle fracture associated with subclavian vein compression: A case report. Orthop Rev 18:431-434, 1989.

224. Pipkin G: Tardy shoulder hand syndrome following ununited fracture of clavicle: A case report. J Mo Med Assoc 48:643-646, 1951.

225. Ghormley RK, Black JR, Cherry JH: Ununited fractures of the clavicle. Am J Surg 51:343-349, 1941.

226. Ledger M, Leeks N, Ackland T, Wang A: Short malunions of the clavicle: An anatomic and functional study. J Shoulder Elbow Surg 14(4):349-354, 2005.

227. Chan KY, Jupiter JB, Leffert RD, Marti R: Clavicle malunion. J Shoulder Elbow Surg 8:287-290, 1999.

228. Basamania CJ: "Clavicwhen" and intramedullary fixation of malunited, shortened clavicle fractures. J Shoulder Elbow Surg 8:540, 1999.

229. Fujita K, Matsuda K, Sakai Y, et al: Late thoracic outlet syndrome secondary to malunion of the fractured clavicle: Case report and review of the literature. J Trauma 50:332-335, 2001.

230. Gebuhr P: Brachial plexus involvement after fractures of the clavicle. Ugeskr Laeger 150:105-106, 1988.

231. Mulder DS, Greenwood FA, Brooks CE: Post-traumatic thoracic outlet syndrome. J Trauma 13:706-713, 1973.

232. Shauffer IA, Collins WV: The deep clavicular rhomboid fossa. JAMA 195:778-779, 1966.

233. Storen H: Old clavicular pseudoarthrosis with late appearing neuralgias and vasomotor disturbances cured by operation. Acta Chir Scand 94:187-191, 1946.

234. Todd TW, D'errico J Jr: The clavicular epiphysis. Am J Anat 41:25-50, 1928.

235. Howard FM, Schafer SJ: Injuries to the clavicle with neurovascular complications: A study of fourteen cases. J Bone Joint Surg Am 47:1335-1346, 1965.

236. Rosati LM, Lord JW Jr: Neurovascular Compression Syndromes of the Shoulder Girdle. New York: Grune & Stratton, 1961.

237. Karwasz RR, Kutzner M, Krammer WG: Late brachial plexus lesion following clavicular fracture. Unfallchirurg 91:45-47, 1988.

238. Lusskin R, Weiss CA, Winer J: The role of the subclavius muscle in the subclavian vein syndrome (costoclavicular syndrome) following fracture of the clavicle. Clin Orthop Relat Res 54:75-84, 1967.

239. Falconer MA, Weddell G: Costoclavicular compression of the subclavian artery and vein. Lancet 2:539-543, 1943.

240. Sampson JJ, Saunders JB, Capp CS: Compression of the subclavian vein by the first rib and clavicle with reference to prominence of the chest veins as a sign of collaterals. Am Heart J 19:292-315, 1940.

241. Stone PW, Lord JW: The clavicle and its relation to trauma to the subclavian artery and vein. Am J Surg 98:834-839, 1955.

242. Das NK, Deb HK: Synovioma of the clavicle: Report of a case. J Int Coll Surg 35:776-780, 1961.

243. Guilfoil PH, Christiansen T: An unusual vascular complication of fractured clavicle. JAMA 200:72-73, 1967.

244. Siffrey PN, Aulong TL: Thrombose post-traumatique de l'artère sousclavière gauche. Lyon Chir 51:479-481, 1956.

245. Rockwood CA: Don't throw away the clavicle. Orthop Trans 16:763, 1992-1993.

246. Gryska PF: Major vascular injuries. N Engl J Med 266:381-385, 1982.

247. Natali J, Maraval M, Kieffer E, et al: Fractures of the clavicle and injuries of the subclavian artery: Report of 10 cases. J Cardiovasc Surg 16:541-547, 1975.

248. Yates AG, Guest D: Cerebral embolus due to ununited fracture of the clavicle and subclavian thrombosis. Lancet 2:225-226, 1928.

249. Caspi I, Ezra E, Nerubay J, et al: Musculocutaneous nerve injury after coracoid process transfer for clavicle instability. Acta Orthop Scand 58:294-295, 1987.

250. De Bakey E, Beall C Jr, Ukkasch DC: Recent developments in vascular surgery with particular reference to orthopaedics. Am J Surg 109:134-142, 1965.

251. Nelson HP: Subclavian aneurysm following fracture of the clavicle. St Bartholomew Hosp Rep 65:219-229, 1932.

252. Shih J, Chao E, Chang C: Subclavian pseudoaneurysm after clavicle fracture: A case report. J Formos Med Assoc 82:332-335, 1983.

253. Hansky B, Murray E, Minami K, Korfer R: Delayed brachial plexus paralysis due to subclavian pseudoaneurysm after clavicular fracture. Eur J Cardiothorac Surg 7:497-498, 1993.

254. Enker SH, Murthy KK: Brachial plexus compression by excessive callus formation secondary to a fractured clavicle: A case report. Mt Sinai J Med 37:678-682, 1970.

255. Guattieri G, Frassi G: Late truncal paralysis of the brachial plexus in sequelae of fracture of the clavicle. Arch Ortop 74:840-848, 1961.

256. Kay SP, Eckardt JJ: Brachial plexus palsy secondary to clavicular nonunion: A case report and literature survey. Clin Orthop Relat Res (206):219-222, 1986.

257. Miller DS, Boswick JA: Lesions of the brachial plexus associated with fractures of the clavicle. Clin Orthop Relat Res 64:144-149, 1969.

258. Suso S, Alemany X, Conbalia A, Ramon R: Compression of the anterior interosseous nerve after use of a Robert Jones type bandage for a distal end clavicle fracture: Case report. J Trauma 136:737-739, 1994.

259. Bartosh RA, Dugdale TW, Nielsen R: Isolated musculocutaneous nerve injury complicating closed fracture of the clavicle: A case report. Am J Sports Med 20:356-359, 1992.

260. Rumball KN, DaSilva VF, Preston DN, Carruthers CC: Brachial plexus injury after clavicular fracture: Case report and literature review. Can J Surg 34:264-266, 1991.

261. Ivey N, Britt N, Johnston RV: Reflex sympathetic dystrophy after clavicle fracture: Case report. J Trauma 31:276-279, 1991.

262. Ring D, Holovacs T: Brachial plexus palsy after intramedullary fixation of a clavicular fracture. A report of three cases. J Bone Joint Surg Am 87(8):1834-1837, 2005.

263. Eilanberger K, Janousek A, Poigenfurst J: Heart arrest as a sequela of clavicular fracture. Unfallchirurgie 18:186-188, 1992.

264. Jackson DW (ed): Shoulder Surgery in the Athlete. Rockville, Md: Aspen, 1985.

265. Middleton SB, Foley SJ, Foy NA: Partial excision of the clavicle for nonunion in National Hunt Jockeys. J Bone Joint Surg Br 77:778-780, 1995.

266. Dela Santo DR, Narakas AO, Bonnard C: Late lesions of the brachial plexus after fracture of the clavicle. Ann Hand Surg 10:531-540, 1991.

267. Neer CS II: Impingement lesions. Clin Orthop Relat Res (173):70-77, 1983.

268. Kreisinger V: Sur le traitement des fractures de le clavicule. Rev Chir Paris 43:376-384, 1927.

269. Lester CW: The treatment of fractures of the clavicle. Ann Surg 89:600-606, 1929.

270. Nordqvist A, Petersson CJ, Redlund-Johnell I: Mid-clavicle fractures in adults: End result study after conservative treatment. J Orthop Trauma 12:572-576, 1998.

271. Bonnett J: Fracture of the clavicle. Arch Chir Neerl 27:143-151, 1975.

272. Liechtl R: Fracture of the clavicle and scapula. In Webber BG, Brunner C, Freuler F (eds): Treatment of Fractures in Children and Adolescents. New York: Springer-Verlag, 1988, pp 88-95.

273. Rang M: Clavicle. In Rang M (ed): Children's Fractures, 2nd ed. Philadelphia: JB Lippincott, 1983.

274. Pollen AG: Fractures and Dislocations in Children. Baltimore: Williams & Wilkins, 1973.

275. Quigley TB: The management of simple fracture of the clavicle in adults. N Engl J Med 243:286-290, 1950.

276. Conwell HE: Fractures of the clavicle. JAMA 90:838-839, 1928.

277. Breck L: Partially threaded round pins with oversized threads for intramedullary fixation of the clavicle and the forearm bones. Clin Orthop 11:227-229, 1958.

278. Katznelson A, Nerubay JN, Oliver S: Dynamic fixation of the avulsed clavicle. J Trauma 16:841-844, 1976.

279. Lee HG: Treatment of fracture of the clavicle by internal nail fixation. N Engl J Med 234:222-224, 1946.

280. Lengua F, Nuss J, Lechner R, et al: The treatment of fracture of the clavicle by closed medio-lateral pinning. Rev Chir Orthop 73:377-380, 1987.

281. Moore TO: Internal pin fixation for fracture of the clavicle. Am Surg 17:580-583, 1951.

282. Murray G: A method of fixation for fracture of the clavicle. J Bone Joint Surg 22:616-620, 1940.

283. Neviaser RJ, Neviaser JS, Neviaser TJ, et al: A simple technique for internal fixation of the clavicle. Clin Orthop Relat Res (109):103-107, 1975.

284. Paffen PJ, Jansen EW: Surgical treatment of clavicular fractures with Kirschner wires: A comparative study. Arch Chir Neerl 30:43-53, 1978.

285. Rush LV, Rush HL: Technique of longitudinal pin fixation in fractures of the clavicle and jaw. Miss Doct 27:332-336, 1949.

286. Piterman L: The fractured clavicle. Aust Fam Physician 11:614, 1982.

287. Billington RW: A new (plaster yoke) dressing for fracture of the clavicle. South Med J 24:667-670, 1931.

288. Cook T: Reduction and external fixation of fractures of the clavicle in recumbency. J Bone Joint Surg Am 36:878-880, 1954.

289. Young CS: The mechanics of ambulatory treatment of fractures of the clavicle. J Bone Joint Surg 13:299-310, 1931.

290. Kini MG: A simple method of ambulatory treatment of fractures of the clavicle. J Bone Joint Surg 23:795-798, 1941.

291. Packer BD: Conservative treatment of fracture of the clavicle. J Bone Joint Surg 26:770-774, 1944.

292. Anderson K, Jensen P, Lauritzen J: Treatment of clavicular fractures: Figure-of-eight bandage vs. a simple sling. Acta Orthop Scand 57:71-74, 1987.

293. McCandless DN, Mowbray M: Treatment of displaced fractures of the clavicle: Sling vs. figure-of-eight bandage. Practitioner 223:266-267, 1979.

294. Hackstock H, Hackstock H: Surgical treatment of clavicular fracture. Unfallchirurg 91:64-69, 1988.

295. O'Rourke IC, Middleton RW: The place and efficacy of operative management of fractured clavicle. Injury 6:236-240, 1975.

296. Simpson LA, Kellam J: Surgical management of fractures of the clavicle, scapula, and proximal humerus. Orthop Update Series 4:1-8, 1985.

297. Siebermann RP, Spieler U, Arquint A: Rush pin osteosynthesis of the clavicle as an alternative to the conservation treatment. Unfallchirurgie 13:303-307, 1987.

298. Khan MAA, Lucas HK: Plating of fractures of the middle third of the clavicle. Injury 9:263-267, 1978.

299. Mueller ME, Allgower N, Willenegger H: Manual of Internal Fixation. New York: Springer-Verlag, 1970.

300. Perry B: An improved clavicular pin. Am J Surg 112:142-144, 1966.

301. Rockwood CA, Green DP: Fractures, 4th ed. Philadelphia: Lippincott-Raven, 1996.

302. Schuind F, Pay-Pay E, Andrianne Y, et al: External fixation of the clavicle for fracture or nonunion in adults. J Bone Joint Surg Am 70:692-695, 1988.

303. Ballmer FT, Hertel R: Other applications of the small AO external fixator to the upper limb. Injury 25(suppl 4):S-D64-S-D68, 1994.

304. Xiao XY: [Treatment of clavicular fracture patient with a percutaneous bone-embracing external clavicular microfixer.] Chung Hua Wai Ko Tsa Chih 31:657-659, 1993.

305. Nowak J, Rahme H, Holgersson M, et al: A prospective comparison between external fixation and plates for treatment of midshaft nonunions of the clavicle. Ann Chir Gynaecol 90(4):280-285, 2001.

306. Patel CV, Audenwalla HS: Treatment of fractured clavicle by immediate partial subperiosteal resection. J Postgrad Med 18:32-34, 1972.

307. Rockwood CA: Management of fracture of the clavicle and injuries of the SC joints. Orthop Trans 6:422, 1982.

308. Edwards DJ, Cavanaugh TG, Flannery NC: Fractures of the distal clavicle: A case for fixation. Injury 23:44-46, 1992.

309. Eskola A, Vainionpaa S, Patiala H, et al: Outcome of operative treatment in fresh lateral clavicle fracture. Ann Chir Gynaecol 76:167-168, 1987.

310. Golser K, Sperner G, Thoni H, Resch H: Early and intermediate results of conservatively and surgically treated lateral clavicle fractures. Aktuelle Traumatol 21:148-152, 1991.

311. Winkler H, Schlimp D, Wentzensen A: Treatment of acromioclavicular joint dislocation by tension band and ligament suture. Aktuelle Traumatol 24:133-139, 1994.

312. Poigenfurst J, Baumgarten-Hofmann U, Hofmann J: Unstabile Bruchformen an auberen Schlusselbeinende und Gurndsatze der Behandlung. Unfallchirurgie 17:131-139, 1991.

313. Brunner U, Habermeyer P, Schweiberer L: Die Sonderstellung der lateralen Klavikulafraktur. Orthopade 21:163-171, 1992.

314. Nordqvist A, Petersson C, Redlund-Johnell I: Fractures of the lateral end of the clavicle: A long term study [abstract]. Acta Orthop Scand Suppl 246:25-26, 1991.

315. Lyons FA, Rockwood CA Jr: Migration of pins used in operations on the shoulder. J Bone Joint Surg Am 72:1262-1267, 1990.

316. Der TJ, Davison JN, Dias JJ: Clavicular fracture non-union surgical outcome and complications. Injury 33(2):135-143, 2002.

317. Eberle C, Fodor P, Metzger U: [Hook plate (so-called Balser plate) or tension banding with the Bosworth screw in complete acromioclavicular dislocation and clavicular fracture.] Z Unfallchir Versicherungsmed 85:134-139, 1992.

318. Voigt C, Enes-Gaiao F, Fahimi S: [Treatment of acromioclavicular joint dislocation with the Rah Manzadeh joint plate.] Aktuelle Traumatol 24:128-132, 1994.

319. Haidar SG, Krishnan KM, Deshmukh SC: Hook plate fixation for type II fractures of the lateral end of the clavicle. J Shoulder Elbow Surg 15(4):419-423, 2006.

320. Muramatsu K, Shigetomi M, Matsunaga T, et al: Use of the AO hook-plate for treatment of unstable fractures of the distal clavicle. Arch Orthop Trauma Surg 127(3):191-194, 2007.

321. McConnell, Alison J, Yoo, DJ, et al: Methods of operative fixation of the acromio-clavicular joint: a biomechanical comparison. J Orthop Trauma 21(4):248-253, 2007.

322. Fazal MA, Saksena J, Haddad FS: Temporary coracoclavicular screw fixation for displaced distal clavicle fractures. J Orthop Surg (Hong Kong) 15(1):9-11, 2007.

323. Jin CZ, Kim HK, Min BH: Surgical treatment for distal clavicle fracture associated with coracoclavicular ligament rupture using a cannulated screw fixation technique. J Trauma 60(6):1358-1361, 2006.

324. Macheras G, Kateros KT, Savvidou OD, et al: Coracoclavicular screw fixation for unstable distal clavicle fractures. Orthopedics 28(7):693-696, 2005.

325. Tsou PN: Percutaneous cannulated screw coracoclavicular fixation for acute acromioclavicular dislocations. Clin Orthop Relat Res (243):112-121, 1989.

326. Yamaguchi H, Arakawa H, Kobayashi M: Results of the Bosworth method for unstable fractures of the distal clavicle. Int Orthop 22(6):366-368, 1998.

327. Friedel W, Fritz T: PDS cord fixation of sternoclavicular dislocation and paraarticular clavicular fractures. Unfallchirurg 97:263-265, 1994.

328. Brighton CT, Pollick SR: Treatment of recalcitrant nonunion with a capacitively coupled electrical field: A preliminary report. J Bone Joint Surg Am 67:577-585, 1985.

329. Day L: Electrical stimulation in the treatment of ununited fractures. Clin Orthop Relat Res (161):54-57, 1981.

330. Connolly JF: Electrical treatment of nonunion: Its use and abuse in 100 consecutive fractures. Orthop Clin North Am 15:89-106, 1984.

331. Koelliker F Ganz R: Results of the treatment of clavicular pseudoarthrosis. Unfallchirurg 92:164-168, 1989.

332. Pusitz ME, Davis EV: Bone-drilling in delayed union of fractures. J Bone Joint Surg Am 26:560-565, 1944.

333. Neviaser JS: Acromioclavicular dislocations treated by transference of the coracoacromial ligament. Bull Hosp Jt Dis 12:46-54, 1951.

334. Weaver JK, Dunn HK: Treatment of acromioclavicular injuries, especially acromioclavicular separation. J Bone Joint Surg Am 54:1187-1198, 1972.

335. Connolly JF, Dehne R: Nonunion of the clavicle and thoracic outlet syndrome. J Trauma 29:1127-1132, 1989.

336. Johansen KH, Thomas GI: Late thoracic outlet syndrome secondary to malunion of the fractured clavicle: Case report and review of the literature. J Trauma 52:607-608, 2002.

337. Mayer JH: Nonunion of fractured clavicle. Proc R Soc Med 58:182, 1965.

338. Chou NS, Wu MH, Chan CS, et al: Intrathoracic migration of Kirschner wires. J Formos Med Assoc 93:974-976, 1994.

339. Kremens V, Glauser F: Unusual sequelae following pinning of medial clavicular fracture. AJR Am J Roentgenol 74:1066-1069, 1956.

340. Mazet R: Migration of a Kirschner wire from the shoulder region into the lung: Report of two cases. J Bone Joint Surg 25:477-483, 1943.

341. Norell H, Llewelleyn RC: Migration of a threaded Steinmann pin from an acromioclavicular joint into the spinal canal: A case report. J Bone Joint Surg Am 47:1024, 1965.

342. Unger JN, Schuchmann GG, Grossman JE, Pellatt JR: Tears of the trachea and main bronchi caused by blunt trauma: Radiologic findings. AJR Am J Roentgenol 153:1175-1180, 1989.

343. Watson-Jones R: Fractures and Other Bone and Joint Injuries. Edinburgh: E & S Livingstone, 1940, pp 90-91.

344. Rockwood CA: Fractures of the outer clavicle in children and adults. J Bone Joint Surg Br 64:642-649, 1982.

345. Boehme D, Curtis RJ, DeHaan JT, et al: Non-union of fractures of the mid-shaft of the clavicle: Treatment with a modified Hagie intramedullary and autogenous bone grafting. J Bone Joint Surg Am 73:1219-1226, 1991.

346. Hicks JH: Rigid fixation as a treatment for hypertrophic nonunion. Injury 8:199-205, 1976.

347. Pyper JB: Nonunion of fractures of the clavicle. Injury 9:268-270, 1978.

348. Echtermeyer V, Zwipp H, Oestern HJ: Fehler und Gefahren in der Behandlung der Fracturen und Pseudarthrosen des Schlusselbeins. Langenbecks Arch Chir 364:351-354, 1984.

349. Edvardsen P, Odegard O: Treatment of posttraumatic clavicular pseudoarthrosis. Acta Orthop Scand 48:456-457, 1977.

350. Kabaharjve E, Joukainen J, Peltonen J: Treatment of pseudoarthrosis of the clavicle. Injury 13:400-403, 1982.

351. Raymakers E, Marti R: Nonunion of the clavicle. In Pseudarthroses and Their Treatment. Eighth International Symposium on Topical Problems in Orthopaedic Surgery. Stuttgart, Germany: Thieme, 1979.

352. Thompson AG, Batten RC: The application of rigid internal fixation to the treatment of nonunion and delayed union using AO technique. Injury 8:88, 1977.

353. Weber BG: Pseudoarthrosis of the clavicle. In Pseudoarthrosis: Pathophysiology, Biomechanics, Therapy, Results. New York: Grune & Stratton, 1976, pp 104-107.

354. Herbsthofer B, Schuz W, Mockweitz J: Indications for surgical treatment of clavicular fractures. Aktuelle Traumatol 24:263-268, 1994.

355. Capicotto PN, Heiple KG, Wilbur JH: Midshaft clavicle nonunions treated with intramedullary Steinmann pin fixation and onlay bone graft. J Orthop Trauma 8:88-93, 1994.

356. Mullaji AB, Jupiter J: Low contact dynamic compression plating of the clavicle. Injury 25:41-45, 1994.

357. Poigenfurst J, Rappold G, Fischer W: Plating of fresh clavicular fractures: Results of 122 operations. Injury 23:237-241, 1992.

358. Pedersen N, Poulsen KA, Thomsen F, Kristiansen B: Operative treatment of clavicular nonunion. Acta Orthop Belg 60:303-306, 1994.

359. Dash UN, Handler D: A case of compression of subclavian vessels by a fractured clavicle treated by excision of the first rib. J Bone Joint Surg Am 42:798-801, 1960.

360. Nordqvist A, Redlund-Johnell I, von Scheele A, Petersson CJ: Shortening of clavicle after fracture. Incidence and clinical significance, a 5-year follow-up of 85 patients. Acta Orthop Scand 68:349-351, 1997.

361. Craig EV: Fractures of the clavicle. In Rockwood CA Jr, Buckholz RW, Heckman JD, Green DP (eds): Fractures in Adults, 4th ed. Philadelphia: Lippincott Raven, 1996, pp 1109-1193.

362. Bostman O, Manninen M, Pihlajamaki H: Complications of plate fixation in fresh displaced midclavicular fractures. J Trauma 43:778-783, 1997.

363. Huang JI, Toogood P, Chen MR, et al: Clavicular anatomy and the applicability of precontoured plates. J Bone Joint Surg Am 89(10):2260-2265, 2007.

364. Iannotti MR, Crosby LA, Stafford P, et al: Effects of plate location and selection on the stability of midshaft clavicle osteotomies: A biomechanical study. J Shoulder Elbow Surg 11(5):457-462, 2002.

365. Shahid R, Mushtaq A, Maqsood M: Plate fixation of clavicle fractures: A comparative study between reconstruction plate and dynamic compression plate. Acta Orthop Belg 73(2):170-174, 2007.

366. Shackford SR, Connolly JF: Taming of the screw: A case report and literature review of limb-threatening complications after plate osteosynthesis of a clavicular nonunion. J Trauma 55(5):840-843, 2003.

367. Harnroongroj T, Vanadurongwan V: Biomechanical aspects of plating osteosynthesis of transverse clavicular fracture with and without inferior cortical defect. Clin Biomech (Bristol, Avon) 11(5):290-294, 1996.

368. Brockway A: Use of the intramedullary beef-bone graft in open reductions of the clavicle. J Bone Joint Surg 12:656-662, 1930.

369. Kuntscher, G, Maatz, R: Technik der Marknagelung, New York: Thieme, 1945.

370. Harnroongroj T, Jeerathanyasakun Y: Intramedullary pin fixation in clavicular fractures: A study comparing the use of small and large pins. J Orthop Surg (Hong Kong) 8(2):7-11, 2000.

371. Grassi FA, Tajana MS, D'Angelo F: Management of midclavicular fractures: Comparison between nonoperative treatment and open intramedullary fixation in 80 patients. J Trauma 50(6):1096-1100, 2001.

372. Strauss EJ, Egol KA, France MA, et al: Complications of intramedullary Hagie pin fixation for acute midshaft clavicle fractures. J Shoulder Elbow Surg 16(3):280-284, 2007.

373. Jubel A, Andermahr J, Weisshaar G, Schiffer G, Prokop A, Rehm KE: Intramedullary nailing (ESIN) in clavicular pseudoarthroses. Results of a prospective clinical trial. Unfallchirurg 108(7):544-550, 2005.

374. Jubel A, Andemahr J, Bergmann H, et al: Elastic stable intramedullary nailing of midclavicular fractures in athletes. Br J Sports Med 37(6):480-483, 2003.

375. Meier C, Grueninger P, Platz A: Elastic stable intramedullary nailing for midclavicular fractures in athletes: Indications, technical pitfalls and early results. Acta Orthop Belg 72(3):269-275, 2006.

376. Walz M, Kolbow B, Auerbach F. [Elastic, stable intramedullary nailing in midclavicular fractures—a change in treatment strategies?]. Unfallchirurg 109(3):200-211, 2006.

377. Mueller M, Burger C, Florczyk A, et al: Elastic stable intramedullary nailing of midclavicular fractures in adults: 32 patients followed for 1-5 years. Acta Orthop 78(3):421-423, 2007.

378. Chuang TY, Ho WP, Hsieh PH, et al: Closed reduction and internal fixation for acute midshaft clavicular fractures using cannulated screws. J Trauma 60(6):1315-1320, 2006.

379. Hoe-Hansen CE, Norlin R: Intramedullary cancellous screw fixation for nonunion of midshaft clavicular fractures. Acta Orthop Scand 74(3):361-364, 2003.

380. Proubasta IR, Itarte JP, Lamas CG, Caceres E: Midshaft clavicular non-unions treated with the Herbert cannulated bone screw. J Orthop Surg (Hong Kong) 12(1):71-75, 2004.

381. Thyagarajan DS: Treatment of displaced midclavicle fractures with Rockwood pin: A comparative study. In Proceedings From the 72nd Annual Meeting of the American Academy of Orthopaedic Surgeons. Rosemont, Ill: American Academy of Orthopaedic Surgeons, 2005.

382. Wu CC, Shih CH, Chen WJ, Tai CL: Treatment of clavicular aseptic nonunion: Comparison of plating and intramedullary nailing techniques. J Trauma 45(3):512-516, 1998.

383. Seiler JG, Jupiter J: Intercalary tri-corticol iliac crest bone grafts for the treatment of chronic clavicular nonunion with bony defect. J Orthop Tech 1:19, 1993.

384. Momberger NG, Smith J, Coleman DA. Vascularized fibular grafts for salvage reconstruction of clavicle nonunion. J Shoulder Elbow Surg 9(5):389-394, 2000.

385. Flinkkila T, Ristiniemi J, Lakovaara M, et al: Hook-plate fixation of unstable lateral clavicle fractures: A report on 63 patients. Acta Orthop 77(4):644-649, 2006.

386. Flinkkila T, Ristiniemi J, Hyvonen P, Hamalainen M: Surgical treatment of unstable fractures of the distal clavicle: A comparative study of Kirschner wire and clavicular hook plate fixation. Acta Orthop Scand 73(1):50-53, 2002.

387. Kashii M, Inui H, Yamamoto K: Surgical treatment of distal clavicle fractures using the clavicular hook plate. Clin Orthop Relat Res (447):158-164, 2006.

388. Nadarajah R, Mahaluxmivala J, Amin A, Goodier DW: Clavicular hook-plate: Complications of retaining the implant. Injury 36(5):681-683, 2005.

389. Tambe AD, Motkur P, Qamar A, et al: Fractures of the distal third of the clavicle treated by hook plating. Int Orthop 30(1):7-10, 2006.

390. Charity RM, Haidar SG, Ghosh S, Tillu AB: Fixation failure of the clavicular hook plate: A report of three cases. J Orthop Surg (Hong Kong) 14(3):333-335, 2006.

391. Harris RI, Wallace AL, Harper GD, et al: Structural properties of the intact and the reconstructed coracoclavicular ligament complex. Am J Sports Med 28:103-108, 2000.

BIBLIOGRAPHY

Andrews JR Wilk KE (eds): The Athlete's Shoulder. New York: Churchill Livingstone, 1994.

Baccarani G, Porcellini G, Brunetti E: Fractures of the coracoid process associated with fracture of the clavicle: A description of a rare case. Chir Organi Mov 78:49-51, 1993.

Ballmer FT, Gerber C: Coracoclavicular screw fixation for unstable fractures of the distal clavicle: A report of five cases. J Bone Joint Surg Br 73:291-294, 1991.

Bosch U, Skutek M, Peters G, Tscherne H: Extension osteotomy in malunited clavicular fractures. J Shoulder Elbow Surg 7:402-405, 1998.

Bronz G, Heim D, Posterla C: Die stabile Clavicula Osteosynthese. Unfallheilkunde 84:319-325, 1981.

Brunner U, Habermeyer P, Schweiberer L: Die Sonderstellung der lateralen Klavikulafraktur. Orthopade 21:163-171, 1992.

Campbell E, Howard WB, Breklund CW: Delayed brachial plexus palsy due to ununited fracture of the clavicle. JAMA 139:91-92, 1949.

Chez RA, Carlan S, Greenberg SL, Spellacy WN: Fractured clavicle is an unavoidable event. Am J Obstet Gynecol 171:797-798, 1994.

Coene LN: Mechanisms of brachial plexus lesions. Clin Neurol Neurosurg 95(suppl):S24-S29, 1993.

Connolly JF: Fracture and dislocations of the clavicle. J Musculoskel Med 9:135-148, 1992.

Connolly JF, Ganjianpour M: Thoracic outlet syndrome treated by double osteotomy of a clavicular malunion: A case report. J Bone Joint Surg Am 84:437-440, 2002.

Costa NC, Robbs JV: Nonpenetrating subclavian artery trauma. J Vasc Surg 8:71-75, 1988.

Danbrain R, Raphael B, Dhen A, Labeau J: Radiation osteitis of the clavicle following radiotherapy and radical neck dissection of head and neck cancer. Bull Group Int Rech Sci Stomatol Odontol 33:65-70, 1990.

Dameron TB Jr: External fixation of the clavicle for fractures or nonunion in adults [letter]. J Bone Joint Surg Am 71:1272, 1989.

Dannohl C, Meeder PJ, Weller S: Costoclavicular syndrome: A rare complication of clavicular fracture. Aktuelle Traumatol 18:149-151, 1988.

Dash UN, Handler D: A case of compression of subclavian vessels by a fractured clavicle treated by excision of the first rib. J Bone Joint Surg Am 42:798-801, 1960.

Dela Santo DR, Narakas AO: [Fractures of the clavicle and secondary lesions of the brachial plexus.] Z Unfallchir Versicherungsmed 85:58-65, 1992.

Dolin M: The operative treatment of midshaft clavicular nonunions [letter]. J Bone Joint Surg Am 68:634, 1986.

Domingo-Pech J: El enclavado a compresion de las fracturas de clavicula, con tornillo de esponjosa. Barcelona Quirurgica 15:500-520, 1971.

Finelli PF, Cardi JK: Seizure as a cause of fracture. Neurology 39:858-860, 1989.

Freeland A: Unstable adult midclavicular fracture. Orthopedics 13:1279-1281, 1990.

Freeman BJ, Feldman A, Mackinnon J: Go-cart injuries of the shoulder region. Injury 25:555-557, 1994.

Friedman RJ, Gordon L: False positive indium-111 white blood cell scan in enclosed clavicle fracture. J Orthop Trauma 2:151-153, 1988.

Goddard NJ, Stabler J, Albert JS: Atlanto-axial rotatory fixation in fracture of the clavicle: An association and a classification. J Bone Joint Surg Br 72:72-75, 1990.

Gonik B, Allan R, Sorab J: Objective evaluation of the shoulder dystocia phenomenon: Effect of maternal pelvic orientation on bone reduction. Obstet Gynecol 74:44-48, 1989.

Hackenbouch W, Ragazzoni P, Schwyzer K: Surgical treatment of lateral clavicular fracture with "clavicular hooked plate." Z Unfallchir Versicherungsmed 87:145-152, 1994.

Havet E, Duparc F, Tobenas-Dujardin AC, Muller JM, Delas B, Freger P. Vascular anatomical basis of clavicular non-union. Surg Radiol Anat 30(1):23-28, 2008.

Houston HE: An unusual complication of clavicular fracture. J Ky Med Assoc 75:170-171, 1977.

Jubel A, Andermahr J, Schiffer G, et al: Elastic stable intramedullary nailing of midclavicular fractures with a titanium nail. Clin Orthop Relat Res (408):279-285, 2003.

Kabak S, Halici M, Tuncel M, et al: Treatment of midclavicular nonunion: Comparison of dynamic compression plating and low-contact dynamic compression plating techniques. J Shoulder Elbow Surg 13(4):396-403, 2004.

Key JA, Conwell EH: The Management of Fractures, Dislocations, and Sprains, 2nd ed. St Louis: CV Mosby, 1937, p 437.

Kitsis CK, Marino AJ, Krikler SJ, Birch R: Late complications following clavicular fractures and their operative management. Injury 34(1):69-74, 2003.

Kohler A, Kach K, Platz A, et al: [Extended surgical indications in combined shoulder girdle fracture.] Z Unfallchir Versicherungsmed 85:140-144, 1992.

Kona J, Bosse NJ, Staeheli JW, Rosseau RL: Type II distal clavicle fractures: A retrospective review of surgical treatment. J Orthop Trauma 4:115-120, 1990.

Matsen FA III, Fu F, Hawkins RJ (eds): The Shoulder: A Balance of Mobility and Stability. Chicago: American Academy of Orthopaedic Surgeons, 1993.

Matsen FA, Lippitt SB, Sidles JA, Harryman DT (eds): Practical Evaluation and Management of the Shoulder. Philadelphia: WB Saunders, 1994.

Matz SO, Welliver PS, and Welliver DI: Brachial plexus neurapraxia complicating a comminuted clavicle fracture in a college football player: Case report and review of the literature. Am J Sports Med 17:581-583, 1989.

McKee MD, Wild LM, Schemitsch EH: Midshaft malunions of the clavicle. J Bone Joint Surg Am 85(5):790-797, 2003.

Niemeier U, Zimmermann HG: Die offene Marknagelung der Clavicula nach Kuntscher. Eine Alternative in der Behandlung alter Schlusselbeinbruche. Chirurg 61:464-466, 1990.

Meda PV, Machani B, Sinopidis C, et al: Clavicular hook plate for lateral end fractures: A prospective study. Injury 37(3):277-283, 2006.

Meyer M, Gast T, Raja S, et al: Accumulation in an acute fracture. Clin Nucl Med 19:13-14, 1994.

Moschiniski D, Baumann G, Linke R: Osteosynthesis of distal clavicle fracture with reabsorptive implant. Aktuelle Chir 27:33-35, 1992.

Naert PA, Chipchase LS, Krishnan J: Clavicular malunion with consequent impingement syndrome. J Shoulder Elbow Surg 7:548-550, 1998.

Neer CS II (ed): Shoulder Reconstruction. Philadelphia: WB Saunders, 1990.

Nordqvist A, Petersson C, Redlund-Johnell I: The natural course of lateral clavicle fracture. Acta Orthop Scand 64:87-91, 1993.

Oestreich AE: The lateral clavicle hook—an acquired as well as a congenital anomaly. Pediatr Radiol 11:147-150, 1981.

Olsen BS, Vaesel NT, Srjbjerg JO: Treatment of midshaft clavicle nonunion with plate fixation and autologous bone grafting. J Shoulder Elbow Surg 4:337-344, 1995.

Oppenheim WL, Davis A, Growdon WA, et al: Clavicle fractures in the newborn. Clin Orthop Relat Res (250):176-180, 1990.

Palarcik J: Clavicular fractures (group of patients treated in the Traumatologic Research Institute in 1986-1989). Cvech Med 14:184-190, 1991.

Pellard S, Moss L, Boyce JM, Brown MJ: Diagnostic dilemma of an atraumatic clavicle fracture following radical treatment for laryngeal carcinoma. J Laryngol Otol 119(12):1013-1014, 2005.

Post M: Current concepts in the treatment of fractures of the clavicle. Clin Orthop Relat Res (245):89-101, 1989.

Postacchini F, Gumina S, De SP, Albo F. Epidemiology of clavicle fractures. J Shoulder Elbow Surg 11(5):452-456, 2002.

Rockwood CA, Matsen FA III (eds): The Shoulder. Philadelphia: WB Saunders, 1990.

Rokito AS, Zuckerman JD, Shaari JM, et al: A comparison of nonoperative and operative treatment of type II distal clavicle fractures. Bull Hosp Jt Dis 61(1-2):32-39, 2002.

Sanders A, Rockwood CA Jr: Management of dislocations of both ends of the clavicle. J Bone Joint Surg Am 72:399-402, 1990.

Schwarz N, Hocker K: Osteosynthesis of irreducible fractures of the clavicle with 2.7 mm ASIF plates. J Trauma 33:179-183, 1992.

Stanley D, Norris SH: Recovery following fractures of the clavicle treated conservatively. Injury 19:162-164, 1988.

Steffelaar H, Heim V: Sekundäre Plattenosteosynthesen an der Clavicula. Arch Orthop Unfallchir 79:75-82, 1974.

Tarar MN, Quaba AA: An adipofascial turnover flap for soft tissue cover around the clavicle. Br J Plast Surg 48:161-164, 1995.

Taylor AR: Some observations on fractures of the clavicle. Proc R Soc Med 62:1037-1038, 1969.

Telford ED, Mottershead S: Pressure at the cervico-brachial junction: An operative and an anatomical study. J Bone Joint Surg Br 30:249-265, 1948.

Urist MR: Complete dislocation of the acromioclavicular joint. J Bone Joint Surg 28:813-837, 1946.

Wang SJ, Liang PL, Pai WN, et al: Experience in open reduction and internal fixation of mid shaft fractures of the clavicle. J Surg Assoc ROC 23:7-11, 1990.

Zlowodzki M, Zelle BA, Cole PA, et al: Treatment of acute midshaft clavicle fractures: Systematic review of 2144 fractures: On behalf of the Evidence-Based Orthopaedic Trauma Working Group. J Orthop Trauma 19(7):504-507, 2005.

Disorders of the Acromioclavicular Joint

David N. Collins, MD

In those cases where the acromion has been torn off, the bone which is thus separated appears prominent. The bone is the bond of connection between the clavicle and scapula, for in this respect the constitution of man is different from that of other animals.[1]

HIPPOCRATES

DEVELOPMENTAL ANATOMY

The clavicle and the scapula are joined together by ligamentous structures existing in two separate locations, one a diarthrodial joint and the other a space, partially occupied by a ligament.

Clavicle

As the sixth postgestation week approaches, the clavicle develops two centers of ossification for its body and becomes the first bone to ossify. In contrast to the other bones in the human body, which form from cartilaginous precursors, clavicle ossification evolves from a mesenchymal or precartilaginous stage, sometimes termed *membranous* or *dermal* bone.[2] Not present at birth, a secondary center of ossification appears in the medial end of the clavicle at 18 to 20 years with union to the remaining clavicle before 25 years. A similar ossification center both appearing and uniting in the 20th year at the lateral end of the clavicle was described by Todd and D'Errico.[3]

Acromion and Coracoid Processes

The acromion and coracoid processes are cartilaginous at birth. As many as three secondary ossification centers have been reported for the coracoid process, which phylogenetically is a separate bone.[2] These centers, as well as two for the acromion, appear between 13 and 16 years and typically unite to form a single bond between 14 and 20 years. Nonunions are possible at all sites, but are most commonly seen in the acromion (os acromiale).

ANATOMY AND FUNCTION

Overview

The human torso bears the upper limb by means of suspensory muscles to the scapula, clavicle, and humerus, maximizing the opportunity for movement. The muscles also serve as support for the sternoclavicular joint, the limb's only true articulation to the axial skeleton. The clavicle braces the upper limb at a fixed distance from the axial skeleton that permits optimal movement and power (Fig. 12-1). This is possible only through the clavicle's attachment to the scapula at the acromioclavicular joint and at the coracoid process via the coracoclavicular ligaments.

The acromioclavicular joint is said to be served by branches from the suprascapular, axillary, and pectoral nerves.[4] Its blood supply is derived from the acromial branch of the thoracoacromial artery, the posterior humeral circumflex artery, and the suprascapular (transverse scapular) artery. These vessels converge to form a smaller network (acromial rete) that overlies the acromion and penetrates the joint.[5]

Skin

The innervation of the skin overlying the distal clavicle, acromioclavicular joint, and acromion process is predominantly via the supraclavicular nerves, deriving from cervical roots C3 and C4.[6] From anterolateral to posterolateral, the coverage can overlap with the upper

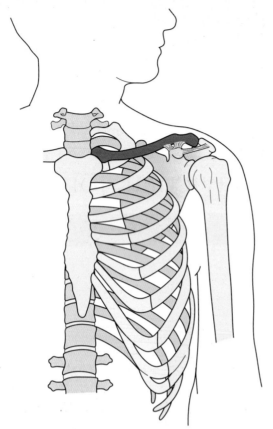

FIGURE 12-1 The clavicle functions as an intercalary strut between the axial skeleton and the upper limb via its interconnecting ligaments with the scapula.

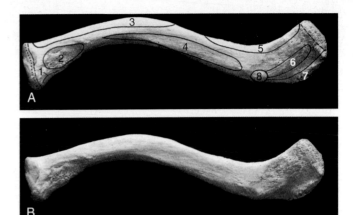

FIGURE 12-2 Osteology of the clavicle, from below. **A,** The attachments for the trapezoid (6) and the conoid (8) ligaments are outlined: 1, sternohyoid; 2, costal tuberosity; 3, pectoralis major; 4, subclavius; 5, deltoid; 7, trapezius muscle. **B,** The inferior aspect of the clavicle is shown. (Adapted from McMinn RMH, Hutchings RT: Color Atlas of Human Anatomy. Chicago: Year Book Medical Publishers, 1985, pp 93 and 94.)

lateral brachial cutaneous nerve, a branch of the axillary nerve derived from cervical root C5.

Muscle Attachments

The anterior head of the deltoid muscle originates from the anterosuperior, anterior, and anteroinferior aspects of the lateral clavicle; the acromioclavicular joint ligaments; and the anterior acromion process. The trapezius inserts onto the posterosuperior aspect of the lateral clavicle, the acromioclavicular joint ligaments, and the medial aspect of the acromion process. The actions of these two muscles contribute to the stability of the acromioclavicular joint and aid the suspension of the upper limb from the clavicle and the axial skeleton. The coracobrachialis and the short head of the biceps brachii originate from the tip of the coracoid process. Proximal and inferomedial to the tip is the insertion of the pectoralis minor. Although not in its immediate vicinity, other muscles, including the pectoralis major, sternocleidomastoid, levator scapulae, rhomboid major and minor, and serratus anterior, have significant action upon the acromioclavicular joint.

Pertinent Osteology

Distal Clavicle

The S-shaped clavicle tapers from being a cylindrical bone medially to a more-flattened bone laterally, where superior and inferior surfaces are distinguishable. The anterior portion of the lateral clavicle articulates with the acromion process of the scapula, hence the acromioclavicular joint. On its inferior surface, points of attachment for the coracoclavicular ligaments are delineated by a slightly prominent tubercle and a more subtle line for the conoid and trapezoid ligaments, respectively (Fig. 12-2).

Coracoid Process

Oriented superior, anterior, and lateral to the axis of the scapula, the coracoid process assumes a hooked shape as it projects from the superior body of the scapula. The coracoid attachments of the coracoacromial ligament as well as the conoid and the trapezoid ligaments, together sometimes referred to as the *coracoclavicular* ligament, though relatively constant in location, lack specific identifying osseous prominences. The distance separating the coracoid's superior aspect from the overlying clavicle's inferior aspect ranges from 1.1 to 1.3 cm.[7,8]

Acromion Process

A rather small, facet-like portion of the anterior medial aspect of the acromion process is the articulation area with the lateral clavicle. The acromial attachment of the coracoacromial ligament is without identifying prominence.[9,10]

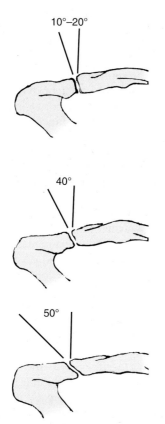

FIGURE 12-3 The sagittal plane orientation of the acromioclavicular joint shows great variability.

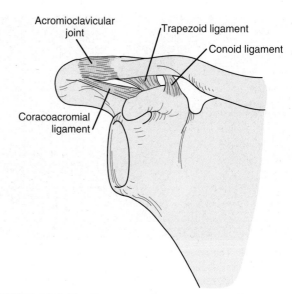

FIGURE 12-4 The ligamentous anatomy around the acromioclavicular joint.

Acromioclavicular Joint Architecture

The hyaline cartilage–covered convex lateral clavicle and the concave medial acromion articulate as a true diarthrodial joint. Whether it remains so throughout life is uncertain. Transitional changes of hyaline cartilage to fibrocartilage have been reported to occur on both sides of the joint between the second and third decades of life.[11]

The joint normally varies in size and shape with respect to adult age, gender, and skeletal morphology.[8,12] Likewise, the orientation of the sagittal plane of the joint is variable, ranging from nearly vertical to angulations from superior lateral to inferior medial approaching 50 degrees, a phenomenon that results in increasingly greater overriding of the lateral clavicle on the medial acromion (Fig. 12-3).[13,14] Although less common, angulations from superior medial to inferior lateral leading to underriding of the clavicle with respect to the acromion have also been reported.[15] It is not unusual for some degree of vertical incongruence of the acromioclavicular joint to exist in the complete absence of pathologic events.[14,16] The relatively lax joint capsule enables essential movement while resisting displacement of the acromion over the clavicle.

Intra-articular Disk

A fibrocartilaginous disk of variable shape and size separates the acromioclavicular joint, either partly (meniscoid)

or completely, into two halves. Although it is presumed to function in a manner similar to a meniscus in the knee (contributions to load distribution, joint stability, motion, and articular cartilage nourishment), its actual role is unknown. In younger patients, it is a structure potentially at risk for an acute injury, including contusion, tearing, or maceration. Structural and functional survival beyond the active years is unlikely as the disk succumbs to age-related degeneration.[17-19]

Ligaments

A relatively weak, thin capsule encloses the acromioclavicular joint. Distinct acromioclavicular ligaments, named by their location—anterior, posterior, superior, and inferior—augment the strength of the capsule.

The coracoclavicular ligament is actually two ligaments, the trapezoid and the conoid (Fig. 12-4). Despite their morphologic differences, the trapezoid and the conoid ligaments have similar dimensional, viscoelastic behavioral, and structural properties.[19-21]

Both ligaments attach to the superior aspect of the angular region of the coracoid process. From a more anterior and lateral site that begins at the angle of the coracoid, courses in the direction of its tip, and ends posterior to the pectoralis minor tendon attachment, the trapezoid ligament is oriented toward the clavicle in a superior, anterior, and slightly lateral direction to attach at the trapezoid line on the inferior clavicle. From a more posterior and medial site on the angle, the conoid ligament expands in circumference as it runs superiorly and slightly medially toward its point of insertion, the conoid tubercle. Here the lateral one third and medial two thirds of the clavicle join to form the posterior curve of the clavicle; at the curve's apex the conoid tubercle can be identified on the posteroinferior clavicle, just posterior

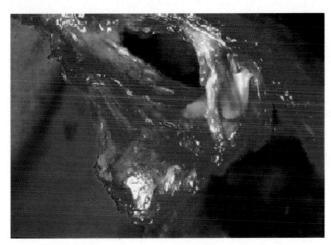

FIGURE 12-5 The coracoacromial ligament attachment to the superolateral aspect of the coracoid process. (From Fealy S, April EW, Khazzam M, et al: The coracoacromial ligament: Morphology and study of acromial enthesopathy. J Shoulder Elbow Surg 14[5]:542-548, 2005, Figure 1).

and medial to the most medial aspect of the trapezoid line (see Fig. 12-2).

Distal to the angle, on the lateral aspect of the more horizontal part of the coracoid is the attachment of the coracoacromial ligament (Fig. 12-5). It joins onto nearly the entire width of the acromion process at its antero-inferior edge.

Rios and colleagues showed that regardless of gender or race, the length of the clavicle can serve as a gauge to the determination of the anatomic attachments of the trapezoid and conoid ligaments.[22] Reliable anatomic points in osteology specimens and fresh specimens were used to measure to the center of the trapezoid ligament and the medial edge of the conoid ligament. The distance from the lateral edge of the clavicle to the respective ligament point of reference was measured and used to express a ratio of the measured distance to the clavicle length. This value was 0.17 for the trapezoid and 0.31 for the conoid. In another cadaver study, Renfree and colleagues determined that there were no gender differences for the measurement from the center of the articular surface to the lateralmost point of trapezoid ligament, but the lateralmost point of the conoid ligament was more medial in men than in women.[23]

By way of its attachments to the clavicle and scapula, and their respective relationship to the axial skeleton and torso, the coracoclavicular ligament helps to link scapulohumeral motion and scapulothoracic motion.[24-26] These two ligaments create a much stronger union of the clavicle to the scapula than the acromioclavicular ligaments. This ensures that the clavicle and scapula will move simultaneously as the acromioclavicular ligaments reach maximum tension, signifying the limits of the natural excursion of the acromioclavicular joint. The functional strength of the acromioclavicular joint increases in the presence of an intact coracoclavicular ligament.[14,27] Thus, the effective suspension of the upper limb from the torso via the sternoclavicular joint and supporting musculature is assured.

Although it is tempting to simplify the function of the acromioclavicular and coracoclavicular ligaments as anterior-to-posterior and superior-to-inferior stabilizers, respectively, displacement resistance of the lateral clavicle is significantly more complex, as borne out in the results of experimental cadaver investigations.[28-35] Not only are the ligaments distinguishable as discrete anatomic structures, the individual roles they play biomechanically is becoming more clear. Collectively, in the midst of a wide range of load, displacement, and restraint variables, these studies have shown that anterior restraint is afforded by the inferior acromioclavicular ligaments, posterior restraint predominantly by the superior and posterior acromioclavicular ligaments and the trapezoid ligament, superior restraint by the conoid ligament, and acromioclavicular joint compression restraint by the trapezoid ligament.[36]

Experimental sectioning of either the conoid or the trapezoid ligaments had no effect on the overall strength of the coracoclavicular ligament.[36] Complete dislocation of the lateral clavicle superior to the acromion process requires the interruption of the integrity of the conoid and the trapezoid ligaments (Fig. 12-6).[14,27,33-35,37] In an experimental study using a high-speed Instron machine and loading shoulders to failure, ligament disruptions were more common than fractures.[38] Age, height, and weight showed no significant relationship to the ligament cross-sectional area or the mechanical properties of the shoulder.

Coracoclavicular Articulation

Although lesser bursae can interdigitate between the layers of the conoid and trapezoid ligaments, a more prominent bursa can exist between the ligaments, sometimes sufficiently expanded to create a coracoclavicular joint between the coracoid process and the clavicle.[39] Twenty cases of such an articulation were documented by dissection or with radiographs in 1939.[40] The gross and histologic appearance is that of a diarthrodial joint with cartilage-covered articulating surfaces and a synovial-lined capsule and correlates with its radiographic properties (Fig. 12-7).[39,40-42] The incidence of this unusual shoulder articulation is probably around 0.5% but, depending upon geographic region, can vary widely from 0.04% to 27%, and it is often bilateral (Fig. 12-8).[43-53] The incidence appears to increase with age.[44] It can develop in response to restricted movement of the scapula caused by variations in the shapes of the scapulae, clavicles, and first ribs.[49]

Symptomatic coracoclavicular joints have been reported in the settings of osteoarthritis and rheumatoid arthritis, trauma, and thoracic outlet syndrome, but the overall clinical significance of the coracoclavicular joint is uncertain (Fig. 12-9).[50,54-56]

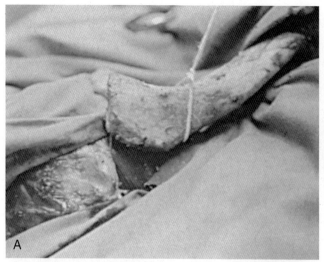

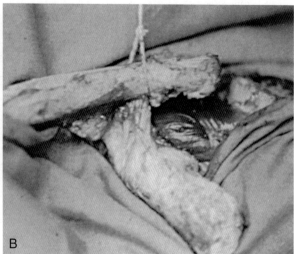

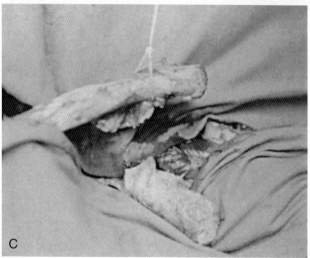

FIGURE 12-6 A fresh cadaver investigation of the stabilizing properties of the acromioclavicular ligament and the coracoclavicular ligaments. **A,** Even with the coracoclavicular ligaments intact, the clavicle can be displaced anterior and posterior to the acromion when the acromioclavicular joint, acromioclavicular ligaments, and surrounding muscles are removed. **B,** The coracoclavicular ligaments prevent significant superior displacement of the clavicle. **C,** Superior displacement of the clavicle occurs when the coracoclavicular ligaments are divided.

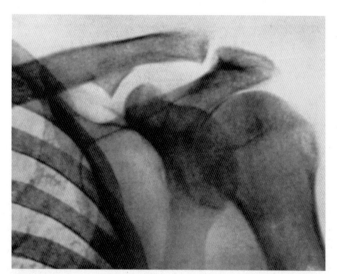

FIGURE 12-7 Coracoclavicular joint seen here as a modest prominence on the inferior clavicle just superior and medial to the coracoid process. (From Rockwood CA, Green DP [eds]: Fractures, 3 vols, 2nd ed. Philadelphia: JB Lippincott, 1984.)

Lehtinen and colleagues recognized resorption of the undersurface of the clavicle and believed it to be an atypical manifestation of rheumatoid arthritis involvement of the coracoclavicular joint.[55] Corticosteroid injection into the joint has been successfully used to treat a painful coracoclavicular articulation.[56] Surgical excision of the joint to resolve pain has been reported.[50,53,57]

EXCISION OF THE DISTAL CLAVICLE

Complete Excision

The surgical removal of the lateral clavicle is the definitive treatment for a multitude of disorders of the acromioclavicular joint. It seems that either Facassini or Morestin first performed the operation about a century ago.[27,58] Subsequently, it has been the subject of many investigations seeking to define the essential yet safe extent of excision. Nearly all recommendations that have been proposed, whether the technique is performed in the

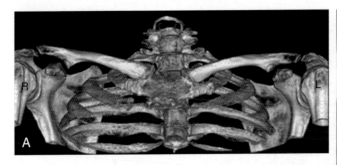

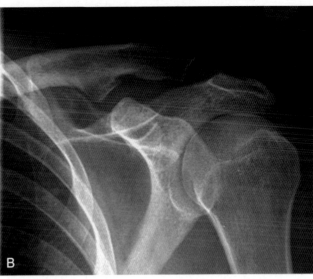

FIGURE 12-8 Coracoclavicular joint. **A,** 3D CT scan of shoulder girdles showing bilateral coracoclavicular joints. **B,** AP radiograph showing the coracoclavicular joint. (From Cheung TF, Boerboom AL, Wolf RF, Diercks RL: Asymptomatic coracoclavicular joint. J Bone Joint Surg Br 88[11]:1519-1520, 2006, Figures 1 and 2.)

traditional open manner or with an arthroscope, take into account the protection of the investing ligamentous support for the acromioclavicular joint and the coracoclavicular ligaments. By doing so, postresection instability that might contribute to discomfort and dysfunction is potentially minimized.

The recommended resection length varies from 0.5 to 2.5 cm. Although the precise amount to be excised in each instance is unknown, it would not be erroneous to suggest removing approximately 1 cm of the lateral clavicle.[59] However, this recommendation lacks a high level of evidence support from the literature.[60] Branch and colleagues suggested that 5 mm is adequate to prevent bony abutment in both rotationally and axially loaded shoulders if the coracoclavicular and acromioclavicular ligaments are intact.[61] Boehm and coworkers advised a resection of no greater than 0.8 cm in women and 1.0 cm in men based upon cadaver studies using magnification and microcalipers.[62] Exceeding the recommended amount consistently resulted in detachment of some portion of the trapezoid ligament. The anatomic study by Renfree and colleagues measured the distance from the center of the articular surface of the distal clavicle to the resected edge of the clavicle.[23] They concluded that resection of less than 11.0 mm should never violate any portion of the trapezoid ligament in 98% of men or women, and resection of less than 24.0 mm should never violate any of the conoid ligament. Resection of more than 7.6 mm of the distal clavicle in men and 5.2 mm in women, performed by an arthroscopic approach, can violate the superior acromioclavicular ligament.[23] Eskola showed that patients with a resection of more than 1.0 cm have more pain than patients with less than 1 cm resection.[63]

In a biomechanical cadaver study, Matthews and associates determined no significant differences in residual acromioclavicular joint stiffness and compressive contact between the acromion and the lateral clavicle when comparing mock 5-mm arthroscopic resection to 10-mm open resection.[64] In a clinical study, Kay and colleagues advised resection of 1.0 to 1.5 cm.[65]

In a cadaver study by Harris and coworkers, 15.3 mm was the average distance between the end of the clavicle and the most lateral fibers of the trapezoid ligament.[20] Rockwood observed cases with persistent pain after lateral clavicle excision that he attributed to inadequate resection and confirmed radiographically.[66] He recommended excision of at least 2 to 2.5 cm of the clavicle,

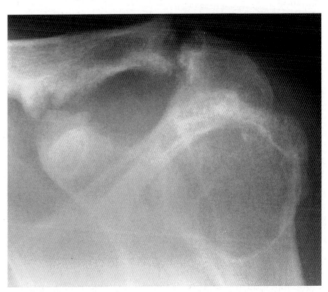

FIGURE 12-9 The coracoclavicular joint in a male patient with ankylosing spondylitis. Note the ipsilateral acromioclavicular joint.

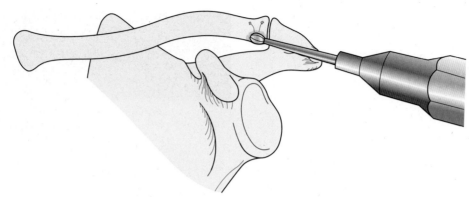

FIGURE 12-10 Demonstrated here is an arthroscopic method for coplaning the clavicle at the time of arthroscopic surgery in the subacromial space. Bone is only removed from the inferior part of the lateral clavicle.

acknowledging that resection to this extent sacrifices the majority of the trapezoid ligament but spares the conoid ligament so that the lateral clavicle remains stabilized. With open techniques for lateral clavicle excision, meticulous closure of the superior capsule and investing acromioclavicular ligaments is extremely important.[67]

Intraoperative ultrasonography has been used for verification of appropriate arthroscopic distal clavicle excision.[68]

Under experimental conditions, it was predicted that when the distal clavicle is resected, higher loads may be borne by the adjacent soft tissues.[69] In the same model, the intact surrounding soft tissues exerted a dampening effect with a reduction in the compressive loads across the acromioclavicular joint. In another study using cadavers, posterior translation of the clavicle was significantly reduced when the coracoacromial ligament was incorporated as an augment to the capsule repair performed at the time of open excision of the distal 1.0 cm of the distal clavicle.[70]

Partial Excision

Concern exists for the fate of the acromial stability at the time of open or arthroscopic subacromial decompression operations, especially when performed with coplaning of the acromioclavicular joint and distal clavicle. The inferior acromioclavicular ligament can extend as far as 10 mm lateral to the joint line.[71,72] In addition, the fibers of the medial-most coracoacromial ligament can be found intimate to the inferior acromioclavicular ligaments and capsule.[19,71,73] It has been shown experimentally that it is impossible to perform the standard subacromial decompression without violating the integrity of the inferior acromioclavicular ligaments on the acromion process.[71] Although the immediate effect in the experimental cadaver model is anteroposterior (AP) and superior compliance increased as much as 32%, in vivo factors such as ligament healing and muscle recovery can dampen the effect of acromioplasty and coplaning. In a cadaveric study by Edwards, coplaning the lateral clavicle together with

acromioplasty contributed to more joint laxity and translations of the lateral clavicle than did acromioplasty alone.[74]

According to studies with 4- to 7-year follow-up data, coplaning of the acromioclavicular joint at the time of arthroscopic subacromial decompression did not contribute to instability, pain, or further surgery at the acromioclavicular joint (Fig. 12-10).[75-79] Contrary to these reports, Fischer and colleagues reported increased osteoarthritis and instances of symptomatic acromioclavicular joint instability, some necessitating reoperation, and expressed their concerns with coplaning at the time of arthroscopic subacromial decompression.[80] This experience led to their recommendation for either resection or preservation of the entire lateral clavicle. Other authors have observed that arthroscopic subacromial decompression accompanied by coplaning or partial excision of the lateral clavicle can result in AP laxity and instability symptoms arising from the modified acromioclavicular joint.[72,81-83] Kuster and associates reported that arthroscopic subacromial decompression did not accelerate the development of osteoarthritic changes in the acromioclavicular joint.[72] The evidence from the literature is conflicting but suggests that coplaning can create or intensify symptoms arising from the acromioclavicular joint.[60]

Results of Excision

Rabalais and McCarty performed a systematic review confirming that the best level of evidence for the excision of the lateral clavicle is level III or level IV.[60] From their careful analysis and identification of low levels of evidence, they concluded that the method with the best results or fewest complications could not be determined. That stated, there is little argument that excision of the lateral clavicle successfully addresses the majority of the pathologic entities encountered at the acromioclavicular joint. However, there are unsatisfactory outcomes because of cosmesis, pain, and dysfunction that have at their root mechanical more than nonmechanical factors. The factors are often interrelated and include improper resection,

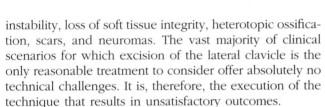

FIGURE 12-11 A proposed mechanism for painful instability after lateral clavicle excision is abutment of the remaining posterolateral clavicle against the posteromedial acromion (*arrow*).

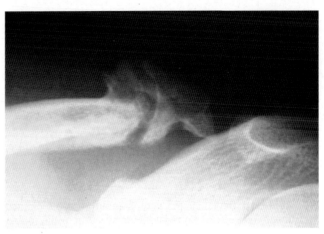

FIGURE 12-12 A more extreme example of heterotopic ossification, nearly complete restoration of the lateral clavicle, following open excision.

instability, loss of soft tissue integrity, heterotopic ossification, scars, and neuromas. The vast majority of clinical scenarios for which excision of the lateral clavicle is the only reasonable treatment to consider offer absolutely no technical challenges. It is, therefore, the execution of the technique that results in unsatisfactory outcomes.

In the orthopaedic literature, there are abundant citations of the results of lateral clavicle excision performed open.[63,84-97] The report by Rabalais and McCarty indicated 76.8% excellent and good results.[60] In the presence of worker's compensation or litigation, the results might not be as predictable.[89]

Arthroscopic excision of the distal clavicle was first described by Johnson in 1986.[98] Snyder and Esch and colleagues reported arthroscopic excision of the distal clavicle in 1988.[99,100] Numerous publications that describe the techniques and the results have followed.[59,65,100-118]

Two studies have compared the results of arthroscopic and open excision of the lateral clavicle with confirmation of the benefits of each method.[105,119] Flatow and coworkers reported earlier recovery of comfort with the arthroscopic method.[105] Freedman and colleagues, using validated outcome measurements tools, showed no significant differences at 1 year ,with the exception that the improvement in visual analogue scores from before surgery to 1 year postoperatively was significant for their arthroscopic group but not their open group.[119] With the arthroscopic method, there is opportunity to diagnose and treat intra-articular lesions.[120]

The direct, or superior, arthroscopic approach to the joint is reported less often than the bursal arthroscopic approach.[105,106] Although the direct approach can yield results similar to those of the bursal approach, a possible disadvantage is that it places the important superior stabilizing structures at risk.[113] Continued pain and instability in the AP plane have been reported after arthroscopic lateral clavicle excision, sometimes necessitating further reconstruction (Fig. 12-11).[80,81,113,115] Inadequate or uneven bone resection has been reported after arthroscopic

lateral clavicle resection.[103,105,108,112] The report by Rabalais and McCarty indicated 92.5% excellent and good results with arthroscopic lateral clavicle excision.[60]

Rabalais and McCarty analyzed level IV evidence reports of lateral clavicle excision performed in conjunction with other procedures and reported 94.7% excellent and good results.[60,65,112,114,116,121-123]

Heterotopic ossification and calcification can occur after an acromioclavicular joint injury or following the excision of the lateral clavicle.[84,85,114,116,124] Symptomatic ossification or calcification is quite uncommon, although it may be an offending lesion when the outcome of distal clavicle excision by either open or arthroscopic methods is not considered satisfactory (Fig. 12-12).[91,116,124] Patients at high risk for developing heterotopic ossification, such as those with previous history of the lesion or patients having either hypertrophic pulmonary osteoarthropathy or spondylitic arthropathy, may be candidates for pharmacologic prophylaxis.

It appears that lateral clavicle excision, regardless of method, following trauma to the acromioclavicular joint produces fewer excellent and good results than when it is performed for nontraumatic conditions.[60,89,90]

Author's Preferred Method

The patient is placed in the beach chair position with the head supported on an adjustable well-padded headrest to allow free access to the superior aspect of the shoulder. The skin incision is made in the relaxed skin tension lines approximately 1 cm medial to the acromioclavicular joint, extending for 3 to 4 cm (Fig. 12-13). A small straight Gelpi retractor is placed into the subcutaneous tissue, which is gently elevated from the underlying fascia.

Beginning 2.0 to 2.5 cm medial to the acromioclavicular joint, electrocautery is used to incise the soft tissue overlying the superior aspect of the clavicle (Fig. 12-14). The incision should be carefully placed to avoid the trapezius and deltoid muscles from their respective insertions. The

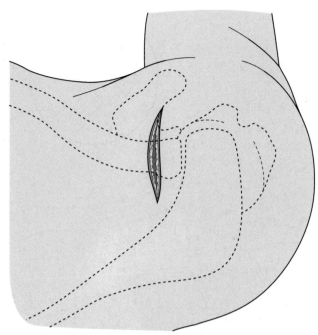

FIGURE 12-13 A superior incision in the relaxed skin tension lines is made slightly medial to the acromioclavicular joint for a distance of 3 to 4 cm.

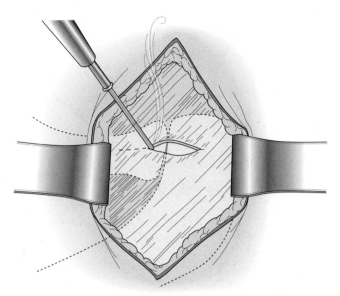

FIGURE 12-14 In line with the clavicle, the deltotrapezius fascia and underlying acromioclavicular joint capsule are divided and reflected from the distal clavicle.

incision is continued laterally through the capsule of the acromioclavicular joint onto the acromion process for a distance of approximately 0.5 to 1 cm. Subperiosteal dissection of the distal clavicle is carried out with electrocautery to create anterior and posterior soft tissue flaps that include the capsule, the superior ligaments of the acromioclavicular joint, and the adjacent muscles. Complete soft tissue dissection is confirmed with a 0.25-inch Key elevator enabling the placement of two small Chandler retractors bent to 90 degrees anterior and posterior to the distal clavicle. A length of 1.25 cm of the distal clavicle is measured, marked, and resected using a microsagittal saw (Fig. 12-15). The resected fragment is grasped with a towel clip or pointed bone-reduction forceps and manipulated to allow access for the release of the remaining soft tissue attachments inferiorly.

Upon removal of the completely resected lateral clavicle, the wound is thoroughly irrigated with normal saline by bulb-syringe technique. The resected clavicular surface is inspected, palpated, and smoothed, if needed, by using a pinecone bur, rasp, or file. Proliferative synovium and abnormal intra-articular disk material is excised. By placing a fingertip into the area of resection and performing extremity adduction, contact between the acromion and the residual distal clavicle is recognized and corrected by additional resection.

The surrounding soft tissues are infiltrated with a local anesthetic solution consisting of equal parts of 0.5% Marcaine with epinephrine and 1% lidocaine. With the medial subcutaneous flap retracted with a bent Army–Navy retractor, a 6-D Mayo trocar needle delivers No. 2 nonabsorbable suture through the anterior and posterior soft

tissue flaps (Fig. 12-16). No more than three sutures placed with a figure-of-eight technique are usually necessary. The sutures are tied with four throws to limit the likelihood of palpable and potentially painful knots beneath the skin at the surgical site. Leaving a small tag further reduces the possibility of palpable suture. For extremely thin patients, an absorbable suture is preferred. The subcutaneous tissue is closed with 2-0 absorbable suture using a buried technique, capturing the dermal layer to ensure excellent superficial soft tissue apposition. Strips of 0.5-in adhesive-backed paper tape cut in half are applied to the skin. A sterile dressing covers the wound and the arm is placed in a sling.

Patients are discouraged from active arm elevation without the assistance of the opposite limb for 3 to 4 weeks to protect the deep soft tissue repair. Heavy use

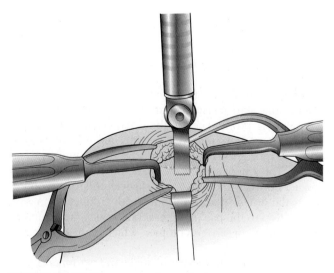

FIGURE 12-15 The surrounding soft tissues are protected as the lateral clavicle is excised with a microsagittal saw.

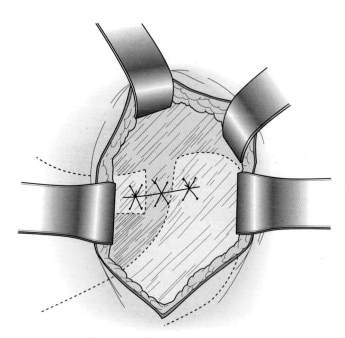

FIGURE 12-16 The residual defect is closed by careful repair of the deltotrapezius fascia and acromioclavicular joint capsule. No more than three sutures placed with a figure-of-eight technique are usually necessary. The sutures are tied with four throws to limit the likelihood of palpable and potentially painful knots beneath the skin at the surgical site. Leaving a small tag further reduces the possibility of palpable suture.

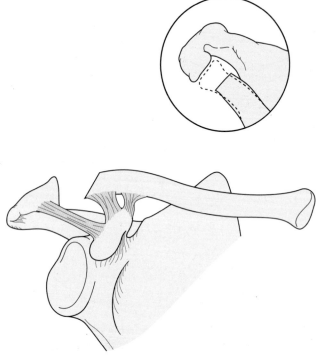

FIGURE 12-17 The plane of resection favors slightly more bone removal superiorly and posteriorly to prevent abutment of the acromion process on the clavicle during extremity adduction. (Adapted from Neer CS II: Shoulder reconstruction. Philadelphia: WB Saunders, 1990, p 435.)

of the extremity is not recommended for 6 to 8 weeks to ensure that sufficient preliminary healing of the acromioclavicular ligaments has taken place and that the residual void created at the time of distal clavicle resection has been filled with scar. Hydrotherapy to obtain range of motion is suitable as soon as the wound is dry. Return of full strength, range of motion, and full function can be expected in most cases by 12 weeks.

Technical Pearls and Pitfalls

Cosmetically unappealing scars may be avoided by carefully placing the incision in the relaxed skin tension lines.

Optimum and safe placement of the saw is enabled by placing the skin incision approximately 1 cm medial to the palpable prominence of the distal clavicle. The angle of resection favors removing slightly more bone superiorly and posteriorly than inferiorly and anteriorly (Fig. 12-17). This orientation of the plane of resection prevents contact between the remaining clavicle and the acromion when the arm is placed in cross-body adduction. A saw is preferred to the use of either a bur, which creates more bone debris, or an osteotome, which can shatter the bone.

The soft tissue sleeve that includes the acromioclavicular joint capsule and its supporting ligaments is carefully closed side to side without an attempt to obliterate the

dead space formed by the absence of the lateral clavicle. It is important that the repair suture engage the entirety of the reflected soft tissue, not just its most superior portion. This effectively reconstructs the superior acromioclavicular ligaments and capsule, which reduces the possibility of iatrogenic acromioclavicular instability. The temptation to create an interposition arthroplasty using the soft tissues adjacent to the joint should be resisted. Their relative immobility risks a closure under tension that can lead to dehiscence of the tissues at the repair site. Overtightening the trapezius or deltoid muscle at the resection site can contribute to focal discomfort. Likewise, an insufficient closure can be painful, cosmetically unappealing, and functionally compromising.

Heterotopic ossification can develop at the surgical site. Preventive measures include subperiosteal dissection with electrocautery rather than sharp or blunt elevation of the soft tissue from the bone, thorough irrigation of the surgical site to remove residual bone debris, and prophylactic administration of pharmacologic agents such as indomethacin.

Summary

Disorders of the distal clavicle that result from internal derangement of the acromioclavicular joint or irreversible deterioration of its articular surface can be effectively treated with excision of the distal clavicle through a limited open surgical approach. It is very important to carefully preserve the soft tissues contiguous with the joint capsule. A sufficient resection requires removal of no less than 1 cm and no more than 2.5 cm of the distal clavicle.

An anatomic approximation of the soft tissues at the time of closure will safeguard the horizontal stability of the acromioclavicular joint. Cosmesis is maintained through the use of proper skin incision orientation and by making no attempt to interpose a large volume of the adjacent soft tissues. Technical ease and swiftness of performance predictably resulting in favorable and durable outcomes are the hallmarks of this operation.

BIOMECHANICS OF ACROMIOCLAVICULAR MOTION

Based upon observations of patients with acromioclavicular joint arthrodesis, observations of the movement of pins drilled into the skeleton under certain conditions, and the data from investigational laboratory models, opinions vary with respect to the amounts and types of movement that takes place at the acromioclavicular joint. With upper limb elevation, Inman and associates recognized 20 degrees of acromioclavicular joint motion and 40 to 50 degrees of clavicle rotation.[25] Codman was the first to suggest that the motion was far less, around 5 degrees.[24] Caldwell's patients with acromioclavicular arthrodesis had excellent range of motion.[125] The studies of Kennedy and Cameron provided the initial description of the downward scapular rotation occurring in conjunction with upward rotation of the clavicle during upper limb elevation.[26,126] Codman's opinion was later supported by the investigations of Rockwood, who detected only 5

to 8 degrees of acromioclavicular joint motion (Fig. 12-18).[24,33-35] Rockwood surmised that in the presence of the diminutive amount of motion at the acromioclavicular joint, full or nearly full elevation of the upper limb was only possible with 40 to 50 degrees of upward rotation of the clavicle and by the simultaneous downward rotation of the scapula. He termed the phenomenon *synchronous scapuloclavicular* motion and acknowledged the earliest description by Codman and later by Kennedy and Cameron (Fig. 12-19).[24,26,126]

Recent studies have enabled a more complete understanding of the complex motion interactions of the upper limb, scapula, clavicle, and thorax and appear to have validated the conclusions of the pioneering investigators. As the upper limb raises, the clavicle elevates 11 to 15 degrees and retracts 15 to 29 degrees.[127] This motion is linked to the movement of the scapula by means of the acromioclavicular joint, the coracoclavicular ligaments, and the deltoid and trapezius muscles, whose attachments the two bones share. When the upper limb is elevated in the scapular plane, the scapula not only rotates 50 degrees upward but also tilts posteriorly 30 degrees around a medial–lateral axis and externally rotates 24 degrees around a vertical axis.[128] Sahara and colleagues performed a three-dimensional (3D) kinematic analysis of the acromioclavicular joint using magnetic resonance imaging (MRI) and observed that the scapula rotated 35 degrees on an axis that passed through the insertions of the acromioclavicular and coracoclavicular ligaments on the acromion and coracoid process, respectively.[129] They also showed that with abduction, the lateral clavicle translated 3.5 mm in the AP and 1 mm in the superior directions.

Changes in the position of the scapula with respect to the clavicle are accompanied by a subtle gliding motion

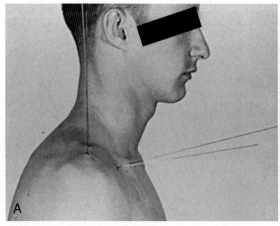
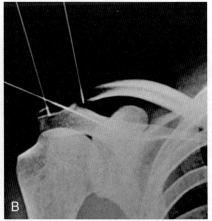

FIGURE 12-18 Pins have been drilled into this volunteer's clavicle, acromion, and coracoid process. Acromial and clavicle pin deviation with movement indicates acromioclavicular joint motion with a maximum of 8 degrees. **A,** Lateral view of a subject with normal shoulders. Pins have been drilled into the coracoid and clavicle and into the acromion process. **B,** Radiograph with the pins in place. When the patient puts his shoulder through a full range of motion, the maximal amount of motion that occurred in the acromioclavicular joint, as determined by deviation of the pins in the clavicle and in the acromion, was 8 degrees. (From Rockwood CA, Green DP [eds]: Fractures, 3 vols, 2nd ed. Philadelphia: JB Lippincott, 1984.)

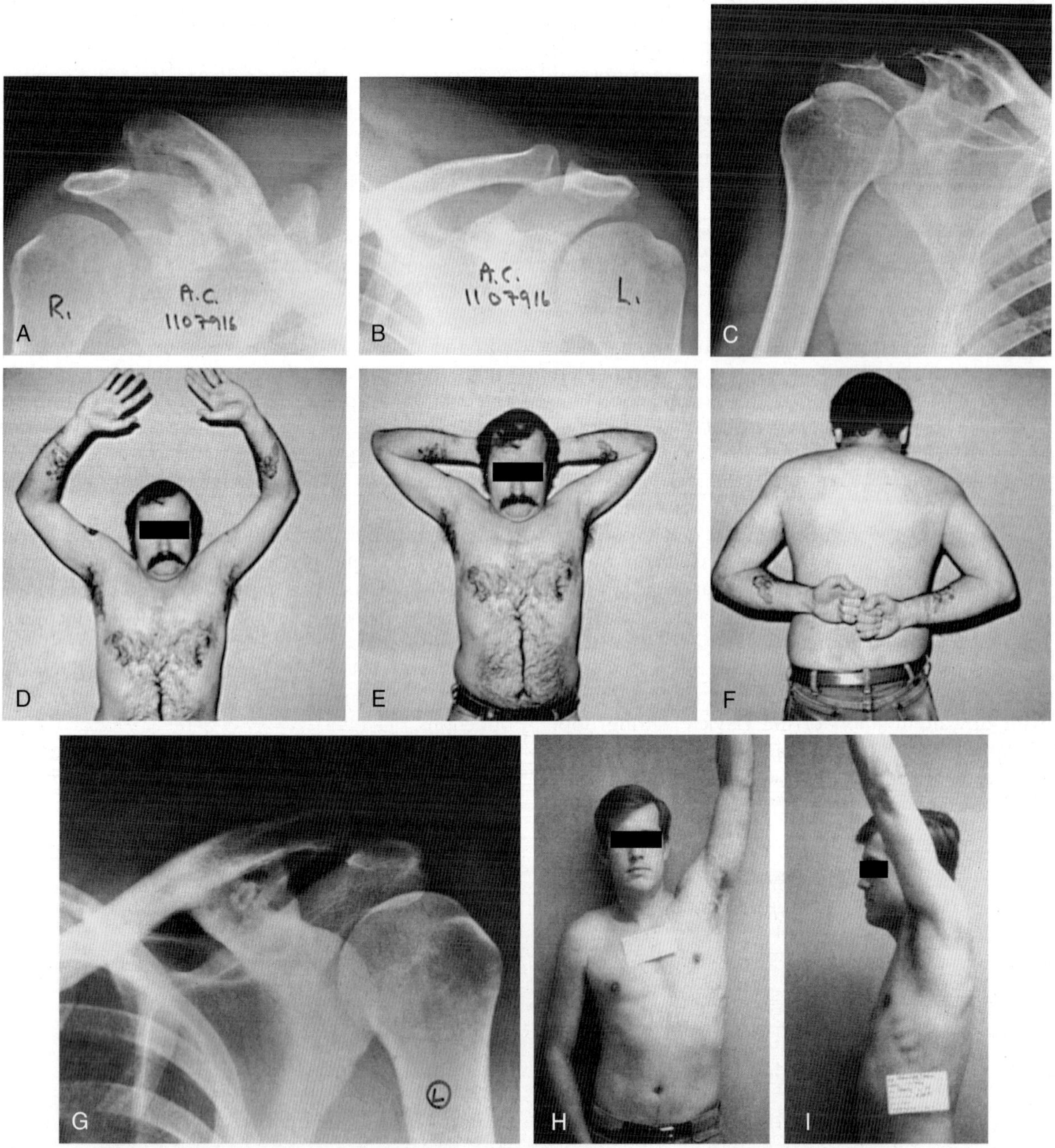

FIGURE 12-19 Motion limitations between the clavicle and scapula (coracoid process) induced either by natural or surgical phenomena have been shown to have no significant effect on range of motion of the upper limb, as shown in these examples. **A** to **F**, Post-traumatic heterotopic ossification essentially fusing the coracoclavicular interval. **G** to **I**, Post-traumatic heterotopic ossification essentially fusing the coracoclavicular interval in another patient.

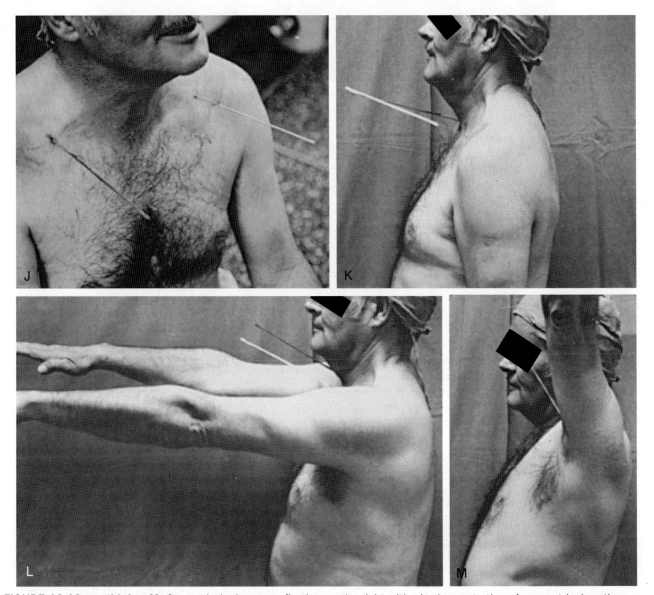

FIGURE 12-19, cont'd J to **M,** Coracoclavicular screw fixation on the right with pin demonstration of symmetrical motion.

Continued

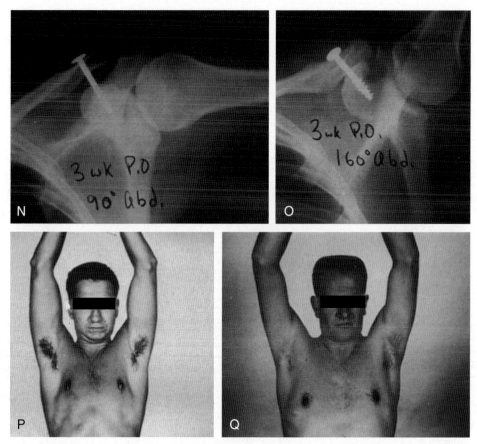

FIGURE 12-19, cont'd N to **Q,** Coracoclavicular screw fixation with symmetrical motion. (**J** to **Q,** From Rockwood CA, Green DP [eds]: Fractures, 3 vols, 2nd ed. Philadelphia: JB Lippincott, 1984.)

between the articular surfaces of the acromioclavicular joint and virtually undetectable motion through the coracoclavicular ligaments. Mazzocca and coworkers considered the mechanical coupling of the clavicle, the scapula, and upper limb elevation vital to upper limb motion and function.[130] They stated, "the acromioclavicular joint should not be fixed, either by fusion, joint-spanning hardware (screws, plates, pins) or by coracoclavicular screws. Motion will be lost, limiting shoulder function, or the hardware can fail."

SPECTRUM OF DISORDERS

The most prevalent disorder of the acromioclavicular joint is degenerative disease. From his classic studies of the aging shoulder, DePalma was able to determine that most persons experience acromioclavicular joint deterioration with advancing age.[131,132] His work revealed a pattern of age-related changes within the joint emerging as early as the third or fourth decade of life and increasing exponentially with time. The incidence in the shoulder is far less than in the hip or knee, but it is notable that the acromioclavicular joint is affected significantly more often than the glenohumeral joint.[133] These pathologic changes

of the joint are recognized radiographically as osteoarthritis.

The acromioclavicular joint is commonly involved with inflammatory arthritis, especially in the more-advanced stages.[134] Superior ascent of the humeral head associated with cuff-tear arthropathy and massive defects in the rotator cuff can erode the acromioclavicular joint, eventually leading to destruction of the joint, sometimes with the formation of large cysts that can mimic a soft tissue tumor.[135-137] Crystal arthropathy with acromioclavicular joint involvement and other forms acromioclavicular arthritis are uncommon. Infections of the acromioclavicular joint are uncommon, even when the general health of the patient is compromised.[138] Neoplasms, both benign and malignant, as well as proliferative disorders of the synovium very rarely affect the acromioclavicular joint.[139]

It is, however, trauma to the acromioclavicular joint and its environs that has garnered the greatest attention, as much due to its relative frequency of occurrence as to the quest to optimize recovery from the lesions thus produced. Evidence supporting this fact is found in literally hundreds of clinical and experimental investigations dealing with acromioclavicular joint trauma. The bulk of the remaining chapter, therefore, is devoted to this topic.

EVALUATION

This section focuses on the assessment of the atraumatic causes of acromioclavicular joint pain and dysfunction.

History

Pain is the most common symptom of an acromioclavicular joint disorder. Without prompting, nearly all patients point directly at the acromioclavicular joint or its vicinity when they begin to describe their symptoms However, the expression of acromioclavicular joint pain may be altogether different as reported in an interesting study by Gerber and colleagues.[140] Hypertonic saline injected into the acromioclavicular joint of otherwise asymptomatic volunteers resulted in variable pain patterns that included not only the acromioclavicular joint but also the area of the anterolateral deltoid, the suprascapular region including the trapezius and the supraspinatus, and the anterolateral aspect of the neck.

The positive value of pain diagrams for detecting and diagnosing acromioclavicular disorders was shown by Walton and colleagues.[141] For the patient exhibiting shoulder pain between the mid clavicle and the deltoid insertion with a positive Paxinos test (described under Physical Examination) and a positive bone scan for uptake at the acromioclavicular joint, the researchers were convinced that the diagnosis of acromioclavicular joint pain was "virtually certain."

Swelling or crepitus arising in or about the joint are not commonly mentioned by patients with a problematic acromioclavicular joint.

Physical Examination

With the patient either sitting or standing and the overlying clothing removed from both shoulders, the examiner looks for asymmetry: shoulder posture at rest, skin color, muscle bulk, and surface topography (Fig. 12-20). Both shoulders are examined for active motion, voluntary provocative maneuvers, skin temperature, tenderness, ligamentous laxity, passive motion, sensation, strength, circulation, and discriminatory maneuvers. The depth of examination of the cervical spine, remaining components of the shoulder girdle, and the upper limb is variable and determined individually.

Asymmetric tenderness well localized to the acromioclavicular joint indicts the acromioclavicular joint as the source of symptoms, especially if the pain so produced is essentially the same in character as the pain experienced by the patient. It is sometimes very difficult to confidently identify and successfully palpate the acromioclavicular joint when the patient is obese or very muscular. In these instances, it might prove helpful to reference the triangle formed by the clavicle, scapular spine and base of the neck. The acromioclavicular joint is directly anterior to an examining fingertip placed just medial to the acromion process at the lateral apex of the triangle (Fig. 12-21).

Several pain-exacerbating examination maneuvers that indicate acromioclavicular joint pathology have been described, including the cross-body adduction stress test, the acromioclavicular resisted-extension test, Buchberger test, the active compression test, and the Paxinos test.[141-145] With the cross-body adduction stress test, the examiner passively elevates the upper limb to 90 degrees in the sagittal plane and, with the elbow either extended or flexed slightly, moves the limb medially (Fig. 12-22).[144] The test is considered positive if it reproduces pain in or near the acromioclavicular joint.

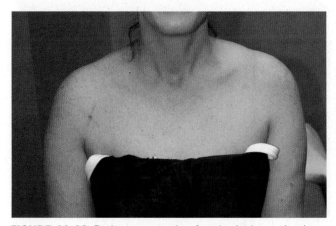

FIGURE 12-20 Patient preparation for physical examination requires unimpeded access to both shoulders.

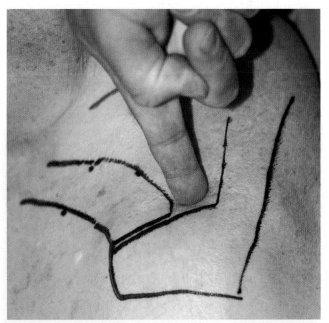

FIGURE 12-21 Surface landmarks helping to identify the acromioclavicular joint, which lies directly anterior to the soft spot at the apex of the isosceles triangle formed by the scapular spine, the clavicle, and the base of the neck.

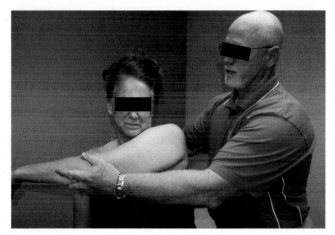

FIGURE 12-22 The cross-body adduction stress test is demonstrated here.

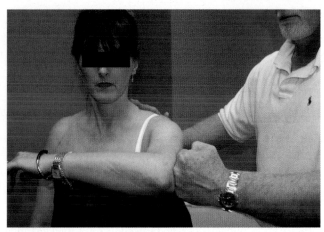

FIGURE 12-23 The acromioclavicular resisted-extension test is performed in this patient with shoulder pain.

The acromioclavicular resisted-extension test starts with the upper limb elevated 90 degrees in the sagittal plane, the elbow flexed to 90 degrees, and internal rotation to 90 degrees (Fig. 12-23).[143] With the examiner's hand fixed in space against the posterior elbow, the patient extends the shoulder in the transverse plane, meeting the examiner's resistance. The test is considered positive if pain is experienced in the acromioclavicular joint.

The Buchberger test combines inferiorly directed force to the lateral clavicle with passive forward elevation of the slightly adducted and externally rotated upper limb.[142] The test is considered positive if pain is invoked or intensified in or near the acromioclavicular joint. To perform the Paxinos test, the examiner places a thumb over the posterolateral acromion and the ipsilateral or contralateral index or long finger (or both) over the superior aspect of the mid-part of the clavicle.[141] Anterosuperior pressure is applied by the thumb while inferior pressure is applied to the acromion. The test is considered positive if pain is produced or intensified in the region of the acromioclavicular joint (Fig. 12-24).

The active compression test is begun by requesting the patient to fully extend the elbow and forward elevate the upper limb 90 degrees in the sagittal plane followed by 10 to 15 degrees medial to the sagittal plane (Fig. 12-25).[145] The thumb is pointed downward by full internal rotation of the shoulder and pronation of the forearm. An inferiorly directed force is applied to the upper limb thus positioned. The force is released, the forearm is fully supinated, and the force is reapplied. The test is considered positive if pain is produced with the first maneuver and reduced or eliminated with the second maneuver. Pain in or near the acromioclavicular joint indicates a problem of the acromioclavicular joint.

I learned the hug test from Douglas Harryman, II, MD, and Frederick A Matsen, III, MD, as an additional clinical tool for assessing the acromioclavicular joint (Fig. 12-26).[146] The examiner stands at a right angle to the patient's symptomatic side, reaches around the patient's shoulders, and locks both hands together. The hug is then performed, compressing both shoulders in the coronal plane between the examiner's chest and hands. The test is

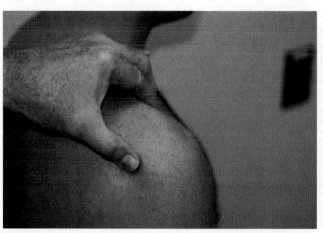

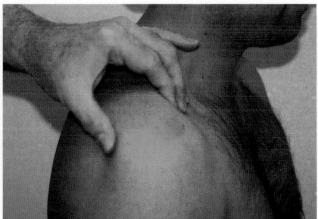

FIGURE 12-24 The Paxinos test. The thumb and finger are squeezed together. (From Walton J, Mahajan S, Paxinos A, et al: Diagnostic values of tests for acromioclavicular joint pain. J Bone Joint Surg Am 86[4]:807-812, 2004.)

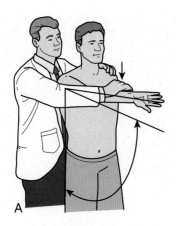

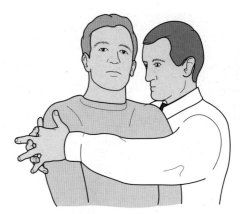

FIGURE 12-26 The hug test squeezes pain out of the affected acromioclavicular joint.

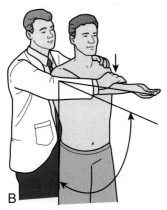

FIGURE 12-25 The active compression test. This two-step maneuver can help to distinguish between acromioclavicular joint and labral lesions. **A,** This maneuver may reproduce pain in the shoulder. Note a downward force being applied to the hyperpronated adducted limb, which has been raised to 90 degrees. **B,** This maneuver may reduce or eliminate shoulder pain. Note the limb in full supination. The test is considered positive if pain produced with maneuver one is reduced or eliminated with maneuver two. Both acromioclavicular joint and labral tears may be discerned by the location of the pain. (Adapted from O'Brien SJ, Pagnani MJ, Fealy S, et al: The active compression test: A new and effective test for diagnosing labral tears and acromioclavicular joint abnormality. Am J Sports Med 26:610-613, 1998.)

abnormality was the Paxinos test. Chronopoulos and coworkers analyzed patients with isolated chronic disorders of the acromioclavicular joint to determine the diagnostic value of physical examination provocative testing techniques.[148] The most sensitive test, the cross-body adduction test, was also the least accurate. The active compression test had the greatest specificity, the least sensitivity, and the most accuracy. The acromioclavicular resisted-extension was between the other two for all diagnostic values. Interestingly, provocative maneuvers described for other shoulder maladies (Neer impingement sign, Hawkins impingement sign, painful arc sign, drop arm sign and Speed's test, Jobe's sign, neck tenderness) are capable of inducing pain in patients with chronic lesions of the acromioclavicular joint.[147,148]

The response to local anesthesia instilled into the acromioclavicular joint can help identify the cause of shoulder pain.[141] This is especially true when provocative testing is performed both before and after the injection.

Despite the very superficial location of the acromioclavicular joint, its relative size, variable anatomy, and pathologic changes often confound arthrocentesis. Successful needle entry into the joint often lacks tactile confirmation (Fig. 12-27). Bisbinas and colleagues reported incorrect

considered positive if pain is produced or aggravated in or near the acromioclavicular joint closest to the examiner.

Maritz and Oosthuizen showed high sensitivity for acromioclavicular joint line tenderness and cross-body adduction stress testing.[147] O'Brien and associates determined that the active compression test exhibited high degree of accuracy (100% sensitive and 96.6% specific) for acromioclavicular joint lesions.[145]

In the study by Walton and colleagues, acromioclavicular joint tenderness to direct palpation had the greatest sensitivity for the detection of acromioclavicular joint disorder in patients with shoulder pain, followed by the Paxinos test.[141] They also reported that the most accurate clinical maneuver for detecting an acromioclavicular

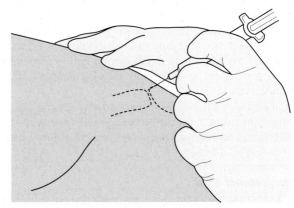

FIGURE 12-27 Even with vast experience, acromioclavicular joint injections are easier said than done.

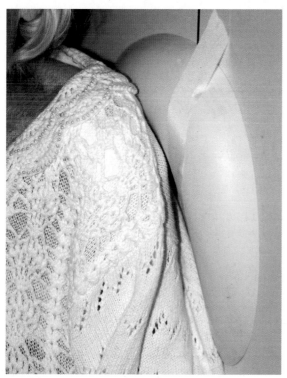

FIGURE 12-28 A type of x-ray filter used to improve visualization of the shoulder area is placed between the patient and the cassette to compensate for local variations in the soft tissue of the shoulder and the density of the proximal humerus.

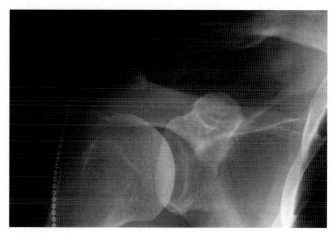

FIGURE 12-29 Over-penetrated (too dark) AP radiograph of a type III injury.

placement more than 60% of the time when orientation to the joint was obtained by palpation alone.[149] When accuracy of injection was deemed critical, they recommended using image guidance. In a cadaver study, acromioclavicular joint injection accuracy was 67%.[150]

Imaging

Plain Radiographs

Due to its composition of less-dense bone and its location in a region of the shoulder with relatively less soft tissue coverage, standard shoulder techniques must be altered to properly delineate the acromioclavicular joint. Depending upon the patient's stature or body habitus, a reduction of x-ray kilovoltage by as much as one half is sometimes necessary in order to gain optimal visualization of the acromioclavicular joint.[66,151]

In addition, a filter can be placed between the patient and the film cassette for further image enhancement (Fig. 12-28). Better techniques decrease the probability of misdiagnosis (Fig. 12-29).

Anteroposterior View

It is preferable to obtain this view with the patient either standing or sitting with the arms unsupported and neutrally positioned in the sagittal plane. Anatomic variations

and technical inconsistencies are effectively dealt with by imaging bilateral acromioclavicular joints simultaneously on a single cassette or on two smaller cassettes for wider patients (Fig. 12-30). A 10- to 15-degree cephalic tilt applied to the x-ray beam optimizes the image of the acromioclavicular joint by eliminating is superimposition on the posterior acromion and lateral scapular spine (Fig. 12-31).[151]

Dimensions and configuration are extremely variable, mandating a cautious approach to interpretation in the setting of injury.[14,152] Acromioclavicular width ranges from 0.5 mm to 7 mm.[151,153,154] The coracoclavicular interval ranges from 1.1 cm to 1.3 cm.[7,8]

Lateral Views

One of two views is selected: either an axillary lateral view or a scapular Y view. The axillary view offers an advantage for determining the anterior or, much more commonly, posterior displacement of the clavicle (Fig.

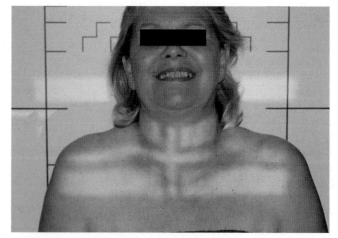

FIGURE 12-30 Positioning and technique for Zanca views. Both shoulders are imaged simultaneously on one or two cassettes, depending upon the width of the shoulders.

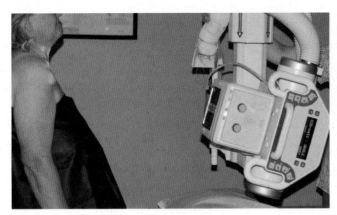

FIGURE 12-31 The Zanca view is taken with the x-ray directed 10 to 15 degrees cephalad.

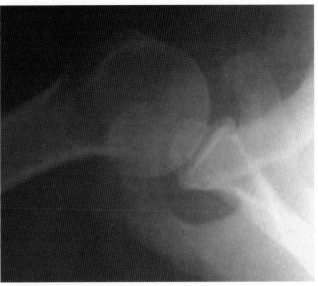

FIGURE 12-32 The axillary lateral view enables assessment for anterior or posterior displacement of the clavicle with respect to the acromion.

12-32). The scapular Y view highlights superior displacement of the clavicle, although posterior displacement can be demonstrated (Fig. 12-33).

Stress Views

It is sometimes possible to subject the acutely injured shoulder to an additional deforming stress as an aid to diagnosis. A radiograph obtained simultaneously with the stress maneuver often captures the critical information sought by the examiner (Fig. 12-34). Stress views can facilitate the diagnosis and characterization of the severity of an acromioclavicular dislocation, although some question their value.[155-157] In a survey of members of the American Shoulder and Elbow Surgeons, 94% responded; 81% indicated that they did not recommend the routine use of stress radiographs in the emergency department[157] and 57% did not use the views. Only 9% changed their treatment plan based upon the outcome of the views. The radiographic assessment for nontraumatic conditions of the acromioclavicular joint does not usually incorporate stress views.

Anteroposterior Stress Views. For standard AP stress views, the technical principles and patient positioning are unchanged from routine AP views of the acromioclavicular joint. Stress of 10 to 15 pounds is applied to both upper limbs while the patient is invited to relax as much as possible (Fig. 12-35). The method of weight attachment to the upper limb, hand-held versus wrist-suspended, might not be important.[158] It may be possible to ascertain avulsion of the anterior deltoid by other forms of stress application, but the accuracy of a weight-lifting view and its role in the routine assessment of suspected acromioclavicular dislocations has yet to be determined.[159]

Lateral Stress Views. It is possible to demonstrate pathological relationships between the acromion and the clavicle by using a shoulder-forward view, obtained like a scapular Y while the patient actively protracts the shoul-

der (Figs. 12-36 and 12-37).[160-162] Although it is anticipated that this stress will displace the acromion anterior and inferior to the clavicle, more comprehensive imaging may be necessary to properly define the severity of injury.[163]

Computed Tomography

The primary purpose of computed tomography (CT) is to obtain a more accurate assessment of the morphology of the distal clavicle, coracoid process, and acromion process and, to a lesser extent, their relationships to one another. It can aid in the analysis of complex injuries, fractures, neoplastic processes, or infections, especially when postprocessing 3D images are generated (see Fig. 12-8A).

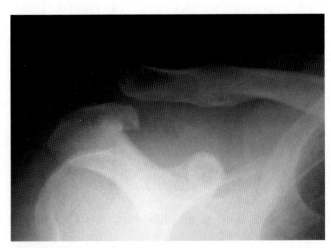

FIGURE 12-33 Scapular Y view showing superior displacement of the clavicle resulting from an injury.

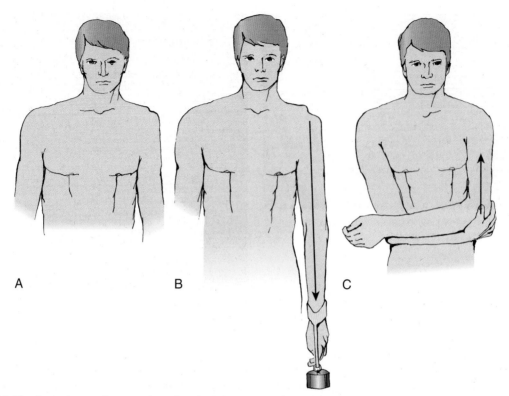

FIGURE 12-34 The importance of stress views for the injured acromioclavicular joint. **A,** Without stress, only mild deformity is observed, suggesting a less-severe injury. **B,** With stress, the deformity is increased, verifying the severity of injury. **C,** A radiograph obtained with the patient in the guarding position can appear normal; hence the rationale for the stress views. (From Rockwood CA, Green DP [eds]: Fractures, 3 vols, 2nd ed. Philadelphia: JB Lippincott, 1984.)

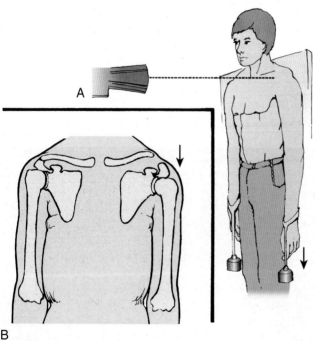

FIGURE 12-35 A and **B,** AP stress views.

Nuclear Medicine

When there are no other clues to a diagnosis in the presence of vague shoulder pain, bone scintigraphy is helpful to rule out an occult osseous lesion of the shoulder girdle. It is an excellent imaging tool to access semiacute injuries to the acromioclavicular joint and acromioclavicular joint arthropathy. The scan is positive when it demonstrates focal increased radioactive tracer uptake when compared to the uninjured contralateral side, especially if the plain radiographs demonstrate bilateral symmetrical acromioclavicular arthrosis (Fig. 12-38). It confirms the ongoing osseous activity in cases of osteolysis. Walton and associates found that bone scanning had a higher degree of accuracy for determining an acromioclavicular abnormality than did MRI or plain radiographs.[141] In this study, it had a higher predictive value (positive and negative) than did clinical testing or local anesthetic injections. Tc-99m leukocyte imaging has proved useful in instances of septic arthritis of the acromioclavicular joint.[164]

Magnetic Resonance Imaging

MRI effectively displays the pathologic changes that result from injuries and nontraumatic disorders that involve the acromioclavicular joint.[165,166] New MRI scan orientations for the acromioclavicular joint have been described and their utility confirmed in a report by Schaefer and col-

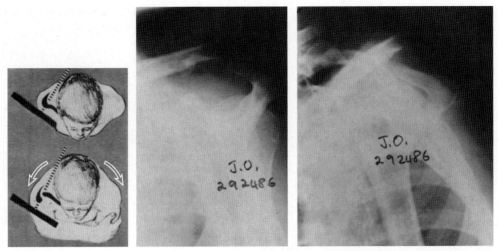

FIGURE 12-36 Lateral stress or Alexander views to assess for injury of the acromioclavicular joint. *Left,* The shoulders are thrust forward while the radiograph is taken. *Center,* Alexander view in the relaxed position. The acromioclavicular joint is only minimally displaced. *Right,* With the shoulders thrust forward, the acromion is displaced anteriorly and inferiorly under the distal end of the clavicle.

leagues.[167] However, plain films usually suffice and do so at significantly less expense.

MRI is the best imaging modality for assessing masses or cysts in the region of the acromioclavicular joint.[138,168,169] In that setting, it can delineate the internal characteristics, margins, and surrounding tissue response to the mass. Concomitant massive rotator cuff tears are identified in many instances.

The value of the routine use of MRI for the diagnosis and management of arthropathy of the acromioclavicular joint has been questioned.[171] One reason is because it is exceedingly rare that an MRI report for a patient with shoulder pain fails to mention an abnormality of the acromioclavicular joint due to its high sensitivity for detecting acromioclavicular abnormalities.[141,171,172] Another is that degenerative findings of the acromioclavicular joint are just as likely to be present in asymptomatic persons.[172] The importance of the clinical evaluation in the presence of this particular imaging abnormality cannot be overemphasized.

In the study by Walton and coworkers, MRI had a higher predictive value (positive and negative) than did clinical tests or local anesthetic injections.[141] It has been shown to be more sensitive for osteoarthritis than conventional radiography.[173] Fiorella and colleagues reported a 12.5% incidence of increased T2 signal in a series of shoulder MRI examinations and stated that it usually was of no clinical significance except in patients with chronic acromioclavicular pain and no other imaging abnormalities.[174] Increased T2 signal intensity representing edema is also a common finding in traumatic and arthropathic conditions of the acromioclavicular joint (Fig. 12-39).[174-176]

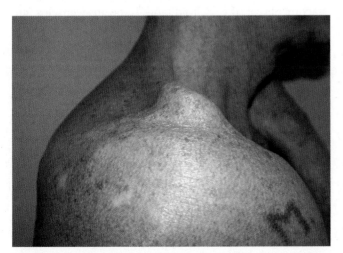

FIGURE 12-37 Clinical appearance of the lateral stress view.

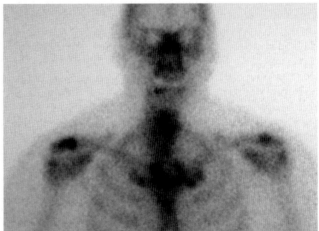

FIGURE 12-38 The two-hour delayed-image Tc-99m bone scan revealing intense uptake in the right acromioclavicular joint.

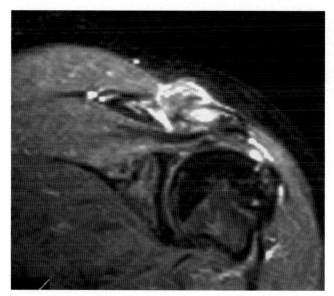

FIGURE 12-39 MRI showing increased T2 signal in the lateral clavicle.

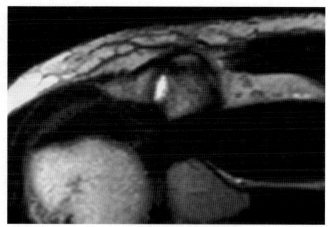

FIGURE 12-40 MRI showing fluid in the acromioclavicular joint.

MRIs of patients with symptomatic acromioclavicular joints are more likely to show edema in the distal clavicle and higher grades of osteoarthritis than in asymptomatic patients. Reactive bone edema in the distal clavicle, medial acromion, or both is a more reliable predictor of acromioclavicular pathology than are degenerative changes.[177] Fluid in the acromioclavicular joint is a common MRI finding in patients with shoulder problems (Fig. 12-40).[178] Advancing age, acromioclavicular joint osteophytes, and glenohumeral joint fluid are notable associated findings that suggest a relationship between acromioclavicular joint fluid and osteoarthritis.

With special techniques, the intra-articular disk may be distinguishable, when present, from the adjacent articular cartilage.[179]

Ultrasonography

Technologic advancements together with the expanding capabilities of ultrasonography have further stimulated an interest in applying this form of imaging to the acromioclavicular joint.[180-184] Its reliability for the injured acromioclavicular joint is well documented.[158,185-190] Heers and Hedtman have demonstrated the advantages of ultrasonography for determining the extent of injury to the deltoid and trapezius muscles and their common fascia.[191] They expressed concern that conventional sagittal plane radiography might have the limitations of either over- or underestimating the extent of soft tissue injury. A simple dynamic provocative maneuver performed with ultrasonography can aid in detecting lesser injuries to the acromioclavicular joint, such as type I injury.[192]

Blankstein and associates favored ultrasonography for assessing patients presenting with atraumatic anterior shoulder pain, citing less pain, negligible ionizing radiation, and the visualization of degenerative changes that can go undetected by conventional radiography.[193]

Ultrasonography has proven utility for diagnosing septic arthritis of the acromioclavicular joint.[194]

TRAUMATIC DISORDERS

Overview

As many as 40% of shoulder injuries involve the acromioclavicular joint.[195] Most injuries to the acromioclavicular joint and its environment are due to minor episodes of trauma that result in nothing more than contusions, minor strains, and sprains and from which full recovery is the norm. However, it is not infrequent that the events that result in injury to the acromioclavicular joint are of sufficient magnitude to damage adjacent soft tissue structures, especially if the conditions of the sustaining force are considered high energy. Under these circumstances, the acromioclavicular and coracoclavicular ligaments and the attachments of the deltoid and trapezius muscles are susceptible to partial or complete tearing or avulsion.

Acromioclavicular joint dislocations represent 12% of all dislocations of the shoulder girdle and 8% of all joint dislocations in the body.[196,197] In a Swedish urban population of nearly one quarter million, taking into account both sexes and all ages, acromioclavicular dislocations represented 4% of all shoulder injuries.[198] Dislocations were eight times more common in male subjects, and the prevalence was highest in the age group younger than 35 years, a finding observed in previous investigations.[93,199-203] Shoulder injuries often happen during alpine skiing, and around 20% affect the acromioclavicular joint.[204,205] In a prospective study of junior hockey players, acromioclavicular joint injuries were second only to facial lacerations in terms of frequency of injury.[206] A recent study of shoulder injuries in competitive rugby players documented a 32% incidence of acromioclavicular joint involvement.[207]

Associated Injuries

Potentially high forces risk damage to other structures in proximity to the acromioclavicular joint. Fractures of the ribs, scapula and clavicle as well as sternoclavicular dislocations and scapulothoracic dissociations have occurred.[66,208,209] Neurologic injuries that can include the brachial plexus are rarely associated with acromioclavicular injuries.[210,211] Pulmonary injuries have been reported.[212]

Classification

The extent and severity of injury to the interconnecting and surrounding soft tissues of the scapula and the clavicle (the acromioclavicular joint capsule with its intimate investing acromioclavicular ligaments and coracoclavicular ligaments and the deltoid and trapezius muscles) define the current and most widely accepted classification of acromioclavicular joint injuries. Zaricznyj suggests that the term *acromioclavicular dislocation* is an incomplete description of the most severe form of injury to the uniting structures of the two bones and that a complete separation of the two bones should be termed *scapuloclavicular dislocation*.[213]

Injuries to the acromioclavicular and coracoclavicular ligaments may be distinguished by the preservation or loss of the gross structural integrity of the ligaments. Incomplete injuries result in no or only slight elongation of the ligament fibers, and complete injuries tear the ligament fibers into at least two separate pieces.[27] By virtue of strength alone, the acromioclavicular ligaments are more vulnerable than the coracoclavicular ligaments. The lowest-energy injuries result in isolated damage to the acromioclavicular ligaments, and higher-energy injuries affect both the acromioclavicular and the coracoclavicular ligaments. The most-severe injuries produce damage to the deltoid and trapezius muscles or attachments. This phenomenon of sequential injury, first mentioned by Cadenat, became the fundamental principle upon which the earliest classification schemes were based.[27,214,215]

Incomplete injury to the acromioclavicular ligaments and no injury to the coracoclavicular ligaments was termed *type I*. Complete injury to the acromioclavicular ligaments with incomplete injury to the coracoclavicular ligaments was termed *type II*. Complete injury to both the acromioclavicular and coracoclavicular ligaments was termed *type III*. Bannister and colleagues and Rockwood astutely recognized certain injuries with displacement sufficiently severe to warrant strong consideration for surgery as the preferred method of treatment and proposed additional classification: type III subcategories A, B, and C by Bannister and separate types IV, V, and VI by Rockwood.[35,159,216] Rockwood's proposal gained widespread acceptance, and together with the original classification it encompassed injuries to the acromioclavicular joint in all recognized forms (Fig. 12-41). Type IV injuries are the result of posteriorly directed forces in which the clavicle

penetrates the trapezius muscle, sometimes completely through its substance. The clavicle in type V injuries is displaced superiorly but, because of disruption of the attachments of the deltoid and trapezius muscles, significantly more than in type III. Type VI injuries feature a clavicle displaced inferior to the acromion or the coracoid process.

Rockwood's classification represents an amalgamation of historical data derived from the analysis of plain and stress radiographs, anatomic dissections, cadaver experiments, and surgical observations infused with extensive, in-depth personal experience. On this basis, and rightly so, the pathoanatomy is often inferred, only to be resolved by direct visualization at the time of operative treatment or by means of more sophisticated imaging such as MRI and ultrasonography.[191,217] The latter concept was applied to four acutely injured patients, two uninjured patients, and one fresh frozen cadaver.[217] In two of the four injured patients, the type of injury based upon classic plain radiographic parameters and Rockwood's classification did not correlate with the pathoanatomy detected by MRI. However, confirmation of findings was only possible in one of the four patients who elected operative treatment. It is intriguing to contemplate the impact of similar investigations with expanded databases upon the classification of these injuries.[191]

Mechanism of Injury

Although any number of physical events may be responsible for an injury, the mechanism of injury is a product of forces characterized by direction, magnitude, and point of application.

Direct

The most common mechanism for injury to the acromioclavicular joint is a direct force that is applied to the superior aspect of the acromion process such as would occur with a fall onto the outer aspect of the shoulder with the upper limb in an adducted position (Fig. 12-42). A falling object or a deliberate blow striking the superior acromion is a rarer mechanism of direct injury.

The acromioclavicular ligaments offer the weakest resistance to the forces that push the acromion inferiorly and medially; stronger resistance is afforded by the intact clavicle and sternoclavicular joint.[218,219] Although isolated injuries are most common, acromioclavicular injuries that occur in conjunction with clavicle fractures or sternoclavicular joint injuries have been reported.[209,220-228] More often, these two structures are spared as the force advances through the acromioclavicular joint to act upon the coracoclavicular ligaments. This is an extremely strong buffer, but should its integrity be overcome, any remaining forces are likely to be dissipated at the attachment sites of the deltoid and trapezius muscle.

An inferiorly directed force acting upon the superior lateral clavicle can cause more damage when the upper limb is abducted and the scapula is retracted and can

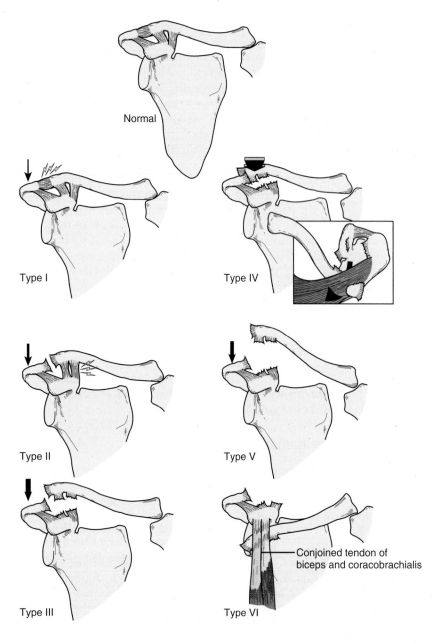

FIGURE 12-41 Classification of ligamentous injuries to the acromioclavicular joint. *Type I,* The acromioclavicular and the coracoclavicular ligaments are intact. *Type II,* The acromioclavicular ligaments are completely torn, but the coracoclavicular ligaments remain intact. *Type III,* The acromioclavicular and coracoclavicular ligaments are disrupted. *Type IV,* The acromioclavicular and coracoclavicular ligaments are disrupted, and the distal end of the clavicle is displaced posteriorly into or through the trapezius muscle. *Type V,* The acromioclavicular and coracoclavicular ligaments are completely torn, and due to the severity of injury, the deltoid and trapezius muscles are detached from the distal clavicle. *Type VI,* The acromioclavicular and coracoclavicular ligaments are completely torn and there is inferior displacement of the clavicle beneath the coracoid process.

result in an inferior dislocation of the clavicle beneath the coracoid process.[229,230]

Indirect

Indirect mechanisms of acromioclavicular joint injury are exceedingly rare. A fall onto the adducted upper limb is apt to drive the humeral head into the inferior aspect of the acromion, subjecting the acromioclavicular joint to variable degrees of injury (Fig. 12-43). The integrity of the acromion process and glenohumeral stability is risked when extremely high superiorly directed forces are encountered. The acromioclavicular joint may be injured by pulling or traction-like forces applied to the upper limb.[48]

Acute Lesions

Type I
Signs and Symptoms

Mild pain is well localized to the acromioclavicular joint and may be aggravated by movement or maneuvers that load the upper limb. Although the acromioclavicular joint may be slightly swollen, the shoulders are not unusually asymmetric in appearance. Active motion through a full range is sometimes hindered due to pain. Tenderness to some degree is appreciated at the acromioclavicular joint but not overlying the coracoclavicular ligaments. Palpable deformity of the joint is not present.

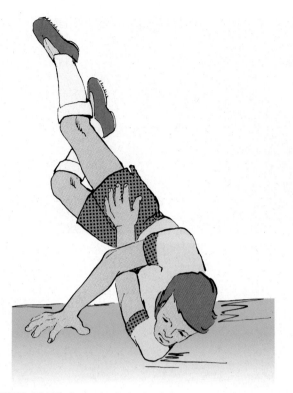

FIGURE 12-42 Acromioclavicular joint injuries most often result from a fall directly onto the point of the shoulder. (From Rockwood CA, Green DP [eds]: Fractures, 3 vols, 2nd ed. Philadelphia: JB Lippincott, 1984.)

Imaging

Sometimes the plain films demonstrate mild soft tissue swelling that accompanies type I injuries. Otherwise, the acromioclavicular joint appears normal and exhibits symmetry to the uninjured shoulder.

Pathoanatomy

The acromioclavicular ligaments sustain a mild to moderate sprain, maintaining the acromioclavicular joint integrity. The coracoclavicular ligaments and the deltoid and trapezius muscles are normal.

Treatment

Virtually all type I injuries should be treated without surgery.[66,214,215,231-242]

Methods. A sling or immobilizer for the upper limb helps to place the shoulder at rest. In the first 24 hours, cryotherapy can help reduce pain and swelling. Non-narcotic analgesics are usually adequate for successful pain management. As pain subsides, motion quickly recovers and external support is discontinued. Although formal physical therapy is usually not necessary, some authors have advised muscle rehabilitation.[243] Participation in contact or collision activities is best avoided until motion has fully recovered, tenderness has disappeared, and manual muscle testing is not painful.

FIGURE 12-43 An indirect mechanism of injury that might occur from a fall onto the adducted upper limb results in complete tearing of the acromioclavicular ligaments while preserving the integrity of the coracoclavicular ligaments. (From Rockwood CA, Green DP [eds]: Fractures, 3 vols, 2nd ed. Philadelphia: JB Lippincott, 1984.)

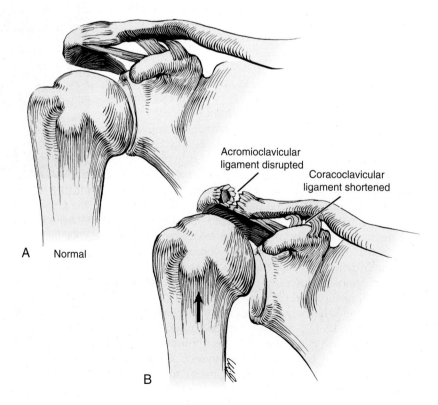

Acromioclavicular ligament disrupted

Coracoclavicular ligament shortened

A   Normal

B

Results. Full recovery of comfort and function is expected for type I injuries treated nonoperatively. This was confirmed in the report by Babe and coworkers[244] On occasion, symptoms are reported anywhere from 6 months to 5 years following injury.[245] More than 90% of the time, the symptoms remain insignificant or reasonably well tolerated.[245,246] Shaw and colleagues determined that patients receiving nonoperative care for type I injuries could expect symptoms to resolve, in most cases, by 12 months.[247] Patients with symptoms at 6 months correlated with those who were symptomatic beyond 1 year.

Mouhsine and associates found a higher incidence of unfavorable outcomes and were concerned that adverse outcomes were underestimated.[235] In their study, operative treatment was necessary in 13% of type I injuries.

Complications. It is possible but quite unlikely that posttraumatic arthrosis would appear following a single type I injury. However, degenerative changes of the acromioclavicular joint were reported in 56% of patients following a type I injury in the study by Mouhsine and colleagues.[235] In some instances degeneration was accompanied by pain and necessitated a reduction in activity. Rarely, osteolysis of the distal clavicle develops as a late phenomenon after this type of injury.[248]

Author's Preferred Method

The patient wears an upper limb sling as long as necessary to provide comfort and protection. Cryotherapy and non-narcotic analgesics are preferred for pain management. Motion recovery is accelerated according to the level of pain. Resolution of acromioclavicular joint tenderness and full, painless range of motion signal complete healing and return to unrestricted activities.

Type II

Signs and Symptoms

Significant pain is present both at rest and with attempted movement of the upper limb. Loss of functional range of motion is an accompanying complaint.

The shoulders might have an asymmetric appearance with slight superior prominence of the distal clavicle. Depending on the interval from injury, ecchymosis in the vicinity of the acromioclavicular joint may be present. Pain limits both active and passive range of motion as well as strength. The acromioclavicular joint may be exquisitely tender, inhibiting reliable instability testing that might otherwise be positive for excessive excursion only in the AP plane. This can be demonstrated with a two-hand maneuver: With the clavicle and the acromion in grasp, opposing forces in the AP plane are applied to each bone, resulting in excessive movement of one with respect to the other when compared to the contralateral shoulder (Fig. 12-44). A subtle rebound phenomenon of the lateral clavicle can result from the application of light inferiorly directed pressure to the superior aspect of the lateral clavicle. Coracoclavicular ligament tenderness is present.

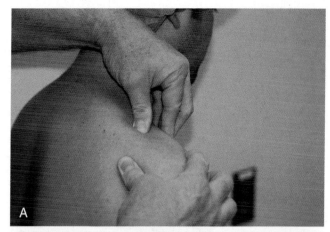
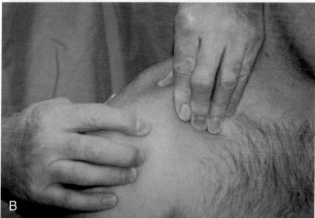
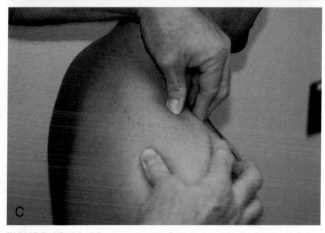

FIGURE 12-44 AP stress test of the acromioclavicular joint. The clavicle is held as stationary as possible (**A**) while straight anterior (**B**) and posterior (**C**) stresses are sequentially applied to the acromion process.

Imaging

Plain films can demonstrate subtle differences from the opposite, uninjured shoulder. The acromioclavicular joint may be widened and have a slight incongruence resulting from the superior displacement of the lateral clavicle. The coracoclavicular interval is normal and remains so when stress is applied (Fig. 12-45).

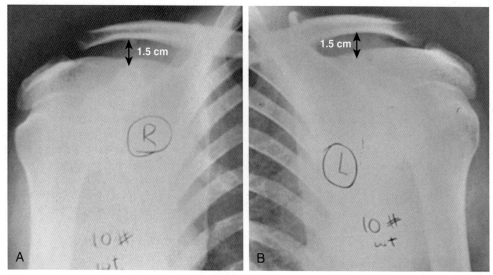

FIGURE 12-45 X-ray appearance of a type II injury to the right shoulder. With stress radiographs, the coracoclavicular distance in both shoulders (**A** and **B**) measures 1.5 cm. However, the injured right shoulder (**A**) has a widened acromioclavicular joint in comparison to the normal left shoulder (**B**).

Pathoanatomy

The acromioclavicular ligaments are completely torn, resulting in disruption of the acromioclavicular joint. The joint widens in the transverse and, less often, coronal planes. The coracoclavicular ligament sustains a mild or moderate sprain that can result in slight widening of the coracoclavicular interval. The deltoid and trapezius muscles are susceptible to partial detachment from the lateral clavicle.

Treatment

Nonoperative treatment is preferred for type II injuries.[66,197,231,233-240,242,246]

Methods. The same fundamental methods for treating a type I injury are used for a type II injury. A sling or immobilizer for the upper limb helps to place the shoulder at rest. In the first 24 hours, cryotherapy can help reduce pain and swelling. Non-narcotic analgesics are usually adequate for successful pain management. As pain subsides, motion quickly recovers and external support is discontinued. Although formal physical therapy is usually not necessary, some authors have advised muscle rehabilitation.[243] Participation in contact or collision activities is best avoided until motion has fully recovered, tenderness has disappeared, and manual muscle testing is not painful. This is usually a bit longer for type II injuries and can require 6 weeks or more.

Some authors have been tempted to treat the deformity associated with type II injuries. These methods use the concept of opposing forces applied to the clavicle and the acromion in a manner that theoretically reduces the subluxation and sustains the congruity of the acromioclavicular joint until healing has been completed. Nearly 40 different methods have been described, all with limitations that include noncompliance, skin breakdown, and loss of reduction.[14,214,249,250] Most authors have abandoned an active form of nonoperative treatment in favor of a simple sling that is worn for a short time. At the risk of further, more serious injury while the ligaments heal, it is generally recommended that forceful maneuvers with the upper limb as well as contact or collision activities be avoided for up to 12 weeks.

Results. Shaw and coworkers determined that patients receiving nonoperative care for type II injuries could expect symptoms to resolve, in most cases, by 12 months.[247] Patients with symptoms at 6 months correlated with those who were symptomatic beyond 1 year.

Even with slight degrees of incongruence of the acromioclavicular joint, full recovery with return to their pre-injury status is expected in most cases.[233,251] Sometimes, however, despite ligament healing, discomfort and dysfunction linger unexpectedly long after the acute event, which is attributable to residual instability, infolded capsule, articular cartilage injury, meniscal injury, residual joint incongruity, and repetitive residual trauma.[237,245,246,252-257]

Weakness has been reported.[253] Factors that can contribute to persistent symptoms include post-traumatic lateral clavicle osteolysis, intra-articular soft tissue entrapment, free-floating chondral or osteochondral bodies, and an unstable intra-articular disk.[221,255,258]

Complications. Reinjuries that occur before the ligament is completely healed can unexpectedly convert a type II into a type III injury. Skin breakdown beneath immobilizing devices forces abandonment of type II injury treatment while the integument heals.

Acromioclavicular joint incongruence, especially in the setting of extreme use, can precipitate symptomatic arthrosis. Such degenerative changes (arthrosis and osteolysis) of the joint been reported with an incidence as high as 70% (Fig. 12-46).[248,258,259]

Author's Preferred Method

Nonoperative treatment is directed toward effective pain management by means of a sling, cryotherapy, and narcotic analgesics. This can require 1 to 2 weeks. Pool therapy is encouraged and hastens the recovery of active, pain-free movement. Once motion fully recovers and tenderness abates, strength rehabilitation is initiated. Forceful use and contact and collision activities are avoided for 12 weeks.

Type III
Signs and Symptoms

The patient has moderate to severe shoulder pain. Pain is not only localized to the acromioclavicular joint but also can emanate from the coracoclavicular and periscapular regions. Motion, either active or passive, in any direction and to any degree exacerbates the pain. Neurologic symptoms are very rare.

The patient appears acutely injured, often with the affected upper limb postured in a protective and stress-relieving manner: supported higher than usual by the opposite hand and arm and braced against the torso. The soft tissue overlying the acromion may be abraded or contused. Ecchymosis might or might not be present. The lateral clavicle is prominent beneath the skin, and the remaining shoulder has a drooped appearance (Fig. 12-47). The clavicles remain relatively level while the weight of the upper limb displaces the clavicle inferiorly (Fig. 12-48).

Motion and strength assessment are unreliable due to pain. Tenderness is more diffuse: acromioclavicular joint, distal clavicle, coracoclavicular region. Pain permitting, global instability of the clavicle is demonstrable. With the clavicle stabilized by one hand, it may be possible to

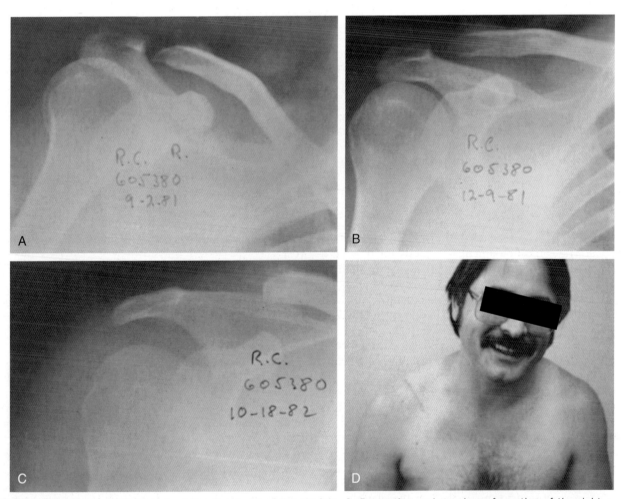

FIGURE 12-46 Traumatic osteolysis of the distal end of the clavicle. **A,** Resorption and new bone formation of the right distal clavicle 3 months after injury. **B,** By 6 months, increasing pain was accompanied by further resorption and new bone formation. **C,** At 14 months, 2.5 cm of the lateral clavicle was excised. Stability was maintained by the conoid ligament. **D,** Skin incision in Langer's lines. (From Rockwood CA, Green DP [eds]: Fractures, 3 vols, 2nd ed. Philadelphia: JB Lippincott, 1984.)

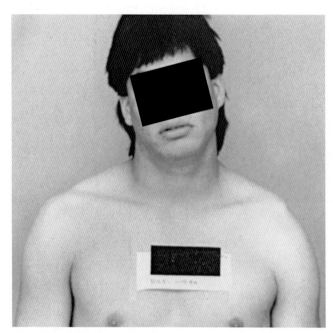

FIGURE 12-47 This type III injury results in an uneven appearance to the shoulders. The injured left shoulder assumes a drooped attitude with respect to the uninjured right shoulder.

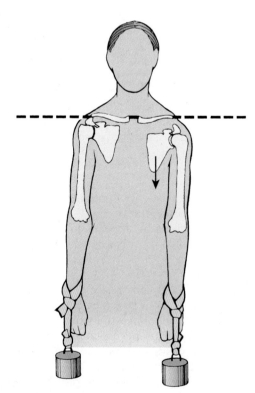

FIGURE 12-48 The type III injury results in deformity due to the downward displacement of the acromion process together with the upper limb, *not* due to superior displacement of the clavicle.

reduce or nearly reduce the dislocated acromioclavicular joint by placing the other hand beneath the flexed elbow and applying a superiorly directed force sufficient to often completely obliterate the visible deformity. The deformity returns when the force is removed.

Imaging

The acromioclavicular joint is incongruent from widening and at least 50% contact loss between the acromion and the clavicle.[215] In the majority of type III injuries, there is no contact between the articular surfaces of the lateral clavicle and the medial acromion. The coracoclavicular interval is widened 20% to 100% (Fig. 12-49).[7,66,216] Stress views are occasionally necessary and demonstrate similar findings (Fig. 12-50).

Pathoanatomy

The acromioclavicular and coracoclavicular ligaments are torn completely, resulting in dislocation of the acromioclavicular joint. In comparison to the normal shoulder, the coracoclavicular interval may be widened by up to 100%. There is a high probability that deltoid and trapezius muscles are detached from the distal clavicle.

Treatment

The treatment of type III injuries has been, is, and will remain in the foreseeable future, a subject of significant controversy. About every 10 to 20 years, certain orthopaedic surgeons are compelled to solicit opinions regarding the treatment of type III injuries from other orthopaedic surgeons, including academic department chairs, by the distribution of survey material.[260-263] Although the purpose of these surveys varies, treatment styles emerge as beacons that divinely light the way for practitioners of the period. This was true in 1974 and it remains true in 2007, as

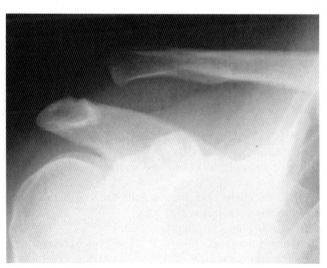

FIGURE 12-49 AP view of a type III injury. The articular surfaces of the acromioclavicular joint are widely displaced. The coracoclavicular interval is significantly increased.

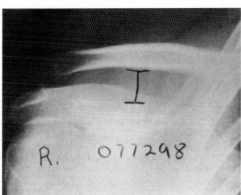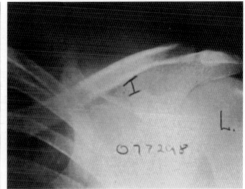

FIGURE 12-50 Type III injury with AP stress views showing incongruity of the acromioclavicular joint and widening of the coracoclavicular interval compared to the uninjured side.

expressed by the conclusions of Nissen and colleagues: Nonoperative symptomatic treatment is preferred, and operative treatment should include resection of the lateral clavicle, reconstruction of at least the coracoclavicular ligaments with either suture or local ligament graft, and protection of the reconstruction with rigid fixation between the coracoid and the clavicle.[262]

Nonoperative Treatment

Nonoperative treatment is recommended by many authors.[232,264-271] For the majority of patients, this is the preferred form of treatment for type III injuries (Fig. 12-51). This specifically includes patients such as contact and collision athletes and cyclists, who remain at high risk for repeated injuries to the acromioclavicular joint. There are no contraindications to nonoperative treatment.

Methods. Taking advantage of the fact that the dislocated joint is easily reducible in the acute setting, some authors have advocated a closed reduction accompanied by external immobilization (Fig. 12-52). Various techniques and methods have been used through decades of experience with the type III injury (Fig. 12-53).[249,272-274] None have proved any better than any other has, and each has its own pitfalls.[26,241,263,271,275]

Recognizing the difficulties with maintaining a satisfactory reduction, many authors have recommended symptomatic treatment only with sling support for the upper limb.[243,265,276] Motion and strengthening exercises are initiated as the resolution of pain permits. Return to higher levels of activity demands enthusiastic participation in a rehabilitation program that emphasizes progressive restoration of strength, function, and sport-specific drills.[265,277]

Results. Excellent and good results are obtainable with nonoperative treatment.[232,233,241,263,265-267,278-283] An earlier return to activities is often possible.[265-267,281,283] At mid- to long-term follow-up, 90% to 100% of patients have very favorable outcomes.[232,233,239,241,263,278,284] At the completion of rehabilitation, strength and endurance approaches that of the opposite upper limb.[271,282]

Overall satisfactory results obtained with nonoperative treatment derived from a meta-analysis review of the literature was 87%.[238] Calvo and colleagues demonstrated that there were no differences in the outcome of nonoperative and operative treatment.[285] Spencer searched 469 publications to identify nine studies with level II and level III evidence that compared nonoperative and operative treatment.[286] From this in-depth analysis of what he considered limited low evidence, he concluded that nonoperative treatment was more appropriate because the results of operative treatment "were not clearly better and were associated with higher complication rates, longer convalescence, and longer time away from work and sport."

Many authors observe that pain, flexibility, range of motion, and strength for nonoperative treatment is at least equal to, if not better than, those for operative treatment.[200,232,253,265,267,269,271,279,280,287-289] If differences exist, they are slight or activity specific.[241,282] A higher rate of complications and a slower return to work has been observed with operative treatment.[279,281] Heavy manual laborers and high-performance overhead athletes such as pitchers might not fare as well with nonoperative treatment because they are less likely to be completely pain free and have normal function.[35,290] In a few studies, pain and weakness have been reported in up to 50% of patients.[271]

After treatment, the extent of congruity or incongruity, the presence of osteoarthritis, and the development of heterotopic ossification appears to have no correlation with the outcome, regardless of the treatment method.

Complications. Although not really a complication, the asymmetry of the shoulder becomes obvious after swelling resolves. The extent of deformity may be unexpected and undesirable, perhaps necessitating treatment. Pressure-related skin breakdown is possible with certain types of external immobilization (Fig. 12-54).

Persistent pain and weakness are the most common late sequelae with type III injuries. Ossification is often present in the coracoclavicular interval at the completion of the period of healing.[14,249,250,258,292-294] The significance of the ossification is uncertain but it does not seem to disturb recovery.[66,258,294]

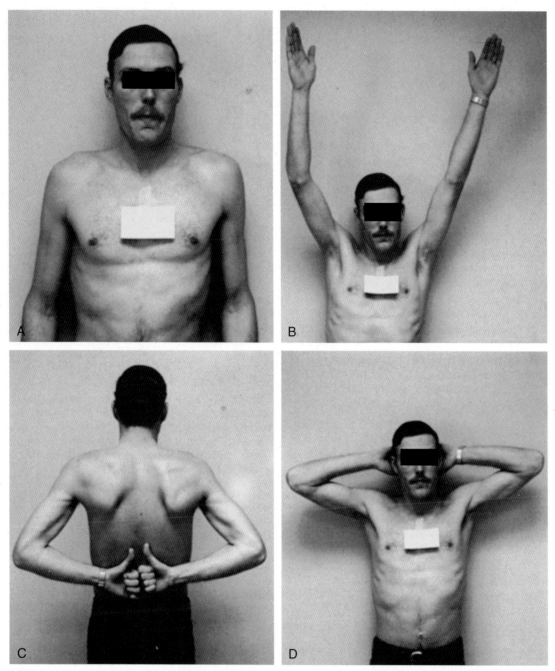

FIGURE 12-51 A to **D,** The results of nonoperative treatment of a type III injury. Prominence of the distal clavicle is noted along with nearly full range of motion. (From Rockwood CA, Green DP [eds]: Fractures, 3 vols, 2nd ed. Philadelphia: JB Lippincott, 1984.)

Osteolysis of the distal clavicle has been reported.[248] The risk of post-traumatic osteoarthritis has been shown to be less after nonoperatively treated injuries, as is the incidence of coracoclavicular ossification.[285]

Author's Preferred Method. Nonoperative treatment of type III injuries differs only slightly from the treatment of type II injuries. The cornerstone is effective pain management by means of a sling, cryotherapy, and narcotic analgesics. This can require 1 to 2 weeks. Pool therapy

is encouraged and hastens the recovery of active, pain-free movement. Once motion fully recovers and tenderness abates, strength rehabilitation is initiated. Protective measures are more relaxed than for type II injuries.

Operative Treatment

Surgical treatment of acromioclavicular joint dislocations has been performed since 1861 and appears to continue to play an important role for some clinicians in the care of carefully selected patients with these injuries.[295]

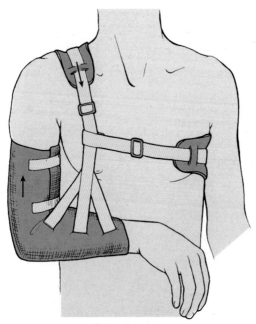

FIGURE 12-52 A method of maintaining a closed reduction with external immobilization: the Kenny–Howard shoulder harness. Sufficient pressure is created between the straps that run over the lateral clavicle and beneath the elbow by sequential tightening to keep the acromioclavicular joint reduced. The strap around the torso keeps the harness from slipping off the shoulder.

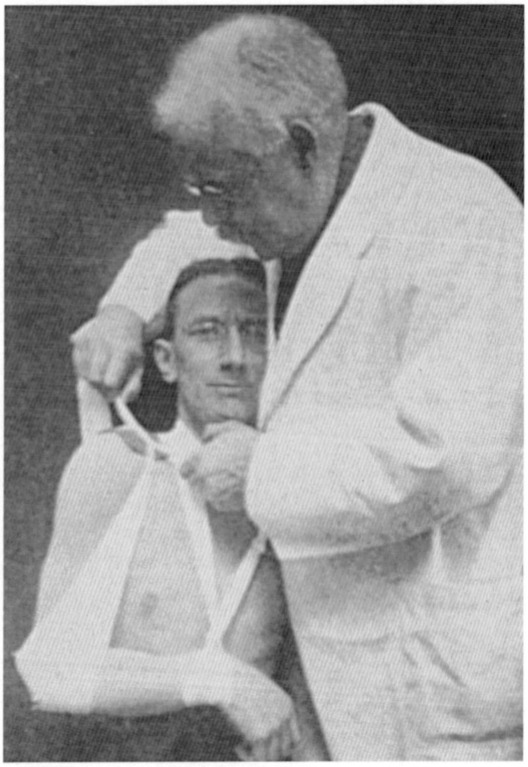

FIGURE 12-53 Sir Robert Jones treats this patient, who has an acromioclavicular dislocation, with a bandage that appears to be a precursor of the method of the Kenny–Howard harness. The clavicle is depressed while the arm is elevated. (From Jones R: Injuries of Joints. London: Oxford University Press, 1917.)

Indications. Operative treatment offers the only opportunity for structural and cosmetic restoration. Reserving it for heavy manual laborers, patients 25 years and younger, athletes, and frequent overhead users has been suggested.[66,281,288] That said, in one review there appeared to be no evidence to support the claim that the outcome of operative treatment is better than that of nonoperative treatment.[286] Currently, proof is lacking that special groups of patients mandate consideration for operative treatment.

Contraindications. Extremely low demand and inactive patients might have nothing to gain with operative treatment. Significant skin abrasions can delay operative treatment.

Methods. The acromioclavicular joint may be reduced by a closed or open technique and repaired with metallic wires or pins that temporarily transgress the articular surfaces of the acromion and the clavicle (Figs. 12-55 and 12-56).* The importance of supplemental techniques performed in conjunction with the method of internal fixations has been emphasized by some authors. These techniques include the additional repair of the acromioclavicular and coracoclavicular ligaments, acromioclavicular and coracoclavicular ligament repair reinforcement with the intra-articular disk, repair or imbrication of the deltoid and trapezius attachments, adjacent soft tissue transfers (coracoacromial ligament, biceps short head), lateral clavicle excision, autologous fascia lata suspension, coracoclavicular suture augmentation, and clavicle osteotomy.† The duration of temporary fixation is typically longer than 6 weeks but varies with the technique. Motion restrictions are mandatory to protect the integrity of the pins or wires until their removal. Thereafter, motion and strengthening programs are introduced.

Open reduction and internal fixation with a hooked plate affords rigid internal fixation and spares the articular surfaces of the joint (Fig. 12-57).[323-339] Implant removal is suggested between 12 and 16 weeks. At that point, efforts toward motion and strength recovery are initiated.

The clavicle and the coracoid process offer secure points of fixation that can be used to maintain either a closed or an open reduction of the acromioclavicular joint. These stabilization techniques may be used independently or as a supplement to other forms of either

*References 13, 14, 25, 86, 93, 201, 241, 252, 267, 280, 281, 291, and 296-322.

†References 93, 252, 263, 296, 297, 301, 302, 306, 308, 310, 311-318, and 320.

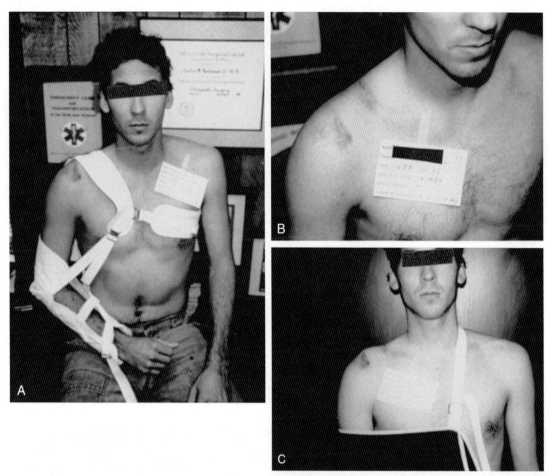

FIGURE 12-54 Skin breakdown is a potential complication of using external immobilization straps that apply continuous pressure over the lateral clavicle. **A** and **B,** The continuous pressure of a strap over the top of the shoulder, which is attempting to depress the clavicle, resulted in a lesion of the integument in this patient. **C,** Treatment was changed to a simple sling.

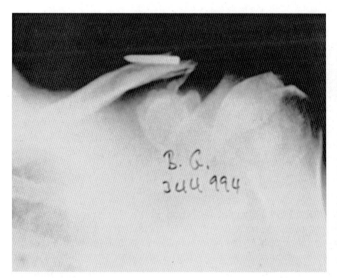

FIGURE 12-55 This type III dislocation was previously fixed with a threaded Steinmann pin. The reduction held satisfactorily but the pin broke, with the tip left embedded in the distal end of the clavicle.

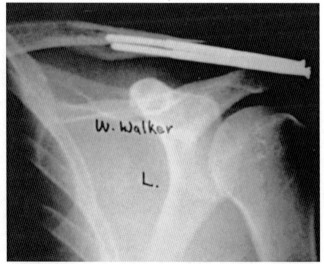

FIGURE 12-56 This type III dislocation was managed by blind pinning of the acromioclavicular joint with two Deyerle hip screws.

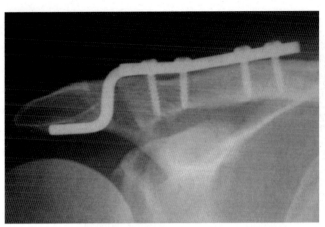

FIGURE 12-57 Hook plate for type III injury enabling excellent restoration of anatomy.

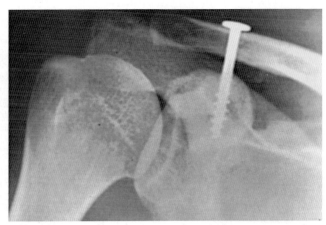

FIGURE 12-58 Satisfactory reduction with the Bosworth screw maintained by coarse threads in the base of the coracoid process. (From Rockwood CA, Green DP [eds]: Fractures, 3 vols, 2nd ed. Philadelphia: JB Lippincott, 1984.)

temporary or permanent means of fixation. In addition, direct repair of the acromioclavicular and coracoclavicular ligaments performed concurrently with the coracoclavicular stabilization can be considered.

Bosworth was the first to describe the use of a screw between the clavicle and the coracoid process to achieve acromioclavicular joint stability.[340] Others have used the technique as described by Bosworth or have made modifications in the technique (Figs. 12-58 and 12-59).[26,126,232,241,267,279,280,283,294,341-346]

The exploration and débridement of the acromioclavicular joint has been advocated,[26,126,294,347] but some

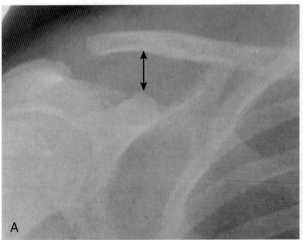

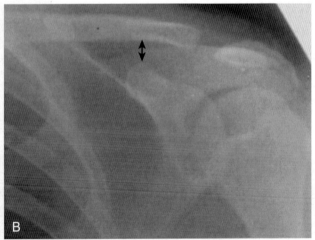

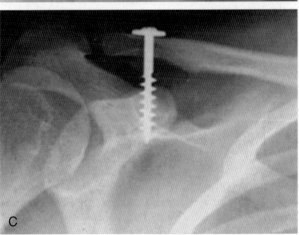

FIGURE 12-59 Excellent reduction with restoration of a normal coracoclavicular interval with a coracoclavicular screw. **A,** AP stress radiograph of the right shoulder in a patient with a type III acromioclavicular dislocation. **B,** A stress film of the left shoulder revealed it to be normal. **C,** Postoperative radiograph showing the acromioclavicular joint reduced and held temporarily in place with a special modified coracoclavicular lag screw. (From Rockwood CA, Green DP [eds]: Fractures, 3 vols, 2nd ed. Philadelphia: JB Lippincott, 1984.)

authors do not consider this an essential component of treatment.[8,340,346,348,349] In the setting of coracoclavicular stabilization, the necessity for the direct repair of the coracoclavicular ligaments is uncertain. Bosworth and others have elected to leave the ligaments unrepaired.[8,26,126,264,340,346,348,349] Some authors have emphasized the importance of supplemental coracoclavicular ligament repair at the time of coracoclavicular stabilization.[347] Repair of the trapezius and deltoid attachments can contribute to the overall strength of the repair and has been emphasized by several authors.[126,294,299,307,347]

There are significant variations in the recommendations for postoperative immobilization, restrictions, rehabilitation, the necessity for implant removal, and the timing of implant removal.[7,126,258,294,340]

Absorbable sutures, nonabsorbable sutures, wires, and synthetic materials have been used for acromioclavicular joint stabilization (Fig. 12-60).[7,242,251,258,308,328,343,350-368] If the material is passed through drill holes in the clavicle, in the coracoid, or in both, the reduction is more accurate and the outcome may be improved (Fig. 12-61).[354,362]

Ryhanen and coauthors have described the use of a coracoclavicular nitinol C-shaped hook implant.[369]

Transposing the coracoacromial ligament into the resected distal clavicle was suggested in 1917 by Cadenet and in 1972 was reported by Weaver and Dunn, who used the technique for both acute and chronic type III injuries.[27,370] Other authors used the coracoacromial ligament in the same or a similar manner.[311,312,314,371-375] Modifications of the Weaver–Dunn method were subsequently described by other authors and were felt to be especially useful for a more-active population.[236,242,289,376-380] The coracoacromial ligament, with or without an accompanying piece of bone, may be transferred to the clavicle and can be supplemented with a Bosworth screw.[381-384] Such concepts of coracoclavicular augmentation in conjunction with the Weaver–Dunn operation have been supported by the results of experimental studies.[385]

In 1941, Gurd described excision of the distal clavicle as a treatment for type III injuries.[386] In the same year, Mumford reported the same operation for type II injuries and advocated that treatment of symptomatic type III injuries should also include coracoclavicular ligament reconstruction as well as distal clavicle excision.[387] The role for excision of the lateral clavicle at the time of surgical treatment of a type III injury is not clear.[242] There were no differences reported between coracoclavicular ligament fixation alone and coracoclavicular fixation with excision of the lateral clavicle.[388] Likewise, when the outcome of acromioclavicular fixation and coracoclavicular ligament repair with and without lateral clavicle excision were compared, no differences were observed with the exception of the more frequent appearance of degenerative changes when the lateral clavicle was retained.[320,389]

In 1965, muscle transfers were suggested as a reasonable treatment for type III injuries.[390,391] The tip of the coracoid process that included the coracobrachialis and the short head of the biceps was osteotomized and attached to the clavicle. Scattered reports appeared later, some with slight modifications of the technique.[328,392-396] Transposition of the biceps long head or a slip of the conjoined tendon have been described as substitution methods for the coracoclavicular ligaments.[397-399]

There appears to be a trend to seek a more anatomic and biological solution for coracoclavicular ligament reconstruction. One method that uses autograft or allograft tendon has been reported by Mazzocca and colleagues (Fig. 12-62).[400]

An arthroscopic method for treating type III injuries was first described by Wolf and associates.[401] In this study, either sutures or allograft semitendinosis were used for coracoclavicular stabilization. Since then, other arthroscopic methods using the coracoacromial ligament, suture, semi-

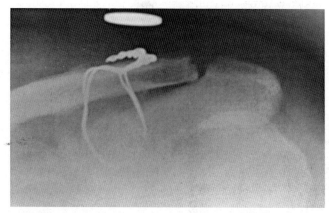

FIGURE 12-60 Shown with an overlying coin marker in preparation for removal, coracoclavicular wire loops proved successful in reduction maintenance in this case.

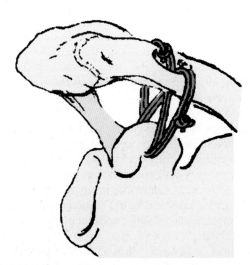

FIGURE 12-61 A method of coracoclavicular reconstruction with loops passing through a prepared hole in the clavicle. (Adapted from Dimakopoulos P, Panagopoulos A: Functional coracoclavicular stabilization for acute acromioclavicular joint disruption. Orthopedics 30[2]:103-108, 2007.)

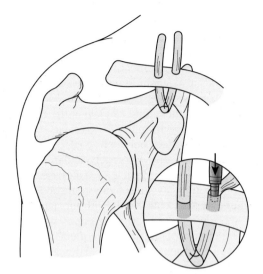

FIGURE 12-62 A coracoclavicular reconstruction that is considered anatomic uses autograft or allograft tendon. (Redrawn from Mazzocca AD, Conway J, Johnson S, et al: The anatomic coracoclavicular ligament reconstruction. Oper Tech Sports Med 12:56-61, 2004.)

tendinosis autograft, or allograft have been described.[402-406] Arthroscopic-assisted percutaneous coracoclavicular screw insertion has been described.[403,405,406]

Further arthroscopic techniques have been investigated, recommended, and performed.[407]

Experimental Investigations. Upon comparing techniques for acromioclavicular fixation, Keifer and colleagues found that the most rigid fixation was provided by the Bosworth screw.[408]

Restoration of acromioclavicular joint congruency using seven different methods of fixation between the clavicle and the coracoid were studied by Jerosch and coworkers.[409] They demonstrated satisfactory vertical stability with all of the techniques. Excessive horizontal translations between the acromion and the clavicle were demonstrated with all of the loop techniques and the Weaver–Dunn reconstruction, whereas the joint anatomy was best restored with the Bosworth screw or bone anchor reconstruction.[409]

In a cadaver model comparing the biomechanical function of different surgical procedures for acromioclavicular joint dislocations, the Rockwood screw resulted in decreased primary and coupled translations and showed increased stiffness.[410] Coracoclavicular sling and coracoacromial ligament transfer resulted in increased primary and coupled translations. In situ forces increased for all three reconstructions.

Harris and colleagues showed that Bosworth screw placement with bicortical purchase provided strength and stiffness as good as or better than the intact coracoclavicular ligaments.[411]

In a cadaver model, McConnell and associates performed reconstructions with coracoclavicular loop (No. 5

polyester fiber [Mersilene]), coracoclavicular screw, and hook plate fixation and subjected the specimens to stiffness and failure testing.[412] Hook plates reproduced physiologic stiffness more closely. The coracoclavicular screw failed at the highest load and was the stiffest reconstruction, and the coracoclavicular loop was the least stiff.

Experimental screw fixation for coracoclavicular ligament reconstruction has been investigated.[413] In this study, coracoclavicular fixation comparing stainless steel and bioabsorbable 4.5-mm screws showed no difference in pull-out strength and fixation strength that exceeded the intact coracoclavicular ligaments. In a study by Motamedi and colleagues, 6.5-mm coracoclavicular screw fixation with one-cortex purchase was significantly weaker and stiffer than the intact coracoclavicular ligaments.[414]

Wickham and coworkers compared the maximum tensile strength and resistance to deformation for one or two strands of Ethibond No. 5 suture, one or two strands of polyester [Mersilene] tape, size 0 polydioxanone braid, and size 2 poly(L-lactic acid) suture braid in a coracoclavicular model and demonstrated the significantly greater tensile strength of poly(L-lactic acid) suture.[415] Two strands of polyester tape, polydioxanone braid, and poly(L-lactic acid) braid exhibited similar resistance to deformation with cyclic loading but significantly better than the other test samples. Failure loads comparable to the intact coracoclavicular ligament (725 N) were observed in the experimental reconstructions performed with braided polydioxanone and braided polyethylene passed around or through the clavicle; failure loads of a 6.5-mm screw with single-cortex purchase in the coracoid were around one half those of the intact coracoclavicular ligaments. The strength and stiffness properties of the braided polyethylene suggested that it could serve effectively as an augmentation for acromioclavicular joint repairs and reconstructions.

In experimental repairs performed by Wellmann and colleagues, loop or button fixation of polydioxanone suture exhibited significantly higher ultimate load than did coracoid suture anchor repairs with No. 2 high-strength polyethylene (Ultrabraid) suture.[407] In a cadaver model, acromioclavicular joint congruity was not restored by any coracoclavicular loop fixation through drill holes in the clavicle but was more closely restored when the drill hole was placed more anteriorly in the calvicle.[416]

The coracoacromial ligament transposition as used in the Weaver–Dunn reconstruction is, experimentally, one fifth the ultimate load of the intact coracoclavicular ligament.[414,417] Deshmukh and associates demonstrated that the Weaver–Dunn method was significantly more lax than native ligaments.[418] In their model, coracoclavicular augmentation was less lax than the Weaver–Dunn reconstruction but more lax than the native ligament. Harris and colleagues showed that coracoacromial ligament transfer in the manner of Weaver–Dunn was the weakest and least stiff experimental reconstruction when compared to the intact coracoclavicular ligament, coracoclavicular screw fixation, woven polyester vascular graft slings, and suture anchor technique with No. 5 braided polyester.[411] The Weaver–Dunn procedure, even with modifications, fails to reproduce the load-to-failure durability of the intact acromioclavicular and coracoclavicular ligament complex.[419,420] In a cadaver model that assessed the motion between two points fixed respectively on the distal clavicle and acromion process, an unaugmented Weaver–Dunn reconstruction demonstrated significant multiplanar laxity when compared to an intact joint.[421] In the same study, a reconstruction augmented with coracoclavicular suture with anchor into the coracoid was neither more nor less mobile than the intact joint.

The rationale for the use of biological coracoclavicular ligament substitutions has been investigated. An experimental anatomic reconstruction with semitendinosis tendon in a cadaver model failed to show significant elongation with cyclic loading in a manner similar to the intact coracoclavicular ligament complex.[422] In addition, the stiffness and ultimate load of the anatomic reconstruction decreased significantly by 40% and 25%, respectively, compared to the intact coracoclavicular ligament complex. Coracoclavicular ligament reconstructions with tendon grafts demonstrate greater stability and less translation in vitro when compared to the Weaver–Dunn procedure in its original or modified forms.[419,420]

Portions of the conjoined tendon have been used for experimental coracoclavicular reconstruction. Sloan and coworkers, in a cadaver model of single load to failure, demonstrated that the strength of the lateral half of the conjoined tendon (265 N) was at least as strong as that of the coracoacromial ligament (246 N) in a simulated reconstruction, although it lacked the strength of the intact coracoclavicular ligaments (621 N).[423] They cited potential advantages of this technique, including retention of the coracoacromial ligament integrity and significantly longer autologous graft material.

The tendon of the pectoralis minor tendon morphology and tensile strength has been investigated in cadavers and compared to the acromioclavicular ligament.[424] It can offer structural properties that render it as suitable as, or even more suitable than, the coracoacromial ligament. Although it has yet to be evaluated clinically, its use for this purpose circumvents the sacrifice of a normal and functionally important part of the coracoacromial archway.

The direction being taken by investigators with interest in acromioclavicular joint stabilization is toward the use of stronger materials or methods. It is not entirely clear at this time whether rigid or nonrigid fixation is better. The greatest attention has focused on direct methods to achieve coracoclavicular stability and, for the most part, indirect methods to achieve acromioclavicular stability. Therein is the challenge. It is intuitive that the preservation of the clavicle in its entirety would afford the best opportunity for preserving strength, motion, and function. However, even with maintenance of a congruent acromioclavicular joint reduction, the necessity for excising the lateral clavicle might not be obviated. Biologically

compatible materials as well as grafts are receiving more attention as are methods considered less invasive.

Results. When compared to nonoperative treatment, operative treatment can result in less pain and better endurance, especially during work.[231,251,287] Operative treatment results in improvement with regard to pain and patient satisfaction both in the short term and long term.[238,289] In high-performance overhead athletes, complete pain relief and return to normal was achieved more with operative treatment, 92% versus 80%.[290]

Methods that transfix the acromioclavicular joint with pins can produce some excellent and good results.[241,263,267,280,281] However, fair and poor results have been reported to be 50% to 100% as common as excellent and good results.[263,280]

Hook plates have been used extensively in Europe, resulting in reports from various centers as far back as 25 years.[323-339] The follow-up period is relatively short, but the results are mixed and inconsistently reported.[323-339,425]

The outcome of the use of coracoclavicular screws is generally excellent and good in more than 77% of patients.[241,267,280,341,342,344,345] This is the case even when ossification between the clavicle and coracoid forms or is encouraged to form.[126,342] Percutaneous screw insertion is more difficult and results in higher complications.[346] Coracoclavicular polydioxanone suture has achieved 89% good or excellent results.[359] Studies that have compared the results of acromioclavicular and coracoclavicular fixation report conflicting outcomes.[426,427]

Favorable results were reported by Weaver and Dunn and subsequently reiterated by other authors who performed the operation as originally described.[370,374,381,428] Modified Weaver–Dunn operations also produced favorable outcomes.[236,242,289,376,377]

Mixed results have been reported for the treatment of type III injuries with transposition of the tip of the coracoid process that includes the short head of the biceps and the coracobrachialis to the clavicle.[369,392,393,429] Skjeldal and colleagues advised that the procedure not be done in patients with acute type III injuries.[429]

It is generally believed that after treatment, the extent of congruity or incongruity, the presence of osteoarthritis, and the development of heterotopic ossification appears to have no correlation with the outcome, regardless of the method.

Complications. Acromioclavicular joint fixation has a higher complication rate than coracoclavicular fixation.[426,427,430]

A high failure rate is expected for soft tissue reconstructions if either acromioclavicular or coracoclavicular fixation techniques are not incorporated as additional protection from deforming forces. A very serious complication of acromioclavicular joint repair or reconstruction is hardware failure. Pins and wires used to stabilize the acromioclavicular joint can break or loosen and subse-

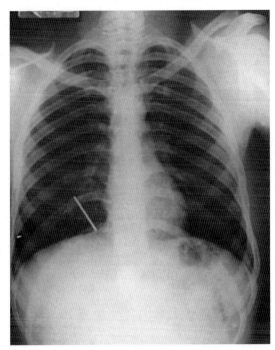

FIGURE 12-63 Steinmann pin fixation was chosen for the acromioclavicular joint. Upon breaking, it migrated to the right lung, shown here. (From Rockwood CA, Green DP [eds]: Fractures, 3 vols, 2nd ed. Philadelphia: JB Lippincott, 1984.)

quently migrate, as reported by Lyons and Rockwood and others (Fig. 12-63).[431-437] Serious injury and death can result from pin migration.[433,438-442] The materials used for coracoclavicular loop techniques, and foreign body reactions to these materials, can result in failures, the majority of which result from the erosion or fracture of either the clavicle or the coracoid process (Figs. 12-64 to 12-66).[353,357,443-448] Screws, wires, cables, or nonmetal synthetics can suffer fatigue breakage, leading to recurrence of the deformity (Fig. 12-67). Screws can lose their purchase in the coracoid and pull through (Fig. 12-68). The engaging hook of the hook plate can lose its purchase beneath the acromion process (Fig. 12-69).

Post-traumatic arthritis has been shown to be more common after operative than after nonoperative treatment.[285] Post-traumatic arthritis can result and is more likely in acromioclavicular joints that remain incongruent at the completion of their treatment.[241,449]

Calvo and associates have shown that the incidence of coracoclavicular ossification is higher after operative treatment.[285] Millbourn reported that the incidence and severity were not different with operative treatment.[293]

At 10 years of follow-up, post-traumatic arthritis was reported to be more common when acromioclavicular fixation, as opposed to coracoclavicular fixation, was used.[241]

Salvage of Failed Coracoclavicular Stabilization. Depending upon the index operation, any number of salvage options may be available. Confounding factors include loss of the integrity of the clavicle or coracoid due to erosion or fracture, clavicle foreshortening, and tissue exhaustion (coracoacromial ligament, conjoined tendon, deltotrapezius fascia). The optimal conditions for revision exist when the clavicle and the coracoid remain intact and specific points for materials anchorage are preserved. Coracoclavicular looping techniques or their variations, with supplemental but temporary rigid fixation, would appear to offer the best option. For these extreme cases there may be advantages to using biological as opposed to synthetic reconstruction techniques. The use of autologous semitendinosis tendon is supported by its strength properties and results in a few cases.[414,450-453]

Author's Preferred Method. I originally used Dacron vascular coracoclavicular loops for type III injuries. When the technique fell out of favor due to erosion, nonabsorbable sutures ranging in size and number were passed in various combinations around and through the clavicle. When this method resulted in frequent failures, a more rigid form of fixation was found with the Rockwood screw. Even with the best visualization for optimal screw placement into the coracoid process, failures continued. A combination of Rockwood screw and modern nonabsorbable suture (FiberWire) did not solve the problem of

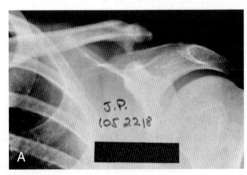
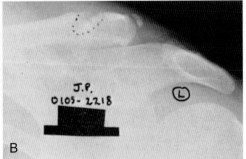

FIGURE 12-64 A and **B,** Erosion of Dacron graft into the clavicle.

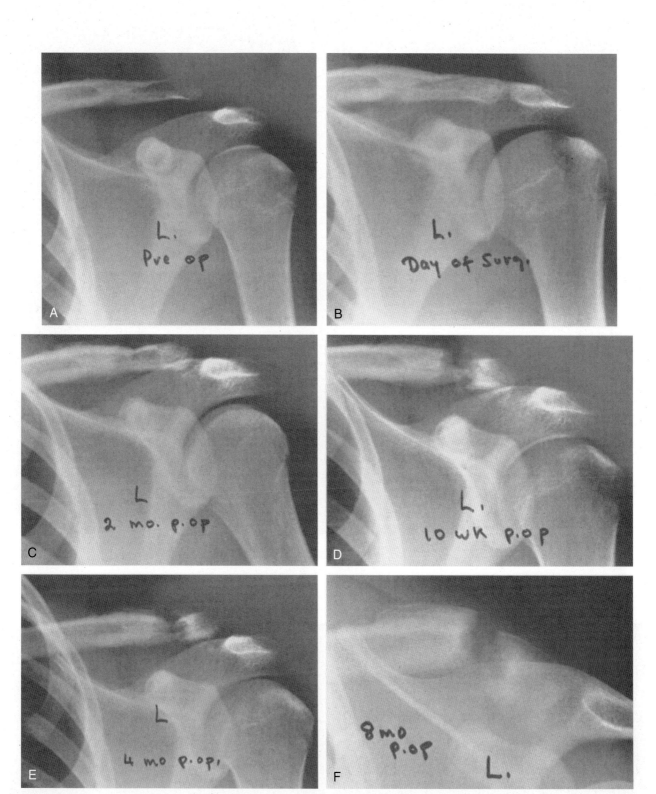

FIGURE 12-65 A to **F,** Erosion of Dacron graft into the clavicle of a patient with a type III dislocation.

Continued

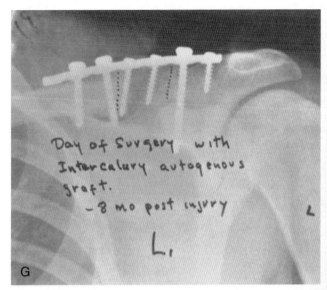

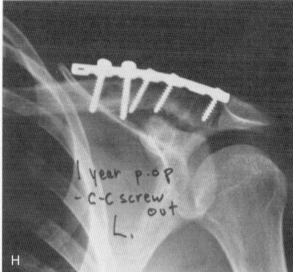

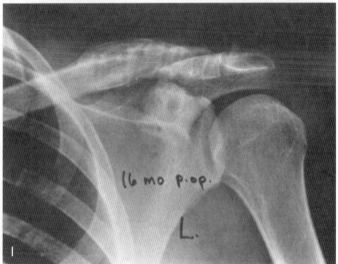

FIGURE 12-65, cont'd G to **I,** Clavicle repaired with screws and plate and autologous bone graft.

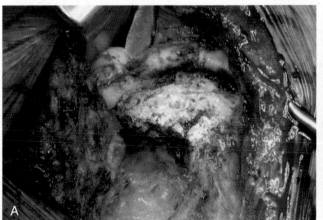

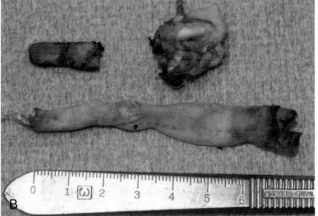

FIGURE 12-66 Coracoclavicular loop fixation with vascular graft. **A,** In situ vascular graft that has eroded into the clavicle. **B,** Bulky vascular graft removed because of painful soft tissue irritation.

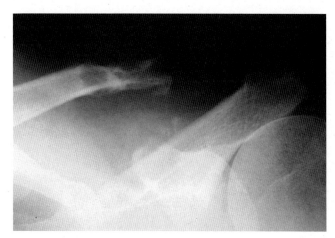

FIGURE 12-67 Failure of nonabsorbable suture used for type III injury with recurrence of deformity and reactive changes within the clavicle.

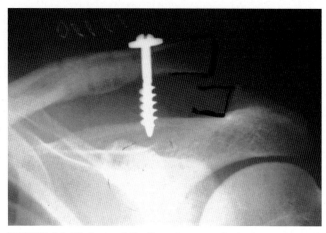

FIGURE 12-68 Loss of fixation of coracoclavicular screw used for type III injury with recurrence of deformity.

failures with recurrent deformity. Since 2004, I have been using a hook plate in conjunction with nonabsorbable coracoclavicular suture (Fig. 12-70).

With the patient in the beach chair position, a skin incision is made in Langer's lines over the clavicle in a line just lateral to the tip of the coracoid process (Figs. 12-71 and 12-72). Generous subcutaneous flaps are raised and the deltotrapezius fascia is incised over the lateral clavicle, extending over its end, where the supporting structures are disrupted and just onto the acromion process (Figs. 12-73 and 12-74). The acromioclavicular joint is inspected and débrided as needed, preserving the entire length of the clavicle (Fig. 12-75). Sufficient subperiosteal exposure of the clavicle is performed to permit application of the shortest plate.

Three 1-mm Cottony Dacron sutures are passed beneath the coracoid process as close as possible to its base, then posterior to the clavicle and back toward the coracoid (Figs. 12-76 to 12-78). They are not tied at this point. Access for the hook portion of the plate is created by

blunt dissection at the junction of the medial acromion and the scapular spine. This important step enables proper placement of the hook beneath the acromion process, advancing it laterally as far as possible (Fig. 12-79). A trial implant is selected based upon the estimated height of the joint and the requirements for adequate screw purchase in the clavicle (Fig. 12-80). The joint is

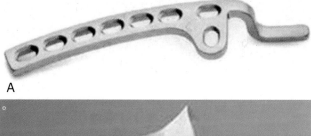

A

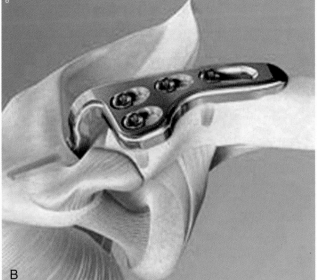

B

FIGURE 12-70 The hook plate that I use (Synthes, Paoli, Penn). **A,** Early. **B,** Current.

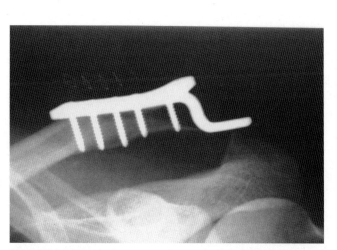

FIGURE 12-69 Hook plate no longer secured beneath the acromion process.

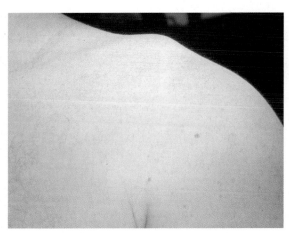

FIGURE 12-71 Acromioclavicular joint deformity is apparent at the time of operation.

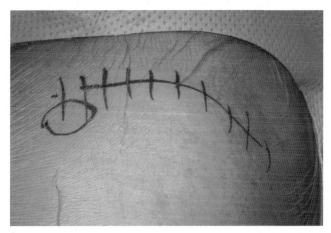

FIGURE 12-72 Skin incision in the relaxed skin tension lines.

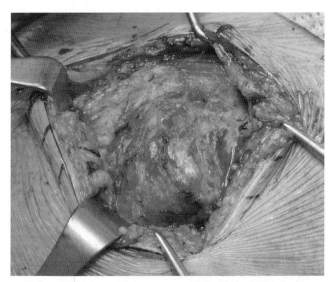

FIGURE 12-73 Superficial dissection to expose the deltoid, the trapezius, the clavicle, and the acromioclavicular joint.

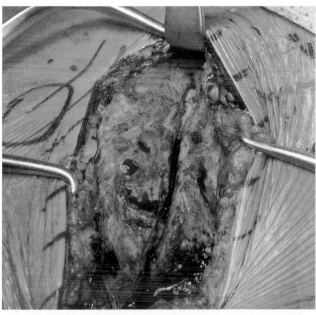

FIGURE 12-74 Deep dissection between the deltoid and the trapezius with entry into the injured acromioclavicular joint.

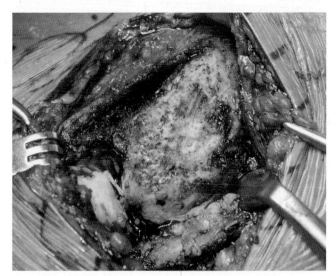

FIGURE 12-75 Exposure of the lateral clavicle. Note the disruption of the intra-articular disk.

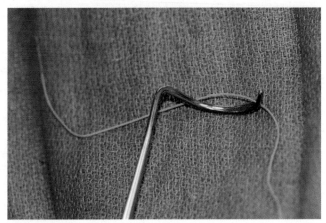

FIGURE 12-76 Curved instrument used to pass the pulling suture beneath the clavicle.

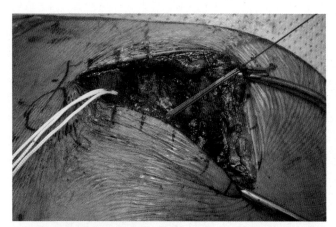

FIGURE 12-77 Three 1-mm cottony Dacron sutures being pulled beneath the coracoid process.

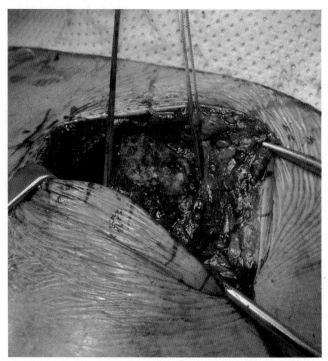

FIGURE 12-78 The sutures are passed posterior to the clavicle.

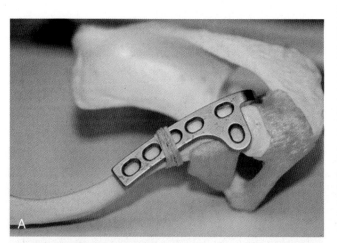

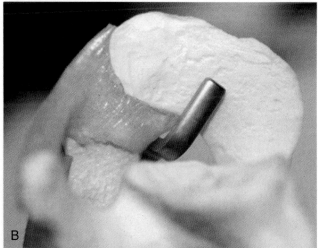

FIGURE 12-79 Positioning the implant. **A** and **B,** Saw bone models demonstrate the proper position of the plate. Note that it is as lateral as possible.

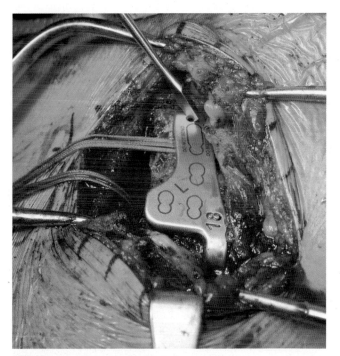

FIGURE 12-80 Implant trial being positioned.

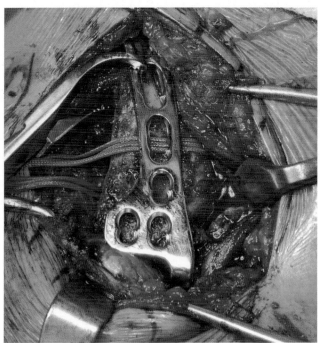

FIGURE 12-81 The definitive implant is provisionally secured.

reduced by manually stabilizing the plate, which now lies superior to the clavicle, while the acromion is brought into proper relationship with the lateral clavicle by axial force delivered through the upper limb. Occasionally at this point, the plate has to be removed and contoured slightly to optimize the fit to the clavicle. It is then held in the reduced position with a bone-holding forceps (Fig. 12-81). Reduction is confirmed. The plate is secured to the clavicle with screws. The sutures, which have come to lie beneath the plate, are tied (Fig. 12-82).

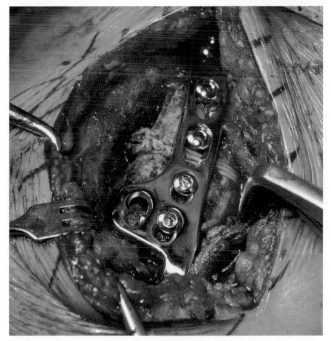

FIGURE 12-82 The definitive implant is secured to the bone with screws and the sutures are tied.

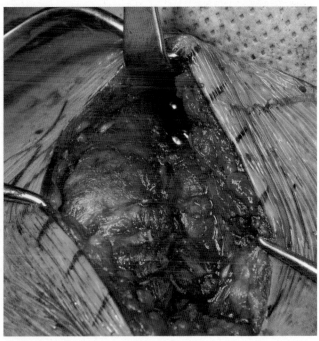

FIGURE 12-83 Deltotrapezius and acromioclavicular joint closure.

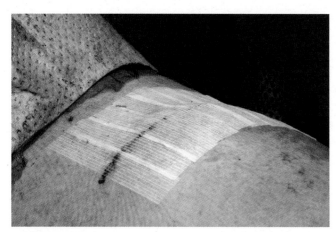

FIGURE 12-84 Skin closure with notable absence of previous deformity.

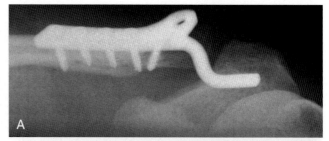

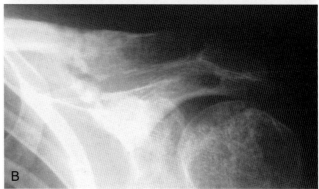

FIGURE 12-85 A, Radiograph after the operation. **B,** Radiograph at final follow-up.

The deltoid, trapezius, and acromioclavicular joint supporting structures are closed anatomically or, where necessary, imbricated (Fig. 12-83). The skin is closed with adhesive strips (Fig. 12-84). The upper limb is immobilized for 6 weeks and used to a very limited extent only below the shoulder for another 6 weeks. The plate is routinely removed between the 12th and the 16th week after the operation (Fig. 12-85).

This technique has produced uniformly excellent results in more than 30 cases with relatively short follow-up, with no recurrences of deformity and no secondary operations except plate removal (Fig. 12-86).

Type III Variants
Pseudodislocation and Physeal Injuries

When exposed to injuring mechanisms and forces sufficient to result in complete acromioclavicular dislocations in adults, skeletally immature patients with open physes and thick periosteum sustain unique injuries generically termed *type III variants*.[454]

Signs and Symptoms. Though the patient appears acutely injured, pain is usually less than with a similar injury in a skeletally mature patient. Guarding is not as strict.

The injured limb is held in a protective manner adjacent to the torso, less often with the assistance of the opposite upper limb. Superior soft tissue abrasion, bruising, and swelling may be present. Active and passive motion is resisted, inhibiting the accurate assessment of motion and strength. Tenderness is confined mostly to the superior aspect of the lateral clavicle.

Imaging. The most obvious finding is complete separation of the acromion and the lateral clavicle that is accompanied by widening of the coracoclavicular interval. A Thurston–Holland fragment may be detectable (Fig. 12-87).

Pathoanatomy. The structural properties of the physeal–metaphyseal interface of the lateral clavicle render it the weakest link of the scapuloclavicular composite in a child or adolescent. Therefore, the forces of injury result in a fracture through the physis (Salter–Harris type I or type II) without disturbing the integrity of the acromioclavicular joint and the adjacent epiphysis of the lateral clavicle. The metaphysis of the lateral clavicle rips through the superior periosteal sleeve, which is then peeled away from the lateral clavicle by any remaining inferiorly directed forces and by the weight of the upper limb (Fig. 12-88).[454-460] The coracoclavicular ligaments remain securely attached to the periosteal sleeve of the lateral clavicle and the coracoid process.

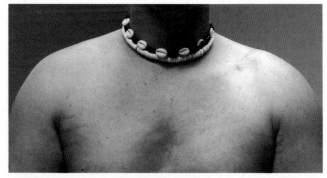

FIGURE 12-86 The clinical appearance after hook plate implantation, healing, and implant removal, with notable lack of deformity and an aesthetically pleasing scar.

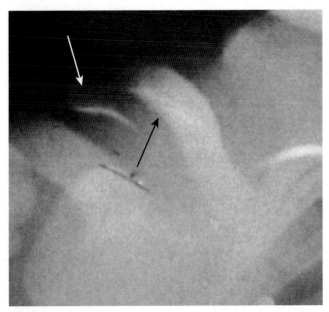

FIGURE 12-87 Type III variant in the immature skeleton. A Thurston–Holland fragment has been created with this injury. *White arrow* indicates Thurston-Holland fragment. *Black arrow* shows apparent coracoclavicular interval widening due to clavicular disruption from the periosteal tube. (From Ogden JA: Distal clavicular physeal injury. Clin Orthop Relat Res [188]:68-73, 1984.)

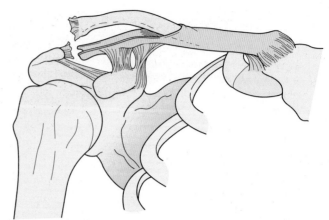

FIGURE 12-88 Type III variant. Shown here is the displaced osseous clavicle leaving behind, inferiorly, a periosteal tube attached to the cartilaginous epiphysis that maintains the integrity of the acromioclavicular joint.

A 2005 report of two cases and the investigation of museum specimens by Edelson and colleagues is the first to describe an even rarer form of this injury whereby the lateral clavicle, having sustained a Salter–Harris II injury, is displaced downward and backward into the supraspinatus outlet toward the spine of the scapula.[461] A case similar to this occurring in an adult was described by Yanagisawa and coworkers.[462] The distal clavicle impaled the supraspinatus muscle.

Treatment. Essentially all of these injuries can be treated nonoperatively. A sling or shoulder immobilizer is used until tenderness resolves. The physeal injury heals within 3 weeks, enabling motion recovery rapidly. When the periosteal healing response is mature, the patients are permitted to return to vigorous activities (Fig. 12-89). The results are usually excellent, with no significant complications. A rare phenomenon of duplication of the clavicle by means of an intense healing within the periosteal tube, especially in cases with wide displacement, has been observed.[463,464]

If, based upon extreme displacement, the lateral clavicle is suspected of spearing the trapezius muscle, it would be appropriate to proceed operatively with the intent of repairing the torn superior periosteal sleeve.[454,457,458] Edelson and colleagues advised operative treatment of the unique injury that they described for children older than 13 years of age.[461]

In the absence of extenuating circumstances, I prefer nonoperative treatment for this injury.

Fracture of the Coracoid Process

Complete dislocation of the acromioclavicular joint combined with fracture of the coracoid process is a very rare injury.[465-473] A similar lesion has been described in the immature skeleton.[474]

Signs and Symptoms. The patient experiences moderate to severe shoulder pain. Pain is not only localized to the acromioclavicular joint but might also emanate more to the anterior aspect of the shoulder. Motion, either active or passive, in any direction and to any degree exacerbates the pain.

The patient appears acutely injured, often with the affected upper limb postured in a protective and stress-relieving manner. The soft tissue overlying the acromion may be abraded or contused. Anterior shoulder ecchymosis resulting from the fracture is possible. Motion and strength assessment are unreliable due to pain. Palpation of the coracoid process induces pain.

Imaging. The most obvious finding on the AP view is complete separation of the acromion and the clavicle, with preservation of a normal coracoclavicular interval. This radiographic feature is most indicative of a fracture at the base of the coracoid, which may be difficult to see unless an axillary view, a Stryker notch view, or a CT scan is obtained (Figs. 12-90 to 12-92).

Pathoanatomy. Although the coracoclavicular ligaments usually maintain their secure attachment to the clavicle and the coracoid fracture fragment, two instances of their concomitant complete rupture resulting in an extraordinary injury triad, or triple lesion, have been reported.[475,476]

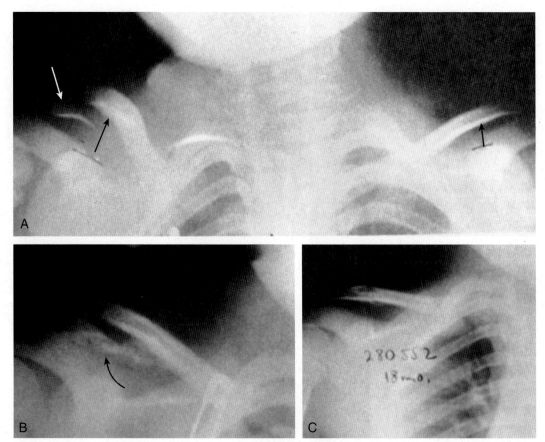

FIGURE 12-89 A to **C,** Type III variant. A brisk healing response is usually observed with remodeling that results in a normal-appearing clavicle. **A,** *White arrow* indicates Thurston-Holland fragment. *Black arrows* show apparent coracoclavicular interval widening due to clavicular disruption from the periosteal tube. **B,** *Arrow* indicates normal coracoclavicular interval now apparent as a result of new bone formation arising from the periosteal sleeve. **C,** Restoration of normal anatomy at the completion of remodeling. (From Ogden JA: Distal clavicular physeal injury. Clin Orthop Relat Res [188]:68-73, 1984.)

Treatment. With little difference reported between the results of operative and nonoperative treatment, the latter is usually preferred.[320,389,466,469-471,475-478] An exception is coracoid fracture extension into the articular surface of the glenoid with significant displacement (Fig. 12-93).[66] Because of the difficulty of open reduction and internal fixation of the base of the coracoid, acromioclavicular joint transfixation pins have been recommended (Figs. 12-94 and 12-95).[66]

Type IV

These rare injuries are characterized by the posterior displacement of the distal clavicle into or through the substance of the adjacent trapezius muscle, sometimes with extreme deformity (Fig. 12-96).[212,479-485] Even more rarely, posterior dislocation of the acromioclavicular joint is accompanied by anterior sternoclavicular dislocation, termed *bipolar clavicle dislocation.*[220-224,226-228,275,486-492]

Signs and Symptoms

The patient experiences moderate to severe shoulder pain. Damage to the trapezius muscle can result in pain

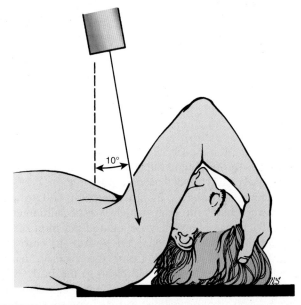

FIGURE 12-90 Fracture of the base of the coracoid process is best seen with the Stryker notch view, demonstrated here. The hand is placed upon the top of the head, placing the humerus in approximately 120 degrees of flexion as the x-ray beam is directed 10 degrees cephalad.

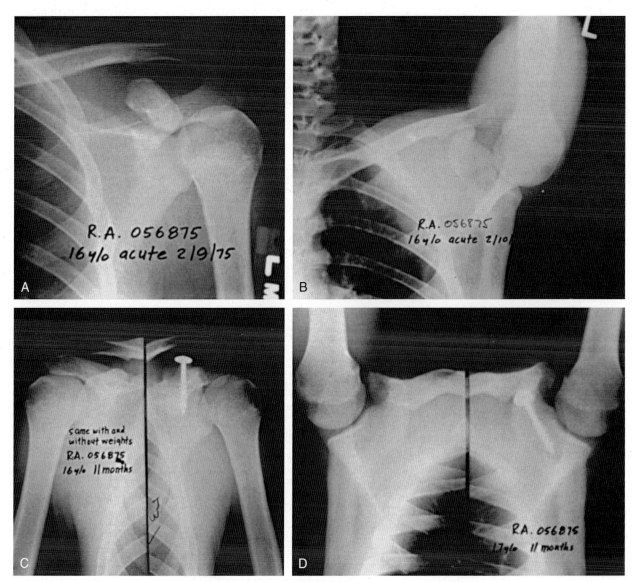

FIGURE 12-91 Type III variant in the skeletally mature patient. **A,** The acromioclavicular joint is dislocated, the coracoclavicular interval is not widened, and the coracoid is not normal. **B,** Fracture of the coracoid base is seen on the Stryker notch view. **C,** Open treatment with a coracoclavicular screw. **D,** Healing demonstrated on the Stryker notch view.

that radiates throughout its substance into the neck, superior shoulder, and medial periscapular region. Motion, either active or passive, in any direction and to any degree exacerbates the pain, which is especially intense if the clavicle has completely penetrated the trapezius.

The patient assumes a guarded posture to ease the significant pain resulting from the acute injury. The affected upper limb is held close to the body with the support of the opposite upper limb. Superior skin abrasions, soft tissue swelling, and ecchymosis are often observed. The acromioclavicular joint is visibly and palpably deformed by superior and posterior displacement of the clavicle (Fig. 12-97). Extreme posterior displacement occurs if the clavicle penetrates the trapezius com-

pletely and comes to lie directly beneath the skin. In this case, it is not likely that the joint is reducible (Fig. 12-98). Like the type III injury, pain inhibits the accurate assessment of motion and strength. The acromioclavicular joint, distal clavicle, coracoclavicular ligament, and trapezius muscle are tender to palpation.

Imaging
The lateral clavicle is displaced, to some degree, above the acromion process, and the coracoclavicular interval is widened. Posterior displacement of the clavicle may be overlooked unless an axillary lateral view is obtained (Fig. 12-99). When this view is not possible because of pain or body habitus, a CT scan might prove helpful. 3D

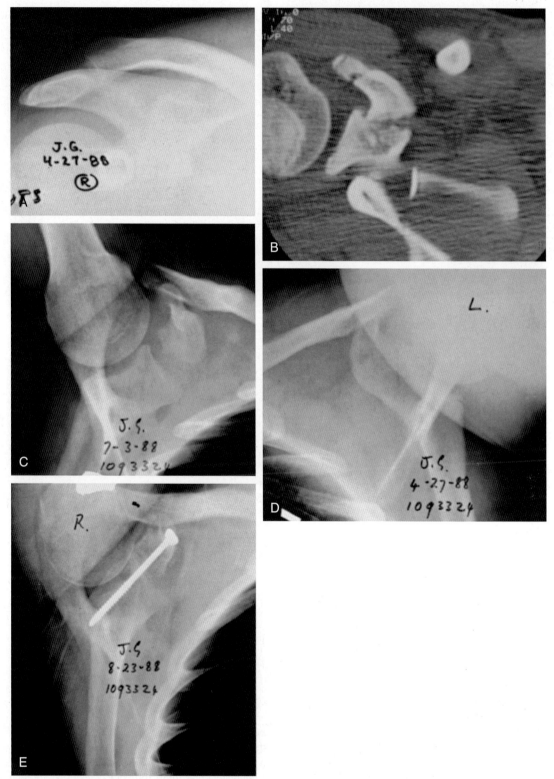

FIGURE 12-92 Nonunion of the base of the coracoid. **A,** The right acromioclavicular joint is unstable. **B,** CT of a fracture of the base of the coracoid process. **C,** Nonunion demonstrated on the Stryker notch view obtained 6 months after the acute injury. **D,** Stryker notch view of the contralateral shoulder. **E,** Nonunion repair with internal fixation and bone graft.

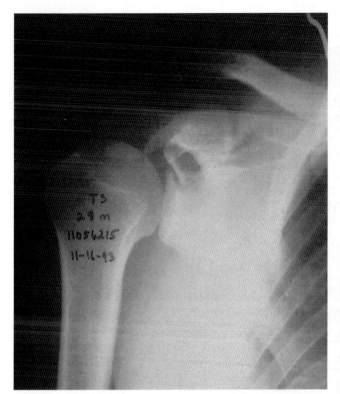

FIGURE 12-93 Type III injury variant with intra-articular extension of the base of the coracoid process fracture and dislocation of the acromioclavicular joint. (From Rockwood CA Jr, Bucholz RW, Heckman JD, Green DP [eds]: Rockwood and Green's Fractures in Adults, 5th ed. Philadelphia: Lippincott Williams & Wilkins, 2001.)

scanning is extremely useful for diagnosis (Fig. 12-100).[493]

Pathoanatomy

The acromioclavicular ligaments are always disrupted. The coracoclavicular ligaments are usually but not always torn. The clavicle is displaced posterior to the acromion, coming to rest in, or sometimes through, the trapezius muscle. This usually changes the orientation of the coracoclavicular interval. There is a high probability that the deltoid and trapezius muscles are detached from the distal clavicle.

Nonoperative Treatment

As a result of the extent of displacement and the severity of soft tissue damage, nonoperative treatment is usually not a consideration for type IV injuries.[223,480,482,483,485] It is such a painful lesion that even the most inactive patient will benefit from operative treatment, even if it is only a closed reduction. Opinions vary with regard to the choice of treatment for bipolar dislocations.[220,228,486,488,494]

Operative Treatment

Indications and Contraindications. With rare exception, all type IV injuries should be considered for operative treat-

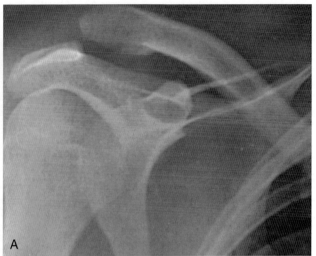

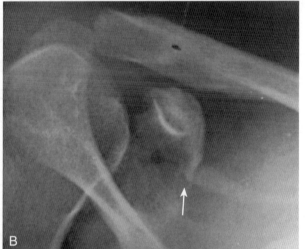

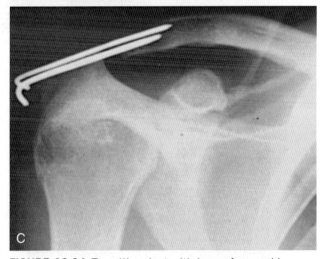

FIGURE 12-94 Type III variant with base of coracoid fracture and acromioclavicular dislocation. **A,** Dislocated acromioclavicular joint; the coracoclavicular interval distance is near normal. **B,** Cephalic tilt rather than Stryker notch demonstrates the fracture through the base of the coracoid process (*arrow*). **C,** Acromioclavicular joint pins, bent to minimize the chance of migration, maintained the reduction. (From Rockwood CA, Green DP [eds]: Fractures, 3 vols, 2nd ed. Philadelphia: JB Lippincott, 1984.)

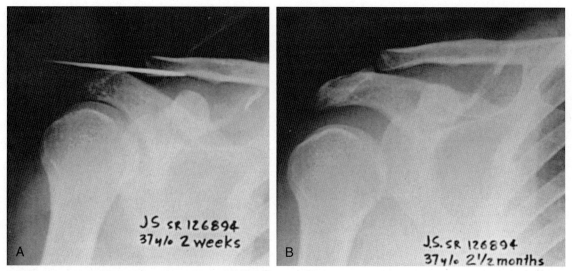

FIGURE 12-95 Type III injury variant with fracture of the base of the coracoid and dislocation of the acromioclavicular joint. **A,** Reduction of the joint and the fracture is maintained by transarticular pins. **B,** At 2.5 months, the pins have been removed, the acromioclavicular joint alignment has been preserved, and the coracoid fracture has healed.

ment.[484] Extremely low demand and inactive patients might have nothing to gain with operative treatment. Significant skin abrasions can delay operative treatment.

Methods. Closed reduction under general anesthesia may be possible and all that is needed for the extremely low demand, frail patient.[236] Otherwise, open treatment is required to disengage the lateral clavicle from the trapezius. It is possible that, immediately after the reduction, the only way to preserve joint congruity is by internal fixation that temporarily transgresses the joint.[480,481,483] Depending upon the findings, acromioclavicular and coracoclavicular ligament repair or reconstruction is con-

sidered. Isolated lateral clavicle excision is reasonable in the presence of intact coracoclavicular ligaments.[482,485]

Results. Successful operative and nonoperative treatment has been reported.[480-483,485]

Complications. No complications have been reported in the extremely few published cases.

Author's Preferred Method
Operative treatment is preferred. A closed reduction would suffice in the most inactive patients. Open reduction allows thorough exploration of the acromioclavicular

FIGURE 12-96 A and **B,** Clinical views of a combined type IV and type V chronic dislocation of the acromioclavicular joint. Not only does the left upper limb droop but also the lateral clavicle is prominent posteriorly. **C,** The acromioclavicular joint is severely displaced.

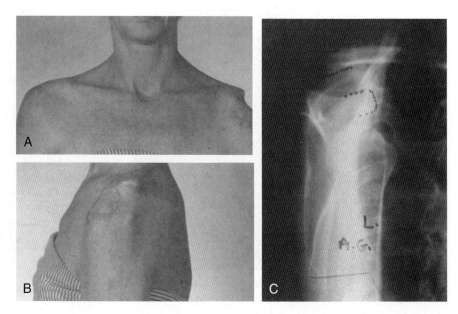

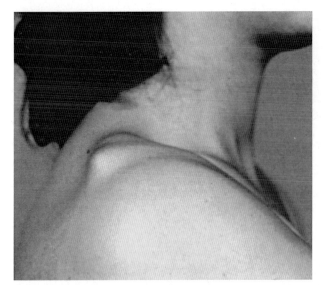

FIGURE 12-97 Patient with a type IV acromioclavicular joint injury. Note that the distal end of the clavicle is displaced posteriorly back into and through the trapezius muscle. (Courtesy of Louis Bigliani, MD.)

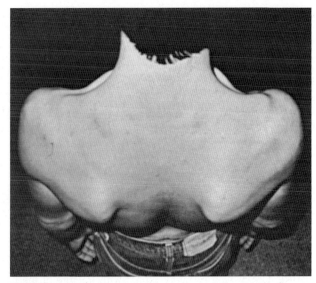

FIGURE 12-98 Type IV injury. The clavicle inclines posteriorly, producing a bump where it penetrates the trapezius muscle. (From Rockwood CA, Green DP [eds]: Fractures, 3 vols, 4th ed. Philadelphia: JB Lippincott, 1995.)

joint and coracoclavicular interval. In the rare instance that the coracoclavicular ligament is only sprained, the trapezius is repaired after acromioclavicular joint reduction. If instability persists, a hook plate is applied and left in place for 12 to 16 weeks. It is then removed under general anesthesia, and rehabilitation commences.

Type V
Signs and Symptoms
The pain of a type V injury is often more intense than the pain in type III or type IV injuries because the damage to the soft tissues is more severe and includes disruption of the muscle attachments from the lateral part of the

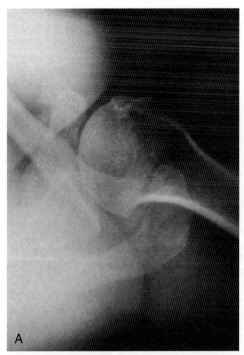

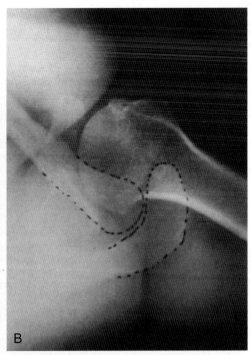

FIGURE 12-99 Type IV posterior dislocation of the acromioclavicular joint. **A,** Axillary lateral view. **B,** The lateral clavicle and acromion have been outlined to better display the injury.

clavicle. For this reason, the pain is widespread and exacerbated by motion, either active or passive, in any direction and to any degree. Neurogenic pain is possible due to the effect of the unsupported weight of the upper limb on the brachial plexus.

The patient holds the affected upper limb close to the torso with the help of the opposite upper limb. The lateral clavicle tents the overlying skin as the unsupported upper limb assumes an extreme inferior attitude (Figs. 12-101 and 12-102). Lateral stress testing can create a remarkable deformity of the shoulder (Fig. 12-103). The soft tissue overlying the acromion is likely to be abraded and contused, and more diffuse swelling and ecchymosis, the result of extensive muscle detachment, is observed. Like the other dislocations, pain inhibits accurate assessment of motion and strength. The shoulder is diffusely tender.

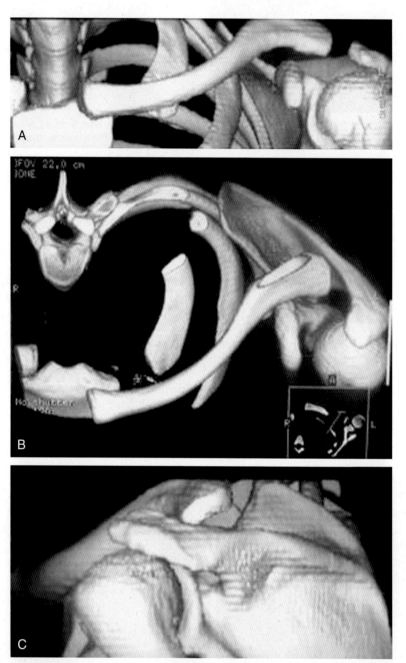

FIGURE 12-100 A to **C,** Type IV injury is clearly demonstrated with 3D CT. The sternoclavicular joint is anteriorly dislocated. **A,** Viewed from the anterior, the acromioclavicular joint appears widened, whereas the coracoclavicular interval appears normal. The medial clavicle is anterior to the manubrium. **B,** From above, the abnormal relationships of the acromioclavicular and sternoclavicular joints and the coracoclavicular interval are obvious. **C,** The lateral clavicle is not only posterior but also superior to the articular surface of the acromion. (From Scapinelli R: Bipolar dislocation of the clavicle: 3D CT imaging and delayed surgical correction of a case. Arch Orthop Trauma Surg 124[6]:421-424, 2004.)

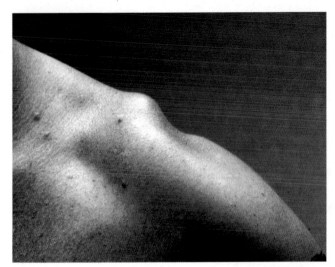

FIGURE 12-101 Type V injury.

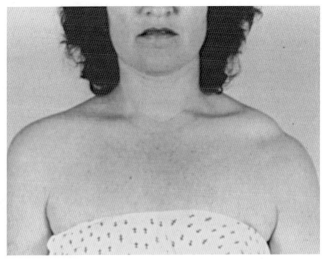

FIGURE 12-102 Type V injury resulting in drooping of the left upper limb. The clavicle, though prominent, is not displaced superiorly.

Imaging

There is extreme incongruity between the lateral clavicle and the acromion process as the scapula, no longer adequately suspended by the clavicle, drops away (Fig. 12-104D). It is not unusual for the coracoclavicular interval to widen by as much as 300% (see Fig. 12-104A and B).

Pathoanatomy

The acromioclavicular and coracoclavicular ligaments are torn completely, resulting in dislocation of the acromioclavicular joint. In comparison to the normal shoulder, the coracoclavicular interval may be widened twofold to threefold. There is the highest probability that the deltoid and trapezius muscles are detached from the lateral half of the clavicle.

Operative Treatment

The extreme displacement and the severity of soft tissue damage precludes nonoperative treatment for type V injuries.

Methods. As in type III injuries, coracoclavicular fixation with synthetic material has been used.[368]

Results. Verhaven reported nearly 30% of patients with fair or poor results.[368] Loss of reduction, osteoarthritis, ossification, or osteolysis did not correlate with outcome.

Experimental Treatment. Ammon and associates created type V injuries in cadavers, compared the failure load and pull-out strengths of fixation, and demonstrated that tita-

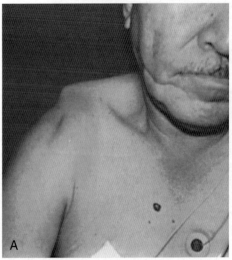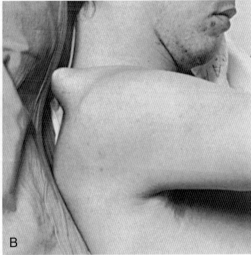

FIGURE 12-103 Type V injury. **A** and **B,** Note the posterior prominence of the clavicle with the lateral stress maneuver.

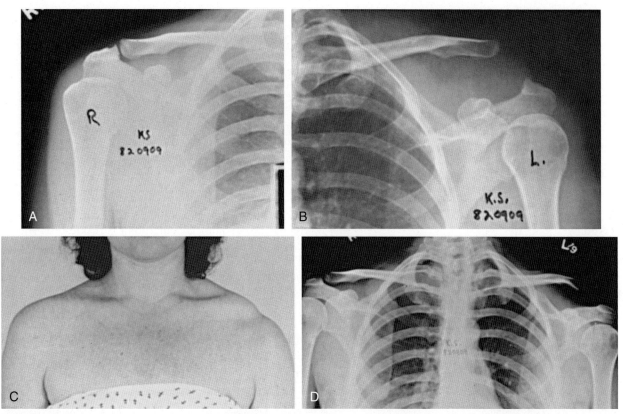

FIGURE 12-104 Type V injury. **A,** The normal right shoulder. **B,** The injured left shoulder with extreme widening of the coracoclavicular interval. **C,** The clavicle is quite prominent as a result of downward displacement of the right upper limb. **D,** Radiograph of this patient. The clavicles are at the same level. Deformity is the result of downward displacement of the upper limb.

nium Bosworth screws were superior to poly(L-lactic acid) screws.[495]

Complications. Early loss of reduction was reported by Verhaven.[368]

Author's Preferred Method
I treat the injury with a hook plate as in type III injuries.

Type VI
Type VI injuries, like type IV, are extremely rare.[229,462,496-502] They are usually produced by high-energy force that results in additional systemic injuries.

Signs and Symptoms
Type VI injuries often occur simultaneously with other musculoskeletal or systemic injuries that affect the overall expression of pain. However, an isolated type VI injury manifests with severe pain localized to the lateral clavicle. The patient typically experiences upper limb paresthesias until the fracture is reduced.[229,496,499]

The patient holds the injured limb in a protective manner adjacent to the torso with the opposite limb, resisting all attempts at movement. With type VI injuries, the normal sloping appearance of the superior shoulder flattens. The acromion becomes unusually prominent, as does the inferiorly distinct coracoid process. However, diffuse swelling and ecchymosis resulting from additional injuries nearby can obscure the deformity of the acromioclavicular joint. Altered peripheral cutaneous sensation is possible. Vascular perfusion of the upper limb remains stable. As with the other high-grade dislocations, pain inhibits the accurate assessment of motion and strength. Diffuse tenderness is the rule.

Imaging
Subacromial dislocations result in narrowing of the coracoclavicular interval as the lateral clavicle is displaced inferior to the acromion process. With subcoracoid dislocations, instead of a coracoclavicular interval superior to the coracoid process, a new coracoclavicular interval is created inferior to the coracoid process (Figs. 12-105 and 12-106). Inferior dislocation accompanied by glenoid

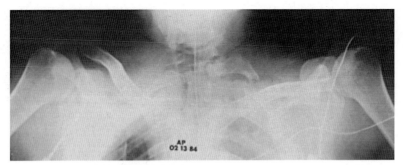

FIGURE 12-105 Type VI injury: subcoracoid dislocation of the left clavicle.

neck fracture and scapulothoracic dissociation has been observed.[497]

Pathoanatomy

The acromioclavicular ligaments are completely torn. The coracoclavicular ligament remains intact with the sub-acromial type but is completely torn with the subcoracoid type. The acromioclavicular joint is dislocated. The clavicle is displaced inferior to the acromion or the coracoid. The coracoclavicular interval is decreased (subacromial) or no longer anatomically exists (subcoracoid). The origin of the conjoined tendon has a deformed appearance

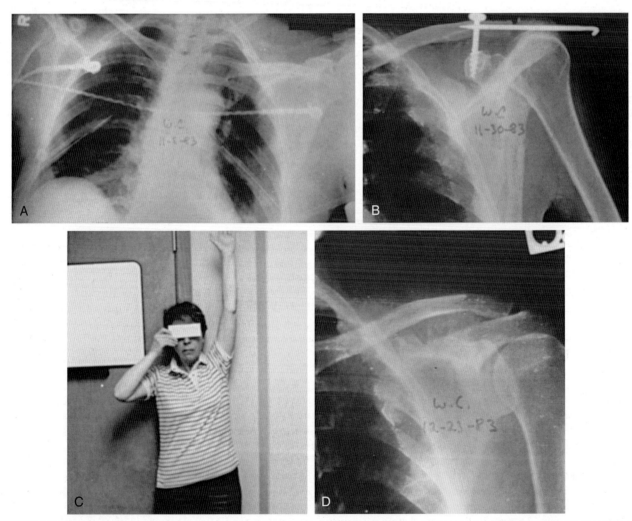

FIGURE 12-106 Type VI acromioclavicular dislocation. **A,** Subcoracoid dislocation of the clavicle. **B,** Open treatment with a coracoclavicular screw and acromioclavicular joint transfixation pins. **C,** At the completion of healing, full range of motion of the injured shoulder was possible. **D,** Heterotopic ossification nearly completely fills the coracoclavicular interval 20 months after the injury. (Courtesy of Robert C. Erickson, II, MD.)

because the lateral clavicle usually rests directly posterior. There is a high probability that deltoid and trapezius muscles are detached from the distal clavicle, but it depends on the extent of displacement. Vascular injuries have not been documented. Multidirectional instability has been observed.[497]

Operative Treatment

The nature and severity of the injury precludes consideration of nonoperative treatment. The preferred treatment for type VI injuries is operative treatment.[187,229,496,499,500,502,503]

Contraindications. There are no specific contraindications to operative treatment. Significant skin abrasions might require a temporary delay.

Methods. A consistent method of operative treatment has not emerged due to the relative rarity of type VI injuries. Closed reduction with various combinations of soft tissue repair, temporary transfixation of the acromioclavicular joint, coracoclavicular screw fixation, immobilization, and lateral clavicle excision have been reported (Fig. 12-107).[187,496,497]

Results. The cases reported in the literature have achieved a successful outcome without complications.

Chronic Lesions

Rockwood's classification scheme of types I to VI facilitates the understanding of acute traumatic lesions more so than chronic ones. From the perspective of treatment, the rudimentary classification espoused by Cadenet is, perhaps, more appropriate: incomplete (excision of the lateral clavicle) and complete (stabilization).[27] Incomplete lesions include Rockwood's types I and II. Practically speaking, complete lesions include only Rockwood type III injuries. The reason for this is that types IV to VI are recognizable as the most severe forms of complete injury, and as such have been treated acutely, in most instances.

Recurrent or habitual forms of complete injury are quite rare. Four cases of recurrent subacromial dislocations of the clavicle that were treated operatively have been reported.[498,500,504] Single cases of bilateral nontraumatic anterior dislocation, one recurrent, were reported separately by Janecki and by Richards and colleagues and can represent a less-severe variant of a type VI injury.[505,506]

Incomplete (Types I and II)
Signs and Symptoms
Mild to moderate pain that is well localized to the acromioclavicular joint is the most common manifestation of a chronic incomplete injury. Movement, which may be slightly diminished, can exacerbate the pain. Pain is sometimes sufficiently intense to contribute to weakness of the upper limb.

The physical findings are often subtle. A slightly more prominent distal clavicle can result in the appearance of an enlarged acromioclavicular joint when compared to the opposite side. The scapula might track abnormally as the upper limb is elevated and lowered. Deficits of internal rotation and cross-body adduction are possible as a result of pain. Crepitus arising from the acromioclavicular joint is usually not appreciated. Provocative testing of the acromioclavicular joint may be beneficial.

Imaging
The plain films are occasionally normal or symmetrical to the opposite acromioclavicular joint. More often a chronic type I injury cannot be distinguished from osteoarthritis and is, in fact, a secondary type of osteoarthritis. Classic findings include eccentric narrowing of the joint space, subchondral cyst formation, densification of the adjacent subchondral bone, and osteophyte formation (Fig. 12-108). One or more loose bodies may be present (Fig. 12-109). At other times, the predominant manifestation is one of osteolysis expressed as a loss of the subchondral bone with radiolucent cysts scattered throughout the epiphysis. Plain films might demonstrate an incongruent acromioclavicular joint with slight superior displacement of the lateral clavicle. A small increase in the coracoclavicular interval is possible.

Pathoanatomy
Depending on the extent of injury, scar tissue can form in the vicinity of the acromioclavicular joint. Slight superior displacement of the lateral clavicle is possible. The findings are those of osteoarthritis of varying degrees. They include capsular and synovial hypertrophy, joint effusion, thinned or absent articular cartilage, eburnated subchondral bone, and perhaps punctate cysts visible within the subchondral bone. The congruency of the joints varies with the amount of displacement and the extent of arthritis. The lateral clavicle may be tapered with an irregular surface as a result of osteolysis. Copious joint fluid can accumulate, sometimes under pressure.

Nonoperative Treatment
Methods. The mainstays of nonoperative treatment are rest, nonsteroidal anti-inflammatory medication, and the liberal use of ice or heat. Judicious use of intra-articular corticosteroid injections is reasonable.

Results. The therapeutic response primarily depends on the severity of the pathologic changes in the acromioclavicular joint. Symptoms can wax and wane or become refractory to all means of treatment.

Complications. The only complications of concern are those related to treatment: side effects of systemic medication and iatrogenic septic arthritis caused by joint injection.

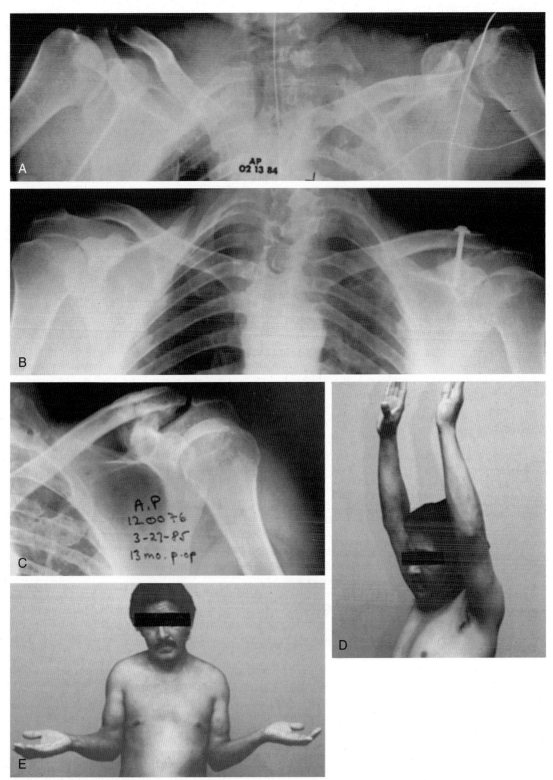

FIGURE 12-107 Type VI injury. **A,** This injury resulted from a train–pedestrian accident. In addition to the type VI subcoracoid dislocation of the clavicle, the patient sustained multiple rib fractures. **B,** Treatment included open reduction and placement of a coracoclavicular screw. **C,** At 6 weeks, the screw was removed. At 13 months, heterotopic ossification has formed in the coracoclavicular interval. **D** and **E,** Even with the coracoclavicular interval heterotopic ossification, essentially full range of motion is possible.

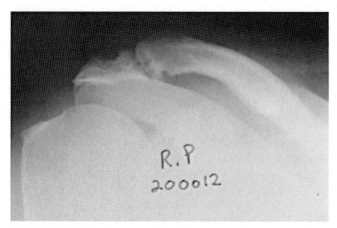

FIGURE 12-108 Osteoarthritis of the acromioclavicular joint, perhaps a sequela to a type I injury. (From Rockwood CA, Green DP [eds]: Fractures, 3 vols, 2nd ed. Philadelphia: JB Lippincott, 1984.)

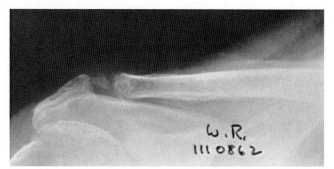

FIGURE 12-109 Loose body in the osteoarthritic acromioclavicular joint.

Operative Treatment

Indications and Contraindications. Intractable pain and dysfunction that has become unresponsive to nonoperative treatment is the indication for operative treatment. There are no specific contraindications to operative treatment.

Methods. The mainstay of operative treatment for chronic type I injuries is excision of the lateral clavicle as described by Mumford in 1941.[387] The techniques have been previously described. There are concerns for its use in occult instability or in patients with generalized ligamentous hypermobility.[103,107]

Results. The results of lateral clavicle resection for chronic type I injuries cannot be discerned from the literature. In theory, the results should not differ from lateral clavicle excision for degenerative disease, which means that comfort and function can be reliably restored.

Complications. Complications of lateral clavicle excision have been described. Heterotopic ossification can develop after excision of the lateral clavicle and is sometimes sufficiently symptomatic to warrant additional operative treatment. Pain can persist because of the excision of too little or too much lateral clavicle. Careless technique can result in the functional loss of the acromioclavicular ligaments, leading to symptomatic instability in the horizontal (AP) plane.

Complete (Types III and V)
Signs and Symptoms

Pain is the predominant feature of a chronic complete injury. As a result of the effect of more extensive soft tissue injury on shoulder mechanics, pain not only is present in the area of the acromioclavicular joint but also can be more widespread. With the loss of the scapula's connection with the clavicle, the sturdiest component of upper limb suspension, the periscapular muscles are pressed into a higher state of activity. Both factors can result in the development of periscapular pain and even pain radiating into the upper limb due to excessive traction on the brachial plexus. A variation of impingement syndrome can result in infra-acromial and subdeltoid pain. Motion is usually normal, though range limitations are possible due to pain. Overall shoulder girdle strength may be diminished on the basis of disuse or because of the mechanical absence of a sturdy articulation between the scapula and the clavicle.

Prominence of the lateral end of the clavicle is the most notable physical feature of a chronic complete injury (Fig. 12-110). As with acute complete injuries, the shoulder girdle and upper limb assume a drooped appearance with respect to the opposite side. Mild disuse muscular

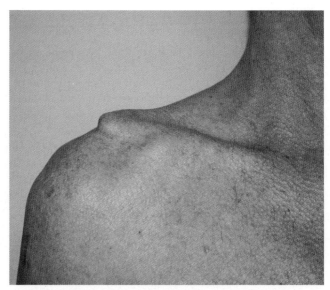

FIGURE 12-110 Clinical appearance of chronic complete acromioclavicular dislocation of the right shoulder.

atrophy is sometimes observed. Range of motion is usually not restricted, but with elevation and lowering of the upper limb, a variation of winging of the scapula, a scapular dyskinesis, is often observed.

Forced internal rotation and cross-body adduction induces acromioclavicular joint pain. Crepitation at the acromioclavicular joint may be produced by upper limb movement or with direct palpation. Manual muscle testing for strength exhibits no significant deficits. The acromioclavicular joint and the periscapular and infra-acromial regions might exhibit tenderness. The joint might or might not be reducible. Due to the disturbance of scapular motion, impingement signs may be positive. The results of acromioclavicular joint provocative testing may be unreliable or misleading in this setting.

Imaging

Chronic and acute complete injuries have a similar radiographic appearance in that there is no contact between the articular surfaces of the lateral clavicle and the medial acromion, and the coracoclavicular interval is widened. Heterotopic ossification is sometimes present in the coracoclavicular interval.

Pathoanatomy

Scarring is present in the region of the acromioclavicular joint and the lateral clavicle, making it difficult to distinguish the acromioclavicular joint capsuloligamentous complex from the healed attachments of the trapezius and deltoid muscles. The gap between the acromion and the clavicle may be filled completely with scar tissue or may be a pseudarthrosis. The intra-articular disk is usually undetectable. In the absence of a coracoclavicular interval that has been obliterated with scar tissue and bone, the coracoclavicular ligament stumps may be palpable. The hyaline cartilage usually remains on the medial acromion and the lateral clavicle but might not be mechanically sound.

Nonoperative Treatment

Methods. Overuse might have provoked a symptomatic flare of the chronic complete injury, necessitating an initial period of rest. It is appropriate to dispense nonsteroidal anti-inflammatory medication or non-narcotic analgesics along with recommendation for the use of ice or heat. Because there is no longer a true articulation, it is not appropriate to consider a corticosteroid injection.

Results. The success of nonoperative treatment of chronic complete injuries depends on compliance with activity modification. Simple modifications are sometimes all that is necessary to render the shoulder both comfortable and functional. If aggravating factors are unavoidable, nonoperative treatment will fail.

Complications. The only complications of concern are those related to treatment with systemic medication.

Operative Treatment

Indications and Contraindications. Intractable pain and dysfunction that has become unresponsive to nonoperative treatment is the indication for operative treatment. There are no specific contraindications to operative treatment.

Methods. Excision of the lateral clavicle will rarely address the symptoms that result from a chronic complete injury and is not advised.[59,66] Reconstructions of the acromioclavicular joint are most successful when the operation incorporates, by some means, fixation between the clavicle and the coracoid process.[507] Biological tissue or synthetic materials have been used to reconstruct the acromioclavicular and the coracoclavicular ligaments simultaneously without excision of the lateral clavicle.[356,508,509]

Dynamic muscle transfers, as described in the treatment of acute type III injuries, have also been performed in chronic cases, with or without excision of the lateral clavicle.[391,393,510]

Transposition of the coracoacromial ligament to the end of the resected clavicle was described by Weaver and Dunn in 1972 and subsequently performed by others as originally described or with subtle technical modifications.[347,370,375,381,382,511,512]

Results. The transposition of the coracoacromial ligament to the end of the resected clavicle yields excellent or good results in a least 80% of patients.[347,511] Biological tissue or synthetic materials have been used to reconstruct the acromioclavicular and the coracoclavicular ligaments simultaneously without excision of the lateral clavicle.[356,508,509] Very favorable results and an extremely high satisfaction rate are reported for reconstructions of the acromioclavicular and the coracoclavicular ligaments performed simultaneously without excision of the lateral clavicle.[356,508,509]

Complications. Essentially the same complications are encountered whether one is treating an acute or a chronic lesion of this type. Isolated excision of the lateral clavicle is significantly more prone to complications in the setting of chronic complete injuries and is best avoided (Fig. 12-111).

Author's Preferred Method. I prefer to use hook plate reconstruction (as described earlier for the treatment of acute type III injury) as a primary treatment for a similar chronic lesion. Greater emphasis is placed on soft tissue dissection inferior to the clavicle to expose the superior aspect of the coracoid. With this method, the deltoid and trapezius are detached more extensively. The end of the clavicle has often undergone attritional changes that would not favor its durability if it is once again apposed to the medial acromion. For this reason, it is unhesitatingly excised even if it has a normal appearance.

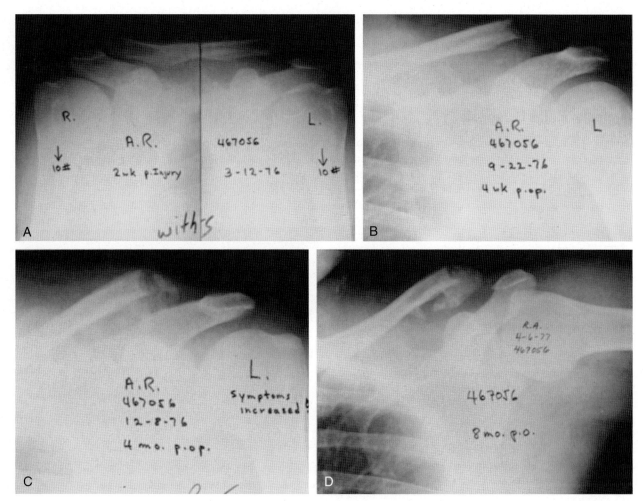

FIGURE 12-111 Complication of instability from lateral clavicle excision for chronic, complete acromioclavicular joint dislocation. **A,** Acute, complete acromioclavicular dislocation on preoperative radiographs. **B,** Six months later, due to continued pain, the lateral clavicle was excised. **C,** Four months after surgical treatment, the patient had increasing pain, heterotopic ossification, and widening of the coracoclavicular interval. **D,** Continued symptoms at 8 months after the index operation. (From Rockwood CA, Green DP [eds]: Fractures, 3 vols, 2nd ed. Philadelphia: JB Lippincott, 1984.)

Success with this technique depends upon the formation of scar tissue in critical locations: between the coracoid process and the clavicle, between the acromion process and the clavicle, and superior to the clavicle. The strength and stiffness of the hook plate maintains the proper osseous relationships during the formation of the stabilizing scar tissue. To avert the possibility of residual acromioclavicular horizontal or medial instability, there are two options to consider. The first option is to strengthen the linkage between the acromion process and the lateral clavicle, which in nearly all cases, has been resected. The coracoacromial ligament can be detached from the coracoid and attached to the lateral clavicle, spanning the acromioclavicular joint (Fig. 12-112). The same reconstruction can be done with tendon graft. The second option is interposition arthroplasty using autografts or allografts or other material that might be considered biologically active (GraftJacket). The method has

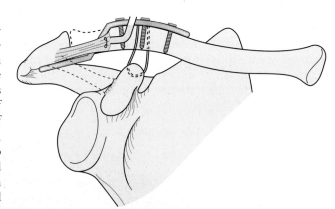

FIGURE 12-112 Chronic complete reconstruction that uses the coracoacromial ligament, detached from the coracoid and attached to the lateral clavicle, spanning the acromioclavicular joint. The hook plate provides rigid internal fixation and the coracoclavicular interval is spanned with nonabsorbable suture.

the benefit of a cushioning effect and, to some extent, a stabilizing effect.

NONTRAUMATIC DISORDERS

Acromioclavicular Osteolysis

The relationship between osteolysis of the distal clavicle and trauma has been well documented. The earliest reports of the condition are found in the non-English literature.[265,513,514] The strong association with trauma was verified by others.[254,515,516] The role for repetitive trauma, perhaps best thought of as overuse, first mentioned by Ehricht more than 5 decades ago, was noted by Seymour in 1977, and subsequently strongly supported by a report of Cahill, who documented an undeniable relationship to weight training.[84,513,517] Other authors have confirmed this relationship to repetitive trauma or overuse, especially weight training.[94,518,519] It is rarely reported in female patients, perhaps due to less risk-activity exposure.[518,520,521]

Various mechanisms for the development of osteolysis under these conditions have been suggested, including vascular compromise, microfractures, nervous system dysfunction, osteoclastic activation, and synovial hyperplasia.[84,254,516,521-525]

The radiographic findings are variable, depending upon the duration of the process, and have been effectively described by all reporting authors. In addition to osteolysis, these can include osteoporosis, irregular or absent subchondral bone, alteration of the distal clavicle morphology such as tapering, cysts of various dimensions, calcification, and osteophytes (see Fig. 12-46). Bone scan activity is usually intense and well localized to the acromioclavicular joint and distal clavicle (Figs. 12-113 and 12-114).[84] MRI, often performed but rarely necessary, might reveal edema within the marrow elements of the distal clavicle, cortical erosions, and cysts.[175,248,526]

Histologic findings obtained at the time of operative treatment were reported by Asano and others and may be extensive: synovial hyperplasia, articular cartilage destruction of the distal clavicle, bone necrosis, vascular

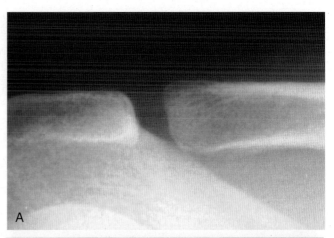
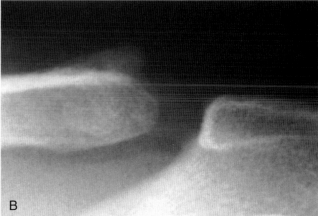

FIGURE 12-113 Osteolysis. **A,** Normal acromioclavicular joint. **B,** Tender, enlarged acromioclavicular joint.

proliferation, reactive woven bone, fibrous tissue invasion, multinucleated giant cells, inflammatory cells within the bone marrow, and preservation of the intra-articular disk.[254,516,522,527-529] Asano also documented noninvolvement of the acromion process.

Another etiologic category has been proposed by Hawkins and coworkers: nontraumatic.[530] They describe the clinical presentation of three healthy patients without exposure to trauma or overuse and without evidence for metabolic disease or any other known cause of osteolysis.

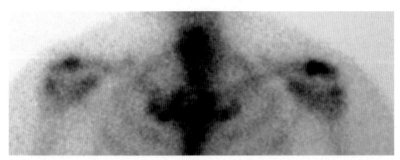

FIGURE 12-114 Bone scan (correlating with plain films in Fig. 12-113) showing intense tracer uptake in the acromioclavicular joint with osteolysis.

The differential diagnosis of atraumatic occurrence is limited. Systemic diseases such as hyperparathyroidism, rheumatoid arthritis, and scleroderma should be given consideration, especially with bilateral involvement. Local processes that can resemble classic osteolysis are massive osteolysis (Gorham's disease), infections, metastatic malignancy, primary bone tumors such as multiple myeloma, and crystal arthropathy, especially gout.

Activity-related pain with local tenderness and perhaps slight swelling are the hallmarks of this disorder. Night pain may be present to a variable degree depending on the intensity of the inflammation that is associated with the process.

A conservative plan of care should be undertaken for osteolysis of the distal clavicle, at least initially. The cornerstone of treatment is rest and activity modification, even going so far as to completely discontinue participation in weight-training programs that are undertaken to maximize athletic performance and vigorously encouraged by coaches and trainers. Nonsteroidal anti-inflammatory medication can be prescribed and from time to time, during the course of recovery, it may be reasonable to perform a corticosteroid injection. Although it can require 6 to 12 months, instances of relatively atraumatic osteolysis of the distal clavicle are capable of recovery of comfort, function, and bone integrity with conservative treatment.[523,531,532]

When nonoperative treatment is deemed a failure, excision of the lateral clavicle will definitively terminate the process and, in nearly all cases, result in an excellent or good outcome.[94,95,530]

Acromioclavicular Arthritis

There are more than 100 different types of arthritis that can involve the acromioclavicular joint. Only three are mentioned here.

Osteoarthritis

Because of the prevalence of osteoarthritis of the acromioclavicular joint in the population, it is near certainty that nearly all providers of musculoskeletal care evaluate and treat the disorder at some point (Fig. 12-115).[533-535] It may be very difficult to ascertain, however, whether the condition is primary or secondary, although the former is not commonly symptomatic and the latter, especially trauma-related osteoarthritis, is more prevalent (Fig. 12-116).[107,241,245]

From their observations of the acromioclavicular joint space narrowing with age, Petersson and Redlund-Johnell concluded that an interval of 0.5 mm or less between the acromion and the clavicle in a patient older than 60 years might not indicate disease.[154] Bonsell and colleagues drew attention to a negative correlation between the age-related radiologic findings of osteoarthritis and symptomatic acromioclavicular joints.[536] The occurrence of traction osteophytes arising from the lateral articular facets of the clavicle significantly correlates with increasing age.[537] It

should be recalled however, that the true incidence of acromioclavicular osteoarthritis is underestimated by plain radiography or tomography.[538] As discussed earlier, the sensitivity of MRI and ultrasonography verifies its presence earlier in life as well as an increasing incidence with age. In addition, the widespread use of MRI of the shoulder has led to the recognition of a high prevalence of age-related changes in the acromioclavicular joint, not infrequently in asymptomatic patients.[169,171,539]

In cadavers, osteoarthritis was also age-related and was especially prevalent after 70 years.[18] Besides age, other risk factors for the development of osteoarthritis are extreme labor and sports participation.[540]

The treatment of osteoarthritis of the acromioclavicular joint differs very little from other joints in the body: activity modification, non-narcotic analgesics, nonsteroidal anti-inflammatory medication, and the liberal use of ice and heat. The results of intra-articular corticosteroid injections vary but usually result, at the least, in short-term pain relief and improvement in range of motion.[106,117,143,541-543] The success of pain relief with intra-articular injection of local anesthetic and corticosteroid has a direct relationship to joint capsule hypertrophy (>3 mm) demonstrated by MRI.[544]

The disease can be definitively treated with excision of the lateral clavicle with predictably satisfactory outcomes if appropriate surgical guidelines are followed.

Rheumatoid Arthritis

The acromioclavicular joint is affected in at least 50% of patients with rheumatoid arthritis; even more commonly than the glenohumeral joint.[92] Only rarely is operative treatment performed.

Crystal Arthritis

Gout and pseudogout of the acromioclavicular joint have been reported.[545-548]

Other Diseases Involving the Acromioclavicular Joint

Synovial chondromatosis has been reported.[549]

Cysts of the Acromioclavicular Joint

The acromioclavicular joint is a common site for the development of cysts or, more accurately, cyst-like structures that are usually the result of massive tears of the rotator cuff. The pathogenesis relates to instability of the humeral head. No longer constrained by sufficient medially directed forces, the humeral head ascends until it makes contact with the fibro-osseous coracoacromial archway. Lacking the protective covering of the rotator cuff, the articular cartilage deteriorates and presents a much rougher surface to the overlying archway. The relatively thin inferior acromioclavicular joint capsule begins to erode while the unusually large effusion that typically accompanies this condition escapes by way of the path

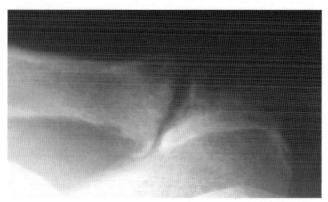

FIGURE 12-115 Osteoarthritis of the acromioclavicular joint seen on the Zanca view. Note eccentric joint space narrowing, osteophytes, and subchondral cysts.

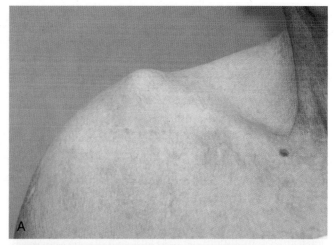

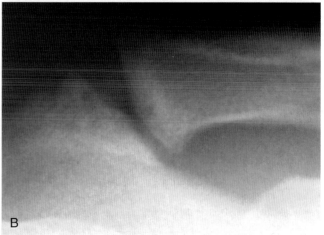

FIGURE 12-116 Osteoarthritis. The patient was asymptomatic. **A,** Clinical appearance. **B,** Radiographic correlation of primary osteoarthritis.

of least resistance into the acromioclavicular joint. The attachments of the deltoid and trapezius muscles act as reinforcements for the anterior and posterior portions of the capsule while exposing the relatively weak superior capsule that bridges them to the ebb and flow of joint fluid under pressure. The capsule eventually fails, permitting the fluid to slowly dissect into the overlying soft tissues. In response, a new, flexible pseudocapsule forms and becomes a discrete permanent enclosure that remains in close proximity to the acromioclavicular joint or, rarely, finds its way into the surrounding muscles (Fig. 12-117). These structures and periarticular ganglions are well documented in the literature and should not be confused with infections or neoplasms.[135,347,550-554] Crystals are sometimes detected in the fluid (Fig. 12-118).

Cysts have been observed in the setting of gouty involvement of the acromioclavicular joint that acquires a characteristic pattern of bony projections from the acromion that give it the name *porcupine shoulder.*[545]

The cysts present no specific threat unless the overlying, protruding skin is threatened by pressure or excessive friction.

Ultrasonography or MRI are the best ways to image the cyst and are sometimes as dramatic as the most extreme form of the geyser sign observed with arthrography (Fig. 12-119).[555,556] Isolated excision of the cyst mandates a soft tissue repair sturdier than originally present to prevent recurrence or, even worse, an arthrocutaneous fistula. Mullett and associates reported successful arthroscopic treatment of a massive cyst.[552] The cuff is usually irreparable and glenohumeral joint arthropathy may be present. In these instances, prosthetic arthroplasty contributes to successful management of the cyst.[546]

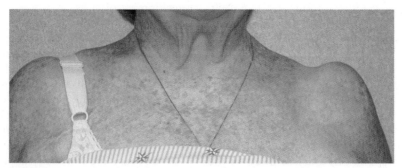

FIGURE 12-117 Acromioclavicular cyst in a patient with a chronic left rotator cuff tear.

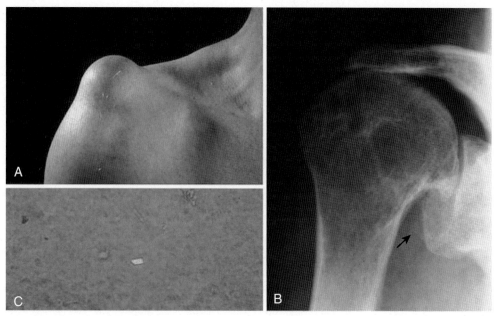

FIGURE 12-118 Acromioclavicular cyst. **A,** Clinical appearance of the cyst. **B,** Accompanying radiograph indicating a massive irreparable rotator cuff tear. Calcific radiodensity within the joint space *(arrow)* indicates crystal deposition within the cyst. **C,** Calcium hydroxyapatite crystals obtained from the fluid-filled cyst.

Infections of the Acromioclavicular Joint

Most infections of the acromioclavicular joint are caused by operations or injections intended to treat a disorder of the joint. Rarely is the infecting organism bloodborne or acquired directly from infected tissue in the vicinity of the joint. A few reports of bacterial arthritis have been published in healthy or compromised persons.[557-560] Non-bacterial infections including tuberculosis and cryptococcosis have been reported.[561,562]

Other Disorders of the Acromioclavicular Joint

Osteonecrosis of the lateral clavicle has been reported.[563] The radiographic, gross, and histologic features allow it to be distinguished from osteolysis.

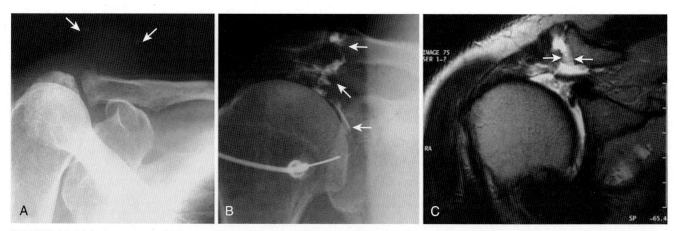

FIGURE 12-119 Acromioclavicular cyst images (cyst in Fig. 12-118). **A,** The humeral head abuts the acromioclavicular joint. The soft tissue outline of the cyst is shown by the *arrows*. **B,** Arthrography demonstrates the Geyser sign *(arrows)*. **C,** MRI shows the rotator cuff tear and the fluid communicating between the acromioclavicular joint and the glenohumeral joint *(arrows)*.

REFERENCES

1. Adams FL: The Genuine Works of Hippocrates, vols 1 and 2. New York: William Wood, 1886.
2. Hollinshead WH: Anatomy for Surgeons, vol. 3, The Back and Limbs. Philadelphia: Harper & Row, 1982, pp 207-208.
3. Todd TW, D'Errico J: The clavicular epiphysis. Am J Anat 41:25-50, 1928.
4. Hollinshead WH: The pectoral region, axilla, and shoulder. In Hollinshead WH: Anatomy for Surgeons, vol. 3, The Back and Limbs. Philadelphia: Harper & Row, 1982, pp 263-264.
5. Hollinshead WH: The pectoral region, axilla, and shoulder. In Hollinshead WH: Anatomy for Surgeons, vol. 3, The Back and Limbs. Philadelphia: Harper & Row, 1982, p 263.
6. Hollinshead WH: General survey of the upper limb. In Hollinshead WH: Anatomy for Surgeons, vol. 3, The Back and Limbs. Philadelphia: Harper & Row, 1982, pp 247-250.
7. Bearden JM, Hughston JC, Whatley GS: Acromioclavicular dislocation: Method of treatment. J Sports Med 1:5-17, 1973.
8. Bosworth BM: Complete acromioclavicular dislocation. N Engl J Med 241:221-225, 1949.
9. Edelson JG, Luchs J: Aspects of coracoacromial ligament anatomy of interest to the arthroscopic surgeon. Arthroscopy 11:715-719, 1995.
10. Fealy S, April EW, Khazzam M, et al: The coracoacromial ligament: Morphology and study of acromial enthesopathy. J Shoulder Elbow Surg 14:542-548, 2005.
11. Tyurina TV: [Age-related characteristics of the human acromioclavicular joint.] Arkh Anat Gistol Embriol 89:75-81, 1985.
12. Poncelet E, Demondion X, Lapegue F, et al: Anatomic and biometric study of the acromioclavicular joint by ultrasound. Surg Radiol Anat 25:439-445, 2003.
13. DePalma AF: Surgery of the Shoulder, 2nd ed. Philadelphia: JB Lippincott, 1973.
14. Urist MR: Complete dislocation of the acromioclavicular joint: The nature of the traumatic lesion and effective methods of treatment with an analysis of 41 cases. J Bone Joint Surg 28:813-837, 1946.
15. Moseley HF: Athletic injuries to the shoulder region. Am J Surg 98:401-422, 1959.
16. Keats TE, Pope TL Jr: The acromioclavicular joint: Normal variation and the diagnosis of dislocation. Skeletal Radiol 17:159-162, 1988.
17. DePalma AF: The role of the disks of the sternoclavicular and acromioclavicular joints. Clin Orthop 13:7-12, 1959.
18. Petersson CJ: Degeneration of the acromioclavicular joint: A morphological study. Acta Orthop Scand 54:434-438, 1983.
19. Salter EG, Nasca RJ, Shelley BS: Anatomical observations on the acromioclavicular joint and supporting ligaments. Am J Sports Med 15:199-206, 1987.
20. Harris RI, Vu DH, Sonnabend DH, et al: Anatomic variance of the coracoclavicular ligaments. J Shoulder Elbow Surg 10:585-588, 2001.
21. Costic RS, Vangura A Jr, Fenwick JA, et al: Viscoelastic behavior and structural properties of the coracoclavicular ligaments. Scand J Med Sci Sports 13:305-310, 2003.
22. Rios CG, Arciero RA, Mazzocca AD: Anatomy of the clavicle and coracoid process for reconstruction of the coracoclavicular ligaments. Am J Sports Med 35:811-817, 2007.
23. Renfree KJ, Riley MK, Wheeler D, et al: Ligamentous anatomy of the distal clavicle. J Shoulder Elbow Surg 12:355-359, 2003.
24. Codman EA: The Shoulder: Rupture of the Supraspinatus Tendon and Other Lesions in or about the Subacromial Bursa. Boston: Thomas Todd, 1934.
25. Inman VT, Saunders JB, Abbott LC: Observations on the function of the shoulder joint. J Bone Joint Surg 26:1-30, 1944.
26. Kennedy JC, Cameron H: Complete dislocation of the acromioclavicular joint. J Bone Joint Surg Br 36:202-208, 1954.
27. Cadenet FM: The treatment of dislocations and fractures of the outer end of the clavicle. Int Clin 1:145-169, 1917.
28. Debski RE, Parsons IM 3rd, Fenwick J, et al: Ligament mechanics during three degree-of-freedom motion at the acromioclavicular joint. Ann Biomed Eng 28:612-618, 2000.
29. Debski RE, Parsons IM, Woo SL, et al: Effect of capsular injury on acromioclavicular joint mechanics. J Bone Joint Surg 83:1344-1351, 2001.
30. Fukuda K, Craig EV, An K-N, et al: Biomechanical study of the ligamentous system of the acromioclavicular joint. J Bone Joint Surg Am 68:434-439, 1986.
31. Klimkiewicz JJ, Williams GR, Sher JS, et al: The acromioclavicular capsule as a restraint to posterior translation of the clavicle: A biomechanical analysis. J Shoulder Elbow Surg 8:119-124, 1999.
32. Lee K, Debski RE, Chen C, et al: Functional evaluation of the ligaments at the acromioclavicular joint during anteroposterior and superoinferior translation. Am J Sports Med 25:858-862, 1997.
33. Rockwood CA Jr: Acromioclavicular dislocation. In Rockwood CA Jr, Greene DD (eds): Fractures, vol 1. Philadelphia: JB Lippincott, 1975, pp 721-756.
34. Rockwood CA Jr: Acromioclavicular separations. In Kane WJ (ed): Current Orthopaedic Management. New York, Churchill Livingstone, 1981, pp 290-311.
35. Rockwood CA Jr: Injuries to the acromioclavicular joint. In Rockwood CA Jr, Green DP (eds): Fractures in Adults, vol 1, 2nd ed. Philadelphia: JB Lippincott, 1984, pp 860-910.
36. Harris RI, Wallace AL, Harper GD, et al: Structural properties of the intact and reconstructed coracoclavicular ligament complex. Am J Sports Med 28:103-108, 2000.
37. Poirier P, Rieffel H: Mechanisme des luxations sur acromiales de la clavicle. Arch Gen Med 1:396-422, 1891.
38. Koh SW, Cavanaugh JM, Leach JP, et al: Mechanical properties of the shoulder ligaments under dynamic loading. Stapp Car Crash J 48:125-53, 2004.
39. Lewis OJ: The coraco-clavicular joint. J Anat 93:296-303, 1959.
40. Gradoyevitch B: Coracoclavicular joint. J Bone Joint Surg 21:918-920, 1939.
41. Cheung TF, Boerboom AL, Wolf RF, et al: Asymptomatic coracoclavicular joint. J Bone Joint Surg Br 88:1519-20, 2006.
42. Cockshott WP: The coracoclavicular joint. Radiology 131:313-316, 1979.
43. Gumina S, Salvatore M, De Santis R, et al: Coracoclavicular joint: Osteologic study of 1020 human clavicles. J Anat 201:513-519, 2002.
44. Cho BP, Kang HS: Articular facets of the coracoclavicular joint in Koreans. Acta Anat (Basel) 163:56-62, 1998.
45. Cockshott WP: The geography of coracoclavicular joints. Skeletal Radiol 21:225-227, 1992.
46. Hamarati N, Cook RA, Raphael B, et al: Coracoclavicular joint: Normal variant in humans. Skeletal Radiol 23:117-119, 1994.
47. Kaur H, Jit I: Coracoclavicular joint in northwest Indians. Am J Phys Anthropol 85:457-460, 1991.
48. Liberson F: The role of the coracoclavicular ligaments in affections of the shoulder girdle. Am J Surg 44:145-157, 1939.
49. Nalla S, Asvat JR: Incidence of the coracoclavicular joint in South African populations. J Anat 186:645-649, 1995.
50. Nehme A: Coracoclavicular joints: Reflections upon incidence, pathophysiology and etiology of the different forms. Surg Radiol Anat 26:33-38, 2004.
51. Nutter PD: Coracoclavicular articulations. J Bone Joint Surg 23:177-179, 1941.
52. Pillay VK: Significance of the coracoclavicular joint (Proceedings). J Bone Joint Surg Br 49:390, 1967.
53. Faraj AA: Bilateral congenital coracoclavicular joint. Case report and review of the literature. Acta Orthop Belg 69:552-554, 2003.
54. Hama H, Matsusue Y, Ito H, et al: Thoracic outlet syndrome associated with an anomalous coracoclavicular joint: A case report. J Bone Joint Surg Am 75:1368-1369, 1993.
55. Lehtinen JT, Kaarela K, Belt EA, et al: Coracoclavicular involvement—an atypical manifestation in rheumatoid arthritis. Scand J Rheumatol 28:252-253, 1999.
56. Nikolaides AP, Dermon AR, Papavasiliou KA, et al: Coracoclavicular joint degeneration, an unusual cause of painful shoulder: A case report. Acta Orthop Belg 72:90-92, 2006.
57. Wertheimer LG: Coracoclavicular joint: Surgical treatment of a painful syndrome caused by an anomalous joint. J Bone Joint Surg Am 30:570-578, 1948.
58. McLaughlin HL: Trauma. Philadelphia: WB Saunders, 1959.
59. Shaffer BS: Painful conditions of the acromioclavicular joint. J Am Acad Orthop Surg 7:176-188, 1999.
60. Rabalais RD, McCarty E: Surgical treatment of symptomatic acromioclavicular joint problems: A systematic review. Clin Orthop Relat Res (455):30-37, 2007.
61. Branch TP, Burdette HL, Shatiriari AS, et al: The role of the acromioclavicular ligaments and the effect of distal clavicle excision. Am J Sports Med 24:293-297, 1996.
62. Boehm TD, Kirschner S, Fischer A, et al: The relation of the coracoclavicular ligament insertion to the acromioclavicular joint: A cadaver study of relevance to lateral clavicle resection. Acta Orthop Scand 74:718-721, 2003.
63. Eskola A, Santaritra S, Viljakka T, et al: The results of operative resection of the lateral end of the clavicle. J Bone Joint Surg Am 78:584-587, 1996.
64. Matthews LS, Parks BG, Paylovich LJ Jr, et al: Arthroscopic versus open distal clavicle resection: A biomechanical analysis on a cadaver model. Arthroscopy 15:237-240, 1999.
65. Kay SP, Dragoo JL, Lee R: Long-term results of arthroscopic resection of the distal clavicle with concomitant subacromial decompression. Arthroscopy 19:805-809, 2003.
66. Rockwood CA Jr, Williams GR Jr, Young DC: Disorders of the acromioclavicular joint. In Rockwood CA Jr, Matsen FA III, Wirth MA, Lippitt SB (eds): The Shoulder, 3rd ed. Philadelphia: Saunders, 2004.
67. Alford W, Bach BR: Open distal clavicle resection. Oper Tech Sports Med 12:9-17, 2004.
68. Boehm TD, Barthel T, Schwemmer U, et al: Ultrasonography for intraoperative control of the amount of bone resection in arthroscopic acromioclavicular joint resection. Arthroscopy 20(Suppl 2):142-145, 2004.

69. Costic RS, Jari R, Rodosky MW, et al: Joint compression alters the kinematics and loading patterns of the intact and capsule-transected AC joint. J Orthop Res 21:379-385, 2003.

70. Corteen DP, Teitge RA: Stabilization of the clavicle after distal resection: A biomechanical study. Am J Sports Med 33:61-67, 2005.

71. Deshmukh AV, Perlmutter GS, Zilberfarb JL, et al: Effect of subacromial decompression on laxity of the acromioclavicular joint: Biomechanical testing in a cadaveric model. J Shoulder Elbow Surg 13:338-343, 2004.

72. Kuster MS, Hales PF, Davis SJ: The effects of arthroscopic acromioplasty on the acromioclavicular joint. J Shoulder Elbow Surg 7:140-143, 1998.

73. Moseley HF: The clavicle: Its anatomy and function. Clin Orthop Relat Res 58:17-27, 1968.

74. Edwards SG: Acromioclavicular stability: A biomechanical comparison of acromioplasty to acromioplasty with coplaning of the distal clavicle. Arthroscopy 19:1079-1084, 2003.

75. Barber FA: Coplaning of the acromioclavicular joint. Arthroscopy 17:913-917, 2001.

76. Barber FA: Long-term results of acromioclavicular joint coplaning. Arthroscopy 22:125-129, 2006.

77. Buford D, Mologne T, McGrath S, et al: Midterm results of arthroscopic coplaning of the acromioclavicular joint. J Shoulder Elbow Surg 9:498-501, 2000.

78. Kharrazi D, Glousman R, Tibone J, et al: Re-operation on the acromioclavicular joint following arthroscopic subacromial decompression [abstract]. Arthroscopy 16:435, 2000.

79. Weber SC: Coplaning the acromioclavicular joint at the time of acromioplasty (A long-term study) [abstract]. Arthroscopy 15:555, 1999.

80. Fischer BW, Gross RM, McCarthy JA, et al: Incidence of acromioclavicular joint complications after arthroscopic subacromial decompression. Arthroscopy 15:241-248, 1999.

81. Blazar PE, Iannotti JP, Williams GR: Anteroposterior instability of the distal clavicle after distal clavicle resection. Clin Orthop Relat Res (348):114-120, 1998.

82. Hazel RM, Tasto JP, Klassen J: Arthroscopic subacromial decompression: A 9-year follow-up [abstract]. Arthroscopy 14:419, 1998.

83. Roberts RM, Tasto JP, Hazel RM: Acromioclavicular joint stability after arthroscopic coplaning. Arthroscopy 14:419-420, 1998.

84. Cahill BR: Osteolysis of the distal part of the clavicle in male athletes. J Bone Joint Surg Am 64:1053-1058, 1982.

85. Cook FF, Tibone JE: The Mumford procedure in athletes: An objective analysis of function. Am J Sports Med 16:97-100, 1988.

86. Eskola A, Vainionpaa O, Korkala S, et al: Four-year outcome of operative treatment of acute acromioclavicular dislocation. J Orthop Trauma 5:9-13, 1991.

87. Grimes DW, Garner RW: The degeneration of the acromioclavicular joint. Orthop Rev 9:41-44, 1980.

88. Neviaser TJ, Neviaser RJ, Neviaser JS, et al: The four-in-one arthroplasty for the painful arc syndrome. Clin Orthop Relat Res (163):107-112, 1982.

89. Novak PJ, Bach BR Jr, Romeo AA, et al: Surgical resection of the distal clavicle. J Shoulder Elbow Surg 4(1 Pt 1):35-40, 1995.

90. Petchell JF, Sonnabend DH, Hughes JS: Distal clavicular excision: A detailed functional assessment. Aust N Z J Surg 65:262-266, 1995.

91. Petersson CJ: Resection of the lateral end of the clavicle: A 3- to 30-year follow-up. Acta Orthop Scand 54:904-907, 1983.

92. Petersson CJ: The acromioclavicular joint in rheumatoid arthritis. Clin Orthop Relat Res (223):86-93, 1987.

93. Sage FP, Salvatore JE: Injuries of acromioclavicular joint: Study of results in 96 patients. South Med J 56:486-495, 1963.

94. Scavenius M, Iversen BF: Nontraumatic clavicular osteolysis in weight lifters. Am J Sports Med 20:463-467, 1992.

95. Slawski DP, Cahill BR: Atraumatic osteolysis of the distal clavicle: Results of open surgical excision. Am J Sports Med 22:267-272, 1994.

96. Wagner C: Partial claviculectomy. Am J Surg 85:259-265, 1953.

97. Worcester JN, Green DP: Osteoarthritis of the acromioclavicular joint. Clin Orthop Relat Res 58:69-73, 1968.

98. Johnson LL: Arthroscopic Surgery: Principles and Practice, vol 2, 3rd ed. St. Louis: CV Mosby, 1986, pp 1356-1404.

99. Esch JC, Ozerkis LR, Helgager JA, et al: Arthroscopic subacromial decompression: Results according to the degree of rotator cuff tear. Arthroscopy 4:241-249, 1988.

100. Snyder SJ: Arthroscopic acromioclavicular joint debridement and distal clavicle resection. Tech Orthop 3:41-45, 1988.

101. Auge WK, Fisher RA: Arthroscopic distal clavicle resection for isolated atraumatic osteolysis in weight lifters. Am J Sports Med 26:189-192, 1998.

102. Bell RH: Arthroscopic distal clavicle resection. Instr Course Lect 47:35-41, 1998.

103. Bigliani LU, Nicholson GP, Flatow EL: Arthroscopic resection of the distal clavicle. Orthop Clin North Am 24:133-141, 1993.

104. Caspari RB, Thal R: A technique for arthroscopic subacromial decompression. Arthroscopy 8:23-30, 1992.

105. Flatow EL, Cordasco FA, Bigliani LU: Arthroscopic resection of the outer end of the clavicle from a superior approach: A critical, quantitative radiographic assessment of bone removal. Arthroscopy 8:55-64, 1992.

106. Flatow EL, Duralde XA, Nicholson GP, et al: Arthroscopic resection of the distal clavicle with a superior approach. J Shoulder Elbow Surg 4:41-50, 1995.

107. Gartsman GM: Arthroscopic resection of the acromioclavicular joint. Am J Sports Med 21:71-77, 1993.

108. Gartsman GM, Combs AH, Davis PF: Arthroscopic acromioclavicular resection: An anatomical study. Am J Sports Med 19:2-5, 1991.

109. Jerosch J, Steinbeck J, Schroder M, et al: Arthroscopic resection of the acromioclavicular joint. Sports Traumatol Arthrosc 1:209-215, 1993.

110. Kay SP, Ellman H, Harris E: Arthroscopic distal clavicle excision. Clin Orthop Relat Res (301):181-184, 1994.

111. Lervick GN: Direct arthroscopic distal clavicle resection: A technical review. Iowa Orthop J 25:149-156, 2005.

112. Levine WN, Barron OA, Yamaguchi K: Arthroscopic distal clavicle resection from a bursal approach. Arthroscopy 14:52-56, 1998.

113. Levine WN, Soong M, Ahmad CS, et al: Arthroscopic distal clavicle resection: A comparison of bursal and direct approaches. Arthroscopy 22:516-520, 2006.

114. Martin SD, Baumgarten TE, Andrews JR: Arthroscopic resection of the distal aspect of the clavicle with concomitant subacromial decompression. J Bone Joint Surg Am 83:328-335, 2001.

115. Nuber GW, Bowen MK: Arthroscopic treatment of acromioclavicular joint injuries and results. Clin Sports Med 22:301-317, 2003.

116. Snyder SJ, Banas MP, Karzel RP: The arthroscopic Mumford procedure. Arthroscopy 11:157-164, 1995.

117. Tolin BS, Snyder SJ: Our technique for the arthroscopic Mumford procedure. Orthop Clin North Am 24:143-151, 1993.

118. Zawadsky M, Marra G, Wiater JM: Osteolysis of the distal clavicle (long-term results of arthroscopic resection). Arthroscopy 16:600-605, 2000.

119. Freedman BA, Javernick MA, O'Brien FP, et al: Arthroscopic versus open distal clavicle excision: Comparative results at 6 months and 1 year from a randomized, prospective clinical trial. J Shoulder Elbow Surg 16(4):413-418, 2007.

120. Brown JN, Roberts SN, Hayes MG, et al: Shoulder pathology associated with symptomatic acromioclavicular joint degeneration. J Shoulder Elbow Surg 9:173-176, 2000.

121. Daluga DJ, Dobozi W: The influence of distal clavicle resection and rotator cuff repair on the effectiveness of anterior acromioplasty. Clin Orthop Relat Res (247):117-123, 1989.

122. Lesko PD: Variation of the arthroscopic Mumford procedure for resecting the distal clavicle. J South Orthop Assoc 10:194-200, 2001.

123. Lozman PR, Hechtman KS, Uribe JW: Combined arthroscopic management of impingement syndrome and acromioclavicular joint arthritis. J South Orthop Assoc 4:177-181, 1995.

124. Berg EE, Ciullo JV: Heterotopic ossification after acromioplasty and distal clavicle resection. J Shoulder Elbow Surg 4:188-193, 1995.

125. Caldwell GD: Treatment of complete permanent acromioclavicular dislocation by surgical arthrodesis. J Bone Joint Surg 25:368-374, 1943.

126. Kennedy JC: Complete dislocation of the acromioclavicular joint: 14 years later. J Trauma 8:311-318, 1968.

127. Ludewig PM, Behrens SA, Meyer SM, et al: Three-dimensional clavicular motion during arm elevation: Reliability and descriptive data. J Orthop Sports Phys Ther 34:140-149, 2004.

128. McClure PW, Michener LA, Sennett BJ, et al: Direct 3-dimensional measurement of scapular kinematics during dynamic movements in vivo. J Shoulder Elbow Surg 10:269-277, 2001.

129. Sahara W, Sugamoto K, Murai M, et al: 3D kinematic analysis of the acromioclavicular joint during arm abduction using vertically open MRI. J Orthop Res 24:1823-1831, 2006.

130. Mazzocca AD, Arciero RA, Bicos J: Evaluation and treatment of acromioclavicular joint injuries. Am J Sports Med 35:316-329, 2007.

131. DePalma A: Degenerative Changes of the Sternoclavicular and Acromioclavicular Joints in Various Decades. Springfield, Ill: Charles C Thomas, 1957.

132. DePalma AF, Callery G, Bennett GA: Variational anatomy and degenerative lesions of the shoulder joint. Instr Course Lect 6:255-281, 1949.

133. Peyron JG: Osteoarthritis. The epidemiologic viewpoint. Clin Orthop Relat Res (213):13-9, 1986.

134. Lehtinen JT, Kaarela K, Belt EA, et al: Incidence of acromioclavicular joint involvement in rheumatoid arthritis: A 15-year endpoint study. J Rheumatol 26:1239-1241, 1999.

135. Montet X, Zamorani-Bianchi MP, Mehdizade A, et al: Intramuscular ganglion arising from the acromioclavicular joint. Clin Imaging 28:109-112, 2004.

136. Neer CS II, Craig EV, Fukuda H: Cuff-tear arthropathy. J Bone Joint Surg Am 65:1232-1244, 1983.

137. Tshering Vogel DW, Steinbach LS, Hertel R, et al: Acromioclavicular joint cyst: Nine cases of a pseudotumor of the shoulder. Skeletal Radiol 34:260-265, 2005.

138. Laktasic-Zerjavic N, Babic-Naglic D, Curkovic B, et al: Septic acromioclavicular arthritis in a patient with diabetes mellitus. Coll Anthropol 29:743-746, 2005.

139. Lohmann CH, Koster G, Klinger HM, Kunze E: Giant synovial osteochondromatosis of the acromio-clavicular joint in a child. A case report and review of the literature. J Pediatr Orthop B 14:126-128, 2005.

140. Gerber C, Galantay RV, Hersche O: The pattern of pain produced by irritation of the acromioclavicular joint and the subacromial space. J Shoulder Elbow Surg 7:352-355, 1998.

141. Walton J, Mahajan S, Paxinos A, et al: Diagnostic values of tests for acromioclavicular joint pain. J Bone Joint Surg Am 86:807-812, 2004.

142. Buchberger DJ: Introduction of a new physical examination procedure for the differentiation of acromioclavicular joint lesions and subacromial impingement. J Manipulative Physiol Ther 22:316-321, 1999.

143. Jacob AK, Sallay PI: Therapeutic efficacy of corticosteroid injections in the acromioclavicular joint. Biomed Sci Instrum 34:380-385, 1997.

144. McLaughlin HL: On the frozen shoulder. Bull Hosp Jt Dis Orthop Inst 12:383-393, 1951.

145. O'Brien SJ, Pagnani MJ, Fealy S, et al: The active compression test: A new and effective test for diagnosing labral tears and acromioclavicular joint abnormality. Am J Sports Med 26:610-613, 1998.

146. Harryman DT II, Matsen FA III: Personal communication. 1990.

147. Maritz NG, Oosthuizen PJ: Diagnostic criteria for acromioclavicular joint pathology. J Bone Joint Surg Br 78(suppl 1):78, 2002.

148. Chronopoulos E, Kim TK, Park HB, et al: Diagnostic value of physical tests for isolated chronic acromioclavicular lesions. Am J Sports Med 32:655-661, 2004.

149. Bisbinas I, Belthur M, Said HG, et al: Accuracy of needle placement in ACJ injections. Knee Surg Sports Traumatol Arthrosc 14:762-765, 2006.

150. Partington PF, Broome GH: Diagnostic injection around the shoulder: Hit and miss? A cadaveric study of injection accuracy. J Shoulder Elbow Surg 7:147-150, 1998.

151. Zanca P: Shoulder pain: Involvement of the acromioclavicular joint: Analysis of 1,000 cases. AJR Am J Roentgenol 112:493-506, 1971.

152. Karn JW, Harris JH: Case report 752: Normal variant of the acromioclavicular separation. Skeletal Radiol 21:419-420, 1992.

153. Oppenheimer A: Arthritis of the acromioclavicular joint. J Bone Joint Surg 25:867-870, 1943.

154. Petersson CJ, Redlund-Johnell I: Radiographic joint space in normal acromioclavicular joints. Acta Orthop Scand 54:431-433, 1983.

155. Bossart PJ, Joyce SM, Manaster BJ, et al: Lack of efficacy of "weighted" radiographs in diagnosing acute acromioclavicular separation. Ann Emerg Med 17:47-51, 1988.

156. Clarke HD, McCann PD: Acromioclavicular joint injuries. Orthop Clin North Am 31:177-186, 2000.

157. Yap JJ, Curl LA, Kvitne RS, et al: The value of weighted views of the acromioclavicular joint. Results of a survey. Am J Sports Med 27:806-809, 1999.

158. Sluming VA: A comparison of the methods of distraction for stress examination of the acromioclavicular joint. Br J Radiol 68:1181-1184, 1995.

159. Bannister GC, Wallace WA, Stableforth PG, et al: A classification of acute acromioclavicular dislocation: A clinical, radiological, and anatomical study. Injury 23:194-196, 1992.

160. Alexander OM: Radiography of the acromio-clavicular joint. Radiography 14:139, 1948.

161. Alexander OM: Dislocation of the acromio-clavicular joint. Radiography 15:260, 1949.

162. Alexander OM: Radiography of the acromio-clavicular articulation. Med Radiogr Photogr 30:34-39, 1954.

163. Waldrop JI, Norwood LA, Alvarez RG: Lateral roentgenographic projections of the acromioclavicular joint. Am J Sports Med 9:337-341, 1981.

164. Zicat B, Rahme DM, Swaraj K, et al: Septic arthritis of the acromioclavicular joint: Tc-99m leukocyte imaging. Clin Nucl Med 31:145-146, 2006.

165. Antonio GE, Cho JH, Chung CB, et al: Pictorial essay. MR imaging appearance and classification of acromioclavicular joint injury. AJR Am J Roentgenol 180:1103-1110, 2003.

166. Gordon BH, Chew FS: Isolated acromioclavicular joint pathology in the symptomatic shoulder on magnetic resonance imaging: A pictorial essay. J Comput Assist Tomogr 28:215-222, 2004.

167. Schaefer FK, Schaefer PJ, Brossmann J, et al: Experimental and clinical evaluation of acromioclavicular joint structures with new scan orientations in MRI. Eur Radiol 16:1488-1493, 2006.

168. Echols PG, Omer GE Jr, Crawford MK: Juxta-articular myxoma of the shoulder presenting as a cyst of the acromioclavicular joint: A case report. J Shoulder Elbow Surg 9:157-159, 2000.

169. Sher JS, Iannotti JP, Williams GR, et al: The effect of shoulder magnetic resonance imaging on clinical decision making. J Shoulder Elbow Surg 7:205-209, 1998.

170. Mohtadi NG, Mohtadi NG, Hollinshead RM, et al: A prospective, double-blind comparison of magnetic resonance imaging and arthroscopy in the evaluation of patients presenting with shoulder pain. J Shoulder Elbow Surg 13:258-265, 2004.

171. Needell SD, Zlatkin MB, Sher JS, et al: MR imaging of the rotator cuff: Peritendinous and bone abnormalities in an asymptomatic population. AJR Am J Roentgenol 166:863-867, 1996.

172. Stein BE, Wiater JM, Pfaff HC, et al: Detection of acromioclavicular joint pathology in asymptomatic shoulders with magnetic resonance imaging. J Shoulder Elbow Surg 10:204-208, 2001.

173. de Abreu MR, Chung CB, Wessely M, et al: Acromioclavicular joint osteoarthritis: Comparison of findings derived from MR imaging and conventional radiography. Clin Imaging 29:273-277, 2005.

174. Fiorella D, Helms CA, Speer KP: Increased T2 signal intensity in the distal clavicle: Incidence and clinical implications. Skeletal Radiol 29:697-702, 2000.

175. de la Puente R, Boutin RD, Theodorou DJ, et al: Post-traumatic and stress-induced osteolysis of the distal clavicle: MR imaging findings in 17 patients. Skeletal Radiol 28:202-208, 1999.

176. Jordan LK, Kenter K, Griffiths HL: Relationship between MRI and clinical findings in the acromioclavicular joint. Skeletal Radiol 31:516-521, 2002.

177. Shubin Stein BE, Ahmad CS, Pfaff CH, et al: A comparison of magnetic resonance imaging findings of the acromioclavicular joint in symptomatic versus asymptomatic patients. J Shoulder Elbow Surg 15:56-59, 2006.

178. Schweitzer ME, Magbalon MJ, Frieman BG, et al: Acromioclavicular joint fluid: Determination of clinical significance with MR imaging. Radiology 192:205-207, 1994.

179. Fialka C, Krestan CR, Stampfl P, et al: Visualization of intraarticular structures of the acromioclavicular joint in an ex vivo model using a dedicated MRI protocol. AJR Am J Roentgenol 185:1126-1131, 2005.

180. Ferri M, Finlay K, Popowich T, et al: Sonographic examination of the acromioclavicular and sternoclavicular joints. J Clin Ultrasound 33:345-355, 2005.

181. Heers G, Hedtmann A: Ultrasound diagnosis of the acromioclavicular joint. Orthopade 31:255-261, 2002.

182. Iovane A, Midiri M, Galia M, et al: Acute traumatic acromioclavicular joint lesions: Role of ultrasound versus conventional radiography. Radiol Med (Torino) 107:367-375, 2004.

183. Martinoli C, Bianchi S, Prato N, et al: US of the shoulder: Non-rotator cuff disorders. Radiographics 23:381-401, 2003.

184. Papatheodorou A, Ellinas P, Takis F, et al: US of the shoulder: Rotator cuff and non-rotator cuff disorders. Radiographics 26:e23, 2006.

185. Alasaarela E, Tervonen O, Takalo R, et al: Ultrasound evaluation of the acromioclavicular joint. J Rheumatol 24:1959-1963, 1997.

186. Fenkl R, Gotzen L: [Sonographic diagnosis of the injured acromioclavicular joint: A standardized examination procedure.] Unfallchirurgie 95:393-400, 1992.

187. Koka SR, D'Arcy JC: Inferior (subacromial) dislocation of the outer end of the clavicle. Injury 24:210-211, 1993.

188. Matter HP, Gruber G, Harland U: [Possibilities of ultrasound diagnosis in Tossy type III acromioclavicular joint injuries in comparison with loaded roentgen images.] Sportverletzung Sportschaden 9:14-20, 1995.

189. Schmid A, Schmid F: [Use of arthrosonography in the diagnosis of Tossy injuries of the shoulder joint.] Aktuelle Traumatol 18:134-138, 1988.

190. Sluming VA: Technical note: Measuring the coracoclavicular distance with ultrasound—a new technique. Br J Radiol 68:189-193, 1995.

191. Heers G, Hedtmann A: Correlation of ultrasonographic findings to Tossy's and Rockwood's classification of acromioclavicular joint injuries. Ultrasound Med Biol 31:725-732, 2005.

192. Peetrons P, Bedard JP: Acromioclavicular joint injury: Enhanced technique of examination with dynamic maneuver. J Clin Ultrasound 35(5):262-267, 2007.

193. Blankstein A, Ganel A, Givon U, et al: Ultrasonography as a diagnostic modality in acromioclavicular joint pathologies. Isr Med Assoc J 7:28-30, 2005.

194. Widman DS, Craig JG, van Holsbeeck MT: Sonographic detection, evaluation and aspiration of infected acromioclavicular joints. Skeletal Radiol 30:388-392, 2001.

195. Rollo J, Raghunath J, Porter K: Injuries of the acromioclavicular joint and current treatment options. Trauma 7:217-223, 2005.

196. Cave EF (ed): Fractures and Other Injuries. Chicago: Year Book, 1961.

197. Riand N, Sadowski C, Hoffmeyer P: [Acute acromioclavicular dislocations.] Acta Orthop Belg 65:393-403, 1999.

198. Nordqvist A, Petersson CJ: Incidence and causes of shoulder girdle injuries in an urban population. J Shoulder Elbow Surg 4:107-112, 1995.

199. Daly PH, Sim FH, Simonet WT: Ice hockey injuries: A review. Sports Med 10:122-131, 1990.

200. Dias JJ, Gregg PJ: Acromioclavicular joint injuries in sport: Recommendations for treatment. Sports Med 11:125-132, 1991.

201. Rowe CR: Symposium on surgical lesions of the shoulder: Acute and recurrent dislocation of the shoulder. J Bone Joint Surg Am 44:977-1012, 1962.

202. Thorndike A Jr, Quigley TB: Injuries to the acromioclavicular joint: A plea for conservative treatment. Am J Surg 55:250-261, 1942.

203. Webb J, Bannister G: Acromioclavicular disruption in first class rugby players. Br J Sports Med 26:247-248, 1992.

204. Kocher MS, Feagin JA Jr: Shoulder injuries during alpine skiing. Am J Sports Med 24:665-669, 1996.

205. Weaver JK: Skiing-related injuries to the shoulder. Clin Orthop Relat Res (216):24-28, 1987.

206. Stuart MJ, Smith A: Injuries in junior A ice hockey: A three-year prospective study. Am J Sports Med 23:458-461, 1995.

207. Headey J, Brooks JH, Kemp SP: The epidemiology of shoulder injuries in English professional rugby union. Am J Sports Med 35(9):1537-1543, 2007.

208. Juhn MS, Simonian PT: Type VI acromioclavicular separation with middle-third clavicle fracture in an ice hockey player. Clin J Sport Med 12:315-317, 2002.

209. Wurtz LO, Lyons FA, Rockwood CA Jr: Fracture of the middle third of the clavicle and dislocation of the acromioclavicular joint. J Bone Joint Surg Am 74:183-186, 1992.

210. Meislin RJ, Zuckerman JD, Nainzadeh N: Type III acromioclavicular joint separation associated with late brachial plexus neuropraxia. J Orthop Trauma 6:370-372, 1992.

211. Sturm JT, Perry JF Jr: Brachial plexus injuries from blunt trauma—a harbinger of vascular and thoracic injury. Ann Emerg Med 16:404-406, 1987.

212. Barber FA: Complete posterior acromioclavicular dislocation: A case report. Orthopedics 10:493-496, 1987.

213. Zaricznyj B: Late reconstruction of the ligaments following acromioclavicular separation. J Bone Joint Surg Am 58:792-795, 1976.

214. Allman FL Jr: Fractures and ligamentous injuries of the clavicle and its articulation. J Bone Joint Surg Am 49:774-784, 1967.

215. Tossy JD, Mead NC, Sigmond HM: Acromioclavicular separations: Useful and practical classification for treatment. Clin Orthop 28:111-119, 1963.

216. Williams GR, Nguyen VD, Rockwood CA Jr: Classification and radiographic analysis of acromioclavicular dislocations. Appl Radiol 18:29-34, 1989.

217. Barnes CJ, Higgins LD, Major NM, et al: Magnetic resonance imaging of the coracoclavicular ligaments: Its role in defining pathoanatomy at the acromio-clavicular joint. J Surg Orthop Adv 13:69-75, 2004.

218. Bearn JG: Direct observations on the function of the capsule of the sterno-clavicular joint in clavicle support. J Anat 101:159-170, 1967.

219. Wolin I: Acute acromioclavicular dislocation: A simple effective method of conservative treatment. J Bone Joint Surg 26:589-592, 1944.

220. Arenas AJ, Pampliega T, Iglesias J: Surgical management of bipolar clavicular dislocation. Acta Orthop Belg 59:202-205, 1993.

221. Beckman T: A case of simultaneous luxation of both ends of the clavicle. Acta Chir Scand 56:156-163, 1924.

222. Cook F, Horowitz M: Bipolar clavicular dislocation: Report of a case. J Bone Joint Surg Am 64:145-147, 1987.

223. Echo BS, Donati RB, Powell CE: Bipolar clavicular dislocation treated surgically: A case report. J Bone Joint Surg Am 70:1251-1253, 1988.

224. Gearen PF, Perry W: Panclavicular dislocation: Report of a case. J Bone Joint Surg Am 64:454-455, 1982.

225. Heinz WM, Misamore GW: Midshaft fracture of the clavicle with grade III acromioclavicular separation. J Shoulder Elbow Surg 4:141-142, 1995.

226. Jain AS: Traumatic floating clavicle: A case report. J Bone Joint Surg Br 66:560-561, 1984.

227. Porral MA: Observation d'une double luxation de la clavicle droite. J Univ Habd Med Chir Prat 2:78-82, 1831.

228. Sanders JO, Lyons FA, Rockwood CA Jr: Management of dislocations of both ends of the clavicle. J Bone Joint Surg Am 72:399-402, 1990.

229. McPhee IB: Inferior dislocation of the outer end of the clavicle. J Trauma 20:709-710, 1980.

230. Patterson WR: Inferior dislocation of the distal end of the clavicle. J Bone Joint Surg Am 49:1184-1186, 1967.

231. Bakalim G, Wilppula E: Surgical or conservative treatment of total dislocation of the acromioclavicular joint. Acta Chir Scand 141:43-47, 1975.

232. Bannister GC, Wallace WA, Stableforth PG, et al: The management of acute acromioclavicular dislocation: A randomized prospective controlled trial. J Bone Joint Surg Br 71:848-850, 1989.

233. Bjerneld H, Hovelius L, Thorling J: Acromio-clavicular separations treated conservatively: A 5-year follow-up study. Acta Orthop Scand 54:743-745, 1983.

234. Lemos MJ: The evaluation and treatment of the injured acromioclavicular joint in athletes. Am J Sports Med 26:137-144, 1998.

235. Mouhsine E, Garofalo R, Crevoisier X, et al: Grade I and II acromioclavicular dislocations: Results of conservative treatment. J Shoulder Elbow Surg 12:599-602, 2003.

236. Nuber GW, Bowen MK: Acromioclavicular joint injuries and distal clavicle fractures. J Am Acad Orthop Surg 5:11-18, 1997.

237. Nuber GW, Bowen MK: Disorders of the acromioclavicular joint: Pathophysiology, diagnosis, and management. In Iannotti JP, Williams GR Jr (eds): Disorders of the Shoulder: Diagnosis and Management. Philadelphia: Lippincott Williams & Wilkins, 1999, pp 739-762.

238. Phillips AM, Smart C, Groom AF: Acromioclavicular dislocation. Conservative or surgical therapy. Clin Orthop Relat Res (353):10-17, 1998.

239. Rawes ML, Dias JJ: Long-term results of conservative treatment for acromioclavicular dislocation. J Bone Joint Surg Br 78:410-412, 1996.

240. Rockwood CA, Williams GR, Young DC: Disorders of the acromioclavicular joint. In Rockwood CA Jr, Matsen FA III (eds): The Shoulder. Philadelphia: Saunders, 1998, pp 483-553.

241. Taft TN, Wilson FC, Oglesby JW: Dislocation of the acromioclavicular joint: An end-result study. J Bone Joint Surg Am 69:1045-1051, 1987.

242. Weinstein DM, McCann PD, McIlveen SJ, et al: Surgical treatment of complete acromioclavicular dislocations. Am J Sports Med 23:324-331, 1995.

243. Glick J: Acromioclavicular dislocation in athletes: Auto arthroplasty of the joint. Orthop Rev 1:31-34, 1972.

244. Babe JG, Valle M, Couceiro J: Trial of a simple surgical approach. Injury 19:159-161, 1988.

245. Bergfeld JA, Andrish JT, Clancy WG: Evaluation of the acromioclavicular joint following first- and second-degree sprains. Am J Sports Med 6:153-159, 1978.

246. Cox JS: The fate of the acromioclavicular joint in athletic injuries. Am J Sports Med 9:50-53, 1981.

247. Shaw MB, McInerney JJ, Dias JJ, et al: Acromioclavicular joint sprains: The post-injury recovery interval. Injury 34:438-442, 2003.

248. Yu JS, Dardani M, Fischer RA: MR observations of post-traumatic osteolysis of the distal clavicle after traumatic separation of the acromioclavicular joint. J Comput Assist Tomogr 24:159-164, 2000.

249. Urist MR: The treatment of dislocation of the acromioclavicular joint. Am J Surg 98:423-431, 1959.

250. Urist MR: Complete dislocation of the acromioclavicular joint (follow-up notes). J Bone Joint Surg Am 45:1750-1753, 1963.

251. Park JP, Arnold JA, Coker TP, et al: Treatment of acromioclavicular separations: A retrospective study. Am J Sports Med 8:251-256, 1980.

252. Bateman JE: Athletic injuries about the shoulder in throwing and body-contact sports. Clin Orthop 23:75-83, 1962.

253. Hedtmann A, Fett H, Ludwing J: Management of old neglected posttraumatic acromioclavicular joint instability and arthrosis. Orthopade 27:556-566, 1998.

254. Madsen B: Osteolysis of the acromial end of the clavicle following trauma. Br J Radiol 36:822-828, 1963.

255. Stohr H, Geyer M, Volle E: [Osteolysis of the lateral clavicle after Tossy II injury in ice hockey players]. Sportverletz Sportschaden. 10:70-73, 1996.

256. Walsh WM, Peterson DA, Shelton G, et al: Shoulder strength following acromioclavicular injury. Am J Sports Med 13:153-158, 1985.

257. Wilson PD, Cochrane WA: Immediate management, after care, and convalescent treatment, with special reference to the conservation and restoration of function. In Fractures and Dislocations. Philadelphia: JB Lippincott, 1925.

258. Alldredge RH: Surgical treatment of acromioclavicular dislocation. Clin Orthop Relat Res 63:262-263, 1969.

259. Reichkendler M, Rangger C, Dessl A, et al: [Comparison and outcome of grade II and III acromioclavicular joint injuries]. Unfallchirurg 99:778-783, 1996.

260. Cox JS: Current method of treatment of acromioclavicular dislocations. Orthopedics 15:1041-1044, 1992.

261. McFarland EG, Blivin SJ, Doehring CB, et al: Treatment of grade III acromioclavicular separations in professional throwing athletes: Results of a survey. Am J Orthop 26:771-774, 1997.

262. Nissen CW, Chatterjee A: Type III acromioclavicular separation: Results of a recent survey on its management. Am J Orthop 36:89-93, 2007.

263. Powers JA, Bach PJ: Acromioclavicular separations—closed or open treatment. Clin Orthop Relat Res (104):213-223, 1974.

264. Anzel SH, Streitz WL: Acute acromioclavicular injuries: A report of nineteen cases treated non-operatively employing dynamic splint immobilization. Clin Orthop Relat Res (103):143-149, 1974.

265. Glick JM, Milburn LJ, Haggerty JF, et al: Dislocated acromioclavicular joint: Follow-up study of 35 unreduced acromioclavicular dislocations. Am J Sports Med 5:264-270, 1977.

266. Jakobsen BW: [Acromioclavicular dislocation: Conservative or surgical treatment?] Ugeskr Laeger 151:235-238, 1989.

267. MacDonald PB, Alexander MJ, Frejuk J, et al: Comprehensive functional analysis of shoulders following complete acromioclavicular separation. Am J Sports Med 16:475-480, 1988.

268. Mulier T, Stuyek J, Fabry G: Conservative treatment of acromioclavicular dislocation: Evaluation of functional and radiological results after six years follow-up. Acta Orthop Belg 59:255-262, 1993.

269. Tibone J, Sellers R, Tonino P: Strength testing after third-degree acromioclavicular dislocations. Am J Sports Med 20:328-331, 1992.

270. Van Fleet TA, Bach B: Injuries to the acromioclavicular joint: Diagnosis and management. Orthop Rev 23:123-129, 1994.

271. Wojtys EM, Nelson G: Conservative treatment of grade III acromioclavicular dislocations. Clin Orthop Relat Res (268):112-114, 1991.

272. Darrow JC, Smith JA, Lockwood RC: A new conservative method for treatment of type III acromioclavicular separations. Orthop Clin North Am 11:727-733, 1980.

273. Spigelman L: A harness for acromioclavicular separation. J Bone Joint Surg Am 51:585-586, 1969.

274. Varney JH, Coker JK, Cawley JJ: Treatment of acromioclavicular dislocation by means of a harness. J Bone Joint Surg Am 34:232-233, 1952.

275. Lazcano MA, Anzel SH, Kelly PJ: Complete dislocation and subluxation of the acromioclavicular joint: End result in seventy-three cases. J Bone Joint Surg Am 43:379-391, 1961.

276. Nicoll EE: Annotation: Miners and mannequins [editorial]. J Bone Joint Surg Br 36:171-172, 1954.

277. Gladstone R, Wilk K, Andrews J: Nonoperative treatment of acromioclavicular joint injuries. Oper Tech Sports Med 5:78-87, 1997.

278. Dias JJ, Steingold RA, Richardson RA, et al: The conservative treatment of acromioclavicular dislocation: Review after five years. J Bone Joint Surg Br 69:719-722, 1987.

279. Galpin RD, Hawkins RJ, Grainger RW: A comparative analysis of operative versus nonoperative treatment of grade III acromioclavicular separations. Clin Orthop Relat Res (193):150-155, 1985.

280. Imatani RJ, Hanlon JJ, Cady GW: Acute complete acromioclavicular separation. J Bone Joint Surg Am 57:328-332, 1975.

281. Larsen E, Bjerg-Nielsen A, Christensen P: Conservative or surgical treatment of acromioclavicular dislocation: A prospective, controlled, randomized study. J Bone Joint Surg Am 68:552-555, 1986.

282. Schlegel TF, Burks RT, Marcus RL, et al: A prospective evaluation of untreated acute grade III acromioclavicular separations. Am J Sports Med 29:699-703, 2001.

283. Rosenorn M, Pedersen EB: A comparison between conservative and operative treatment of acute acromioclavicular dislocation. Acta Orthop Scand 45:50-59, 1974.

284. Sleeswijk Visser SV, Haarsma SM, Speeckaert MTC: Conservative treatment of acromioclavicular dislocation: Jones strap versus mitella [abstract]. Acta Orthop Scand 55:483, 1984.

285. Calvo E, Lopez-Franco M, Arribas IM: Clinical and radiologic outcomes of surgical and conservative treatment of type III acromioclavicular joint injury. J Shoulder Elbow Surg 15:300-305, 2006.

286. Spencer EE Jr: Treatment of grade III acromioclavicular joint injuries: A systematic review. Clin Orthop Relat Res (455):38-44, 2007.

287. Indrekvam K, Störkson R, Langeland N, et al: [Acromioclavicular joint dislocation: Surgical or conservative treatment?] Tidsskr Nor Laegeforen 106:1303-1305, 1986.

288. Larsen E, Hede A: Treatment of acute acromioclavicular dislocation: Three different methods of treatment prospectively studied. Acta Orthop Belg 53:480-484, 1987.

289. Press J, Zuckerman JD, Gallagher M, et al: Treatment of grade III acromioclavicular separations. Bull Hosp Jt Dis 56:77-83, 1997.

290. McFarland EG, Blivin SJ, Doehring CB, et al: Treatment of grade III acromioclavicular separations in professional throwing athletes: Results of a survey. Am J Orthop 26:771-774, 1997.

291. Paavolainen P, Björkenheim JM, Paukku P, Slätis P: Surgical treatment of acromioclavicular dislocation: A review of 39 patients. Injury 14:415-420, 1983.

292. Arner O, Sandahl U, Ohrling H: Dislocation of the acromioclavicular joint: Review of the literature and a report of 56 cases. Acta Chir Scand 113:140-152, 1957.

293. Millbourn E: On injuries to the acromioclavicular joint: Treatment and results. Acta Orthop Scand 19:349-382, 1950.

294. Weitzman G: Treatment of acute acromioclavicular joint dislocation by a modified Bosworth method: Report on twenty-four cases. J Bone Joint Surg Am 49:1167-1178, 1967.

295. Cooper ES: New method of treating long standing dislocations of the scapulo-clavicular articulation. Am J Med Sci 41:389-392, 1861.

296. Ahstrom JP Jr: Surgical repair of complete acromioclavicular separation. JAMA 217:785-789, 1971.

297. Augereau B, Robert H, Apoil A: Treatment of severe acromioclavicular dislocation: A coracoclavicular ligamentoplasty technique derived from Cadenat's procedure. Ann Chir 35:720-722, 1981.

298. Avikainen V, Ranki P, Turunen M, et al: Acromioclavicular complete dislocation. Ann Chir Gynaecol 68:117-120, 1979.

299. Bartonicek J, Jehlicka D, Bezvoda Z: [Surgical treatment of acromioclavicular luxation.] Acta Chir Orthop Traumatol Cech 55:289-309, 1988.

300. Bateman JE: The Shoulder and Neck. Philadelphia: WB Saunders, 1972.

301. Bundens WD Jr, Cook JI: Repair of acromioclavicular separations by deltoid–trapezius imbrication. Clin Orthop 20:109-114, 1961.

302. Dannohl CH: [Angulation osteotomy at the clavicle in old dislocations of the acromioclavicular joint.] Aktuelle Traumatol 14:282-284, 1984.

303. Eskola A, Vainionpaa S, Korkala O, et al: Acute complete acromioclavicular dislocation: A prospective randomized trial of fixation with smooth or threaded Kirschner wires or cortical screw. Ann Chir Gynaecol 76:323-326, 1987.

304. Fama G, Bonaga S: [Safety pin synthesis in the cure of acromioclavicular luxation.] Chir Organi Mov 73:227-235, 1988.

305. Inman VT, McLaughlin HD, Neviaser J, et al: Treatment of complete acromioclavicular dislocation. J Bone Joint Surg Am 44:1008-1011, 1962.

306. Linke R, Moschinski D: [Combined method of operative treatment of ruptures of the acromioclavicular joint.] Unfallheilkunde 87:223-225, 1984.

307. Lizaur A, Marco L, Cebrian R: Acute dislocation of the acromioclavicular joint. Traumatic anatomy and the importance of deltoid and trapezius. J Bone Joint Surg Br 76:602-606, 1994.

308. Mayr E, Braun W, Eber W, et al: Treatment of acromioclavicular joint separations. Central Kirschner-wire and PDS-augmentation Unfallchirurg 102:278-286, 1999.

309. Mikusev IE, Zainulli RV, Skvortso AP: [Treatment of dislocations of the acromial end of the clavicle.] Vestn Khir 139:69-71, 1987.

310. Moshein J, Elconin KB: Repair of acute acromioclavicular dislocation, utilizing the coracoacromial ligament (Proceedings). J Bone Joint Surg Am 51:812, 1969.

311. Neviaser JS: Acromioclavicular dislocation treated by transference of the coracoacromial ligament. Bull Hosp Jt Dis Orthop Inst 12:46-54, 1951.

312. Neviaser JS: Acromioclavicular dislocation treated by transference of the coracoacromial ligament. Arch Surg 64:292-297, 1952.

313. Neviaser JS: Complicated fractures and dislocations about the shoulder joint. J Bone Joint Surg Am 44:984-998, 1962.

314. Neviaser JS: Acromioclavicular dislocation treated by transference of the coraco-acromial ligament: A long-term follow-up in a series of 112 cases. Clin Orthop Relat Res 58:57-68, 1968.

315. Neviaser JS: Injuries of the clavicle and its articulations. Orthop Clin North Am 11:233-237, 1980.

316. Neviaser RJ: Injuries to the clavicle and acromioclavicular joint. Orthop Clin North Am 18:433-438, 1987.

317. O'Donoghue DH: Treatment of Injuries to Athletes. Philadelphia: WB Saunders, 1970.

318. Probst A, Hegelmaier C: Die Stabilisierung des verletzten Schultereckgelenkes durch PDS-Kordel. Aktuelle Traumatol 22:61-64, 1992.

319. Simmons EH, Martin RF: Acute dislocation of the acromioclavicular joint. Can J Surg 11:479, 1968.

320. Smith MJ, Stewart MJ: Acute acromioclavicular separations. Am J Sports Med 7:62-71, 1979.

321. Stephens HEG: Stuck nail fixation for acute dislocation of the acromioclavicular joint. J Bone Joint Surg Br 51:197, 1969.

322. Vainionpaa S, Kirves P, Laike E: Acromioclavicular joint dislocation—surgical results in 36 patients. Ann Chir Gynaecol 70:120-123, 1981.

323. Albrecht F: The Balser plate for acromioclavicular fixation. Chirurg 53:732-734, 1982.

324. Broos P, Stoffelen D, Van de Sijpe, et al: Surgical management of complete Tossy III acromioclavicular joint dislocation with the Bosworth screw or the Wolter plate: A critical evaluation. Unfallchirugie 23:153-159, 1997.

325. De Baets T, Truijen J, Driesen R, et al: The treatment of acromioclavicular joint dislocation Tossy grade III with a clavicle hook plate. Acta Orthop Belg 70:515-519, 2004.

326. Dittel KK, Pfaff G, Metzger H: [Results after operative treatment of complete acromioclavicular separation (Tossy III injury).] Aktuelle Traumatol 17:16-22, 1987.

327. Dittmer H, Jauch KW, Wening V: [Treatment of acromioclavicular separations with Balser's hookplate.] Unfallheilkunde 87:216-222, 1984.

328. Gohring H, Matusewicz A, Friedl W, et al: Results of treatment after different surgical procedures for management of acromioclavicular joint dislocation. 64:565-571, 1993.

329. Graupe F, Daver U, Eyssel J: Spatergibnisse nach operativer Behandlung der Schultereckgelenksprengung Tossy III durch die Balser-platte. Unfallchirug 98:422-426, 1995.

330. Habernek H, Weinstabl R, Schmid L, et al: A crook plate for treatment of acromioclavicular joint separations. J Trauma 35:893-901, 1993.

331. Henkel T, Oetiker R, Hackenbruch W: Treatment of fresh Tossy III acromioclavicular joint dislocation by ligament suture and temporary fixation with the clavicular hooked plate. Swiss Surg 3:160-166, 1997.

332. Kaiser W, Ziemer G, Heymann H: [Treatment of acromioclavicular luxations with the Balser hookplate and ligament suture.] Chirurg 55:721-724, 1984.

333. Nadarajah R, Mahaluxmivala J, Amin A, et al: Clavicular hook-plate: Complications of retaining the implant. Injury 36:681-683, 2005.

334. Schindler A, Schmid JP, Heyse C: [Hookplate fixation for repair of acute complete acromioclavicular separation: Review of 41 patients.] Unfallchirurg 88:533-540, 1985.

335. Schmittinger K, Sikorski A: [Experiences with the Balser plate in dislocations of the acromioclavicular joint and lateral fractures of the clavicle]. Aktuelle Traumatol 13:190-193, 1983.

336. Sim E, Schwarz N, Hocker K, et al: Repair of complete acromioclavicular separations using the acromioclavicular-hook plate. Clin Orthop Relat Res (314):134-142, 1995.

337. Voigt C, Enes-Gaiao F, Fahimi S: [Treatment of acromioclavicular joint dislocation with the Rahmanzadeh joint plate]. Aktuelle Traumatol 24:128-132, 1994.

338. Wolter D, Eggers C: [Reposition and fixation of acromioclavicular luxation using a hooked plate.] Hefte Unfallheilkd 170:80-86, 1984.

339. Wu JH, Liao QD, Chen G, et al: [Clavicular hook plate in the treatment of dislocation of acromioclavicular joint and fracture of distal clavicle.] Zhong Nan Da Xue Xue Bao Yi Xue Ban 31:595-598, 2006.

340. Bosworth BM: Acromioclavicular separation: New method of repair. Surg Gynecol Obstet 73:866-871, 1941.

341. Armbrecht A and Graudins J: [Temporary extra-articular Bosworth fixation in complete shoulder joint separation. Follow-up results of 41 surgically treated patients.] Aktuelle Traumatol 20:283-287, 1990.

342. Lowe GP, Fogarty MJP: Acute acromioclavicular joint dislocation: Results of operative treatment with the Bosworth screw. Aust N Z J Surg 47:664-667, 1977.

343. Pfahler M, Krodel A, Refior HJ: Surgical treatment of acromioclavicular dislocation. Arch Orthop Trauma Surg 113:308-311, 1994.

344. Sundaram N, Patel N, Porter DS: Stabilization of acute acromioclavicular dislocation by a modified Bosworth technique: A long-term follow-up study. Injury 3:189-193, 1992.

345. Tanner A, Hardegger F: Die korakoklavikulare Verschraubung: Eine einfache Behandlung der Schulterechgelenksprengung. Unfallchirurg 98:518-521, 1995.

346. Tsou PM: Percutaneous cannulated screw coracoclavicular fixation for acute acromioclavicular dislocations. Clin Orthop Relat Res (243):112-121, 1989.
347. Guy DK, Wirth MA, Griffin JL, et al: Reconstruction of chronic and complete dislocations of the acromioclavicular joint. Clin Orthop Relat Res (347):138-149, 1998.
348. Bosworth BM: Calcium deposits in the shoulder and subacromial bursitis: A survey of 12,122 shoulders. JAMA 116:2477-2482, 1941.
349. Bosworth BM: Acromioclavicular dislocation: End-results of screw suspension treatment. Ann Surg 127:98-111, 1948.
350. Chen SK, Chou PPH, Cheng YM, et al.: Surgical treatment of complete acromioclavicular separations. Koahsiung J Med Sci 13:175-181, 1997.
351. Clayer M, Slavotinek J, Krishnan J: The results of coraco-clavicular slings for acromio-clavicular dislocation. Aust N Z J Surg 67:343-346, 1997.
352. Dahl E: Follow-up after coracoclavicular ligament prosthesis for acromioclavicular joint dislocation [abstract]. Acta Chir Scand Suppl 506:96, 1981.
353. Dahl E: Velour prosthesis in fractures and dislocations in the clavicular region. Chirurg 53:120-122, 1982.
354. Dimakopoulos P, Panagopoulos A: Functional coracoclavicular stabilization for acute acromioclavicular joint disruption. Orthopedics 30:103-108, 2007.
355. Dimakopoulos P, Panagopoulos A, Syggelos SA, et al: Double-loop suture repair for acute acromioclavicular joint disruption. Am J Sports Med 34:1112-1119, 2006.
356. Fleming RE, Tomberg DN, Kiernan HA: An operative repair of acromioclavicular separation. J Trauma 18:709-712, 1978.
357. Goldberg JA, Viglione W, Cumming WJ, et al: Review of coracoclavicular ligament reconstruction using Dacron graft material. Aust N Z J Surg 57:441-445, 1987.
358. Gollwitzer M: [Surgical management of complete acromioclavicular joint dislocation (Tossy III) with PDS cord cerclage.] Aktuelle Traumatol 23:366-370, 1993.
359. Hessmann H, Gotzen L, Gehling H, et al: Reconstruction of complete acromioclavicular separations (Tossy III) using PDS-banding as augmentation: Experience in 64 cases. Acta Chir Belg 95:147-151, 1995.
360. Kappakas GS, McMaster JH: Repair of acromioclavicular separation using a Dacron prosthesis graft. Clin Orthop Relat Res (131):247-251, 1978.
361. Monig SP, Burger C, Helling HJ, et al: Treatment of complete acromioclavicular dislocation: Present indications and surgical technique with biodegradable cords. Int J Sports Med 20:560-562, 1999.
362. Morrison DS, Lemos MJ: Acromioclavicular separation: Reconstruction using synthetic loop augmentation. Am J Sports Med 23:105-110, 1995.
363. Nelson CL: Repair of acromio-clavicular separations with knitted Dacron graft. Clin Orthop Relat Res (143):289-292, 1979.
364. Rustemeier M, Kulenkampff HA: Die operative Behandlung der Akromioklavikulargelenk-Sprengung mit einer resorbierbaren PDS-Kordel. Unfallchirurgie 16:70-74, 1990.
365. Stam L, Dawson I: Complete acromioclavicular dislocations: Treatment with a Dacron ligament. Injury (Netherlands) 22:173-176, 1991.
366. Su EP, Vargas JH III, Boynton MD: Using suture anchors for coracoclavicular fixation in treatment of complete acromioclavicular separation. Am J Orthop 33:256-257, 2004.
367. Tagliabue D, Riva A: [Current approaches to the treatment of acromioclavicular joint separation in athletes.] Ital J Sports Traumatol 3:15-24, 1981.
368. Verhaven E, Casteleyn PP, De Boeck H, et al: Surgical treatment of acute type V acromioclavicular injuries. A prospective study. Acta Orthop Belg 58:176-182, 1992.
369. Ryhanen J, Leminen A, Jamsa T, et al: A novel treatment of grade III acromioclavicular joint dislocations with a C-hook implant. Arch Orthop Trauma Surg 126:22-27, 2006.
370. Weaver JK, Dunn HK: Treatment of acromioclavicular injuries, especially complete acromioclavicular separation. J Bone Joint Surg Am 54:1187-1197, 1972.
371. De la Caffinière JY, de la Caffinière M, Lacaze F: Traitement des dislocations acromio-claviculaires au moyen d'une plastie coraco-clavi-acromiale (CCA). Rev Chir Orthop 84:9-16, 1998.
372. Dumontier C, Sautet A, Man M, et al: Acromioclavicular dislocations: Treatment by coracoacromial ligamentoplasty. J Shoulder Elbow Surg 4:130-134, 1995.
373. Kawabe N, Watanabe R, Sato M: Treatment of complete acromioclavicular separation by coracoacromial ligament transfer. Clin Orthop Relat Res (185):222-227, 1984.
374. Rauschning W, Nordesjö LO, Nordgren B, et al: Resection arthroplasty for repair of complete acromioclavicular separations. Arch Orthop Traumatol Surg 97:161-164, 1980.
375. Shoji H, Roth C, Chuinard R: Bone block transfer of coracoacromial ligament in acromioclavicular injury. Clin Orthop Relat Res (208):272-277, 1986.
376. Lemos MJ: The evaluation and treatment of the injured acromioclavicular joint in athletes. Am J Sports Med 26:137-144, 1998.
377. McCann PD, Gibbons JM: Current concepts in acromioclavicular joint injuries. Curr Opin Orthop 9:66-71, 1998.

378. Ponce BP, Millett PJ, Warner JP: Acromioclavicular joint instability: Reconstruction indications and techniques. Oper Tech Sports Med 12:35-42, 2004.
379. Rokito AS, Oh YH, Zuckerman JD: Modified Weaver–Dunn procedure for acromioclavicular joint dislocations. Orthopedics 27:21-28, 2004.
380. Tienen TG, Oyen JF, Eggen PJ: A modified technique of reconstruction for complete acromioclavicular dislocation: A prospective study. Am J Sports Med 31:655-659, 2003.
381. Burton ME: Operative treatment of acromioclavicular dislocations. Bull Hosp Jt Dis 36:109-120, 1975.
382. Copeland S, Kessel L: Disruption of the acromioclavicular joint: Surgical anatomy and biological reconstruction. Injury 11:208-214, 1980.
383. Kumar S, Sethi A, Jain AK: Surgical treatment of complete acromioclavicular dislocation using the coracoacromial ligament and coracoclavicular fixation: Report of a technique in 14 patients. J Orthop Trauma 9:507-510, 1996.
384. Kutschera HP, Kotz RI: Bone–ligament transfer of coracoacromial ligament for acromioclavicular dislocation. Acta Orthop Scand 68:246-248, 1997.
385. Deshmukh AV, Wilson DR, Zilberfarb JL, et al: Stability of acromioclavicular joint reconstruction: Biomechanical testing of various surgical techniques in a cadaveric model. Am J Sports Med 32:1492-1498, 2004.
386. Gurd FB: The treatment of complete dislocation of the outer end of the clavicle: A hitherto undescribed operation. Ann Surg 113:1094-1098, 1941.
387. Mumford EB: Acromioclavicular dislocation. J Bone Joint Surg 23:799-802, 1941.
388. Browne JE, Stanley RF Jr, Tullos HS: Acromioclavicular joint dislocations. Am J Sports Med 5:258-263, 1977.
389. Smith DW: Coracoid fracture associated with acromioclavicular dislocation. Clin Orthop Relat Res (108):165, 1975.
390. Bailey RW: A dynamic repair for complete acromioclavicular joint dislocation [abstract]. J Bone Joint Surg Am 47:858, 1965.
391. Dewar FP, Barrington TW: The treatment of chronic acromioclavicular dislocation. J Bone Joint Surg Br 47:32-35, 1965.
392. Bailey RW, O'Connor GA, Tilus PD, et al: A dynamic repair for acute and chronic injuries of the acromioclavicular area [abstract]. J Bone Joint Surg Am 54:1802, 1972.
393. Berson BL, Gilbert MS, Green S: Acromioclavicular dislocations: Treatment by transfer of the conjoined tendon and distal end of the coracoid process to the clavicle. Clin Orthop Relat Res (135):157-164, 1978.
394. Brunelli G, Brunelli F: The treatment of acromioclavicular dislocation by transfer of the short head of the biceps. Int Orthop 12:105-108, 1988.
395. Cozma T, Alexa O, Georgescu N: [Dewar–Barrington technique original adaptation used in the treatment of acromioclavicular dislocations.] Rev Med Chir Soc Med Nat Iasi 108:420-423, 2004.
396. Glorian B, Delplace J: [Dislocations of the acromioclavicular joint treated by transplant of the coracoid process.] Rev Chir Orthop 59:667-679, 1973.
397. Budoff JE, Rodin D, Ochiai D, et al: Conjoined tendon transfer for chronic acromioclavicular dislocation in a patient with paraplegia: A case report with 38-year follow-up. Am J Orthop 34:189-191, 2005.
398. Laing PG: Transplantation of the long head of the biceps in complete acromioclavicular separations (Proceedings). J Bone Joint Surg Am 51:1677-1678, 1969.
399. Vargas L: Repair of complete acromioclavicular dislocation, utilizing the short head of the biceps. J Bone Joint Surg 24:772-773, 1942.
400. Mazzocca AD, Conway J, Johnson S et al: The anatomic coracoclavicular ligament reconstruction. Oper Tech Sports Med 12:56-61, 2004.
401. Wolf EM, Pennington WT: Arthroscopic reconstruction for acromioclavicular joint dislocation. Arthroscopy 17:558-563, 2001.
402. Baumgarten KM, Altchek DW, Cordasco FA: Arthroscopically assisted acromioclavicular joint reconstruction. Arthroscopy 22:228, e1-228.e6, 2006.
403. Chernchujit B, Tischer T, Imhoff AB: Arthroscopic reconstruction of the acromioclavicular joint disruption: Surgical technique and preliminary results. Arch Orthop Trauma Surg 126(9):575-581, 2006.
404. Lafosse L, Baier GP, Leuzinger J: Arthroscopic treatment of acute and chronic acromioclavicular joint dislocation. Arthroscopy 21:1017.e1-1017.e8, 2005.
405. Rolla PR, Surace MF, Murena L: Arthroscopic treatment of acute acromioclavicular joint dislocation. Arthroscopy 20:662-668, 2004.
406. Trikha SP, Acton D, Wilson AJ, et al: A new method of arthroscopic reconstruction of the dislocated acromio-clavicular joint. Ann R Coll Surg Engl 86:161-164, 2004.
407. Wellmann M, Zantop T, Weimann A, et al: Biomechanical evaluation of minimally invasive repairs for complete acromioclavicular joint dislocation. Am J Sports Med 35(6):955-961, 2007.
408. Kiefer H, Claes L, Burri C, et al: The stabilizing effect of various implants on the torn acromioclavicular joint: A biomechanical study. Arch Orthop Trauma Surg 106:42-46, 1986.
409. Jerosch J, Filler T, Peuker E, et al: Which stabilization technique corrects anatomy best in patients with AC separation. Knee Surg Sports Traumatol Arthrosc 7:365-372, 1999.
410. Jari R, Costic RS, Rodosky MW, et al: Biomechanical function of surgical procedures for acromioclavicular joint dislocations. Arthroscopy 20(3):237-245, 2004.

411. Harris RI, Wallace AL, Harper GD, et al: Structural properties of the intact and reconstructed coracoclavicular ligament complex. Am J Sports Med 28:103-108, 2000.

412. McConnell AJ, Yoo DJ, Zdero R, et al: Methods of operative fixation of the acromio-clavicular joint: A biomechanical comparison. J Orthop Trauma 21:248-253, 2007.

413. Talbert TW, Green JR 3rd, Mukherjee DP, et al: Bioabsorbable screw fixation in coracoclavicular ligament reconstruction. J Long Term Eff Med Implants 13:319-323, 2003.

414. Motamedi AR, Blevins FT, Willis MC: Biomechanics of the coracoclavicular ligament complex and augmentations used in its repair and reconstruction. Am J Sports Med 28:380-384, 2000.

415. Wickham MQ, Wyland DJ, Glisson RR, et al: A biomechanical comparison of suture constructs used for coracoclavicular fixation. J South Orthop Assoc 12:143-148, 2003.

416. Baker JE, Nicandri GT, Young DC, et al: A cadaveric study examining acromioclavicular joint congruity after different methods of coracoclavicular loop repair. J Shoulder Elbow Surg 12:595-598, 2003.

417. Lee SJ, Nicholas SJ, Akizuki KH, et al: Reconstruction of the coracoclavicular ligaments with tendon grafts: A comparative biomechanical study. Am J Sports Med 31:648-655, 2003.

418. Deshmukh AV, Wilson DR, Zilberfarb JL, et al: Stability of acromioclavicular joint reconstruction: Biomechanical testing of various surgical techniques in a cadaveric model. Am J Sports Med 32:1492-1498, 2004.

419. Grutter PW, Petersen SA: Anatomical acromioclavicular ligament reconstruction: A biomechanical comparison of reconstructive techniques of the acromioclavicular joint. Am J Sports Med 33:1723-1728, 2005.

420. Mazzocca AD, Santangelo SA, Johnson ST, et al: A biomechanical evaluation of an anatomical coracoclavicular ligament reconstruction. Am J Sports Med 34:236-246, 2006.

421. Wilson DR, Moses JM, Zilberfarb JL, et al: Mechanics of coracoacromial ligament transfer augmentation for acromioclavicular joint injuries. J Biomech 38:615-619, 2005.

422. Costic RS, Labriola JE, Rodosky MW, et al: Biomechanical rationale for development of anatomical reconstructions of coracoclavicular ligaments after complete acromioclavicular joint dislocations. Am J Sports Med 32:1929-1936, 2004.

423. Sloan SM, Budoff JE, Hipp JA, et al: Coracoclavicular ligament reconstruction using the lateral half of the conjoined tendon. J Shoulder Elbow Surg 13:186-190, 2004.

424. Moinfar AR, Murthi AM: Anatomy of the pectoralis minor tendon and its use in acromioclavicular joint reconstruction. J Shoulder Elbow Surg 16(3):339-346, 2007.

425. Chaudry SN, Waseem M: Clavicular hook plate: Complications of retaining the implant. Injury 37(7):665, 2006.

426. Bargren JH, Erlanger S, Dick HM: Biomechanics and comparison of two operative methods of treatment of complete acromioclavicular separation. Clin Orthop Relat Res (130):267-272, 1978.

427. Lancaster S, Horowitz M, Alonso J: Complete acromioclavicular separations: A comparison of operative methods. Clin Orthop Relat Res (216):80-88, 1987.

428. Warren-Smith CD, Ward MW: Operation for acromioclavicular dislocation: A review of 29 cases treated by one method. J Bone Joint Surg Br 69:715-718, 1987.

429. Skjeldal S, Lundblad R, Dullerud R: Coracoid process transfer for acromioclavicular dislocation. Acta Orthop Scand 59:180-182, 1988.

430. Pulles HJW: Operative treatment of acromio-clavicular dislocation [abstract]. Acta Orthop Scand 55:483, 1984.

431. Eaton R, Serletti J: Computerized axial tomography—a method of localizing Steinmann pin migration: A case report. Orthopedics 4:1357-1360, 1981.

432. Lindsey RW, Gutowski WT: The migration of a broken pin following fixation of the acromioclavicular joint: A case report and review of the literature. Orthopedics 9:413-416, 1986.

433. Lyons FA, Rockwood CA Jr: Migration of pins used in operations on the shoulder. J Bone Joint Surg Am 72:1262-1267, 1990.

434. Mazet RJ: Migration of a Kirschner wire from the shoulder region into the lung: Report of two cases. J Bone Joint Surg Am 25:477-483, 1943.

435. Norrell H, Llewellyn RC: Migration of a threaded Steinmann pin from an acromioclavicular joint into the spinal canal: A case report. J Bone Joint Surg Am 47:1024-1026, 1965.

436. Urban J, Jaskiewicz A: [Idiopathic displacement of Kirschner wire to the thoracic cavity after the osteosynthesis of acromioclavicular joint.] Chir Narzadow Ruchu Ortop Pol 49:399-402, 1984.

437. Wirth MA, Lakoski SG, Rockwood CA Jr.: Migration of broken cerclage wire from the shoulder girdle into the heart: A case report. J Shoulder Elbow Surg 9:543-544, 2000.

438. Foster GT, Chetty KG, Matutte K, et al: Hemoptysis due to migration of a fractured Kirschner wire. Chest 119:1285-1286, 2001.

439. Grauthoff VH, Klammer HL: [Complications due to migration of a Kirschner wire from the clavicle.] Fortschr Rontgenstr 128:591-594, 1978.

440. Kumar S, Sethi A, Jain AK: Surgical treatment of complete acromioclavicular dislocation using the coracoacromial ligament and coracoclavicular fixation: Report of a technique in 14 patients. J Orthop Trauma 9:507-510, 1996.

441. Retief PJ, Meintjes FA: Migration of a Kirschner wire in the body—a case report. S Afr Med J 53:557-558, 1978.

442. Sethi GK, Scott SM: Subclavian artery laceration due to migration of a Hagie pin. Surgery 80:644-646, 1976.

443. Boldin C, Fankhauser F, Ratschek M, et al: Foreign-body reaction after reconstruction of complete acromioclavicular dislocation using PDS augmentation. J Shoulder Elbow Surg 13:99-100, 2004.

444. Dust WN, Lenczner EM: Stress fracture of the clavicle leading to non-union secondary to coracoclavicular reconstruction with Dacron. Am J Sports Med 17:128-129, 1989.

445. Fullerton LR Jr: Recurrent third degree acromioclavicular joint separation after failure of a Dacron ligament prosthesis. Am J Sports Med 18:106-107, 1990.

446. Martell JR Jr: Clavicular nonunion. Complications with the use of Mersilene tape. Am J Sports Med 20:360-362, 1992.

447. Moneim MS, Balduini FC: Coracoid fractures as a complication of surgical treatment by coracoclavicular tape fixation. Clin Orthop Relat Res (168):133-135, 1982.

448. Stewart AM, Ahmad CS: Failure of acromioclavicular reconstruction using Gore-Tex graft due to aseptic foreign-body reaction and clavicle osteolysis: A case report. J Shoulder Elbow Surg 13:558-561, 2004.

449. Cook DA, Heiner JP: Acromioclavicular joint injuries. J Orthop Rev 19:510-516, 1990.

450. Hamner DL, Brown CH, Steiner ME: Hamstring tendon grafts for reconstruction of the anterior cruciate ligament: Biomechanical evaluation of the use of multiple strands and tensioning techniques. J Bone Joint Surg Am 81:549-557, 1999.

451. Jones HP, Lemos MJ, Schepsis AA: Salvage of failed acromioclavicular joint reconstruction using autogenous semitendinosis tendon from the knee: Surgical technique and case report. Am J Sports Med 29:234-237, 2001.

452. LaPrade RF, Hilger B: Coracoclavicular ligament reconstruction using a semitendinosis graft for failed acromioclavicular separation surgery. Arthroscopy 21:1279.e1-1279.e5, 2005.

453. Tauber M, Eppel M, Resch H: Acromioclavicular reconstruction using autogenous semitendinosis tendon graft: Results of revision surgery in chronic cases. J Shoulder Elbow Surg 16(4):429-433, 2007.

454. Ogden JA: Distal clavicular physeal injury. Clin Orthop Relat Res (188):68-73, 1984.

455. Black GB, McPherson JAM, Reed MH: Traumatic pseudodislocation of the acromioclavicular joint in children: A fifteen year review. Am J Sports Med 19:644-646, 1991.

456. Curtis RJ: Operative management of children's fractures of the shoulder region. Orthop Clin North Am 21:315-324, 1990.

457. Eidman DK, Siff SJ, Tullos HS: Acromioclavicular lesions in children. Am J Sports Med 9:150-154, 1981.

458. Falstie-Jensen S, Mikkelsen P: Pseudodislocation of the acromioclavicular joint. J Bone Joint Surg Br 64:368-369, 1982.

459. Havranek P: Injuries of the distal clavicular physis in children. J Pediatr Orthop 9:213-215, 1989.

460. Katznelson A, Nerubay J, Oliver S: Dynamic fixation of the avulsed clavicle. J Trauma 16:841-844, 1976.

461. Edelson G, Ganayem M, Saffuri H, et al: Unusual lateral clavicle fracture dislocation: Case reports and museum specimens. Clin Orthop Relat Res (439):274-279, 2005.

462. Yanagisawa K, Hamada K, Gotoh M, et al: Posteroinferior acromioclavicular dislocation with supraspinatus tear. A case report. Clin Orthop Relat Res (353):134-137, 1998.

463. Golthamer CR: Duplication of the clavicle; (os subclaviculare). Radiology 68(4):576-578, 1957.

464. Tyler GT: Acromioclavicular dislocation fixed by a Vitallium screw through the joint. Am J Surg 58:245-247, 1942.

465. Barentsz JH, Driessen AP: Fracture of the coracoid process of the scapula with acromioclavicular separation: Case report and review of the literature. Acta Orthop Belg 55:499-503, 1989.

466. Bernard TN Jr, Bruent ME, Haddad RJ: Fractured coracoid process in acromioclavicular dislocations. Clin Orthop Relat Res (175):227-232, 1983.

467. Carr AJ, Broughton NS: Acromioclavicular dislocation associated with fracture of the coracoid process. J Trauma 29:125-126, 1989.

468. Gunes T, Demirhan M, Atalar A, et al: [A case of acromioclavicular dislocation without coracoclavicular ligament rupture accompanied by coracoid process fracture.] Acta Orthop Traumatol Turc 40(4):334-337, 2006.

469. Hak DJ, Johnson EE: Avulsion fracture of the coracoid associated with acromioclavicular dislocation: Case report and review of the literature. J Orthop Trauma 7:381-383, 1993.

470. Kumar A: Management of coracoid process fracture with acromioclavicular joint dislocation. Orthopedics 13:770-772, 1990.

471. Martin-Herrero T, Rodriquez-Merchan C, Munuera-Martinez L: Fracture of the coracoid process: Presentation of seven cases and review of the literature. J Trauma 30:1597-1599, 1993.

472. Montgomery SP, Loyd RD: Avulsion fracture of the coracoid epiphysis with acromioclavicular separation. J Bone Joint Surg Am 59:963-965, 1977.

473. Santa S: [Acromioclavicular dislocation associated with fracture of the coracoid process.] Magyar Traumatol 35:162-167, 1992.

474. Combalia A, Arandes JM, Alemany X, et al: Acromioclavicular dislocation with epiphyseal separation of the coracoid process: Report of a case and review of the literature. J Trauma 38:812-815, 1995.

475. Wang K, Hsu K, Shih C: Coracoid process fracture combined with acromioclavicular dislocation and coracoclavicular ligament rupture: A case report and review of the literature. Clin Orthop Relat Res (300):120-122, 1994.

476. Wilson KM, Colwill JC: Combined acromioclavicular dislocation with coracoclavicular ligament disruption and coracoid process fracture. Am J Sports Med 17:324-327, 1989.

477. Ishizuki M, Yamaura I, Isobe Y: Avulsion fracture of the superior border of the scapula. J Bone Joint Surg Am 63:820-822, 1981.

478. Lasda NA, Murray DG: Fracture separation of the coracoid process associated with acromioclavicular dislocation: Conservative treatment—a case report and review of the literature. Clin Orthop Relat Res (134):222-224, 1978.

479. Capelli R, Avai A: An unusual case of posterior acromioclavicular dislocation. J Sports Traumatol Rel Res 14:249-253, 1992.

480. Hastings DE, Horne JG: Anterior dislocation of the acromioclavicular joint. Injury 10:285-288, 1979.

481. Lee A, Bismil Q, Allom R, et al: Missed type IV AC joint dislocation: A case report. Injury Extra 37(8):283-285, 2006.

482. Malcapi C, Grassi G, Oretti D: Posterior dislocation of the acromioclavicular joint: A rare or an easily overlooked lesion? Ital J Orthop Traumatol 4:79-83, 1978.

483. Nieminen S, Aho AJ: Anterior dislocation of the acromioclavicular joint. Ann Chir Gynaecol 73:21-24, 1984.

484. Sahara W, Sugamoto K, Miwa T, et al: Atraumatic posterior dislocation of the acromioclavicular joint with voluntary reduction. Clin J Sports Med 15:104-106, 2005.

485. Sondergard-Petersen P, Mikkelsen P: Posterior acromioclavicular dislocation. J Bone Joint Surg Br 64:52-53, 1982.

486. Benabdallah O: Luxation bipolaire de la clavicule. A propos d'un cas. Rev Chir Orthop 77:265-266, 1991.

487. Dieme C, Bousso A, Sane A, et al: [Bipolar dislocation of the clavicle or floating clavicle. A report of 3 cases.] Chir Main 26(2):113-116, 2007.

488. Ebrheim NA, An HS, Jackson WT: Scapulothoracic disassociation. J Bone Joint Surg Am 70:428-432, 1988.

489. Eni-Olotu DO, Hobbs NJ: Floating clavicle: Simultaneous dislocation of both ends of the clavicle. Injury 28:319-320, 1997.

490. Neer CS II: Shoulder Reconstruction. Philadelphia: WB Saunders, 1990, p 362.

491. Pang KP, Yung SW, Lee TS, et al: Bipolar clavicular injury. Med J Malaysia 58:621-624, 2003.

492. Rockwood CA Jr: Fractures and dislocations of the shoulder. Part II. Subluxations and dislocations about the shoulder. In Rockwood CA, Green DP (eds): Fractures in Adults, vol 1, 2nd ed. Philadelphia: J B Lippincott, 1984, pp 722-985.

493. Scapinelli R: Bipolar dislocation of the clavicle: 3D CT imaging and delayed surgical correction of a case. Arch Orthop Trauma Surg 124(6):421-424, 2004.

494. Salter EG, Shelley BS, Nasca R: A morphological study of the acromioclavicular joint in humans [abstract]. Anat Rec 211:353, 1985.

495. Ammon JT, Voor MJ, Tillett ED: A biomechanical comparison of Bosworth and poly-L lactic acid bioabsorbable screws for treatment of acromioclavicular separations. Arthroscopy 21:1443-1446, 2005.

496. Gerber C, Rockwood CA Jr: Subcoracoid dislocation of the lateral end of the clavicle: A report of three cases. J Bone Joint Surg Am 69:924-927, 1987.

497. Harvey EJ, Reindl R, Berry GK: Surgical images: Musculoskeletal. Multidirectional acromioclavicular joint instability posttrauma. Can J Surg 49:434, 2006.

498. Naumann T: [A rare case of habitual lateral clavicular dislocation in the dorsal subacromial direction (case report).] Z Orthop Ihre Grenzgeb 124:34-35, 1986.

499. Patterson WR: Inferior dislocation of the distal end of the clavicle. J Bone Joint Surg Am 49:1184-1186, 1967.

500. Sage J: Recurrent inferior dislocation of the clavicle at the acromioclavicular joint. A case report. Am J Sports Med 10:145-146, 1982.

501. Schwarz N, Kuderna H: Inferior acromioclavicular separation: Report of an unusual case. Clin Orthop Relat Res (234):28-30, 1988.

502. Torrens C, Mestre C, Perez P, et al: Subcoracoid dislocation of the distal end of the clavicle. A case report. Clin Orthop Relat Res (348):121-123, 1998.

503. Namkoong S, Zuckerman JD, Rose DJ: Traumatic subacromial dislocation of the acromioclavicular joint: A case report. J Shoulder Elbow Surg 16(1):e8-e10, 2007.

504. Leppilahti J, Jalovaara P: Recurrent inferior dislocation of the acromioclavicular joint: A report of two cases. J Shoulder Elbow Surg 10:387-388, 2001.

505. Janecki CJ: Voluntary subluxation of the acromioclavicular joint. Clin Orthop Relat Res (125):29-31, 1977.

506. Richards RR, Herzenberg JE, Goldner JL: Bilateral nontraumatic anterior acromioclavicular joint dislocation: A case report. Clin Orthop Relat Res (209):255-258, 1986.

507. Saranglia D, Julliard R, Marcone L, et al: [The results of the modified Cadenat procedure in old acromioclavicular dislocations: 26 cases.] Rev Chir Orthop 73:187-190, 1987.

508. Bednarek J, Kaczan Z, Krochmalski M: [Results of treatment in acromioclavicular dislocations.] Chir Narzadow Ruchu Ortop Pol 46:13-16, 1981.

509. Zaricznyj B: Reconstruction for chronic scapuloclavicular instability. Am J Sports Med 11:17-25, 1983.

510. Ferris BD, Bhamra M, Paton DF: Coracoid process transfer for acromioclavicular dislocations: A report of 20 cases. Clin Orthop Relat Res (242):184-187, 1989.

511. Boussaton M, Julia F, Horvath E, et al: [Transposition of the coracoacromial ligament according to the technique of Weaver and Dunn in the treatment of old acromioclavicular luxations: A report of 15 cases.] Acta Orthop Belg 51:80-90, 1985.

512. Larsen E, Petersen V: Operative treatment of chronic acromioclavicular dislocation. Injury 18:55-56, 1987.

513. Ehricht HG: Die Osteolyse im lateralen Claviculaende nach Pressluftschaden. Arch Orthop Unfallchirurg 50:576-589, 1959.

514. Werder H: Posttraumatische Osteolyse des Schlusselbeinendes. Schweiz Med Wochenschr 80:912-913, 1950.

515. Jacobs P: Post-traumatic osteolysis of the outer end of the clavicle. J Bone Joint Surg Br 46:705-707, 1964.

516. Murphy OB, Bellamy R, Wheeler W, et al: Posttraumatic osteolysis of the distal clavicle. Clin Orthop Relat Res (109):108-114, 1975.

517. Seymour EQ: Osteolysis of the clavicular tip associated with repeated minor trauma to the shoulder. Radiology 123:56, 1977.

518. Matthews LS, Simonson BG, Wolock BS: Osteolysis of the distal clavicle in a female body builder. A case report. Am J Sports Med 21:50-52, 1993.

519. Scavenius M, Iversen BF, Sturup J: Resection of the lateral end of the clavicle following osteolysis, with emphasis on non-traumatic osteolysis of the acromial end of the clavicle in athletes. Injury 18:261-263, 1987.

520. Merchan EC: Osteolysis of the distal clavicle in a woman: Case report and review of the literature. Ital J Orthop Traumatol 18:561-563, 1992.

521. Orava S, Virtanen K, Holopainen YVO: Posttraumatic osteolysis of the distal ends of the clavicle. Ann Chir Gynaecol 73:83-86, 1984.

522. Asano H, Mimori K, Shinomiya K: A case of post-traumatic osteolysis of the distal clavicle: Histologic lesion of the acromion. J Shoulder Elbow Surg 11(2):182-187, 2002.

523. Brunet ME, Reynolds MC, Cook SD, et al: Atraumatic osteolysis of the distal clavicle: Histologic evidence of synovial pathogenesis: A case report. Orthopedics 9:557-559, 1986.

524. Levin AH, Pais MJ, Schwartz EE: Post-traumatic osteolysis of the distal clavicle with emphasis on early radiographic changes. AJR Am J Roentgenol 127:781-784, 1976.

525. Quinn SF, Glass TA: Posttraumatic osteolysis of the clavicle. South Med J 76:307-308, 1983.

526. Patten RM: Atraumatic osteolysis of the distal clavicle: MR findings. J Comput Assist Tomogr 19:92-95, 1995.

527. Griffiths CJ, Glucksman E: Posttraumatic osteolysis of the clavicle: A case report. Arch Emerg Med 3:129-132, 1986.

528. Lamont MK: Letter to the editor re "Osteolysis of the outer end of the clavicle." N Z Med J 95:241-242, 1982.

529. Zsernaviczky J, Horst M: Kasuistischer Beitrag zur Osteolyse am distalen Klavikulaende. Arch Orthop Unfallchirurg 89:163-167, 1977.

530. Hawkins BJ, Covey DC, Thiel BG: Distal clavicle osteolysis unrelated to trauma, overuse, or metabolic disease. Clin Orthop Relat Res (370):208-211, 2000.

531. Gajeski BL, Kettner NW: Osteolysis of the distal clavicle: Serial improvement and normalization of acromioclavicular joint space with conservative care. J Manipulative Physiol Ther 27(7):e12, 2004.

532. Levine AH, Pais MJ, Schwartz EE: Posttraumatic osteolysis of the distal clavicle with emphasis on early radiologic changes. AJR Am J Roentgenol 127:781-784, 1976.

533. Buttaci CJ, Stitik TP, Yonclas PP, et al: Osteoarthritis of the acromioclavicular joint: A review of anatomy, biomechanics, diagnosis, and treatment. Am J Phys Med Rehabil 83(10):791-797, 2004.

534. Henry MH, Liu SH, Loffredo AH: Arthroscopic management of the acromioclavicular joint disorder. Clin Orthop Relat Res (316):276-283, 1995.

535. Mehrberg RD, Lobel SM, Gibson WK: Disorders of the acromioclavicular joint. Phys Med Rehabil Clin N Am 15:v, 537-555, 2004.

536. Bonsell S, Pearsall AWT, Heitman RJ, et al: The relationship of age, gender, and degenerative changes observed on radiographs of the shoulder in asymptomatic individuals. J Bone Joint Surg Br 82:1135-1139, 2000.

537. Mahakkanukrauh P, Surin P: Prevalence of osteophytes associated with the acromion and acromioclavicular joint. Clin Anat 16:506-510, 2003.

538. Stenlund B, Marions O, Engstrom KF, Goldie I: Correlation of macroscopic osteoarthrotic changes and radiographic findings in the acromioclavicular joint. Acta Radiol 29:571-576, 1988.

539. Shubin Stein BE, Wiater JM, Pfaff HC, et al: Detection of acromioclavicular joint pathology in asymptomatic shoulders with magnetic resonance imaging. J Shoulder Elbow Surg 10:204-208, 2001.

540. Stenlund B, Goldie I, Hagberg M, et al: Radiographic osteoarthritis in the acromioclavicular joint resulting from manual work or exposure to vibration. Br J Sports Med 49:588-593, 1992.

541. Kurta I, Datir S, Dove M, et al: The short term effects of a single corticosteroid injection on the range of motion of the shoulder in patients with isolated acromioclavicular joint arthropathy. Acta Orthop Belg 71:656-661, 2005.

542. Meyers JF: Arthroscopic debridement of the acromioclavicular joint and distal clavicle resection. In McGinty JB, Caspari RB, Jackson RW, et al (eds): Operative Arthroscopy. New York, Raven Press, 1991, pp 557-560.

543. Waxman J: Acromioclavicular disease in rheumatologic practice—the forgotten joint. J La State Med Soc 129:1-3, 1977.

544. Strobel K, Pfirrmann CW, Zanetti M, et al: MRI features of the acromioclavicular joint that predict pain relief from intraarticular injection. AJR Am J Roentgenol 181:755-760, 2003.

545. De Santis D, Palazzi C, D'Amico E, et al: Acromioclavicular cyst and "porcupine shoulder" in gout. Rheumatology (Oxford) 40(11):1320-1321, 2001.

546. Groh GL, Badwey B, Rockwood CA: Treatment of cysts of the acromioclavicular joint with shoulder hemiarthroplasty. J Bone Joint Surg Am 75:1790-1794, 1993.

547. Huang GS, Bachmann D, Taylor JAM, et al: Calcium pyrophosphate dihydrate crystal deposition disease and pseudogout of the acromioclavicular joint: Radiographic and pathologic features. J Rheumatol 20:2077-2082, 1993.

548. Miller-Blair D, White R, Greenspan A: Acute gout involving the acromioclavicular joint following treatment with gemfibrozil. J Rheumatol 19:166-168, 1992.

549. Pattee GA, Snyder SJ: Synovial chondromatosis of the acromioclavicular joint: A case report. Clin Orthop Relat Res (233):205-207, 1988.

550. Burns SJ, Zvirbulis RA: A ganglion arising over the acromioclavicular joint: A case report. Orthopedics 7:1002-1004, 1984.

551. Craig EV: The acromioclavicular joint cyst: An unusual presentation of a rotator cuff tear. Clin Orthop Relat Res (202):189-192, 1986.

552. Mullett H, Benson R, Levy O: Arthroscopic treatment of a massive acromioclavicular joint cyst. Arthroscopy Apr;23(4):446.e1-e4, 2007.

553. Ozaki J, Tomita Y, Nakagawa Y, et al: Synovial chondromatosis of the acromioclavicular joint. Arch Orthop Trauma Surg 112:152-154, 1993.

554. Postacchini F, Perugia D, Gumina S: Acromioclavicular joint cyst associated with rotator cuff tear. Clin Orthop Relat Res (294):111-113, 1993.

555. Craig EV: The geyser sign and torn rotator cuff: Clinical significance and pathomechanics. Clin Orthop Relat Res (191):213-215, 1984.

556. Tshering Vogel DW, Steinbach LS, Hertel R, et al: Acromioclavicular joint cyst: Nine cases of a pseudotumor of the shoulder. Skeletal Radiol 34:260-265, 2005.

557. Blankstein A, Amsallem JL, Rubinstein E, et al: Septic arthritis of the acromioclavicular joint. Arch Orthop Trauma Surg 103:417-418, 1985.

558. Griffith PH III, Boyadjis TA: Acute pyarthrosis of the acromioclavicular joint: A case report. Orthopedics 7:1727-1728, 1984.

559. Hammel JM, Kwon N: Septic arthritis of the acromioclavicular joint. J Emerg Med 29:425-427, 2005.

560. Laktasic-Zerjavic N, Babic-Naglic D, Curkovic B, et al: Septic acromioclavicular arthritis in a patient with diabetes mellitus. Coll Antropol 29(2):743-746, 2005.

561. Adams R, McDonald M: Cryptococcal arthritis of the acromioclavicular joint. N C Med J 45:23-24, 1984.

562. Richter R, Hahn H, Naaubling W, et al: [Tuberculosis of the shoulder girdle.] Z Rheumatol 44:87-92, 1985.

563. Nehme A, Bone S, Gomez-Brouchet A, et al: Bilateral aseptic necrosis of the outer end of the clavicle. J Bone Joint Surg Br 85:275-277, 2003.

Disorders of the Sternoclavicular Joint

Michael A. Wirth, MD, and Charles A. Rockwood, Jr, MD

The first detailed case report of a sternoclavicular joint injury appeared as early as 1843,[1] and numerous related articles appeared in the late 19th century. However, it was not until the 1920s and 1930s that such articles appeared in the American literature.[2-4]

Injuries to the sternoclavicular joint are an uncommon problem and many authors apologize for reporting only three or four cases. The rarity of these injuries and the lack of standardized methods for treatment, measuring outcomes, and reporting complications increases methodologic flaws in structured literature reviews and often precludes a meaningful meta-analysis. From a review of the literature and in our combined 50 years of clinical experience, anterior dislocations are best treated nonoperatively, and posterior dislocations, which have accounted for deaths, need to be promptly diagnosed and reduced. Anterior and posterior injuries in adults up to age 23 years are usually physeal injuries and heal without specific treatment. Special radiographs are usually required to make the diagnosis. In our experience, high definition three-dimensional computed tomography (CT) images are the gold standard for evaluating these injuries (Fig. 13-1).

SURGICAL ANATOMY

Because less than half of the medial clavicle articulates with the upper angle of the sternum, the sternoclavicular joint has the distinction of having the least amount of bony stability of the major joints of the body.

The sternoclavicular joint is a diarthrodial joint and is the only true articulation between the upper extremity and the axial skeleton. The articular surface of the clavicle is much larger than that of the sternum, and both are covered with fibrocartilage. The enlarged bulbous medial end of the clavicle is concave front to back and convex vertically and therefore creates a saddle-type joint with the clavicular notch of the sternum. The clavicular notch of the sternum is curved, and the joint surfaces are not congruent. In 2.5% of patients there is a small facet on the inferior aspect of the medial clavicle, which articulates with the superior aspect of the first rib at its synchondral junction with the sternum.[5]

Ligaments of the Sternoclavicular Joint

The sternoclavicular joint has so much incongruity that integrity of the joint has to come from its surrounding ligaments, that is, the intra-articular disk ligament, the extra-articular costoclavicular ligament (rhomboid ligament), the capsular ligament, and the interclavicular ligament.

Intra-articular Disk Ligament

The intra-articular disk ligament is a very dense, fibrous structure that arises from the synchondral junction of the first rib with the sternum and passes through the sternoclavicular joint. This ligament divides the joint into two separate joint spaces. The upper attachment is on the superior and posterior aspects of the medial clavicle. DePalma[6] has shown that the disk is perforated only rarely; the perforation allows a free communication between the two joint compartments (Fig. 13-2). Anteriorly and posteriorly, the disk blends into the fibers of the capsular ligament. The disk acts as a checkrein against medial displacement of the medial clavicle.

Costoclavicular Ligament

The costoclavicular ligament, also called the *rhomboid ligament*, consists of an anterior and a posterior fasciculus. The costoclavicular ligament attaches inferiorly to the upper surface of the first rib and to the synchondral junction of the first rib and sternum; it attaches superiorly to

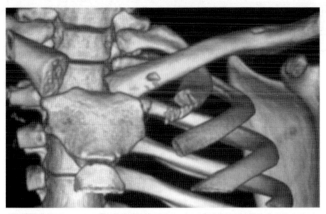

FIGURE 13-1 Three-dimensional CT scan revealing a posterior left sternoclavicular joint dislocation. Note the medial aspect of the clavicle posterior to the manubrium.

the margins of the impression on the inferior surface of the medial end of the clavicle, sometimes known as the rhomboid fossa.[7,8]

The fibers of the anterior fasciculus arise from the anteromedial surface of the first rib and are directed upward and laterally. The fibers of the posterior fasciculus are shorter and arise lateral to the anterior fibers on the rib and are directed upward and medially. The fibers of the anterior and posterior components cross and allow stability of the joint during rotation and elevation of the clavicle. The anatomy of the costoclavicular ligament is in many ways similar to the structural configuration of the coracoclavicular ligament on the outer end of the clavicle (Fig. 13-3).

Bearn[9] has shown experimentally that the anterior fibers resist excessive upward rotation of the clavicle and

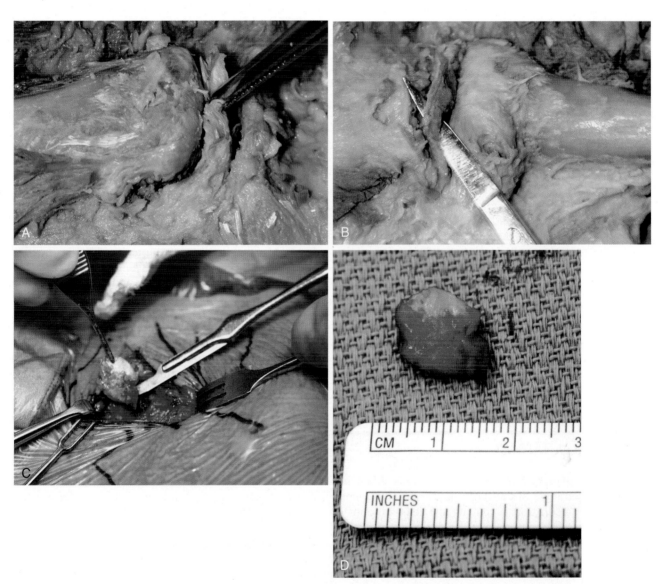

FIGURE 13-2 A, Normal-appearing articular disk ligament (held by forceps). **B,** Degenerative articular disk ligament with a central perforation. **C,** Intraoperative photograph demonstrating excision of a symptomatic articular disk ligament. **D,** Surgical specimen of excised articular disk ligament.

that the posterior fibers resist excessive downward rotation. Specifically, the anterior fibers also resist lateral displacement and the posterior fibers resist medial displacement (Fig. 13-4).

Interclavicular Ligament

The interclavicular ligament connects the superomedial aspects of each clavicle with the capsular ligaments and the upper part of the sternum. The interclavicular ligament assists the capsular ligaments in producing *shoulder poise*, that is, holding the shoulder up. The function of this ligament can be tested by putting a finger in the superior sternal notch; with elevation of the arm, the ligament is quite lax, but as soon as both arms hang at the sides, the ligament becomes tight.

Capsular Ligament

The capsular ligament covers the anterosuperior and posterior aspects of the joint and represents thickenings of the joint capsule (Fig. 13-5). This structure is the strongest of all the sternoclavicular ligaments and is the first line of defense against the upward displacement of the medial clavicle caused by a downward force on the distal end of the shoulder. We have observed that the clavicular attachment of the ligament is primarily onto the epiphysis of the medial clavicle, with some secondary blending of the fibers into the metaphysis. Although some authors report that the intra-articular disk ligament greatly assists the costoclavicular ligament in preventing upward displacement of the medial clavicle, Bearn[9] has shown that the capsular ligament is the most important structure in preventing upward displacement of the medial clavicle (see Fig. 13-4). In experimental postmortem studies, he determined, after cutting the costoclavicular, intra-articular disk, and interclavicular ligaments, that they had no effect on clavicle poise. However, the division of the capsular ligament alone resulted in a downward depression of the distal end of the clavicle. Bearn's findings have many clinical implications for the mechanisms of injury of the sternoclavicular joint.

Through a cadaveric study Spencer and coworkers[10] measured anterior and posterior translation of the sternoclavicular joint. Anterior and posterior translation was measured in intact specimens and following transection of randomly chosen ligaments about the sternoclavicular joint. Cutting the posterior capsule resulted in a significant increase in both anterior and posterior translation. Cutting the anterior capsule produced a significant increase in anterior translation. This study demonstrated that the posterior sternoclavicular joint capsule is the most important structure for preventing both anterior and posterior translation of the sternoclavicular joint, with the anterior capsule acting as an important secondary stabilizer.

Range of Motion of the Sternoclavicular Joint

The sternoclavicular joint is freely movable and functions almost like a ball-and-socket joint in that the joint has

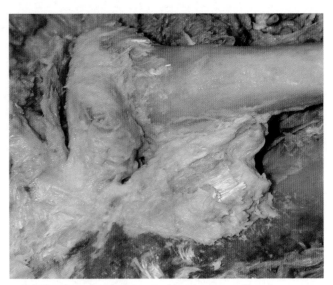

FIGURE 13-3 Left medial clavicle demonstrating the rhomboid appearance of the costoclavicular ligament and the anterior sternoclavicular capsular ligament.

motion in all planes, including rotation. The clavicle and therefore the sternoclavicular joint in normal shoulder motion is capable of 30 to 35 degrees of upward elevation, 35 degrees of combined forward and backward movement, and 45 to 50 degrees of rotation around its long axis (Fig. 13-6). It is most likely to be the most frequently moved joint of the long bones in the body because almost any motion of the upper extremity is transferred proximally to the sternoclavicular joint.

Epiphysis of the Medial Clavicle

Although the clavicle is the first long bone of the body to ossify (intrauterine week 5), the epiphysis at the medial end of the clavicle is the last of the long bones in the body to appear and the last epiphysis to close (Fig. 13-7). The medial clavicular epiphysis does not ossify until the 18th to 20th year, and it fuses with the shaft of the clavicle around the 23rd to 25th year. Webb and Suchey,[11] in an extensive study of the medial clavicular physis in 605 male and 254 female cadavers at autopsy, reported that complete union might not be present until 31 years of age. This knowledge of the epiphysis is important because we believe that many of the so-called sternoclavicular dislocations are fractures through the physeal plate.

Applied Surgical Anatomy

Surgeons planning an operative procedure on or near the sternoclavicular joint should be completely knowledgeable about the vast array of anatomic structures immediately posterior to the sternoclavicular joint. A curtain of muscles—the sternohyoid, sternothyroid, and scaleni—

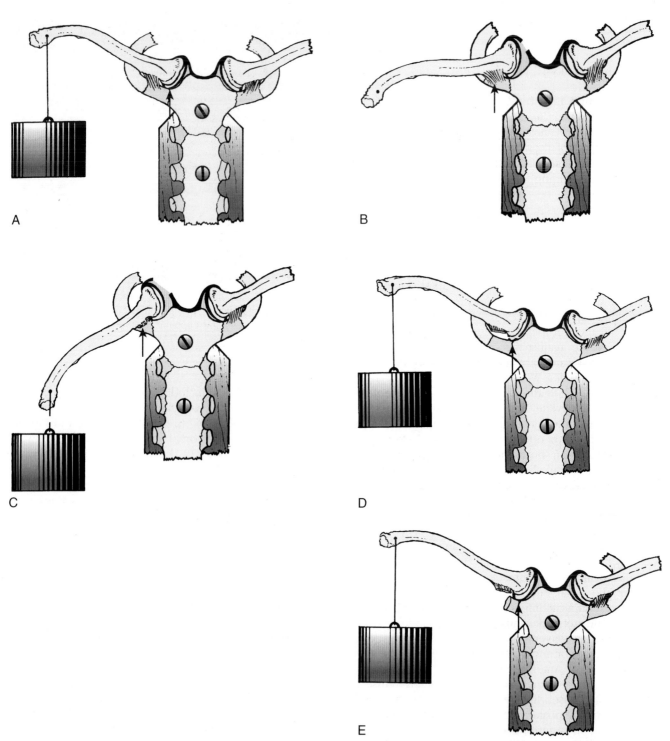

FIGURE 13-4 The importance of the various ligaments around the sternoclavicular joint in maintaining normal shoulder poise. **A,** The lateral end of the clavicle is maintained in an elevated position through the sternoclavicular ligaments. The *arrow* indicates the fulcrum. **B,** When the capsule is divided completely, the lateral end of the clavicle descends under its own weight without any loading. The clavicle seems to be supported by the intra-articular disk ligament. **C,** After division of the capsular ligament, it was determined that a weight less than 5 lb was enough to tear the intra-articular disk ligament from its attachment on the costal cartilage junction of the first rib. The fulcrum was transferred laterally so that the medial end of the clavicle hinged over the first rib in the vicinity of the costoclavicular ligament. **D,** After division of the costoclavicular ligament and the intra-articular disk ligament, the lateral end of the clavicle could not be depressed as long as the capsular ligament was intact. **E,** After resection of the medial first costal cartilage along with the costoclavicular ligament, there was no effect on the poise of the lateral end of the clavicle, as long as the capsular ligament was intact. (From Bearn JG: Direct observation on the function of the capsule of the sternoclavicular joint in clavicular support. J Anat 101:159-170, 1967.)

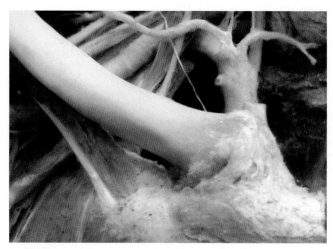

FIGURE 13-5 Normal anatomy around the sternoclavicular joint. Note that the tendon of the subclavius muscle arises in the vicinity of the costoclavicular ligament from the first rib and has a long tendon structure.

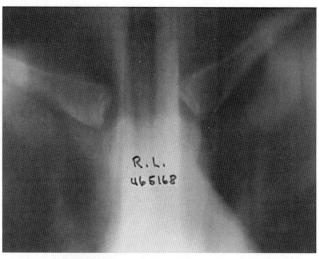

FIGURE 13-7 Tomogram demonstrating the thin, wafer-like disk of the epiphysis of the medial part of the clavicle. (From Rockwood CA, Green DP [eds]: Fractures [3 vols], 2nd ed. Philadelphia: JB Lippincott, 1984.)

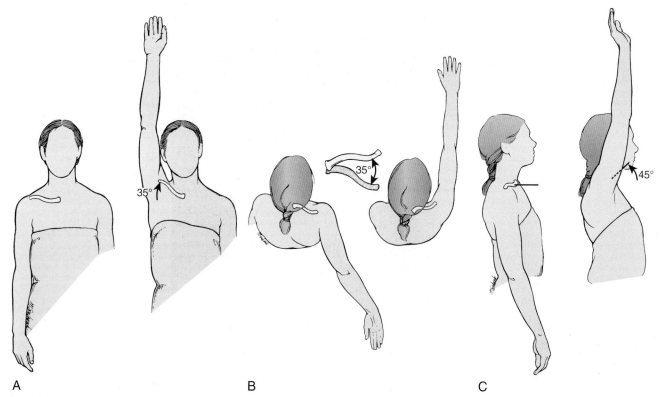

A   B   C

FIGURE 13-6 Motions of the clavicle and the sternoclavicular joint. **A,** With full overhead elevation, the clavicle elevates 35 degrees. **B,** With adduction and extension, the clavicle displaces anteriorly and posteriorly 35 degrees. **C,** The clavicle rotates on its long axis 45 degrees as the arm is elevated to the full overhead position.

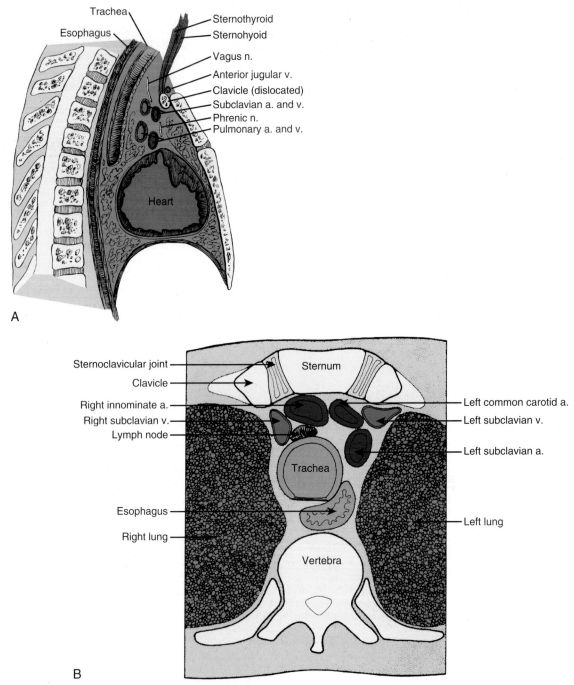

FIGURE 13-8 Applied anatomy of the vital structures posterior to the sternoclavicular joint. **A** and **B,** Sagittal view and cross section demonstrating the structures posterior to the sternoclavicular joint.

are located posterior to the sternoclavicular joint and the inner third of the clavicle and block the view of vital structures. Some of these vital structures include the innominate artery, innominate vein, vagus nerve, phrenic nerve, internal jugular vein, trachea, and esophagus. If one is considering the possibility of stabilizing the sterno-

clavicular joint by running a pin down from the clavicle into the sternum, it is important to remember that the arch of the aorta, the superior vena cava, and the right pulmonary artery are also very close at hand (Fig. 13-8).

Another structure to be aware of is the anterior jugular vein, which is between the clavicle and the curtain of

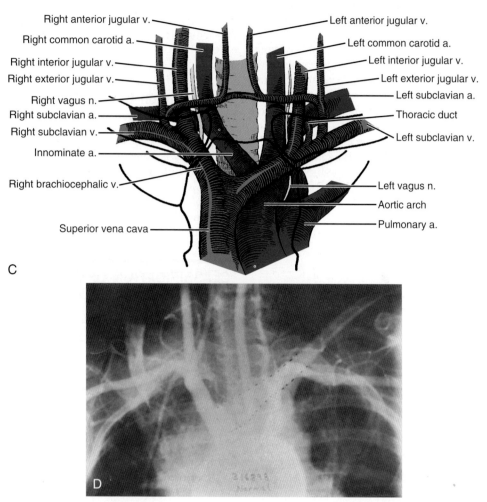

FIGURE 13-8, cont'd **C,** A diagram demonstrates the close proximity of the major vessels that are posterior to the sternoclavicular joint. **D,** Aortogram showing the relationship of the medial end of the clavicle to the major vessels in the mediastinum. (From Bucholz RW, Heckman JD [eds]: Rockwood and Green's Fractures in Adults, 5th ed. Philadelphia: Lippincott Williams & Wilkins, 2001, p 1260.)

muscles. Anatomy books state that this vein can be quite variable in size. We have seen it as large as 1.5 cm in diameter. This vein has no valves, and when it is nicked, it looks like someone has opened up the floodgates.

MECHANISM OF INJURY

Either direct or indirect force can produce a dislocation of the sternoclavicular joint. Because the sternoclavicular is so small and incongruous, one would think that it would be the most commonly dislocated joint in the body. However, the ligamentous supporting structure is so strong and has evolved in such a manner that it is one of the least commonly dislocated joints in the body. Traumatic dislocation of the sternoclavicular joint usually

occurs only after tremendous force, either direct or indirect, has been applied to the shoulder.

Direct Force

When force is applied directly to the anteromedial aspect of the clavicle, the clavicle is pushed posteriorly behind the sternum into the mediastinum. This injury can occur in a variety of ways:

- An athlete lying supine on the ground is jumped on, and the knee of the jumper lands directly on the medial end of the clavicle.
- A kick is delivered to the front of the medial clavicle.
- A person is run over by a vehicle.
- A person is pinned between a vehicle and a wall.

Indirect Force

A force can be applied indirectly to the sternoclavicular joint from the anterolateral or posterolateral aspects of the shoulder (Fig. 13-9). This is the most common mechanism of injury to the sternoclavicular joint. Mehta and colleagues[12] reported that three of four posterior sternoclavicular dislocations were produced by indirect force, and Heinig[13] reported that indirect force was responsible for eight of nine cases of posterior sternoclavicular dislocations. Indirect force was the most common mechanism of injury in our 185 patients as well. If the shoulder is compressed and rolled forward, an ipsilateral posterior dislocation results; if the shoulder is compressed and rolled backward, an ipsilateral anterior dislocation results.

Most Common Cause of Injury to the Sternoclavicular Joint

The most common cause of dislocation of the sternoclavicular joint is vehicular accidents; the second is an injury sustained during participation in sports.[14-16] Omer,[16] in his review of patients from 14 military hospitals, found 82 cases of sternoclavicular joint dislocations. He reported that almost 80% of these occurred as the result of vehicular accidents (47%) and athletics (31%).

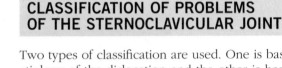

CLASSIFICATION OF PROBLEMS OF THE STERNOCLAVICULAR JOINT

Two types of classification are used. One is based on the etiology of the dislocation and the other is based on the anatomic position that the dislocation assumes.

Classification Based on Anatomy

Detailed classifications are confusing and difficult to remember, and the following classification is suggested.

Anterior Dislocation

An anterior dislocation is the most common type of sternoclavicular dislocation. The medial end of the clavicle is displaced anteriorly or anterosuperiorly to the anterior margin of the sternum (Fig. 13-10).

Posterior Dislocation

Posterior sternoclavicular dislocation is uncommon. The medial end of the clavicle is displaced posterior, posteroinferior, or posterosuperior with respect to the sternum.

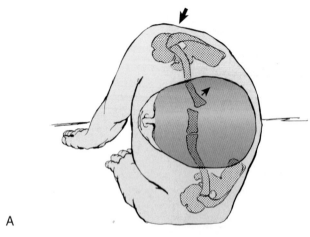

A

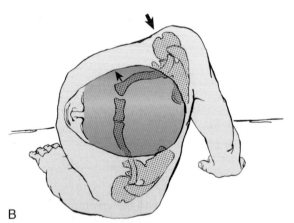

B

FIGURE 13-9 Mechanisms that produce anterior or posterior dislocation of the sternoclavicular joint. **A,** If the patient is lying on the ground and a compression force is applied to the posterolateral aspect of the shoulder, the medial end of the clavicle will be displaced posteriorly. **B,** When the lateral compression force is directed from the anterior position, the medial end of the clavicle is dislocated posteriorly. (From Bucholz RW, Heckman JD [eds]: Rockwood and Green's Fractures in Adults, 5th ed. Philadelphia: Lippincott Williams & Wilkins, 2001, p 1247.)

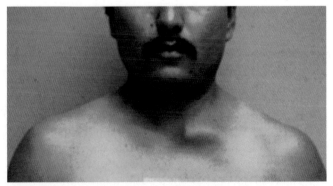

FIGURE 13-10 Clinical view demonstrating anterior dislocation of the left sternoclavicular joint.

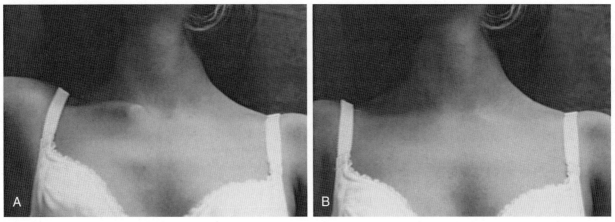

FIGURE 13-11 Spontaneous anterior subluxation of the sternoclavicular joint. **A,** With the arms in the overhead position, the medial end of the right clavicle spontaneously subluxes out anteriorly without any trauma. **B,** When the arm is brought back down to the side, the medial end of the clavicle spontaneously reduces. Such subluxation and reduction are not usually associated with any significant discomfort.

Classification Based on Etiology

Traumatic Injury

Sprain or Subluxation

Acute sprains of the sternoclavicular joint can be classified as mild, moderate, or severe. In a *mild* sprain, all the ligaments are intact and the joint is stable. A *moderate* sprain is characterized by subluxation of the sternoclavicular joint. The capsular, intra-articular disk, and costoclavicular ligaments may be partially disrupted. The subluxation may be anterior or posterior. A *severe* sprain involves complete disruption of the sternoclavicular ligaments, and the dislocation may be anterior or posterior.

Acute Dislocation

In a dislocated sternoclavicular joint, the capsular and intra-articular ligaments are ruptured. Occasionally, the costoclavicular ligament is intact but stretched out enough to allow the dislocation.

Recurrent Dislocation

If the initial acute traumatic dislocation does not heal, mild to moderate force may produce recurrent dislocations. However, this is rare.

Atraumatic Problems

For a variety of nontraumatic reasons, the sternoclavicular joint can sublux or enlarge.

Spontaneous Subluxation or Dislocation

Although both sternoclavicular joints can be affected, usually one joint is more symptomatic. It usually occurs in patients who have generalized ligament laxity of other joints (Fig. 13-11). In some patients, the anterior dislocation of the sternoclavicular joint is painful and is associated with a snap or pop as the arm is elevated overhead,

and another snap occurs when the arm is returned to the patient's side. The condition usually occurs in the late teens and young adulthood.

Arthritis

Arthritis involving the sternoclavicular joint can come in many forms:

- Osteoarthritis
- Arthropathies
- Condensing osteitis of the medial clavicle
- Sternocostoclavicular hyperostosis
- Postmenopausal arthritis

Osteoarthritis. Osteoarthritis is characterized by narrowing of the joint space, osteophytes, subchondral sclerosis, and cysts on both sides of the joint (Fig. 13-12). Because most of the wear occurs in the inferior part of the head of the

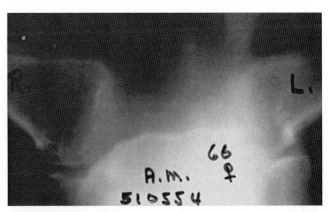

FIGURE 13-12 Tomogram of the sternoclavicular joints in a 66-year-old patient with degenerative arthritis of the sternoclavicular joint.

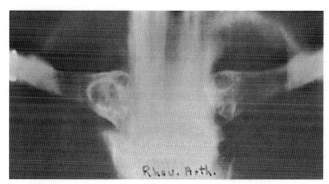

FIGURE 13-13 Tomogram of a patient with rheumatoid arthritis and bilateral degenerative changes in the medial aspect of the clavicles. (From Rockwood CA, Green DP [eds]: Fractures [3 vols], 2nd ed. Philadelphia: JB Lippincott, 1984.)

medial clavicle, most of the degenerative changes occur in that region. The sometimes discrete degenerative changes are best seen on tomograms and CT scans. Sternoclavicular joint arthritis and hypertrophy can develop after radical neck surgery, particularly when the spinal accessory nerve is sacrificed.[17,18] The incidence is reported to be as high as 54%.[17]

Arthropathies. Some of the disease processes that produce degenerative changes in the sternoclavicular joint are rheumatoid arthritis, rheumatoid spondylitis, scleroderma, Reiter's syndrome, psoriasis, polymyalgia rheumatica, secondary hyperparathyroidism, gout, pseudogout, leprosy, syringomyelia, metastatic carcinoma, condensing osteitis, Friedreich's disease (aseptic necrosis of the medial end of the clavicle), and sternoclavicular hyperostosis (Fig. 13-13).

Condensing Osteitis of the Medial Clavicle. Condensing osteitis of the medial clavicle is an uncommon condition that usually develops in women older than 40 years and can occur secondary to chronic stress on the joint.[59,60] The joint is swollen and tender, and radionuclide studies reveal increased uptake of the isotope.

Radiographs show sclerosis and slight expansion of the medial third of the clavicle. The inferior portion of the sternal end of the clavicle shows sclerotic changes. Some osteophytes may be present, but the joint space is preserved. The changes in the medial clavicle are best detected by CT. The differential diagnosis includes Paget's disease, sternoclavicular hyperostosis, Friedreich's avascular necrosis of the medial clavicular epiphysis, infection, Tietze's syndrome, and osteoarthritis. More recently, Vierboom and coworkers[19] described the use of magnetic resonance imaging (MRI) as an adjunctive method for diagnosing this entity. Most patients do well with conservative treatment, that is, with antiinflammatory medications. However, Kruger and associates[20] recommend incisional or excisional biopsy in refractory cases.

Sternocostoclavicular Hyperostosis. First described by Sonozaki,[21,22] sternocostoclavicular hyperostosis involves adults of both genders between 30 and 50 years of age and is usually bilateral. The process begins at the junction of the medial clavicle, the first rib, and the sternum as an ossification in the ligaments and later involves the bones. In some cases, the hyperostosis is extensive and forms a solid block of bone consisting of the sternum, ribs, and clavicle. Patients may have peripheral arthritis. Subperiosteal bone changes have been noted on the radiographs of other bones of the skeleton, specifically, the humerus, pelvis, tibia, ribs, and vertebral bodies.

The condition has been graded into stages I, II, and III by Sonozaki and colleagues.[21,22] Stage I consists of mild ossification in the costoclavicular ligaments. Stage II is characterized by an ossific mass between the clavicle and the first rib. In stage III, a bone mass exists between the clavicle, sternum, and first rib.

As might be expected with fusion of the sternoclavicular joint, shoulder motion is severely restricted. Sternoclavicular hyperostosis is a seronegative and HLA-B27–negative rheumatic disease. In this condition, hypostosis can appear in the spine, long bones, sacroiliac joints, and the sternoclavicular region. This entity is also associated with palmoplantar pustulosis. Tamai and Saotome have described a patient with palmar and plantar lesions associated with bilateral osseous fusion of both the acromioclavicular and sternoclavicular joints.[23]

Postmenopausal Arthritis. Postmenopausal arthritis is seen primarily in postmenopausal women. Sadr and Swann[24] reported on 22 patients with this problem who were seen in a 5-year study; 20 of the patients were women, and the majority of cases involved the sternoclavicular joint of the dominant arm. Nonoperative treatment was recommended.

The condition is the result of normal degeneration of a frequently moved joint. It is almost without symptoms; a lump develops at the sternoclavicular joint and, occasionally, a vague ache (Fig. 13-14). Patients have no previous history of injury or disease. Radiographs reveal sclerosis and enlargement of the medial end of the clavicle, reactive sclerosis of the sternum, and subluxation of the joint. The pathologic changes are those of degenerative arthritis.

Infection

Spontaneous swelling with the appearance of joint subluxation may be associated with acute, subacute, or chronic bacterial arthritis. Predisposing conditions include intravenous (IV) drug addiction, bacteremia, rheumatoid arthritis, alcoholism, chronic debilitating diseases, and human immunodeficiency virus (HIV) infection.[25,26] Sternoclavicular joint sepsis and osteomyelitis have also been reported in patients undergoing subclavian vein catheterization and in dialysis patients.[27,28] CT is very helpful in making an early diagnosis of a septic sternoclavicular joint (Fig. 13-15).

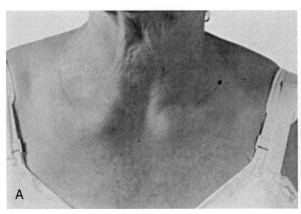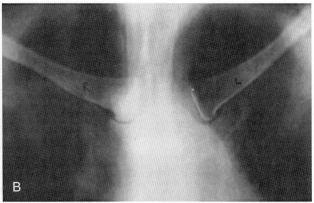

FIGURE 13-14 A, Bilateral anterior swelling of the sternoclavicular joints in a 67-year-old woman. The right medial clavicle was more prominent because she was right handed. **B,** A tomogram demonstrates sclerosis and degenerative changes in the right sternoclavicular joint consistent with ordinary degenerative arthritis. (From Rockwood CA, Green DP [eds]: Fractures [3 vols], 2nd ed. Philadelphia: JB Lippincott, 1984.)

In 2002, Song and coworkers[29] presented seven patients who had sternoclavicular joint infections. Predisposing factors included diabetes mellitus, HIV infection, immunosuppression, and pustular skin disease. All patients had local symptoms, including a medial clavicular mass and swelling. Antibiotic therapy and simple drainage and débridement were generally ineffective, with recurrence of infection in five of six patients. The patients were subsequently treated by resection of the sternoclavicular joint and the involved portions of adjacent ribs with an advancement flap from the pectoralis major muscle. The response to therapy was excellent in all patients and there were no wound complications.

Richter and coauthors[30] reported on nine patients with infection of the sternoclavicular joint secondary to tuberculosis. The average time from onset of the disease to diagnosis was 1.4 years.

Higoumenakis[31] has stated that unilateral enlargement of the sternoclavicular joint is a diagnostic sign of congenital syphilis. The enlargement of the sternoclavicular joint can be mistaken for an anterior dislocation. He reported the sign to be positive in 170 of 197 patients with congenital syphilis. The enlargement is attributed to hyperostosis of the medial aspect of the clavicle occurring in the sternoclavicular joint of the dominant extremity, which reaches its permanent stage and size at puberty.

INCIDENCE OF INJURY TO THE STERNOCLAVICULAR JOINT

The incidence of sternoclavicular dislocation, based on the series of 1603 injuries of the shoulder girdle reported by Cave and colleagues,[5] is 3%. (Specific incidences of dislocation in the study were glenohumeral, 85%; acromioclavicular, 12%; and sternoclavicular, 3%.) In the series by Cave's group, and in our experience, dislocation of the sternoclavicular joint is not as rare as posterior dislocation of the glenohumeral joint.

In a study of 3451 injuries during alpine skiing, Kocher and Feagin[32] showed that injuries involving the shoulder complex accounted for 39% of upper extremity injuries and 11.4% of all alpine skiing injuries. Of the 393 injuries involving the shoulder complex, sternoclavicular separations accounted for 0.5%.

The largest series from a single institution is reported by Nettles and Linscheid,[14] who studied 60 patients with sternoclavicular dislocations (57 anterior and 3 posterior). However, in our series of 185 traumatic sternoclavicular injuries, 135 patients had anterior dislocation and 50 patients had posterior dislocation.

Dislocations of Both Ends of the Clavicle

Dislocation of both ends of the clavicle is a rare, high-energy injury with fewer than 30 cases reported in the literature. In 1990, Sanders and associates[33] reported six patients who sustained a dislocation of both ends of the clavicle (anterior dislocation of the sternoclavicular joint and posterior dislocation of the acromioclavicular joint). Two patients who had fewer demands on the shoulder did well with only minor symptoms after nonoperative management. The other four patients had persistent symptoms that were localized to the acromioclavicular joint. Each of these patients underwent reconstruction of the acromioclavicular joint that resulted in painless full range of motion and return to normal activity.

Combinations of Sternoclavicular Fractures and Dislocations of the Clavicle

Elliot[34] reported on a tripartite injury about the clavicular region in which the patient sustained an anterior subluxation of the right sternoclavicular joint, a type II injury to the right acromioclavicular joint, and a fracture of the

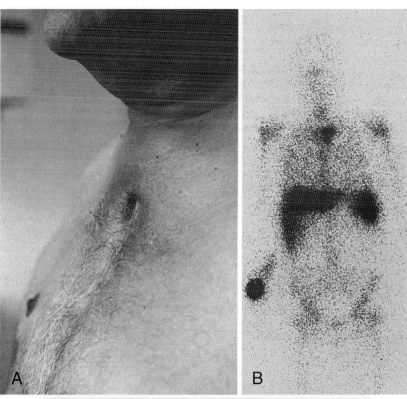

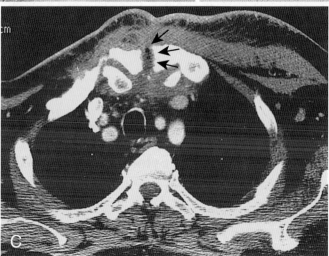

FIGURE 13-15 **A,** This patient had long-standing insulin-dependent diabetes and a coronary artery bypass procedure that was complicated by a postoperative wound infection. **B,** Indium-enhanced white blood cell scan consistent with infection in the region of the left sternoclavicular joint. **C,** CT scan revealing significant soft tissue swelling, interspersed locules of air (*arrows*) within the sternal osteotomy site, and focal irregularity of the posterior aspect of the sternum consistent with an infectious process. (From Rockwood CA, Green DP, Bucholz RW, Heckman JD [eds]: Fractures in the Adult. Philadelphia: JB Lippincott, 1996.)

right midclavicle. Velutini and Tarazona[35] reported a bizarre case of posterior dislocation of the left medial clavicle, the first rib, and a section of the manubrium. Others have reported fracture of the clavicle associated with posterior sternoclavicular dislocation, anterior sub-luxation, and injury to the long thoracic nerve.[36] All of these injuries involving the sternoclavicular joint and the clavicle were associated with severe trauma to the shoulder region: The involved shoulder struck an immovable object or was severely compressed (Fig. 13-16).

Combination of Sternoclavicular Dislocation and Scapulothoracic Dissociation

Tsai and colleagues[37] reported a patient with a sternocla-vicular dislocation associated with a scapulothoracic dissociation. The patient had also sustained a transection of the axillary artery, an avulsion of the median nerve, and a complete brachial plexopathy. Surgical manage-ment included vascular repair and an above-elbow amputation.

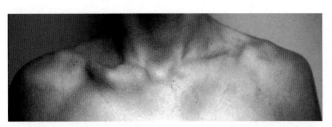

FIGURE 13-16 Clinical view of a patient with fracture of the medial clavicle and partial ligamentous injury to the sternoclavicular joint following a motor vehicle accident.

SIGNS AND SYMPTOMS OF INJURIES TO THE STERNOCLAVICULAR JOINT

Atraumatic Subluxation and Dislocations

Atraumatic subluxation and dislocations are usually anterior and are usually not associated with a great deal of pain. As the patient raises the arm forward, the medial clavicle spontaneously displaces anteriorly and superiorly, and, when the arm is returned to the patient's side, the medial clavicle is reduced. Occasionally, the displacement and reduction are associated with a sharp pain. Rockwood and Odor[38] reported on this condition in 37 patients and urged nonoperative treatment.

Traumatic Subluxation

In a mild sprain, the ligaments of the joint are intact. The patient complains of mild to moderate pain, particularly with movement of the upper extremity. The joint may be slightly swollen and tender to palpation, but instability is not noted. A moderate sprain results in a subluxation of the sternoclavicular joint. The ligaments are either partially disrupted or severely stretched. Swelling is noted and pain is marked, particularly with any movement of the arm. Anterior or posterior subluxation may be obvious to the examiner when the injured joint is compared with the normal sternoclavicular joint.

Signs Common to Anterior and Posterior Dislocations

The patient with a sternoclavicular dislocation has severe pain that is increased with any movement of the arm, particularly when the shoulders are pressed together by a lateral force. The patient usually supports the injured arm across the trunk with the normal arm. The affected shoulder appears to be shortened and thrust forward when compared with the normal shoulder. The head may be tilted toward the side of the dislocated joint. The discomfort increases when the patient is placed in the supine position, at which time it will be noted that the involved shoulder does not lie back flat on the table.

Signs and Symptoms of Anterior Dislocations

With an anterior dislocation, the medial end of the clavicle is visibly prominent anterior to the sternum and can be palpated anterior to the sternum. It may be fixed anteriorly or be quite mobile.

Signs and Symptoms of Posterior Dislocations

The patient with a posterior dislocation has more pain than a patient with an anterior dislocation. The anterosuperior fullness of the chest produced by the clavicle is less prominent and visible when compared with the normal side. The usually palpable medial end of the clavicle is displaced posteriorly. The corner of the sternum is easily palpated compared with the normal sternoclavicular joint. Venous congestion may be present in the neck or in the upper extremity. Symptoms can also include a dry, irritating cough and hoarseness. Breathing difficulties or shortness of breath may be secondary to a pneumothorax. Circulation to the ipsilateral arm may be decreased. The patient might complain of difficulty swallowing, a tight feeling in the throat, or a choking sensation.

We have seen a number of patients who clinically appeared to have an anterior dislocation of the sternoclavicular joint but on x-ray studies were shown to have a posterior dislocation. The point is that one cannot always rely on the clinical findings of observing and palpating the joint to make a distinction between anterior and posterior dislocations.

RADIOGRAPHIC FINDINGS OF INJURY TO THE STERNOCLAVICULAR JOINT

Anteroposterior Views

Occasionally, routine radiographs of the chest or sternoclavicular joint suggest something is wrong with one of the clavicles, because it appears to be displaced compared with the normal side (Fig. 13-17). For example, a difference in relative craniocaudal positions of the medial clavicles greater than 50% of the width of the heads of the clavicles suggests dislocation.

It would be ideal to take a view at right angles to the anteroposterior plane, but because of our anatomy, it is impossible to take a true 90-degree cephalic-to-caudal lateral view. Lateral x-rays of the chest are at right angles to the anteroposterior plane, but they cannot be interpreted because of the density of the chest and the overlap of the medial clavicles with the first rib and the sternum. Regardless of a clinical impression that suggests an anterior dislocation, radiographs and preferably a CT scan must be obtained to confirm one's suspicions (Fig. 13-18).

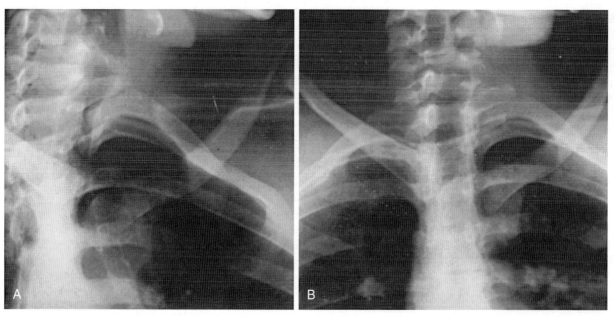

FIGURE 13-17 A and **B,** Routine radiographs of the sternoclavicular joint are difficult to interpret, even though this patient has a classic posterior dislocation of the left sternoclavicular joint. (From Rockwood CA, Green DP [eds]: Fractures [3 vols], 2nd ed. Philadelphia: JB Lippincott, 1984.)

Heinig View[13]

For the Heinig view, with the patient in a supine position, the x-ray tube is placed approximately 30 inches from the involved sternoclavicular joint and the central ray is directed tangential to the joint and parallel to the opposite clavicle. The cassette is placed against the opposite shoulder and centered on the manubrium (Fig. 13-19).

Hobbs View[39]

For the Hobbs view, the patient is seated at the x-ray table, high enough to lean forward over the table. The cassette is on the table, and the lower anterior rib cage is against the cassette (Fig. 13-20). The patient leans forward so that the base of the neck is almost parallel to the table. The flexed elbows straddle the cassette and support the head and neck. The x-ray source is above the nape of the neck, and the beam passes through the cervical spine to project the sternoclavicular joints onto the cassette.

Serendipity View

One of us (CAR) accidentally noted that the next best thing to having a true cephalocaudal lateral view of the

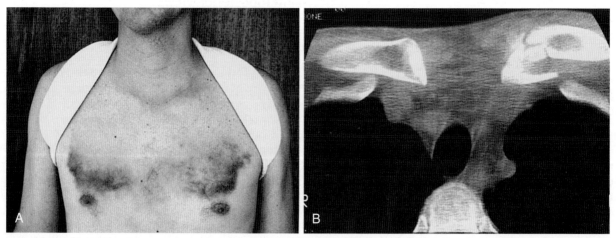

FIGURE 13-18 A, A 34-year-old patient was involved in a motorcycle accident and sustained an anterior blow to the chest. Note the symmetrical anterior chest wall ecchymosis. **B,** CT reveals a left medial clavicular fracture without disruption of the sternoclavicular joint. (From Bucholz RW, Heckman JD [eds]: Rockwood and Green's Fractures in Adults, 5th ed. Philadelphia: Lippincott Williams & Wilkins, 2001, p 1249.)

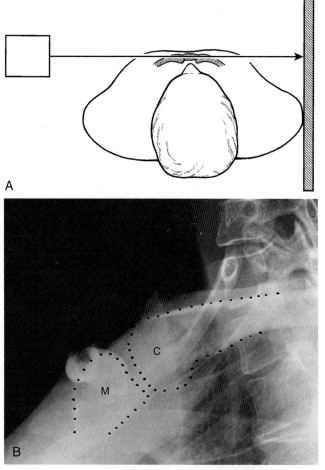

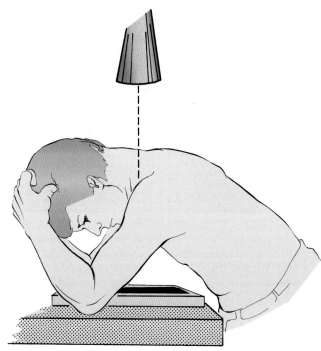

FIGURE 13-20 Positioning of the patient for x-ray evaluation of the sternoclavicular joint, as recommended by Hobbs. (Modified from Hobbs DW: The sternoclavicular joint: A new axial radiographic view. Radiology 90:801-802, 1968.)

FIGURE 13-19 A, Positioning of the patient for radiographic evaluation of the sternoclavicular joint, as described by Heinig. **B,** Heinig view demonstrating a normal relationship between the medial end of the clavicle (C) and the manubrium (M). (From Bucholz RW, Heckman JD [eds]: Rockwood and Green's Fractures in Adults, 5th ed. Philadelphia: Lippincott Williams & Wilkins, 2001, p 1250.)

Lucet and colleagues[40] used CT scans to evaluate the sternoclavicular joints in 60 healthy subjects homogeneously distributed by gender and decade of life from 20 to 80 years old. They reported that 98% of the subjects had at least one sign of abnormality, such as sclerosis, osteophytes, erosion, cysts, or joint narrowing. The number of signs increased with age, and the number of signs in the clavicle was greater than those in the sternum.

Magnetic Resonance Imaging

MRI has been correlated with anatomic sections in sternoclavicular joints and is an excellent method for evaluating the anatomy of the sternoclavicular joint and surrounding soft tissues in great detail. The sagittal plane is useful to assess the integrity of the costoclavicular ligament and the attachments of the intra-articular disk to the sternoclavicular ligaments. This view is also helpful in assessing the location of the great vessels, trachea, and esophagus. MR arthrography allows the delineation of perforations in the intra-articular disk. In children and young adults, MRI is especially helpful in distinguishing between a dislocation of the sternoclavicular joint and a physeal injury (Fig. 13-24). MRI is far superior to CT in its ability to detect bone marrow abnormalities, cartilage injury, effusions, and surrounding soft tissues.

sternoclavicular joint was a 40-degree cephalic tilt view, hence, the *serendipity view.* The patient is positioned supine on the x-ray table. The tube is tilted at a 40-degree angle off the vertical and is centered directly on the sternum (Fig. 13-21).

Computed Tomography Scans

Without question, the CT scan is the best means to study injuries of the sternoclavicular joint (Fig. 13-22). It is important to image both sides, because comparison is often helpful in assessing pathology. The ability to reformat CT data to reconstruct various imaging planes has been very helpful, particularly in preoperative planning (Fig. 13-23).

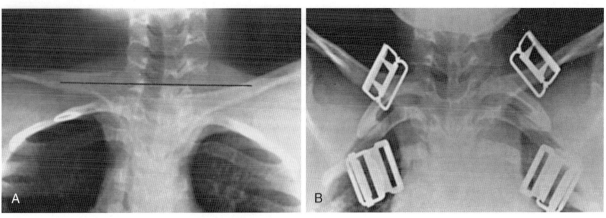

FIGURE 13-21 **A,** Posterior dislocation of the left sternoclavicular joint as seen on the 40-degree cephalic tilt radiograph in a 12-year-old boy. The left clavicle is displaced inferiorly to a line drawn through the normal right clavicle. **B,** After closed reduction, the medial ends of both clavicles are in the same horizontal position. The buckles are a part of the figure-of-eight clavicular harness that is used to hold the shoulders back after reduction. (From Rockwood CA, Green DP [eds]: Fractures [3 vols], 2nd ed. Philadelphia: JB Lippincott, 1984.)

Ultrasound

The role of ultrasound is limited in comparison to CT and MRI except in the case of intraoperative evaluation, where it can be nearly impossible to precisely determine the adequacy of reduction. In this setting, the value of ultrasound is unsurpassed in accurately confirming whether a closed reduction has been successful.[41]

TREATMENT

Traumatic Injuries: Anterior

Nonoperative Treatment
Subluxation

For subluxation of the sternoclavicular joint, application of ice is recommended for the first 24 hours, followed by

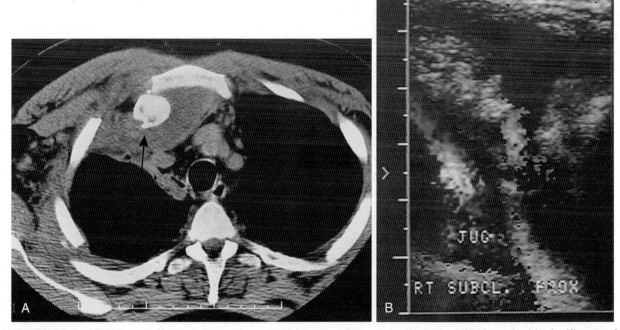

FIGURE 13-22 **A,** CT scan revealing a posterior fracture-dislocation of the sternoclavicular joint (*arrow*) with significant soft tissue swelling and compromise of the hilar structures. **B,** Duplex ultrasound study revealing a large pseudoaneurysm of the right subclavian artery. Note the large neck of the pseudoaneurysm, which measured approximately 1 cm in diameter. (From Bucholz RW, Heckman JD [eds]: Rockwood and Green's Fractures in Adults, 5th ed. Philadelphia: Lippincott Williams & Wilkins, 2001, p 1285.)

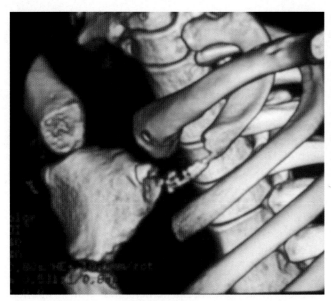

FIGURE 13-23 Reformatted three-dimensional CT revealing a left posterior sternoclavicular dislocation in a trauma patient with shortness of breath.

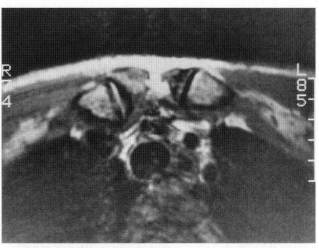

FIGURE 13-24 MRI of the sternoclavicular joint. The epiphysis on the medial aspect of both clavicles is clearly visible. (From Bucholz RW, Heckman JD [eds]: Rockwood and Green's Fractures in Adults, 5th ed. Philadelphia: Lippincott Williams & Wilkins, 2001, p 1253.)

heat for the next 36 to 48 hours. The joint may be reduced by drawing the shoulders backward as if reducing and holding a fracture of the clavicle. For anterior subluxations that are stable, a clavicle strap may be used to hold the reduction. A sling and swath also could be used to hold up the shoulder and to prevent motion of the arm. The patient is protected from further injury for 4 to 6 weeks. Immobilization can be accomplished with a soft figure-of-eight bandage with a sling for temporary support.

Dislocation

There still is some controversy regarding the treatment of acute or chronic anterior dislocation of the sternoclavicular joint. A large series of sternoclavicular injuries was published in 1988 by Fery and Sommelet.[42] They reported on 40 anterior dislocations, 8 posterior dislocations, and 1 unstable sternoclavicular joint dislocation. Fery and Sommelet ended up treating 15 injuries closed, but, because of problems, had to operate on 17 patients; 17 patients were not treated. They had good and excellent results with the closed and operative treatments, but they recommended that closed reduction initially be undertaken.

In 1990, de Jong and Sukul[43] reported long-term follow-up results in 10 patients with traumatic anterior sternoclavicular dislocations. All patients were treated nonoperatively with analgesics and immobilization. The results of treatment were good in 7 patients, fair in 2 patients, and poor in 1 patient at an average follow-up of 5 years.

Method of Closed Reduction. Closed reduction of anterior dislocation of the sternoclavicular joint may be accomplished with local or general anesthesia or, in stoic patients, without anesthesia. Most authors recommend using narcotics or muscle relaxants.

The patient is placed supine on the table, lying on a 3- to 4-inch-thick pad between the shoulders. In this position, the joint might reduce with direct gentle pressure over the anteriorly displaced clavicle. However, when the pressure is released, the clavicle usually dislocates again. Occasionally, the clavicle remains reduced. Sometimes the physician needs to push both the patient's shoulders back to the table while an assistant applies pressure to the anteriorly displaced clavicle.

Postreduction Care. After reduction, to allow ligament healing, the shoulders are held back for 4 to 6 weeks with a figure-of-eight dressing or one of the commercially available figure-of-eight straps used to treat fractures of the clavicle.

Operative Treatment

Most acute anterior dislocations are unstable after reduction, and many operative procedures have been described to repair or reconstruct the joint. Although some authors have recommended operative repair of anterior dislocations of the sternoclavicular joint, we believe that the operative complications are too great and the end results are too unsatisfactory to consider an open reduction.

Traumatic Injuries: Posterior

Nonoperative Treatment
Subluxation

In mild sprains, the ligaments remain intact and the patient complains of moderate discomfort. The joint may be swollen and tender to palpation. Care must be taken

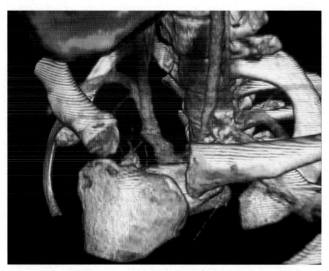

FIGURE 13-25 Three-dimensional CT with vascular contrast demonstrating posterior displacement of the left medial clavicle and the close proximity of the left internal carotid artery.

to rule out the more significant posterior dislocation, which might have initially occurred and spontaneously reduced. When in doubt, it is best to protect the sternoclavicular joint with a figure-of-eight bandage for 2 to 6 weeks. As with all injuries to the sternoclavicular joint, the joint must be carefully evaluated by CT scan.

Dislocation

As a general rule, when a posterior dislocation of the sternoclavicular joint is suspected, the physician must examine the patient very carefully to rule out damage to the structures posterior to the joint, such as the trachea, esophagus, brachial plexus, great vessels, and lungs. Not only is a careful physical examination important, but special x-rays must be obtained. A CT scan of both medial clavicles allows the physician to compare the injured side with the normal side. Occasionally, when vascular injuries are suspected, the CT scan needs to be combined with an arteriogram of the great vessels (Fig. 13-25).

General anesthesia is usually required for reduction of a posterior dislocation of the sternoclavicular joint because the patient has considerable pain and muscle spasms. However, for the stoic patient, some authors have performed the reduction with the patient under IV narcotics and muscle relaxants.

Methods of Closed Reduction

Most posterior sternoclavicular dislocations are successfully reduced if reduction is accomplished within 48 hours of injury. Different techniques have been described for closed reduction of a posterior dislocation of the sternoclavicular joint.

Abduction Traction Technique. For the abduction traction technique, the patient is placed on his or her back, with the dislocated shoulder near the edge of the table. A 3- to 4-inch-thick roll is placed between the shoulders (Fig.

13-26). Lateral traction is applied to the abducted arm, which is then gradually brought back into extension. This may be all that is necessary to accomplish the reduction. The clavicle usually reduces with an audible snap or pop, and it is almost always stable. Too much extension can bind the anterior surface of the dislocated medial clavicle on the back of the manubrium.

Occasionally, it may be necessary to grasp the medial clavicle with one's fingers to dislodge it from behind the sternum. If this fails, the skin is prepared, and a sterile towel clip is used to grasp the medial clavicle to apply lateral and anterior traction (Fig. 13-27).

Adduction Traction Technique. In this technique, the patient is supine on the table with a 3- to 4-inch bolster between the shoulders. Traction is then applied to the arm in adduction, while a posterior pressure is exerted on the shoulder. The clavicle is levered over the first rib into its normal position. Buckerfield and Castle[44] reported that this technique was successful in seven patients when the abduction traction technique had failed.

Postreduction Care

After reduction, to allow ligament healing, the shoulders are held back for 4 to 6 weeks with a figure-of-eight dressing or one of the commercially available figure-of-eight straps used to treat fractures of the clavicle.

Operative Treatment

The operative procedure needs to be performed in a manner that disturbs as few anterior ligament structures as possible. If all the ligaments are disrupted, an important decision has to be made regarding an attempt to stabilize the sternoclavicular joint or resect the medial 2 to 3 cm of the clavicle and stabilize the remaining clavicle to the first rib.

Several basic procedures can be used to maintain the medial end of the clavicle in its normal articulation with the sternum. Fascia lata, suture, internal fixation across the joint, subclavius tendons, osteotomy of the medial clavicle, and resection of the medial end of the clavicle have been advocated.

Fascia Lata

Bankart[45] used fascia lata between the clavicle and the sternum. Lowman[4] used a loop of fascia in and through the sternoclavicular joint so that it acts like the ligamentum teres in the hip. Key and Conwel[46] reported on the use of a fascial loop between the clavicle and the first rib ligament

Subclavius Tendon

Burrows[47] recommended that the subclavius tendon be used to reconstruct a new costoclavicular ligament. The insertion of the tendon is to the inferior surface of the junction of the middle third and outer third of the clavicle, and the muscle fibers arising from the tendon insert into the inferior surface of the middle third of the clavicle. The muscle fibers coming off the tendon look like feath-

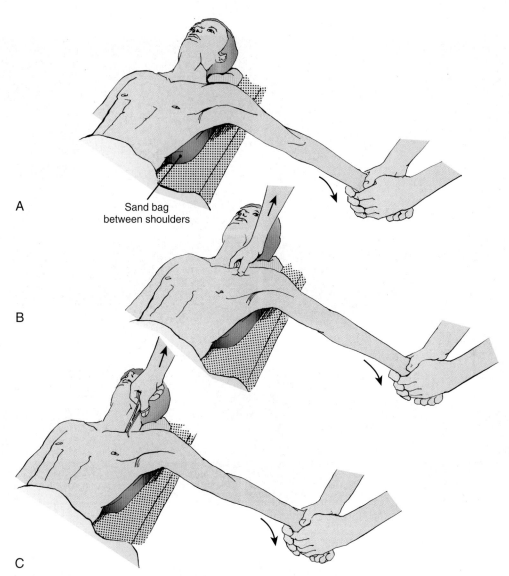

A

Sand bag
between shoulders

B

C

FIGURE 13-26 Technique of closed reduction of the sternoclavicular joint. **A,** The patient is positioned supine with a sandbag placed between the shoulders. Traction is then applied to the arm against countertraction in an abducted and slightly extended position. With anterior dislocations, direct pressure over the medial end of the clavicle can reduce the joint. **B,** With posterior dislocations, in addition to traction it might be necessary to manipulate the medial end of the clavicle with the fingers to dislodge the clavicle from behind the manubrium. **C,** In stubborn cases of posterior dislocation, it may be necessary to sterilely prepare the medial end of the clavicle and use a towel clip to grasp around the medial clavicle to lift it back into position. (From Bucholz RW, Heckman JD [eds]: Rockwood and Green's Fractures in Adults, 5th ed. Philadelphia: Lippincott Williams & Wilkins, 2001, p 1264.)

ers on a bird's wing. Burrows detaches the muscle fiber from the tendon, does not disturb the origin of the tendon, and then passes the tendon through drill holes in the anterior aspect of the proximal end of the clavicle. When comparing his operation with the use of free strips of fascia, Burrows said that it is "safer and easier to pick up a mooring than to drop anchor; the obvious mooring is the tendon of the subclavius separated from its muscle fiber and suitably realigned."

Semitendinosus Tendon

Spencer and Kuhn,[48] through a biomechanical analysis, evaluated three different reconstruction techniques with use of a cadaveric model. An intramedullary ligament reconstruction, a subclavius tendon reconstruction, and a reconstruction with the use of a semitendinosus graft placed in a figure-of-eight fashion through drill holes in the clavicle and manubrium were used to reconstruct the sternoclavicular joint.

Each of the three reconstruction methods was subjected to anterior and posterior translation to failure, and the changes in stiffness compared with the intact state were analyzed statistically. The figure-of-eight semitendinosus reconstruction showed superior initial mechanical properties to the other two techniques. Spencer and Kuhn stated that this method reconstructs both the anterior and

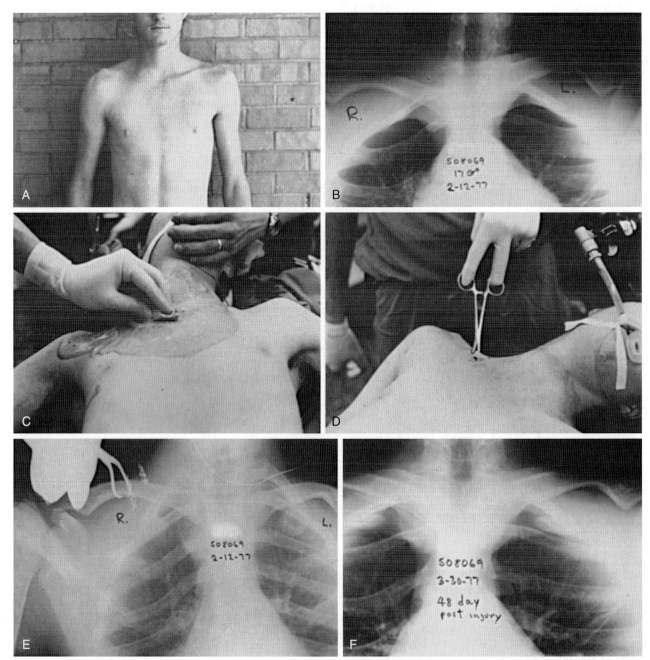

FIGURE 13-27 Posterior dislocation of the right sternoclavicular joint. **A,** A 16-year-old boy had a 48-hour-old posterior displacement of the right medial clavicle that occurred as a result of direct trauma to the anterior aspect of the right clavicle. He noted an immediate onset of difficulty swallowing and some hoarseness in his voice. **B,** The 40-degree cephalic tilt radiograph confirmed the presence of posterior displacement of the right medial clavicle by comparison with the left clavicle. Because of the patient's age, it was considered most likely to be a physeal injury of the right medial clavicle. **C,** Because the injury was 48 hours old, we were unable to reduce the dislocation with simple traction on the arm. The right shoulder was surgically cleansed so that a sterile towel clip could be used. **D,** With the towel clip securely around the clavicle and with continued lateral traction, a visible and audible reduction occurred. **E,** Postreduction radiographs showed that the medial part of the clavicle had been restored to its normal position. The reduction was quite stable, and the patient's shoulders were held back with a figure-of-eight strap. **F,** The right clavicle has remained reduced. In particular, note the periosteal new bone formation along the superior and inferior borders of the right clavicle. This bone formation is the result of a physeal injury whereby the epiphysis remains adjacent to the manubrium while the clavicle is displaced out of a split in the periosteal tube. (From Bucholz RW, Heckman JD [eds]: Rockwood and Green's Fractures in Adults, 5th ed. Philadelphia: Lippincott Williams & Wilkins, 2001, p 1265.)

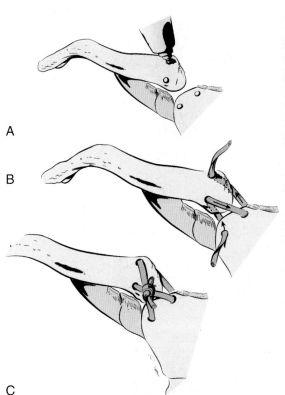

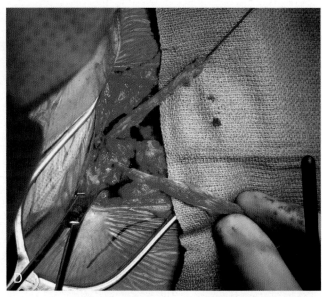

FIGURE 13-28 A, Drill holes in the clavicle and manubrium. **B,** Placement of a semitendinosus graft. **C,** Final reconstruction. **D,** Operative photograph of a sternoclavicular reconstruction using a semitendinosus graft.

posterior joint capsules, providing an initial stiffness that is closer to that of the intact sternoclavicular joint (Fig. 13-28).

Osteotomy of the Medial Clavicle

As described by Omer,[16] the sternoclavicular ligaments are repaired and a step-cut osteotomy is made lateral to the sternoclavicular joint to minimize stress on the reconstruction. The author also recommends releasing the clavicular head of the sternocleidomastoid muscle from the proximal fragment.

Resection of the Medial Clavicle

Several authors have recommended excision of the medial clavicle when degenerative changes are noted in the joint.[49-51] If the medial end of the clavicle is to be removed because of degenerative changes, the surgeon must be careful to not damage the costoclavicular ligament.

Arthrodesis

Arthrodesis was once reported[52] in the treatment of habitual dislocation of the sternoclavicular joint. However, this procedure should *not* be performed because it prevents the previously described normal elevation, depression, and rotation of the clavicle. The end result would be severe restriction of shoulder movement (Fig. 13-29).

Plate Fixation

Franck and colleagues[53] reported an alternative treatment for traumatic sternoclavicular instability that employs a Balser plate for stabilization. The plate was contoured to match the shape of the clavicle, and the hook of the plate was used for sternal fixation. A retrosternal hook position was used for 7 anterior dislocations, and an intrasternal position was used for 3 posterior dislocations. For each patient, the plate was attached to the clavicle with screws and the torn ligaments were repaired. All plates were removed by 3 months. At 1-year follow-up, 9 of 10 patients had excellent results with no cases of redislocation. One patient developed a postoperative seroma that required surgical drainage, and 1 patient developed arthrosis (Fig. 13-30).

Physeal Injuries

This epiphysis does not appear on radiographs until about the 18th year and does not unite with the clavicle until the 23rd to 25th year.

This information is important to remember because many "dislocations of the sternoclavicular joint" are not dislocations but physeal injuries. Most of these injuries heal with time and without surgical intervention. The remodeling process eliminates any bone deformity or displacement. Anterior physeal injuries can certainly be

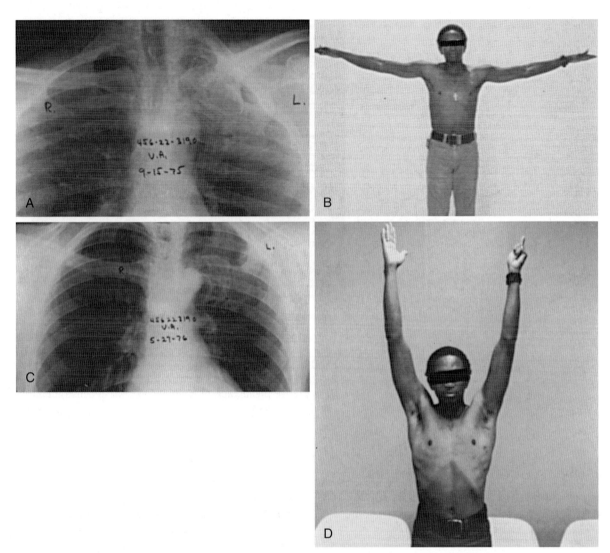

FIGURE 13-29 The effect of arthrodesis of the sternoclavicular joint on shoulder function. **A,** As a result of a military gunshot wound to the left sternoclavicular joint, this patient had a massive bony union of the left medial clavicle to the sternum and upper three ribs. **B,** Shoulder motion was limited to 90 degrees of flexion and abduction. **C,** Radiograph after resection of the bony mass to free up the medial part of the clavicle. **D,** Function of the left shoulder was essentially normal after elimination of the sternoclavicular arthrodesis. (From Bucholz RW, Heckman JD [eds]: Rockwood and Green's Fractures in Adults, 5th ed. Philadelphia: Lippincott Williams & Wilkins, 2001, p 1271.)

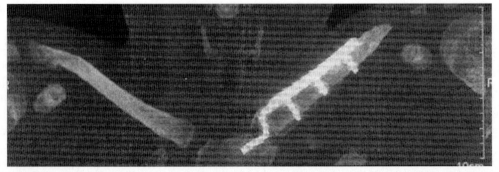

FIGURE 13-30 CT of the chest showing intrasternal placement of a Balser plate. (From Franck WM, Jannasch O, Siassi M, et al: Balser plate stabilization: An alternate therapy for traumatic sternoclavicular instability. J Shoulder Elbow Surg 12:276-281, 2003).

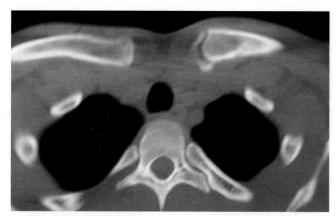

FIGURE 13-31 CT scan at 3 months following closed reduction of a posterior sternoclavicular dislocation in a 17-year-old patient.

left alone without problem. Posterior physeal injuries are reduced (Fig. 13-31). If the posterior dislocation cannot be reduced and the patient is having no significant symptoms, the displacement can be observed while remodeling occurs. If the posterior displacement is symptomatic and cannot be reduced by closed means, the displacement must be reduced during surgery.

Atraumatic Problems

Spontaneous Subluxation or Dislocation

As with glenohumeral joint instability, the importance of distinguishing between traumatic and atraumatic instability of the sternoclavicular joint must be recognized if complications are to be avoided. Rowe[54] described several patients who have undergone one or more unsuccessful attempts to stabilize the sternoclavicular joint. In all cases the patient could voluntarily dislocate the clavicle after surgery. In a conversation, Rowe has also described several young patients who could "flip the clavicle out and back in" without elevating the arms (June 27, 1988).

Martin and colleagues[55] described a case of spontaneous atraumatic posterior dislocation of the sternoclavicular joint. This occurred in a 50-year-old previously healthy woman who awoke one morning with a painful sternoclavicular joint. CT scan confirmed the posterior dislocation. She later developed dysphagia, and a closed reduction was unsuccessful. At 1 year without any other treatment, she was back to playing golf and was asymptomatic.

Martinez and colleagues[56] reported on the operative treatment of a 19-year-old woman with a symptomatic spontaneous posterior subluxation. The posteriorly displaced medial clavicle was stabilized with a figure-of-eight suture technique with the use of a gracilis autograft. At follow-up the patient was pain free; however, a repeat CT scan demonstrated posterior subluxation of the medial

clavicle, with erosion of the clavicle and manubrium. The authors recommended conservative treatment of atraumatic posterior subluxation of the sternoclavicular joint.

Crosby and Rubino[57] reported a case of spontaneous atraumatic anterior dislocation secondary to pseudarthrosis of the first and second ribs. Despite a 6-month course of conservative treatment, this 14-year-old girl was still experiencing pain. A CT scan of the chest with three-dimensional reconstruction was performed. The scan revealed a pseudarthrosis anteriorly between the first and second ribs underlying the medial part of the clavicle. Resection of the anterior portions of the first and second ribs containing the pseudarthrosis relieved her symptoms and allowed her to return to her normal activities. The authors recommended chest x-rays and a possible CT scan with three-dimensional reconstruction to completely evaluate an underlying congenital condition if the subluxation is rigid and unresponsive to nonoperative care.

In our experience, spontaneous subluxations and dislocations of the sternoclavicular joint are seen most often in patients younger than 20 years and more often in female patients. Without significant trauma, one or both of the medial clavicles can spontaneously displace anteriorly during abduction or flexion to the overhead position. The clavicle reduces when the arm is returned to the side. Such voluntary displacement is usually associated with laxity in other joints of the extremities. Rockwood and Odor reviewed 37 cases and found it to be a self-limited condition.[38] Surgical reconstruction should *not* be attempted because the joint will continue to subluxate or dislocate and surgery can indeed cause more pain, discomfort, and an unsightly scar (Fig. 13-32).

Arthritis

Management of patients with osteoarthritis and women with postmenopausal osteoarthritis can usually be accomplished with conservative nonoperative treatment: heat, antiinflammatory agents, and rest. However, the patient must be thoroughly evaluated to rule out other conditions that mimic changes in the sternoclavicular joint (i.e., tumor or metabolic, infectious, or collagen disorders). Patients with post-traumatic arthritic changes in the sternoclavicular joint after fracture and previous attempts at reconstruction might require formal arthroplasty of the joint and careful stabilization of the remaining clavicle to the first rib.

Pingsmann and coauthors[58] reported on the midterm results in eight women who did not respond to conservative therapy and underwent surgical treatment for primary arthritis of the sternoclavicular joint. After limited resection of the medial clavicle and preservation of the coracoclavicular and interclavicular ligaments, they reported improvement in the Constant and Rockwood score and concluded that the arthroplasty was effective and safe for the treatment of chronic symptomatic degenerative arthritis of the sternoclavicular joint.

Patients with collagen disorders, such as rheumatoid arthritis, and some patients with condensing osteitis of

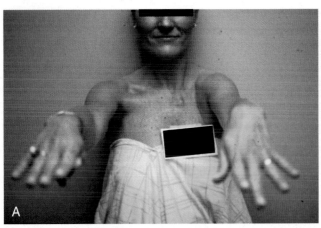 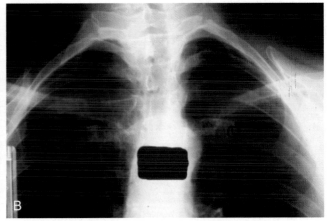

FIGURE 13-32 A, This patient was treated with surgery for spontaneous atraumatic subluxation of the sternoclavicular joint. Postoperatively she noted increased pain, limitation of activity, alteration in lifestyle, persistent instability of the joint, and a significant scar. Note the medial displacement of the entire right shoulder girdle. **B,** Anteroposterior radiograph demonstrating excision of the medial clavicle which extended lateral to the costoclavicular ligament.

the medial clavicle require an arthroplasty. In operating on the sternoclavicular joint, care must be taken to evaluate the residual stability of the medial clavicle.

It is the same analogy as used when resecting the distal clavicle for a complete old acromioclavicular joint problem. If the coracoclavicular ligaments are intact, excision of the distal end of the clavicle is indicated. If the coracoclavicular ligaments are gone, in addition to excision of the distal clavicle, the coracoclavicular ligaments must be reconstructed. If the costoclavicular ligaments are intact, the portion of clavicle medial to the ligaments are resected and beveled smooth. If the ligaments are irreparable, the clavicle must be stabilized to the first rib. If too much clavicle is resected or the clavicle is not stabilized to the first rib, symptoms can increase (Fig. 13-33).

Infection

Infections of the sternoclavicular joint are managed as they are in other joints, except that during aspiration and surgical drainage, great care and respect must be directed to the vital structures that lie posterior to the joint. If aspiration demonstrates purulent material in the joint or

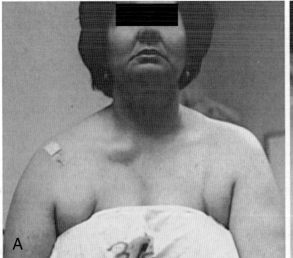 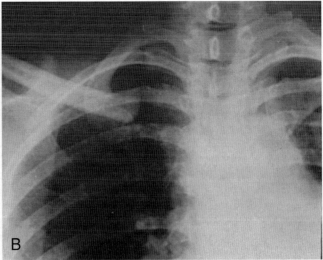

FIGURE 13-33 A, This postmenopausal right-hand–dominant woman underwent medial clavicular resection because of a preoperative diagnosis of "possible tumor." The postoperative microscopic diagnosis was degenerative arthritis of the right medial clavicle. After surgery, the patient complained of pain and discomfort, marked prominence, and gross instability of the right medial clavicle. **B,** A radiograph confirms that excision of the medial clavicle extended lateral to the costoclavicular ligaments; hence, the patient had an unstable medial clavicle. (From Bucholz RW, Heckman JD [eds]: Rockwood and Green's Fractures in Adults, 5th ed. Philadelphia: Lippincott Williams & Wilkins, 2001, p 1275.)

the orthopaedist has a high index of suspicion, formal arthrotomy is carried out. Arthrotomy is especially important with sternoclavicular septic arthritis because of the significant risk of abscess formation and subsequent spread of infection to the mediastinal structures.

The need for arthrotomy is supported by Wohlgethan and Newberg's review of the literature,[26] which documented a 20% incidence of abscess formation after infection of the sternoclavicular joint. The anterior sternoclavicular ligament will need to be removed, but the posterior and interclavicular ligaments are spared. Occasionally, the infection arises in the medial end of the clavicle or the manubrium, which necessitates resection of some of the dead bone. Depending on the status of the wound after débridement, one can either close the wound loosely over a drain or pack the wound open and close it at a later time.

AUTHORS' PREFERRED METHOD OF TREATMENT

Type I Injury (Mild Sprain)

For mild sprains, we recommend the use of cold packs for the first 12 to 24 hours and a sling to rest the joint. Ordinarily, after 5 to 7 days the patient may use the arm for everyday living activities.

Type II Injury (Subluxation)

In addition to the cold pack, we might use a soft, padded, figure-of-eight clavicle strap to gently hold the shoulders back to allow the sternoclavicular joint to rest. The figure-of-eight harness may be removed after a week or so, and then the patient either uses a sling for a week or so or is allowed to gradually return to everyday living activities.

Type III Injury (Dislocation)

In general, we manage almost all dislocations of the sternoclavicular joint in children and adults by either closed reduction or a nonoperative skillful-neglect form of treatment. Acute traumatic posterior dislocations are reduced by closed means and become stable when the shoulders are held back in a figure-of-eight dressing. Most anterior dislocations are unstable, but we accept the deformity because it is less of a problem than the potential difficulty of operative repair and internal fixation.

Anterior Dislocation
Method of Reduction

In most instances, knowing that the anterior dislocation will be unstable, we still try to reduce the anterior displacement. Muscle relaxants and narcotics are administered via IV, and the patient is placed supine on the table with a stack of three or four towels between the shoulder blades. While an assistant gently applies downward pressure on the anterior aspect of both of the patient's shoulders, the medial end of the clavicle is pushed posteriorly. On some occasions, rare as they may be, the anterior sternoclavicular dislocation reduces in a stable fashion. However, in most cases, either with the shoulders still held back or when they are relaxed, the anterior displacement promptly recurs. We explain to the patient that the joint is unstable and that the hazards of internal fixation are too great. In these cases we prescribe a sling for a couple of weeks and allow the patient to begin using the arm as soon as the discomfort is gone.

Most of the anterior injuries that we have treated in patients up to 25 years of age are not dislocations of the sternoclavicular joint but rather type I or II physeal injuries, which heal and remodel without operative treatment. Patients who are older than 23 to 25 years and who have anterior dislocations of the sternoclavicular joint do have persistent prominence of the anterior clavicle. However, this does not seem to interfere with usual activities and, in some cases, has not even interfered with heavy manual labor.

We wish to reemphasize that *we do not recommend open reduction* of the joint and would *never* recommend transfixing pins across the sternoclavicular joint.

Postreduction Care

If the reduction happens to be stable, we place the patient in either a figure-of-eight dressing or whatever device or position the clavicle is most stable in. If the reduction is unstable, the arm is placed in a sling for a week or so, and then the patient may begin to use the arm for gentle daily activities.

Posterior Dislocation

It is important to obtain a careful history and perform a careful physical examination in the patient with a posterior sternoclavicular dislocation. For every patient, the physician should obtain x-rays and a CT scan. If the patient has distention of the neck vessels, swelling of the arm, a bluish discoloration of the arm, or difficulty swallowing or breathing, the patient ideally is evaluated by using a CT scan with contrast. It is also important to determine if the patient has a feeling of choking or hoarseness. If any of these symptoms are present, indicating pressure on the mediastinum, the appropriate cardiovascular or thoracic specialist needs to be consulted.

We do not believe that operative techniques are usually required to reduce acute posterior sternoclavicular joint dislocations. Furthermore, once the joint has been reduced by closed means, it is usually stable.

Although we used to think that the diagnosis of an anterior or posterior injury of the sternoclavicular joint could always be made on physical examination, one cannot rely on the anterior swelling and firmness as being diagnostic of an anterior injury. Therefore, we recommend that the clinical impression always be documented with appropriate imaging studies, preferably a CT scan, before a decision is made to treat or not to treat.

Method of Closed Reduction

The patient is placed in the supine position with a 3- to 4-inch-thick sandbag or three or four folded towels between the scapulae to extend the shoulders. The dislocated shoulder is positioned near the edge of the table so that the arm and shoulder can be abducted and extended. If the patient is having extreme pain and muscle spasm and is quite anxious, we use general anesthesia; otherwise, narcotics, muscle relaxants, or tranquilizers are given through an established IV route in the normal arm. First, gentle traction is applied on the abducted arm in line with the clavicle while countertraction is applied by an assistant who steadies the patient on the table. The traction on the abducted arm is gradually increased while the arm is brought into extension. If reduction cannot be accomplished with the patient's arm in abduction, then we use the adduction technique of Buckerfield and Castle[44] that is described earlier.

Reduction of an acute injury may occur with an audible pop or snap, and the relocation can be noted visibly and by palpation. If the traction techniques are not successful, an assistant grasps or pushes down on the clavicle in an effort to dislodge it from behind the sternum.

Occasionally, in a stubborn case, especially in a thick-chested person or a patient with extensive swelling, it is impossible to obtain a secure grasp on the clavicle with the assistant's fingers. The skin is then surgically prepared and a sterile towel clip used to gain purchase on the medial clavicle percutaneously. The towel clip is used to grasp completely around the shaft of the clavicle. The dense cortical bone prevents the purchase of the towel clip into the clavicle. Then the combined traction through the arm plus the anterior lifting force on the towel clip will reduce the dislocation. Following the reduction, the sternoclavicular joint is usually stable, even with the patient's arm at the side. However, we always hold the shoulders back in a well-padded figure-of-eight clavicle strap for 3 to 4 weeks to allow for soft tissue and ligamentous healing.

Technique of Open Reduction

The complications of an unreduced posterior dislocation are numerous: thoracic outlet syndrome, vascular compromise, and erosion of the medial clavicle into any of the vital structures that lie posterior to the sternoclavicular joint. Therefore, in adults older than 23 years, if closed reduction fails, an open reduction should be performed.

The patient is supine on the table, and the three or four towels or a sandbag are placed between the scapulae. The upper extremity is draped out free so that lateral traction can be applied during the open reduction. In addition, a folded sheet around the patient's thorax is left in place so that it can be used for countertraction while traction is applied to the involved extremity. An anterior incision is used that parallels the superior border of the medial 5 to 7 cm of the clavicle and then extends downward over the sternum just medial to the involved ster-

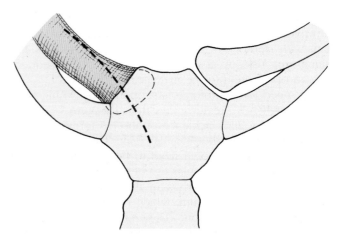

FIGURE 13-34 Proposed skin incision for open reduction of a posterior sternoclavicular dislocation.

noclavicular joint (Fig. 13-34). As previously stated, the operation is usually done with a thoracic surgeon. The trick is to try to remove sufficient soft tissue to expose the joint but to leave the anterior capsular ligament intact. The reduction can usually be accomplished with traction and countertraction while lifting up anteriorly with a clamp around the medial clavicle. Along with the traction and countertraction, it may be necessary to use an elevator to pry the clavicle back to its articulation with the manubrium.

When the reduction has been obtained, and with the shoulders held back, the reduction will be stable if the anterior capsule has been left intact. If the anterior capsule is damaged or is insufficient to prevent anterior displacement of the medial end of the clavicle, we recommend excision of the medial 2 to 3 cm of the clavicle and securing the residual clavicle anatomically to the first rib with 1-mm Dacron tape. The medial clavicle is exposed by careful subperiosteal dissection (Fig. 13-35). When possible, any remnants of the capsular or intra-articular disk ligaments are identified and preserved because these structures can be used to help stabilize the medial clavicle.

The capsular ligament covers the anterosuperior and posterior aspects of the joint and represents thickenings of the joint capsule. This ligament is primarily attached to the epiphysis of the medial clavicle and is usually avulsed from this structure with posterior sternoclavicular dislocations. The intra-articular disk ligament is a very dense, fibrous structure and may be intact. It arises from the synchondral junction of the first rib and sternum and is usually avulsed from its attachment site on the medial clavicle (Fig. 13-36). If the sternal attachment site of the intra-articular or capsular ligaments are intact, a nonabsorbable 1-mm Cottony Dacron suture is woven back and forth through the ligament so that the ends of the suture exit through the avulsed free end of the tissue.

The medial 2 to 3 cm of the clavicle is resected, with the surgeon being careful to protect the underlying vas-

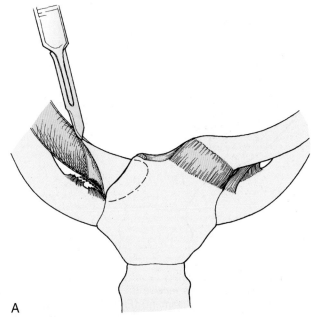

A

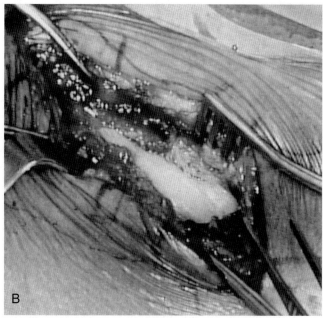

B

FIGURE 13-35 A and **B,** Subperiosteal exposure of the medial end of the clavicle. Note the posteriorly displaced medial clavicle. (**A,** From Bucholz RW, Heckman JD [eds]: Rockwood and Green's Fractures in Adults, 5th ed. Philadelphia: Lippincott Williams & Wilkins, 2001, p 1276.)

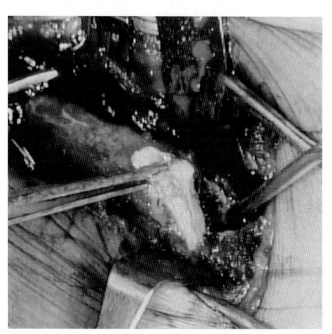

FIGURE 13-36 Forceps holding the superior portion of the articular disk ligament, which was avulsed from its attachment on the medial clavicle. The sternal attachment site of this ligament was intact.

cular structures and being careful not to damage any of the residual costoclavicular (rhomboid) ligament. The vital vascular structures are protected by passing a curved Crego or ribbon retractor around the posterior aspect of the medial clavicle, which isolates them from the operative field during the bony resection.

Excision of the medial clavicle is facilitated by creating drill holes through both cortices of the clavicle at the intended site of clavicular osteotomy (Fig. 13-37). Follow-

ing this step, an air drill with a side-cutting bur is used to complete the osteotomy. The anterior and superior corners of the clavicle are beveled smooth with an air bur for cosmetic purposes. The medullary canal of the medial clavicle is drilled and curetted to receive the transferred intra-articular disk ligament (Fig. 13-38). Two small drill holes are then placed in the superior cortex of the medial clavicle, approximately 1 cm lateral to the site of resection (Fig. 13-39). These holes communicate with the medullary canal and will be used to secure the suture in the transferred ligament. The free ends of the suture are passed into the medullary canal of the medial clavicle and out the two small drill holes in the superior cortex of the clavicle (Fig. 13-40). While the clavicle is held in a reduced anteroposterior position in relationship to the first rib and sternum, the sutures are used to pull the ligament tightly into the medullary canal of the clavicle. The suture is tied, thus securing the transferred ligament into the clavicle (Fig. 13-41).

The stabilization procedure is completed by passing five or six 1-mm Cottony Dacron sutures around the reflected periosteal tube, the clavicle, and any of the residual underlying costoclavicular ligament and periosteum on the dorsal surface of the first rib (Fig. 13-42). The intent of the sutures around the periosteal tube and clavicle and through the costoclavicular ligament and periosteum of the first rib is to anatomically restore the normal space between the clavicle and the rib. To place sutures around the clavicle and the first rib and pull them tight would decrease the space and could lead to a

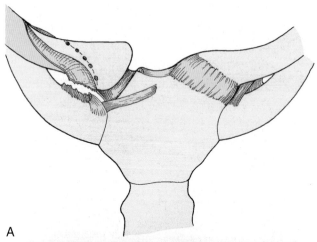

A

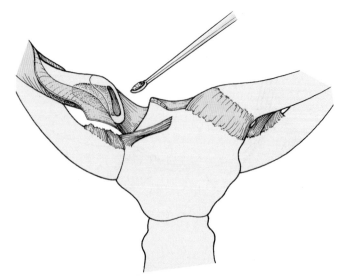

FIGURE 13-38 The medullary canal of the medial clavicle is prepared with a curet to receive the transferred sternoclavicular capsular ligament. (From Bucholz RW, Heckman JD [eds]: Rockwood and Green's Fractures in Adults, 5th ed. Philadelphia: Lippincott Williams & Wilkins, 2001, p 1276.)

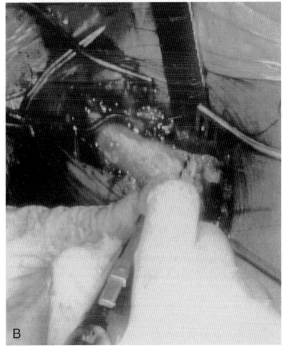

B

FIGURE 13-37 A and **B,** Excision of the medial clavicle is facilitated by drilling holes at the intended site of osteotomy.

painful problem. We usually detach the clavicular head of the sternocleidomastoid, which temporarily eliminates the superior pull of the muscle on the medial clavicle

Postoperatively, the shoulders are held back in a figure-of-eight dressing for 4 to 6 weeks to allow healing of the soft tissues. If the repair is tenuous, we have been pleased with the reconstruction method described by Spencer and Kuhn, which uses a semitendinosus figure-of-eight technique.[10] However, as a note of caution, one must be aware that the drill holes required for this technique weaken the bone and can lead to a stress fracture (Fig. 13-43).

Postreduction Care of Posterior Dislocations

If open reduction is required, a figure-of-eight dressing is used for 6 weeks, and this is followed by a sling for

another 6 weeks. During this time, patients are instructed to avoid using the arm for any strenuous activities of pushing, pulling, or lifting. They should not elevate or abduct the arm more than 60 degrees during the 12-week period. They may use the involved arm to care for bodily needs, such as eating, drinking, dressing, and toilet care. This prolonged immobilization will allow the soft tissues a chance to consolidate and stabilize the medial clavicle to the first rib. After 12 weeks, the patient is allowed to gradually use the arm for usual daily living activities, including over-the-head use of the arm. However, we do not recommend that patients, after resection of the medial clavicle and ligament reconstruction, return to heavy labor activities.

In 1997, Rockwood and associates[8] reported on a series of 15 patients who had undergone a resection of the medial end of the clavicle. The patients were divided into two groups:

Group I: Those who underwent resection of the medial end of the clavicle with maintenance or reconstruction of the costoclavicular ligament (7 patients)
Group II: Those who had a resection without maintaining or reconstructing the costoclavicular ligament (8 patients)

The outcome in all but 1 of the 7 patients in group II was poor, with persistence or worsening of preoperative symptoms (Fig. 13-44). The only patient of this group with a successful result suffered a posterior epiphyseal separation in which the costoclavicular ligament remained attached to the periosteum, thus preventing instability.

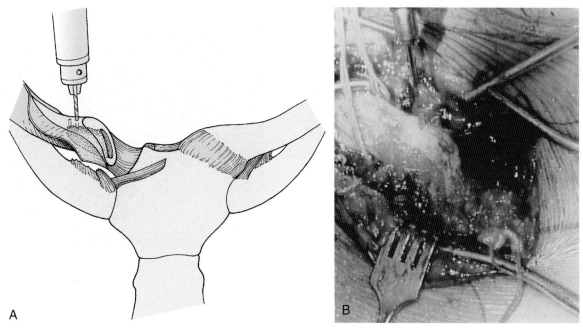

FIGURE 13-39 A and **B,** Drill holes are placed in the superior cortex of the clavicle, approximately 1 cm lateral to the osteotomy site. (**A,** From Bucholz RW, Heckman JD [eds]: Rockwood and Green's Fractures in Adults, 5th ed. Philadelphia: Lippincott Williams & Wilkins, 2001, p 1277.)

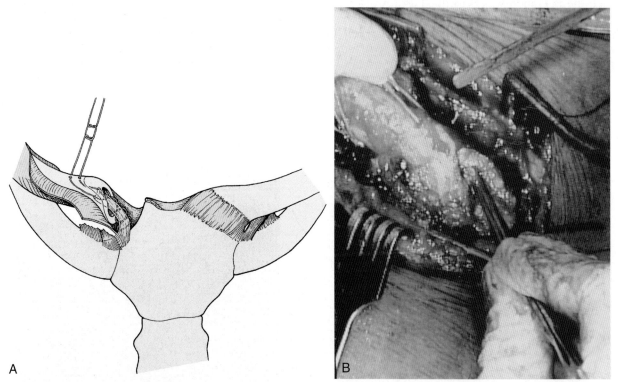

FIGURE 13-40 A and **B,** The free ends of the suture are passed into the medullary canal and out the two holes in the superior cortex. (**A,** From Bucholz RW, Heckman JD [eds]: Rockwood and Green's Fractures in Adults, 5th ed. Philadelphia: Lippincott Williams & Wilkins, 2001, p 1277.)

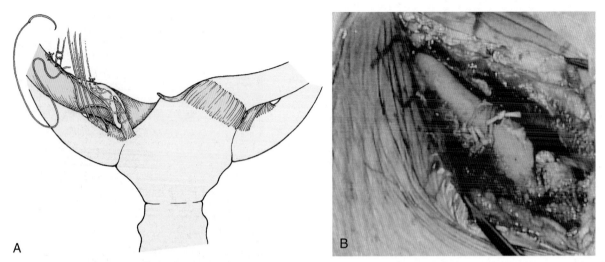

FIGURE 13-41 A and **B,** The transferred capsular ligament is secured in the medial clavicle by tying the sutures exiting from the superior cortex of the clavicle. (**A,** From Bucholz RW, Heckman JD [eds]: Rockwood and Green's Fractures in Adults, 5th ed. Philadelphia: Lippincott Williams & Wilkins, 2001, p 1277.)

All of the 8 patients in group I who had a primary surgical resection of the medial end of the clavicle with maintenance of the costoclavicular ligaments had an excellent result.

When the operation was performed as a revision of a previous procedure with reconstruction of the costoclavicular ligaments, the results were less successful, but only 1 patient of 7 was not satisfied with the outcome of treatment.

Physeal Injuries of the Medial Clavicle

We still perform the closed reduction maneuvers as described earlier for a suspected anterior or posterior injury. Open reduction of the physeal injury is seldom indicated, except for an irreducible posterior displacement in a patient with significant symptoms of compression of the vital structures in the mediastinum. After reduction, the shoulders are held back with a figure-of-eight strap or dressing for 3 to 4 weeks.

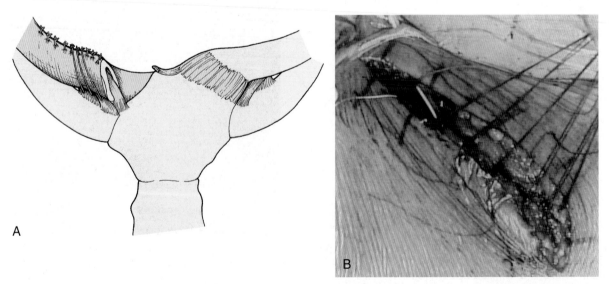

FIGURE 13-42 A and **B,** Closure of the periosteal sleeve around the medial clavicle and secure fixation of these structures to the costoclavicular ligament. (**A,** From Bucholz RW, Heckman JD [eds]: Rockwood and Green's Fractures in Adults, 5th ed. Philadelphia: Lippincott Williams & Wilkins, 2001, p 2377.)

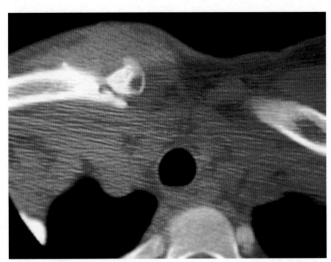

FIGURE 13-43 CT scan of a 16-year-old patient whose sternoclavicular reconstruction was complicated by fracture of the medial clavicle in the early postoperative period.

Before the epiphysis ossifies at the age of 18, one cannot be sure whether a displacement about the sternoclavicular joint is a dislocation of the sternoclavicular joint or a fracture through the physeal plate. Although there is significant displacement of the shaft with either a type I or type II physeal fracture, the periosteal tube remains in its anatomic position and the attaching ligaments are intact (i.e., the costoclavicular ligaments inferiorly and the capsular and intra-articular disk ligaments medially) (Fig. 13-45).

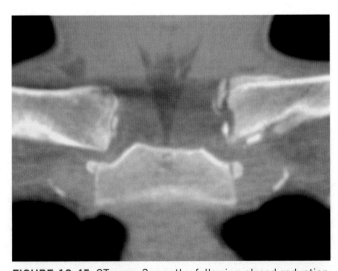

FIGURE 13-45 CT scan 3 months following closed reduction of a left posterior sternoclavicular dislocation in an 18-year-old patient. New bone formation is readily apparent within the periosteal sleeve of the medial clavicle.

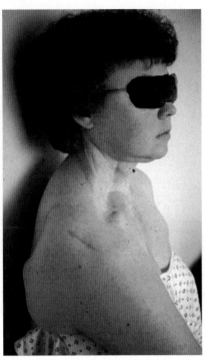

FIGURE 13-44 A 46-year-old patient with increased pain and an unsightly scar following medial clavicle resection that compromised the costoclavicular ligament. Note the postoperative scapular winging, which was associated with fatigue and spasm of the scapular stabilizing musculature.

COMPLICATIONS OF INJURIES TO THE STERNOCLAVICULAR JOINT

A physician treating sternoclavicular instability faces many challenges. Complications of the injury itself, improper selection of treatment, potential intraoperative misadventures, and postoperative problems such as migration of hardware and iatrogenic instability can all threaten the surgical outcome and, at times, even the patient's life. Thorough knowledge of the potential pitfalls is necessary if they are to be avoided.[61-64]

The serious complications that occur at the time of dislocation of the sternoclavicular joint are primarily limited to posterior injuries. About the only complication that occurs with anterior dislocation of the sternoclavicular joint is a cosmetic bump or late degenerative changes.

Many complications have been reported secondary to retrosternal dislocation:

- Pneumothorax and laceration of the superior vena cava[65]
- Venous congestion in the neck
- rupture of the esophagus with abscess and osteomyelitis of the clavicle[66]
- Pressure on the subclavian artery in an untreated patient[67]

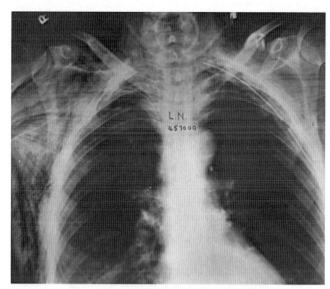

FIGURE 13-46 Complications of sternoclavicular dislocation. As a result of posterior dislocation of the sternoclavicular joint, the patient had a lacerated trachea, and massive subcutaneous emphysema developed. (From Bucholz RW, Heckman JD [eds]: Rockwood and Green's Fractures in Adults, 5th ed. Philadelphia: Lippincott Williams & Wilkins, 2001, p 1285.)

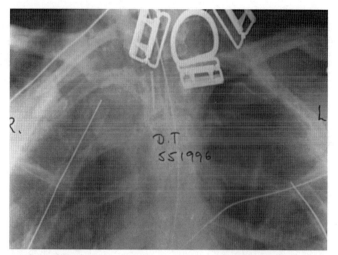

FIGURE 13-47 Complications of sternoclavicular joint dislocation. This patient had an anterior dislocation on the right and a posterior dislocation on the left. As a result of the posterior dislocation, he had sufficient pressure on the mediastinal structures to cause significant hypotension. When the posterior dislocation was reduced, blood pressure on the continuous monitor promptly returned to normal. (From Bucholz RW, Heckman JD [eds]: Rockwood and Green's Fractures in Adults, 5th ed. Philadelphia: Lippincott Williams & Wilkins, 2001, p 1286.)

- Occlusion of the subclavian artery[68]
- Compression of the right common carotid artery by a fracture-dislocation of the sternoclavicular joint[69]
- Brachial plexus compression[70]
- Hoarseness of the voice, onset of snoring, and voice changes from normal to falsetto with movement of the arm[66,70-73]

Associated injuries have also included the following[74-77]:

- Fatal tracheoesophageal fistula
- Severe thoracic outlet syndrome with swelling and cyanosis of the upper extremity
- Chronic brachial plexopathy
- Severe great vessel injuries (innominate, carotid, and subclavian arteries)
- Stridor
- Dysphagia

Several of our patients have had unusual complications that have resulted from traumatic injuries to the sternoclavicular joint. In one patient, massive subcutaneous emphysema developed as a result of posterior dislocation and rupture of the trachea (Fig. 13-46). Another patient sustained an anterior dislocation on the right and a posterior dislocation on the left. When first seen, his blood pressure was very low. After reduction of the posterior dislocation, his blood pressure, as recorded on his monitor, instantly returned to normal. It was theorized that the posteriorly displaced clavicle was irritating some

of the vital structures of the mediastinum. Another patient, who had vascular compromise, was discussed in the section on treatment of posterior dislocations. Still another patient had a traumatic injury to both sternoclavicular joints—the left was posterior and the right was anterior. After reduction of the left posterior dislocation, the right side remained unstable. However, he eventually had a painless full range of motion (Fig. 13-47).

Worman and Leagus,[78] in an excellent review of the complications associated with posterior dislocation of the sternoclavicular joint, reported that 16 of 60 patients reviewed from the literature had suffered complications of the trachea, esophagus, or great vessels.

COMPLICATIONS OF OPERATIVE PROCEDURES

Complications of surgery are listed in Table 13-1. Because of the degree of motion at the sternoclavicular joint, tremendous torque is applied to pins that cross the sternoclavicular joint; such force causes migration of hardware and fatigue breakage of the pins. We are aware of eight deaths[14,72,79-83] and four near-deaths,[78,84-86] from complications of transfixing the sternoclavicular joint with Kirschner wires or Steinmann pins. Numerous reports document migration of pins, either intact or broken, into the heart, pulmonary artery, subclavian artery, innominate artery, or the aorta.[81,84,85,87-92] *We do not recommend any type of transfixing pins—large or small—across the sternoclavicular joint.*

TABLE 13-1 Complications of Operative Procedures

Author	No. of Patients	Procedure	Complications
Brown (1961)	10	Kirschner wire transfixation pin	2 arthritic symptoms 2 broken pins (required sternotomy for retrieval) 1 pulmonary artery injury (required a thoracotomy secondary to pericardial tamponade)
Eskola et al (1989)	12	Reconstruction with a tendon graft Resection of sternal end of clavicle	4 poor (painful restriction of motion and weakness) 1 loss of reduction (local tenderness; pain radiating to the arm)
Lunseth et al (1975)	4	Stabilization with fascial loop Threaded Steinmann transfixation pin	1 loss of reduction
Omer (1967)	4	Horizontal Z or step-cut transverse osteotomy	1 postoperative infection

Brown JE: Anterior sternoclavicular dislocation—a method of repair. Am J Orthop 31:184-189, 1961.
Eskola A, Vainionpaa S, Vastamaki M, et al: Operation for older sternoclavicular dislocation. Results in 12 cases. J Bone Joint Surg Br 71(1):53-55, 1989.
Lunseth PA, Chapman KW, Frankel VH: Surgical treatment of chronic dislocation of the sterno-clavicular joint. J Bone Joint Surg Br 57:193-196, 1975.
Omer GE: Osteotomy of the clavicle in surgical reduction of anterior sternoclavicular dislocation. J Trauma 7:584-590, 1967.

REFERENCES

1. Rodrigues H: Case of dislocation, inwards, of the internal extremity of the clavicle. Lancet 1:309-310, 1843.
2. Cooper AP: The Lectures of Sir Astley Cooper on the Principles and Practices of Surgery. Philadelphia: EL Carey & A Hart, 1935, p 559.
3. Duggan N: Recurrent dislocation of sternoclavicular cartilage. J Bone Joint Surg 13:365, 1931.
4. Lowman CL: Operative correction of old sternoclavicular dislocation. J Bone Joint Surg 10:740-741, 1928.
5. Cave EF: Fractures and Other Injuries. Chicago: Year Book, 1958.
6. DePalma AF: The role of the disks of the sternoclavicular and the acromio-clavicular joints. Clin Orthop 13:222-233, 1959.
7. Gray H: Anatomy of the Human Body, 28th ed, Goss CM (ed). Philadelphia: Lea & Febiger, 1966, pp 324-326.
8. Rockwood CA, Groh GI, Wirth MA, Grassi FA: Resection arthroplasty of the sternoclavicular joint. J Bone Joint Surg Am 79:387-393, 1997.
9. Bearn JG: Direct observations on the function of the capsule of the sterno-clavicular joint in clavicular support. J Anat 101:159-170, 1967.
10. Spencer EE, Kuhn JE, Huston LJ, et al: Ligamentous restraints to anterior and posterior translation of the sternoclavicular joint. J Shoulder Elbow Surg 11:43-47, 2002.
11. Webb PAO, Suchey JMM: Epiphyseal union of the anterior iliac crest and medial clavicle in a modern multiracial sample of American males and females. Am J Phys Anthropol 68:457-466, 1985.
12. Mehta JC, Sachdev A, Collins JJ: Retrosternal dislocation of the clavicle. Injury 5:79-83, 1973.
13. Heinig CF: Retrosternal dislocation of the clavicle: Early recognition, x-ray diagnosis, and management [abstract]. J Bone Joint Surg Am 50:830, 1968.
14. Nettles JL, Linscheid R: Sternoclavicular dislocations. J Trauma 8:158-164, 1968.
15. Waskowitz WJ: Disruption of the sternoclavicular joint: An analysis and review. Am J Orthop 3:176-179, 1961.
16. Omer GE: Osteotomy of the clavicle in surgical reduction of anterior sterno-clavicular dislocation. J Trauma 7:584-590, 1967.
17. Cantlon GE, Gluckman JL: Sternoclavicular joint hypertrophy following radical neck dissection. Head Neck Surg 5:218-221, 1983.
18. Searle AB, Gluckman R, Sanders R, Breach NM: Sternoclavicular joint swellings: Diagnosis and management. Br J Plast Surg 44:403-405, 1991.
19. Vierboom MAC, Steinberg JDJ, Mooyaart EL, Rijswijk MHV: Condensing osteitis of the clavicle: Magnetic resonance imaging as an adjunct method for differential diagnosis. Ann Rheum Dis 51:539-541, 1992.
20. Kruger GD, Rock MG, Munro TG: Condensing osteitis of the clavicle: A review of the literature and report of three cases. J Bone Joint Surg Am 69:550-557, 1987.
21. Sonozaki H, Azuma A, Okai K, et al: Clinical features of 22 cases with "inter-sterno-costo-clavicular ossification." Arch Orthop Trauma Surg 95:13-22, 1979.
22. Sonozaki H, Azuma A, Okai K, et al: Inter-sterno-costoclavicular ossification with a special reference to cases of unilateral type. Kanto J Orthop Traumatol 9:196-200, 1978.
23. Tamai K, Saotome K: Panclavicular ankylosis in pus-tulotic arthrosteitis. A case report. Clin Orthop Relat Res (359):146-150, 1999.
24. Sadr B, Swann M: Spontaneous dislocation of the sterno-clavicular joint. Acta Orthop Scand 50:269-274, 1979.
25. Covelli M, Lapadula G, Pipitone N, et al: Isolated sternoclavicular joint arthritis in heroin addicts and/or HIV positive patients: A report of three cases. Clin Rheumatol 12:422-425, 1993.
26. Wohlgethan JR, Newberg AH: Clinical analysis of infection of the sternocla-vicular joint [abstract]. Clin Res 32:666A, 1984.
27. Lindsey RW, Leach JA: Sternoclavicular osteomyelitis and pyoarthrosis as a complication of subclavian vein catheterization: A case report and review of the literature. Orthopedics 7:1017-1021, 1984.
28. Renoult B, Lataste A, Jonon B, et al: Sternoclavicular joint infection in hemo-dialysis patients. Nephron 56:212-213, 1990.
29. Song HK, Sloane G, Kaiser LR, Shrager JB: Current pre-sentation and optimal surgical management of sterno-clavicular joint infections. Ann Thorac Surg 73:427-431, 2002.
30. Richter R, Hahn H, Nübling W, Kohler G: [Tuberculosis of the shoulder girdle.] Z Rheumatol 44:87-92, 1985.
31. Higoumenakis GK: Neues Stigma der kongenitalen Lues. Die Vergrösserung des sternalen Endes des rechten Schlüsselbeins, seine Beschreibung, Deutung and Ätiologie. Dtsche Z Nervenh 114:288-299, 1930.
32. Kocher MS, Feagin JA Jr: Shoulder injuries during alpine skiing. Am J Sports Med 24:665-669, 1996.
33. Sanders JO, Lyons FA, Rockwood CA: Management of dislocations of both ends of the clavicle. J Bone Joint Surg Am 72:399-402, 1990.
34. Elliott AC: Tripartite injury of the clavicle. A case report. S Afr Med J 70:115, 1986.
35. Velutini JA, Tarazona PF: Fracture of the manubrium with posterior displace-ment of the clavicle and first rib. A case report. Int Orthop 22(4):269-271, 1998.
36. Pearsall AW, Russell GV: Ipsilateral clavicle fracture, sternoclavicular joint subluxation, and long thoracic nerve injury: An unusual constellation of injuries sustained during wrestling. Am J Sports Med 28:904-908, 2000.
37. Tsai DW, Swiontkowski MF, Kottra CL: A case of sternoclavicular dislocation with scapulothoracic dissociation. AJR Am J Roentgenol 167:332, 1996.
38. Rockwood CA, Odor JM: Spontaneous anterior subluxation of the sternocla-vicular joint. J Bone Joint Surg Am 71:1280-1288, 1989.

39. Hobbs DW: Sternoclavicular joint: A new axial radiographic view. Radiology 90:801-802, 1968.
40. Lucet L, Le Loet X, Menard JF, et al: Computed tomography of the normal sternoclavicular joint. Skeletal Radiol 25:237-241, 1996.
41. Siddiqui A, Turner SM: Posterior sternoclavicular joint dislocation: The value of intra-operative ultrasound. Injury 34(6):448-453, 2003.
42. Fery A, Sommelet J: Dislocation of the sternoclavicular joint: A review of 49 cases. Int Orthop 12:187-195, 1988.
43. de Jong KP, Sukul DM: Anterior sternoclavicular dislocation: A long-term follow-up study. J Orthop Trauma 4:420-423, 1988.
44. Buckerfield CT, Castle ME: Acute traumatic retrosternal dislocation of the clavicle. J Bone Joint Surg Am 66:379-384, 1984.
45. Bankart ASB: An operation for recurrent dislocation (subluxation) of the sternoclavicular joint. Br J Surg 26:320-323, 1938.
46. Key JA, Conwell HE: The Management of Fractures, Dislocations, and Sprains, 5th ed. St Louis: CV Mosby, 1951, pp 458-461.
47. Burrows HJ: Tenodesis of subclavius in the treatment of recurrent dislocation of the sternoclavicular joint. J Bone Joint Surg Br 33:240-243, 1951.
48. Spencer EE, Kuhn JE: Biomechanical analysis of reconstructions for sternoclavicular joint instability. J Bone Joint Surg Am 86:98-105, 2004.
49. Breitner S, Wirth CJ: [Resection of the acromial and sternal ends of the clavicula.] Z Orthop 125:363-368, 1987.
50. Bateman JE: The Shoulder and Neck, 2nd ed. Philadelphia: WB Saunders, 1978.
51. Milch H: The rhomboid ligament in surgery of the sternoclavicular joint. J Int Coll Surg 17:41-51, 1952.
52. Rice EE: Habitual dislocation of the sternoclavicular articulation—a case report. J Okla State Med Assoc 25:34-35, 1932.
53. Franck WM, Jannasch O, Siassi M, et al: Balser plate stabilization: An alternate therapy for traumatic sternoclavicular instability. J Shoulder Elbow Surg 12:276-281, 2003.
54. Rowe CR: The Shoulder. New York: Churchill Livingstone, 1988, pp 313-327.
55. Martin SD, Altchek D, Erlanger S: Atraumatic posterior dislocation of the sternoclavicular joint. Clin Orthop Relat Res (292):159-164, 1993.
56. Martinez A, Rodriguez A, Gonzalez G, et al: Atraumatic spontaneous posterior subluxation of the sterno-clavicular joint. Arch Orthop Trauma Surg 119:344-346, 1999.
57. Crosby LA, Rubino LJ: Subluxation of the sternoclavicular joint secondary to pseudoarthrosis of the first and second ribs. J Bone Joint Surg Am 84:623-626, 2002.
58. Pingsmann A, Patsalis T, Ivo M: Resection arthroplasty of the sternoclavicular joint for treatment of primary degenerative sternoclavicular arthritis. J Bone Joint Surg Br 84:513-517, 2002.
59. Kruger GD, Rock MG, Munro TG: Condensing osteitis of the clavicle: A review of the literature and report of three cases. J Bone Joint Surg Am 69:550-557, 1987.
60. Gerster JC, Lagier R, Nicod L: Case report 311: Sternocostoclavicular hyperostosis (SCCH). Skeletal Radiol 14:53-60, 1985.
61. Wirth MA, Rockwood CA: Chronic conditions of the acromioclavicular and sternoclavicular joints. In Chapman MW (ed): Operative Orthopaedics, part XI, 2nd ed. Philadelphia: JB Lippincott, 1992, pp 1683-1693.
62. Wirth MA, Rockwood CA: Complications following repair of the sternoclavicular joint. In Bigliani LU (ed): Complications of the Shoulder. Baltimore: Williams & Wilkins, 1993, pp 139-153.
63. Wirth MA, Rockwood CA: Complications of treatment of injuries to the shoulder. In Epps CH (ed): Complications in Orthopaedic Surgery, 3rd ed. Philadelphia: JB Lippincott, 1994, pp 229-253.
64. Wirth MA, Rockwood CA: Acute and chronic traumatic injuries of the sternoclavicular joint. J Am Acad Orthop Surg 4:268-278, 1996.
65. Paterson DC: Retrosternal dislocation of the clavicle. J Bone Joint Surg Br 43:90-92, 1961.
66. Borowiecki B, Charow A, Cook W, et al: An unusual football injury (posterior dislocation of the sternoclavicular joint). Arch Otolaryngol 95:185-187, 1972.
67. Howard FM, Shafer SJ: Injuries to the clavicle with neurovascular complications: A study of fourteen cases. J Bone Joint Surg Am 47:1335-1346, 1965.
68. Stankler L: Posterior dislocation of clavicle: A report of 2 cases. Br J Surg 50:164-168, 1962.
69. McKenzie JMM: Retrosternal dislocation of the clavicle: A report of two cases. J Bone Joint Surg Br 45:138-141, 1963.
70. Kennedy JC: Retrosternal dislocation of the clavicle. J Bone Joint Surg Br 31:74-75, 1949.
71. Mitchell WJ, Cobey MC: Retrosternal dislocation of clavicle. Med Ann Dist Columbia 29:546-549, 1960.
72. Salvatore JE: Sternoclavicular joint dislocation. Clin Orthop Relat Res 58:51-54, 1968.
73. Tyler HDD, Sturrock WDS, Callow FM: Retrosternal dislocation of the clavicle. J Bone Joint Surg Br 45:132-137, 1963.
74. Gangahar DM, Flogaites T: Retrosternal dislocation of the clavicle producing thoracic outlet syndrome. J Trauma 18:369-372, 1978.
75. Gardner NA, Bidstrup BP: Intrathoracic great vessel injury resulting from blunt chest trauma associated with posterior dislocation of the sternoclavicular joint. Aust N Z J Surg 53:427-430, 1983.
76. Rayan GM: Compression brachial plexopathy caused by chronic posterior dislocation of the sternoclavicular joint. J Okla State Med Assoc 87:7-9, 1994.
77. Wasylenko MJ, Busse EF: Posterior dislocation of the clavicle causing fatal tracheoesophageal fistula. Can J Surg 24:626-627, 1981.
78. Worman LW, Leagus C: Intrathoracic injury following retrosternal dislocation of the clavicle. J Trauma 7:416-423, 1967.
79. Clark RL, Milgram JW, Yawn DH: Fatal aortic perforation and cardiac tamponade due to a Kirschner wire migrating from the right sternoclavicular joint. South Med J 67:316-318, 1974.
80. Gerlach D, Wemhöner SR, Ogbuihi S: [On two cases of fatal heart tamponade due to migration of fracture nails from the sternoclavicular joint.] Z Rechtsmed 93:53-60, 1984.
81. Leonard JW, Gifford RW: Migration of a Kirschner wire from the clavicle into pulmonary artery. Am J Cardiol 16:598-600, 1965.
82. Richman KM, Boutin RD, Vaughan LM, et al: Tophaceous pseudogout of the sternoclavicular joint. AJR Am J Roentgenol 172:1587-1589, 1999.
83. Smolle-Juettner FM, Hofer PH, Pinter H, et al: Intracardiac malpositioning of a sternoclavicular fixation wire. J Orthop Trauma 6:102-105, 1992.
84. Brown JE: Anterior sternoclavicular dislocation—a method of repair. Am J Orthop 31:184-189, 1961.
85. Pate JW, Wilhite J: Migration of a foreign body from the sternoclavicular joint to the heart: A case report. Am Surg 35:448-449, 1969.
86. Song HK, Sloane G, Kaiser LR, Shrager JB: Current presentation and optimal surgical management of sternoclavicular joint infections. Ann Thorac Surg 73:427-431, 2002.
87. Nordback I, Markkula H: Migration of Kirschner pin from clavicle into ascending aorta. Acta Chir Scand 151:177-179, 1985.
88. Jelesijevic V, Knoll D, Klinke F, et al: Penetrating injuries of the heart and intrapericardial blood vessels caused by migration of a Kirschner pin after osteosynthesis. Acta Chir Iugosl 29:274, 1982.
89. Liu HP, Chang CH, Lin PJ, et al: Migration of Kirschner wire for the right sternoclavicular joint into the main pulmonary artery: A case report. Chang Gung Med J 15:49-53, 1992.
90. Rubenstein ZR, Moray B, Itzchak Y: Percutaneous removal of intravascular foreign bodies. Cardiovasc Intervent Radiol 5:64-68, 1982.
91. Schechter DC, Gilbert L: Injuries of the heart and great vessels due to pins and needles. Thorax 24:246-253, 1969.
92. Sethi GK, Scott SM: Subclavian artery laceration due to migration of a Hagie pin. Surgery 80:644-646, 1976.

Sepsis of the Shoulder: Molecular Mechanisms and Pathogenesis

Robin R. Richards, MD, FRCSC

Shoulder sepsis can have a devastating impact on shoulder function, particularly if diagnosis and treatment are delayed or inadequate. The general principles in the pathogenesis of shoulder sepsis are similar to those pertaining to all intra-articular infections. There are three fundamental pathways for pathogens to enter a joint:

1. Spontaneous hematogenous seeding via the synovial blood supply
2. Contiguous spread from adjacent metaphyseal osteomyelitis via the intra-articular portion of the metaphysis
3. Penetration of the joint by trauma, therapy, or surgery (Fig. 14-1)

Susceptibility to infection is determined by the adequacy of the host defenses. Spontaneous bacteremia, trauma, and surgery present opportunities for inoculation of the joint, particularly if local or systemic conditions are favorable for infection to develop. Shoulder sepsis is relatively uncommon due to the normal defense mechanisms, the use of antibiotic prophylaxis, and a good local blood supply.

Certain patient groups with immune system depression or aberrations are at increased risk for infection. Patients with rheumatoid disease can manifest a spontaneous and somewhat cryptic sepsis in joints.[1,2] Diabetics, infants, children, the aged, patients with vascular disease, drug abusers, and patients with HIV infection have an increased susceptibility to specific organisms, as are patients with hematologic dyscrasias and neoplastic disease.

Joint infection requires a threshold inoculum of bacteria and can be facilitated by damaged tissue, foreign body substrata, and the acellularity of cartilage surfaces. Total joint arthroplasties are at potential risk because of the presence of metal and polymer biomaterials and the decreased phagocytic ability of macrophages in the presence of methylmethacrylate. Biomaterials and adjacent damaged tissues and substrates are readily colonized by bacteria in a polysaccharide biofilm that is resistant to macrophage attack and antibiotic penetration.[3,4] With antibiotic prophylaxis, published infection rates of total joint arthroplasty are low: 1% to 5%, depending on the device and the location.[5,6] However, once infected, biomaterials and damaged tissues are exceedingly resistant to treatment.

Clinical infection in immunosuppressed patients involves the maturation of an inoculum of known pathogens (e.g., *Staphylococcus aureus* or *Pseudomonas aeruginosa*) or the transformation of nonpathogens (*Staphylococcus epidermidis*) to a septic focus of adhesive virulent organisms. This transformation can occur in the presence of, and be potentiated by, the surface of biomaterials,[7,8] damaged tissue, and defenseless cartilage matrix surfaces.[9]

HISTORY

Experiences in shoulder infection have paralleled those of other large joints, although with less frequency. The work of outstanding scientists, such as Louis Pasteur (1822-1895), Joseph Lister (1827-1912), and Robert Koch (1843-1910), in the last quarter of the 19th century, ushered in the modern age of bacteriology and an early understanding of intra-articular sepsis. Koch's experiments with culture media at the Berlin Institute for Infectious Disease verified the role of the tubercle bacillus in musculoskeletal infection.

The latter part of the 19th century also saw the development of the concept of antisepsis. Lister maintained that sepsis was the main obstacle to significant advances in surgery. He documented a dramatic drop in cases of empyema, erysipelas, hospital gangrene, and surgical infection through the use of antiseptic techniques.

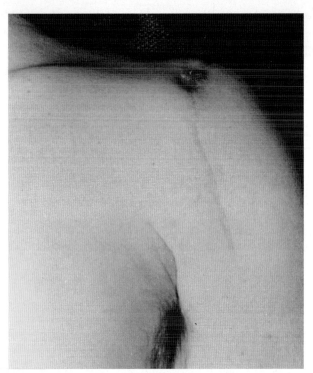

FIGURE 14-1 Sinus communicating with a prosthetic shoulder joint. This patient developed a chronic low-grade infection after undergoing a total shoulder arthroplasty.

Although the popularization of antiseptic technique in the surgical theater greatly reduced the rate of complications resulting from infection, it was not until the 1930s that specific antimicrobial therapy was discovered. In 1935, a German bacteriologist, Gerhard Domagk, discovered that sulfonamides protected mice against fatal doses of hemolytic staphylococci. Sulfonamides were soon employed for infections in patients, with excellent results.

Although the history of bacteriology, antiseptic techniques in surgery, and the development of antibiotics are well documented, very little of the early literature relates specifically to infections about the shoulder. In Codman's book, *The Shoulder*, first published in 1934, infection of the shoulder and, in particular, osteomyelitis of the proximal humerus were considered very rare lesions.[10] Codman cited a report by King and Holmes in 1927 in which a review of 450 consecutive symptomatic shoulders evaluated at the Massachusetts General Hospital revealed 5 cases of tuberculosis of the shoulder, 1 luetic infection of the shoulder, 3 unspecified shoulder infections, and 2 cases of osteomyelitis of the proximal humerus. The rarity of tubercular lesions of the shoulder was documented through the results of four large series of tuberculosis involving the musculoskeletal system (Townsend, 21 of 3244 cases; Whitman, 38 of 1833 cases; Young, 7 of 5680 cases; Billroth, 14 of 1900 cases). As microbial culturing and identification techniques developed in the early 20th century, streptococcal and staphylococcal species were more often identified as the causative agents in shoulder infection.

SEPTIC ANATOMY OF THE SHOULDER

A review of shoulder anatomy reveals specific structural relationships that are intimately linked to the pathogenesis of joint sepsis and osteomyelitis. The circulation of the proximal humerus and periarticular structures (particularly the synovium) and the intricate system of bursae about the shoulder are critical factors.

Classically, the age-dependent presentations of hematogenous osteomyelitis and septic arthritis of the shoulder (and other large joints such as the hip and knee) have been attributed to the vascular development about the growth plate and epiphysis. The most detailed studies of the vascular development in this area have been done on the proximal femur but are analogous to the same development about the proximal humerus. Experimental work by Trueta[11] demonstrated that before 8 months of age, there are direct vascular communications across the growth plate between the nutrient artery system and the epiphyseal ossicle. This observation was believed to account for the frequency of infection involving the epiphyseal ossicle and subsequent joint sepsis in infants. At some point between 8 months and 18 months of age (an average of 1 year), the growth plate forms a complete barrier to direct vascular communication between the metaphysis and epiphysis. The last vestiges of the nutrient artery turn down acutely at the growth plate and reach sinusoidal veins. At this point the blood flow slows down, creating an ideal medium for the proliferation of pathogenic bacteria.[12]

In the adult shoulder, the intra-articular extent of the metaphysis is located in the inferior sulcus and is intracapsular for approximately 10 to 12 mm.[13] Infection of the proximal metaphysis, once established, can gain access to the shoulder joint via the haversian and Volkmann canals at the nonperiosteal zone (Fig. 14-2). With obliteration of the growth plate at skeletal maturity, anastomoses of the metaphyseal and epiphyseal circulation are again established.

In his study of the vascular development of the proximal femur, Chung did not find evidence of direct communications between the metaphyseal and epiphyseal circulation across the growth plate in any age group.[14] Chung's work demonstrated a persistent extraosseous anastomosis between metaphyseal and epiphyseal circulation on the surface of the perichondral ring. He found no evidence of vessels penetrating the growth plate in the infant population and attributed apparent changes in the arterial supply with age to enlargement of the neck and ossification center.

Branches of the suprascapular artery and the circumflex scapular branch of the subscapular artery from the scapular side of the shoulder anastomose with the anterior and posterior humeral circumflex arteries from the humeral side of the shoulder. This anastomotic system supplies the proximal humerus by forming an extra-articular and extracapsular arterial ring. Vessels from this

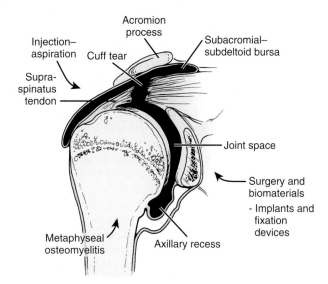

FIGURE 14-2 Routes of infection for intra-articular sepsis.

ring traverse the capsule and form an intra-articular synovial ring. This fine anastomosis of vessels in the synovial membrane is located at the junction of the synovium and the articular cartilage. This subsynovial ring of vessels was first described by William Hunter in 1743 and named the *circulus articuli vasculosus*.[15] At the transitional zone, synovial cells become flattened over this periarticular vascular fringe. Fine arterioles at this boundary acutely loop back toward the periphery. Again, blood flow at this level can decrease, which provides a site for establishing an inoculum of pathogenic organisms. Rather than hemodynamic changes, however, it is more probable that receptor-specific, microbe–to–cell surface interactions potentiate the infectious process.

Another consideration in the septic anatomy of the shoulder is the communication between the joint space and capsule and the system of bursae about the shoulder. Anteriorly, there is direct communication between the capsule and the subscapular bursa located just below the coracoid process. Posteriorly, the capsule communicates with the infraspinatus bursa. A third opening in the capsule occurs at the point at which the tendon of the long head of the biceps enters the shoulder. From the transverse humeral ligament to its entry into the shoulder capsule, the tendon of the long head of the biceps is enveloped in folds of synovium. Intentional or inadvertent injection of the subscapular bursa, the infraspinatus bursa, or the tendon of the long head of the biceps provides the potential for intra-articular bacterial inoculation. Injection of the subacromial or subdeltoid bursa in the presence of a rotator cuff tear (degenerative or traumatic) provides another potential setting for bacterial contamination of the joint.

Ward and Eckardt[16] reported on four subacromial or subdeltoid bursa abscesses. Three of the four patients were chronically ill and debilitated, and in these patients

the bursal abscesses coexisted with clinically diagnosed mild to resolving glenohumeral pyarthrosis. The symptoms and signs of these abscesses were minimal in all four patients. Ward and Eckardt found that computed tomography (CT) or magnetic resonance imaging (MRI) can help to detect abscesses and plan treatment.

MICROANATOMY AND CELL BIOLOGY

The hyaline cartilage of the articular surface is essentially acellular and consists of horizontally arranged collagen fibers in proteoglycan macromolecules. The boundaries of the joint cavity are composed of a richly vascularized cellular synovial tissue. It has been suggested that collagen fibers and the glycoprotein matrix, rather than the synovium, are the target substrata for microbial adhesion and colonization.[9,17]

Some synovial cells are phagocytic and appear to combat infection as part of the inflammatory response. Microscopic examination of infected joints in a lupine animal model indicated predominant colonization of cartilaginous, rather than synovial, surfaces.[9] Receptors for collagen have been identified on the cell surfaces of certain strains of *S. aureus*.[17] The infrequent occurrence of bacteria on synovial tissue might reflect innate resistance of synovial cells to colonization, the lack of appropriate synovial ligands, or functional host defense mechanisms at a synovial level.[18] The subintimal vascularized layer contains fibroadipose tissue, lymphatic vessels, and nerves. Ultrastructural studies of the synovial subintimal vessels reveal that gaps between endothelial cells are bridged by a fine membrane. There is no epithelial tissue in the synovial lining and, therefore, no structural barrier (basement membrane) to prevent the spread of infection from synovial blood vessels to the joint. The synovial lining in the transition zone is rarely more than three or four cell layers thick, placing the synovial blood vessels in a superficial position. Intra-articular hemorrhage caused by trauma, combined with transient bacteremia, may be implicated as a factor in the pathogenesis of joint sepsis. Hematogenous seeding can allow bacterial penetration of synovial vessels, producing an effusion consisting primarily of neutrophils that release cartilage-destroying lysosomal enzymes.

Articular (hyaline) cartilage varies from 2 to 4 mm in thickness in the large joints of adults. This avascular, aneural tissue consists of a relatively small number of cells and chondrocytes and an abundant extracellular matrix. The extracellular matrix contains collagen and a ground substance composed of carbohydrate and noncollagenous protein and has a high water content. The chondrocytes are responsible for the synthesis and degradation of matrix components and are therefore ultimately responsible for the biomechanical and biologic properties of articular cartilage. Collagen produced by the chondrocytes accounts for more than half of the dry weight of adult articular cartilage (type II). Individual collagen fibers, with a characteristic periodicity of 640 Å, vary from 300 to 800 Å in diameter, depending on their distance from the articular surface.

The principal component of the ground substance produced by chondrocytes is a protein polysaccharide complex termed *proteoglycan*. The central organizing molecule of proteoglycan is hyaluronic acid. Numerous glycosaminoglycans (mainly chondroitin sulfate and keratan sulfate) are covalently bound from this central strand. Glycosaminoglycans carry considerable negative charge. The highly ordered array of electronegativity on the proteoglycan molecule interacts with large numbers of water molecules (small electric dipole). Approximately 75% of the wet weight of articular cartilage is water, the majority of which is structured by the electrostatic forces of the proteoglycan molecule.

The structure of articular cartilage varies relative to its distance from the free surface. For purposes of description, the tissue has been subdivided into zones that run parallel to the articular surface. Electron microscopy of the free surface reveals a dense network of collagen fibers (40-120 Å in diameter) that is arranged tangentially to the load-bearing surface and at approximately right angles to each other. This dense, mat-like arrangement, the lamina obscurans, is acellular.

Zone 1 contains large bundles of collagen fibers that are approximately 340 Å thick and lie parallel to the joint surface and at right angles to each other (Fig. 14-3). This zone, the lamina splendins, has little or no intervening ground substance and contains the highest density of collagen. Chondrocytes in zone 1 are ellipsoid and are oriented parallel to the articular surface. They show little electron microscopic evidence of metabolic activity.

In zone 2, the collagen consists of individual randomly oriented fibers of varying diameters. The chondrocytes in zone 2 tend to be more spherical and larger than those of zone 1, with abundant mitochondria and extensive endoplasmic reticulum, suggesting greater metabolic activity. The proteoglycan-to-collagen ratio in zone 2 is much higher than that near the surface.

In zone 3, the collagen fibers are thicker, often in the range of 1400 Å, and tend to form a more orderly meshwork that lies radial to the articular surface. The chondrocytes in zone 3 are larger and tend to be arranged in columns, often appearing in groups of two to eight cells. The cells are noted to have enlarged Golgi complexes, many mitochondria, and an extensively developed endoplasmic reticulum, indicating a high degree of metabolic activity.

Bone is a composite structure incorporating calcium hydroxyapatite crystals in a collagen matrix grossly similar to synthetic composites or to partially crystalline polymers. Devitalized bone provides a passive substratum for bacterial colonization and the ultimate incorporation of its proteinaceous and mineral constituents as bacterial metabolites.[3] *S. aureus* binds to bone sialoprotein, a glycoprotein found in joints, and it produces chondrocyte proteases that hydrolyze synovial tissue.[19]

CLASSIFICATION

Intra-articular sepsis may be classified in order of pathogenesis and frequency as direct hematogenous; secondary to contiguous spread from osteomyelitis; or secondary to trauma, surgery, or intra-articular injection (Fig. 14-4 and Box 14-1). Most joint infections are caused by hematogenous spread, although direct contamination is not uncommon with trauma. Inoculation of the joint with bacteria can occur in association with intra-articular injection of steroid, local anesthetic, or synthetic joint fluid. Infection rates following arthroscopy are also low, ranging

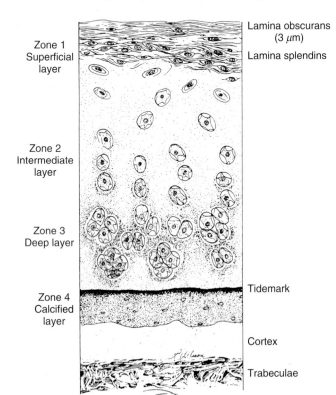

Zone 1
Superficial
layer

Zone 2
Intermediate
layer

Zone 3
Deep layer

Zone 4
Calcified
layer

Lamina obscurans
(3 μm)

Lamina splendins

Tidemark

Cortex

Trabeculae

FIGURE 14-3 The zones of adult articular cartilage. (Modified with permission from Turek SL: Orthopaedics: Principles and Their Application. Philadelphia: JB Lippincott, 1977.)

BOX 14-1 Classification of Osteomyelitis and Intra-articular Sepsis

Hematogenous

Contiguous spread
- Osteomyelitis
- Soft tissue sepsis
- Vascular insufficiency

Direct inoculation
- Surgery with or without a foreign body or biomaterials
- Trauma with or without a foreign body or biomaterials

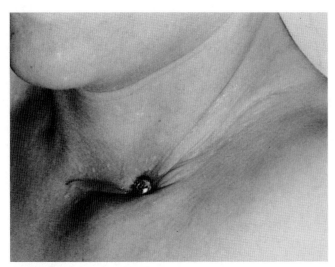

FIGURE 14-4 Internal fixation visible over the clavicle. The patient had a clavicular nonunion that was treated with internal fixation and bone grafting. Infection occurred, resulting in wound breakdown and exposure of the internal fixation. The patient was treated by removal of the internal fixation and dressing changes. The wound healed with this treatment, and there has been no recurrence of drainage over 6 years. Infection is not uncommon in the area of the clavicle and the acromioclavicular joint due to the thin soft tissue envelope that overlies the clavicle and the acromioclavicular joint.

from 0.4% to 3.4%.[20] Armstrong and Bolding report that sepsis following arthroscopy can be associated with inadequate arthroscope disinfection and the use of intraoperative intra-articular corticosteroids.[21]

Osteomyelitis of the humerus can spread intra-articularly, depending on the age of the patient, the type of infecting organism, and the severity of infection. Osteomyelitis of the clavicle or scapula is uncommon, although it can occur after surgery and internal fixation, from retained shrapnel fragments, or in heroin addicts.[22-25] Brancos and associates reported that *S. aureus* and *P. aeruginosa* were the etiologic agents in 75% and 11% of episodes, respectively, of septic arthritis in heroin addicts.[26] The sternoclavicular joint was involved more commonly than the shoulder joint. Septic arthritis of the shoulder has been reported by Chaudhuri and associates following mastectomy and radiotherapy for breast carcinoma.[27] Lymphedema was present in all cases. The infection had a subacute onset in all cases, and delays in diagnosis led to destruction of the joint in all but one patient.

Hematogenous osteomyelitis, although common in children,[28] is uncommon in adults until the sixth decade or later and is usually associated with a compromised immune system. Intravenous (IV) drug use is associated with the development of osteomyelitis in adults. Direct spread from wounds or foreign bodies, including total joint and internal fixation devices, is the most common etiology of shoulder sepsis in adults. Gowans and Granieri noted the

relationship between intra-articular injections of hydrocortisone acetate and the subsequent development of septic arthritis in 1959.[29] Kelly and associates noted that two of their six patients had a history of multiple intra-articular injections of corticosteroid.[30] Ward and Goldner reported that chronic disease was present in more than half of their 30 cases of glenohumeral pyarthrosis and that 4 cases were associated with ipsilateral forearm arteriovenous dialysis fistulas.[31] Soft tissue infection about the shoulder can also manifest in the form of pyomyositis, sometimes occurring as a result of hematogenous spread.[32] Aglas and associates reported sternoclavicular joint arthritis as a complication of subclavian venous catheterization.[33] Their two cases responded to antibiotic treatment. Glenohumeral pyarthrosis has been observed following acupuncture.[34] Lossos and coworkers reported that associated medical conditions were present in the majority of their patients with septic arthritis of the shoulder.[35]

PATHOGENIC MECHANISMS OF SEPTIC ARTHRITIS AND OSTEOMYELITIS

Surfaces as Substrata for Bacterial Colonization

The pathogenesis of bone and joint infections is related, in part, to preferential adhesive colonization of inert substrata whose surfaces are not integrated with healthy tissue composed of living cells and intact extracellular polymers such as the articular surface of joints or damaged bone (Fig. 14-5).[3,36-39] Almost all natural biologic surfaces are lined by a cellular epithelium or endothelium. The exceptions are intra-articular cartilage and the surface of teeth. Mature enamel is the only human tissue that is totally acellular; it is primarily composed of inorganic hydroxyapatite crystals (96% by weight), with a small amount of water (3%) and organic matrix (<1%).[40] Proteins in the organic matrix are distributed between the hydroxyapatite crystals, forming a framework that strengthens the enamel by decreasing its tendency to fracture or separate. These proteins are unique among mineralized tissue because they are not a fibrous collagen protein like that found in bone, dentin, and cementum or in cartilage but are similar to the keratin family of proteins.

Cartilage and enamel are readily colonized by bacteria because they lack the protection by natural desquamation or by intact extracapsular polysaccharides that is provided by an active cellular layer. Their acellular surfaces are similar to many of those in nature for which bacteria have developed colonizing mechanisms. Certain strains of *S. aureus* adhere to specific sites on collagen fibrils, a process that is mediated by specific surface receptor proteins. Dissimilarities in surface structure are probably responsible for the specificity of the colonization of bacterial species on these surfaces.

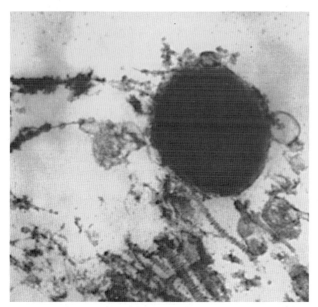

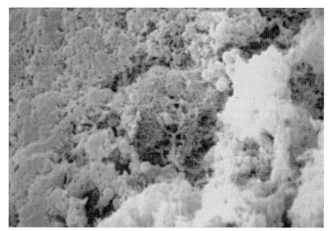

FIGURE 14-6 A photoelectromicrograph of articular cartilage at 7 days demonstrates destructive changes occurring beneath matrix-enclosed cocci. (From Voytek A, Gristina AG, Barth E, et al: Staphylococcal adhesion to collagen in intra-articular sepsis. Biomaterials 9:107-110, 1988.)

FIGURE 14-5 A photoelectromicrograph of rabbit articular cartilage illustrating direct bacteria-to-collagen fiber contact. (From Voytek A, Gristina AG, Barth E, et al: Staphylococcal adhesion to collagen in intra-articular sepsis. Biomaterials 9:107-110, 1988.)

Enamel is mostly crystalline and inorganic, and cartilage is organic and noncrystalline. Enamel contains no collagen, whereas collagen is ubiquitous in cartilage and bone. *S. aureus* is the natural colonizer of cartilage but not of enamel, because it contains collagen receptors.[41,42] The specificity of colonization is also modulated in part by lectins and the host-derived synovial fluid, blood, and serum; conditioning films of protein; and polysaccharide macromolecules. The colonization of teeth by *Streptococcus mutans* and other organisms is a natural polymicrobial process and may be symbiotic or slowly destructive, but bacterial colonization of articular cartilage is unnatural and rapidly destructive.

The acellular cartilage matrix and inanimate biomaterial surfaces offer no resistance to colonization by *S. aureus* and *S. epidermidis*, respectively. The observed invasion and gradual destruction of the cartilage over time supports clinical observations of the course of untreated septic arthritis (Fig. 14-6).[43,44] The acellular cartilaginous surfaces of joints are particularly vulnerable to sepsis because they allow direct exposure to bacteria from open trauma, surgical procedures, or hematogenous spread. This mechanism parallels previous observations on the mechanism of osteomyelitis, which suggest that the adhesion of bacteria to dead bone or cartilage (surfaces not protected by living cells) via receptors and extracellular polysaccharides is a factor in pathogenesis.[3,45]

Intra-articular Sepsis

The articular cavity is a potential dead space that can provide a favorable environment for bacterial growth. In this avascular and relatively acellular space, host defense mechanisms are at a disadvantage. Synovial cells are not actively antibacterial, although they are somewhat phagocytic. White blood cells (WBCs) must be delivered to the area and lack a surface for active locomotion. Under such conditions it is expected that phagocytic action is impaired, especially against encapsulated organisms.

Spontaneous intra-articular sepsis of the shoulder is derived from random hematogenous bacterial seeding. The synovial vasculature is abundant, and the vessels lack a limiting basement membrane. Bacteremia, especially *Neisseria gonorrhoeae*, increases the risk of intra-articular spread. Nosocomial infections in neonatal intensive care units are usually related to the presence of intravascular devices.[46] Contiguous spread from adjacent and intracapsular metaphyseal osteomyelitis also occurs. Surgery, arthroscopy, total joint replacement, aspirations, and steroid injections also can result in direct inoculation of bacteria into the intra-articular space. The presence of foreign bodies from trauma or after surgery (stainless steel, chrome-cobalt alloys, ultra-high molecular weight polyethylene, and methylmethacrylate) increases the possibility of infection by providing a foreign body nidus for colonization, allowing antibiotic-resistant colonization to occur.[3,7] The presence of a foreign body also decreases the size of the inoculant required for sepsis and perturbs host defense mechanisms.

Septic arthritis of the shoulder most often involves the glenohumeral joint. The acromioclavicular and sternoclavicular joints are occasionally infected in specific patient groups or after steroid injections in arthritis. Direct contamination from open wounds is also possible. Sternoclavicular sepsis is more common in drug addicts and usually involves gram-negative organisms, specifically *P. aeruginosa*. The involvement of *S. aureus*, *Escherichia coli*, *Brucella* species, and *N. gonorrhoeae* has also been reported.

Septic arthritis of the shoulder represents up to 14% of all septic arthritis cases.[47] In earlier studies, the incidence was 3.4%.[48] Caksen and associates report shoulder involvement in 2 of 49 joints involved in their series of pediatric patients with septic arthritis.[49] A more elderly population, increased trauma, and the common use of articular and periarticular steroids may be factors in this epidemiology (Fig. 14-7). The primary causal organism of shoulder sepsis is *S. aureus*. Sepsis in immunocompromised patients may be polyarticular as well as polymicrobial. Ten percent of septic arthritis involves more than one joint and is likely to occur in children.

Osteomyelitis

Hematogenous osteomyelitis accounts for most cases of osteomyelitis in children. Contiguous osteomyelitis is more common in adults, secondary to surgery and direct inoculation. In persons older than 50 years, contiguous osteomyelitis and disease related to vascular insufficiency are predominant. Of the bones of the shoulder, the humerus is most commonly involved in osteomyelitis. The clavicle is occasionally involved in drug addicts by hematogenous spread. The scapula is rarely involved; usually infection occurs by direct inoculation or contiguous spread (Table 14-1).

Epps and associates reviewed 15 patients who had sickle cell disease and osteomyelitis affecting 30 bones.[50] *S. aureus* was isolated on culture of specimens of bone

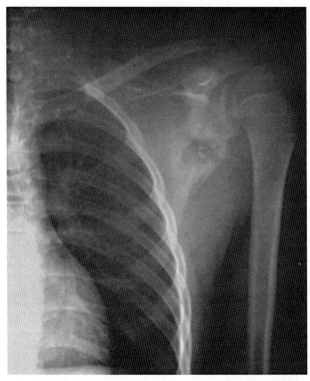

FIGURE 14-7 Staphylococcal osteomyelitis of the scapula secondary to closed trauma and hematologic seeding with abscess formation. The shoulder joint is not involved. (From the Department of Radiology, Wake Forest University Medical Center, Winston-Salem, NC.)

TABLE 14-1 Frequency of Joint Involvement in Infectious Arthritis (%)

Joint	Bacterial (Suppurative)		Mycobacterial[‡]	Viral
	*Children**	*Adults[†]*		
Knee	41	48	24	60
Hip	23	24	20	4
Ankle	14	7	12	30
Elbow	12	11	8	20
Wrist	4	7	20	55
Shoulder	4	15	4	5
Interphalangeal and metacarpal	1.4	1	12	75
Sternoclavicular	0.4	8	0	0
Sacroiliac	0.4	2	0	0

Note: *More than one joint may be involved; therefore, the percentage exceeds 100%.*
Compiled from Nelson JD, Koontz WC: Septic arthritis in infants and children: A review of 117 cases. Pediatrics 38:966-971, 1966; and Jackson MA, Nelson JD: Etiology and medical management of acute suppurative bone and joint infections in pediatric patients. J Pediatr Orthop 2:313-323, 1982.
†Compiled from Kelly PJ, Martin WJ, Coventry MD: Bacterial (suppurative) arthritis in the adult. J Bone Joint Surg Am 52:1595-1602, 1970; Argen RJ, Wilson DH Jr, Wood P: Suppurative arthritis. Arch Intern Med 117:661-666, 1966; Gifford DB, Patzakis M, Ivler D, Swezey RL: Septic arthritis due to Pseudomonas in heroin addicts. J Bone Joint Surg Am 57:631-635, 1975.*
‡Compiled from Smith JW, Sanford JP: Viral arthritis. Ann Intern Med 67:651-659, 1967; Medical Staff Conference: Arthritis caused by viruses. Calif Med 199:38-44, 1973.*
From Mandell L, Douglas KG Jr, Bennett JE (eds): Principles and Practice of Infectious Diseases, 2nd ed. New York: John Wiley, 1985, p 698.

from 8 of the 15 patients; *Salmonella* species from 6; and *Proteus mirabilis* from 1. Accordingly it appears that *Salmonella* species are not always the principle causative organisms of osteomyelitis in patients who have sickle cell disease.

MICROBIAL ADHESION AND INTRA-ARTICULAR SEPSIS

An understanding of microbial adhesion is required for complete clinical and therapeutic insights in joint sepsis. Studies of bacteria in marine ecosystems indicate that they tend to adhere in colonies to surfaces or substrata. The number of bacteria that can exist in a given environment is related directly to stress and nutrient supply.[51] Because surface attachment, rather than a floating or suspension population, is a favored survival strategy, it is the state of the major portion of bacterial biomasses in most natural environments and is a common mode of microbial life in humans.

Bacterial attachment to surfaces is influenced by proteinaceous bacterial receptors and by an extracapsular exopolysaccharide substance within which bacteria aggregate and multiply.[52] Once bacteria have developed a biofilm-enclosed adhesive mode of growth, they become more resistant to antiseptics,[53] antibiotics,[54] and host defense systems.[39,54,55] Free-floating, nonadhesive bacteria or microbes that lack a well-developed outer layer or exopolysaccharide are more susceptible to host-clearing mechanisms[56] and to lower concentrations of antibacterial agents.[54] Gibbons and van Houte first described the significance of this adhesive phenomenon in the formation of dental plaque.[57] In diseases such as gonococcal urethritis,[58] cystic fibrosis,[59] and endocarditis, bacterial colonization and propagation occur along endothelial and epithelial surfaces. The association between bacterial growth on biomaterial surfaces and infection was first described in 1963.[60]

Microbial adhesion and associated phenomena also explain the foreign-body effect, an increased susceptibility to infection experienced in the presence of a foreign body. Infections centered on foreign bodies are resistant to host defenses and treatment and tend to persist until the infecting locus is removed. Foreign bodies include implanted biomaterials, fixation materials, prosthetic monitoring and delivery devices, traumatically acquired penetrating debris and bone fragments, and compromised tissues.

Initial bacterial attachment or adhesion depends on the long-range physical force characteristics of the bacterium,

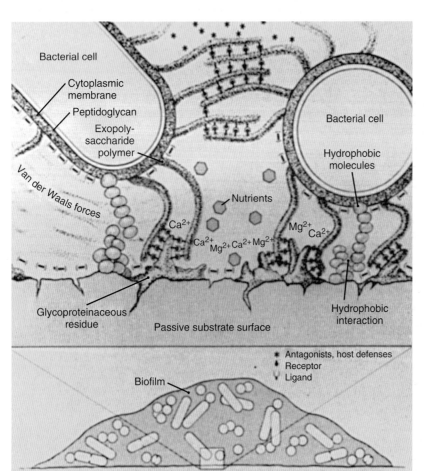

FIGURE 14-8 Mechanism of bacterial adherence. At specific distances, the initial repelling forces between like charges on the surfaces of bacteria and substrate are overcome by attracting Van der Waals forces, and there are hydrophobic interactions between molecules. Under appropriate conditions, extensive development of exopolysaccharide polymers occurs, allowing ligand–receptor interaction and proteinaceous binding of the bacteria to the substrate. (From Gristina AG, Oga M, Webb LX, Hobgood CD: Adherent bacterial colonization in the pathogenesis of osteomyelitis. Science 228:990-993, 1985. Copyright 1985 by the American Association for the Advancement of Science.)

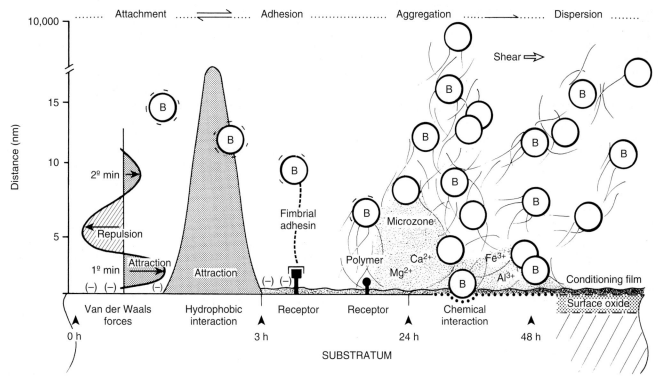

FIGURE 14-9 Molecular sequence in bacterial (*B*) attachment, adhesion, aggregation, and dispersion at the substratum surface. A number of possible interactions can occur, depending on the specificities of the bacteria or substratum system (graphics, nutrients, contaminants, macromolecules, species, and materials). (From Gristina AG: Biomaterial-centered infection: Microbial adhesion versus tissue integration. Science 237:1588-1595, 1987. Copyright 1987 by the American Association for the Advancement of Science.)

the fluid interface, and the substratum. Specific irreversible adhesion, which occurs after initial attachment, is based on time-dependent adhesin–receptor interactions and on extracapsular polysaccharide synthesis.[61] Biomaterial surfaces present sites for environmental interactions derived from their atomic structures (Fig. 14-8).[62] Metal alloys have a thin (100-200 Å) oxide layer that is the true biological interface.[63,64] The surfaces of polymers and metals are modified by texture, manufacturing processes, trace chemicals, and debris and also by host-derived ionic, polysaccharide, and glycoproteinaceous constituents (conditioning films). The finite surface structure of conditioning film in a human is specific for each individual biomaterial, type of tissue cell, and local host environment.[65] Tissue cells and matrix macromolecules also provide substrata for bacterial colonization. Bacteria have developed adhesins or receptors that interact with tissue cell surface structures (Fig. 14-9).

Subsequent to or concomitant with initial attachment, fimbrial adhesins (*E. coli*) and substratum receptors can interact, as in bacteria–to–tissue cell pathogenesis or for the glycoproteinaceous conditioning films that immediately coat implants.[65] The production and composition of the extracellular polysaccharide polymer, which tends to act like a glue, is a pivotal factor.[51] After colony maturation, cells on the periphery of the expanding biomass can

separate or disaggregate and disperse, a process that is moderated by colony size, nutrient conditions, and hemodynamic or mechanical shear forces. In natural environments, disaggregation is a survival strategy; in humans, however, it is involved in the pathogenesis of septic emboli. Disaggregation (dispersion) and its parameters might explain the phenomenon of intermittent or short-term bacterial showers or disseminated bacterial emboli.

BACTERIAL PATHOGENS

Organisms involved in septic arthritis and osteomyelitis of the shoulder (in order of frequency)[30] include *S. aureus, S. epidermidis, Streptococcus* group B, *E. coli, P. aeruginosa, Haemophilus influenzae* type B, *N. gonorrhoeae, Mycobacterium tuberculosis, Salmonella* and *Pneumococcus* species, and *Yersinia enterocolitica*.[66] Reported associations[67-72] and other etiologic pathogens are listed in Box 14-2.

H. influenzae type B is most commonly isolated in children younger than 2 years and is rarely found in children older than 5 years. Group B *Streptococcus*, gram-negative bacilli, and *S. aureus* are common infecting organisms in the neonatal period. *S. aureus* is most common in adults; *N. gonorrhoeae* is common in adults

BOX 14-2 Organisms Involved in Septic Arthritis and Osteomyelitis of the Shoulder

Bacteria

Staphylococcus aureus

Staphylococcus epidermidis, Streptococcus group B

Escherichia coli, Pseudomonas aeruginosa, Haemophilus influenzae type B, *Neisseria gonorrhoeae, Mycobacterium tuberculosis,* and *Salmonella* and *Pneumococcus* species

Yersinia enterocolitica[66]

Fungi

Actinomyces species

Blastomyces species

Coccidioides species

Candida albicans

Sporothrix schenckii

Reported Associations

Rheumatoid arthritis: *Listeria monocytogenes*[67]

Renal transplant: *Aspergillus fumigatus*[68]

Newborns and pregnant women: Group B β-hemolytic *Streptococcus agalactiae*[69]

Lymphedema: *Pasteurella multocida*[70]

Systemic lupus erythematosus septic arthritis: *Mycobacterium xenopi*[71]

Chronic vesicoureteral reflux: *Escherichia coli*[72]

younger than 30 years.[73] Hemolytic streptococci are the most common streptococci in adults and children. Hematogenous septic arthritis in infants is primarily streptococcal, whereas hospital-acquired infections are primarily staphylococcal but can also feature *Candida* and gram-negative organisms, especially in infants.[74]

Lavy and associates reported on 19 children under the age of 2 years with *Salmonella* septic arthritis of the shoulder.[75] The authors concluded that low nutritional status was a factor in the development of bacteremia in their patients. Rarely group B β-hemolytic streptococcal infection may be associated with necrotizing fasciitis and death.[76] Necrotizing fasciitis has also been reported to be caused by *Staphylococcus aureus*.[77] *Clostridium* septic arthritis has been reported to develop spontaneously and following intra-articular steroid injection.[78]

Gram-negative bacilli such as *E. coli* and *P. aeruginosa* are found in approximately 15% of joints, especially in association with urinary tract infections, diabetes,[79] or debilitating disease. *Pseudomonas* sternoclavicular pyarthrosis is associated with IV drug use.[80] *M. tuberculosis* involves the knee, hip, ankle, and wrist more commonly than the shoulder. *Mycobacterium marinum* is found in marine environments. *Blastomyces* usually spreads from osteomyelitis to the intra-articular space. *Candida albi-*

cans can spread via the hematogenous route in debilitated patients or directly from steroid injections. Shoulder girdle abscess formation due to *Streptococcus agalactiae* has been described as a complication of esophageal dilation.[81] *Aspergillus* arthritis of the glenohumeral joint has been reported in a renal transplant patient with associated neurologic involvement. Neutropenia and corticosteroid therapy were associated immunodeficiency–inducing risk factors. *Pneumococcal* septic arthritis seems to be predominantly a disease affecting the elderly.[82]

S. aureus is often the major pathogen in biometal, bone, joint, and soft tissue infections and is the most common pathogen isolated in osteomyelitis when damaged bone or cartilage acts as a substratum.[3] The predominance of *S. aureus* in adult intra-articular sepsis may be explained by its ubiquity as a tissue pathogen seeded from remote sites, its natural invasiveness and toxicity, and its receptors for collagen, fibronectin, fibrinogen, and laminin. *S. epidermidis* is most often involved when the biomaterial surface is a polymer or when a polymer is a component of a complex device (extended-wear contact lenses,[38] vascular prostheses,[39] and total joint prostheses). *S. epidermiidis, S. aureus,* and *Propionibacterium* species are the most common organisms associated with deep infection following rotator cuff repair.[83]

Studies of chronic adult osteomyelitis have revealed polymicrobial infections in more than two thirds of cases.[3] The most common pathogens isolated included *S. aureus* and *S. epidermidis* and *Pseudomonas, Enterococcus, Streptococcus, Bacillus,* and *Proteus* species. Polymicrobial infections, therefore, appear to be an important feature of substratum-induced infections, are probably present more often than is realized, and can be a feature of chronic intra-articular sepsis and sinus formation.

In summary, *S. aureus* is the most common organism in septic infections and is usually spread via hematogenous seeding. *S. epidermidis* is the principal organism in biomaterial-related infections, especially those centered on polymers. Mixed (polymicrobial), gram-negative, and anaerobic infections are often associated with open wounds and sinus tracts.

CLINICAL PRESENTATION

Symptoms and Signs

Pain, loss of motion, and effusion are early signs of infection. Shoulder effusion is difficult to detect and is often missed. Motion is painful, and the arm is adducted and internally rotated. X-rays might show a widened glenohumeral joint space and later signs of osteomyelitis (Fig. 14-10). Systemic signs include fever, leukocytosis, and sedimentation rate changes. The symptoms of immunosuppressed and rheumatoid patients may be muted. Nolla and colleagues reported that the mean diagnostic delay in their patients with pyarthrosis and rheumatoid arthritis was 7.3 days.[84]

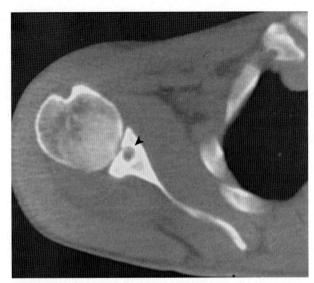

FIGURE 14-10 Staphylococcal osteomyelitis of the scapula. The *arrowhead* indicates an abscess secondary to infection caused by intra-articular steroid injection. (Courtesy of Mark Warburton, MD, High Point, NC.)

The sternoclavicular joint may be involved and should be suspected in unilateral enlargement without trauma in patients younger than 50 years. Gonococcal and staphylococcal infections have been reported. IV drug addicts are susceptible to infection by gram-negative organisms, especially *P. aeruginosa* and *Serratia marcescens*. The acromioclavicular joint is rarely involved in sepsis but may be contaminated by steroid injections. Wound infection is not uncommon after surgical resection of the distal clavicle for osteoarthritis, probably due to the proximity of the joint to the overlying skin and lack of an intervening muscle layer. Chanet and associates reported that a past history of radiation for breast cancer was a risk factor for the development of septic arthritis of the glenohumeral and sternoclavicular joints.[85] The mean time elapsed since radiation was 16 years (range, 3-34).

Gabriel and colleagues reported on a 5-week-old boy who had a brachial plexus neuropathy and paralysis of the upper extremity secondary to septic arthritis of the glenohumeral joint and osteomyelitis of the proximal part of the humerus.[86] They point out that pseudoparalysis of a limb associated with sepsis is a well-documented phenomenon. Similarly, muscular spasm associated with pain caused by infection can lead to apparent weakness. True nerve paralysis associated with osteomyelitis is uncommon, and documentation by electrodiagnostic studies is rare. Permanent weakness persisted in their patient even though the glenohumeral joint and proximal humerus were surgically drained. The possible causes of plexus neuropathy associated with infection include ischemic neuropathy from thrombophlebitis of the vasa nervorum, arterial embolism, hyperergic or hypersensitivity reactions, and local compression due to abscess formation.

Rankin and Rycken reported bilateral dislocations of the proximal humerus as a result of septic arthritis.[87] Miron and colleagues have also reported transient brachial plexus palsy associated with suppurative arthritis of the shoulder.[88]

Total Shoulder Replacement

Sepsis after total joint replacement of the shoulder is relatively rare because of prophylactic antibiotic use and the excellent blood supply of the surrounding soft tissues. Symptoms of infection include pain, loss of motion, and subluxation. Pain relief is so universal after total shoulder replacement that infection should be suspected if pain or lucency around the cement mantle are present.

Rheumatoid Arthritis

Patients with chronic rheumatoid arthritis are susceptible to spontaneous septic arthritis.[1,2] Because the active destructive process of the rheumatoid arthritis masks the septic condition, detection of infection is often delayed. The onset of septic arthritis should be suspected when the clinical course of the rheumatoid patient worsens acutely, especially if the disease is long term. When infection is present, the patient experiences a sudden aggravation of pain and swelling and increased temperature in the joint. Sudden chills can also occur. The physician should emphasize to patients with chronic rheumatoid arthritis (and to caregivers) that a sudden exacerbation of symptoms warrants investigation.

Differential Diagnosis

Roentgenograms are not very useful in the early diagnosis because septic arthritis does not significantly alter the bone destruction resulting from rheumatoid arthritis and because bone and joint radiographic changes are delayed. Other acute arthritic disorders can imitate or mask sepsis, including gout, pseudogout, rheumatic fever, juvenile rheumatoid arthritis, neuropathic arthropathy,[89] and the oligoarthritic syndromes. Trauma and tumors can cause adjacent joint effusions and must be considered.

LABORATORY EVALUATION

Culture and analysis of synovial fluid is critical for diagnosis. The joint should always be aspirated when sepsis is suspected. X-ray control is indicated if the approach is difficult about total joints. The injection of saline or simultaneous arthrogram of the glenohumeral joint may be helpful in certain cases. When the results of cultures are negative and the diagnosis is difficult to make, an arthroscopic biopsy can be useful. A synovial biopsy and culture for acid-fast organisms and fungi should be performed in patients with chronic monarticular arthritis, especially those with tenosynovitis.

Viral infection must be considered when bacteria cannot be identified. Smith and Percy report that viral arthritis is associated with rubella, parvovirus, mumps, hepatitis B, and lymphocytic choriomeningitis.[19] For a person who presents with multiple joint involvement and systemic manifestations consistent with a viral infection, serologic confirmation of the infection should be obtained because it is not usually possible to isolate the virus from joint fluid.

Synovial Fluid Analysis

If septic arthritis is suspected, the synovial fluid should be examined. Septic arthritis is probable if the leukocyte count is more than 50,000 cells/mm[3], the glucose level is low, and more than 75% of the cells are polymorphonuclear. These findings are beyond the range compatible with uncomplicated rheumatoid arthritis. In bacterial infections, aspiration can yield 10 mL or more of fluid. Synovial joint fluid is usually opaque or brownish, turbid, and thick, but it may be serosanguineous in 15% of cases with poor mucin clot. Proteins are elevated, primarily because of an elevated WBC count (usually >50,000 and often as great as 100,000, primarily neutrophils). Half of adults and a less than half of children have a joint fluid glucose level of 40 mg less than serum glucose drawn at the same time.[90-92] These findings are more common later in infection. Polymorphonuclear leukocytes are dominant (90%). Counts greater than 100,000/mm[3] are typical of staphylococcal and acute bacterial infection. Mehta and associates noted positive cultures in 96% of aspirates from patients with suspected septic arthritis when the polymorphonuclear differential count was greater than 85% of the total aspirate WBC count.[93] Monocytes are more predominant in mycobacterial infections. Rheumatoid, rheumatic, and crystalline joint diseases also elevate leukocytes, but the presence of these diseases does not exclude concomitant sepsis. Crystal examination is needed to rule out gout or pseudogout.

The results of Gram stains are positive approximately 50% of the time, but false-positive results do occur. Positive joint cultures occur in 90% of patients with established bacterial septic arthritis and in 75% of patients with tubercular arthritis.[94] Blood cultures should also be obtained, and the results are positive in approximately 50% of patients with acute infection. Some prosthesis-centered infections are difficult to detect unless tissue is biopsied and prepared for culture (Table 14-2). Culture specimens should be taken for gram-positive, gram-negative, aerobic, and anaerobic bacteria, mycobacteria, and fungi. Laboratory technique and media selection should be based on the type of antibiotic given to the patient and on the special nutrient requirements of suspected bacteria. The magnitude of anaerobic septic arthritis has been underestimated in the past.[95]

Imaging Studies

X-rays and CT scans of the septic shoulder can indicate changes ranging from widening to subluxation and from bone destruction to new bone formation (Figs. 14-11 to 14-13). Ultrasound is useful in assisting aspiration and in assessing the infected shoulder joints.[96] Positive technetium bone scanning has been reported in 75% to 100% of septic arthritis cases, but technetium, gallium, and indium scans are not always consistent.[97-99] Schmidt and colleagues found that the results of technetium bone scans performed on children with septic arthritis were

TABLE 14-2 Synovial Fluid Findings in Acute Pyogenic Arthritis

Joint Fluid Examination	Noninflammatory Fluids	Inflammatory Fluids	
		Noninfectious	*Infectious*
Color	Colorless, pale yellow	Yellow to white	Yellow
Turbidity	Clear, slightly turbid	Turbid	Turbid, purulent
Viscosity	Not reduced	Reduced	Reduced
Mucin clot	Tight clot	Friable	Friable
Cell count (per mm[3])	200-1000	3000-10,000	10,000-100,000
Predominant cell type	Mononuclear	PMN	PMN
Synovial fluid–to–blood glucose ratio	0.8-1.0	0.5-0.8	<0.5
Lactic acid	Same as plasma	Higher than plasma	Often very high
Gram stain for organism	None	None	Positive*
Culture	Negative	Negative	Positive*

*In some cases, especially in gonococcal infection, no organisms may be demonstrated.
PMN, polymorphonuclear leukocyte.
From Schmid FR: principles of diagnosis and treatment of bone and joint infections. In McCarty DJ (ed): Arthritis and Allied Conditions: A Textbook of Rheumatology. Philadelphia: Lea & Febiger, 1985, p 1638.

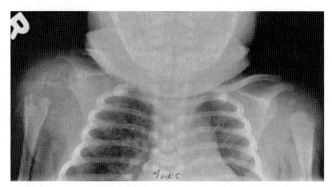

FIGURE 14-11 Septic arthritis of the right shoulder with destruction and widening of the proximal humerus. Also note healing of a right clavicle fracture. Organism is β-hemolytic streptococcus. (From the Department of Radiology, Wake Forest University Medical Center, Winston-Salem, NC.)

often negative.[74] Indium scans may be more accurate indicators of sepsis, but conclusive data are lacking. Indium scintigraphy for osteomyelitis should be preceded by a positive result on a technetium scan. If the result of an indium scan is negative, infection is unlikely. A positive result on an indium scan increases the specificity of the diagnosis. Indium uptake should be evaluated against the normal reticuloendothelial background.[99] False-negative results can occur in neonates and during the acute phase of osteomyelitis.[100]

Gupta and Prezio[101] found that the specificity of nuclear scintigraphy using ^{99m}Tc phosphonates, ^{67}Ga citrate or ^{111}In-labeled leukocytes for diagnosing musculoskeletal infection could be improved if two nucleotide studies were used in conjunction. The main limitation of scintigraphic investigations is their limited spatial resolution,

making the results inexact. Furthermore, such studies can take hours to days to complete.

CT is useful in identifying small early lytic lesions caused by osteomyelitis that might be obscured in ordinary x-rays. Diagnosis of sternoclavicular joint sepsis and clavicular osteomyelitis infections may be improved using CT, because it overcomes the tissue-overlap problem that occurs with ordinary x-rays; however, CT does not offer much advantage in imaging the humerus.

MRI can facilitate differentiation of acute from chronic osteomyelitis and can help to detect evidence of active infection in the presence of chronic inflammation or post-traumatic lesions.[102,103] Early changes of osteomyelitis cause fluid, inflammatory cell, and exudate accumulation in the marrow, producing a focus of low signal intensity within bright, fatty marrow. In chronic osteomyelitis, large areas of abnormal or low signals with MRI can indicate an area of possible sequestration and hyperemia, especially along sinus tracts.[104] Capsular distention of articular cartilage and fluid-filled spaces are clearly visible on MRI, as are damaged surfaces, loose bodies, and avascular regions. MRI can be sensitive in early detection and specific for localizing and identifying sequestra.[105-107]

De Boeck and colleagues reported on the usefulness of MRI in detecting pyomyositis.[108] MRI was useful in excluding other pathologic processes such as infectious arthritis, osteomyelitis, hematoma, thrombophlebitis, and malignant tumor. MRI is helpful in pregnant patients because it provides a highly sensitive method of detecting skeletal infection without exposing the fetus to ionizing radiation.

Ultrasound can also be used to advantage in defining abscess formation.[109] Widman and associates reported

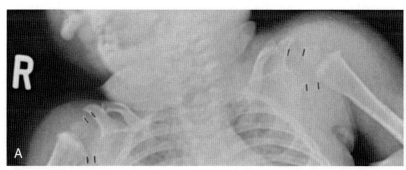

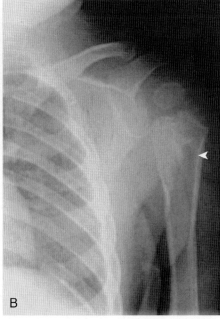

FIGURE 14-12 A, Early intra-articular sepsis of the left shoulder. Note the widening of the joint space (*markers*) compared with the opposite side. **B,** Late intra-articular sepsis. Note the lucent lesion and osteomyelitis of the proximal humerus (*arrowhead*). Organisms are *Staphylococcus epidermidis*, β-hemolytic streptococcus, and *Bacillus subtilis*.

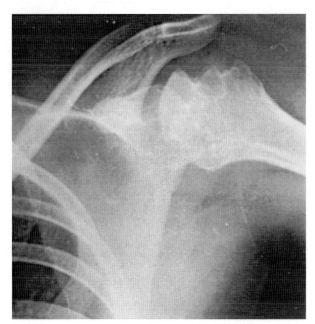

FIGURE 14-13 Cystic lesions in the humeral head consistent with tuberculosis sicca in a 19-year-old woman. (From DePalma AF [ed]: Surgery of the Shoulder, 3rd ed. Philadelphia: JB Lippincott, 1983.)

that ultrasound can be used to differentiate septic arthritis of the acromioclavicular joint from septic arthritis of the shoulder joint.[110]

Hopkins and colleagues assessed the role of gadolinium-enhanced MRI in providing diagnostic information beyond that given by nonenhanced MRI in the evaluation of musculoskeletal infectious processes.[111] They found that gadolinium-enhanced MRI was a highly sensitive technique that was especially useful in distinguishing abscesses from surrounding cellulitis or myositis. Lack of contrast enhancement ruled out infection with a high degree of certainty. However, these authors point out that contrast enhancement cannot be used to reliably distinguish infectious from noninfectious inflammatory conditions. In their study, gadolinium-enhanced MRI was found to have a very high sensitivity (89%-100%) and accuracy (79%-88%) in the diagnosis of various infectious lesions in the musculoskeletal system. However, the specificities (46%-88%) were not as high.

Tehranzadeh and colleagues have reported on the use of MRI in diagnosing osteomyelitis.[103] In several comparative studies MRI has been more advantageous in detecting the presence and determining the extent of osteomyelitis over scintigraphy, CT, and conventional radiography.

COMPLICATIONS

Inadequately treated intra-articular sepsis or osteomyelitis can result in recurrent infection, contiguous spread, bacteremia, distant septic emboli, anemia, septic shock, and death. Delayed diagnosis with adequate treatment can result in joint surface destruction, contractures, subluxation, arthritis, and growth aberrations (Fig. 14-14).[112] Inflammation, bacterial products, and lysosomal enzymes break down cartilage.[113] Within weeks, bacterial antigens stimulate destructive inflammation that can persist after

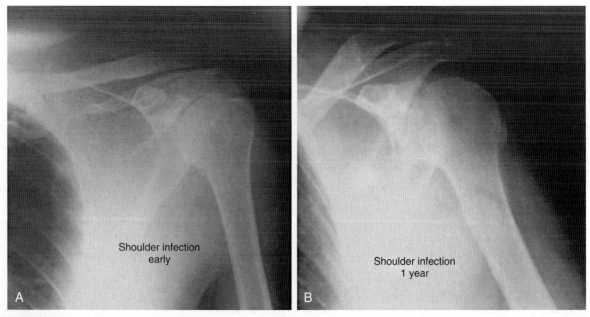

FIGURE 14-14 Hematogenous osteomyelitis secondary to intra-articular sepsis. **A,** Minimal lucency of the proximal humerus at 2 weeks after probable onset of infection. **B,** After arthrotomy, antibiotic treatment, and resolution of infection, the x-ray reveals periosteal new bone formation and joint contracture. Organism is *Staphylococcus aureus.*

the infection is treated. Bacterial endotoxins are chemo-tactic, and bacterial proteolytic enzymes further destroy surfaces. Increased intra-articular pressure also causes ischemia. Thrombotic events are also stimulated by burgeoning infection, further destroying the joint and adjacent bone. Long-term complications of chronic osteomyelitis can include amyloidosis, the nephrotic syndrome, and epidermal carcinoma.

TREATMENT

Most clinicians agree that systemic antibiotic therapy should begin immediately after the diagnosis of septic arthritis, but there is less agreement on subsequent therapy. Repeated needle aspiration has been recommended as a primary treatment.[92,114] In my opinion, drainage by urgent arthroscopy or arthrotomy is the treatment of choice, especially for the shoulder.[115,116] Forward and Hunter report the use of a small arthroscope in the treatment of septic arthritis of the shoulder in infants.[117] They recommended insertion of the arthroscope posteriorly and reported full recovery in 3 patients with a single intervention. Stutz and colleagues reported that septic arthritis in 78 joints (including 10 shoulders) could be treated with arthroscopic irrigation and systemic antibiotic therapy in 91% of the affected joints.[118] Jerosch and associates reported the successful treatment of septic arthritis by arthroscopy in 12 patients ranging between 4 and 57 years of age.[119] Jeon and colleagues reported on 19 patients who had arthroscopic irrigation and débridement for septic arthritis of the glenohumeral joint.[120] Fifteen patients had had injection into the joint preceding the development of infection. The infection was eradicated completely with a single procedure in 14 patients. Patients who had the procedure with less than 2 weeks of symptoms had better results.

In general, the literature suggests that treatment of septic arthritis with repeated needle aspiration and appropriate IV antibiotics may be adequate except for the hip. However, conclusive studies of initial surgical drainage versus needle aspiration are lacking. A retrospective study comparing 55 infected joints treated by needle aspiration with 18 joints treated surgically concluded that 60% of surgically treated patients had sequelae, whereas 80% of medically treated patients recovered completely.[121] However, it must be noted that in the only randomized prospective study comparing aspiration to arthrotomy[122] there was no difference in outcome. These authors studied 61 children in Malawi who had septic arthritis of the shoulder. Both groups received antibiotics for 6 weeks, and most of the infections were due to *Salmonella*.

Most orthopaedic surgeons believe that the anatomy of the shoulder and the nature of shoulder sepsis demand surgical treatment. Septic arthritis that does not rapidly and progressively respond to medical management should be surgically drained. Sternoclavicular joint infections in drug abusers usually involve bone and joint. For these patients, needle aspiration has not been useful in establishing the diagnosis. However, surgical drainage has been useful in providing the pathogen. It also allows débridement of necrotic bone and permits drainage of abscesses, which are often present.[123,124] Intra-articular sepsis should be treated in a timely manner.[41] Variables that influence the selection of treatment methods include the duration of infection, host immune status, types of infecting organisms, and presence of foreign bodies or adjacent osteomyelitis. The most critical factors in treatment are the infecting organism and the presence of a foreign body.

Osteomyelitis of the proximal metaphysis can precede or be secondary to septic arthritis of the glenohumeral joint (Fig. 14-15). Therefore, drilling of the metaphysis has been recommended for pediatric septic glenohumeral arthritis to rule out osteomyelitis and to allow adequate decompression of the bone.

Immobilization is usually recommended for septic arthritis. However, the study by Salter and colleagues of septic arthritis in a rabbit model indicated that the use of continuous passive motion was superior to immobilization or to intermittent active motion.[125] Possible explanations for these results include prevention of bacterial adhesion, enhanced diffusion of nutrients, improved clearance of lysosomal enzymes and debris from the infected joints, and stimulation of chondrocytes to synthesize the various components of the matrix.

Gonococcal septic arthritis may be polyarticular. Fever is low grade, usually below 102°F. Articular and periarticular structures are swollen, stiff, and painful, followed by desquamation of skin over the joints. During septicemia, a macular rash or occasionally a vesicular rash occurs in one third of patients but is also caused by *Neisseria meningitidis*, *Haemophilus* species, and *Streptobacillus* species Organisms are not common in joint fluid and therefore are not isolated in most cases. The general picture of gonococcal septic arthritis is less acute than that of staphylococcal infection. Gonococcal arthritis responds well to systemic antibiotic therapy and needle aspiration; however, in refractory cases, arthrocentesis may be required.

Antimicrobial agents used to treat joint infections generally achieve levels intra-articularly equal to or greater than serum levels except for erythromycin and gentamicin (Table 14-3). Accordingly, intra-articular antibiotics are generally not advocated. In osteomyelitis, antibiotic penetration into bone is unreliable.[126] Clindamycin achieves higher bone levels than cephalothin or methicillin. When healthy (nonsequestrated) bone in children is being treated, delivery of antibiotics to the infected site is likely. The opposite situation exists in adults, the aged, vascularly compromised patients, and patients with chronic osteomyelitis, sequestration, and sinus formation. Animal studies have suggested that antibiotic combinations (e.g., oxacillin and aminoglycosides) may be more effective in osteomyelitis.[126] The quinolone group of antibiotics may be useful because of its broad spectrum of

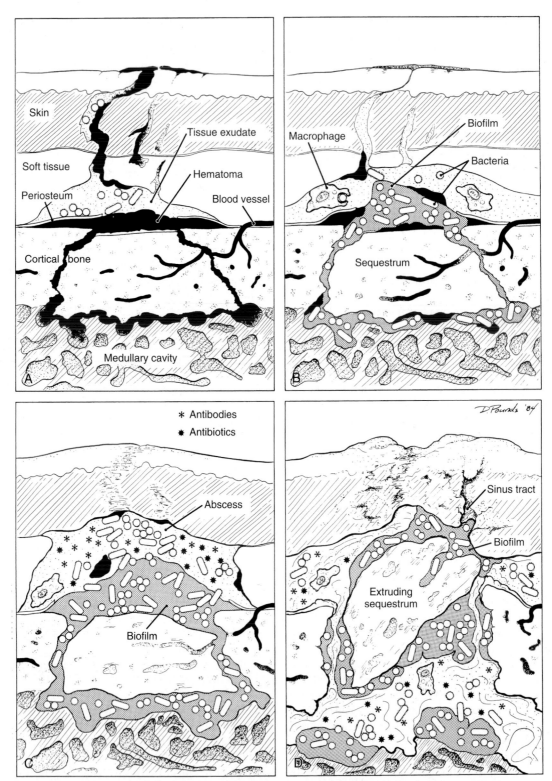

FIGURE 14-15 The sequence of pathogenesis in osteomyelitis. **A,** Initial trauma produces soft tissue destruction and bone fragmentation as well as wound contamination by bacteria. In closed wounds, contamination can occur by hematogenous seeding. **B,** As the infection progresses, bacterial colonization occurs within a protective exopolysaccharide biofilm. The biofilm is particularly abundant on the devitalized bone fragment, which acts as a passive substratum for colonization. **C,** Host defenses are mobilized against the infection but are unable to penetrate or be effective in the presence of the biofilm. **D,** Progressive inflammation and abscess formation eventually result in the development of a sinus tract and, in some cases, ultimate extrusion of the sequestrum that is the focus of the resistant infection. (From Gristina AG, Barth E, Webb LX: Microbial adhesion and the pathogenesis of biomaterial-centered infections. In Gustilo RB, Gruninger RP, Tsukayama DT [eds]: Orthopaedic Infection: Diagnosis and Treatment. Philadelphia: WB Saunders, 1989, pp 3-25.)

TABLE 14-3 Empirical Antibiotic Therapy for Septic Arthritis

	Antibiotic	
Pathology	*Preferred*	*Alternative*
<2 Months		
No organism	Oxacillin and aminoglycoside	Cefazolin and aminoglycoside
Gram-positive cocci	Oxacillin *or* nafcillin	Cephalothin *or* cephapirin
Gram-negative bacilli	Aminoglycoside	Cefotaxime
2 Months to 5 Years		
No organism	Nafcillin and chloramphenicol	Cefuroxime
Gram-positive cocci	Nafcillin or oxacillin	Cefazolin, cephalothin, vancomycin, clindamycin
Gram-negative bacilli	Aminoglycoside	Cefotaxime
Gram-negative coccobacilli	Cefotaxime *or* ampicillin and chloramphenicol	Chloramphenicol alone; trimethoprim-sulfamethoxazole
5 to 15 Years		
No organism	Nafcillin *or* oxacillin	Cefazolin *or* vancomycin
Gram-positive cocci	Nafcillin *or* oxacillin	Cefazolin, cephalothin, vancomycin, clindamycin
Gram-negative bacilli*	Aminoglycoside	Cefotaxime
Gram-negative cocci	Treat for *Neisseria gonorrhoeae*	
>40 Years		
No organism	Nafcillin ± aminoglycoside	Cefazolin ± aminoglycoside
Gram-positive cocci	Nafcillin or oxacillin	Cefazolin, cephalothin, vancomycin, clindamycin
Gram-negative bacilli	Ticarcillin + aminoglycoside	Cefotaxime ± aminoglycoside

*To 40 years.
Adapted from American Medical Association, Division of Drugs and Toxicology: Anti-microbial therapy for common infectious diseases. In American Medical Association: Drug Evaluations Annual 1995. Chicago: American Medical Association, 1995, pp 1277-1282.

activity against staphylococci, *Pseudomonas* species, and gram-negative bacteria.[127] These agents achieve excellent local levels in living and dead bone. Mutant strains can emerge but they can be reduced by intelligent use of quinolones in combination with other antibiotics.

Mader and colleagues reported that antibiotic selection should be based on in vitro sensitivity testing and that the drug exhibiting the highest bactericidal activity with the least toxicity and lowest cost should be chosen.[128] Surgical treatment must convert an infection with dead bone to a situation with well-vascularized tissues that are readily penetrated by blood-borne antibiotics. The length of antibiotic therapy is empirical and depends on the clinical response of the patient. Several (4-6) weeks of treatment has become a standard length for empirical reasons. Dirschl and Almekinders reported that combined IV and oral antibiotic therapy has become accepted as a standard treatment for osteomyelitis in children.[129] The duration of IV antibiotic therapy ranges from 3 to 14 days in various series. Close outpatient follow-up is imperative, and treatment should be continued for 4 to 6 weeks.

Treatment should be prolonged if the erythrocyte sedimentation rate does not fall below 20 mm/hour after 6 weeks. Oral antibiotic therapy has obvious economic advantages over IV therapy. The route of antibiotic delivery is probably not important as long as the infecting organism is susceptible to the antibiotic and the antibiotic is delivered to the tissues in adequate concentration to eradicate infection. The decision to use oral or parenteral antibiotics should be based on microorganism sensitivity, patient compliance, infectious disease consultation, and the surgeon's experience.[130]

Antibiotic therapy is generally continued for more than 3 weeks in septic arthritis and for more than 4 to 6 weeks in osteomyelitis and is monitored by systemic signs, WBC count, and sedimentation rate.[131] Surgical débridement is the mainstay of treatment for septic arthritis and osteomyelitis of the shoulder. The logic is as follows: Toxic products, damaged tissue, and foreign bodies must be removed to prevent damage and to treat infection effectively; laboratory studies have shown that the minimum inhibitory concentration (MIC) and minimum bactericidal concentration (MBC) levels needed to treat surface-adherent bacterial populations are 10 to 100 times higher than those for suspension populations.[8,112,132] These findings suggest that it is possible to clear a bacteremia or bacteria suspended in synovial fluid but very difficult to sterilize an infected cartilaginous joint surface or sequestrum covered with debris without administering toxic levels of antibiotics.

Antibiotic-impregnated beads (gentamicin or tobramycin) may be indicated in certain cases of osteomyelitis and articular sepsis.[133,134] Removal at 6 to 12 weeks is suggested. Closed suction and irrigation may be used for short periods (<3 days) if necessary in special cases in septic joints, provided the system does not allow retrograde contamination. However, the literature does not indicate a definite advantage with this treatment, and it is seldom required in de novo joint sepsis because adequate antibiotic levels can be achieved systemically. IV amphotericin B remains the preferred drug in patients with deep systemic fungal infections.[129] Chronic osteomyelitis requires débridement to healthy viable tissue. Débridement should be performed until punctate bleeding is noted. Local muscle flaps or vacuum-assisted closure systems may be helpful if there is associated soft tissue deficiency.

OUTCOME

The prognosis for adults with septic arthritis of the shoulder is poor, but shoulders treated soon after the onset of symptoms may do well. Poor results are associated with delayed diagnosis, virulent (gram-negative) infecting organisms, persistent pain, drainage, osteomyelitis, and destruction of the joint. Bos and associates concluded that in their series of eight children who had neonatal septic arthritis of the shoulder, early diagnosis and treatment was associated with a more favorable outcome.[135]

In a series of 16 shoulders, Gelberman and associates reported a satisfactory outcome in 8 of 10 patients with septic arthritis of the shoulder when treatment was begun 4 weeks or less after symptoms appeared.[73] Six of the 8 satisfactory results from Gelberman's series were in patients who had either infection with *Streptococcus* or coagulase-negative *Staphylococcus* species. Gelberman attributed poor results in 8 patients to delay in diagnosis, although 6 of the poor results were in patients who were infected with *S. aureus*. Pfeiffenberger and Meiss reported that in their series of 28 patients with bacterial infections of the shoulder, favorable results could only be obtained if the diagnosis was made early.[136] Bettin and colleagues found early diagnosis to be the most important determining factor concerning the final outcome of septic arthritis in their 35 elderly patients.[137]

Leslie and colleagues reviewed 18 cases of septic arthritis of the shoulder in adults.[138] The patients ranged in age from 42 to 89 years. All except 1 patient had at least one serious associated disease. Eight patients had an injection or aspiration of the shoulder before the infection developed. The diagnosis was delayed in 17 of the 18 patients. At the time of admission to the hospital, the erythrocyte sedimentation rate was always elevated but the body temperature and WBC count were not. After treatment, the functional result was usually poor. Only 5 patients regained forward flexion to 90 degrees or more; 8 patients had no active motion of the glenohumeral joint, and 2 patients died. Arthrotomy appeared to have a better result than did repeated aspiration.

Leslie and colleagues noted that five of six patients with septic arthritis who had rotator cuff tears had a marked discrepancy between active and passive shoulder motion.[138] They noted that the poor functional results recorded in these six patients may have been more of a reflection of the rotator cuff tear than of damage to the articular cartilage as a result of infection. Septic arthritis following rotator cuff surgery rarely results in exposure of the humeral head and formation of sinus tracts. In such cases, interposition of a muscle flap may be required, as has been described for the closure of infected sternotomy wounds.[139]

Smith and Piercy reported that the characteristics of patients with bacterial arthritis for whom a poor outcome is expected include age greater than 60 years, preexisting rheumatoid arthritis, infection in the shoulder, duration of symptoms before treatment for more than 1 week, involvement of more than four joints, and persistently positive cultures after a 7-day course with appropriate antibiotic therapy.[19] Smith and associates reported mortality in 3 of 15 rheumatoid patients with sepsis of the shoulder.[140] Nine patients had multiple joint infections. Unsatisfactory shoulder function was common, and mean forward elevation was 100 degrees.

Deep infection following rotator cuff repair is uncommon. Nevertheless, when such infection occurs, numerous procedures are usually required in order to eradicate the infection. Such patients are often afebrile with normal WBC counts but do have elevated erythrocyte sedimentation rates. Patients rarely recover overhead shoulder function. Extensive débridement, often combined with a muscle transfer and antibiotics, were required to control the infection in the series of Mirzayan and associates.[83]

Haidukewych and Sperling reported on the treatment of 15 infected humeral nonunions, of which 4 were proximal.[141] All patients were treated with débridement and antibiotics, and 10 patients had attempts to achieve bony union. Only 7 of these 10 patients achieved bony union, although pain relief was predictable in most patients.

Duncan and associates reviewed six patients who had infection following a clavicle fracture.[142] Five of the six infections occurred in association with open reduction and internal fixation. Three infections were polymicrobial and three were single-organism infections. Only two patients went on to bony union of their fractures. Infection following clavicle fracture is extremely difficult to treat and has a poor prognosis. Sperling and associates reviewed six patients who developed infection following shoulder instability surgery.[143] Three patients had late infections manifesting more than 8 months after surgery. Each of these three patients had a sinus leading to a retained nonabsorbable suture. Three patients had polymicrobial infections and three had single-organism infections. None of the patients developed recurrent shoulder instability. Infection may be acute or significantly delayed following surgery for shoulder instability, and if it occurs late, it may be associated with a nidus of infection surrounding nonabsorbable sutures.

Ross and Shamsuddin reviewed 180 cases of sternoclavicular septic arthritis.[144] Risk factors included IV drug use, distant site of infection, diabetes mellitus, trauma, and an infected central line. No risk factor was found in 23% of the cases. The mean age of the patients was 45 years, and 73% of the patients were male. *S. aureus* was isolated in 49% of the cases. Sternoclavicular septic arthritis accounts for 1% of septic arthritis in the general population and 17% in IV drug users, possibly due to attempted local injections with inadequate antisepsis. CT or MRI should be performed to rule out associated abscess formation or mediastinitis. Surgical drainage, antibiotics and, in some cases, pectoralis major muscle flap procedures were required to control the infection.

The majority of children do well after treatment for septic shoulder arthritis. In a study of nine children with glenohumeral arthritis, Schmidt and associates suggested surgical treatment with exploration of the biceps tendon sheath.[74] Growth center damage is possible. Lejman and colleagues reported that almost all patients had reduced motion as a sequela of septic arthritis occurring during the first 18 months of life.[145] Although only 7% of the humeral heads were normal in their series of 42 patients, the range of motion could not be predicted from the shape of the humeral head. Saisu and associates noted humeral shortening and inferior subluxation as sequelae of septic arthritis of the shoulder in neonates and infants when arthrotomy was performed more than 10 days after the onset of the infection.[146]

Mileti and colleagues reported on 13 patients who underwent shoulder arthroplasty for the treatment of postinfectious glenohumeral arthritis.[147] No patient had a recurrence of infection; mean follow-up was 9.7 years. Pain decreased and motion improved in their patients. Shoulder abduction improved from 75 degrees to 117 degrees, and mean external rotation improved from 13 degrees to 36 degrees. They concluded that shoulder arthroplasty for the treatment of the sequelae of an infected shoulder can be performed with a low risk of reinfection.

Refractory clavicular infection may require clavicular resection. Krishnan and associates report a high complication rate following claviculectomy, although functional outcome was good in their group of six patients.[148]

Wick and colleagues treated 15 patients with septic arthritis by shoulder arthrodesis.[149] Antibiotics were administered for 6 weeks. A positive outcome was more common in patients younger than 50 years and in patients who had fewer than four previous procedures. I have rarely performed shoulder arthrodesis to treat infection.

Resection arthroplasty is a rare option for failed shoulder replacement and/or chronic infection of the shoulder joint. Risploi and colleagues reported on 18 patients who underwent resection arthroplasty with a mean follow-up of 8.3 years.[150] Although pain was decreased by the procedure, 15 patients continued to have moderate to severe pain. Mean active elevation was 70 degrees. Most shoulders were comfortable at rest with profound functional limitations.

PREVENTION

Antibiotic prophylaxis is effective because bacteria are cleared before they establish surface-adherent, rapidly growing populations at sites deep within bone or on biomaterials. I suggest using antibiotic prophylaxis, such as cefazolin 2 g IV at anesthesia.[151] The use of prophylactic antibiotics is suggested for all implant surgery, including both prosthetic and internal fixation of fractures. The antibiotic used varies according to the special conditions of each case and patient.[152] Treatment for 24 hours in clean cases is believed to be sufficient.

Open wounds involving joints are by definition contaminated, even though bacteria are not always detected. Type 3 open fractures, especially those involving joints, have a very high rate of infection. Open fractures should be treated either with cefazolin or with a combination of cefazolin and gentamicin.[152]

AUTHOR'S PREFERRED METHOD OF TREATMENT

Either an arthroscopic or an open approach can be used to drain the shoulder joint. If arthroscopy is used, the surgeon should use multiple portals to facilitate drainage and insert instruments for débridement.

When performing open drainage, I use an anterior deltopectoral approach. The deltoid and coracoid are not detached. Infected surfaces are débrided of adherent clot and other debris. Lavage of the joint with saline or saline mixed with bacitracin is an appropriate technique. In most cases, the wound may be loosely closed and a large Hemovac is inserted for 24 hours to remove postsurgical accumulations. In cases of chronic sepsis or infection by gram-negative organisms, the wound is packed open and allowed to close spontaneously, with daily packing changes. Adequate intra-articular concentrations of antibiotics can be achieved by IV administration.[153] The duration of antibiotic treatment varies, depending on the host and organism; 3 weeks of IV therapy followed by 3 weeks of oral treatment is a reasonable base. The patient's response is the key to duration of treatment.

SUMMARY

Intra-articular shoulder sepsis presents many challenges in diagnosis and treatment. Sepsis following shoulder arthroplasty is seen more often now due to the number of arthroplasties inserted. The shoulder anatomy is unique in that bursae communicating with the joint can provide a pathway for bacteria for which cartilage is the target substratum. Successful treatment depends on the immune system response, the type of infecting organism, early surgical débridement, and effective antibiotic treatment.

REFERENCES

1. Gristina AG, Rovere GD, Shoji H: Spontaneous septic arthritis complicating rheumatoid arthritis. J Bone Joint Surg Am 56:1180-1184, 1974.
2. Kellgren JH, Ball J, Fairbrother RW, Barnes KL: Suppurative arthritis complicating rheumatoid arthritis. BMJ 1:1193-1200, 1958.
3. Gristina AG, Oga M, Webb LX, Hobgood CD: Adherent bacterial colonization in the pathogenesis of osteomyelitis. Science 228:990-993, 1985.
4. Gristina AG: Biomaterial-centered infection: Microbial adhesion versus tissue integration. Science 237:1558-1595, 1987.
5. Gristina AG, Romano RL, Kammire GC, Webb LX: Total shoulder replacement. Orthop Clin North Am 18:445-453, 1987.
6. Neer CS, Kirby RM: Revision of humeral head and total shoulder arthroplasties. Clin Orthop Relat Res 170:189-195, 1982.
7. Gristina AG, Costerton JW: Bacterial adherence to biomaterials and tissue. The significance of its role in clinical sepsis. J Bone Joint Surg Am 67:264-273, 1985.
8. Gristina AG, Hobgood CD, Webb LX, Myrvik QN: Adhesive colonization of biomaterials and antibiotic resistance. Biomaterials 8:423-426, 1987.
9. Voytek A, Gristina G, Barth E, et al: Staphylococcal adhesion to collagen in intra-articular sepsis. Biomaterials 9:107-110, 1988.
10. Codman EA: The Shoulder. Rupture of the Supraspinatus Tendon and Other Lesions in or About the Subacromial Bursa, 2nd ed. Malabar, Fla: Robert E. Kreiger, 1984.
11. Trueta J: The normal vascular anatomy of the human femoral head during growth. J Bone Joint Surg Br 39:358-394, 1957.
12. Trueta J: The three types of acute hematogenous osteomyelitis: A clinical and vascular study. J Bone Joint Surg Br 41:671-680, 1959.
13. Clemente C (ed): Gray's Anatomy of the Human Body, 5th ed. Philadelphia: Lea & Febiger, 1985.
14. Chung SMK: The arterial supply of the developing proximal end of the human femur. J Bone Joint Surg Am 58:961-970, 1976.
15. Hunter W: Of the structures and diseases of articulating cartilage. Philos Trans R Soc Lond 42:514-521, 1743.
16. Ward WG, Eckardt JJ: Subacromial/subdeltoid bursa abscesses: An overlooked diagnosis. Clin Orthop Relat Res (288):189-194, 1993.
17. Speziale P, Raucci G, Visai L, et al: Binding of collagen to Staphylococcus aureus Cowan 1. J Bacteriol 167:77-81, 1986.
18. Bhawan J, Das Tandon H, Roy S: Ultrastructure of synovial membrane in pyogenic arthritis. Arch Pathol 96:155-160, 1973.
19. Smith JW, Piercy EA: Infectious arthritis. Clin Infect Dis 20:225-231, 1995.
20. Bigliani LU, Flatow EL, Deliz ED: Complications of shoulder arthroscopy. Orthop Rev 20(9):743-751, 1991.
21. Armstrong RW, Bolding F: Septic arthritis after arthroscopy: The contributing roles of intraarticular steroids and environmental factors. Am J Infect Control 22(1):16-18, 1994.
22. Broadwater JR, Stair JM: Sternoclavicular osteomyelitis: Coverage with a pectoralis major muscle flap. Surg Rounds Orthop 2:47-50, 1988.
23. Manny J, Haruzi I, Yosipovitch Z: Osteomyelitis of the clavicle following subclavian vein catheterization. Arch Surg 106:342-343, 1973.
24. Srivastava KK, Garg LD, Kochhar VL: Tuberculous osteomyelitis of the clavicle. Acta Orthop Scand 45:668-672, 1974.
25. Wray TM, Bryant RE, Killen DA: Sternal osteomyelitis and costochondritis after median sternotomy. J Thorac Cardiovasc Surg 65:227-233, 1973.
26. Brancos MA, Peris P, Miro JM, et al: Septic arthritis in heroin addicts. Semin Arthritis Rheum 21(2):81-87, 1991.
27. Chaudhuri K, Lonergan D, Portek I, McGuigan L: Septic arthritis of the shoulder after mastectomy and radiotherapy for breast carcinoma. J Bone Joint Surg Br 75(2):318-321, 1993.
28. Morrey BF, Bianco AJ: Hematogenous osteomyelitis of the clavicle in children. Clin Orthop Relat Res 125:24-28, 1977.
29. Gowans JDC, Granieri PA: Septic arthritis, its relation to intra-articular injections of hydrocortisone acetate. N Engl J Med 261:502-504, 1959.
30. Kelly PJ, Fitzgerald RH Jr: Bacterial arthritis. In Braude AI, Davis CE, Fierer J (eds): Infectious Diseases and Medical Microbiology, 2nd ed. Philadelphia: WB Saunders, 1986, pp 1468-1472.
31. Ward WG, Goldner RD: Shoulder pyarthrosis: A concomitant process. Orthopedics 17(7):591-595, 1994.
32. Ejlertsen T, Dossing K: Pneumococcal pyomyositis secondary to pneumonia. Scand J Infect Dis 29(5):520-521, 1997.
33. Aglas F, Gretler J, Rainer F, Krejs GJ: Sternoclavicular septic arthritis: A rare but serious complication of subclavian venous catheterization. Clin Rheumatol 13(3):507-512, 1994.
34. Kirschenbaum AE, Rizzo C: Glenohumeral pyarthrosis following acupuncture treatment. Orthopedics 20(12):1184-1186, 1997.
35. Lossos IS, Yossepowitch O, Kandel L, et al: Septic arthritis of the glenohumeral joint. A report of 11 cases and review of the literature. Medicine (Baltimore) 77(3):177-187, 1998.
36. Birinyi LK, Douville C, Lewis SA, et al: Increased resistance to bacteremic graft infection after endothelial cell seeding. J Vasc Surg 5:193-197, 1987.
37. Hamill RJ, Vann JM, Proctor RA: Phagocytosis of Staphylococcus aureus by cultured bovine aortic endothelial cells: Model for postadherence events in endovascular infections. Infect Immun 54:833-836, 1986.
38. Slusher MM, Myrvik QN, Lewis JC, Gristina AG: Extended-wear lenses, biofilm, and bacterial adhesion. Arch Ophthalmol 105:110-115, 1987.
39. Webb LX, Myers RT, Cordell AR, et al: Inhibition of bacterial adhesion by antibacterial surface pretreatment of vascular prostheses. J Vasc Surg 4:16-21, 1986.
40. Avery JK (ed): Oral Development and Histology. Baltimore: Williams & Wilkins, 1987.
41. Holderbaum D, Spech T, Ehrhart L, et al: Collagen binding in clinical isolates of Staphylococcus aureus. J Clin Microbiol 25:2258-2261, 1987.
42. Switalski LM, Ryden C, Rubin K, et al: Binding of fibronectin to Staphylococcus strains. Infect Immun 42:628-633, 1983.
43. Smith RL Schurman DJ: Comparison of cartilage destruction between infectious and adjuvant arthritis. J Orthop Res 1:136-143, 1983.
44. Smith RL, Schurman DJ, Kajiyama G, et al: The effect of antibiotics on the destruction of cartilage in experimental infectious arthritis. J Bone Joint Surg Am 69:1063-1068, 1987.
45. Speers DJ, Nade SML: Ultrastructural studies of adherence of Staphylococcus aureus in experimental acute haematogenous osteomyelitis. Infect Immun 49:443-446, 1985.
46. Eggink BH, Rowen JL: Primary osteomyelitis and suppurative arthritis caused by coagulase-negative staphylococci in a preterm neonate. Pediatr Infect Dis J 22:572-573, 2003.
47. Master R, Weisman MH, Armbuster TG, et al: Septic arthritis of the glenohumeral joint. Unique clinical and radiographic features and a favorable outcome. Arthritis Rheum 10:1500-1506, 1977.
48. Kelly PJ, Conventry MB, Martin WJ: Bacterial arthritis of the shoulder. Mayo Clin Proc 40:695-699, 1965.
49. Caksen H, Ozturk MK, Uzum K, et al: Septic arthritis in childhood. Pediatr Int 42(5):534-540, 2000.
50. Epps CH Jr, Bryant DD 3rd, Coles MJ, Castro O: Osteomyelitis in patients who have sickle-cell disease. Diagnosis and management. J Bone Joint Surg Am 73(9):1281-1294, 1991.
51. Wrangstadh M, Conway PL, Kjelleberg S: The production and release of an extracellular polysaccharide during starvation of a marine Pseudomonas sp. and the effect thereof on adhesion. Arch Microbiol 145:220-227, 1986.
52. Costerton JW, Geesey GG, Cheng K-J: How bacteria stick. Sci Am 238:86-95, 1978.
53. Marrie TJ, Costerton JW: Prolonged survival of Serratia marcescens in chlorhexidine. Appl Environ Microbiol 42:1093-1102, 1981.
54. Govan JRW, Fyfe JAM: Mucoid Pseudomonas aeruginosa and cystic fibrosis: Resistance of the mucoid form to carbenicillin, flucloxacillin and tobramycin and the isolation of mucoid variants in vitro. J Antimicrob Chemother 4:233-240, 1978.
55. Baltimore RS, Mitchell M: Immunologic investigations of mucoid strains of Pseudomonas aeruginosa: Comparison of susceptibility to opsonic antibody in mucoid and nonmucoid strains. J Infect Dis 141:238-247, 1980.
56. Schwarzmann S, Boring JR III: Antiphagocytic effect of slime from a mucoid strain of Pseudomonas aeruginosa. Infect Immun 3:762-767, 1971.
57. Gibbons RJ, Van Houte J: Dental caries. Annu Rev Med 26:121-136, 1975.
58. Watt PJ, Ward ME: Adherence of Neisseria gonorrhoeae and other Neisseria species to mammalian cells. In Beachey EH (ed): Bacterial Adherence. Receptors and Recognition, series B, vol 6. London: Chapman & Hall, 1980, pp 251-288.
59. Woods DE, Bass JA, Johanson WG Jr, Straus DC: Role of adherence in the pathogenesis of Pseudomonas aeruginosa lung infection in cystic fibrosis patients. Infect Immun 30:694-699, 1980.
60. Gristina AG, Rovere GD: An in vitro study of the effects of metals used in internal fixation on bacterial growth and dissemination. J Bone Joint Surg Am 45:1104, 1963.
61. Jones GW, Isaacson RE: Proteinaceous bacterial adhesins and their receptors. Crit Rev Microbiol 10:229-260, 1984.
62. Tromp RM, Hamers RJ, Demuth JE: Quantum states and atomic structure of silicon surfaces. Science 234:304-309, 1986.

63. Albrektsson T: The response of bone to titanium implants. Crit Rev Biocompat 1:53-84, 1985.

64. Kasemo B, Lausmaa J: Surface science aspects on inorganic biomaterials. Crit Rev Biocompat 2:335-380, 1986.

65. Baier RE, Meyer AE, Natiella JR, et al: Surface properties determine bioadhesive outcomes: Methods and results. J Biomed Mater Res 18:337-355, 1984.

66. Tiddia F, Cherchi GB, Pacifico L, Chiesa C: *Yersinia enterocolitica* causing suppurative arthritis of the shoulder. J Clin Pathol 47(8):760-761, 1994.

67. Ukkonen HJ, Vuori KP, Lehtonen OP, Kotilainen PM: *Listeria monocytogenes* arthritis of several joints. Scand J Rheumatol 24(6):392-394, 1995.

68. Franco M, Van Elslande L, Robino C, et al: *Aspergillus* arthritis of the shoulder in a renal transplant recipient. Failure of itraconazole therapy. Rev Rhum Engl Ed 62(3):215-218, 1995.

69. Garcia S, Combalia A, Segur JM: Septic arthritis of the shoulder due to *Streptococcus agalactiae*. Acta Orthop Belg 62(1):66-68, 1996.

70. Fellows L, Boivin M, Kapusta M: *Pasteurella multocida* arthritis of the shoulder associated with postsurgical lymphedema. J Rheumatol 23(10):1824-1825, 1996.

71. Rutten MJ, van den Berg JC, van den Hoogen FH, Lemmens JA: Nontuberculous mycobacterial bursitis and arthritis of the shoulder. Skeletal Radiol 27(1):33-35, 1998.

72. Egan SC, LaSalle MD, Stock JA, Hanna MK: Septic arthritis secondary to vesicoureteral reflux into single ectopic ureter. Pediatr Nephrol 13(9):932-933, 1999.

73. Gelberman RH, Menon J, Austerlitz S, Weisman MH: Pyogenic arthritis of the shoulder in adults. J Bone Joint Surg Am 62:550-553, 1980.

74. Schmidt D, Mubarak S, Gelberman R: Septic shoulders in children. J Pediatr Orthop 1:67-72, 1981.

75. Lavy CB, Lavy VR, Anderson I: Salmonella septic arthritis of the shoulder in Zambian children. J R Coll Surg Edinb 41(3):197-199, 1996.

76. Batalis, NI, Caplan MJ, Schandl CA: Acute deaths in nonpregnant adults due to invasive streptococcal infections. Am J Forensic Med Pathol 28:63-68, 2007.

77. Lee YT, Chou TD, Peng MY, Chang FY: Rapidly progressive necrotizing fasciitis caused by *Staphylococcus aureus*. Microbiol Immunol Infect 38:361-364, 2005.

78. Goon PK, O'Brien M, Titley OG: Spontaneous *clostridium septicum* arthritis of the shoulder and gas gangrene: A case report. J Bone Joint Surg Am 87:874-877, 2005.

79. Barzaga RA, Nowak PA, Cunha BA: *Escherichia coli* septic arthritis of a shoulder in a diabetic patient. Heart Lung 20(6):692-693, 1991.

80. Kaw D, Yoon Y: *Pseudomonas* sternoclavicular pyarthrosis. South Med J 97:705-706, 2004.

81. Popa A, Fenster J, Jacob H, Gleich S: Shoulder girdle abscess due to *Streptococcus agalactiae* complicating esophageal dilatation. Am J Gastroenterol 94(5):1410-1411, 1999.

82. Bertone C, Rivera F, Avallone F, et al: Pneumococcal septic arthritis of the shoulder. Case report and literature review. Panminerva Med 44(2):151-154, 2002.

83. Mirzayan R, Itamura JM, Vangsness CT Jr, et al: Management of chronic deep infection following rotator cuff repair. J Bone Joint Surg Am 82:1115-1121, 2000.

84. Nolla JM, Gomez-Vaquero C, Fiter J, et al: Pyarthrosis in patients with rheumatoid arthritis: A detailed analysis of 10 cases and literature review. Semin Arthritis Rheum 30:121-126, 2000.

85. Chanet V, Soubrier M, Ristori JM, et al: Septic arthritis as a late complication of carcinoma of the breast. Rheumatology 44:1157-1160, 2005.

86. Gabriel SR, Thometz JG, Jaradeh S: Septic arthritis associated with brachial plexus neuropathy. J Bone Joint Surg Am 78:103-105, 1996.

87. Rankin KC, Rycken JM: Bilateral dislocation of the proximal humeral epiphyses in septic arthritis: A case report. J Bone Joint Surg Br 75(2):329, 1993.

88. Miron D, Bor N, Cutai M, Horowitz J: Transient brachial palsy associated with suppurative arthritis of the shoulder. Pediatr Infect Dis J 16(3):326-327, 1997.

89. Louthrenoo W, Ostrov BE, Park YS, et al: Pseudoseptic arthritis: An unusual presentation of neuropathic arthropathy. Ann Rheum Dis 50(10):717-721, 1991.

90. Jackson MA, Nelson JD: Etiology and medical management of acute suppurative bone and joint infections in pediatric patients. J Pediatr Orthop 2:313-323, 1982.

91. Sharp JT, Lidsky MD, Duffey J, Duncan MW: Infectious arthritis. Arch Intern Med 139:1125-1130, 1979.

92. Ward JR, Atcheson SG: Infectious arthritis. Med Clin North Am 61:313-329, 1977.

93. Mehta P, Schnall SB, Zalavras CG: Septic arthritis of the shoulder, elbow and wrist. Clin Orthop Relat Res (451):42-45, 2006.

94. Wallace R, Cohen AS: Tuberculous arthritis. A report of two cases with review of biopsy and synovial fluid findings. Am J Med 61:277-282, 1976.

95. Fitzgerald RH, Rosenblatt JE, Tenney JH, Bourgault A-M: Anaerobic septic arthritis. Clin Orthop Relat Res 164:141-148, 1982.

96. Gompels BM, Darlington LG: Septic arthritis in rheumatoid disease causing bilateral shoulder dislocation: Diagnosis and treatment assisted by grey scale ultrasonography. Ann Rheum Dis 40:609-611, 1981.

97. Gentry LO: Osteomyelitis: Options for diagnosis and management. J Antimicrob Chemother 21(Suppl):115-128, 1988.

98. Merkel KD, Brown ML, DeWanjee MK, Fitzgerald RH: Comparison of indium-labeled leukocyte imaging with sequential technetium–gallium scanning in the diagnosis of low-grade musculoskeletal sepsis. J Bone Joint Surg Am 67:465-476, 1985.

99. Wukich DK, Abreu SH, Callaghan JJ, et al: Diagnosis of infection by preoperative scintigraphy with indium-labeled white blood cells. J Bone Joint Surg Am 69:1353-1360, 1987.

100. Garnett ES, Cockshott WP, Jacob J: Classical acute osteomyelitis with a negative bone scan. Br J Radiol 50:757-760, 1977.

101. Gupta NC, Prezio JA: Radionuclide imaging in osteomyelitis. Semin Nucl Med 18:287-299, 1988.

102. Berquist TH, Brown M, Fitzgerald R, et al: Magnetic resonance imaging: Application in musculoskeletal infection. Magn Reson Imaging 3:219-230, 1985.

103. Tehranzadeh J, Wang F, Mesgarzadeh M: Magnetic resonance imaging of osteomyelitis. Crit Rev Diagn Imaging 33:495-534, 1992.

104. David R, Barron BJ, Madewell JE: Osteomyelitis, acute and chronic. Radiol Clin North Am 25:1171-1201, 1987.

105. Fletcher BD, Scoles PV, Nelson AD: Osteomyelitis in children: Detection by magnetic resonance. Radiology 150:57-60, 1984.

106. Hendrix RW, Fisher MR: Imaging of septic arthritis. Clin Rheum Dis 12:459-487, 1986.

107. Sartoris DJ, Resnick D: Magnetic resonance imaging for musculoskeletal disorders. Western J Med 148:102-109, 1988.

108. De Boeck H, Noppen L, Desprechins B: Pyomyositis of the adductor muscles mimicking an infection of the hip. Diagnosis by magnetic resonance imaging: A case report. J Bone Joint Surg Am 76:747-750, 1994.

109. Steiner GM, Sprigg A: The value of ultrasound in the assessment of bone. Br J Radiol 65(775):589-593, 1992.

110. Widman DS, Craig JG, van Holsbeeck MT: Sonographic detection, evaluation and aspiration of infected acromioclavicular joints. Skeletal Radiol 30(7):388-392, 2001.

111. Hopkins KL, Li KC, Bergman G: Gadolinium-DTPA-enhanced magnetic resonance imaging of musculoskeletal infectious processes. Skeletal Radiol 24:325-330, 1995.

112. O'Meara PM, Bartal E: Septic arthritis: Process, etiology, treatment outcome: A literature review. Orthopedics 11:623-628, 1988.

113. Klein RS: Joint infection, with consideration of underlying disease and sources of bacteremia in hematogenous infection. Clin Geriatr Med 4:375-394, 1988.

114. Kelly PJ, Martin WJ, Coventry MD: Bacterial (suppurative) arthritis in the adult. J Bone Joint Surg Am 52:1595-1602, 1970.

115. Karten I: Septic arthritis complicating rheumatoid arthritis. Ann Intern Med 70:1147-1151, 1969.

116. Rimoin DL, Wennberg JE: Acute septic arthritis complicating chronic rheumatoid arthritis. JAMA 196:617-621, 1966.

117. Forward DP, Hunter JB: Arthroscopic washout of the shoulder for septic arthritis in infants. A new technique. J Bone Joint Surg Br 84(8):1173-1175, 2002.

118. Stutz G, Kuster MS, Kleinstuck F, Gachter A: Arthroscopic management of septic arthritis: Stages of infection and results. Knee Surg Sports Traumatol Arthrosc 8(5):270-274, 2000.

119. Jerosch J, Hoffstetter I, Schroder M, Castro WH: Septic arthritis: Arthroscopic management with local antibiotic treatment. Acta Orthop Belg 61(2):126-134, 1995.

120. Jeon IH, Choi CH, Seo KJ, et al: Arthroscopic management of septic arthritis of the shoulder joint. J Bone Joint Surg Am 88:1802-1806, 2006.

121. Goldenberg DL, Reed JI: Bacterial arthritis. N Engl J Med 312:764-771, 1985.

122. Smith SP, Thyoka M, Lavy CB, Pitani A: Septic arthritis of the shoulder in children in Malawi. A randomised, prospective study of aspiration versus arthrotomy and washout. J Bone Joint Surg Br 84(8):1167-1172, 2002.

123. Bayer AS, Chow AW, Louie JS, et al: Gram-negative bacillary septic arthritis: Clinical, radiologic, therapeutic, and prognostic features. Semin Arthritis Rheum 7:123-132, 1977.

124. Roca RP, Yoshikawa TT: Primary skeletal infections in heroin users: A clinical characterization, diagnosis and therapy. Clin Orthop Relat Res (144):238-248, 1979.

125. Salter RB, Bell RS, Keeley FW: The protective effect of continuous passive motion in living articular cartilage in acute septic arthritis: An experimental investigation in the rabbit. Clin Orthop Relat Res 159:223-247, 1981.

126. Norden C: Experimental osteomyelitis. IV. Therapeutic trials with rifampin alone and in combination with gentamicin, sisomicin, and cephalothin. J Infect Dis 132:493-499, 1975.

127. Desplaces N, Acar JF: New quinolones in the treatment of joint and bone infections. Rev Infect Dis 10(Suppl 1):S179-S183, 1988.

128. Mader JT, Landon GC, Calhoun J: Antimicrobial treatment of osteomyelitis. Clin Orthop Relat Res 295:87-95, 1993.

129. Dirschl DR, Almekinders LC: Osteomyelitis: Common causes and treatment recommendations. Drugs 45:29-43, 1993.

130. Lazzarini L, Mader JT, Calhoun JH: Osteomyelitis in long bones. J Bone Joint Surg Am 86:2305-2318, 2004.

131. Norden CW: A critical review of antibiotic prophylaxis in orthopedic surgery. Rev Infect Dis 5:928-932, 1983.

132. Ladd TI, Schmiel D, Nickel JC, Costerton JW: Rapid method for detection of adherent bacteria on Foley urinary catheters. J Clin Microbiol 21:1004-1006, 1985.

133. Flick AB, Herbert JC, Goodell J, Kristiansen T: Noncommercial fabrication of antibiotic-impregnated polymethylmethacrylate beads. Technical note. Clin Orthop Relat Res 223:282-286, 1987.

134. Goodell JA, Flick AB, Hebert JC, Howe JG: Preparation and release characteristics of tobramycin-impregnated polymethylmethacrylate beads. Am J Hosp Pharm 43:1454-1460, 1986.

135. Bos CF, Mol LJ, Obermann WR, Tjin a Ton ER: Late sequelae of neonatal septic arthritis of the shoulder. J Bone Joint Surg Br 80(4):645-650, 1998.

136. Pfeiffenberger J, Meiss L: Septic conditions of the shoulder—an updating of treatment strategies. Arch Orthop Trauma Surg 115(6):325-331, 1996.

137. Bettin D, Schul B, Schwering L: Diagnosis and treatment of joint infections in elderly patients. Acta Orthop Belg 64(2):131-135, 1998.

138. Leslie BM, Harris JM, Driscoll D: Septic arthritis of the shoulder in adults. J Bone Joint Surg Am 71:1516-1522, 1989.

139. Fansa H, Handstein S, Schneider W: Treatment of infected median sternotomy wounds with a myocutaneous latissimus dorsi muscle flap. Scand Cardiovasc J 32(1):33-39, 1998.

140. Smith AM, Sperling JW, Cofield RH: Outcomes are poor after treatment of sepsis in the rheumatoid shoulder. Clin Orthop Relat Res (439):68-73, 2005.

141. Haidukewych GJ, Sperling KW: Results of treatment of infected humeral nonunions: The Mayo Clinic experience. Clin Orthop Relat Res (414):25-30, 2003.

142. Duncan SF, Sperling JW, Steinmann S: Infection after clavicular fracture. Clin Orthop Relat Res (439):74-78, 2005.

143. Sperling JW, Cofield RH, Torchia ME, Hanssen AD: Infection after shoulder instability surgery. Clin Orthop Rel Res (414):61-64, 2003.

144. Ross JJ, Shamsuddin H: Sternoclavicular septic arthritis: Review of 180 cases. Medicine (Baltimore) 83:139-148, 2004.

145. Lejman T, Strong M. Michno P, Hayman M: Septic arthritis of the shoulder during the first 18 months of life. J Pediatr Orthop 15(2):172-175, 1995.

146. Saisu T, Kawashima A, Kamegaya M, et al: Humeral shortening and inferior subluxation as sequelae of septic arthritis of the shoulder in neonates and infants. J Bone Joint Surg Am 89:1784-1793, 2007.

147. Mileti J, Sperling JW, Cofield RH: Shoulder arthroplasty for the treatment of postinfectious glenohumeral arthritis. J Bone Joint Surg Am 85:609-614, 2003.

148. Krishnan SG, Schiffern SC, Pennington SD, et al: Functional outcome after total claviculectomy as a salvage procedure. A series of six cases. J Bone Joint Surg Am 89:1215-1219, 2007.

149. Wick M, Muller EJ, Ambacher T, et al: Arthrodesis of the shoulder after septic arthritis. Long term results. J Bone Joint Surg Br 85:666-670, 2003.

150. Rispoli DM, Sperling JW, Athwal, et al: Pain relief and functional results after resection arthroplasty of the shoulder. J Bone Joint Surg Br 89:184-187, 2007.

151. Neu HC: Cephalosporin antibiotics as applied in surgery of bones and joints. Clin Orthop Relat Res 190:50-64, 1984.

152. Patzakis MJ, Wilkins M, Moore TM: Use of antibiotics in open tibial fractures. Clin Orthop Relat Res 178:31-35, 1983.

153. Nelson JD: Antibiotic concentrations in septic joint effusions. N Engl J Med 284:349-353, 1971.

Fractures, Dislocations, and Acquired Problems of the Shoulder in Children

Paul D. Choi, MD, Gilbert Chan, MD, David L. Skaggs, MD, and John M. Flynn, MD

FRACTURES OF THE PROXIMAL HUMERUS

Anatomy

Embryology and Development

The formation of the humerus begins with the appearance of the cartilage anlage, which is present by the fifth week. The primary ossification center for the humerus appears at about the sixth week.[1] By birth the entire humeral shaft is completely ossified.

The proximal humerus is primarily cartilaginous at birth; however, the ossification centers can be detected through ultrasonography as early as the 38th week of gestation and are generally present between the 38th and 42nd week of gestation.[2,3]

The three proximal humeral ossification centers consist of the greater and lesser tuberosities and the humeral head. The ossification center for the humeral head is usually present at birth; the one for the greater tuberosity appears by 1 to 3 years of age, and the lesser tuberosity ossification center appears by 5 years of age.[4-6] These ossification centers fuse by 5 to 7 years of age to form the head of the humerus. The proximal humeral ossification center fuses with the humeral shaft by 14 to 17 years of age in girls and 16 to 18 years in boys.[4,7-9]

Humeral retroversion likewise gradually develops over time. The normal adult value for humeral retroversion is highly variable based on anatomic and imaging studies.[10-16] Humeral retroversion averages 65 degrees in infants and young children and gradually decreases, approaching adult values by 11 years of age.[17]

At birth, the body or shaft of the humerus is completely ossified.[4] The proximal and distal ends allow longitudinal growth of the humerus. Eighty percent of humeral growth is secondary to the proximal humeral physis, accounting for approximately 40% of growth of the entire upper extremity.[9,18] Growth derived from the proximal humerus likewise varies with age: less than 75% of growth occurs before 2 years of age and more than 85% occurs by age 8 years.[7-9] This growth continues until physeal closure, which occurs at 14 years of age in girls and 17 years of age in boys.

Surgical Anatomy

The capsule of the glenohumeral joint extends from the glenoid rim, progressing laterally toward the surgical neck of the humerus and blending with the tendons of the rotator cuff musculature, where it surrounds the articular surface of the proximal humerus. The posterior medial metaphysis, a portion of the physis, and the epiphysis are intracapsular. A large portion of the physis is extracapsular, making it susceptible to injury. The proximal humeral physis is irregularly shaped, with its apex located on the posteromedial portion of the proximal humerus. The periosteum is also thicker in the posteromedial portion of the proximal humerus as opposed to the anterolateral portion, which is quite thin.[19] The posteromedial periosteum is stronger compared to the anterolateral periosteum; hence, the tendency for the fracture to penetrate the periosteum anterolaterally.

The proximal humerus is also the insertion site for numerous muscles around the shoulder girdle; this anatomic fact greatly influences the fracture configuration due to the forces exerted on the humerus both proximally and distally. The muscles of the rotator cuff, which act as stabilizers of the shoulder, run transverse, anterior, superior, and posterior to the glenohumeral joint.[20-23] The subscapularis, which originates from the undersurface of the scapula, inserts into the lesser tuberosity. The greater tuberosity provides attachment superiorly and posteriorly for the supraspinatus, the infraspinatus, and teres minor, all of which originate from the posterior portion of the scapula. The deltoids, which act as flexors and abductors, run from the clavicle and acromion inserting into the lateral portion of the upper third of the humeral shaft. Other muscles of importance include the pectoralis major, which inserts into the lateral lip of the bicipital groove.

Important neurovascular structures also course through the glenohumeral joint and the proximal humerus. The proximal humerus receives its blood supply from the axillary artery. The anterior and posterior humeral circumflex arteries supply the proximal humerus. The arcuate artery, which ascends from the anterior humeral circumflex artery, supplies the humeral head.[24-27] The subscapular artery also branches from the axillary artery, which supplies the rotator cuff muscles. Close proximity of the proximal humerus to the brachial plexus makes the brachial plexus prone to injury when the proximal humerus is injured in dislocations or fractures. The axillary nerve in particular passes inferior to the glenohumeral joint and posterior to the proximal humerus.[28-31]

Incidence

Numerous studies have reported on the incidence of fractures in children. However, these studies are affected by multiple factors, which include cultural differences, climate, and environmental factors; patient factors such as age and gender likewise exert an influence on the occurrence of the different fracture types.

Fractures of the proximal humerus have been reported to be about 5% of all children's fractures.[32-36] The incidence of fractures of the proximal humerus show a linear increase with age, with Salter–Harris type I fractures predominating in younger children, metaphyseal fractures more common in children 5 to 11 years, and Salter–Harris type II fractures in children older than 11 years. Fractures of the proximal humeral epiphysis represent 2% to 7% of all growth plate injuries in children.[37-39]

Mechanism of Injury

Shoulder dystocia is an infrequent cause of birth injuries in children. Shoulder dystocia is usually associated with conditions such as maternal diabetes, macrosomia, postterm pregnancy, and a previous history of shoulder dystocia. Gherman and colleagues reported on the incidence of birth injuries and found the incidence of birth injuries associated with shoulder dystocia to be 24.9%, with a 4.2% incidence of proximal humeral fractures.[40] The mechanism of injury is also related to arm position during delivery. Abnormal positions implicated in birth fractures, such as separation of the proximal humeral physis, include hyperextension and external rotation of the humerus.[41-44]

In the older child, both direct and indirect trauma to the proximal humerus has been implicated. Injuries from sports, vehicular or traffic accidents, and falls are the most common cause of proximal humerus fractures in children.[45] Six mechanisms of injury have been reported by Williams: forced extension, forced flexion, flexion with lateral rotation or with medial rotation, and forced extension with lateral rotation or with medial rotation.[46]

Repetitive injury can also cause damage to the proximal humeral physis (Fig. 15-1). Slipping of the proximal humeral growth plate has been reported to occur in gymnasts.[47] Stress-related injuries have likewise been reported secondary to gymnastics, baseball pitching, and various sporting activities, causing stress secondary to upper extremity loading.[48-55]

Pathologic fractures occurring through benign lesions have been reported infrequently (Fig. 15-2), particularly common benign lesions causing pathologic fractures through the proximal humerus, including aneurysmal and unicameral bone cysts.[56-59] Malignant lesions have been reported to cause pathologic fractures through the proximal humerus.[59-62]

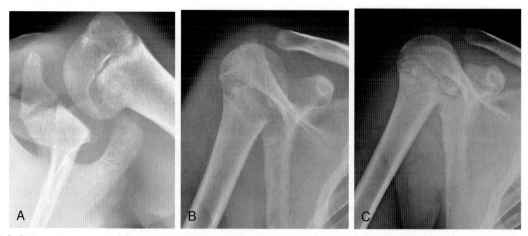

FIGURE 15-1 Epiphysiolysis in a 12-year-old right hand–dominant male baseball pitcher who came in for evaluation of right shoulder pain. **A** and **B,** On initial evaluation, radiographs showed widening of the proximal humeral growth plate. **C,** The patient was managed conservatively with activity modification for 3 months and went on to heal uneventfully.

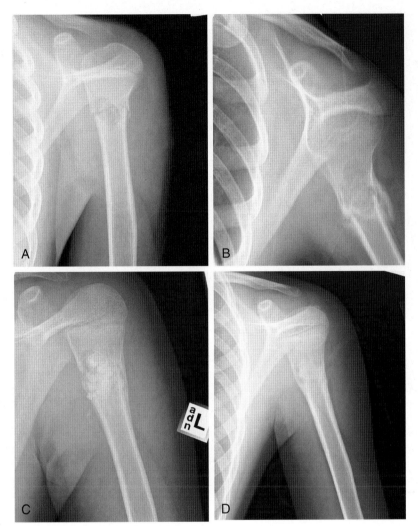

FIGURE 15-2 A, A 7-year-old boy who sustained a pathologic fracture through a simple bone cyst. This fracture was treated conservatively with a shoulder immobilizer. **B,** Follow-up radiographs show healing of the pathologic fracture with the presence of residual cystic lesion. **C,** The residual cystic lesion was treated with percutaneous biopsy, curettage, and bone grafting with Osteoset calcium sulfate pellets. **D,** Latest follow-up films showing progressive healing and remodeling through the lesion.

Metabolic conditions such as pituitary gigantism can cause weakening of the growth plate, leading to development of deformity.[63] Underlying neuromuscular conditions such as Arnold–Chiari malformation, syringomyelia, myelomeningocele, and cerebral palsy have been identified as risk factors or etiologic agents in the development of growth plate injuries and fractures about the proximal humerus.[64-67]

Nonaccidental injury should also be considered when children present with the proximal humerus fracture, particularly if the underlying cause is unclear and multiple injuries are noted.[68-72]

Classification

Fractures of the proximal humerus in children may be classified according to the location of the injury. Growth plate injuries in children are classified according to the Salter–Harris classification.[18] In younger children (<5 years), Salter–Harris type I injuries predominate (Fig. 15-3). In children older than 11 years, Salter–Harris type II fracture patterns predominate (Fig. 15-4).[39] The other three types Salter–Harris—types III, IV, and V—are very rare, particularly in the proximal humerus. However, cases of Salter–Harris type III injuries have been reported in the literature.[73]

The location of the fracture may also be used to define the fracture. This is a broad categorization, dividing the fractures according to area of involvement, such as the proximal humeral metaphysis (Fig. 15-5), growth plate, and lesser and greater tuberosities. Fractures can also be classified based on the degree of deformity as well as the degree of displacement. Neer and Horwitz classified proximal humeral fractures according to degree of displacement.[74] They divided the fractures into four types based on degree of displacement:

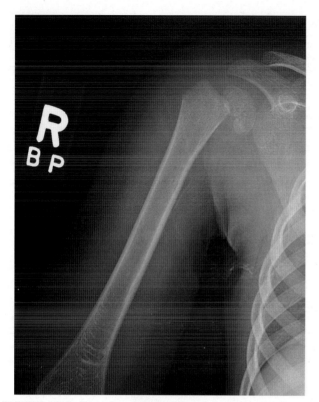

FIGURE 15-3 AP radiograph of a 2 year old who sustained a displaced Salter–Harris type I fracture through the proximal humeral growth plate.

Type 1 fractures have less than 5 mm of displacement.

Type 2 fractures are displaced greater than 5 mm to less than one third of the humeral shaft.

Type 3 fractures are displaced up to two thirds of the width of the shaft.

Type 4 fractures are displaced greater than two thirds of the shaft width.

Open fractures of the proximal humerus, although uncommon, also occur and can be classified using the Gustilo–Anderson classification for open fractures.[75,76]

Signs and Symptoms

In neonates and infants, evaluation of the shoulder for injuries may be very difficult. An infant who presents with the inability to move the shoulder should raise suspicion of a fracture or injury about the shoulder girdle or proximal humerus. A detailed history should be obtained, including any abnormalities throughout the prenatal period such as maternal diabetes or other maternal conditions that can predispose to macrosomia. Inability to move the shoulder and upper extremity should always raise the suspicion of an injury or pathologic condition in and about the shoulder girdle. Useful differential diagnosis includes fractures, dislocations, fracture-dislocations, infection, and brachial plexus injury. The neonate should have a thorough physical evaluation. Palpation of the upper extremity should likewise be performed for any warmth, direct tenderness, or deformity. Gentle range of motion (ROM) should be done to examine for any possible limitation of motion; abnormal motion likely points to a fracture or dislocation.

In the older child, a history consistent with a traumatic event can usually be elicited. The most common presenta-

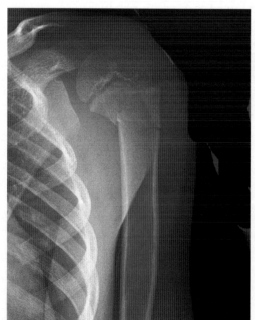
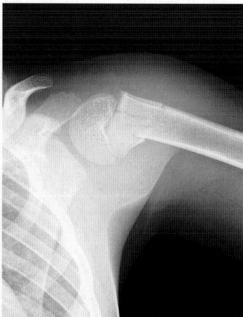

FIGURE 15-4 Radiographs of an 8 year old who sustained a Salter–Harris type II growth plate injury secondary to a fall.

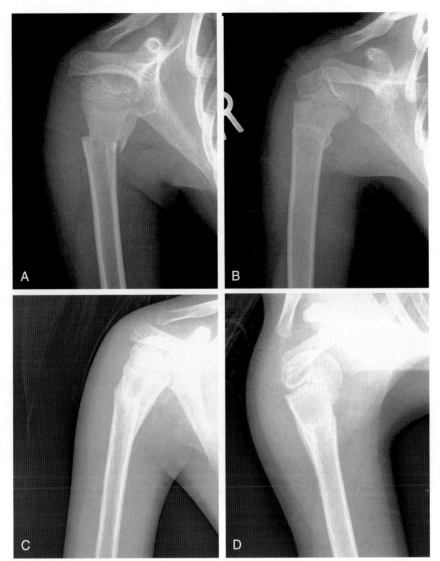

FIGURE 15-5 A and **B,** Radiographs taken of an 8-year-old boy who sustained a metaphyseal fracture through the proximal humerus. This fracture was treated conservatively. **C** and **D,** Radiographs taken at 7 weeks after injury show complete healing of the fracture.

tion is limited ROM of the shoulder, with abnormal fullness or deformity of the affected shoulder as compared to the contralateral extremity. Depending on the degree of trauma, other signs of injury are likewise present, including soft tissue injuries, ecchymosis, and swelling. The affected extremity is usually carried in an internally rotated posture. In posterior fracture-dislocations there is painful limited external rotation of the shoulder. In lesser tuberosity fractures there is limited abduction and external rotation of the shoulder.[77-79] Greater tuberosity fractures manifest with luxatio erecta.[80-82] The shoulder is in abduction with the elbow flexed and the hand above the head.

Radiographic Evaluation

Imaging of the proximal humerus can be challenging in neonates and infants because the proximal humerus is primarily cartilaginous. Generally, in neonates and infants with a suspected fracture of the proximal humerus or proximal humeral growth plate, a single anteroposterior (AP) view of the chest and upper extremities may be used to screen for injuries. On plain radiographs, the relationship of the proximal humeral metaphysis, scapula, and acromion are evaluated. These structures are compared with the contralateral side (Fig. 15-6). The abnormal relationship of the scapula and humerus has been described to denote a proximal humeral physeal injury with a posteriorly displaced proximal humeral fragment. This has been termed the *vanishing epiphysis sign.*[44,83] Ultrasound examination may be a valuable imaging tool.[84-88] Ultrasonography is quick and noninvasive, and the injury may be directly visualized, with the contralateral side serving as a comparison. Arthrography can also be valuable.[89,90] Computed tomography (CT) may also be useful in evaluating the shoulder injuries missed at birth, particularly those with posterior dislocation.[91]

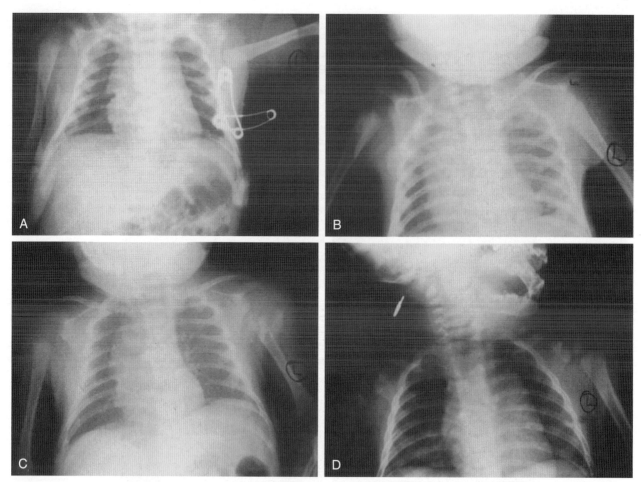

FIGURE 15-6 In a newborn, injury to the proximal part of the humerus is usually a completely displaced physeal injury, a pseudodislocation. **A,** Radiographs in the newborn are sometimes misleading because of lack of ossification in the proximal epiphysis. **B,** Closed manipulation can be performed by applying longitudinal traction and gentle posterior pressure over the proximal end of the humerus. **C,** At 2.5 weeks, abundant callus is present and the patient is clinically asymptomatic. **D,** A 6-month follow-up radiograph shows no asymmetry when compared with the opposite side.

Plain radiographs are still the mainstay in the initial evaluation of shoulder injuries in older children. Well-performed radiographs obtained in orthogonal views should be adequate in providing information on the pathology. A true AP and lateral view of the shoulder are usually sufficient for assessing the injury. A true AP image of the shoulder is taken in the scapular plane with the beam parallel to the glenohumeral joint. The axillary lateral view is preferred, although it may be difficult to obtain in the setting of an acutely injured child. In lieu of the axillary lateral view, alternative views such as the transthoracic axillary view or the scapular Y view may be obtained. The apical oblique view is also valuable in some cases.

Treatment

The treatment of fractures of the proximal humerus generally depends on the age of the patient and on the fracture type and location. In general, the prognosis for most proximal humerus fractures in children is good, with the vast majority amenable to nonoperative management. Because the proximal humeral physis contributes the most growth of the upper extremity and closes late, there is tremendous remodeling potential for the proximal humerus (Fig. 15-7). The location of the fracture likewise exerts a great influence on the management, whether the fracture involves the growth plate or extends through the metaphysis.

In neonates with birth injuries, the prognosis is generally good; only the most severely displaced fractures require any attempt at reduction. If reduction is performed, gentle maneuvers without anesthesia generally work well. These maneuvers may be monitored using ultrasonography. In the vast majority of cases, the shoulder can be immobilized efficiently by pinning the shirt sleeve or soft dressing to the shirt. These fractures heal very quickly, usually within 2 to 3 weeks.[19,43]

Children with a slipped proximal humeral epiphysis usually do not need any form of reduction. These injuries generally respond well to nonoperative management.

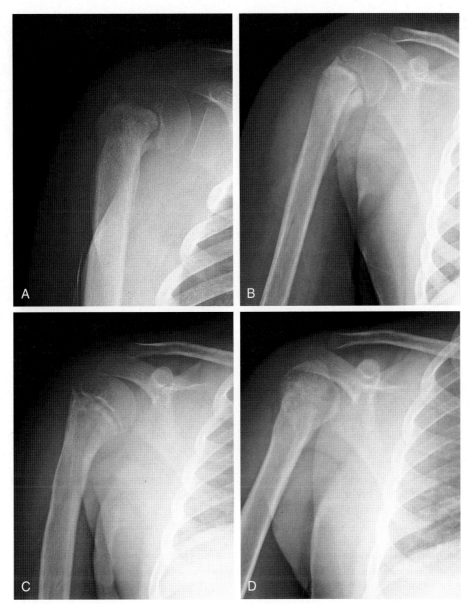

FIGURE 15-7 A, Radiographs of a 9-year-old boy who had sustained a Salter–Harris II fracture of the proximal humerus, showing angulation of the proximal fragment in the AP plane. **B,** The child was treated conservatively, and follow-up radiographs taken 6 weeks after injury show excellent callus formation and healing of the fracture. **C** and **D,** Radiographs taken 9 months after injury show full healing of the previous fracture with remodeling of the proximal humerus.

In general, fracture treatment is determined by the degree of displacement and the amount of remodeling potential. Beaty recommended treatment guidelines based on the patient's age (Table 15-1).[92] In young children, excellent outcomes have been reported with nonoperative management.[19,74,93] In older children, nonoperative management has been reported to have good results, particularly in Neer type 1 and type 2 cases. Reduction, however, was required more often in Neer type 3 and 4 fractures.[19,74,93,94]

Reduction

In general, reduction is reserved for severely displaced or angulated fractures in older children. Potential barriers to reduction include periosteum, capsule, and biceps tendon.[92,95-97] Numerous reduction maneuvers have been recommended. Most fractures can be treated with gentle traction coupled with abduction, external rotation, and flexion of the shoulder. Neer and Horwitz recommended reduction with 90 degrees of forward flexion, abduction, and external rotation.[74] Others recommend reduction with 135 degrees of abduction and 30 degrees of flexion and external rotation; the fracture is manipulated directly to obtain reduction.[98,99]

Once acceptable or adequate reduction is obtained, any of several immobilization techniques may be used. Immobilization methods described in the literature include sling and swathe (Fig. 15-8), two-prong splint,

TABLE 15-1 Guidelines for Reduction

Age	Acceptable Angulation	Acceptable Displacement
<5 yr	70 degrees	100%
5-12 yr	40-70 degrees	—
>12 yr	40 degrees	50%

Based on Beaty JH: Fractures of the proximal humerus and shaft in children. Instr Course Lect 41:369-372, 1992.

thoracobrachial bandage, shoulder spica cast, Statue of Liberty cast, and hanging arm cast.[19,74,93,100,101] It is important for the surgeon and family to understand that very displaced proximal humerus fractures in older children are generally quite unstable. Some loss of reduction is common if internal fixation is not used.

Operative Treatment

Operative management is rarely indicated for children with fractures of the proximal humerus. However, occasionally, some fractures are not amenable to reduction due to soft tissue interposition. More often, these fractures require an open reduction and possible internal fixation. The operative consent for internal fixation of proximal humerus fractures should include the possibility of open reduction, should interposed tissue cause an obstacle to reduction. Other indications for operative management include segmental fractures to obtain adequate stabilization, the rare displaced, intra-articular fracture, open fractures requiring débridement, fracture-dislocations, and fracture of the proximal humerus with concomitant neurovascular injury. Open reduction of proximal humeral fractures is generally carried through a deltopectoral approach. A limited skin incision may be used to gain direct access into the joint space. The significant advantage of performing a reduction is that it lessens the amount of time needed for remodeling.

There are numerous options for internal fixation of proximal humerus fractures. Displaced fractures may be treated with closed reduction and percutaneous techniques or open reduction and internal fixation.[102-104]

Percutaneous pin fixation may be performed once adequate reduction has been obtained (Fig. 15-9).[105,106] Percutaneous pinning can be done under image intensification. The patient is placed supine on the operating table. A closed reduction is performed under image intensification. Once adequate reduction has been obtained, the pins are inserted laterally through the metaphysis, in an inferior-to-superior fashion. The surgeon should be careful to avoid the axillary nerve laterally and anteriorly, as well as the other neurovascular structures more medially. The pinning technique can be challenging because the optimal trajectory is quite steep and the cortex of the proximal humerus can be very hard. Smooth pins can be

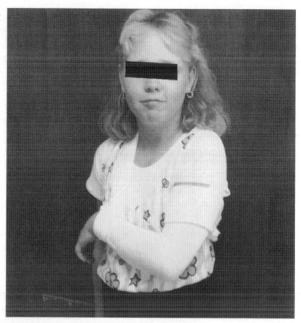

FIGURE 15-8 Clinical photograph of a 9-year-old girl wearing a homemade sling and swathe used in the treatment of proximal humerus fractures. A stockinette is padded at pressure points with cast padding and held in position with safety pins.

used, or the small external fix-it or pins with threaded tips can be used instead, if there are concerns about pin migration.

Depending on the stability of the fracture after reduction, two or more pins may be used. In younger children, when smooth pins are used, they can be left in the percutaneous position and removed in the office. In older children with threaded pins, the pins should be buried in the subcutaneous tissue and removed in the operating room once the fracture has healed.

Flexible intramedullary nails have also been used to manage proximal humerus fractures in children (Fig. 15-10).[107]

Treatments for Specific Fracture Patterns

The lesser tuberosity is the site of the insertion of the subscapularis. Good results have been reported with nonoperative management of lesser tuberosity fractures.[77,79,108] However, several authors advocate open reduction and internal fixation in acute fractures.[78,109,110] Ogawa and Takahashi reported better results with operative management of lesser tuberosity fractures.[111] Options for fracture fixation depend on the size of the avulsed fragment. In most cases suture fixation is adequate. Screw fixation may be performed in fractures with larger fragments. Good results have been reported after arthroscopic treatment.[112]

Greater tuberosity fractures in the young child can often be treated nonoperatively with good outcomes. In a child who is approaching maturity, a displaced greater tuberosity fracture often requires open reduction and internal fixation with subsequent repair of the rotator cuff.

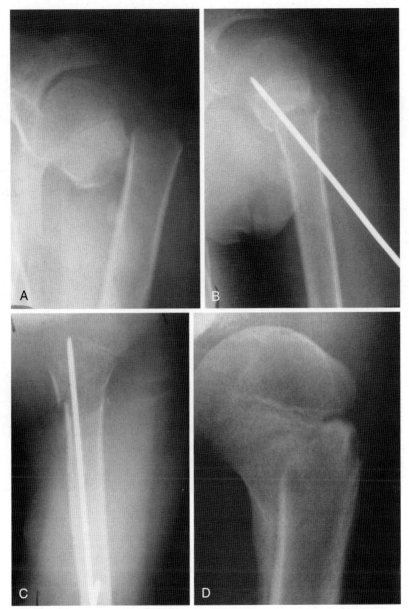

FIGURE 15-9 Technique of percutaneous pinning of a proximal humeral metaphyseal fracture from a distal approach to avoid the axillary nerve. **A,** AP radiograph demonstrating a displaced proximal humerus metaphyseal fracture. **B** and **C,** Once satisfactory reduction is obtained, pins are inserted distally through the deltoid and advanced in an inferior-to-superior direction. **D,** AP radiograph after pin removal showing a healed fracture, which has started to remodel. (From Rockwood CA, Wilkins KE, Beaty J [eds]: Fractures in Children. Philadelphia: JB Lippincott, 1996.)

Fracture-dislocations of the proximal humerus are not very common injuries. Proper treatment of the injury consists of stabilizing the fracture and reducing the glenohumeral joint.[113,114]

Authors' Preferred Treatment

Nonoperative

Most proximal humerus fractures, including physeal fractures, can be managed nonoperatively. Our preferred method for treatment depends on the age of the patient. In the neonate and infant, we manage most fractures with simple immobilization often by safety-pinning the shirt-sleeve to the front of the shirt. In the older child with a proximal humerus fracture, we follow the displacement guidelines of Beaty (see Table 15-1). Most fractures can be treated with immobilization alone. We usually start with a coaptation splint and an elastic (Ace) wrap, then, at 10 to 14 days after injury, change to a shoulder immobilizer or hanging cast once the child is more comfortable (see Fig. 15-8).

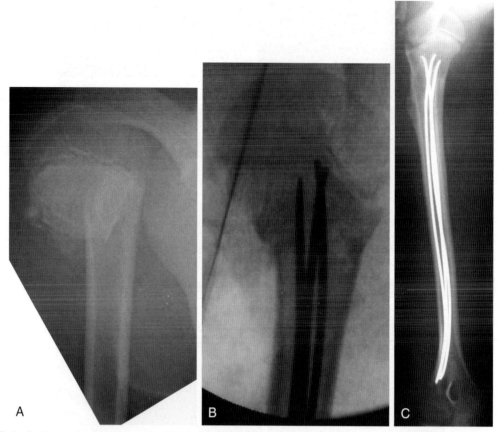

FIGURE 15-10 A, Radiograph of an 11-year-old boy with multiple trauma, including bilateral femoral fractures and a contralateral proximal humeral fracture. The left side was treated in closed fashion. **B,** The proximal end of the right humerus was treated by closed reduction with flexible nails (Synthes titanium elastic intramedullary nails) to facilitate mobilization. **C,** The fracture was well maintained with this internal splint. (Courtesy of Richard L. Munk, MD.)

Operative

Fractures that exceed the Beaty guidelines are treated with closed reduction and possibly internal fixation. The patient is placed supine on a radiolucent table. A bump may be placed under the scapula to allow greater ROM of the shoulder. The fracture is reduced using fluoroscopic guidance, using the maneuvers described earlier. If closed reduction is unsuccessful, the deltopectoral interval can be opened to facilitate reduction.

Once adequate reduction is achieved, percutaneous pins are inserted through the lateral cortex. We prefer the small external fixator or pins with a threaded tip to minimize the risk of migration. These pins are directed across the fracture site and into the head of the humerus, stopping short of the subchondral bone. Two or three pins are inserted until the fracture has been satisfactorily stabilized (Fig. 15-11). In older children (perhaps 13 years old and older), it is best to cut the pins and bury them beneath the skin, because fracture healing can take 4 to 6 weeks. The pins are cut to appropriate length. The extremity is placed in a shoulder immobilizer for 2 to 3 weeks.

Postfracture Care and Rehabilitation

Birth injuries and fractures in very young children tend to heal rapidly. Usually the healing is observed within 2 to 3 weeks. No rehabilitation is required in this age group.

In older children, injuries take longer to heal. In growth plate injuries, the fracture is usually stable in 3 weeks, after which gentle ROM and pendulum exercises can be instituted. After 6 weeks, active range-of-motion exercises, which include flexion and extension, abduction, and internal and external rotation, can be started. This is followed by strengthening of the deltoids and rotator cuff muscles.

Metaphyseal fractures may take 4 to 6 weeks to heal. Rehabilitation should start with gentle ROM exercises, followed by strengthening exercises once motion is restored.

Complications

Proximal humerus fracture complications may be divided into early and late. Early complications result directly

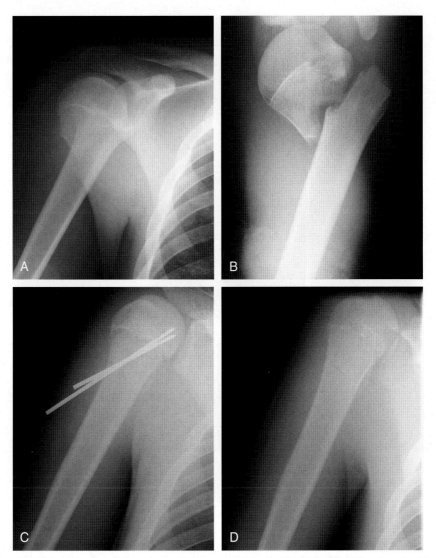

FIGURE 15-11 A 14-year-old male quarterback who sustained an injury to his right shoulder when tackled. AP (**A**) and lateral (**B**) radiographs show a displaced and angulated fracture of the proximal humerus. Attempt at treatment in a hanging cast failed. A closed reduction was performed under anesthesia. **C,** The fracture was deemed unstable even after reduction and percutaneous pinning was performed. Postoperative course was uneventful. **D,** Radiograph taken 6 weeks into his postoperative period show excellent healing of the fracture.

from the fracture. These complications can be serious and develop into potentially limb-threatening injuries. Neurologic injuries have been reported to occur with proximal humerus fractures.[115-118] Typically, these are injuries to the brachial plexus from fracture dislocation. They can often be diagnosed early after injury, with loss of strength and sensation in the nerve distribution. Most of these injuries are neurapraxias that recover within 4 to 6 months. If no sign of recovery is noted, an EMG study is warranted to document whether there is actual improvement in the status of the nerve palsy. No improvement at this time is an indication for surgical exploration and possible repair or nerve grafting of the involved structure.[115]

Vascular injuries are uncommon but have been reported.[119-121] Implant-related complications such as hardware migration have also been reported after internal

fixation of proximal humerus fractures.[107,122-124] Loss of motion is also another complication that is seen, particularly in patients who were treated surgically.

Late complications are often sequelae of the original injury. Humerus varus usually occurs in children and neonates after a history of trauma, infection, or metabolic or hematologic conditions (Fig. 15-12).[125-130] This usually results in a decrease in the humeral neck-shaft angle accompanied by shortening of the humerus. The deformity results in slight limitation of ROM and often does not require surgical intervention. However, in some cases surgical management is needed to properly realign the humerus.[121,127,130-132]

Growth arrest has been reported in children who have growth plate fractures and in some pathologic conditions that cross the physis, such as chondroblastomas and bone

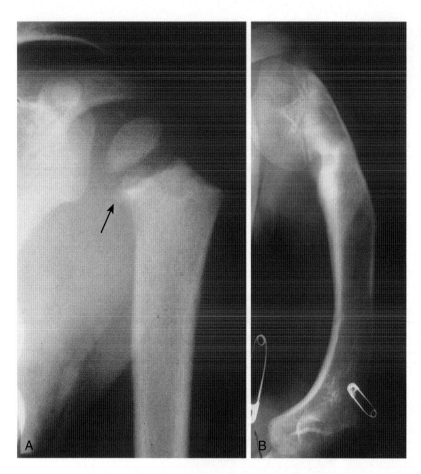

FIGURE 15-12 Proximal humeral varus resulting from an infection at 11.5 years of age. **A,** Marked shortening (*arrow*). **B,** Varus. (From Rockwood CA, Wilkins KE, Beaty J [eds]: Fractures in Children. Philadelphia: JB Lippincott, 1996.)

cysts.[45,133-139] Complete physeal arrest has been reported but is relatively rare. More often these cases do not produce any functional deficit, and most children do not need any form of surgical intervention.

Hypertrophic scar formation is a complication seen after surgical management.[19,140,141] To avoid this, some authors have reported a more cosmetic axillary approach for treatment of these injuries.[142] Osteonecrosis of the humeral head is a rare complication; however, even with osteonecrosis, good outcomes have been reported.[143] Glenohumeral subluxation has also been reported in children with proximal humerus fractures.[73,114] These often respond well to a period of nonoperative management, which includes supporting the extremity in a sling and instituting early rehabilitation.

FRACTURES OF THE CLAVICLE

Anatomy

Embryology and Development
The clavicle is one of the first bones to ossify. The clavicle begins ossification from two primary ossification centers (medial and lateral) by 5 to 6 weeks of gestation. By 7 to 8 weeks of gestation, the clavicle already has assumed its overall contour and typical S shape. Most growth (80%) occurs from the medial physis. Despite its early appearance, the clavicle is one of the last bones to complete ossification. The lateral epiphysis forms and fuses in a remarkably short time around 18 to 19 years of age. The medial epiphysis is the last in the body to ossify, at age 18 to 20 years, and the last to complete ossification, at age 23 to 25 years of age.[144,145]

Relevant Anatomy
The clavicle is an S-shaped bone that articulates medially with the sternum and laterally with the scapula at the acromion process. Through the sternoclavicular and acromioclavicular joints, the clavicle functionally links the axial skeleton and upper extremity. The medial two thirds of the bone is round and tubular; the lateral third is flat. The anterosuperior aspect of the clavicle is subcutaneous. The subclavian vessels and brachial plexus lie posterior to the clavicle near the junction of the medial two thirds and lateral one third (Fig. 15-13).

Numerous muscles and ligaments attach to the clavicle. Anteriorly, the pectoralis major originates on the medial two thirds of the clavicle and the deltoid on the lateral third. Posteriorly, the trapezius muscle inserts on to the

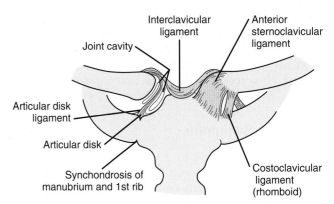

FIGURE 15-14 Anatomy of the sternoclavicular joint.

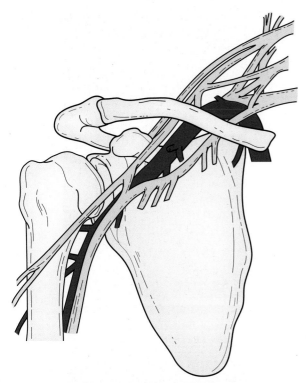

FIGURE 15-13 Relationship of the clavicle and scapula to the brachial plexus and subclavian artery. (From Sarwark JF, King EC, Luhmann SJ: Proximal humerus, scapula, and clavicle. In Beaty JH, Kasser JR [eds]: Fractures in Children, 6th ed. Philadelphia: Lippincott Williams & Wilkins, 2006, pp 703-771.)

lateral third of the clavicle. The clavicular head of the sternocleidomastoid muscle originates on the superior surface. The subclavius muscle and enveloping clavipectoral fascia attach to the inferior surface.

By providing these muscular and ligamentous attachment sites, in particular to the principal mobilizers of the upper arm, the pectoralis major and deltoid muscles, the clavicle plays a significant part in overall motion and function of the upper extremity. In addition, through the sternoclavicular joint, the clavicle itself is responsible for limited motion.[146-148] Upward elevation of the clavicle approximately 30 to 35 degrees contributes to shoulder abduction. The clavicle can also protract and retract approximately 35 degrees in the anterior-to-posterior plane. Lastly, the clavicle can rotate 45 to 50 degrees about the long axis of the clavicle.

Laterally, the clavicle articulates with the acromion of the scapula through the acromioclavicular joint. The acromioclavicular joint is a diarthrodial joint, surrounded by a relatively weak capsule and supported superiorly and inferiorly by the acromioclavicular ligaments. In a child, the lateral third of the clavicle is surrounded circumferentially by thick periosteum that acts as a protective tube. The capsule and acromioclavicular ligaments blend with the periosteum of the lateral part of the clavicle. The

primary stabilizing ligaments, the conoid and trapezoid portions of the coracoclavicular ligaments, arise from the coracoid and attach to the lateral end of the clavicle and its periosteum.

Medially, the clavicle articulates with the manubrium of the sternum and the first rib through the sternoclavicular joint. The sternoclavicular joint is also diarthrodial, and similar to the acromioclavicular joint, it lacks inherent structural stability. The joint is stabilized by a group of ligaments, including the intra-articular disk ligament, the anterior and posterior capsular ligaments, the interclavicular ligament, and the costoclavicular ligament (Fig. 15-14). The anterior portion of the capsular ligament is heavier and stronger than the posterior portion.[149] The capsular ligaments attach mainly to the epiphysis of the medial clavicle; therefore, the physis is extra-articular and susceptible during injuries to the medial clavicle. The sternoclavicular joint lies anterior to many important mediastinal structures such as the great vessels, the vagus and phrenic nerves, and the trachea and esophagus.

Incidence

Fractures of the clavicle occur in 1% to 13% of all births.[150] The clavicle is also commonly injured during childhood, and clavicle fractures represent between 8% and 15.5% of all pediatric fractures.[151] Most fractures of the clavicle involve the middle third (76%-85%). The lateral third is second most commonly involved (10%-21%); the incidence of lateral fractures increases with age. Fractures in the medial third are less common and account for only 1% to 5% of clavicle injuries in children.

Mechanism of Injury

The clavicle is the most commonly fractured bone during childbirth. The risk of birth-related clavicle fractures is increased for infants of larger birth weight (>4500 g), increased height (>52 cm), and shoulder dystocia.[152] However, the majority of birth-related clavicle fractures occur in uneventful deliveries of average-birth-weight infants.

In children, falls, especially onto the shoulder, are the most common cause of fractures of the clavicle.[151] Fractures of the clavicle can also occur in motor vehicle accidents and secondary to direct trauma sustained in sports such as football. Nonaccidental trauma can also be a cause. Stress fractures are rare but do occur.

Signs and Symptoms

Fractures of the clavicle in newborns may be difficult to diagnose. One of the more reliable signs is difficulty with palpation of the margins of the injured clavicle due to generalized edema. Pain is usually present with forced movement about the shoulder or direct palpation of the clavicle. Presumably to lessen pain, newborns with clavicle fractures sometimes voluntarily splint or immobilize the ipsilateral arm. This pseudoparalysis can at times be misdiagnosed as a brachial plexus injury. To minimize pain related to the pull of the sternocleidomastoid muscle across the fracture site, affected infants might turn their head toward the side of the fracture. Infants with acute clavicle fractures generally have an asymmetric Moro reflex.

In older children, the diagnosis of a clavicle injury is typically straightforward. Pain is present around the area of the fracture. Ecchymosis, swelling, and tenderness can also be present around the fracture site. Children with fractures of the clavicle resist and stop movement of the affected arm. A bony prominence or deformity may be noted with severely displaced fractures.

Associated Injuries

Fractures involving the clavicle are at risk for serious vascular injuries, including subclavian and axillary artery disruption; subclavian vessel compression, thrombosis, and pseudoaneurysm; and arteriovenous fistulas.[153-155] Brachial plexus neuropathy has also been reported in association with injuries to the clavicle.[156-158] Thorough neurovascular examination of the upper extremity is warranted. Onset of neurologic deficits related to brachial plexus neuropathy can be early or late. Open reduction and stabilization of the fractured clavicle may be required.

Fractures of the clavicle can be secondary to high-energy injuries and so can be associated with injuries to the ipsilateral lung and chest wall such as pneumothorax, hemothorax, pulmonary contusion, and rib fractures. Additional injuries to the ipsilateral upper extremity and shoulder girdle are also common.

Posterior displaced fractures of the medial clavicle and posterior dislocations of the sternoclavicular joint are at particular risk for concomitant injury to the retrosternal structures in the mediastinum, including the great vessels, the esophagus, and the trachea.[159-165] The index of suspicion should be raised in children who are choking or having difficulty with speaking, breathing, or swallowing. Signs of venous congestion and diminished distal pulses

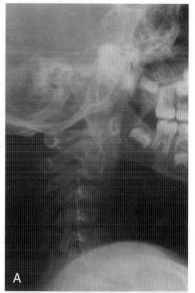
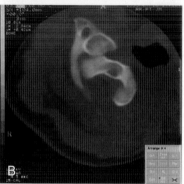
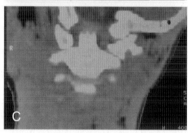

FIGURE 15-15 A, Lateral radiograph of the cervical spine with increased atlantodental interval and anterolisthesis of the atlas. **B,** Axial CT showing significant atlantoaxial rotatory subluxation. **C,** Coronal CT reconstruction showing the eccentric axis of the dens in relation to lateral masses of the atlas. (From Nannapaneni R, Nath FP, Papastefanou SL: Fracture of the clavicle associated with a rotatory atlantoaxial subluxation. Injury 32:71-73, 2001.)

can also suggest associated injury. These associated injuries can be life threatening. Associated injury to the brachial plexus can also occur.

Fractures of the clavicle are rarely associated with atlantoaxial (C1-C2) rotatory subluxation (Fig. 15-15).[166,167] Clinically, the head is tilted laterally toward and rotated away from the fractured clavicle. The diagnosis of C1-C2 rotatory subluxation is difficult because of the masking of the torticollis by the acute symptoms of the fractured

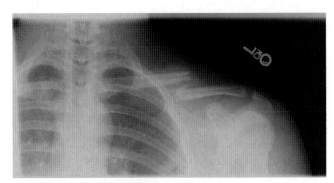

FIGURE 15-16 AP radiograph of the left clavicle showing a midshaft fracture of the clavicle.

clavicle, but it should be suspected by asymmetrical ROM. The diagnosis is best confirmed by dynamic CT.

Radiographic Evaluation

An AP radiograph of the clavicle is the standard initial study (Fig. 15-16). In newborns, ultrasound examination is a reasonable alternative to conventional radiography in the diagnosis of fractures involving the clavicle.[168-170] Ultrasonographic imaging is particularly sensitive in detecting occult clavicle fractures and sternoclavicular injuries in this young age group. Ultrasound is also useful during follow-up to assess fracture healing.

Additional radiographic views are necessary for complete assessment and characterization. For fractures of the clavicle shaft, a view oblique to the AP radiograph is

useful. Cephalad-directed views, an apical oblique view, and an apical lordotic view have been described. The cephalad-directed views, taken with the x-ray beam directed 20 to 45 degrees cephalad to the clavicle, aid in defining the degree and direction of displacement (Fig. 15-17). The apical oblique view, taken with the x-ray beam directed 45 degrees lateral to the axial axis of the body and 20 degrees cephalad to the clavicle, also offers an additional oblique view of the clavicle shaft and is particularly effective for fractures involving the middle third of the clavicle. The apical lordotic view is a true perpendicular view to the AP radiograph (Fig. 15-18). Because the view is taken laterally with the shoulder abducted more than 130 degrees, the technique can cause significant discomfort and can be difficult for the patient in the acute setting.

For injuries to the lateral aspect of the clavicle and acromioclavicular joint, an AP radiograph centered on the acromioclavicular joint is recommended. In addition, cephalad-directed (15-20 degrees) and axillary lateral views are helpful for further fracture delineation. The Stryker notch view (AP radiograph of the shoulder with the patient's hand resting on top of the head) is helpful in detecting concomitant fractures of the coracoid (Fig. 15-19). Stress views, AP radiographs with distraction applied to the ipsilateral upper extremity, can reveal subtle injuries to the lateral clavicle or acromioclavicular joint. Stress views, however, are not routinely indicated. CT scan is indicated if additional detailed evaluation of the physis and acromioclavicular joint is needed.

Radiographic evaluation of injuries involving the medial third of the clavicle and sternoclavicular joint is difficult.

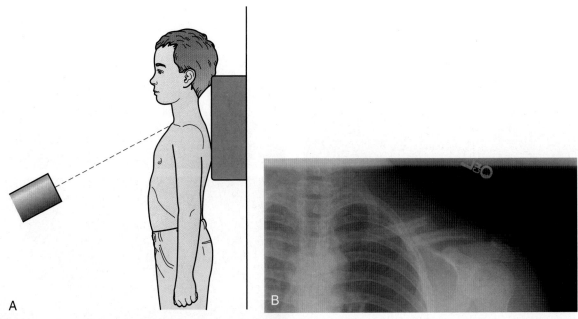

FIGURE 15-17 A, Technique for cephalad-directed view of the clavicle. **B,** Cephalad-directed radiograph of left clavicle, showing midshaft fracture of the clavicle. (**A** from Sarwark JF, King EC, Luhmann SJ: Proximal humerus, scapula, and clavicle. In Beaty JH, Kasser JR [eds]: Fractures in Children, 6th ed. Philadelphia: Lippincott Williams & Wilkins, 2006, pp 703-771.)

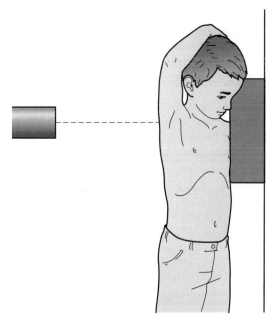

FIGURE 15-18 Technique for apical lordotic view of the clavicle. (From Sarwark JF, King EC, Luhmann SJ: Proximal humerus, scapula, and clavicle. In Beaty JH, Kasser JR [eds]: Fractures in Children, 6th ed. Philadelphia: Lippincott Williams & Wilkins, 2006, pp 703-771.)

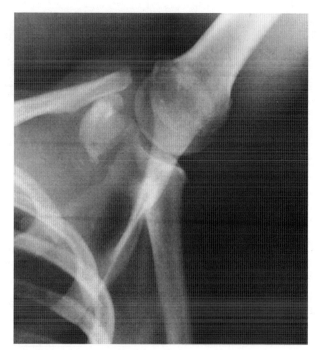

FIGURE 15-19 Stryker notch view showing a fracture of the base of the coracoid.

A serendipity view, taken with the x-ray beam directed 40 degrees cephalad to the clavicle, can be helpful (Fig. 15-20). CT, however, has become the imaging modality of choice (Fig. 15-21). In addition to providing a more comprehensive assessment of the fracture or dislocation, CT allows evaluation of possible associated injuries to the underlying mediastinal structures.

Differential Diagnosis

The differential diagnosis for fractures of the clavicle includes congenital pseudarthrosis of the clavicle.[171] Congenital pseudarthrosis of the clavicle is rare and usually asymptomatic. Involvement is generally right-sided. When involvement is left-sided, dextrocardia or situs inversus is

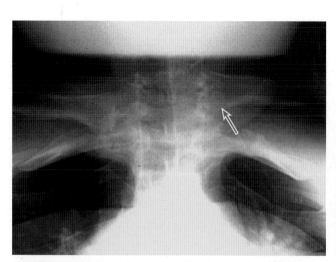

FIGURE 15-20 Serendipity view showing an anteriorly displaced left sternoclavicular dislocation (*arrow*). (From Linnau KF, Blackmore CC: Bony injuries of the shoulder. Curr Probl Diagn Radiol 31:29-47, 2002.)

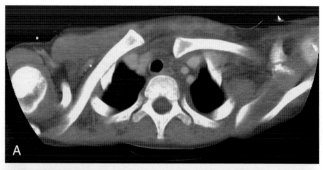

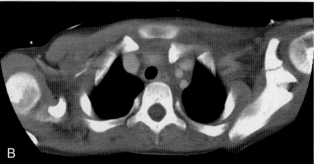

FIGURE 15-21 A and **B,** Axial CT of a posteriorly displaced fracture of the medial end of the left clavicle.

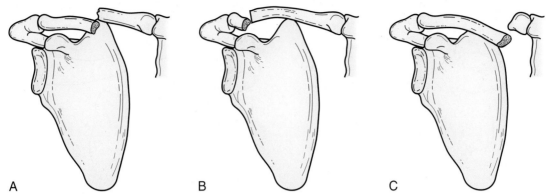

FIGURE 15-22 Anatomic classification scheme for fractures of the clavicle. **A,** Type I, fracture of the middle third of the clavicle. **B,** Type II, fracture of the lateral third of the clavicle. **C,** Type III, fracture of the medial third of the clavicle. (From Sarwark JF, King EC, Luhmann SJ: Proximal humerus, scapula, and clavicle. In Beaty JH, Kasser JR [eds]: Fractures in Children, 6th ed. Philadelphia: Lippincott Williams & Wilkins, 2006, pp 703-771.)

usually present. Bilateral involvement occurs but is rare. Clavicular abnormalities can also be secondary to benign or malignant tumors, metabolic disorders such as hyperparathyroidism, and renal osteodystrophy. Idiopathic hyperostosis may be difficult to differentiate from a fracture of the clavicle. Osteomyelitis of the clavicle is uncommon but can produce a periosteal reaction mimicking fracture healing.

Classification

The most common classification scheme for fractures of the clavicle is based on the anatomic location of the fracture (Fig. 15-22).[172] Type I fractures involve the middle third of the clavicle, lateral to the sternocleidomastoid muscle and medial to the coracoclavicular ligaments. Type II fractures involve the lateral third, including and lateral to the coracoclavicular ligaments. Type III fractures involve the medial third, medial to the sternocleidomastoid muscle. Other classification schemes have been developed to categorize injuries involving the lateral and medial ends of the clavicle.

Lateral Clavicle Injuries

The most widely used classification scheme for injuries involving the lateral end of the clavicle and acromioclavicular joint in children is based on the adult system for lateral clavicle injuries (Fig. 15-23).[173] In a child, displacement of the lateral clavicle occurs through the periosteal sleeve and not through the coracoclavicular ligaments. True acromioclavicular dislocations are uncommon in children, but they do occur in older adolescents. Instead, most injuries to the lateral end of the clavicle in the immature skeleton are fractures involving the metaphyseal or physeal regions (Salter–Harris type I or II fractures) (Fig. 15-24). The lateral epiphysis of the clavicle does not ossify until age 18 or 19 years; therefore, these metaphyseal and physeal injuries involving the lateral

clavicle can radiographically manifest more as an acromioclavicular dislocation than a fracture (described as *pseudodislocation*).[174,175]

Type I injuries are caused by low-energy trauma, with mild strain of the acromioclavicular ligaments and no disruption of the periosteal tube. Radiographs are normal.

In type II injuries, the acromioclavicular ligaments are completely disrupted with partial damage to the superolateral aspect of the periosteal sleeve. These injuries result in mild instability of the lateral end of the clavicle. Minimal widening of the acromioclavicular joint may be seen on radiographs.

In type III injuries, complete disruption of the acromioclavicular ligaments occurs in addition to a larger disruption of the periosteal sleeve, resulting in gross instability of the distal end of the clavicle. Superior displacement of the lateral clavicle is seen on an AP radiograph, with an increase in the coracoid–clavicle interval by 25% to 100% compared to the contralateral uninjured side.

In type IV injuries, the soft tissue disruptions are similar. The lateral clavicle, however, displaces posteriorly and can pierce the trapezius muscle. Little displacement is noted on the AP radiograph, and the axillary lateral view is best to appreciate the posterior displacement of the clavicle relative to the acromion.

Type V injuries are similar to type III injuries but more severe. The superior aspect of the periosteal sleeve is completely disrupted in type V injuries, resulting in displacement of the distal clavicle into the subcutaneous tissues. The deltoid and trapezius muscles may be detached from the clavicle as well. On an AP radiograph, the coracoid–clavicle interval is increased 100% more than on the contralateral uninjured side.

In type VI injuries, the distal clavicle is displaced inferiorly, with the distal end displaced inferior to the coracoid process.

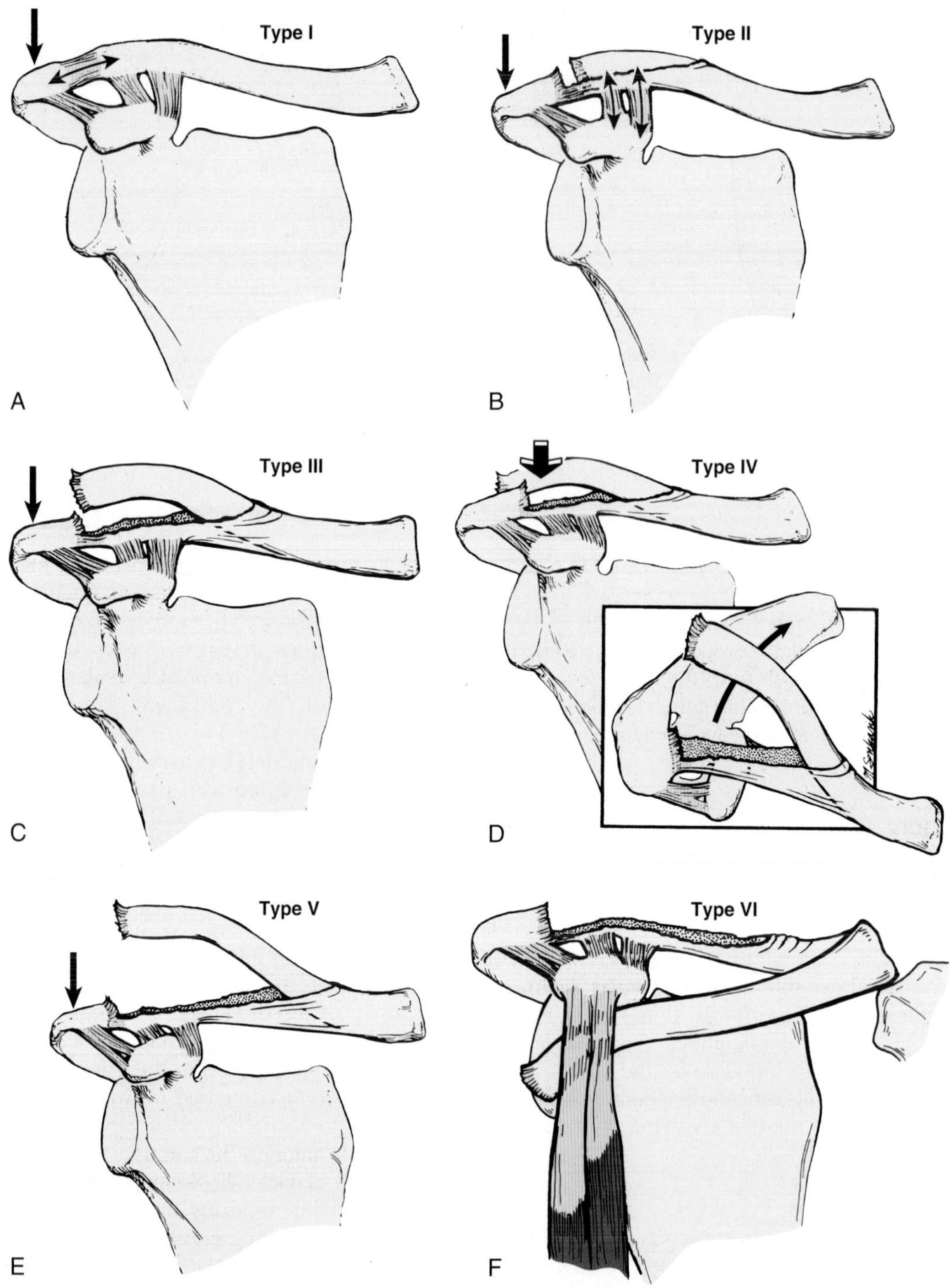

FIGURE 15-23 Dameron and Rockwood classification of fractures involving the lateral end of the clavicle and acromioclavicular joint in children (see text for description).

Medial Clavicle Injuries

Injuries to the medial end of the clavicle and sternoclavicular joint are classified by the direction of displacement of the clavicle—anterior or posterior. Anterior displacement occurs more commonly than posterior displacement.[176-178] In addition, most injuries to the medial end of the clavicle in the immature skeleton are fractures through the physis and metaphysis (Salter–Harris type I and II fractures) rather than true dislocations through the sternoclavicular joint (Fig. 15-25). The medial physis of the clavicle is the last in the body to close, and the medial epiphysis of the clavicle does not fuse completely to the

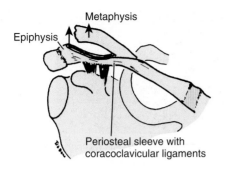

FIGURE 15-24 Most injuries to the lateral end of the clavicle in children are Salter–Harris type I or II fractures.

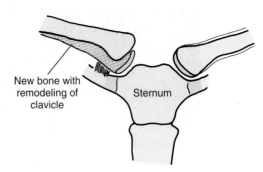

FIGURE 15-25 Similar to injuries to the lateral end of the clavicle, most injuries to the medial end of the clavicle are also Salter–Harris type I or II fractures.

shaft until age 23 to 25 years. Also, because the sternoclavicular ligaments attach primarily to the epiphysis, the medial physis is extracapsular and left relatively unprotected.

Treatment

Fractures of the Clavicle Shaft

The treatment for birth-related fractures of the clavicle is nonoperative. Minimal to no treatment is needed. In an infant who appears uncomfortable, the affected arm should be immobilized for 10 to 14 days.[179] A stockinette stretch bandage may be used to immobilize the affected arm to the chest wall. Otherwise, the shirtsleeve of the affected arm can be safety-pinned to the shirt.

Nonoperative treatment is also effective for most clavicle shaft fractures in older children (Fig. 15-26). Treatment of nondisplaced and displaced clavicle shaft fractures with a figure-of-eight splint or sling is effective and results in excellent outcomes. Caution is required with the use of a figure-of-eight splint, because too much tightening can lead to excessive swelling, compression of the axillary vessels, pain, and brachial plexus neuropathy.[180-182] If a figure-of-eight splint is chosen, close follow-up at weekly intervals is required to monitor the skin and neurovascular status. There is no evidence that use of a figure-of-eight splint leads to healing of the clavicle with less shortening than with sling treatment.[181,183] If a sling is used, inadvertent migration around the neck (choking) must be prevented.

Operative intervention is not usually needed. Indications for operative treatment include open fractures, severely displaced and irreducible clavicle fractures at risk for skin perforation, associated vascular injury requiring repair, irreducible displaced fractures causing compression of mediastinal structures such as the trachea and esophagus, and possibly compromise of the brachial plexus.[184,185] Concomitant displaced fractures of the scapula (acromion, coracoid, or scapular neck)—a floating shoulder injury pattern—might necessitate operative treatment, although this view is controversial.[186] More recently, in the older adolescent nearing skeletal maturity, the relative indications for operative treatment have been

broadened to include high-energy closed fractures with greater than 1.5 to 2.0 cm of shortening, fractures with complete displacement, and fractures with comminution.[181,187-189] Fixation options include plate-and-screw fixation and intramedullary fixation with elastic nails (Fig. 15-27).[185,190] Fixation with percutaneous smooth Kirschner wires should be avoided because this technique has been associated with migration into vital structures and an overall high complication rate.[123,190,191]

Lateral Clavicle Injuries

Given the exceptional healing and remodeling potential for these fractures, most fractures involving the lateral end

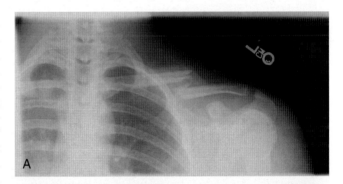

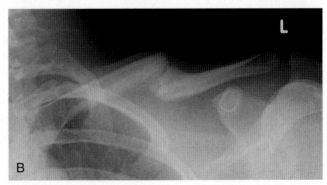

FIGURE 15-26 A, AP radiograph of the left clavicle showing a midshaft fracture of the clavicle. **B,** AP radiograph of the left clavicle 4 months after injury and nonoperative treatment with sling, showing significant callus formation and healing of the clavicle fracture.

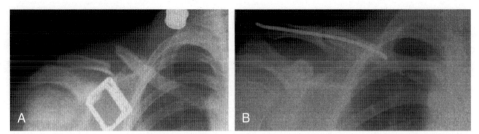

FIGURE 15-27 This 12-year-old boy who sustained a midshaft fracture of the right clavicle. **A,** AP radiograph demonstrates no signs of callus formation after 10 days of treatment using a figure-of-eight brace. **B,** Fixation with stable intramedullary nailing (2.0 mm) after open reduction and removal of impinged soft tissue. (From Kubiak R, Slongo T: Operative treatment of clavicle fractures in children. J Pediatr Orthop 22:736-739, 2002.)

of the clavicle in children can be treated nonoperatively. Injuries to the lateral clavicle in the immature skeleton are typically physeal injuries. Moreover, the enhanced capacity to heal and remodel is related to the retained periosteal sleeve and the usually undamaged and intact acromioclavicular joint and coracoclavicular ligaments.

Most agree that nondisplaced or minimally displaced injuries of the lateral clavicle (types I, II, and III) can be treated effectively without surgery in a sling or a figure-of-eight splint (Fig. 15-28). Nonoperative treatment results in predictably excellent outcomes without long-term functional disability.[173,175,192-194] The treatment of displaced types IV, V, and VI lateral clavicle fractures is controversial. Historically, recommendations have varied widely from nonoperative treatment to treatment with open

reduction and internal fixation.[175,192,194-196] At present, most are advocating open reduction and stable fixation.[194-197] In many cases, the lateral end of the clavicle can be reduced into its periosteal sleeve, and stable fixation can be achieved after repair of the periosteum.

Although rare, true acromioclavicular dislocations can occur in the pediatric population. The vast majority affect adolescents, however, and treatment recommendations overlap with those for the adult population.

Medial Clavicle Injuries

The potential for satisfactory healing and subsequent remodeling is also significant for fractures involving the medial end of the clavicle; therefore, nonoperative treatment is typically appropriate for most fractures of the

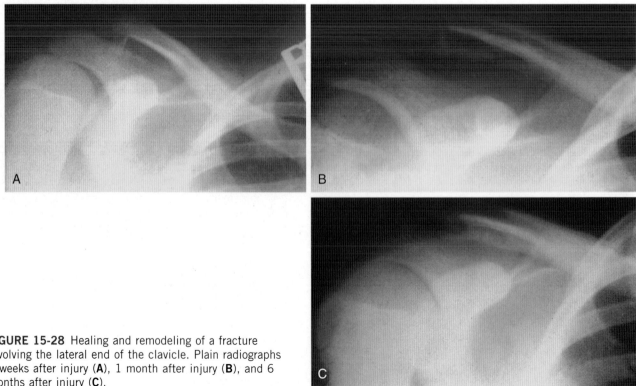

FIGURE 15-28 Healing and remodeling of a fracture involving the lateral end of the clavicle. Plain radiographs 2 weeks after injury (**A**), 1 month after injury (**B**), and 6 months after injury (**C**).

medial clavicle. Injuries to the medial clavicle in the immature skeleton are also usually physeal injuries and not true dislocations of the sternoclavicular joint. Symptomatic treatment is usually adequate for nondisplaced or minimally displaced fractures of the medial clavicle.[95,154] A sling can be worn for comfort, and early motion is recommended.

Remodeling of anterior displaced medial clavicle injuries is expected; therefore, reduction is not warranted routinely. If reduction is attempted, reduction can be safely performed in the emergency department or operating room under local or general anesthesia. The reduction maneuver consists of longitudinal traction of the ipsilateral upper extremity while the shoulder is abducted to 90 degrees. Gentle posterior pressure is applied over the fracture. Limited immobilization with a figure-of-eight splint is recommended for 3 to 4 weeks. The reduction can be unstable, and redisplacement is not uncommon. Open reduction with internal fixation, however, is usually unnecessary.

With posterior displaced medial clavicle injuries, evaluation for concomitant injuries of the airway and great vessels should be initiated immediately. In the absence of significant associated injuries, minimally displaced fractures and dislocations may be treated without reduction. Fractures and dislocations with significant displacement should be reduced. If the airway or great vessels are compromised, the need for reduction is urgent.

Reduction should be attempted under general anesthesia in an operating room setting, preferably with a thoracic or general surgeon readily available. The patient is positioned supine with a bolster placed in the midline between the scapulae. Gentle longitudinal traction of the ipsilateral arm is applied while drawing the ipsilateral shoulder posteriorly and into abduction.

If attempts at closed reduction are unsuccessful, a sterile towel clip can aid reduction. After sterile preparation of the skin, the medial end of the clavicle is grasped and manipulated with a towel clip while longitudinal traction is applied to the ipsilateral upper arm (Fig. 15-29). If attempts at percutaneous reduction fail, open reduction is performed. Open reduction is also indicated for open fractures. The reduction is generally stable, and internal fixation is not usually necessary. If the reduction is unstable, however, stable fixation can be achieved with suture repair of the overlying periosteum or ligaments. Internal fixation with metal implants is inadvisable because they can migrate into the mediastinum.

Complications

Malunions

Malunions, especially of initially displaced fractures, are common, but significant deformity and long-term disability are unlikely given the remodeling potential of children. Clavicular reduplication and cleidoscapular synostosis can occur but are rare.[175,197] If the malunion is symptomatic, operative excision is recommended.

Nonunions

Nonunions following traumatic fractures of the clavicle are uncommon; rates of nonunion are reported to be 0.1% to 5.9%.[181,198-202] In most cases, nonunions are asymptomatic. Rarely, operative intervention with bone grafting and stable fixation is required for unacceptable cosmetic deformity or pain.

Neurovascular Injuries

Numerous neurovascular complications have been reported in association with injuries to the clavicle: injury to the subclavian, axillary, and great vessels and brachial plexus palsy.[153-158] The majority of these neurovascular injuries occur concomitantly at the time or near the time of injury. Neurovascular complications, however, also occur later following nonoperative and operative treatment. Vascular complications include subclavian artery and vein compression, thrombosis, pseudoaneurysm, transection, or laceration; arteriovenous fistulas; and thoracic outlet syndrome. Neurologic deficits related to brachial plexus neuropathy can also occur. Brachial plexus palsy has been reported in association with inappropriate use of a figure-of-eight splint. Most brachial plexus neuropathies are self-limited and resolve spontaneously, but permanent deficits have been reported.

Implant Complications

Implants for fractures of the clavicle have been associated with numerous complications, including implant

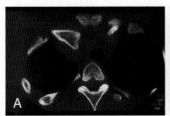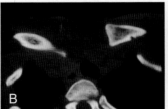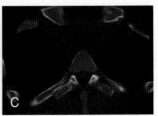

FIGURE 15-29 CT of a left posterior epiphyseal fracture of the medial clavicle. **A,** On the first cut of the scan, the injury appears to be a posterior dislocation. **B,** Another cut shows the epiphyseal fragment. **C,** After closed reduction with a towel clip, the epiphysis is realigned with the metaphysis. (From Bishop JY, Flatow AL: Pediatric shoulder trauma. Clin Orthop Relat Res [432]:41-48, 2005.)

migration, infection, and nonunion.[123,191,203] Smooth Kirschner-wire fixation, in particular, has been associated with an overall high complication rate and with death secondary to pin migration.[123] Whenever possible, fixation of pediatric clavicle injuries should use minimal or no implants.

FRACTURES OF THE SCAPULA

Anatomy

Embryology and Development

During development, the scapula begins to form in the fifth week of fetal life.[6,204] The scapula first develops at the C4 to C5 level, and then descends to its final position overlying the first through fifth ribs. Failure of the scapula to descend results in Sprengel's deformity.[204,205] The majority of the scapula forms by intramembranous ossification and develops from multiple centers of ossification throughout the scapula: three for the body, two to five for the acromion, two for the coracoid process, and one for the glenoid (Fig. 15-30).

Relevant Anatomy

The scapula is a triangular flat bone that links the upper extremity to the axial skeleton. Seventeen distinct muscles attach to the scapula, and this overlying musculature leaves the scapula relatively protected. The scapular spine separates the inferior and superior fossae. The acromion is the lateral projection of the spine. The coracoid process is on the anterolateral portion of the scapular neck, and the glenoid is the lateral extension of the scapular neck. The scapula articulates with the clavicle at the acromioclavicular joint, with the humerus at the glenohumeral joint, and functionally with the chest wall at the scapulothoracic articulation (not a true joint). The scapula is highly mobile and provides approximately 60 degrees of shoulder elevation.

While passing posterior to the clavicle, the brachial plexus and axillary artery course across the anterosuperior aspect of the scapula. These neurovascular structures continue and pass the tip of the coracoid process first medially, then inferiorly. The suprascapular nerve and artery pass under and over the transverse scapular ligament, respectively, which overlies the suprascapular notch medial to the base of the coracoid process. The axillary nerve travels immediately inferior to the glenoid.

The superior shoulder suspensory complex (SSSC) is a bone and soft tissue ring comprising the glenoid, coracoid process, coracoclavicular ligament, lateral part of the clavicle, acromioclavicular joint, acromion process, and coracoacromial ligament (Fig. 15-31).[186,206-208] The complex can be divided into three components: the clavicular–acromioclavicular joint–acromial strut; the clavicular–coracoclavicular ligamentous–coracoid (C-4) linkage; and the three-process–scapular body junction (Fig. 15-32). The SSSC is secured to the trunk by superior and inferior struts from which the upper extremity is suspended. The superior strut is the middle clavicle, and the inferior strut is the junction of the lateral scapular body and medial scapular neck. Functionally, the SSSC links the upper extremity and axial skeleton.

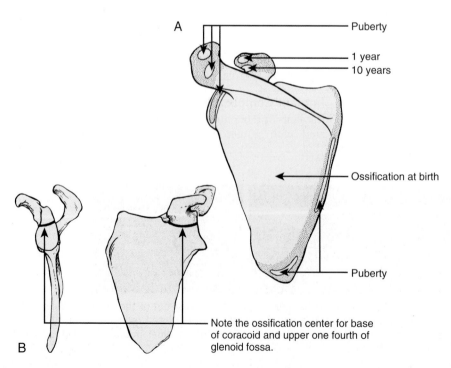

A — Puberty
— 1 year
— 10 years
— Ossification at birth
— Puberty
Note the ossification center for base of coracoid and upper one fourth of glenoid fossa.
B

FIGURE 15-30 Multiple ossification centers of the scapula. **A,** Posterior view. **B,** Lateral and anterior views.

Incidence

Fractures of the scapula are rare and constitute only 1% of all fractures and 5% of shoulder fractures.[206,209] Fractures of the body and spine of the scapula are most common, and fractures of the coracoid are least common. According to one series in adults, the distribution of scapula fracture types is 35% body, 27% neck, 12% acromion, 11% spine, 10% glenoid, and 7% coracoid.[209]

Mechanism of Injury

Injury to the scapula usually is a result of severe, high-energy trauma; therefore, scapular injuries are rarely isolated. Scapular body fractures usually occur as a result of direct impact. In the absence of clear traumatic cause, nonaccidental trauma must be excluded. Injury to the scapula, especially the coracoid process, can also occur as a result of an avulsion mechanism. Stress fractures are rare. Fractures of the glenoid typically occur secondary to a fall onto the upper extremity. Scapulothoracic dissociations usually result from high-energy trauma with massive, direct force to the chest and shoulder regions accompanied by traction forces applied to the shoulder girdle.

Signs and Symptoms

Fractures of the scapula are characterized clinically by significant pain, swelling, ecchymosis, and tenderness around the shoulder girdle. The overall surface anatomy of the shoulder may be hidden by the localized swelling. Children with fractures of the scapula typically resist movement of the injured arm. Massive swelling about the shoulder girdle, especially in the setting of an abnormal vascular examination and neurologic deficit, is seen following scapulothoracic dissociation. The presence of associated, sometimes life-threatening, injuries often leads to late diagnosis and delayed treatment.

Associated Injuries

About 80% to 95% of fractures involving the scapula are associated with additional injuries, which may be life-threatening.[206,209-211] The most common injuries are to the head, chest, kidneys, and especially the ipsilateral lung, chest wall, and ipsilateral shoulder girdle. Mortality associated with scapula fractures in one series exceeded 14%.[211] Given the close anatomic relationship between the scapula and numerous neurovascular structures, associated neurovascular injury, particularly to the brachial plexus and axillary artery, can also occur. Scapulothoracic dissociations in particular are highly associated with ipsilateral neurovascular injury.[212,213]

Radiographic Evaluation

Fractures involving the scapula are often first seen on the AP chest radiograph from a trauma series. If a scapula fracture is visible or suspected, AP and lateral radiographs of the scapula are necessary to define the fracture (Fig. 15-33). Additional radiographic views can further characterize the scapula injury. Most trauma series to evaluate the shoulder region should include the axillary lateral view to confirm location of the humeral head within the glenoid. The axillary lateral view also allows better assessment of fractures involving the glenoid. A 20-degree caudal tilt lateral view with the shoulder adducted may be helpful for injuries involving the acromion. The Stryker notch view (AP radiograph of the shoulder with the patient's hand resting on top of the head) may be helpful for coracoid injuries (Fig. 15-34). Given the complex anatomy of the scapula, CT with reconstructions is often

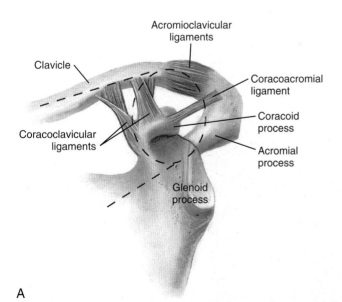

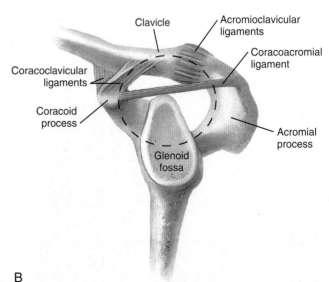

A   B

FIGURE 15-31 The superior shoulder suspensory complex. AP (**A**) and lateral (**B**) views of the bone–soft-tissue ring and the superior and inferior bone struts.

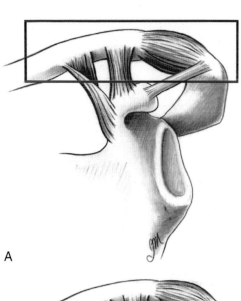

A

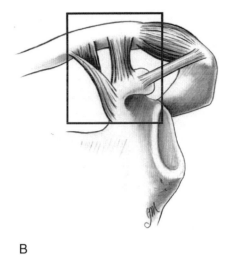

B

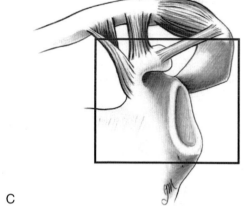

C

FIGURE 15-32 The three units of the superior shoulder suspensory complex. **A,** The clavicular–acromioclavicular joint–acromial strut. **B,** The clavicular–coracoclavicular ligamentous–coracoid (C-4) linkage. **C,** The three-process–scapular body junction. (From Goss TP: Fractures of the scapula. In Rockwood CA, Matsen FA, Wirth MA, et al [eds]: The Shoulder, 3rd ed. Philadelphia: Saunders, 2004, p 413.)

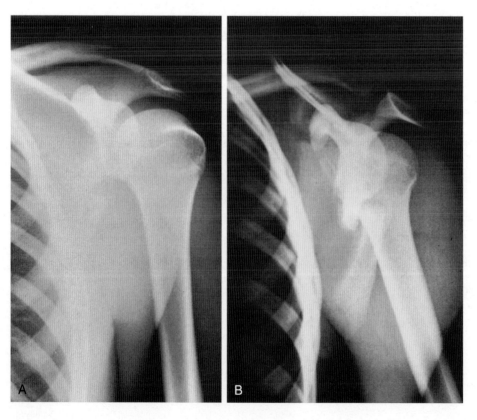

A   B

FIGURE 15-33 AP (**A**) and scapulolateral (**B**) views of the scapula define most scapular fractures.

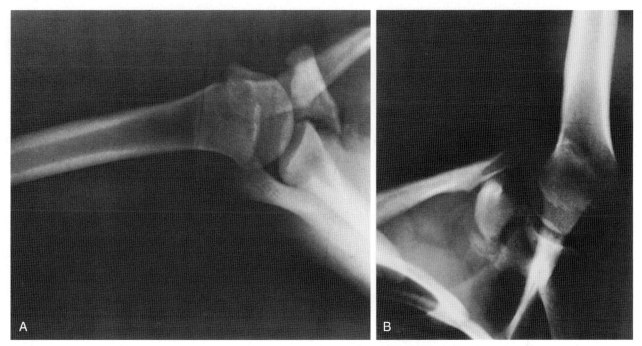

FIGURE 15-34 A and **B,** A Stryker notch view may be helpful in defining fractures of the coracoid process.

necessary and particularly useful for intra-articular glenoid fractures (Fig. 15-35).

Scapulothoracic dissociations are also identified initially on the AP chest radiograph. Index of suspicion for these injuries should be high, especially with high-energy injuries. Lateral displacement of the scapula (relative to the uninjured side) is pathognomonic (Fig. 15-36).[206,214] In addition to lateral scapular displacement, severely displaced clavicle fractures, acromioclavicular joint injuries, and sternoclavicular injuries may be present.

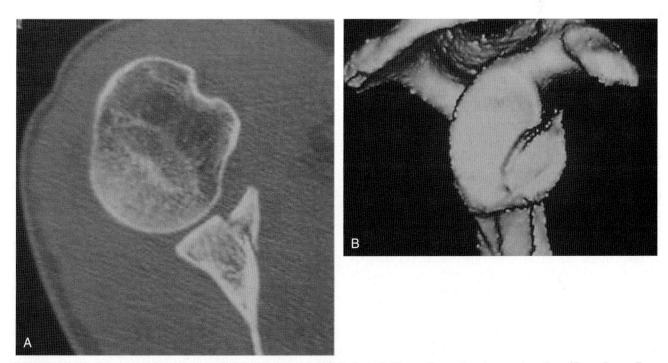

FIGURE 15-35 CT of an intra-articular glenoid fracture. **A,** Axial view, **B,** Three-dimensional reconstruction. (From Bauer T, Abadie O, Hardy P: Arthroscopic treatment of glenoid fractures. Arthroscopy 22:569.e1-e6, 2006.)

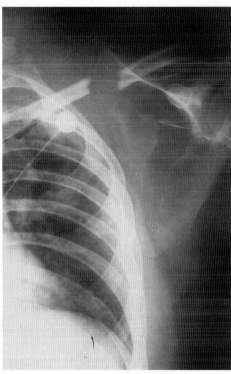

FIGURE 15-36 AP radiograph showing scapulothoracic dissociation with concomitant fractures of the clavicle and scapula. (From Masmejean EH, Asfazadourian H, Alnot JY: Brachial plexus injuries in scapulothoracic dissociation. J Hand Surg Br 25:336-340, 2000.)

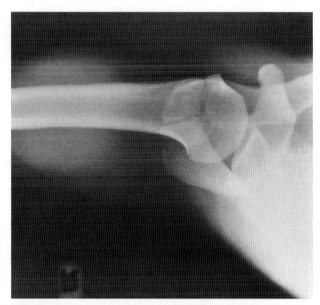

FIGURE 15-37 Axillary lateral radiograph showing one of several possible patterns of os acromiale.

Differential Diagnosis

Developmental variations in scapular anatomy must be distinguished from a fracture or injury to the scapula. A failure of the ossification centers in the acromion to unite, called *os acromiale,* can be confused with a fracture (Fig. 15-37).[215] Other scapular anomalies that can mimic a fracture include Sprengel's deformity, absent acromion, bipartite or tripartite acromion, bipartite coracoid, and coracoid duplication.[6,205,216,217]

Classification

Numerous classification schemes have been described for fractures of the scapula; none are specific for the pediatric population. The majority are based on the anatomic location of the fracture. According to Ada and Miller, scapula fractures are classified into fractures involving the scapular body, neck, acromion, spine, glenoid, and coracoid.[209] Thompson and colleagues relied on broader anatomic categories: fractures of the body, fractures of the acromion and the coracoid, and fractures of the glenoid and scapular neck.[211]

Fractures of the body and spine of the scapula are broadly divided into those with and without displacement. Fractures of the scapular neck are similarly classified into those with and without displacement. Fractures involving the scapular neck have also been classified by the anatomic location of the fracture: anatomic neck (lateral to the base of the coracoid) and surgical neck (medial to the base of the coracoid) (Fig. 15-38).[218]

Isolated scapular neck fractures should be distinguished from those associated with an ipsilateral fracture of the clavicle. This latter injury pattern (ipsilateral fractures of the scapular neck and clavicle) was first described by Ganz and Noesberger in 1975 and termed *floating shoulder* (Fig. 15-39).[186,207,219] The definition of a floating shoulder has subsequently evolved and has expanded to include injuries that result in a scapular neck fracture and additional disruption to the superior shoulder suspensory complex (SSSC): coracoid base fracture, acromion fracture, coracoacromial and coracoclavicular ligament disruption, and coracoclavicular and acromioclavicular ligament disruption (Fig. 15-40).[219] The significance of these double-disruption injuries to the SSSC is the risk of increased displacement and instability.

Fractures of the coracoid process are divided into those with and without associated injury to the lateral end of the clavicle or acromioclavicular joint.[220,221] The latter injury pattern is considered a double-disruption injury to the SSSC. Fractures of the acromion are classified into those with and without displacement.[220,222] If displacement is present, an additional disruption of the SSSC is usually present—commonly an associated fracture of the coracoid process. Displaced fractures of the acromion are further categorized based on the presence or absence of subacromial narrowing.

Fractures of the glenoid are divided into five groups based on their location and the course of the fracture through the rest of the scapula (Fig. 15-41).[206,223,224] Type I fractures are isolated glenoid rim fractures, with Ia involving the anterior rim and Ib involving the posterior

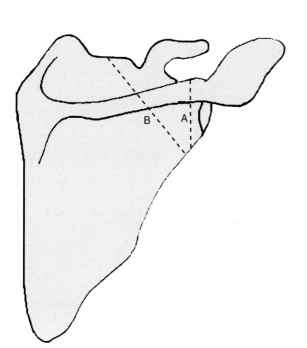

FIGURE 15-38 Classification of fractures of the scapular neck: Fracture through the anatomic neck (*A*) and fracture through the surgical neck (*B*). (From van Noort A, van der Werken C: The floating shoulder. Injury 37:218-227, 2006.)

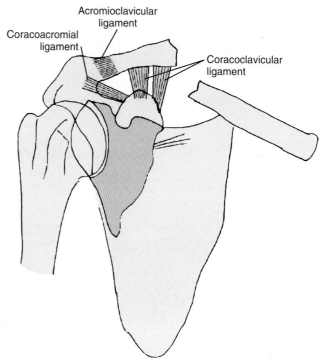

FIGURE 15-39 Diagram of a floating shoulder. Ipsilateral fractures of the clavicle and scapular neck. The glenoid has lost its attachment to the axial skeleton. (From van Noort A, van der Werken C: The floating shoulder. Injury 37:218-227, 2006.)

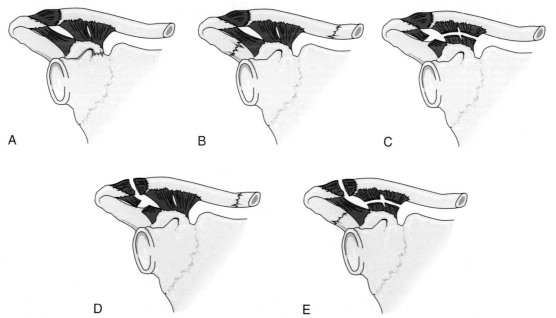

FIGURE 15-40 Floating shoulder injury patterns. Purely osseous injuries: Type IA (*A*): scapular neck fracture combined with a coracoid base fracture; type IB (*B*): scapular neck fracture combined with a clavicle fracture and scapular spine or acromion fracture. Purely ligamentous injury: Type II (*C*): scapular neck fracture combined with coracoacromial and coracoclavicular ligament disruption. Combined osseoligamentous injuries: Type IIIA (*D*): scapular neck fracture combined with a clavicle shaft fracture plus coracoacromial and acromioclavicular ligament disruption; type IIIB (*E*): scapular neck fracture combined with an acromion or scapular spine fracture plus coracoclavicular and acromioclavicular ligament disruption. (Reproduced with permission from Wong KL, Ramsey ML, Williams GR Jr: Scapular fractures. In *Orthopaedic Knowledge Update Shoulder and Elbow* 2. Rosemont, IL, American Academy of Orthopaedic Surgeons, 2002, pp 227-236.)

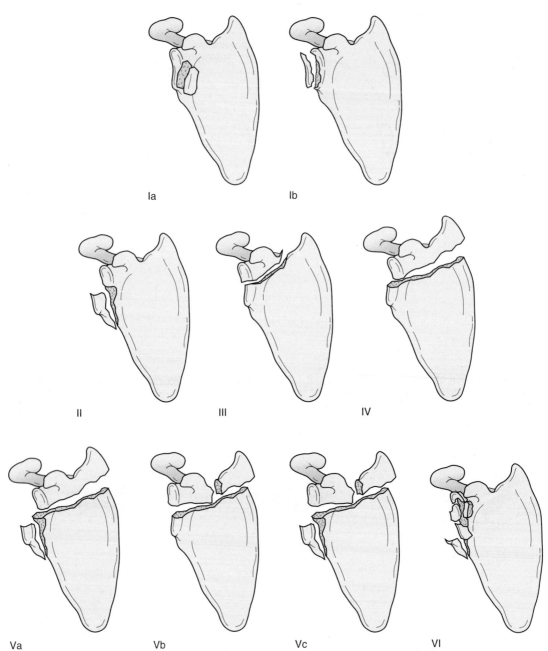

FIGURE 15-41 Classification of fractures of the glenoid (see text for description). (From Sarwark JF, King EC, Luhmann SJ: Proximal humerus, scapula, and clavicle. In Beaty JH, Kasser JR [eds]: Fractures in Children, 6th ed. Philadelphia: Lippincott Williams & Wilkins, 2006, pp 703-771.)

rim. Type II fractures are glenoid fractures with the fracture line through the glenoid fossa and exiting at the lateral border of the scapula. Type III fractures are glenoid fractures with the fracture line exiting at the superior aspect of the scapula. Type IV fractures are glenoid fractures with the fracture line exiting at the medial border of the scapula. Type V fractures are various combinations of type II, III, and IV fractures. Type Va is a combination of types II and IV; type Vb is a combination of types III and IV; and type Vc is a combination of types II, III, and

IV. Type VI fractures are glenoid fractures with severe comminution of the glenoid fossa.

Scapulothoracic dissociations are characterized by complete disruption of the scapulothoracic articulation with severe damage to the soft tissue supporting structures, including the deltoid, pectoralis minor, rhomboids, levator scapulae, trapezius, and latissimus dorsi. In the presence of a severe ipsilateral neurovascular injury, scapulothoracic dissociations effectively are termed *closed forequarter amputations.*

Treatment

Most scapular body fractures can be successfully treated nonoperatively—usually with sling immobilization.[210,225-227] Isolated fractures of the scapular body are inherently stable due to the overlying musculature, and so most fractures tend to be nondisplaced or minimally displaced. In adults, scapular body fractures with significant displacement greater than 10 mm are at risk for pain and disability when treated nonoperatively.[210] Operative treatment, therefore, may be indicated for widely displaced fractures of the scapular body in children.

Isolated nondisplaced or minimally displaced fractures of the scapular neck can be treated nonoperatively with satisfactory long-term outcomes.[210,228,229] Significantly displaced fractures of the scapular neck, however, appear to be at risk for limited glenohumeral motion and glenohumeral instability.[206,210,230-232] In adults, significant displacement has traditionally been defined as displacement greater than 10 mm or angulation greater than 40 degrees in either the axial or coronal plane. More recently, angular displacement has been determined more accurately by a glenopolar angle less than 20 degrees.[229,232,233] The glenopolar angle, measured on an AP radiograph, is the angle between the line connecting the most cranial with the most caudal point of the glenoid cavity and the line connecting the most cranial point of the glenoid cavity with the most caudal point of the scapular body (normal range, 30-45 degrees) (Fig. 15-42). Operative treatment should be considered for significantly displaced scapular neck fractures in children. A posterior approach to the scapular neck is recommended. After reduction, fixation can usually be achieved with a 3.5-mm contoured reconstruction plate or interfragmentary compression screws.

The treatment for scapular neck fractures in the presence of associated injury to the clavicle is controversial. Historically, this combination of injuries necessitated operative intervention with open reduction and internal fixation of the scapular neck or clavicle fracture (or both).[206,209,234] Currently, nonoperative treatment is recommended for nondisplaced or minimally displaced fractures involving the scapular neck and clavicle. Significant fracture displacement and ligament disruption, however, lead to less-predictable outcomes. Therefore, operative intervention should be strongly considered.[235] Operative intervention should also be considered for all floating shoulder injury patterns.

Isolated fractures of the coracoid process typically are nondisplaced or minimally displaced. Nonoperative treatment with sling immobilization followed by early functional shoulder exercises is effective in most cases. Displaced coracoid fractures are commonly associated with injury to the acromioclavicular joint or lateral clavicle and consequently double disruption of the SSSC. Displaced coracoid fractures near the suprascapular notch can also be associated with injury to the suprascapular nerve. Therefore, for most displaced fractures of the

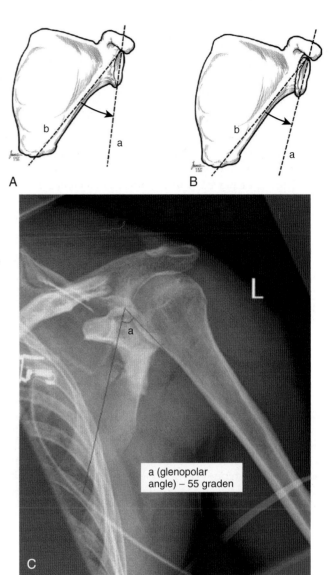

FIGURE 15-42 Normal (**A**) and abnormal (**B**) glenopolar angle (measure of obliquity of glenoid articular surface in relation to the scapular body). The normal range for the glenopolar angle is 30 to 45 degrees. **C,** Plain radiograph demonstrating abnormal glenopolar angle of 55 degrees. (**A** and **B** from DeFranco MJ, Patterson BM: The floating shoulder. J Am Acad Orthop Surg 14:499-509, 2006. **C** from van Noort A, van der Werken C: The floating shoulder. Injury 37:218-227, 2006.)

coracoid, open reduction and internal fixation is recommended.[221,226,227]

Isolated fractures of the acromion in children are usually nondisplaced or minimally displaced; therefore, they can be treated nonoperatively.[222] Indications for open reduction and internal fixation include displaced acromial fractures with narrowing of the subacromial space or with concomitant injury to the SSSC.[206,222] In adults, displaced acromial fractures with narrowing of the subacromial space have resulted in problems with subacromial impingement.

Nondisplaced or minimally displaced glenoid rim fractures (types I and II) not associated with glenohumeral instability can be treated nonoperatively, typically with sling immobilization. Open reduction and internal fixation should be considered for glenoid rim fractures associated with glenohumeral instability. The surgical approach is anterior for fractures of the anterior rim and posterior for fractures of the posterior rim. Fixation options include interfragmentary compression screw or small plate fixation. Based on studies in adults, the risk of glenohumeral instability is increased with fracture displacement greater than 10 mm or with involvement of at least one fourth of the anterior portion or one third of the posterior portion of the glenoid.[218,223,236]

Nondisplaced or minimally displaced glenoid fossa fractures (types III-VI) can also be treated nonoperatively. Open reduction and internal fixation should be considered for glenoid fossa fractures with intra-articular displacement greater than 5 to 10 mm; significant separation between fracture fragments, making nonunion likely; and significant displacement of glenoid fragments, resulting in an incongruent relationship between the humeral head and glenoid cavity.[206,237] Fractures of the glenoid fossa are typically best approached posteriorly. The goals of operative intervention are anatomic restoration of the articular surface and stable fixation, usually by interfragmentary compression screw or contoured reconstruction plate, to allow early functional shoulder exercises. For severely displaced fractures of the glenoid fossa with significant comminution (type VI), nonoperative treatment should be considered because acceptable operative reduction and fixation is difficult to achieve.

Because of the high-energy nature of these injuries, massive trauma to the entire extremity occurs with scapulothoracic dissociations. Initial management should focus on airway, breathing, and circulation, following trauma protocols. Thorough neurovascular examination is critical. Vascular consultation or evaluation may be necessary. Once the patient is stabilized, focus should shift to stabilization and repair of the neurovascular injury. If the injuries to the axillary artery and brachial plexus are beyond repair or reconstruction, early amputation should be considered.[214,238] On the other hand, if the neurovascular injuries appear reparable, an attempt at limb salvage is recommended. If vascular injuries are identified, vascular repair should be prioritized to avoid either life-threatening hemorrhage or prolonged upper extremity ischemia. Immediate exploration of brachial plexus injuries is not required. However, in the presence of a concomitant vascular injury needing repair, a combined primary vascular repair and nerve reconstruction should be considered in the same operative setting.[214,239] With persistent brachial plexus palsy, nerve reconstruction or musculotendinous transfer should be performed within 6 months to minimize muscle atrophy and fibrosis.[238,240-242] Operative stabilization of injuries to the clavicle, scapula, acromioclavicular joint, or sternoclavicular joint is necessary only if the bony instability endangers the integrity of the neurovascular structures.[214,243,244]

Complications

Neurovascular injuries often occur concomitantly in association with scapula fractures. All or portions of the brachial plexus are susceptible to injury, especially in association with scapulothoracic dissociations. Given their proximity, the subclavian and axillary vessels are also at risk for injury. Also, given the high-energy nature of these injuries, multisystem trauma is not uncommon, and injuries occur to other organ systems, including the brain and especially the lungs, such as pneumothorax, hemothorax, and pulmonary contusion.

Fractures of the scapula can lead to disability of the shoulder complex and poor functional outcome of the upper extremity.[206,209,210] Fractures with initial significant displacement and subsequent residual scapular deformity are at increased risk for long-term upper extremity weakness and pain. Displaced acromion fractures in particular are at risk for pain and stiffness secondary to narrowing and impingement of the subacromial space.[220,222] Displaced intra-articular glenoid fractures are also at risk given the risk of glenohumeral instability and early-onset degenerative arthritis.[206,236] Symptomatic nonunion of fractures involving the scapular body and acromion can also occur.[245-247]

REFERENCES

1. Gray DJ, Gardner E: The prenatal development of the human humerus. Am J Anat 124:431-445,1969.
2. Donne HD, Faundes A, Tristao EG, et al: Sonographic identification and measurement of the epiphyseal ossification centers as markers of fetal gestational age. J Clin Ultrasound 33:394-400, 2005.
3. Nazario AC, Tanaka CI, Novo NF: Proximal humeral ossification center of the fetus: Time of appearance and the sensitivity and specificity of this finding. J Ultrasound Med 12:513-515, 1993.
4. Gray H: Anatomy of the human body, ed W Lewis. Philadelphia: Lea & Febiger, 2000.
5. Ogden JA, Conlogue GJ, Jensen PS: Radiology of postnatal skeletal development. The proximal humerus. Skeletal Radiol 2:153-160, 1978.
6. Samilson RL: Congenital and developmental anomalies of the shoulder girdle. Orthop Clin North Am 11:219-231, 1980.
7. Bortel DT, Pritchett JW: Straight-line graphs for the prediction of growth of the upper extremities. J Bone Joint Surg Am 75:885-892, 1993.
8. Pritchett JW: Growth and predictions of growth in the upper extremity. J Bone Joint Surg Am 70:520-525, 1988.
9. Pritchett JW: Growth plate activity in the upper extremity. Clin Orthop Relat Res (268):235-242, 1991.
10. Boileau P, Walch G: The three-dimensional geometry of the proximal humerus. Implications for surgical technique and prosthetic design. J Bone Joint Surg Br 79:857-865, 1997.
11. Cassagnaud X, Maynou C, Petroff E, et al: A study of reproducibility of an original method of CT measurement of the lateralization of the intertubercular groove and humeral retroversion. Surg Radiol Anat 25:145-151, 2003.
12. Edelson G: Variations in the retroversion of the humeral head. J Shoulder Elbow Surg 8:142-145, 1999.
13. Hernigou P, Duparc F, Filali C: [Humeral retroversion and shoulder prosthesis]. Rev Chir Orthop Reparatrice Appar Mot 81:419-427, 1995.
14. Hernigou P, Duparc F, Hernigou A: Determining humeral retroversion with computed tomography. J Bone Joint Surg Am 84:1753-1762, 2002.
15. Krahl VE: The phylogeny and ontogeny of humeral torsion. Am J Phys Anthropol 45:595-599, 1976.
16. Robertson DD, Yuan J, Bigliani LU, et al: Three-dimensional analysis of the proximal part of the humerus: Relevance to arthroplasty. J Bone Joint Surg Am 82:1594-1602, 2000.
17. Edelson G: The development of humeral head retroversion. J Shoulder Elbow Surg 9:316-318, 2000.

18. Salter R, Harris W: Injuries involving the epiphyseal plate. J Bone Joint Surg Am 45:587-622, 1963.
19. Dameron TB, Reibel DB: Fractures involving the proximal humeral epiphyseal plate. J Bone Joint Surg Am 51:289-297, 1969.
20. Cain PR, Mutschler TA, Fu FH, et al: Anterior stability of the glenohumeral joint. A dynamic model. Am J Sports Med 15:44-48, 1987.
21. Howell SM, Galinat BJ: The glenoid-labral socket. A constrained articular surface. Clin Orthop Relat Res 243:122-125, 1989.
22. Howell SM, Galinat BJ, Renzi AJ, et al: Normal and abnormal mechanics of the glenohumeral joint in the horizontal plane. J Bone Joint Surg Am 70:227-232, 1988.
23. Howell SM, Imobersteg AM, Seger DH, et al: Clarification of the role of the supraspinatus muscle in shoulder function. J Bone Joint Surg Am 68:398-404, 1986.
24. Brooks CH, Revell WJ, Heatley FW: Vascularity of the humeral head after proximal humeral fractures. An anatomical cadaver study. J Bone Joint Surg Br 75:132-136, 1993.
25. Duparc F, Muller JM, Freger P: Arterial blood supply of the proximal humeral epiphysis. Surg Radiol Anat 23:185-190, 2001.
26. Gerber C, Schneeberger AG, Vinh TS: The arterial vascularization of the humeral head. An anatomical study. J Bone Joint Surg Am 72:1486-1494, 1990.
27. Meyer C, Alt V, Hassanin H, et al: The arteries of the humeral head and their relevance in fracture treatment. Surg Radiol Anat 27:232-237, 2005.
28. Bono CM, Grossman MG, Hochwald N, et al: Radial and axillary nerves. Anatomic considerations for humeral fixation. Clin Orthop Relat Res (373):259-264, 2000.
29. Gardner MJ, Griffith MH, Dines JS, et al: The extended anterolateral acromial approach allows minimally invasive access to the proximal humerus. Clin Orthop Relat Res (434):123-129, 2005.
30. Kamineni S, Ankem H, Sanghavi S: Anatomical considerations for percutaneous proximal humeral fracture fixation. Injury 35:1133-1136, 2004.
31. Zlotolow DA, Catalano LW, Barron OA, et al: Surgical exposures of the humerus. J Am Acad Orthop Surg 14:754-765, 2006.
32. Hohl JC: Fractures of the humerus in children. Orthop Clin North Am 7:557-571, 1976.
33. Horak J, Nilsson BE: Epidemiology of fracture of the upper end of the humerus. Clin Orthop Relat Res (112):250-253, 1975.
34. Iqbal QM: Long bone fractures among children in Malaysia. Int Surg 59:410-415, 1974.
35. Landin LA: Fracture patterns in children. Analysis of 8,682 fractures with special reference to incidence, etiology and secular changes in a Swedish urban population 1950-1979. Acta Orthop Scand Suppl 202:1-109, 1983.
36. Rose SH, Melton LJ, Morrey BF, et al: Epidemiologic features of humeral fractures. Clin Orthop Relat Res (168):24-30, 1982.
37. Mann DC, Rajmaira S: Distribution of physeal and nonphyseal fractures in 2,650 long-bone fractures in children aged 0-16 years. J Pediatr Orthop 10:713-716, 1990.
38. Mizuta T, Benson WM, Foster BK, et al: Statistical analysis of the incidence of physeal injuries. J Pediatr Orthop 7:518-523, 1987.
39. Peterson HA, Madhok R, Benson JT, et al: Physeal fractures: Part 1. Epidemiology in Olmsted County, Minnesota, 1979-1988. J Pediatr Orthop 14:423-430, 1994.
40. Gherman RB, Ouzounian JG, Goodwin TM: Obstetric maneuvers for shoulder dystocia and associated fetal morbidity. Am J Obstet Gynecol 178:1126-1130, 1998.
41. Cumming WA: Neonatal skeletal fractures. Birth trauma or child abuse? J Can Assoc Radiol 30:30-33, 1979.
42. Harris BA: Shoulder dystocia. Clin Obstet Gynecol 27:106-111, 1984.
43. Madsen ET: Fractures of the extremities in the newborn. Acta Obstet Gynecol Scand 34:41-74, 1955.
44. Scaglietti O: The obstetrical shoulder trauma. Surg Gynecol Obstet 66:868-877, 1938.
45. Kohler R, Trillaud JM: Fracture and fracture separation of the proximal humerus in children: Report of 136 cases. J Pediatr Orthop 3:326-332, 1983.
46. Williams DJ: The mechanisms producing fracture-separation of the proximal humeral epiphysis. J Bone Joint Surg Br 63:102-107, 1981.
47. Dalldorf PG, Bryan WJ: Displaced Salter–Harris type I injury in a gymnast. A slipped capital humeral epiphysis? Orthop Rev 23:538-541, 1994.
48. Caine DJ, Nassar L: Gymnastics injuries. Med Sport Sci 48:18-58, 2005.
49. Cooney WP: Sports injuries to the upper extremity. How to recognize and deal with some common problems. Postgrad Med 76:45-50, 1984.
50. Davidson PL, Mahar B, Chalmers DJ, et al: Impact modeling of gymnastic back-handsprings and dive-rolls in children. J Appl Biomech 21:115-128, 2005.
51. Gainor BJ, Piotrowski G, Puhl J, et al: The throw: Biomechanics and acute injury. Am J Sports Med 8:114-118, 1980.
52. Perry J: Anatomy and biomechanics of the shoulder in throwing, swimming, gymnastics, and tennis. Clin Sports Med 2:247-270, 1983.
53. Richardson AB: Overuse syndromes in baseball, tennis, gymnastics, and swimming. Clin Sports Med 2:379-390, 1983.
54. Sabick MB, Kim YK, Torry MR, et al: Biomechanics of the shoulder in youth baseball pitchers: Implications for the development of proximal humeral epiphysiolysis and humeral retrotorsion. Am J Sports Med 33:1716-1722, 2005.
55. Sinha AK, Kaeding CC, Wadley GM: Upper extremity stress fractures in athletes: Clinical features of 44 cases. Clin J Sport Med 9:199-202, 1999.
56. Deyoe L, Woodbury DF: Unicameral bone cyst with fracture. Orthopedics 8:529-531, 1985.
57. Haims AH, Desai P, Present D, et al: Epiphyseal extension of a unicameral bone cyst. Skeletal Radiol 26:51-54, 1997.
58. Keret D, Kumar SJ: Unicameral bone cysts in the humerus and femur in the same child. J Pediatr Orthop 7:712-715, 1987.
59. Ortiz EJ, Isler MH, Navia JE, et al: Pathologic fractures in children. Clin Orthop Relat Res (432):116-126, 2005.
60. De Boeck H, Handelberg F, Otten J: Unusual evolution of a benign-looking cortical defect of the proximal humerus. A case of intracortical osteosarcoma? Acta Orthop Belg 64:96-99, 1998.
61. Ebeid W, Amin S, Abdelmegid A: Limb salvage management of pathologic fractures of primary malignant bone tumors. Cancer Control 12:57-61, 2005.
62. Harrington KD: Orthopedic surgical management of skeletal complications of malignancy. Cancer 80:1614-1627, 1997.
63. Robin G, Kedar S: Separation of the upper humeral epiphysis in pituitary gigantism. J Bone Joint Surg Am 44:189-192, 1962.
64. Aroojis AJ, Gajjar SM, Johari AN: Epiphyseal separations in spastic cerebral palsy. J Pediatr Orthop B 16:170-174, 2007.
65. Gray B, Hsu JD, Furumasu J: Fractures caused by falling from a wheelchair in patients with neuromuscular disease. Dev Med Child Neurol 34:589-592, 1992.
66. Lock TR, Aronson DD: Fractures in patients who have myelomeningocele. J Bone Joint Surg Am 71:1153-1157, 1989.
67. Torwalt CR, Balachandra AT, Youngson C, et al: Spontaneous fractures in the differential diagnosis of fractures in children. J Forensic Sci 47:1340-1344, 2002.
68. Caviglia H, Garrido CP, Palazzi FF, et al: Pediatric fractures of the humerus. Clin Orthop Relat Res (432):49-56, 2005.
69. Conradi S, Brissie R: Battered child syndrome in a four-year-old with previous diagnosis of Reye's syndrome. Forensic Sci Int 30:195-203, 1986.
70. King J, Diefendorf D, Apthorp J, et al: Analysis of 429 fractures in 189 battered children. J Pediatr Orthop 8:585-589, 1988.
71. Leventhal JM, Thomas SA, Rosenfield NS, et al: Fractures in young children. Distinguishing child abuse from unintentional injuries. Am J Dis Child 147:87-92, 1993.
72. Shaw BA, Murphy KM, Shaw A, et al: Humerus shaft fractures in young children: Accident or abuse? J Pediatr Orthop 17:293-297, 1997.
73. Wang P, Koval KJ, Lehman W, et al: Salter–Harris type III fracture-dislocation of the proximal humerus. J Pediatr Orthop B 6:219-222, 1997.
74. Neer CS, Horwitz BS: Fractures of the proximal humeral epiphysial plate. Clin Orthop Relat Res 41:24-31, 1965.
75. Gustilo RB: Management of open fractures and complications. Instr Course Lect 31:64-75, 1982.
76. Gustilo RB, Mendoza RM, Williams DN: Problems in the management of type III (severe) open fractures: A new classification of type III open fractures. J Trauma 24:742-746, 1984.
77. Le Huec JC, Schaeverbeke T, Moinard M, et al: Isolated avulsion fracture of the lesser tubercle of the humerus in children. Acta Orthop Belg 60:427-429, 1994.
78. Levine B, Pereira D, Rosen J: Avulsion fractures of the lesser tuberosity of the humerus in adolescents: Review of the literature and case report. J Orthop Trauma 19:349-352, 2005.
79. Ross GJ, Love MB: Isolated avulsion fracture of the lesser tuberosity of the humerus: Report of two cases. Radiology 172:833-834, 1989.
80. Freundlich BD: Luxatio erecta. J Trauma 23:434-436, 1983.
81. Kothari K, Bernstein RM, Griffiths HJ, et al: Luxatio erecta. Skeletal Radiol 11:47-49, 1984.
82. Yamamoto T, Yoshiya S, Kurosaka M, et al: Luxatio erecta (inferior dislocation of the shoulder): A report of 5 cases and a review of the literature. Am J Orthop 32:601-603, 2003.
83. Kleinman PK, Akins CM: The "vanishing" epiphysis: Sign of Salter type I fracture of the proximal humerus in infancy. Br J Radiol 55:865-867, 1982.
84. Broker FH, Burbach T: Ultrasonic diagnosis of separation of the proximal humeral epiphysis in the newborn. J Bone Joint Surg Am 72:187-191, 1990.
85. Fisher NA, Newman B, Lloyd J, et al: Ultrasonographic evaluation of birth injury to the shoulder. J Perinatol 15:398-400, 1995.
86. Jones GP, Seguin J, Shiels WE, et al: Salter–Harris II fracture of the proximal humerus in a preterm infant. Am J Perinatol 20:249-253, 2003.
87. Schmit P, Hautefort P, Raison-Boulley AM. [Ultrasonographic diagnosis of an epiphyseal detachment of the upper end of the humerus due to birth injury]. J Radiol 80:466-468, 1999.
88. Zieger M, Dorr U, Schulz RD: Sonography of slipped humeral epiphysis due to birth injury. Pediatr Radiol 17:425-426, 1987.

89. DeSimone DP, Morwessel RM: Diagnostic arthrogram of a Salter I fracture of the proximal humerus in a newborn. Orthop Rev 17:782-785, 1988.

90. White SJ, Blane CE, DiPietro MA, et al: Arthrography in evaluation of birth injuries of the shoulder. Can Assoc Radiol J 38:113-115, 1987.

91. Troum S, Floyd WE, Waters PM: Posterior dislocation of the humeral head in infancy associated with obstetrical paralysis. A case report. J Bone Joint Surg Am 75:1370-1375, 1993.

92. Beaty JH: Fractures of the proximal humerus and shaft in children. Instr Course Lect 41:369-372, 1992.

93. Larsen CF, Kiaer T, Lindequist S: Fractures of the proximal humerus in children. Nine-year follow-up of 64 unoperated on cases. Acta Orthop Scand 61:255-257, 1990.

94. Sherk HH, Probst C: Fractures of the proximal humeral epiphysis. Orthop Clin North Am 6:401-413, 1975.

95. Curtis RJ: Operative management of children's fractures of the shoulder region. Orthop Clin North Am 21:315-324, 1990.

96. Lentz W, Meuser P: The treatment of fractures of the proximal humerus. Arch Orthop Trauma Surg 96:283-285, 1980.

97. Visser JD, Rietberg M: Interposition of the tendon of the long head of biceps in fracture separation of the proximal humeral epiphysis. Neth J Surg 32:12-15, 1980.

98. Bourdillon J: Fracture-separation of the proximal humeral epiphysis of the humerus. J Bone Joint Surg Br 32:35-37, 1950.

99. Jeffrey C: Fracture-separation of the upper humeral epiphysis. Surg Gynecol Obstet 96:205-209, 1953.

100. Haliburton RA, Barber JR, Fraser RL: Pseudodislocation: An unusual birth injury. Can J Surg 10:455-462, 1967.

101. Karatosun V, Unver B, Alici E, et al: Treatment of displaced, proximal, humeral, epiphyseal fractures with a two-prong splint. J Orthop Trauma 17:578-581, 2003.

102. Burgos-Flores J, Gonzalez-Herranz P, Lopez-Mondejar JA, et al: Fractures of the proximal humeral epiphysis. Int Orthop 17:16-19, 1993.

103. Dobbs MB, Luhmann SL, Gordon JE, et al: Severely displaced proximal humeral epiphyseal fractures. J Pediatr Orthop 23(2):208-215, 2003.

104. Schwendenwein E, Hajdu S, Gaebler C, et al: Displaced fractures of the proximal humerus in children require open/closed reduction and internal fixation. Eur J Pediatr Surg 14:51-55, 2004.

105. Chen CY, Chao EK, Tu YK, et al: Closed management and percutaneous fixation of unstable proximal humerus fractures. J Trauma 45:1039-1045, 1998.

106. Rowles DJ, McGrory JE: Percutaneous pinning of the proximal part of the humerus. An anatomic study. J Bone Joint Surg Am 83:1695-1699, 2001.

107. Wachtl SW, Marti CB, Hoogewoud HM, et al: Treatment of proximal humerus fracture using multiple intramedullary flexible nails. Arch Orthop Trauma Surg 120:171-175, 2000.

108. Shibuya S, Ogawa K: Isolated avulsion fracture of the lesser tuberosity of the humerus. A case report. Clin Orthop Relat Res (211):215-218, 1986.

109. Klasson SC, Vander Schilden JL, Park JP: Late effect of isolated avulsion fractures of the lesser tubercle of the humerus in children. Report of two cases. J Bone Joint Surg Am 75:1691-1694, 1993.

110. White GM, Riley LH: Isolated avulsion of the subscapularis insertion in a child. A case report. J Bone Joint Surg Am 67:635-636, 1985.

111. Ogawa K, Takahashi M: Long-term outcome of isolated lesser tuberosity fractures of the humerus. J Trauma 42:955-959, 1997.

112. Scheibel M, Martinek V, Imhoff AB: Arthroscopic reconstruction of an isolated avulsion fracture of the lesser tuberosity. Arthroscopy 21:487-494, 2005.

113. Jaschke W, Hopf G, Gerstner C, et al: [Proximal humerus fracture with dislocation in childhood. Transacromial percutaneous osteosynthesis using Kirschner wires]. Zentralbl Chir 106:618-621, 1981.

114. Obremskey W, Routt ML: Fracture-dislocation of the shoulder in a child: Case report. J Trauma 36:137-140, 1994.

115. Artico M, Salvati M, D'Andrea V, et al: Isolated lesion of the axillary nerve: Surgical treatment and outcome in 12 cases. Neurosurgery 29:697-700, 1991.

116. Drew SJ, Giddins GE, Birch R: A slowly evolving brachial plexus injury following a proximal humeral fracture in a child. J Hand Surg Br 20:24-25, 1995.

117. Vastamaki M, Solonen KA: Posterior dislocation and fracture-dislocation of the shoulder. Acta Orthop Scand 51:479-484, 1980.

118. Visser CP, Coene LN, Brand R, et al: Nerve lesions in proximal humeral fractures. J Shoulder Elbow Surg 10:421-427, 2001.

119. Baxter MP, Wiley JJ: Fractures of the proximal humeral epiphysis. Their influence on humeral growth. J Bone Joint Surg Br 68:570-573, 1986.

120. Linson MA: Axillary artery thrombosis after fracture of the humerus. A case report. J Bone Joint Surg Am 62:1214-1215, 1980.

121. Wera GD, Friess DM, Getty PO, et al: Fracture of the proximal humerus with injury to the axillary artery in a boy aged 13 years. J Bone Joint Surg Br 88:1521-1523, 2006.

122. Liebling G, Bartel HG: [Unusual migration of a Kirschner wire following drill wire fixation of a subcapital humerus fracture]. Beitr Orthop Traumatol 34:585-587, 1987.

123. Lyons FA, Rockwood CA: Migration of pins used in operations on the shoulder. J Bone Joint Surg Am 72:1262-1267, 1990.

124. Tristan TA, Daughtridge TG: Migration of a metallic pin from the humerus into the lung. N Engl J Med 270:987-989, 1964.

125. Bollini G, Rigault P: [Humerus varus (author's transl)]. Chir Pediatr 21:369-376, 1980.

126. Cho TJ, Choi IH, Chung CY, et al: Humerus varus in a patient with pseudohypoparathyroidism. J Korean Med Sci 20:158-161, 2005.

127. Ellefsen BK, Frierson MA, Raney EM, et al: Humerus varus: A complication of neonatal, infantile, and childhood injury and infection. J Pediatr Orthop 14:479-486, 1994.

128. Lawson JP, Ablow RC, Pearson HA: Premature fusion of the proximal humeral epiphyses in thalassemia. AJR Am J Roentgenol 140:239-244, 1983.

129. Ogden JA, Weil UH, Hempton RF: Developmental humerus varus. Clin Orthop Relat Res (116):158-165, 1976.

130. Russo R, Vernaglia Lombardi L, Giudice G, et al: Surgical treatment of sequelae of fractures of the proximal third of the humerus. The role of osteotomies. Chir Organi Mov 90:159-169, 2005.

131. Benegas E, Zoppi Filho A, Ferreira Filho AA, et al: Surgical treatment of varus malunion of the proximal humerus with valgus osteotomy. J Shoulder Elbow Surg 16:55-59, 2007.

132. Gill TJ, Waters P: Valgus osteotomy of the humeral neck: A technique for the treatment of humerus varus. J Shoulder Elbow Surg 6:306-310, 1997.

133. Schopler SA, Lawrence JF, Johnson MK: Lengthening of the humerus for upper extremity limb length discrepancy. J Pediatr Orthop 6:477-480, 1986.

134. Von Laer L: [Surgical correction of the upper and lower arm of children]. Unfallchirurg 107:552-562, 2004.

135. Kraus R, Schnettler R: [Distraction osteogenesis for adjusting humeral length difference due to premature closure of the proximal growth plate in a simple bone cyst.]. Chirurg 77:376-380, 2006.

136. Pazzaglia UE, Ceciliani L: Periosteal chondroma of the humerus leading to shortening. A case report. J Bone Joint Surg Br 67:290-292, 1985.

137. Ramappa AJ, Lee FY, Tang P, et al: Chondroblastoma of bone. J Bone Joint Surg Am 82:1140-1145, 2000.

138. Stanton RP, Abdel-Mota'al MM: Growth arrest resulting from unicameral bone cyst. J Pediatr Orthop 18:198-201, 1998.

139. Violas P, Salmeron F, Chapuis M, et al: Simple bone cysts of the proximal humerus complicated with growth arrest. Acta Orthop Belg 70:166-170, 2004.

140. Fraser RL, Haliburton RA, Barber JR: Displaced epiphyseal fractures of the proximal humerus. Can J Surg 10:427-430, 1967.

141. Giebel G, Suren EG: [Injuries of the proximal humeral epiphysis. Indications for surgical therapy and results]. Chirurg 54:406-410, 1983.

142. Leslie J, Ryan T: The anterior axillary incision to approach the shoulder joint. J Bone Joint Surg Am 44:1193-1196, 1962.

143. Barra JA, Le Saout J, Gaultier Y: [Late signs of vascular complications of closed trauma of the shoulder (author's transl)]. J Chir (Paris) 115:151-157, 1978.

144. Garner E: The embryology of the clavicle. Clin Orthop 58:9-16, 1968.

145. Webb LX, Mooney JF: Fractures and dislocations about the shoulder. In Green NE, Swiontkowski MF (eds): Skeletal trauma in children. Philadelphia: Saunders, 2003, pp 322-343.

146. Abbott LC, Lucas DB: Function of the clavicle: Its surgical significance. Ann Surg 140:583-599, 1954.

147. Inman VT, Saunders JB, Abbott LC: Observations on the function of the shoulder joint. J Bone Joint Surg 26:1-30, 1944.

148. Moseley HF: The clavicle: Its anatomy and function. Clin Orthop 58:17-27, 1968.

149. Rowe CR: An atlas of anatomy and treatment of midclavicular fractures. Clin Orthop 58:29-42, 1968.

150. Cohen AW, Otto SR: Obstetric clavicular fractures. J Reprod Med 25:119-122, 1980.

151. Nordqvist A, Petersson C: The incidence of fractures of the clavicle. Clin Orthop Relat Res (300):127-132, 1994.

152. Beall MH, Ross MG: Clavicle fracture in labor: risk factors and associated morbidities. J Perinatol 21:513-515, 2001.

153. Howard FM, Shafer SJ: Injuries to the clavicle with neurovascular complications: A study of fourteen cases. J Bone Joint Surg Am 47:1335-1346, 1965.

154. Serrano JA, Rodriguez P, Castro L, et al: Acute subclavian artery pseudoaneurysm after closed fracture of the clavicle. Acta Orthop Belg 69:555-557, 2003.

155. Taitsman LA, Nork SE, Coles CP, et al: Open clavicle fractures and associated injuries. J Orthop Trauma 20:396-399, 2006.

156. Barbier O, Malghem J, Delaere O, et al: Injury to the brachial plexus by a fragment of bone after fracture of the clavicle. J Bone Joint Surg Br 79:534-536, 1997.

157. Della Santa D, Narakas A, Bonnard C: Late lesions of the brachial plexus after fracture of the clavicle. Ann Chir Main Memb Super 10:531-540, 1991.

158. Watanabe K, Matsumura T: Late-onset brachial plexus paresis caused by subclavian pseudoaneurysm formation after clavicular fracture. J Trauma 58:1073-1074, 2005.

159. Buckerfield CT, Castle ME: Acute traumatic retrosternal dislocation of the clavicle. J Bone Joint Surg Am 66:379-385, 1984.

160. Garner MA, Bidstrup BP: Intrathoracic great vessel injury resulting from blunt chest trauma associated with posterior dislocation of the sternoclavicular joint. Aust N Z J Surg 53:427-430, 1983.

161. Lehnert M, Maier B, Jakob H, et al: Fracture and retrosternal dislocation of the medial clavicle in a 12-year-old child. J Pediatr Surg 40:E1-E3, 2005.

162. Lewonowski K, Bassett GS: Complete posterior sternoclavicular epiphyseal separation. Clin Orthop Relat Res (281):84-88, 1992.

163. Noda M, Shiraishi H, Mizuno K: Chronic posterior sternoclavicular dislocation causing compression of a subclavian artery. J Shoulder Elbow Surg 6:564-569, 1997.

164. Rockwood CA: Dislocations of the sternoclavicular joint. Instr Course Lect 24:144-159, 1975.

165. Worman LW, Leaus C: Intrathoracic injury following retrosternal dislocation of the clavicle. J Trauma 7:416-423, 1967.

166. Bowen RE, Mah JY, Otsuka NY: Midshaft clavicle fractures associated with atlantoaxial rotatory displacement: A report of two cases. J Orthop Trauma 17:444-447, 2003.

167. Nannapaneni R, Nath FP, Papastefanou SL: Fracture of the clavicle associated with a rotatory atlantoaxial subluxation. Injury 32:71-73, 2001.

168. Blab E, Geibler W, Rokitansky A: Sonographic management of infantile clavicular fractures. Pediatr Surg Int 15:251-254, 1999.

169. Katz R, Landman J, Dulitzy F, et al: Fracture of the clavicle in the newborn: An ultrasound diagnosis. J Ultrasound Med 7:21-23, 1988.

170. Kayser R, Mahlfeld K, Heyde C, et al: Ultrasonographic imaging of fractures of the clavicle in newborn infants. J Bone Joint Surg Br 85:115-116, 2003.

171. Beslikas TA, Dadoukis DJ, Gigis IP, et al: Congenital pseudoarthrosis of the clavicle: A case report. J Orthop Surg 15:87-90, 2007.

172. Allman FL: Fractures and ligamentous injuries of the clavicle and its articulations. J Bone Joint Surg Am 49:774-784, 1967.

173. Rockwood CA: The shoulder: Facts, confusions, and myths. Int Orthop 15:401-405, 1991.

174. Falstie-Jensen S, Mikkelsen P: Pseudodislocation of the acromioclavicular joint. J Bone Joint Surg Br 64:368-369, 1982.

175. Ogden JA: Distal clavicular physeal injury. Clin Orthop Relat Res (188):68-73, 1984.

176. Mehta JC, Sachdev A, Collins JJ: Retrosternal dislocation of the clavicle. Injury 5:79-83, 1973.

177. Waters PM, Bae DS, Kadiyala RK: Short-term outcomes after surgical treatment of traumatic posterior sternoclavicular fracture-dislocations in children and adolescents. J Pediatr Orthop 23:464-469, 2003.

178. Wirth MA, Rockwood CA: Acute and chronic traumatic injuries of the sternoclavicular joint. J Am Acad Orthop Surg 4:268-278, 1996.

179. Joseph PR, Rosenfeld W: Clavicular fractures in neonates. Am J Dis Child 144:165-167, 1990.

180. Fowler AW: Treatment of fractured clavicle. Lancet 1:46-47, 1968.

181. Jeray KJ: Acute midshaft clavicular fractures. J Am Acad Orthop Surg 15:239-248, 2007.

182. Leffert RD: Brachial plexus injuries. N Engl J Med 291:1059-1067, 1974.

183. Andersen K, Jensen PO, Lauritzen J: Treatment of clavicular fractures. Figure-of-eight bandage versus a simple sling. Acta Orthop Scand 58:71-74, 1987.

184. Howard FM, Shafer SJ: Injuries to the clavicle with neurovascular complications: A study of fourteen cases. J Bone Joint Surg Am 47:1335-1346, 1965.

185. Kubiak R, Slongo T: Operative treatment of clavicle fractures in children: A review of 21 years. J Pediatr Orthop 22:736-739, 2002.

186. DeFranco MJ, Patterson BM: The floating shoulder. J Am Acad Orthop Surg 14:499-509, 2006.

187. Canadian Orthopaedic Trauma Society: Nonoperative treatment compared with plate fixation of displaced midshaft clavicular fractures. A multicenter, randomized clinical trial. J Bone Joint Surg Am 89(1):1-10, 2007.

188. Hill JM, McGuire MH, Crosby LA: Closed treatment of displaced middle-third fractures of the clavicle gives poor results. J Bone Joint Surg Br 79(4):537-539, 1997.

189. Wick M, Müller EJ, Kollig E, Muhr G: Midshaft fractures of the clavicle with a shortening of more than 2 cm predispose to nonunion. Arch Orthop Trauma Surg 121(4):207-211, 2001.

190. Jubel A, Andermahr J, Bergmann H, et al: Elastic stable intramedullary nailing of midclavicular fractures in athletes. Br J Sports Med 37:480-484, 2003.

191. Fowler AW: Migration of a wire from the sternoclavicular joint to the pericardial cavity. Injury 13:261-262, 1981.

192. Black GH, McPherson JA, Reed MH: Traumatic pseudodislocation of the acromioclavicular joint in children. A 15-year review. Am J Sports Med 19:644-646, 1991.

193. Eidman DK, Siff SJ, Tullos HS: Acromioclavicular lesions in children. Am J Sports Med 9:150-154, 1981.

194. Havranek P: Injuries of distal clavicular physis in children. J Pediatr Orthop 9:213-215, 1989.

195. Daroy C, Fenoll B, Hra B, et al: Epiphyseal fracture-avulsion of the distal extremity of the clavicle. Ann Radiol (Paris) 36:125-128, 1993.

196. Roper BA, Levack B: The surgical treatment of acromioclavicular dislocations. J Bone Joint Surg Am 69:1045-1051, 1982.

197. Qureshi AA, Kuo KN: Posttraumatic cleidoscapular synostosis following a fracture of the clavicle: A case report. J Bone Joint Surg Am 81:256-258, 1999.

198. Manske DJ, Szabo RM: The operative treatment of mid-shaft clavicular nonunions. J Bone Joint Surg Am 67:1367-1371, 1985.

199. Neer CS II: Nonunion of the clavicle. JAMA 49:774-784, 1967.

200. Nogi J, Heckman JD, Hakala M, et al: Non-union of the clavicle in a child: A case report. Clin Orthop Relat Res (110):19-21, 1975.

201. Pyper JB: Non-union of fractures of the clavicle. Injury 9:268-270, 1978.

202. Zlowodzki M, Zelle BA, Cole PA, et al: Evidence-based Orthopaedic Trauma Working Group: Treatment of acute midshaft clavicle fractures. J Orthop Trauma 19:504-507, 2005.

203. Tavitian JD, Davison JNS, Dias JJ: Clavicular fracture non-union surgical outcome and complications. Injury 33:135-143, 2002.

204. Horwitz AE: Congenital elevation of the scapula—Sprengel's deformity. J Bone Joint Surg Am 6:260-311, 1908.

205. Khairouni A, Bensahel H, Csukonyi Z, et al: Congenital high scapula. J Pediatr Orthop Br 11:85-88, 2002.

206. Goss TP: Scapular fractures and dislocations: Diagnosis and treatment. J Am Acad Orthop Surg 3:22-33, 1995.

207. Owens BD, Goss TP: The floating shoulder. J Bone Joint Surg Br 88:1419-1424, 2006.

208. Williams GR, Naranja J, Kliemkiewicz J, et al: The floating shoulder: A biomechanical basis for classification and management. J Bone Joint Surg Am 83:1182-1187, 2001.

209. Ada JR, Miller ME: Scapular fractures. Clin Orthop Relat Res (269):174-180, 1991.

210. Nordqvist A, Petersson C: Fracture of the body, neck, or spine of the scapula. Clin Orthop Relat Res (283):139-144, 1992.

211. Thompson DA, Flynn TC, Miller PW, et al: The significance of scapular fractures. J Trauma 25:974-977, 1985.

212. Katsamouris AN, Kafetzakis A, Kostas T, et al: The initial management of scapulothoracic dissociation: A challenging task for the vascular surgeon. Eur J Vasc Endovasc Surg 24:547-549, 2002.

213. Masmejean EH, Asfazadourian H, Alnot JY: Brachial plexus injuries in scapulothoracic dissociation. J Hand Surg Br 25:336-340, 2000.

214. Brucker PU, Gruen GS, Kaufmann RA: Scapulothoracic dissociation: Evaluation and management. Injury 36:1147-1155, 2005.

215. Andrews JR, Byrd JW, Kupferman SP, et al: The profile view of the acromion. Clin Orthop Relat Res (263):142-146, 1991.

216. McClure JG, Raney RB: Anomalies of the scapula. Clin Orthop Relat Res (110):22-31, 1975.

217. Sarwark JF, King EC, Luhmann SJ: Proximal humerus, scapula, and clavicle. In Beaty JH, Kasser JR (eds): Rockwood and Wilkins' Fractures in Children. Philadelphia: Lippincott Williams & Wilkins, 2006, pp 703-771.

218. Hardegger FH, Simpson LA, Weber BG: The operative treatment of scapular fractures. J Bone Joint Surg Br 66:725-731, 1984.

219. Ganz R, Noesberger B: [Treatment of scapular fractures]. Hefte Unfallheilkd 126:59-62, 1975.

220. Goss TP: The scapula: Coracoid, acromial, and avulsion fractures. Am J Orthop 25:106-115, 1996.

221. Montgomery SP, Loyd RD: Avulsion fracture of the coracoid epiphysis with acromioclavicular separation. J Bone Joint Surg Am 29:963-965, 1977.

222. Kuhn JE, Blasier RB, Carpenter JE: Fractures of the acromion process: A proposed classification system. J Orthop Trauma 8:6-13, 1994.

223. Goss TP: Current concept review: Fractures of the glenoid cavity. J Bone Joint Surg Am 72:299-305, 1992.

224. Ideberg R: Unusual glenoid fractures. Acta Orthop Scand 58:191-192, 1987.

225. Imatani RJ: Fractures of the scapulae: A review of 53 fractures. J Trauma 15:473-478, 1975.

226. Rowe CR: Fractures of the scapula. Surg Clin North Am 43:1565-1571, 1963.

227. Wilber MC, Evans EB: Fractures of the scapula. J Bone Joint Surg Am 59:358-362, 1977.

228. Lindblom A, Leven H: Prognosis in fractures of body and neck of the scapula. Acta Chir Scand 140:33-47, 1974.

229. van Noort A, van Kampen A: Fractures of the scapula surgical neck: Outcome after conservative treatment in 13 cases. Arch Orthop Trauma Surg 125:696-700, 2005.

230. Khallaf F, Mikami A, Al-Akkad M: The use of surgery in displaced scapular neck fractures. Med Princ Pract 15:443-448, 2006.

231. Pace AM, Stuart R, Brownlow H: Outcome of glenoid neck fractures. J Shoulder Elbow Surg 14:585-590, 2005.

232. Romero J, Schai P, Imhoff AB: Scapular neck fracture—the influence of permanent malalignment of the glenoid neck on clinical outcome. Arch Orthop Trauma Surg 121:313-316, 2001.

233. Bozkurt M, Can F, Kirdemir V, et al: Conservative treatment of scapular neck fracture: The effect of stability and glenopolar angle on clinical outcome. Injury 36:1176-1181, 2005.

234. Leung KS, Lam TP: Open reduction and internal fixation of ipsilateral fractures of the scapular neck and clavicle. J Bone Joint Surg Am 75:1015-1018, 1993.

235. Herscovici D Jr, Fiennes AG, Allgower M, et al: The floating shoulder: Ipsilateral clavicle and scapular neck fractures. J Bone Joint Surg Br 74:362-364, 1992.

236. Guttentag IJ, Rechtine GR: Fractures of the scapula: A review of the literature. Orthop Rev 17:147-158, 1988.

237. Lee S, Meinhard B, Schultz E, et al: Open reduction and internal fixation of a glenoid fossa fracture in a child: A case report and review of the literature. J Orthop Trauma 11:452-454, 1997.

238. Oreck SL, Burgess A, Levine AM: Traumatic lateral displacement of the scapula: A radiographic sign of neurovascular disease. J Bone Joint Surg Am 66:748-763, 1984.

239. Shaw AD, Milne AA, Christie J, et al: Vascular trauma of the upper limb and associated nerve injuries. Injury 8:515-518, 1995.

240. Fogarty BJ, Brennen MD: Upper root brachial plexus trauma: Patient selection and reconstruction. Injury 33:57-62, 2000.

241. Nagano A: Treatment of brachial plexus injury. J Orthop Sci 3:71-80, 1998.

242. Narakas AO: The treatment of brachial plexus injuries. Int Orthop 9:29-36, 1985.

243. Clements RH, Reisser JR: Scapulothoracic dissociation: A devastating injury. J Trauma 40:146-149, 1996.

244. Damschen DD, Cogbill TH, Siegel MJ: Scapulothoracic dissociation caused by blunt trauma. J Trauma 42:537-540, 1997.

245. Ferraz I, Papadimitriou N, Sotreanos D: Scapular body nonunion: A case report. J Shoulder Elbow Surg 11:98-100, 2002.

246. Kaminsky S, Pierce V: Nonunion of a scapula body fracture in a high school football player. Am J Orthop 31:456-457, 2002.

247. Mick CA, Weiland AJ: Pseudoarthrosis of a fracture of the acromion. J Trauma 23:248-249, 1983.

Glenohumeral Instability

Frederick A. Matsen, III, MD, Steven B. Lippitt, MD, Alexander Bertlesen, PAC,
Charles A. Rockwood, Jr, MD, and Michael A. Wirth, MD

It deserves to be known how a shoulder which is subject to frequent dislocations should be treated. For many persons owing to this accident have been obliged to abandon gymnastic exercises, though otherwise well qualified for them; and from the same misfortune have become inept in warlike practices, and have thus perished. And this subject deserves to be noticed, because I have never known any physician [to] treat the case properly; some abandon the attempt altogether, and others hold opinions and practice the very reverse of what is proper.

HIPPOCRATES, 5TH CENTURY BCE

In every case the anterior margin of the glenoid cavity will be found to be smooth, rounded, and free of any attachments, and a blunt instrument can be passed freely inwards over the bare bone on the front of the neck of the scapula.

PERTHES,[1] 1906

The only rational treatment is to reattach the glenoid ligament (or the capsule) to the bone from which it has been torn.

BANKART,[2] 1939

HISTORICAL REVIEW

Early Descriptions

The first report of a shoulder dislocation is found in humankind's oldest book, the Edwin Smith Papyrus (3000-2500 BCE).[3] Hussein[4] reported that in 1200 BCE in the tomb of Upuy, an artist and sculptor to Ramses II, there was a drawing of a scene that was strikingly similar to Kocher's method of reduction (Fig. 16-1).

The most detailed early description of anterior dislocations came from the Father of Medicine, Hippocrates, who was born in 460 BCE on the island of Cos.[5] Hippocrates described the anatomy of the shoulder, the types of dislocations, and the first surgical procedure. In one of his classic procedures for reduction, he stressed the need for suitably sized, leather-covered balls to be placed into the axilla, for without them the heel could not reach the head of the humerus in his reduction maneuver. Other Hippocratic techniques are described by Brockbank and Griffiths (Fig. 16-2).[6]

Hippocrates criticized his contemporaries for improper burning of the shoulder, a treatment popular at the time. In this first description of a surgical procedure for recurrent dislocation of the shoulder, he described how physicians had burned the top, anterior, and posterior aspects of the shoulder, which only caused scarring in those areas and promoted downward dislocation. He advocated the use of cautery in which an oblong, red-hot iron was inserted through the axilla to make eschars, but only in the lower part of the joint. Hippocrates displayed considerable knowledge of the anatomy of the shoulder, and he warned the surgeon to not let the iron come in contact with the major vessels and nerves because it would cause great harm. Following the burnings, he bound the arm to the side, day and night for a long time, "for thus more especially will cicatrization take place, and the wide space into which the humerus used to escape will become contracted."[32]

Interested readers are referred to the text by Moseley,[7] which has a particularly good section on the historical aspects of management of shoulder instability.

Humeral Head Defect

In 1861, Flower[8] described the anatomic and pathologic changes found in 41 traumatically dislocated shoulders

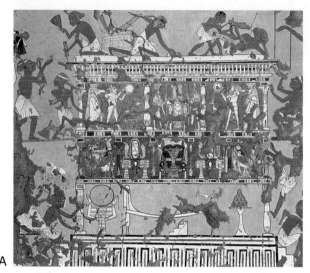

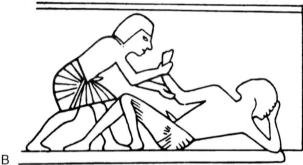

FIGURE 16-1 The Kocher technique is 3000 years old.
A, Drawing from the tomb of Upuy in 1200 BCE.
B, Schematic drawing of the picture in the upper right corner of the tomb painting depicting a patient on the ground while a man—possibly a physician—is manipulating a dislocated shoulder in the technique of Kocher. (From Hussein MK: Kocher's method is 3000 years old. J Bone Joint Surg Br 50:669-671, 1968.)

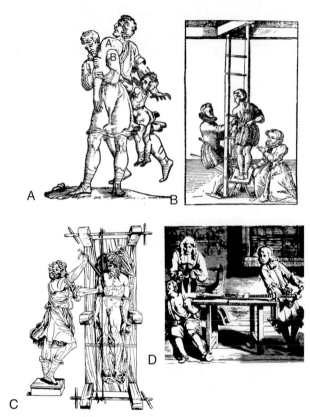

FIGURE 16-2 Modified techniques of Hippocrates to reduce dislocations of the shoulder. **A,** Reduction over the operator's shoulder. (From the Venice edition of Galen in 1625.) **B,** Reduction over the rung of a ladder. When the stepstool on which the patient is standing is withdrawn, the weight of the patient's body reduces the dislocation. (From deCruce in 1607.) **C,** Use of the rack to reduce a shoulder dislocation (Vidius). **D,** Reduction of a dislocation by a medieval type of screw traction (From Scultetus in 1693). (From Brockbank W, Griffiths DL: Orthopaedic surgery in the 16th and 17th centuries. J Bone Joint Surg Br 30:365-375, 1948.)

from specimens in London museums. He wrote that "where the head of the humerus rests upon the edge of the glenoid fossa absorption occurs, and a groove is evacuated, usually between the articular head and the greater tuberosity."[8] In 1880, Eve[9] reported an autopsy of a patient who died 12 hours after an acute anterior dislocation in which he found a deep groove in the posterolateral aspect of the head. Joessel[10] also observed the defect. According to Hill and Sachs,[11] beginning in 1882, publications by Kuster,[12] Cramer,[13] Löbker,[14] Schüller,[15] Staffel,[16] and Francke[17] described the finding of a posterolateral defect in humeral heads resected for relief of chronic or recurrent dislocation.

In 1887, Caird[18] of Edinburgh concluded that a true subcoracoid dislocation must have an indentation fracture of the humeral head that is produced by the dense, hard anterior lip of the glenoid fossa. In cadaver experiments, he was able to produce the head defect. He said that the hard, dense glenoid lip would cut into the soft cancellous bone like a knife (Fig. 16-3).

Roentgen's discovery of x-rays in 1895 ushered in new evaluations and studies of the anatomy of the anterior glenoid and humeral head defects. The first description of the radiographic changes in the humeral head associated with recurrent instability is attributed to Francke[17] in 1898, only 3 years after Roentgen's discovery.[19] Hermodsson demonstrated that the posterolateral humeral head defect is the result of a compression fracture caused by the anterior glenoid rim following the exit of the humeral head from the glenoid fossa.[19] He also observed that the defect is seen in the majority of cases; the longer the head is dislocated, the larger the defect will be; the defects are generally larger in anteroinferior dislocations than in anterior dislocations; and the defect is usually larger in recurrent anterior dislocations of the shoulder.

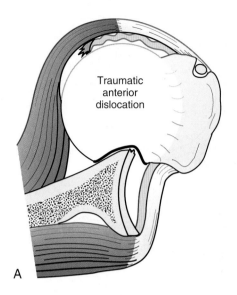

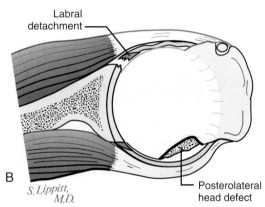

FIGURE 16-3 **A,** Anterior dislocation shown in an axillary projection with a posterolateral humeral head defect (Hill–Sachs defect) and a tear of the anterior capsule and labrum from the glenoid lip (Bankart lesion). **B,** The dislocation is reduced, but the humeral head and capsular lesions remain.

In 1925, Pilz[20] reported the first detailed radiographic examination of recurrent dislocation of the shoulder and stated that routine radiographs were of little help. He stressed the need for an angled-beam projection to observe the defect. In 1940, Hill and Sachs[11] published a very clear and concise review of the available information on the humeral head compression fracture defect that now carries their names.

Anterior Capsule and Muscle Defects

According to the Hunterian Lecture given by Reeves in 1967, Roger of Palermo in the 13th century taught that the lesion in an acute dislocation was a capsular rupture. Bankart,[21] following the concepts of Broca and Hartmann,[22] Perthes,[1] Flower,[8] and Caird,[18] claimed that

the essential lesion was detachment of the labrum and capsule from the anterior glenoid as a result of forward translation of the humeral head (referred to by subsequent authors as the *Bankart lesion*) (see Fig. 16-3). Later experimental and clinical work by Reeves[23] and Townley[24] suggested that other lesions might be responsible for recurrent dislocation, such as failure of the initial injury to incite a healing response, detachment of the subscapularis tendon, and variance in attachment of the inferior glenohumeral ligament.

Moseley and Overgaard[25] found laxity in 25 consecutive cases, and DePalma and associates[26] reported subscapularis laxity, rupture, and decreased muscle tone in 38 consecutive cases. Several of their cases and some from Hauser[27] revealed a definite defect along the anterior or inferior aspect of the subscapularis tendon, as though it had been partially torn from its bone attachment, along with separation of the muscle fibers that insert into the humerus directly below the lesser tuberosity. McLaughlin,[28] DePalma and associates,[26] Jens,[29] and Reeves[30] have noted at the time of surgery before arthrotomy that with abduction and external rotation, the humeral head would dislocate under the lower edge of the subscapularis tendon. Symeonides[31] took biopsy samples of the subscapularis muscle-tendon unit at the time of surgery and found microscopic evidence of "healed post-traumatic lesions." He stated that instability results because traumatic lengthening of the subscapularis muscle leads to loss of the power necessary to stabilize the shoulder.

Rotator Cuff Injuries

In 1880, Joessel[10] reported on his careful postmortem studies of four cases of known recurrent dislocation of the shoulder. In all cases he found a rupture of the posterolateral portion of the rotator cuff from the greater tuberosity and a greatly increased shoulder joint capsule volume (Fig. 16-4). He also noted fractures of the humeral head and the anterior glenoid rim (Figs. 16-5 and 16-6). Joessel concluded that cuff disruptions that did not heal predisposed to recurrence of the problem, that recurrences were facilitated by the enlarged capsule, and that fractures of the glenoid or the head of the humerus resulted in a smaller articular surface, which can tend to produce recurrent dislocation. However, his four patients were elderly and might have had the degenerative cuff changes common in older people.

Treatment of Acute Traumatic Dislocations

Hippocrates[32] discussed in detail at least six different techniques to reduce a dislocated shoulder. From century to century the literature has included woodcuts, drawings, and redrawings illustrating modifications of Hippocrates' teachings by such investigators as Paré, de Cruce, Vidius, and Scultetus. Hippocrates' original technique[5] is still used on occasion. The stockinged foot of

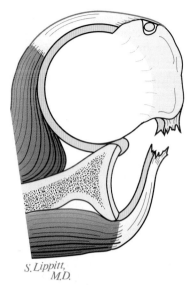

FIGURE 16-4 An anterior dislocation shown in an axillary projection with a tear in the posterior rotator cuff.

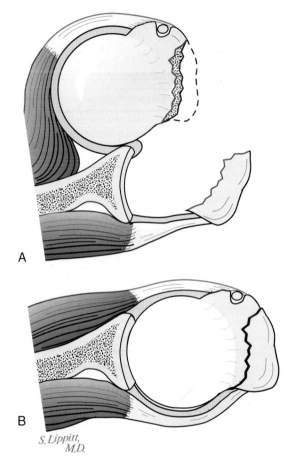

FIGURE 16-5 This anterior dislocation is shown in the axillary projection with a displaced fracture of the greater tuberosity. **A,** Anterior dislocation with displaced tuberosity fracture. **B,** Tuberosity fracture reduced when dislocation is reduced.

the physician is used as countertraction. The heel should not go into the axilla (i.e., between the anterior and posterior axillary folds) but should extend across the folds and against the chest wall. Traction should be slow and gentle; as with all traction techniques, the arm may be gently rotated internally and externally to disengage the head.

In 1870, Theodore Kocher,[33] who won the Nobel Prize for medicine in 1909, gave a somewhat confusing report of his technique for levering in an anteriorly dislocated shoulder. Had Kocher not been so famous as a thyroid surgeon, his article might have received only scant attention. In the Kocher technique, the humeral head is levered on the anterior glenoid and the shaft is levered against the anterior thoracic wall until the reduction is completed.

In 1938, Milch[34] described a technique for reduction in the supine position whereby the arm is abducted and externally rotated and the thumb is used to gently push the head of the humerus back into place. Lacey[35] modified the technique by performing the maneuver with the patient prone on an examining table. Russell and associates[36] reported on the ease and success of this technique.

DePalma[37] warned that with the Kocher technique, undue forces used in rotation leverage can damage the soft tissues of the shoulder joint, the vessels, and the brachial plexus. Beattie and coworkers[38] reported a fracture of the humeral neck during a Kocher procedure. Other authors have described spiral fractures of the upper shaft of the humerus and further damage to the anterior capsular mechanism when the Kocher leverage technique of reduction was used. McMurray[39] reported that of 64 dislocations reduced by the Kocher method, 40% became

recurrent, whereas of 112 dislocations reduced by gently lifting the head into place, only 12% became recurrent.

Since 1975, numerous articles have described simple techniques to reduce a dislocated shoulder: the forward

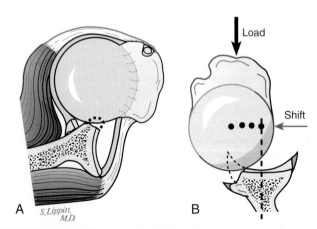

FIGURE 16-6 A, This anterior dislocation is shown in the axillary projection with a displaced fracture of the anterior glenoid rim. **B,** This fracture reduces the intrinsic stability provided by the glenoid concavity.

elevation maneuver,[40,41] the external rotation method,[42,43] scapular manipulation,[44] the modified gravity method,[45] the crutch and chair technique,[46] the chair and pillow technique,[47] and others.[48,49]

Operative Reconstructions for Anterior Instability

Most of the published literature on shoulder dislocations is concerned with the problem of recurrent anterior dislocations. As mentioned previously, Hippocrates[32] described the use of a white-hot poker to scar the antero-inferior part of the capsule. Since then, hundreds of operative procedures have been described for the management of recurrent anterior dislocations. Readers who have a yearning for the detailed history should read the classic texts by Moseley[7] and Hermodsson.[19]

Various operative techniques have been based on the posterolateral defect and soft tissue disruptions on the front of the shoulder. Bardenheuer[50] in 1886 and Thomas[51,52] in 1909 and 1921 discussed capsular plication or shrinking. In 1898, Albert[53] performed arthrodesis, and in 1902, Hildebrand[54] deepened the glenoid socket.

In 1906, Perthes[1] wrote a classic paper on the operative treatment of recurrent dislocations. He stated that the operation should be directed at repairing the underlying lesion (i.e., repair of the capsule, the glenoid labrum detachment from the anterior bony rim, and the rotator cuff tear). He repaired the capsule with suture to the anterior glenoid rim through drill holes, and in several cases he used staples to repair the anterior capsular structures. This report gave the first description of repair of the anterior labrum and capsule to the anterior glenoid rim. Two patients were monitored for 17 years, one for 12 years, two for 3 years, and one for 1 year and 9 months. All had excellent function with no recurrence.

The muscle sling myoplasty operation was used in 1909 by Clairmont and Ehrlich.[55] The posterior third of the deltoid, with its innervation left intact, was removed from its insertion on the humerus, passed through the quadrilateral space, and sutured to the coracoid process. When the arm was abducted, the deltoid contracted, which held up the humeral head. Finsterer,[56] in a similar but reversed procedure, used the coracobrachialis and the short head of the biceps from the coracoid and transferred them posteriorly. Both operations failed, with high recurrence rates.

In 1923, Bankart[21] first published his operative technique and noted that only two classes of operations were used at that time for recurrent dislocation of the shoulder: those designed to decrease the size of the capsule by plication or pleating[51,52] and those designed to give inferior support to the capsule.[55,57] Bankart condemned both in preference to his procedure. He stated that the essential lesion was detachment or rupture of the capsule from the glenoid ligament. He recommended repair with interrupted sutures of silkworm gut passed between the free edge of the capsule and the glenoid ligament. At that time he did not repair the lateral capsule to the bone of the anterior glenoid rim.

In his 1939 article, Bankart[2] described the essential lesion as "detachment of the glenoid ligament from the anterior margin of the glenoid cavity" and stated, "the only rational treatment is to reattach the glenoid ligament (or the capsule) to the bone from which it has been torn." He further wrote that "the glenoid ligament may be found lying loose either on the head of the humerus or the margin of the glenoid cavity." He recommended repair of the lateral capsule down to the raw bone of the anterior glenoid and that it be held in place with suture through drill holes made in the anterior glenoid rim with sharp, pointed forceps. Although no references were listed in either article, Bankart must have been greatly influenced by the previously published work of Broca and Hartmann[22] and particularly that of Perthes,[1] which described virtually identical pathology and repair.

Beginning in 1929, Nicola[58-62] published a series of articles on management of recurrent dislocation of the shoulder. He used the long head of the biceps tendon and the coracohumeral ligament as a suspension checkrein to the front of the shoulder. Henderson[63,64] described another checkrein operation that looped half the peroneus longus tendon through drill holes in the acromion and the greater tuberosity. In 1927, Gallie and LeMesurier[65] described the use of autogenous fascia lata suture in treating recurrent dislocation of the shoulder. This procedure has been modified by Bateman.[66]

Posterior Glenohumeral Instability

In 1839 in a Guy's Hospital report,[67] Sir Astley Cooper described in detail a dislocation of the os humeri on the dorsum scapulae. This report is a classic, for Cooper presented most of the characteristics associated with posterior dislocations: the dislocation occurred during an epileptic seizure; the pain was greater than with the usual anterior dislocation; external rotation of the arm was entirely impeded, and the patient could not elevate his arm from his side; the shoulder had an anterior void or flatness and a posterior fullness; and the patient was "unable to use or move his arm to any extent." In this report of a case in which Cooper had acted as a consultant, reduction could not be accomplished and the patient never recovered the use of his shoulder. Postmortem examination of the shoulder, performed 7 years later, revealed that the subscapularis tendon was detached and the infraspinatus muscles were stretched posteriorly about the head of the humerus. The report suggested that the detached subscapularis was "the cause of the symptoms." Cooper further described resorption of the anterior aspect of the humeral head where it was in contact with the posterior glenoid, probably the first description of the reverse Hill–Sachs lesion.

Another classic article on the subject was published in 1855 by Malgaigne,[68] who reported on 37 cases of posterior dislocation of the shoulder; 3 cases were his own

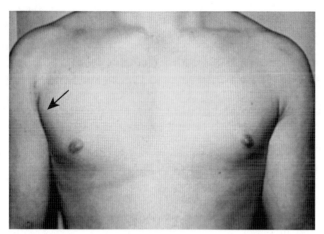

FIGURE 16-7 A cosmetic anterior approach on the patient's right shoulder. The incision is made in the axillary skin crease.

and 34 were reviewed from the literature. This series of cases was collected 40 years before the discovery of x-rays, and it points out that with adequate physical examination of the patient, the correct diagnosis can be made.

RELEVANT ANATOMY

Skin

Shoulder stabilization surgery can usually be accomplished through cosmetically acceptable incisions in the lines of the skin (see Chapter 2). Anteriorly, the surgeon can identify and mark the prominent anterior axillary crease by adducting the shoulder. An incision placed in the lower part of this crease provides excellent access to the shoulder for anterior repair and yet heals nicely with subcuticular closure (Figs. 16-7 and 16-8). When cosmesis is a concern, the incision can be made more into the axilla, as described by Leslie and Ryan.[69]

Posteriorly, an analogous vertical incision in line with the extended posterior axillary crease (best visualized by extending the shoulder backward) also heals well (Fig. 16-9). Fortuitously, these creases lie directly over the joint to which the surgeon needs access.

First Muscle Layer

The shoulder is covered by the deltoid muscle arising from the clavicle, acromion, and scapular spine. The anterior deltoid extends to a line running approximately from the midclavicle to the midlateral portion of the humerus. This line passes over the cephalic vein, the anterior venous drainage of the deltoid, and the coracoid process. The deltoid is innervated by the axillary nerve, whose branches swoop upward as they extend anteriorly (Fig. 16-10). The commonly described safe zone 5 cm distal to the acromion does not take into account these

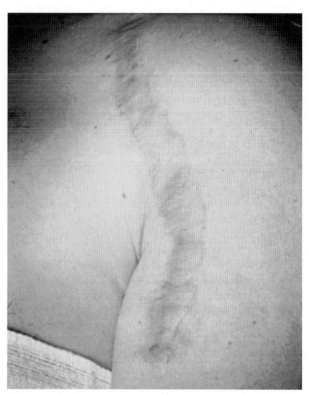

FIGURE 16-8 A noncosmetic approach across the front of the shoulder.

anterior branches, which can come as close as 2 cm to the acromion.

At the deltopectoral groove, the deltoid meets the clavicular head of the pectoralis major, which assists the anterior deltoid in forward flexion. The medial and lateral

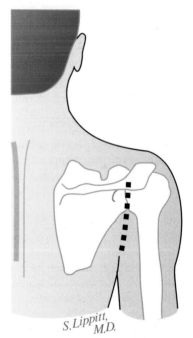

S. Lippitt, M.D.

FIGURE 16-9 A posterior approach for treatment of posterior glenohumeral instability. The incision (*dashed line*) is centered over the posterior glenoid rim.

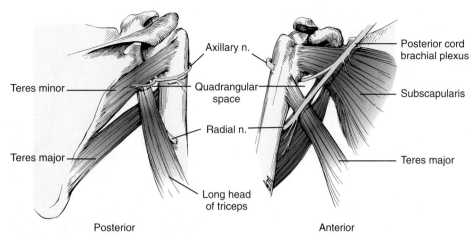

FIGURE 16-10 Relationships of the axillary nerve to the subscapularis muscle, the quadrangular space, and the neck of the humerus. With anterior dislocations, the subscapularis is displaced forward, which creates a traction injury in the axillary nerve. The nerve cannot move out of the way because it is held above by the brachial plexus and below where it wraps around behind the neck of the humerus. *Left,* Posteroanterior view. *Right,* AP view. (From Rockwood CA, Green DP [eds]: Fractures, 3 vols, 2nd ed. Philadelphia: JB Lippincott, 1984.)

pectoral nerves are not in the surgical field of shoulder stabilization. Splitting the deltopectoral interval just medial to the cephalic vein preserves the deltoid's venous drainage and takes the surgeon to the next layer. Extension of the shoulder tightens the pectoralis major and the anterior deltoid, as well as the coracoid muscles, and thus compromises the exposure. Accordingly, surgical assistants must be reminded to hold the shoulder in slight flexion to relax these muscles and facilitate access to the joint.

Posteriorly, the medial edge of the deltoid is too medial to provide useful access to the glenohumeral joint. Access must be achieved by splitting the deltoid, which is most conveniently done at the junction of its middle and pos-

terior thirds. This junction is marked by the posterior corner of the acromion. The site is favorable for a split because it overlies the joint and also because the axillary nerve exiting the quadrangular space divides into two trunks (its anterior and posterior branches) near the inferior aspect of the split.

The Coracoacromial Arch and Clavipectoral Fascia

The coracoacromial arch provides a concavity that articulates with the proximal humeral convexity (Figs. 16-11 to 16-13). The center of this articulation is identical to the

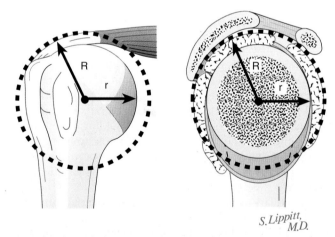

FIGURE 16-11 The proximal humeral convexity. *Left,* The rotational center of the proximal humeral convexity is the center of the sphere that best fits the tuberosities and the cuff tendons near their insertion. *Right,* The radius of the proximal humeral convexity (*R*) should be equal to the radius of the humeral articular surface sphere (*r*) plus the thickness of the rotator cuff tendons. (From Matsen FA III, Lippitt SB: Shoulder Surgery: Principles and Procedures. Philadelphia: WB Saunders, 2004, p 81.)

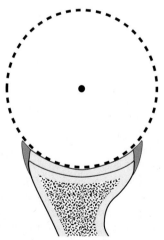

FIGURE 16-12 The glenoid concavity. The center of rotation of the glenoid (*dot*) is the center of the spherical concavity that best fits the glenoid articular surface. (From Matsen FA III, Lippitt SB: Shoulder Surgery: Principles and Procedures. Philadelphia: WB Saunders, 2004, p 82.)

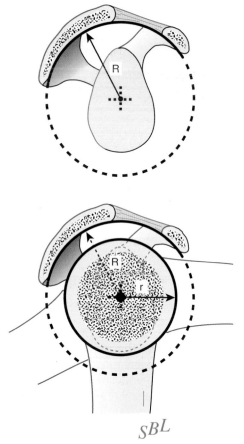

SBL

FIGURE 16-13 The coracoacromial concavity. The center of the coroacoacromial concavity is the center of the sphere that best fits the concave undersurface of the coracoacromial arch. *R*, radius of the proximal humeral convexity; *r*, radius of the humeral articular surface sphere. (From Rockwood CA, Matsen FA (eds): The Shoulder 2nd ed. Philadelphia: WB Saunders, 1998, p 764.)

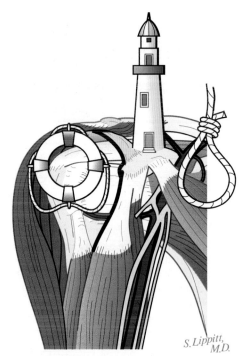

S. Lippitt, M.D.

FIGURE 16-14 Safe side/suicide. The coracoid serves as a lighthouse for proper orientation in a scarred shoulder. It divides the lateral (safe side) from the medial side (suicide), where the brachial plexus and vascular structures are located. (From Matsen FA III, Lippitt SB: Shoulder Surgery: Principles and Procedures. Philadelphia: WB Saunders, 2004, p 663.)

center of the glenohumeral articulation in the normal shoulder. The radii of these two articulations differ by the thickness of the rotator cuff and tuberosity. The concentricity of the coracoacromial and glenohumeral spheres provides stable centering of the normal shoulder through an extremely wide range of positions.

The coracoid process is the lighthouse of the anterior aspect of the shoulder in that it provides a palpable guide to the deltopectoral groove, a locator for the coracoacromial arch, and an anchor for the coracoid muscles (the coracobrachialis and short head of the biceps) that separate the lateral "safe side" from the medial "suicide" where the brachial plexus and major vessels lie (Fig. 16-14). The surgeon comes to full appreciation of the value of such a lighthouse when it is lacking—for example, when re-exploring a shoulder for complications of a coracoid transfer procedure. The clavipectoral fascia covers the floor of the deltopectoral groove. Rotating the humerus enables the surgeon to identify the subscapularis moving beneath this fascial layer. Incising the fascia up to but

not through the coracoacromial ligament preserves the stabilizing function of the coracoacromial arch.

The Humeroscapular Motion Interface

The humeroscapular motion interface (Fig. 16-15) separates the structures that do not move on humeral rotation (the deltoid, coracoid muscles, acromion, and coracoacromial ligament) from those that do (the rotator cuff, long head of the biceps tendon, and humeral tuberosities). During shoulder motion, substantial gliding takes place at this interface (Fig. 16-16). The humeroscapular motion interface provides a convenient plane for medial and lateral retractors and is also the plane in which the principal nerves lie.

The axillary nerve runs in the humeroscapular motion interface, superficial to the humerus and cuff and deep to the deltoid and coracoid muscles (Fig. 16-17; see also Fig. 16-10). Sweeping a finger in a superior-to-inferior direction along the anterior aspect of the subscapularis muscle catches the axillary nerve, which hangs like a watch chain across the muscle belly. Tracing this nerve proximally and medially leads the finger to the bulk of the brachial plexus. Tracing it laterally and posteriorly leads the finger beneath the shoulder capsule toward the quadrangular space. From a posterior vantage, the axil-

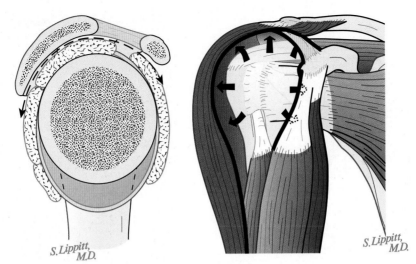

FIGURE 16-15 The humeroscapular motion interface (*arrows*) is an important location of motion between the humerus and the scapula. The deltoid, acromion, coracoacromial ligament, coracoid process, and tendons attaching to the coracoid lie on the superficial side of this interface, whereas the proximal end of the humerus, rotator cuff, and biceps tendon sheath lie on the deep side. (Modified from Matsen FA III, Lippitt SE, Sidles JA, Harryman DT II: Practical Evaluation and Management of the Shoulder. Philadelphia: WB Saunders, 1994.)

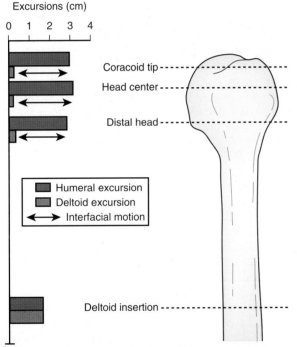

FIGURE 16-16 Mean humeroscapular interface motion recorded in vivo from five normal subjects with the use of MRI. The humerus at the *right* shows the levels at which the motions were measured. The excursion (in centimeters) of the humerus (*blue*) and the deltoid (*orange*) from maximal internal to maximal external rotation is indicated by the *horizontal bars.* The magnitudes of motion at the interface between the deltoid and the humerus are indicated by the *double-headed arrows.* The mean excursion at the humerothoracic motion interface was approximately 3 cm proximally and 0 cm at the deltoid insertion. (From Matsen FA III, Lippitt SB, Sidles JA, Harryman DT II: Practical Evaluation and Management of the Shoulder. Philadelphia: WB Saunders, 1994.)

lary nerve is seen to exit the quadrangular space beneath the teres minor and extend laterally, where it is applied to the deep surface of the deltoid muscle. By virtue of its prominent location in close proximity to the shoulder joint anteriorly, inferiorly, and posteriorly, the axillary nerve is the most commonly injured structure in shoulder surgery.

The musculocutaneous nerve lies on the deep surface of the coracoid muscles and penetrates the coracobrachialis with one or more branches lying a variable distance distal to the coracoid. (The often-described 5-cm safe zone for the nerve beneath the process refers only to the average position of the main trunk and not to an area that can be entered recklessly.) The musculocutane-

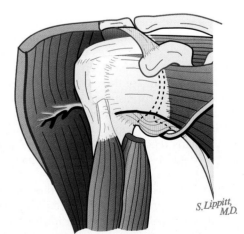

FIGURE 16-17 The axillary nerve in the humeroscapular motion interface between the cuff and the humerus on the inside and the coracoid muscles and the deltoid on the outside. (From Matsen FA III, Lippitt SB, Sidles JA, Harryman DT II: Practical Evaluation and Management of the Shoulder. Philadelphia: WB Saunders, 1994.)

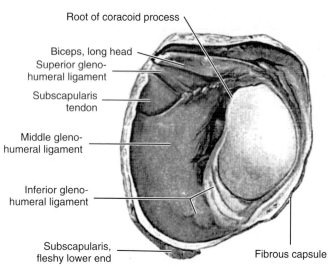

Root of coracoid process

Biceps, long head
Superior gleno-
humeral ligament

Subscapularis
tendon

Middle gleno-
humeral ligament

Inferior gleno-
humeral ligament

Subscapularis,
fleshy lower end

Fibrous capsule

FIGURE 16-18 Anterior glenohumeral ligaments. This drawing shows the anterosuperior, anterior middle, and anteroinferior glenohumeral ligaments. The middle and inferior anterior glenohumeral ligaments are often avulsed from the glenoid or the glenoid labrum in traumatic anterior instability. (From Grant JCB: Grant's Atlas of Anatomy, 4th ed. Baltimore: Williams & Wilkins, 1956.)

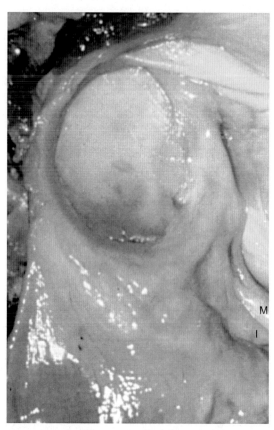

FIGURE 16-19 Cadaver dissection of the glenoid, biceps tendon insertion, and associated glenohumeral ligaments. This dissection demonstrates the anterior glenohumeral ligaments. Note the relationship of the anterior inferior (I) and the anterior middle (M) glenohumeral ligaments to the anterior rim of the glenoid.

ous nerve is vulnerable to injury from retractors placed under the coracoid muscles and to traction injury during coracoid transfer. Knowledge of the position of these nerves can make the shoulder surgeon both more comfortable and more effective.

The Rotator Cuff

The next layer of the shoulder is the rotator cuff. The tendons of these muscles blend in with the capsule as they insert into the humeral tuberosities.[70] Thus, in reconstructions that require splitting of these muscles from the capsule, such splitting is more easily accomplished medially, before the blending becomes complete. The nerves to these muscles run on their deep surfaces: the upper and lower subscapular to the subscapularis and the suprascapular to the supraspinatus and infraspinatus. Medial dissection on the deep surface of these muscles can jeopardize their nerve supply.[71] The superior portion of the subscapularis tendon has been found to have significantly higher stiffness and ultimate load than its inferior portion has.[72]

The capsule is relatively thin between the supraspinatus and the subscapularis (the rotator interval). This thinness allows the cuff to slide back and forth around the coracoid process as the arm is elevated and lowered. Splitting this interval toward the base of the coracoid may be helpful when mobilization of the subscapularis is needed.

The tendon of the long head of the biceps originates from the supraglenoid tubercle (Figs. 16-18 and 16-19).

It runs beneath the cuff in the area of the rotator interval and exits the shoulder beneath the transverse humeral ligament and between the greater and lesser tuberosities. It is subject to injury when incising the upper subscapularis from the lesser tuberosity. In the bicipital groove of the humerus, this tendon is endangered by procedures that involve lateral transfer of the subscapularis tendon across the groove.

The Scapulohumeral Ligaments

Though often suggested as the primary stabilizers of the glenohumeral joint, the scapulohumeral ligaments are now recognized to play a primary role only in positions near the extremes of the allowed range of motion. The thickness of the capsule decreases as it nears the humerus. The capsule is thickest in the inferior pouch at 2.8 mm, 2.4 mm in its anterior portion, and 2.2 mm in the posterior portion. The thickness ranges from 1.3 to 4.5 mm in cadaveric specimens.[73] The glenohumeral joint capsule is normally large, loose, and redundant, which allows full and free range of motion of the shoulder. By virtue of their mandatory redundancy, the capsule and its ligaments are lax throughout most of the range of joint motion. Thus, they can exert major stabilizing effects only when they come under tension as the joint approaches the limits of its range of motion. In the midrange of shoulder motion, the center of the humeral head remains within 2.2 mm of the center of the glenoid on magnetic resonance imaging (MRI).[74] This limited stabilizing effect shows the importance of mechanisms of glenohumeral stability other than the capsule and its ligaments. The capsular structures are also believed to contribute to stability through their proprioceptive functions.[75]

The three anterior glenohumeral ligaments were first described by Schlemm in 1853.[76] Since then, many observers have described their anatomy and role in limiting glenohumeral rotation and translation (see Figs. 16-18 and 16-19).[23,25,28,77-81]

Codman[82] and others pointed out the variability of the ligaments (see Fig. 16-19).[25,37,77,79,83,84] These authors also demonstrated great variation in the size and number of synovial recesses that form in the anterior capsule above, below, and between the glenohumeral ligaments. They observed that if the capsule arises at the labrum, few if any synovial recesses are present (in this situation, because of generalized blending of all three ligaments, no room is left for synovial recesses or weaknesses, and hence the anterior glenohumeral capsule is stronger). However, the more medially the capsule arises from the glenoid (i.e., from the anterior scapular neck), the larger and more numerous the synovial recesses are. The end result is a thin, weak anterior capsule. In an embryologic study involving 52 specimens, Uhthoff and Piscopo[85] demonstrated that the anterior capsule inserted into the glenoid labrum in 77% and into the medial neck of the scapula in 23%. This variation in anatomy was later classified into two different types, I and II. A type I attachment occurs when the fibers primarily originate from the labrum, with some fibers attaching to the glenoid, and it is seen 80% of the time. A type II origin of the capsuloligamentous structures occurs solely from the glenoid neck and is seen in 20% of cadaveric specimens.[86]

The superior glenohumeral ligament (SGHL) is identified as the most consistent capsular ligament.[87] It crosses the rotator interval capsule and lies between the supraspinatus and subscapularis tendons. Another interval capsular structure, the coracohumeral ligament, originates at the base of the coracoid, blends into the cuff tendons, and inserts into the greater and lesser tuberosities.[88-93]

Harryman and colleagues pointed out that these two ligaments and the rotator interval capsule come under tension with glenohumeral flexion, extension, external rotation, and adduction.[89] When they are under tension, these structures resist posterior and inferior displacement of the humeral head. Clinical and experimental data have shown that releasing or surgically tightening the rotator interval capsule increases or decreases the allowed posterior and inferior translational laxity, respectively.[89,94-97]

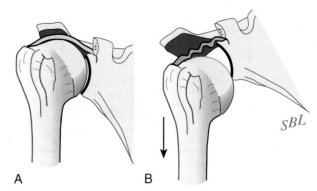

FIGURE 16-20 Scapular dumping. With the scapula in a normal position (**A**), the superior capsular mechanism is tight and supporting the head in the glenoid concavity. Drooping of the lateral aspect of the scapula (**B**) relaxes the superior capsular structures and rotates the glenoid concavity so that it does not support the head of the humerus. (From Matsen FA III, Lippitt SB, Sidles JA, Harryman DT II: Practical Evaluation and Management of the Shoulder. Philadelphia: WB Saunders, 1994.)

It is these ligaments and capsule, as well as the inferior glenoid lip, that provide static restraint against inferior translation.[94] It is of anatomic interest and clinical significance that when the lateral aspect of the scapula is allowed to droop inferiorly, the resulting passive abduction of the humerus relaxes the rotator interval capsule and the superior ligaments; as a result, the humeral head can be dumped out of the glenoid fossa (Fig. 16-20).[98] Drooping of the lateral part of the scapula is normally prevented by the postural action of the scapular stabilizers, particularly the trapezius and serratus. Elevation of the lateral aspect of the scapula with the arm at the side enhances inferior stability in two ways: the resulting glenohumeral adduction tightens the superior capsule and ligaments, and the scapular rotation places more of the inferior glenoid lip beneath the humeral head.[97,99]

The SGHL and coracohumeral ligament come under tension with external rotation in adduction, whereas the middle glenohumeral ligament (MGHL) is tensioned by external rotation when the humerus is abducted to 45 degrees.[31,100,101] The MGHL originates anterosuperiorly on the glenoid and inserts midway along the anterior humeral articular surface adjacent to the lesser tuberosity. In more than a third of shoulders, the MGHL is absent or poorly defined, a situation that can place the shoulder at greater risk for anterior glenohumeral instability.[102]

With greater degrees of shoulder abduction, for example, in the apprehension position, the inferior glenohumeral ligament (IGHL) and the inferior capsular sling come into play.[100,101] The IGHL originates below the sigmoid notch and courses obliquely between the anteroinferior glenoid and its humeral capsular insertion.[83] O'Brien and coworkers have described an anterior thickening of the IGHL, the anterior superior band.[83] The anterior and posterior aspects of the IGHL are said to

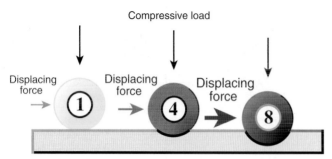

FIGURE 16-21 Concavity and compression. In the absence of a concavity, only a minimal translational force is required to displace the sphere. As the concavity becomes deeper, a greater displacing force is required for a given compressive load. (From Matsen FA III, Lippitt SB: Shoulder Surgery: Principles and Procedures. Philadelphia: WB Saunders, 2004, p 83.)

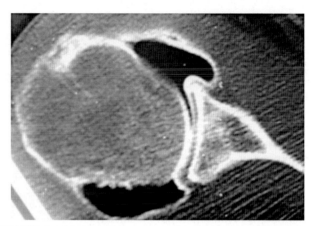

FIGURE 16-22 CT arthrogram of the glenohumeral joint. The depth of the bony glenoid is enhanced by contributions of the articular cartilage and the glenoid labrum, which further increases the stability of the glenohumeral joint. Note that in this position, the anterior and posterior capsuloligamentous structures are relaxed and cannot contribute to stability.

function as a cruciate construct in which they alternately tighten in external and internal rotation.[83,97,103] These ligaments can be stretched out with repeated use. The dominant shoulders of handball athletes were placed in 90 degrees of abduction and external rotation and then brought into extension while being observed in a computed tomography (CT) scanner. The dominant shoulders were seen to have more external rotation of the humeral head and more of a shift from the posterior aspect of the glenoid to its center than noted in normal shoulders when brought into the late cocking position.[104]

When the humerus is elevated anteriorly in the sagittal plane (flexion), the posterior-inferior capsular pouch and the rotator interval capsule come into tension.[83,89,97,105,106] If the humerus is internally rotated while elevated in the sagittal plane, the interval capsule slackens but the posterior inferior pouch tightens. Posteroinferior capsular tension also limits flexion, internal rotation, and horizontal adduction.[89,105,106] Excessive tightness of this portion of the capsule is a well-recognized clinical entity (see Chapter 17 on the rotator cuff).

Coracoacromial Ligament

Resection of the coracoacromial ligament in cadaveric shoulders was found to result in significantly greater anterior translation of the humeral head with the shoulder in 0 and 30 degrees of abduction. At 0 degrees of abduction, significantly greater inferior translation occurred after resection of the coracoacromial ligament.[107] This observation should encourage caution with needless resection of the ligament.

Glenoid Concavity and Labrum

The predominant method for centering the humeral head in the glenoid fossa is concavity compression.[108] The glenoid concavity provides the essential concavity (see Figs. 16-18 and 16-19). The deeper the concavity, the more stability results from compression of the humeral

head in it (Fig. 16-21). The glenoid concavity is provided by the shape of the bony socket, which is functionally deepened by the fact that the articular cartilage at the periphery is thicker than at the center (Fig. 16-22). Weldon and colleagues[109] showed that removal of the glenoid cartilage dramatically compromised the intrinsic stability offered by the glenoid fossa, especially in the posterior-inferior direction, where the balance stability angle was reduced almost 50% by cartilage removal.

The socket is further deepened by the presence of the labrum around the rim of the socket (Fig. 16-23). The glenoid labrum is a fibrous rim that serves to deepen the glenoid fossa and allow attachment of the glenohumeral ligaments and the biceps tendon to the glenoid. Anatomically, it is the interconnection of the periosteum of the glenoid, the glenoid bone, the glenoid articular cartilage, the synovium, and the capsule. Although microscopic studies have shown that a small amount of fibrocartilage is located at the junction of the hyaline cartilage

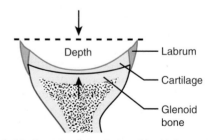

FIGURE 16-23 Components of the glenoid fossa. The glenoid fossa results from the relatively small concavity of the glenoid bone, deepened by the glenoid cartilage and by the labrum at its periphery. (From Matsen FA III, Lippitt SB: Shoulder Surgery: Principles and Procedures. Philadelphia: WB Saunders, 2004, p 88.)

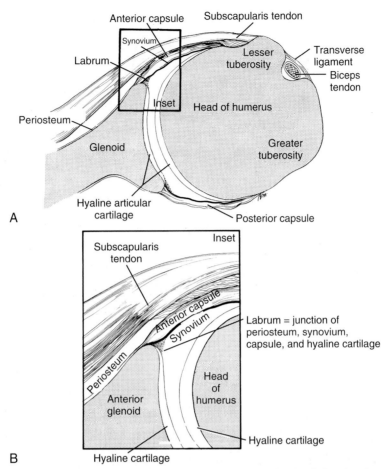

FIGURE 16-24 Normal shoulder anatomy. **A,** Horizontal section through the middle of the glenohumeral joint demonstrating normal anatomic relationships. Note the close relationship of the subscapularis tendon to the anterior capsule. **B,** Close-up view in the area of the labrum. The labrum consists of tissues from the nearby hyaline cartilage, capsule, synovium, and periosteum. (From Rockwood CA, Green DP [eds]: Fractures, 3 vols, 2nd ed. Philadelphia: JB Lippincott, 1984.)

of the glenoid and the fibrous capsule, the vast majority of the labrum consists of dense fibrous tissue with a few elastic fibers (Fig. 16-24).[24,25,110] The posterosuperior portion of the labrum is continuous with the tendon of the long head of the biceps. Anteriorly, it is continuous with the IGHL (see Fig. 16-19).[111-114] Hertz and colleagues[115] detailed the microanatomy of the labrum, and Prodromos and associates,[116] DePalma,[37] and Olsson[117] described changes in the glenoid labrum with age.

In cadavers, isolated labral lesions are not usually sufficient to allow complete glenohumeral dislocation.[24,30,118,119] However, cadaveric studies have shown diminished stability with labral lesions. Fehringer and colleagues have demonstrated that a simple incision in its attachment to the glenoid uncenters the humeral head.[120] Resection of the labrum was found to decrease the stability ratio of cadaveric shoulders by 9.6%.[121] Lazarus and coworkers[122] demonstrated that resection of the cartilage and labrum from the anteroinferior glenoid reduced the height of the glenoid by approximately 80% and the stability ratio by approximately 65% for translation in the direction of the defect. Halder and colleagues[121] again demonstrated the stabilizing effect of the labrum in a cadaver model.

Clinical studies reveal a high incidence of labral deficiency in patients with recurrent traumatic instability.[2,123-127] In our experience, it is rare to see a shoulder with recurrent anterior traumatic instability without a detachment of the glenoid labrum from the glenoid lip.

For a review of the gross anatomy of the glenohumeral joint surfaces, ligaments, labrum, and capsule, see Chapter 2.

MECHANICS OF GLENOHUMERAL STABILITY

The most remarkable feature of the glenohumeral joint is its ability to precisely stabilize the humeral head in the center of the glenoid on the one hand and to allow a vast range of motion on the other. This balance of stability and mobility is achieved by a combination of mechanisms particular to this articulation.[128]

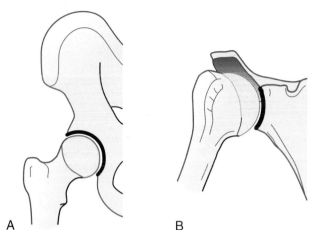

FIGURE 16-25 In contrast to the hip (**A**), the shallow glenoid captures relatively little of the articulating ball (**B**). (From Matsen FA III, Lippitt SB, Sidles JA, Harryman DT II: Practical Evaluation and Management of the Shoulder. Philadelphia: WB Saunders, 1994.)

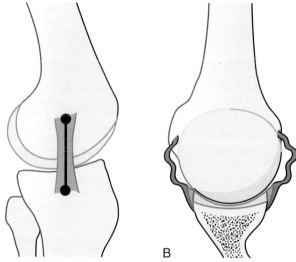

FIGURE 16-26 In contrast to the knee, where the ligaments remain isometric during joint motion (**A**), the glenohumeral ligaments must be slack in most of the joint's positions (**B**). (Modified from Matsen FA III, Lippitt SB, Sidles JA, Harryman DT II: Practical Evaluation and Management of the Shoulder. Philadelphia: WB Saunders, 1994.)

In contrast to the hip joint, the glenohumeral joint does not offer a deep stabilizing socket. An acetabulum-like socket would limit motion by contact of the anatomic neck of the humerus with its rim. Instead, the small arc of the glenoid captures relatively little of the humeral articular surface, thus neck-to-rim contact is avoided for a wide range of positions (Fig. 16-25).[98,101,129-131]

In contrast to hinge-like joints with shallow sockets, such as the knee, interphalangeal joints, elbow, and ankle, the glenohumeral joint does not offer isometric articular ligaments that provide stability as the joint is flexed around a defined anatomic axis. Instead, the glenohumeral ligaments play important stabilizing roles only at the extremes of motion; they are lax and relatively ineffectual in most functional positions of the joint (Fig. 16-26).[97,98]

In spite of its lack of a deep socket or isometric ligaments, the normal shoulder precisely constrains the humeral head to the center of the glenoid cavity throughout most of the arc of movement.[74,131-135] It is remarkable that this seemingly unconstrained joint can provide such precise centering, resist the gravitational pull on the arm hanging at the side for long periods, remain located during sleep, allow the lifting of large loads, permit throwing a baseball at speeds exceeding 100 miles per hour, and maintain stability during the application of an almost infinite variety of forces of differing magnitude, direction, duration, and abruptness.

The mechanics of glenohumeral stability can be most easily understood in terms of the relationship between the net force acting on the humeral head and the shape of the glenoid fossa. A working familiarity with the mechanics of glenohumeral stability will greatly enhance one's understanding of the workings of the normal joint, laboratory models of instability, clinical problems of instability, and clinical strategies for managing glenohumeral instability.

The basic law of glenohumeral stability is that the glenohumeral joint will not dislocate as long as the net humeral joint reaction force* (Fig. 16-27) is directed within the effective glenoid arc† (Figs. 16-28 and 16-29).[132,136] If the net humeral joint reaction force passes outside the effective glenoid arc, the joint becomes unstable. The effective glenoid arc in a given direction is also known as the *balance stability angle,* the maximal angle that the net humeral joint reaction force can make with the glenoid center line in a given direction before dislocation (see Fig. 16-28). Balance stability angles vary for different directions around the glenoid (Fig. 16-30). The requisite for a stable glenohumeral joint is that the net humeral joint reaction force be maintained within the balance stability angles. The balance stability angle may be compromised by congenital deficiency (glenoid hypoplasia), excessive compliance, traumatic lesions (rim fractures or Bankart defects), or wear (Fig. 16-31).[10,53,98,121,125,126,132,137-145] The balance stability angle may be restored or augmented by anatomic repair of fractures or Bankart lesions (Fig. 16-32), by rim augmentation,[146] by congruent glenoid bone grafting,[147] and by glenoid osteotomy.[122]

The net humeral joint reaction force is the resultant of all muscular, ligamentous, inertial, gravitational, and other external forces applied to the head of the humerus (other than the force applied by the glenoid).

†*Because the rim of the glenoid is deformable under load, the effective glenoid arc is the arc of the glenoid available to support the humeral head under the specified loading conditions.*

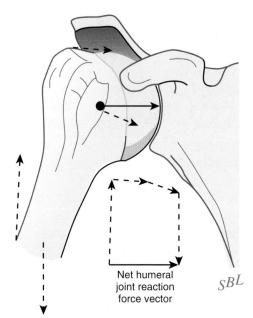

FIGURE 16-27 The net humeral joint reaction force is the vector sum of all forces acting on the head of the humerus relative to the glenoid fossa. (From Matsen FA III, Lippitt SB, Sidles JA, Harryman DT II: Practical Evaluation and Management of the Shoulder. Philadelphia: WB Saunders, 1994.)

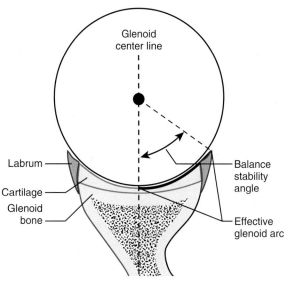

FIGURE 16-28 The effective glenoid arc is the arc of the glenoid able to support the net humeral joint reaction force. The balance stability angle is the maximal angle that the net humeral joint reaction force can make with the glenoid center line before dislocation occurs. The shape of the bone, cartilage, and labrum all contribute to the effective glenoid arc and the balance stability angle.

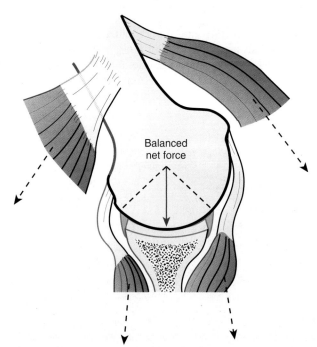

FIGURE 16-29 The deltoid and cuff muscle forces (*dotted arrows*) maintain the net humeral joint reaction force (*solid arrow*) within the balance stability angle (*dotted lines*). (Modified from Matsen FA III, Lippitt SB, Sidles JA, Harryman DT II: Practical Evaluation and Management of the Shoulder. Philadelphia: WB Saunders, 1994.)

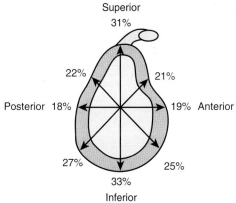

FIGURE 16-30 The balance stability angle varies around the face of the glenoid. For a normal glenoid, the superior and inferior balance stability angles are greater than the anterior and posterior balance stability angles. This figure shows the balance stability angles (*solid arrows*) measured in eight directions around the face of the glenoid. Values are means for 10 cadaver shoulders with a compressive load of 50 N. (Modified from Matsen FA III, Lippitt SB, Sidles JA, Harryman DT II: Practical Evaluation and Management of the Shoulder. Philadelphia: WB Saunders, 1994.)

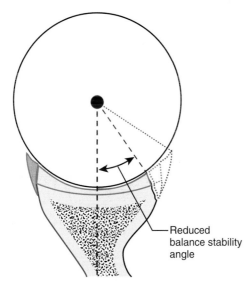

FIGURE 16-31 The balance stability angle and the effective glenoid arc are reduced by a fracture of the glenoid rim. (Modified from Matsen FA III, Lippitt SB, Sidles JA, Harryman DT II: Practical Evaluation and Management of the Shoulder. Philadelphia: WB Saunders, 1994.)

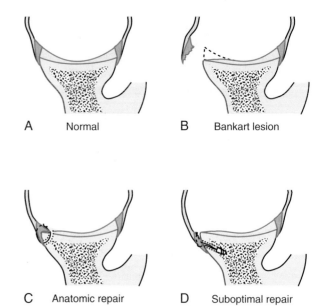

FIGURE 16-32 **A,** Normally, the capsule and labrum deepen the effective glenoid fossa. **B,** This effect is lost in the presence of a Bankart lesion, particularly if the articular cartilage is worn away. **C,** Anatomic repair of the detached glenoid labrum and glenohumeral ligaments to the glenoid rim helps restore the effective glenoid arc. **D,** By contrast, when the labrum and capsule heal to the neck, the effective glenoid arc is not restored. (Modified from Matsen FA III, Lippitt SB, Sidles JA, Harryman DT II: Practical Evaluation and Management of the Shoulder. Philadelphia: WB Saunders, 1994.)

The Net Humeral Joint Reaction Force

The direction of the net humeral joint reaction force is controlled actively by elements of the rotator cuff and other shoulder muscles along with the weight of the arm and externally applied forces. Each active muscle generates a force whose direction is determined by the effective origin and insertion of that muscle (Fig. 16-33). Neural control of the magnitude of these muscle forces provides the mechanism by which the direction of the net humeral joint reaction force is controlled. For example, by increasing the force of contraction of muscles whose force directions are close to the glenoid center line, the direction of the net humeral joint reaction force can be aligned more closely with the glenoid fossa (Fig. 16-34). The elements of the rotator cuff are well positioned to contribute to this muscle balance.[118,148-162]

In addition to the compression provided by the rotator cuff musculature, the deltoid assists in this capacity as well. The middle and posterior portions of the deltoid have been shown to be more important than the anterior portion in producing concavity compression.[163,164] The long head of the biceps muscle might also contribute to shoulder stability.[165]

In the healthy shoulder, strengthening and neuromuscular training help optimize neuromuscular control of the net humeral joint reaction force. Conversely, the net humeral joint reaction force is difficult to optimize when muscle control is impaired by injury, disuse, contracture, paralysis, loss of coordination, or tendon defects or when the glenoid concavity is compromised (Fig. 16-35). Neuromuscular training may be guided by proprioceptors in the labrum and ligaments.[166-169] Blasier and

coworkers[170] and Kronberg and colleagues[171] showed that persons with generalized joint laxity have less-acute proprioception and altered muscle activation. Zuckerman and associates demonstrated that motion and position sense are compromised in the presence of traumatic

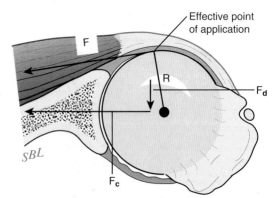

FIGURE 16-33 Each active muscle generates a force (*F*) whose direction is determined by the effective origin and insertion of that muscle. Note that the rotator cuff tendons wrap around the head of the humerus, so their effective point of attachment is on the humeral articular surface. Note also that each muscle force has a compressive (F_c) and a displacing (F_d) component. The product of the force multiplied by the radius (*R*) is the torque (F • R). (Modified from Matsen FA III, Lippitt SB, Sidles JA, Harryman DT II: Practical Evaluation and Management of the Shoulder. Philadelphia: WB Saunders, 1994.)

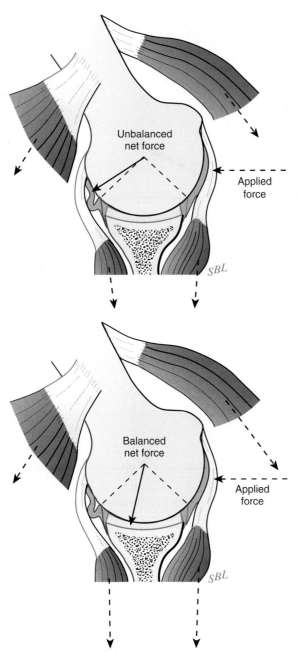

FIGURE 16-34 Stabilizing the glenohumeral joint against an applied translational force. *Top,* Weak contraction of cuff muscles results in an unbalanced net force and risk instability. *Bottom,* Strong contraction of the cuff muscles provides an increased compression force into the glenoid concavity. As a result, the net humeral force is balanced within the glenoid concavity.

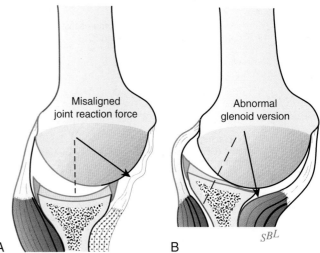

FIGURE 16-35 **A,** Stability is compromised by muscle imbalance. In this example, the humerus is aligned with the glenoid center line (*dotted line*), but the net humeral joint reaction force (*arrow*) is misaligned because of weakness of the posterior cuff musculature. **B,** Balance stability is compromised with abnormal glenoid version. In this example, the humerus is aligned with the plane of the scapula, but severe glenoid retroversion results in a posteriorly directed glenoid center line (*dotted line*) that is divergent from the net humeral joint reaction force (*arrow*). (Modified from Matsen FA III, Lippitt SB, Sidles JA, Harryman DT II: Practical Evaluation and Management of the Shoulder. Philadelphia: WB Saunders, 1994.)

The Balance Stability Angle and the Stability Ratio

The balance stability angle is the maximal angle that the net humeral joint reaction force can make with the glenoid center line before glenohumeral dislocation occurs. The tangent of this balance stability angle is the ratio between its displacing component (perpendicular to the glenoid center line) and its compressive component (parallel to the glenoid center line), which is known as the *stability ratio* (Fig. 16-36). The stability ratio is the maximal displacing force in a given direction that can be stabilized by a specified compressive load, assuming frictional effects to be minimal.* The effective glenoid arc, the balance stability angle, and stability ratios vary around the perimeter of the glenoid (see Fig. 16-30). It is handy to note that for small angles, the stability ratio can be

anterior instability and are restored 1 year after surgical reconstruction.[172]

The reader is referred to reviews of neuromuscular stabilization of the shoulder by Lieber and Friden[128(Ch4)] and by Speer and Garrett.[128(Ch8)] In the same reference are found reviews of the role of capsular feedback and pattern generators in shoulder kinematics by Grigg[128(Ch9)] and the role of muscle optimization by Flanders.[128(Ch39)]

Measured stability ratios may be influenced by the friction of the joint surfaces and by other stabilizing mechanisms such as adhesion and cohesion and the glenoid suction cup (discussed later). These effects tend to increase the displacing force necessary to dislocate the humeral head for a given compressive load. It is essential to control for these effects in the laboratory. Specifically, the underlubricated, aged cadaver joints available to the laboratory can have substantially greater coefficients of friction in vitro than the exquisitely lubricated and smooth joint of a young person in vivo.

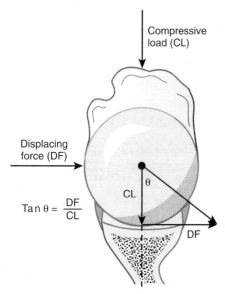

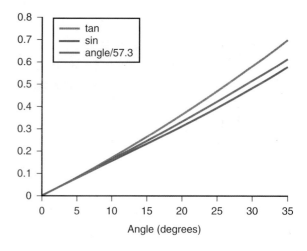

FIGURE 16-36 The relationship of the maximum local stability ratio to the balance stability angle. The tangent of the balance stability angle is equal to the ratio of the displacing force and the compressive load. (From Matsen FA III, Lippitt SB: Shoulder Surgery: Principles and Procedures. Philadelphia: WB Saunders, 2004, p 108.)

estimated by dividing the balance stability angle by 57 degrees (Fig. 16-37).*

The stability ratio is often used in the laboratory because it is relatively easy to measure: A compressive load is applied, and the displacing force is progressively increased until dislocation occurs. For example, Lippitt and colleagues[137] found that a compressive load of 50 N resisted displacing loads of up to 30 N and that the effectiveness of this stabilization mechanism varied with the depth of the glenoid (Fig. 16-38). Investigation of these parameters provides important information on stability mechanics; for example, resection of the labrum has been shown to reduce the stability ratio by 20%.[137] Furthermore, a 3-mm anterior glenoid defect has been shown to reduce the balance stability angle more than 25% from 18 to 13 degrees.[98] Bony defects of 21% of the anterior glenoid rim were noted to reduce the balance stability angle by 50%.[147,173]

Clinically, the stability ratio can be sensed by using the load and shift test, wherein the examiner applies a compressive load pressing the humeral head into the glenoid while noting the amount of translating force necessary to move the humeral head from its centered position.[174] This test gives the examiner an indication of the adequacy of the glenoid concavity and is one of the most practical ways to detect deficiencies of the glenoid rim.

At small angles, the tangent of an angle is approximately equal to the angle expressed in radians. Thus, the stability ratio (tangent of the balance stability angle) is approximately the balance stability angle divided by 57 degrees per radian.

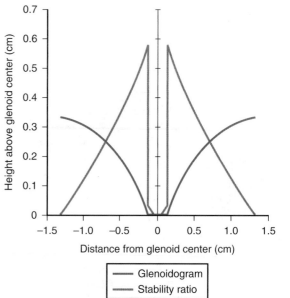

FIGURE 16-37 Small angle approximation. For small angles, the sine, the tangent, and the angle expressed in radians (57.3°) are all approximately the same, making it easy to predict the balance stability angle (BSA) without trigonometry calculations (BSA ≅ 57.3 × W/R, where W is width and R is radius of the glenoid). (From Matsen FA III, Lippitt SB: Shoulder Surgery: Principles and Procedures. Philadelphia: WB Saunders, 2004, p 97.)

The Glenoidogram

The effective shape of the glenoid is revealed by the *glenoidogram*, which, rather than showing how the glenoid *looks*, shows how it *works*.[122,125] The glenoidogram is the path taken by the center of the humeral head as it is translated away from the center of the glenoid fossa in a specified direction. The shape of the glenoidogram indicates the extent of the effective glenoid arc in that direction. The glenoidogram is oriented with respect to the *glenoid center line*, a reference line perpendicular to the center of the glenoid fossa (Figs. 16-39 and 16-40). As the humeral head is translated from the center of the

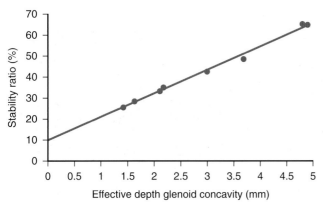

FIGURE 16-38 A nearly linear relationship exists between the effective depth of the glenoid concavity and the stability ratio with a 50-N compressive load. These data include points representing superior, inferior, anterior, and posterior translation before and after excision of the glenoid labrum. (From Matsen FA III, Lippitt SB, Sidles JA, Harryman DT II: Practical Evaluation and Management of the Shoulder. Philadelphia: WB Saunders, 1994.)

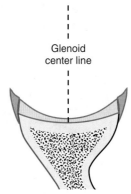

FIGURE 16-39 The glenoid center line is a line perpendicular to the surface of the glenoid fossa at its midpoint. (Modified from Matsen FA III, Lippitt SB, Sidles JA, Harryman DT II: Practical Evaluation and Management of the Shoulder. Philadelphia: WB Saunders, 1994.)

glenoid to the rim in a given direction, the center of the humeral head traces the glenoidogram, which has a characteristic gullwing shape (Figs. 16-41 and 16-42). The glenoidogram is different for different directions of translation (Fig. 16-43) and presents data recorded for the superior, inferior, anterior, and posterior directions in a typical shoulder.

The shape of the glenoidogram can be predicted given the radius of curvature of the humeral head (R_h), the radius of curvature of the glenoid fossa (R_g), the effective glenoid width (W), the effective glenoid depth (D), and the balance stability angle (BSA) in radians. For each value of x (the distance away from the glenoid center line), the perpendicular distance of the center of the humeral head away from the glenoid bottom, y, is given by

$$D - R_h + (R_h \times R_h - [W - x] \times [W - x])^{1/2}$$

The sample spreadsheet (Table 16-1) displays the case in which $R_g = R_h = 25$ mm and the BSA = 30 degrees = 0.5236 radians. In this case, the effective glenoid width (W) = $R_g \times \sin(\text{BSA})$, and the effective glenoid depth (D) = $R_g \times (1 - \cos[\text{BSA}])$. The results of this prediction are shown in Table 16-1 and Fig. 16-44.

Predicted glenoidograms are qualitatively similar to glenoidograms measured experimentally (compare Figs. 16-43 and 16-44). The glenoidogram also reveals another important aspect of shoulder stability: The slope of the glenoidogram at any point is equal to the stability ratio at that point. For most glenoidograms it can be seen that the stability ratio is maximal when the humeral head is centered in the glenoid (see Fig. 16-44). Thus, the joint has the highly desirable property of being most stable when the head is centered. As the humeral head is moved

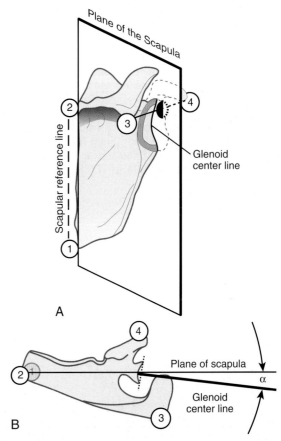

FIGURE 16-40 The glenoid center line can be related to scapular coordinates and the plane of the scapula. **A,** The plane of the scapula is the plane passing through the inferior pole of the scapula (*1*), through the medial extent of the spine of the scapula (*2*), and halfway between the coracoid tip (*4*) and the posterior angle of the acromion (*3*). **B,** The glenoid center line lies laterally approximately 10 degrees (α) posterior to this plane and perpendicular to the line connecting the inferior pole and the medial spine (the scapular reference line). (From Matsen FA III, Lippitt SB: Shoulder Surgery: Principles and Procedures. Philadelphia: WB Saunders, 2004, p 89.)

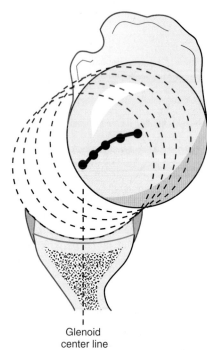

Glenoid
center line

FIGURE 16-41 Glenoidogram. The glenoidogram is the path taken by the center of the humeral head as it translates across the face of the glenoid in a specified direction away from the glenoid center line. The height of the glenoidogram reflects the amount of work needed to dislocate the humeral head for a given compressive load. (From Matsen FA III, Lippitt SB: Shoulder Surgery: Principles and Procedures. Philadelphia: WB Saunders, 2004, p 100.)

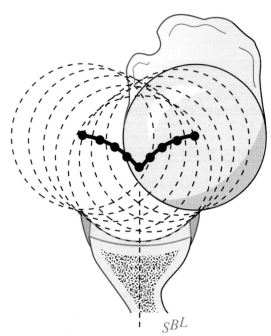

SBL

FIGURE 16-42 Paired glenoidograms. When the glenoidograms in two opposite directions are similar, they form a gull-wing shape together. The most stable position for the humeral head is that in which the two halves of the gull wing come together: at the center of the glenoid. (From Matsen FA III, Lippitt SB: Shoulder Surgery: Principles and Procedures. Philadelphia: WB Saunders, 2004, p 101.)

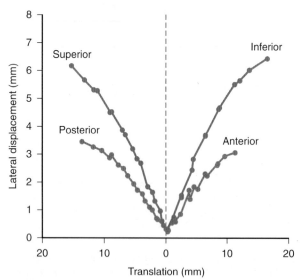

FIGURE 16-43 Measured glenoidograms for four different directions of translation in a young cadaver shoulder. The *dotted vertical line* represents the glenoid center line. The effective glenoid depth in this shoulder was 3.4 mm for translation in the posterior direction, 3.2 mm in the anterior direction, 6.2 mm in the superior direction, and 6.4 mm in the inferior direction. Note the high degree of symmetry about the glenoid center line and the deep valley when the head is exactly centered in the glenoid socket. (From Matsen FA III, Lippitt SB, Sidles JA, Harryman DT II: Practical Evaluation and Management of the Shoulder. Philadelphia: WB Saunders, 1994.)

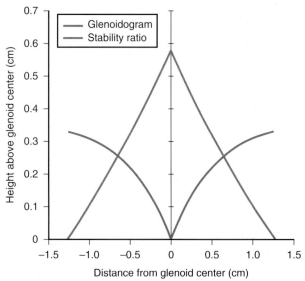

FIGURE 16-44 Local stability ratio: head and glenoid of the same radius. The stability ratio does not remain constant across the glenoid. The local stability ratio is maximal where the glenoidogram has the greatest slope. When the glenoid and humerus have the same radius, there is a peak in the local stability ratio at the center of the glenoid: The humerus is most stable in the center of the glenoid. (From Matsen FA III, Lippitt SB: Shoulder Surgery: Principles and Procedures. Philadelphia: WB Saunders, 2004, p 106.)

TABLE 16-1 Predicted Coordinates of the Glenoidogram

Effective Glenoid Width (*W*) $R_g \times$ sine(BSA)	Effective Glenoid Depth (D) $R_g \times (1 - \cos[\text{BSA}])$	*X*	*y* $D - R_h + (R_h \times R_h - [W - X] \times [W - X])^{1/2}$
12.5	3.35	0	0
12.5	3.35	0.1	0.057428086
12.5	3.35	0.2	0.114245197
12.5	3.35	0.3	0.170456105
12.5	3.35	0.4	0.226065482
12.5	3.35	0.5	0.281077905
12.5	3.35	0.6	0.335497855
12.5	3.35	0.7	0.38932972
12.5	3.35	0.8	0.442577799
12.5	3.35	0.9	0.495246303
12.5	3.35	1.0	0.547339357

BSA, balance stability angle.

away from the center, the slope of the glenoidogram and the stability ratio become less. Accordingly, as the head is displaced from the glenoid center, it becomes progressively more unstable. Once enough force is applied to displace the head from the center, that same amount of force easily displaces the humeral head over the glenoid lip. When the humeral head is translated to the lip of the glenoid, the stability ratio is, as expected, zero. These observations are consistent with the clinical jerk tests described for anterior[175] and posterior[89] instability; in these tests, there is no translation of the humeral head until the point of instability, at which sudden and substantial translation occurs (Figs. 16-45 and 16-46).[122,137]

Glenoid Version

Glenoid version is the angle that the glenoid center line makes with the plane of the scapula. The glenoid center line usually points a few degrees posterior to the plane of the scapula (see Fig. 16-40). Changing the version of the glenoid articular surface imposes a corresponding change in the humeroscapular positions in which the net humeral joint reaction force will be contained by the effective glenoid arc. Glenoid version may be altered by

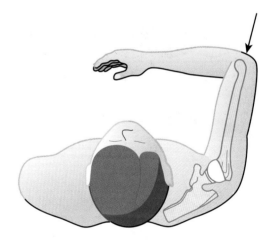

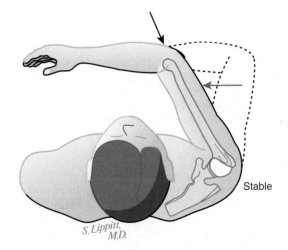

FIGURE 16-45 *Top,* Negative jerk test: The humeral head of the axially loaded arm remains centered in the glenoid fossa even with axial loading of humerus (*black arrow*). *Bottom,* Positive jerk test: The humeral head of the axillary loaded arm slides out the back of the shoulder when the arm is adducted across the body and clunks back in when the arm position is aligned with the scapula. (From Matsen FA III, Lippitt SB: Shoulder Surgery: Principles and Procedures. Philadelphia: WB Saunders, 2004, p 115.)

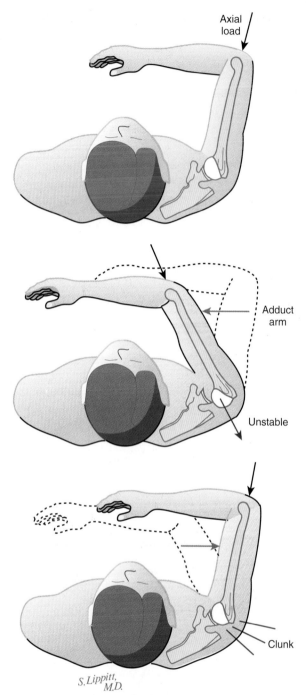

Axial
load

Adduct
arm

Unstable

Clunk

S. Lippitt,
M.D.

FIGURE 16-46 Positive jerk test: The humeral head of the axially loaded arm slides out the back of the shoulder when the arm is adducted across the body and clunks back in when the arm position is aligned with the scapula. (From Matsen FA III, Lippitt SB: Shoulder Surgery: Principles and Procedures. Philadelphia: WB Saunders, 2004, p 115.)

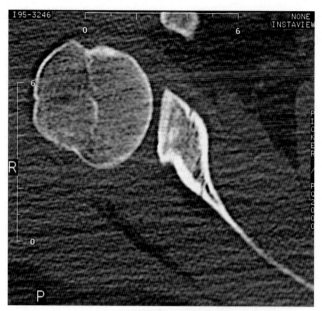

FIGURE 16-47 A CT scan of a shoulder with glenoid dysplasia manifested as absence of the posterior glenoid lip and glenoid retroversion. When the glenoid rim is hypoplastic, it cannot contribute normally to the glenoidogram.

version is often a critical step in glenohumeral reconstruction.

Apparent changes in glenoid version can arise from loss of part of the glenoid rim (see Figs. 16-31 and 16-35).[178-180] Dias and colleagues did not find any difference in apparent glenoid version between normal subjects and recurrent anterior dislocators.[181] Dowdy and O'Driscoll[182] found only minor variance in radiographic glenoid version among patients with and without recurrence after stabilization surgery. However, Hirschfelder and Kirsten[183] detected increased glenoid retroversion in both the symptomatic and asymptomatic shoulders of patients with posterior instability, and Grasshoff and coworkers[184] found increased anteversion in shoulders with recurrent anterior instability. It has been shown that the dominant shoulder of throwing athletes has an average of 17 degrees of retroversion of the humeral head and 3 degrees of retroversion of the glenoid.[185] It was demonstrated in a cadaveric study by Churchill and colleagues that black men and women have less glenoid retroversion than white men and women do: 0.2 and 2.65 degrees, respectively.[186] No significant difference was found between men and women. Patients with posterior instability were found to be more likely to have glenoid rim deficiency than were those with normal or anteriorly unstable shoulders.[187]

Changes in version may be difficult to quantitate on axillary radiographs unless the view is carefully standardized (Fig. 16-49). Even with optimal radiographic technique, the important contributions of cartilage and labrum to the depth and orientation of the fossa[132,136] cannot be seen on plain radiographs or CT scans. When it is important to know the orientation of the cartilaginous joint

glenoid dysplasia (Fig. 16-47),[176] glenoid osteotomy,[176,177] and glenoid arthroplasty.[109] Abnormal glenoid version positions the glenoid fossa in an abnormal relationship to the forces generated by the scapulohumeral muscles and changes the intrinsic stability provided by the glenoid concavity (Fig. 16-48). Normalization of abnormal glenoid

FIGURE 16-48 Glenoid hypoplasia. When the glenoid rim is hypoplastic, it cannot contribute normally to the glenoidogram. (From Matsen FA III, Lippitt SB: Shoulder Surgery: Principles and Procedures. Philadelphia: WB Saunders, 2004, p 111.)

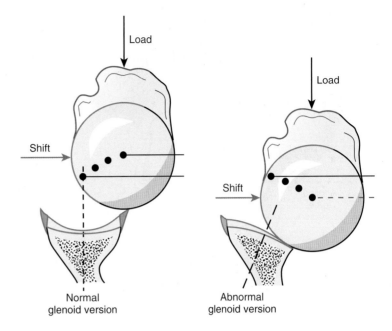

surface in relation to the scapular body, a double-contrast CT scan may be necessary (see Fig. 16-22).

Scapular Positioning

A special feature of the glenohumeral joint is that the glenoid can be positioned on the thorax (in contrast to the fixed acetabulum of the hip). This scapular alignment greatly increases the range of positions in which the criteria for glenohumeral stability can be met (Fig. 16-50). Consider the arm to be elevated 90 degrees in the sagittal thoracic plane. This position can be achieved with the scapula protracted or retracted. If the scapula is protracted, the humerus is closely aligned with the glenoid center line. When the humerus is in this position, most of the humeroscapular muscles are oriented to compress the humeral head into the glenoid fossa (Fig. 16-51). Alternatively, if the scapula is maximally retracted, the humerus is almost at right angles to the glenoid center line. In this position, the net humeral joint reaction force is directed posteriorly and might not be contained within the balance stability angle.[136,188-192]

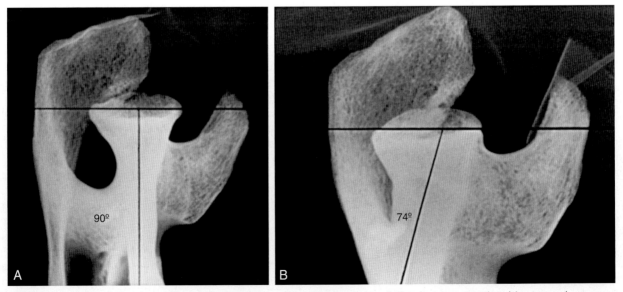

FIGURE 16-49 Two radiographs of the same cadaver scapula showing the variation in apparent glenoid retroversion, depending on the radiographic projection. **A,** Proper orientation. **B,** Oblique orientation.

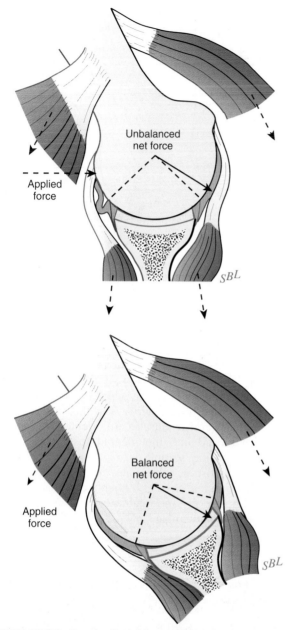

FIGURE 16-50 *Top,* Applied force results in an unbalanced net force. *Bottom,* Stabilization against an applied translational force by repositioning the glenoid concavity to support the net humeral force.

Scapular position also affects the tension in the glenohumeral capsule and ligaments (see Fig. 16-20). Which humeroscapular position is used to achieve a given humerothoracic position is a question of habit and training. Coordination of scapular position and glenohumeral muscle balance is an important element of the neuromuscular control of glenohumeral stability.

Atwater[193] has documented that in most throwing and striking skills, the shoulder abduction angle is usually 100 degrees. Higher and lower release points are achieved by tilting the trunk rather than by increasing or decreasing the shoulder abduction angle relative to the trunk.

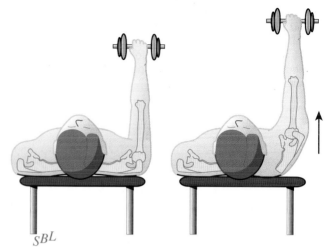

FIGURE 16-51 The glenoid can be moved to support the net humeral joint reaction force. Protraction of the scapula, for example in the bench press, places the glenoid fossa squarely beneath the force exerted on it by the loaded humerus. (From Matsen FA III, Lippitt SB: Shoulder Surgery: Principles and Procedures. Philadelphia: WB Saunders, 2004, p 91.)

Ligaments

Properties of Ligaments

Each glenohumeral ligament has clinically important properties that can be characterized by the relationship of the distance between its origin and insertion and its tension.[194] These properties include its resting length, its elastic deformability, and its plastic deformability. Resting length is how far a ligament's origin and insertion can be separated with minimal force. Elastic deformability is how much additional separation of the origin and insertion can be achieved by the application of larger forces without permanently changing the ligament's properties. Plastic deformability is deformability beyond the ligament's elastic limit: how much additional separation between the origin and insertion can be achieved by applying larger forces that permanently deform the ligament up to the point where the ligament fails.

These properties can be demonstrated as a plot of the ligament's tension versus the distance between the ligament's origin and insertion. The same relationship pertains whether the ligament's origin and insertion are separated by translation of the humeral head or by rotation (Fig. 16-52).

At point *A*, the origin and insertion of the ligament are closely approximated. At point *B*, the origin and insertion have been separated enough to initiate tension in the ligament. Thus, the resting length of the ligament is shown as A–B. Stefko and coworkers[195] found the length of the anterior band of the IGHL to be 37 mm.

Additional separation of the origin and insertion causes increasing ligament tension. Up to point *C*, this separation is elastic (i.e., it does not result in permanent change in the ligament). Further separation of the origin and inser-

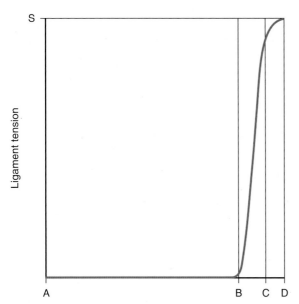

FIGURE 16-52 The properties of the glenohumeral ligament include its resting length, its elastic deformability, and its plastic deformability. These properties can be demonstrated as a plot of the ligament's tension versus the distance between the ligament's origin and insertion. At point *A*, the origin and insertion of the ligament are closely approximated. At point *B*, the origin and insertion have been separated enough to initiate tension in the ligament. Thus, the resting length of the ligament is shown as A–B. Additional separation of the origin and insertion causes increasing ligament tension. Up to point *C*, this separation is elastic. Further separation of the origin and insertion plastically deforms the ligament up to point *D*, where the ligament fails at a tension of *S*.

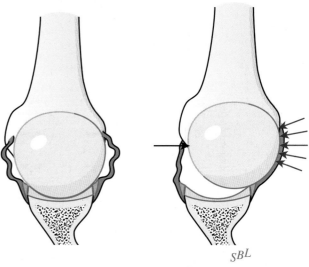

FIGURE 16-53 Glenohumeral translation is movement of the center of the humeral head with respect to the face of the glenoid. *Left*, The humeral head in mid glenoid with lax ligaments. *Right*, The amount of translation allowed (*black arrow*) is determined by the initial position of the joint and the length of the ligament that becomes tight (*red arrows*).

tion plastically deforms the ligament up to point *D*, where the ligament fails at a tension of *S*. The midsubstance strain to failure has been measured as 7% to 11%.[195]

Such graphs are helpful in describing the properties of ligaments. The *strength* of a ligament is the amount of tension that it can take before failure (*S* in Fig. 16-52). The *laxity* of a ligament is the amount of translation (Fig. 16-53) or rotation (Fig. 16-54) that it allows from a specified starting position when a small load is applied. Ligaments with long A–B distances demonstrate substantial laxity if the starting point for laxity testing is close to A. Laxity is diminished when the joint is positioned near the extremes of motion (Fig. 16-55), that is, when the starting point for the laxity measurement is close to B (see Fig. 16-52). Ligaments with small A–B distances are short or contracted. *Translational laxity and rotational laxity are closely correlated*: They both reflect the ability to separate the attachment points of the ligament.

A typical relationship between humeroscapular position and torque (capsular tension times humeral head radius) is shown in Figure 16-56.[98] Note that the greatest part of glenohumeral motion and function takes place in the area where no tension is being placed on the capsule

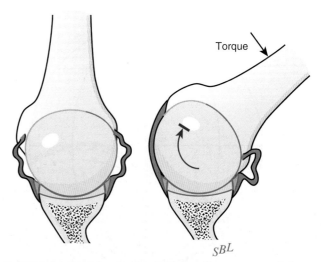

FIGURE 16-54 Glenohumeral rotation is movement of the humerus around the center of the humeral head, which remains centered in the glenoid fossa. *Left*, The humeral head in mid glenoid with lax ligaments. *Right*, The amount of rotation allowed (*red arrow*) in response to an applied torque (*black arrow*) is determined by the initial position of the joint and the length of the ligament that becomes tight.

Mean translational laxity in intact shoulders

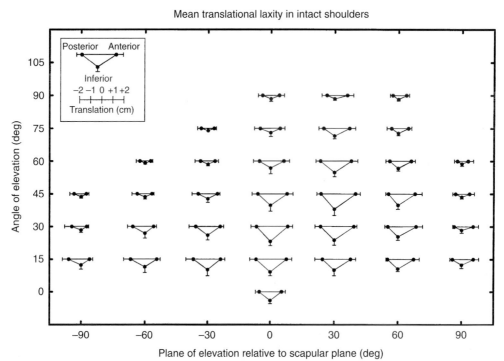

FIGURE 16-55 Mean translational laxity as measured in eight cadaveric shoulders. The applied translational force was 30 N (~6 lb), and it was applied along the anterior, posterior, and inferior axes. The planes of elevation are measured relative to the plane of the scapula (see Fig. 16-40), not the thoracic plane. The angles of elevation are measured relative to the scapular reference line (see Fig. 16-40). Standard deviations are shown at the vertex of each triangle. (From Matsen FA III, Lippitt SB, Sidles JA, Harryman DT II: Practical Evaluation and Management of the Shoulder. Philadelphia: WB Saunders, 1994.)

(corresponding to zone A–B in Fig. 16-52). Also note that at the limits of motion (corresponding to zone B–C), the torque increases rapidly with changes in position, as suggested by the rapid increase in tension shown in Figure 16-52.

These diagrams help distinguish laxity from instability. Normally stable shoulders can demonstrate substantial laxity; consider the very lax but very stable glenohumeral joints of gymnasts. In a most important study, Emery and Mullaji[196] found that of 150 asymptomatic shoulders

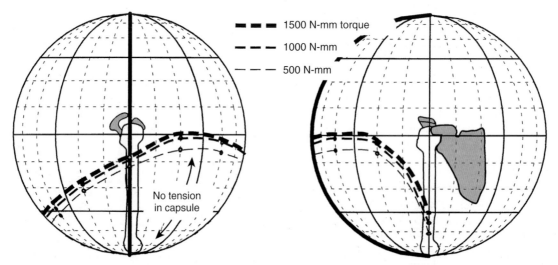

FIGURE 16-56 The range of humeroscapular elevation with no capsular tension. This global diagram represents data from a cadaver experiment in which the humerus was elevated in various scapular planes with free axial rotation. Elevation was performed until the torque reached 500, 1000, and 1500 N • mm. The positions associated with these torque levels are indicated by the isobars. The area within the inner isobars indicates the range of positions in which no tension is placed on the capsuloligamentous structures. (From Matsen FA III, Lippitt SB, Sidles JA, Harryman DT II: Practical Evaluation and Management of the Shoulder. Philadelphia: WB Saunders, 1994.)

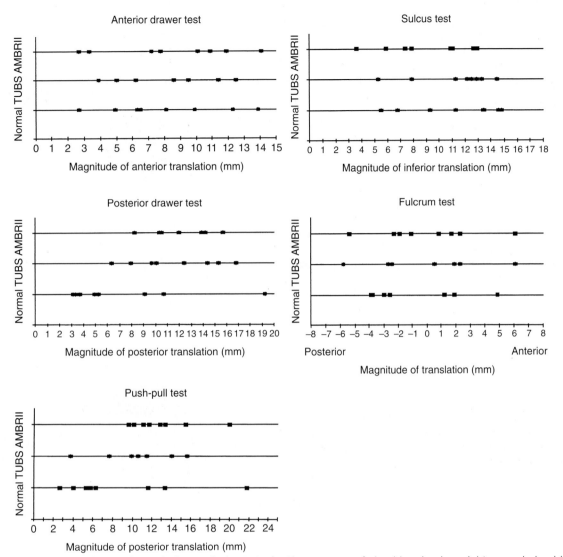

FIGURE 16-57 The magnitude of translation on laxity tests for three groups of shoulders in vivo: eight normal shoulders, eight shoulders with symptomatic atraumatic instability (AMBRII), and eight shoulders with symptomatic traumatic instability (TUBS). Each shoulder is represented by a mark on the horizontal lines. Note that for each of these laxity tests, the range of translations for the normal subjects is essentially the same as the range of translations for subjects with symptomatic instability requiring surgical repair. (From Matsen FA III, Lippitt SB, Sidles JA, Harryman DT II: Practical Evaluation and Management of the Shoulder. Philadelphia: WB Saunders, 1994.)

in schoolchildren, 50% demonstrated positive signs of increased laxity.

Some investigators have measured increased laxity in patients with glenohumeral instability.[197-201] However, recent evidence indicates that these differences are not always significant.[98,202,203] Starting in a neutral position, the translational laxity of eight normal living subjects was found to be 8 ± 4 mm, 8 ± 6 mm, and 11 ± 4 mm in the anterior, posterior, and inferior directions, respectively. Interestingly, virtually identical laxity was measured in 16 patients who required surgery for symptomatic recurrent instability (Fig. 16-57), thus indicating that in these subjects, the measured laxity was not the determinant of glenohumeral stability.[98,203] Sperber and Wredmark[204] found no differences in joint volume or capsular elasticity

between healthy and unstable shoulders. These results indicate that the amount of laxity cannot be used to distinguish clinically stable shoulders from those that are unstable.

The *stretchiness* of a ligament is its elasticity. Ligaments with long B-C distances (see Fig. 16-52) are stretchy and have "soft" end points on clinical laxity tests. Ligaments with short B-C distances are stiff and have "firm" end points on clinical laxity tests. It is also evident that ligaments that are stretchy require more displacement before tension sufficient for failure is developed in them.

Biochemical composition (as in Ehlers–Danlos syndrome), anatomic variation (anomalies of attachment), use (or disuse), age, disease (e.g., diabetes, frozen shoulder), injury, and surgery (e.g., capsulorrhaphy) can affect the strength, laxity, and stretchiness of glenohumeral ligaments. See reviews of the material properties of the IGHL by Mow and colleagues[128 (Ch 2)] and the role of ligaments in glenohumeral stability by Lew and associates.[128 (Ch 3)]

Ligamentous Stabilization

The glenohumeral ligaments exert two stabilizing effects: as checkreins and as countervailing forces.

The glenohumeral ligaments serve as *checkreins* in which the range of joint positions is restricted to those that can be stabilized by muscle balance. This function is important because at extreme glenohumeral positions, the net humeral joint reaction force becomes increasingly difficult to balance within the glenoid (Fig. 16-58). For example, excessive abduction, extension, and external rotation of the shoulder may allow the net humeral joint reaction force vector to point beyond the anterior-inferior balance stability angle. Similarly, excessive posterior capsular laxity allows the net humeral joint reaction force to achieve large angles with the glenoid center line; these angles can exceed the posterior balance stability angle. At the extremes of motion, the muscles tend to be near their maximal extension, a position in which their force-generating capacity is diminished.[205] In these positions where muscles are disadvantaged, ligamentous forces can provide the necessary compression (Fig. 16-59).

The patient can modify the checkrein function by altering the position of the scapula (see Fig. 16-20). Surgeons can likewise modify the checkrein function: Capsular tightening moves points B, C, and D closer to point A, thereby reducing laxity (see Fig. 16-52). The checkrein function is inoperant when the ligament is not under tension, that is, when the humeroscapular position is within the tension-free zone (see Fig. 16-52 [points *A* and *B*] and Fig. 16-56).

When torque is applied to the humerus so that a ligament comes under tension, this ligament applies a force to the proximal end of the humerus. Because of the attachments of the ligament, this *countervailing force* both compresses the humeral head into the glenoid fossa and resists displacement in the direction of the tight ligament (Fig. 16-60).

An analysis of ligament function* demonstrates the limits of the stability provided by ligaments acting alone. For example, such an analysis suggests that if the torque resulting from a modest 20-lb force applied to the arm at a distance of 30 inches from the center of a humeral head with a 1-inch radius were resisted only by the tension in the IGHL, the IGHL would need to be able to withstand a tension of 600 lb (Fig. 16-61).

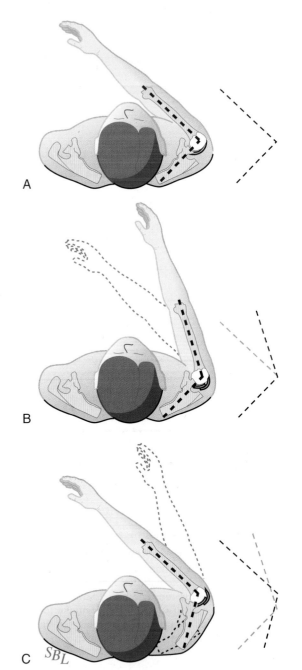

FIGURE 16-58 A, Excessive posterior capsular laxity allows an excessively small angle between the humerus and the plane of the scapula; as a result, posterior stability is challenged. **B,** Normal tightness appropriately limits the allowed angular position to the range that can be stabilized. **C,** Cross-body adduction is achieved by scapular protraction as well as by humeroscapular angulation.

---

*The magnitude of the countervailing force is determined by the applied torque and limited by the strength of the ligament. The direction of this force is tangent to the humeral head at the point of its contact with the glenoid rim.

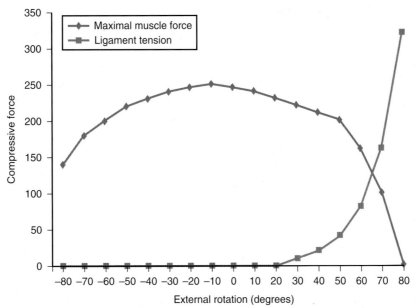

FIGURE 16-59 Hypothetical graph showing the interplay between muscular and capsular tension. As the humerus is passively externally rotated, the force that the subscapularis can generate drops off and the force generated by the anterior capsular ligaments increases in a complementary manner. (From Matsen FA III, Chebli C, Lippitt S: Principles for the Evaluation and Management of Shoulder Instability. J Bone Joint Surg Am 88:648-659, 2006.)

The countervailing force mechanism operates in the arc, where the ligament is elastically deformed. If the ligament behaves perfectly elastically, the tension in the ligament provides a stabilizing force T in which

$$T = (Angle) \times Diameter\ of\ humeral\ head \times \pi/360° \times Spring\ constant\ of\ the\ ligament$$

This relationship predicts the following:

- Until the ligament becomes taut, no force is generated by it.
- The larger the angle past the point where the ligament becomes taut, the more force that is generated (up to the elastic limit).
- Stiffer ligaments generate more force for a given angular displacement.

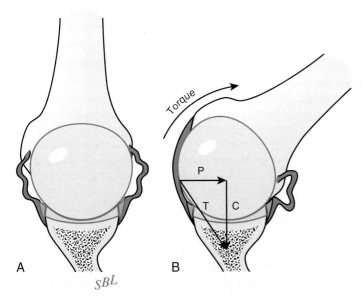

FIGURE 16-60 A, When the glenohumeral ligaments are slack, they exert no force. **B,** When torque is applied, the ligaments come under tension (*T*). This ligament tension exerts a compressive force (*C*) directed into the glenoid and a displacing force (*P*) pushing the humeral head away from the tight ligament.

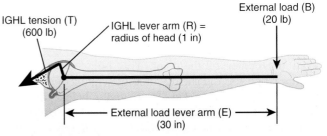

FIGURE 16-61 Mechanism of ligamentous avulsion. A load applied to the outstretched arm results in a much greater tension in the ligaments that restrain the rotation of the joint. If a load of 20 lb applied at a distance of 30 in from the center of the humeral head is opposed by a ligament acting 1 in from the humeral head center, the necessary tension in the ligament would be 600 lb, a tension sufficient to avulse the ligament attachment. If a load of 600 pounds were applied directly to the shoulder, other injuries such as fractures may well result. IGHL, inferior glenohumeral ligament. (From Matsen FA III, Lippitt SB: Shoulder Surgery: Principles and Procedures. Philadelphia: WB Saunders, 2004, p 122.)

- Larger humeral heads generate more force for each degree of angular displacement.

Ligament tension results from applied torque. When an externally applied force B acts at a distance E from the center of the humeral head, it creates a torque (Q) that is the product of B and E (see Fig. 16-61). If this torque is resisted by a ligament closely applied to the humeral head (i.e., the effective moment arm equals the head radius [R]), the tension in the ligament (T) is

$$T = Q/R = B \times E/R$$

If tension in the ligament exceeds the strength of the ligament, the ligament breaks. A few investigations have attempted to measure the strength of the glenohumeral capsular ligaments. Kaltsas[206] has studied some of the material properties of the shoulder capsule and found it to be more elastic and stronger than the capsule of the elbow. He noted that the entire glenohumeral capsule ruptured at 2000 N of distraction (450 lb). Stefko and colleagues[195] found the average load to failure of the entire IGHL to be 713 N, or 160 lb.

Bigliani and coworkers[207] noted in 16 cadaver shoulders that the IGHL could be divided into three anatomic regions: a superior band, an anterior axillary pouch, and a posterior axillary pouch, the thickest of which was the superior band (2.8 mm). With relatively low strain rates, the stress at failure was found to be nearly identical for the three regions of the ligament, an average of 5.5 mPa, which is 5.5 N/mm². Therefore, to function as the primary stabilizer for a load of 600 lb as in the previous example, the IGHLs of these cadavers would need to be 500 mm² in cross section. Thus, no experimental measurements have demonstrated that the IGHL alone is sufficiently strong to balance the torque resulting from a load of 20 lb applied to the arm at a distance of 30 inches from the center of the humeral head.

Excessive ligament tension can produce obligate translation of the humeral head. Harryman and colleagues[105] demonstrated that certain passive motions of the glenohumeral joint forced translation of the humeral head away from the center of the joint. This obligate translation occurs when the displacing force generated by ligament tension (quantity P in Fig. 16-60) overwhelms the concavity compression stability mechanism (Fig. 16-62). In Harryman's study, anterior humeral translation occurred at the extremes of flexion and cross-body adduction, whereas posterior humeral translation occurred at the extremes of extension and external rotation. Operative tightening of the posterior portion of the capsule increased anterior translation on flexion and cross-body adduction and caused it to occur earlier in the arc of motion than in an intact joint. Operative tightening of the posterior part of the capsule also resulted in significant superior translation with flexion of the glenohumeral joint.

These data indicate that glenohumeral translation can occur in sports when the joint is forced to the extremes of its motion, such as at the transition between late

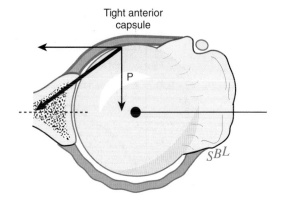

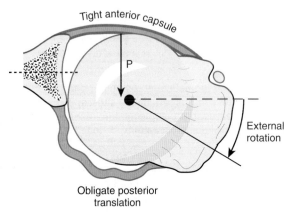

FIGURE 16-62 If the humerus is rotated beyond the point at which the ligaments become tight, the displacing force (P) can push the humeral head out of the glenoid center, a phenomenon known as *obligate translation*. (Modified from Matsen FA III, Lippitt SB, Sidles JA, Harryman DT II: Practical Evaluation and Management of the Shoulder. Philadelphia: WB Saunders, 1994.)

cocking and early acceleration. Such obligate translation can account for the posterior labral tears and calcifications seen at the posterior glenoid in throwers. In addition, these results point to the hazard of overtightening the glenohumeral capsule, which can result in a form of secondary osteoarthritis known as *capsulorrhaphy arthropathy* (Fig. 16-63). Hawkins and Angelo[208] pointed to these complications of obligate translation in overtightened capsular repairs.

Adhesion and Cohesion

Adhesion–cohesion is a stabilizing mechanism by which joint surfaces wet with joint fluid are held together by the molecular attraction of the fluid to itself and to the joint surfaces. Fluids such as water and joint fluid demonstrate the property of cohesion; that is, they tend to stick together. Some surfaces, such as clean glass or articular cartilage, can be wet with water or synovial fluid, which means that the fluid adheres to them. When two surfaces with adherent fluid are brought into contact, the adhesion of the fluid to the surfaces and the cohesion of the fluids

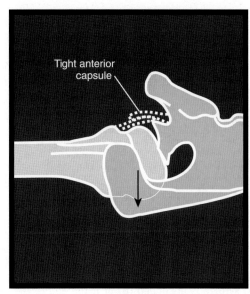

SBL

FIGURE 16-63 Axillary view of capsulorrhaphy arthropathy in which an excessively tight anterior capsular repair is forcing the head of the humerus posteriorly (*arrow*). This effect is accentuated by forced external rotation. Note also the typical posterior glenoid erosion. (Modified from Matsen FA III, Lippitt SB, Sidles JA, Harryman DT II: Practical Evaluation and Management of the Shoulder. Philadelphia: WB Saunders, 1994.)

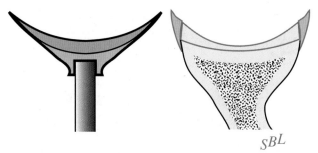

SBL

FIGURE 16-64 In cross section, the glenoid (*right*) looks much like a rubber suction cup (*left*) with respect to its feathered, compliant edges and more rigid center. (Modified from Matsen FA III, Lippitt SB, Sidles JA, Harryman DT II: Practical Evaluation and Management of the Shoulder. Philadelphia: WB Saunders, 1994.)

tend to hold the two surfaces together (like two wetted microscope slides). The amount of stability generated by adhesion–cohesion is related to the adhesive and cohesive properties of the joint fluid, the wetability of the joint surfaces, and the area of contact between the glenoid socket and the humerus. Joint fluid has the highly desirable properties of high tensile strength (difficult to pull apart) and low shear strength (allows easy sliding of the two joint surfaces on each other with low resistance).[209]

The adhesion–cohesion effect is reduced by any factor that lowers the cohesion of joint fluid (such as in inflammatory joint disease), reduces wetability of the joint surfaces (as can occur in degenerative joint disease), or diminishes the glenohumeral contact area (such as in a displaced articular surface fracture or a congenitally small glenoid). It is also noteworthy that adhesion–cohesion forces do not stabilize a prosthetic shoulder replacement because metal and polyethylene are insufficiently compliant to provide the necessary nearly perfect congruence and because water does not adhere to their surfaces.

The Glenohumeral Suction Cup

The glenohumeral suction cup provides stability by virtue of the seal of the labrum and capsule to the humeral head (Fig. 16-64). A suction cup adheres to a smooth surface by expressing the interposed air or fluid and then forming a seal with the surface. A rubber suction cup is noncompliant in the center but becomes more flexible toward its

periphery. In a similar manner, the center of the glenoid is covered with a relatively thin layer of articular cartilage. At greater distances from the center, the articular cartilage becomes thicker and thus provides greater flexibility. More peripherally, the glenoid labrum and, finally, the capsule provide even more flexibility. This graduated flexibility permits the socket to conform and seal to the smooth humeral articular surface. Compression of the head into the glenoid fossa expels any intervening fluid so that a suction is produced that resists distraction.

The glenoid suction cup stabilization mechanism was demonstrated by Harryman and associates.[210] In elderly cadaver shoulders without degenerative changes, the suction cup resisted an average of 20 ± 3 N of lateral traction (about 4 lb). Creating a defect in the labrum completely eliminated the suction cup effect. No suction cup effect could be demonstrated in the two shoulders with mild degenerative change of the joint surface. It is likely that this effect would be even stronger in younger living shoulders in which the articular cartilage, glenoid labrum, and joint capsule are larger, more hydrated, and more compliant. Like stabilization from adhesion–cohesion, the glenoid suction cup centers the head of the humerus in the glenoid without muscle action and is effective in midrange positions in which the ligaments are not under tension and thus do not contribute to stability.

Limited Joint Volume

Limited joint volume is a stabilizing mechanism in which the humeral head is held to the glenoid by the relative vacuum created when they are distracted (Figs. 16-65 and 16-66). Although it is common to speak of the glenohumeral joint space, there is essentially no space and minimal free fluid within the confines of the articular surfaces and the joint capsule of a normal glenohumeral joint. The scarcity of fluid within the joint can be confirmed on MRI scans of normal joints, on inspection of normal joints, and on attempts to aspirate fluid from normal joints. The appearance of the *potential* joint volume can only be demonstrated after instilling fluids

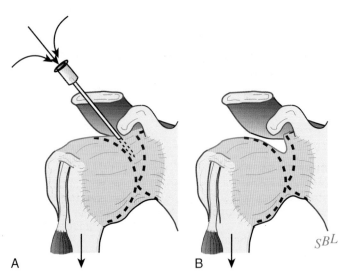

FIGURE 16-65 Normally, the glenohumeral capsule establishes a limited joint volume, so distraction of the humeral head produces a relative vacuum within the capsule that resists further displacement. **A,** Venting of the capsule eliminates the limited joint volume effect. **B,** The limited joint volume effect is reduced if the capsule is excessively compliant and can be displaced into the joint. (From Matsen FA III, Lippitt SB, Sidles JA, Harryman DT II: Practical Evaluation and Management of the Shoulder. Philadelphia: WB Saunders, 1994.)

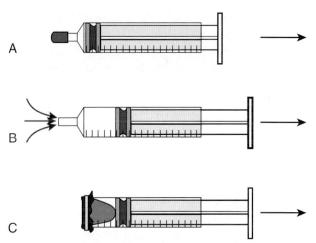

FIGURE 16-66 Limited joint volume effect demonstrated with a syringe model. Substantial force is required to pull the plunger from a plugged syringe (**A**). This stabilizing effect is lost if the syringe is uncapped (**B**) or if the end of the syringe is covered with compliant material (**C**). (From Matsen FA III, Lippitt SB, Sidles JA, Harryman DT II: Practical Evaluation and Management of the Shoulder. Philadelphia: WB Saunders, 1994.)

such as air, saline, or contrast material into the joint. Osmotic action by the synovium removes free fluid, thus keeping slightly negative pressure within a normal joint.[209-211] This negative intra-articular pressure holds the joint together with a force proportional to the joint surface area and the magnitude of the negative intra-articular pressure. For example, if the colloid osmotic pressure of normal synovial fluid is 10 mm Hg and the colloid osmotic pressure of the synovial interstitium is 14 mm Hg, the equilibrium pressure in the joint fluid will be −4 mm Hg.[209] This negative intra-articular pressure adds a small amount of resistance to distraction (about 1 oz/in^2) to the limited joint volume effect. Because a normal joint is sealed, attempted distraction of the joint surfaces lowers the intra-articular pressure even more, thereby progressively adding substantial resistance to greater displacement.[148,212]

The limited joint volume effect is reduced if the joint is vented (opened to the atmosphere) or the capsular boundaries of the joint are very compliant. In the latter circumstance, attempted distraction draws the flexible capsule into the joint and produces a sulcus (see Figs. 16-65 and 16-66). The decreased stability from venting the joint was initially described by Humphry in 1858[213] and subsequently by others.[92,162,214-221] Gibb and colleagues[98,222] found that simply venting the capsule with an 18-gauge needle reduced the force necessary to translate the head of the humerus halfway to the edge of the glenoid by an average of 50%. Wulker and coworkers[223] found that venting the joint increased displacement of the joint with an applied load of 50 N by 50% in all directions.

From these results it is expected that glenohumeral stability from limited joint volume is compromised by arthrography, arthroscopy, articular effusions, hemarthrosis, and other situations in which free fluid is allowed to enter the glenohumeral joint. In a very interesting study, Habermeyer and associates[224,225] found that the mean stabilizing force obtained by atmospheric pressure was 146 N (32 lb). In 15 stable living shoulders, traction on the arm caused negative intra-articular pressure proportionate to the amount of force exerted. In contrast, unstable shoulder joints with a Bankart lesion did not exhibit this phenomenon.

These stabilizing mechanisms may be overwhelmed by the application of traction, as in cracking of the metacarpophalangeal joint. A crack is produced as the joint cavitates: subatmospheric pressure within the joint releases gas (>80% CO_2) from solution in the joint fluid. This release of gas is accompanied by a sudden increase in separation of the joint surfaces. Once a joint has cracked, it cannot be cracked again until about 20 minutes later when all the gas has been reabsorbed.[226,227]

Stability at Rest

It is apparent that a relaxed glenohumeral joint is held together without either active muscle contraction or ligament tension. The intact shoulder of a fresh anatomic specimen,[214] the anesthetized and paralyzed shoulder of a patient in the operating room, and the arm relaxed at the side[94] all maintain the normal relationships of the

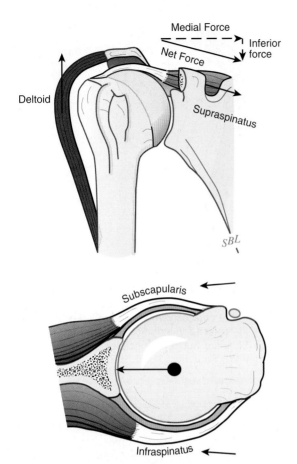

FIGURE 16-67 *Top,* The supraspinatus muscle compresses the humeral head into the glenoid and thereby provides stability against displacement by the force of the deltoid (*arrow*). It is not optimally oriented to depress the head of the humerus because the inferiorly directed component of its force is small. *Bottom,* Similarly, the subscapularis and infraspinatus compress the head into the glenoid, providing additional stability. (From Matsen FA III, Lippitt SB, Sidles JA, Harryman DT II: Practical Evaluation and Management of the Shoulder. Philadelphia: WB Saunders, 1994.)

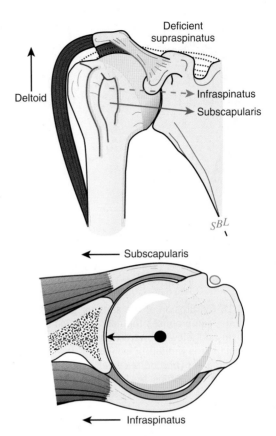

FIGURE 16-68 Compressive force from the infraspinatus and subscapularis can stabilize the humeral head in the absence of a supraspinatus, provided that the glenoid concavity is intact. *Top,* AP view. *Bottom,* Axillary view. (Modified from Matsen FA III, Lippitt SB, Sidles JA, Harryman DT II: Practical Evaluation and Management of the Shoulder. Philadelphia: WB Saunders, 1994.)

glenoid and humeral joint surfaces. This resting stability is due to a group of mechanisms, including adhesion and cohesion, the glenoid suction cup, and limited joint volume. These mechanisms save energy, as pointed out by Humphry in 1858[213]: "We have only to remember that this power is in continual operation to appreciate the amount of animal force that is economized."

Superior Stability: The Same Plus a Unique Addition

Superior stability benefits from all the same mechanisms as anterior, posterior, and inferior stability: socket shape and orientation, muscle balance, ligamentous effects, adhesion and cohesion, the suction cup, and limited joint volume. Compression of the humeral head into the glenoid concavity is an important mechanism by which

the head of the humerus is centered and stabilized in the glenoid fossa to resist superiorly directed loads (Fig. 16-67). Even when a substantial supraspinatus defect is present, compression from the subscapularis and infraspinatus can hold the humeral head centered in the glenoid (Fig. 16-68). More severe cases of chronic rotator cuff deficiency, however, may be associated with superior subluxation of the head of the humerus and wear on the superior lip of the glenoid fossa (Fig. 16-69). This erosive wear flattens the superior glenoid concavity and thereby reduces the effective glenoid depth in that direction. Once the effective superior glenoid depth is lost, repair of the rotator cuff tendons or complex capsular reconstructions cannot completely restore the glenohumeral stability previously provided by concavity compression (see Fig. 16-69).

In addition to mechanisms that stabilize the shoulder in other directions, superior stability has a unique aspect: a ball-in-socket effect provided by the articulation of the proximal humeral convexity into the coracoacromial concavity compressed together by the action of the deltoid (Fig. 16-70)—another example of concavity compression.

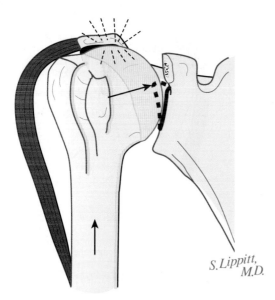

S. Lippitt, M.D.

FIGURE 16-69 Erosion of the superior glenoid concavity (*dotted line*) compromises the concavity compression stability mechanism and allows upward translation (*vertical arrow*). This translation is limited by contact of the humeral head with the acromion (*fine dotted lines*). (Modified from Matsen FA III, Lippitt SB, Sidles JA, Harryman DT II: Practical Evaluation and Management of the Shoulder. Philadelphia: WB Saunders, 1994.)

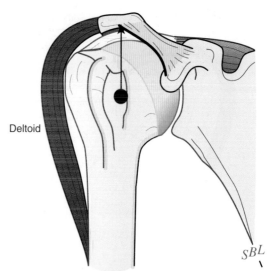

Deltoid

SBL

FIGURE 16-70 Compression into the coracoacromial concavity. The deltoid compresses the proximal humeral convexity into the coracoacromial concavity, keeping the humeral head center (*dot*) stabilized. (From Matsen FA III, Lippitt SB: Shoulder Surgery: Principles and Procedures. Philadelphia: WB Saunders, 2004, p 84.)

As every shoulder surgeon has observed, in a normal shoulder in a resting position, no gap is present between the humeral head, the superior cuff tendon, and the coracoacromial arch. As a result, the slightest amount of superior translation compresses the cuff tendon between the humeral head and the arch. Thus, when the humeral head is pressed upward (for example, when pushing up from an armchair or with isometric contraction of the deltoid), further superior displacement is opposed by a downward force exerted by the coracoacromial arch through the cuff tendon to the humeral head.

Ziegler and coworkers[228] confirmed this stabilizing effect in cadavers by demonstrating acromial deformation when the neutrally positioned humerus was loaded in a superior direction. By attaching strain gauges percutaneously to the acromion, they were able to measure its deformation under load. The acromion thus became an in situ load transducer. By applying known loads to the acromion, they were able to derive calibration load-deformation curves that were essentially linear. Superiorly directed loads applied to the humerus were then correlated with the resulting acromial loads and with superior humeral displacement. In 10 fresh cadaver specimens with the superior cuff tendon intact but not under tension, superiorly directed loads of 80 N produced only 1.7 mm of superior displacement of the humeral head relative to the acromion. When the cuff tendon was excised, a similar load produced superior displacement of 5.4 mm ($P < .0001$). In specimens in which the cuff tendon was

intact, an upward load of 20 N gave rise to an estimated acromial load of 8 N. Greater humeral loads up to 80 N were associated with a linear increase in acromial load of up to 55 N when an upward load of 80 N was applied (Fig. 16-71). In a single in vivo experiment in which the acromion was instrumented and calibrated as in the cadavers, very similar relationships between upward humeral load and acromial load were noted (see Fig. 16-71). These acromial loads must have been transmitted through the intact cuff tendon. When the tendon was excised, the humeral head rose until it contacted and again loaded the acromial undersurface (Fig. 16-72).

Flatow and colleagues[229] used a cadaver model to explore the active and passive restraints to superior humeral translation. Whereas Ziegler's study was conducted with the arm in neutral position with axial loads, Flatow's involved abducting the humerus with simulated deltoid and cuff muscle forces. Both groups noted that the presence of the supraspinatus tendon limited superior translation of the humeral head, even with no tension from simulated muscle action.

Both Ziegler and Flatow cautioned that the effectiveness of the superior stabilizing mechanism depends on an intact coracoacromial arch. Sacrifice of the ceiling of the joint, the coracoacromial ligament, or the undersurface of the acromion can be expected to compromise the superior stability of the humeral head (Fig. 16-73).

The reader is referred to Soslowsky and colleagues' review[128] [Ch 5] of stabilization of the glenohumeral joint surfaces by articular contact and by contact in the subacromial space.

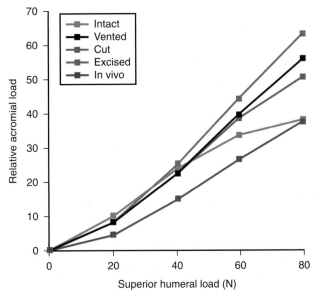

FIGURE 16-71 Relative acromial load as a function of a superiorly directed humeral load. The graph compares loads for intact specimens, after venting of the joint to air, after cutting (but not excising) the cuff tendon, and after excising the superior cuff tendon. Also included are the data from a single in vivo experiment performed with the identical instrumentation. Note that the difference in these acromial load and humeral load relationships is minimal, even after the cuff tendon has been excised. In the latter case, the humeral head loaded the acromion directly rather than through the interposed cuff tendon.

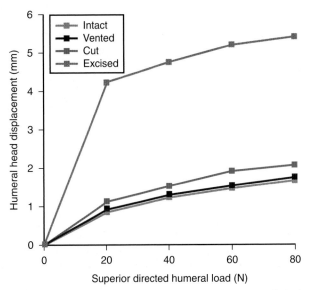

FIGURE 16-72 Mean superior humeral displacement (relative to the scapula) as a function of the superior humeral load. The graph compares displacements for intact specimens, after venting of the joint to air, after cutting (but not excising) the cuff tendon, and after excising the superior cuff tendon.

TYPES OF GLENOHUMERAL INSTABILITY

Glenohumeral instability is an inability of the humeral head to remain centered in the glenoid fossa.[98,128] It is not the same as laxity, which is a physical finding often unassociated with clinical instability. As demonstrated by Largacha and associates[230] it is most commonly a functional disability and rarely a cause of pain in the absence of obvious functional difficulties. Clinical cases of instability can be characterized according to the circumstances under which they occur, the degree of instability, and the direction of instability.

Circumstances of Instability

Congenital instability may result from local anomalies such as glenoid dysplasia[231] or from systemic conditions such as Ehlers–Danlos syndrome. Instability is acute if seen within the first days after its onset; otherwise it is *chronic*. A dislocation is *locked* (or fixed) if the humeral head has been impaled on the edge of the glenoid, thus making reduction of the dislocation difficult. If a glenohumeral joint has been unstable on many occasions, the instability is *recurrent*. Recurrent instability can consist of repeated glenohumeral dislocations, subluxations, or both.

Instability can arise from a *traumatic* episode in which an injury occurs to the bone, rotator cuff, labrum, capsule, or a combination of ligaments. Recurrent traumatic instability typically produces symptoms when the arm is placed in a position near that of the original injury. Conversely, instability can arise from *atraumatic* decompensation of the stabilizing mechanisms. The degree to which the shoulder was "torn loose" as opposed to "born loose" or just "worn loose" is critical in determining the best management strategy.

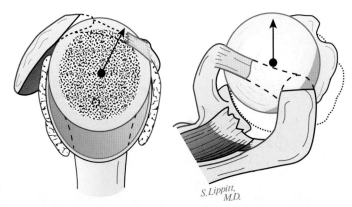

FIGURE 16-73 Anterosuperior escape. Unless the acromion and the coracoacromial ligament are preserved to maintain the anterosuperior stability of the glenohumeral joint, the severe problem of anterosuperior escape may arise. Humeral head center (*dot*) translating anterosuperiorly after acromioplasty. *Left,* Sagittal view. *Right,* Axillary view. (From Matsen FA III, Lippitt SB: Shoulder Surgery: Principles and Procedures. Philadelphia: WB Saunders, 2004, p 391.)

We have found that most patients with recurrent insta-bility fall into one of two groups. On one hand, patients with a *t*raumatic etiology usually have *u*nidirectional instability, often have obvious pathology such as a *B*ankart lesion, and often require *s*urgery when the instability is recurrent, thus the acronym TUBS. On the other hand, patients with *a*traumatic instability often have *m*ultidirec-tional laxity that is commonly *b*ilateral and usually responds to a *r*ehabilitation program. However, should surgery be performed, the surgeon must pay particular attention to performing an *i*nferior capsular shift and closing the rotator *i*nterval, thus the acronym AMBRII. Rowe[232] carefully analyzed 500 dislocations of the gleno-humeral joint and determined that 96% were traumatic (caused by a major injury) and the remaining 4% were atraumatic. DePalma,[233] Rockwood,[234] and Collins and Wilde[235] also recognized the importance of distinguishing between traumatic and atraumatic instability of the shoulder.

Patients with atraumatic instability might have general-ized joint laxity. Imazato[236] and Hirakawa[237] demonstrated that in patients with loose shoulders, the collagen fibers in the capsule, muscles, and skin are relatively immature, more soluble, and less cross-linked than those in controls; presumably, tissues such as the glenoid labrum contain immature collagen as well, thus making them more deformable under load but less likely to tear. Further evidence of constitutional factors is gained from a number of reports of positive family histories and bilateral involve-ment in patients with shoulder dislocations (Fig. 16-74). O'Driscoll and Evans[238] and Dowdy and O'Driscoll[239] found a family history of shoulder instability in 24% of patients who required surgery for anterior glenohumeral instability. Morrey and Janes[240] reported a positive family

history in approximately 15% of patients who were oper-ated on for recurrent anterior shoulder instability. A posi-tive family history was also noted twice as often in patients whose postoperative course was complicated by recurrent instability as in those with successful surgery. Rowe and colleagues[126] reported a positive family history in 27% of 55 patients with anterior shoulder instability who were treated with a Bankart procedure. Bilateral instability was noted in 50% of patients with a positive family history versus 26% of those with a negative family history, which suggests the possibility of genetic predisposition.

When instability develops with no or minimal injury,[241-243] the initial reason for the loss of stability is often unclear. However, it appears that once they are lost, the factors maintaining stability may be difficult to regain. Certain phenomena may be self-perpetuating: When the humeral head rides up on the glenoid rim, the rim becomes flattened and less effective and allows easier translation. Furthermore, when normal neuromuscular control is compromised, the feedback systems that maintain head centering fail to provide effective input. Thus, the joint becomes launched on a cycle of instability leading to loss of the effective glenoid concav-ity and loss of neuromuscular control, leading to more instability.

If a patient intentionally subluxates or dislocates the shoulder, the instability is described as *voluntary*. If the instability occurs unintentionally, it is *involuntary*. Voluntary and involuntary instability can coexist. Volun-tary anterior dislocation can occur with the arm at the side or in abduction and external rotation. Voluntary posterior dislocation can occur with the arm in flexion, adduction and internal rotation or with the arm at the side. The association of voluntary dislocation of the shoulder with emotional instability and psychiatric prob-lems has been noted by several authors (Figs. 16-75 and 16-76).[244,245] The desire to voluntarily dislocate the shoul-der cannot be treated surgically. However, the fact that patients can voluntarily demonstrate their instability does not necessarily mean that they are emotionally impaired.

Neuromuscular causes of shoulder instability have been reported as well. Percy[246] described a woman in whom posterior dislocation developed after an episode of encephalitis. Kretzler and Blue[247] discussed the man-agement of posterior dislocation of the shoulder in chil-dren with cerebral palsy. Sever,[248] Fairbank,[249] L'Episcopo,[250] Zachary,[251] and Wickstrom[252] reported techniques for the management of neurologic dislocation of the shoulder as a result of upper brachial plexus birth injuries. Stroke is another important neurologic cause of instability.[253] Sei-zures, including those from alcoholism, glucose imbal-ance, head injury, and intracranial neoplasms can cause glenohumeral instability, both from the uncontrolled muscle activity at the time of the seizure and afterwards from bone and soft tissue injuries caused by the seizure.

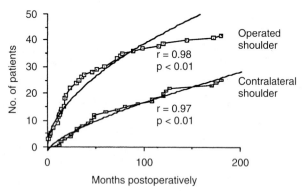

FIGURE 16-74 Incidence of contralateral shoulder instability from the data of O'Driscoll and Evans. In 13% of the patients with normal contralateral shoulders at the time of surgery, contralateral instability developed within the next 15 years. (From O'Driscoll SW, Evans DC: The DuToit staple capsulorrhaphy for recurrent anterior dislocation of the shoulder: Twenty years of experience in six Toronto hospitals. Paper presented at the American Shoulder and Elbow Surgeons 4th Open Meeting, Atlanta, Ga, March 1988.)

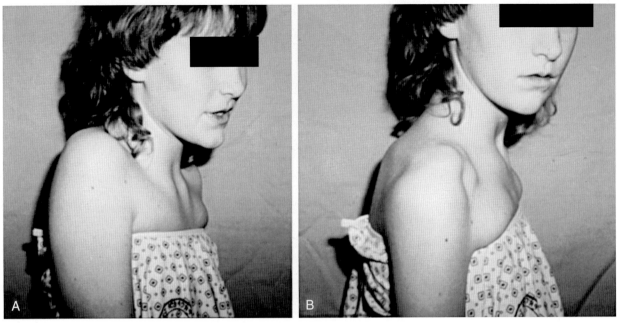

FIGURE 16-75 Voluntary instability. This patient had no significant history of injury but could voluntarily dislocate her shoulder with minimal discomfort. She is shown with the right shoulder reduced (**A**) and posteriorly dislocated (**B**).

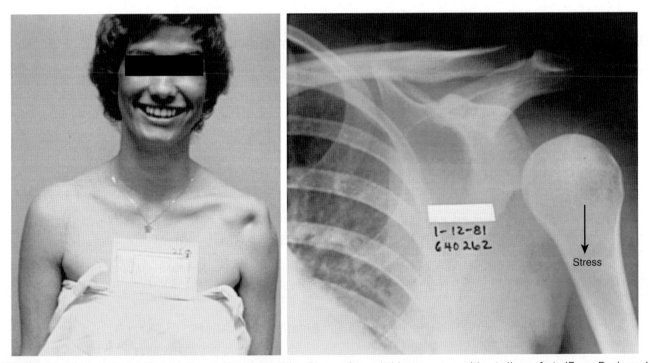

FIGURE 16-76 A patient with voluntary inferior instability. She performed this maneuver without discomfort. (From Rockwood CA, Green DP [eds]: Fractures, 3 vols, 2nd ed. Philadelphia: JB Lippincott, 1984.)

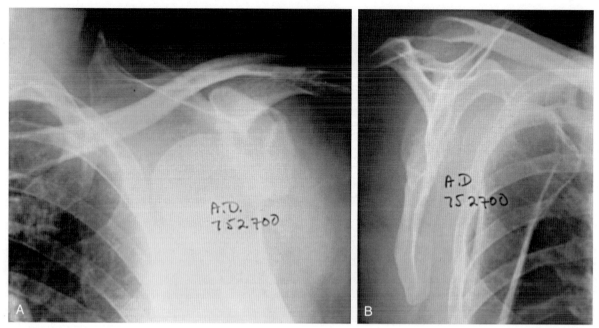

FIGURE 16-77 Subcoracoid dislocation. **A,** This AP view reveals that the head is medially displaced away from the glenoid fossa. With this view it is difficult to be sure whether the head is dislocated anteriorly or posteriorly. **B,** On a true scapular lateral view, the humeral head is completely anterior to the glenoid fossa. (From Rockwood CA, Green DP [eds]: Fractures, 3 vols, 2nd ed. Philadelphia: JB Lippincott, 1984.)

Degree of Instability

Recurrent instability may be characterized as dislocation, subluxation, or apprehension. *Dislocation* of the glenohumeral joint is complete separation of the articular surfaces; immediate, spontaneous relocation might not occur. Glenohumeral *subluxation* is defined as symptomatic translation of the humeral head on the glenoid without complete separation of the articular surfaces. *Apprehension* refers to the fear that the shoulder will subluxate or dislocate. This fear may prevent the person from participating fully in work or sports.

Subluxation of the glenohumeral joint is usually transient: the humeral head returns spontaneously to its normal position in the glenoid fossa. In a series of patients with anterior shoulder subluxation reported by Rowe and Zarins,[243] 87% of cases were traumatic, and more than 50% of patients were not aware that their shoulders were unstable. Like dislocations, subluxations may be traumatic or atraumatic; anterior, posterior, or inferior; or acute or recurrent; or they can occur after previous surgical repairs that did not achieve complete shoulder stability. Recurrent subluxations can coexist with or be initiated by glenohumeral dislocation. Rowe and Zarins[232,254] reported seeing a Hill–Sachs compression fracture in 40% of patients in their series on subluxation of the shoulder, an observation indicating that at some time these shoulders had been completely dislocated.

Traumatic Instability

Traumatic instability may have consequences beyond recurrent dislocation of the shoulder, including inability to return to work, inability to return to sport, or subsequent degenerative conditions. Nine percent of rugby players who stopped playing did so because of dislocation of the shoulder.[255] This figure was higher than the rate in players who abandoned rugby because of concussion, 4%. The likelihood of glenohumeral arthrosis developing has been shown to be 10 to 20 times higher in patients who have had a shoulder dislocation.[256]

Direction of Instability

Dislocations of the shoulder account for approximately 45% of all dislocations.[257] Of these, almost 85% are anterior glenohumeral dislocations.[258]

Anterior Dislocations

Subcoracoid dislocation is the most common type of anterior dislocation. The usual mechanism of injury that causes a subcoracoid dislocation is a combination of shoulder abduction, extension, and external rotation producing forces that can challenge the anterior capsule and ligaments, the glenoid rim, and the rotator cuff mechanism. The head of the humerus is displaced anteriorly with respect to the glenoid and is inferior to the coracoid process (Fig. 16-77).

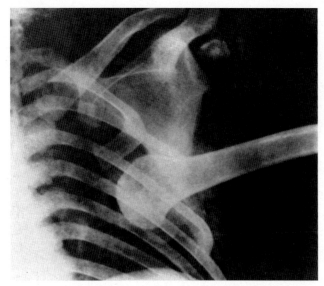

FIGURE 16-78 Intrathoracic anterior dislocation of the left shoulder. Note the wide interspace laterally between the third and fourth ribs and the avulsion fracture of the greater tuberosity, which remained in the vicinity of the glenoid fossa. (From Rockwood CA Jr, Green DP, Bucholz RW [eds]: Fractures in Adults. Philadelphia: JB Lippincott, 1991.)

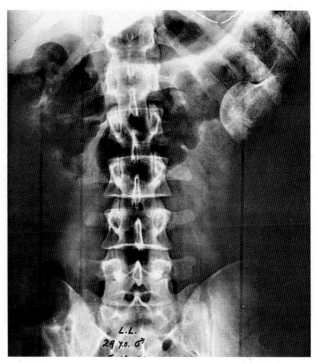

FIGURE 16-79 Abdominal radiograph revealing the proximal end of the humerus in the left upper quadrant.

Other types of anterior dislocation include subglenoid (the head of the humerus lies anterior to and below the glenoid fossa), subclavicular (the head of the humerus lies medial to the coracoid process, just inferior to the lower border of the clavicle), intrathoracic (the head of the humerus lies between the ribs and the thoracic cavity) (Fig. 16-78),[259-263] and retroperitoneal (Figs. 16-79 and 16-80).[264] These rarer types of dislocation are usually associated with severe trauma and have a high incidence of fracture of the greater tuberosity of the humerus and rotator cuff avulsion. Neurologic, pulmonary, and vascular complications can occur, as can subcutaneous emphysema.

West[263] reported a case of intrathoracic dislocation in which on reduction, the humerus was felt to slip out of the chest cavity with a sensation similar to that of slipping a large cork from a bottle. His patient, who had an avulsion fracture of the greater tuberosity and no neurologic deficit, regained functional range of motion and returned to his job as a carpenter.

Posterior Dislocations

Posterior dislocations can leave the humeral head in a subacromial (head behind the glenoid and beneath the acromion), subglenoid (head behind and beneath the glenoid), or subspinous (head medial to the acromion and beneath the spine of the scapula) location. Subacromial dislocation is the most common by far (Fig. 16-81). Posterior dislocations are often locked. Hawkins and coworkers[265] reviewed 41 such cases related to motor vehicle accidents, surgery, and electroshock therapy.

The incidence of posterior dislocations is estimated at 2% but is difficult to ascertain because of the frequency with which this diagnosis is missed. Thomas[266] reported seeing only four cases of posterior shoulder dislocation in 6000 x-ray examinations. The literature reflects that the diagnosis of posterior dislocation of the shoulder is missed in more than 60% of cases.[267-271] A 1982 article by Rowe and Zarins[254] indicated that the diagnosis was missed in 79% of cases! McLaughlin[272] stated that posterior

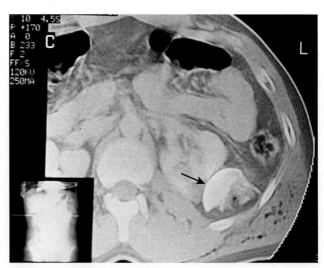

FIGURE 16-80 Enhanced CT scan of the abdomen. Note the retroperitoneal location of the humeral head posterior to the left kidney (*arrow*).

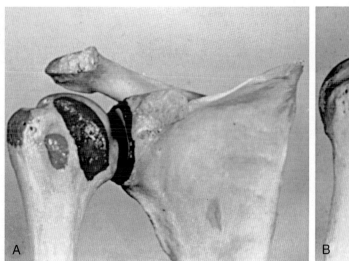
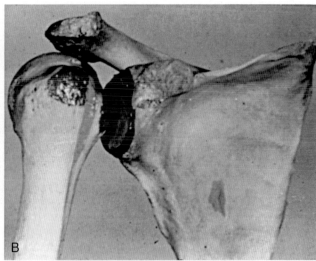

FIGURE 16-81 A subacromial posterior dislocation can appear deceptively normal on radiographs. **A,** Normal position of the humeral head in the glenoid fossa. **B,** In the subacromial type of posterior shoulder dislocation, the arm is in full internal rotation and the articular surface of the head is completely posterior, with only the lesser tuberosity left in the glenoid fossa. This positioning explains why abduction—and particularly external rotation—is blocked in posterior dislocations of the shoulder. (From Rockwood CA, Green DP [eds]: Fractures, 3 vols, 2nd ed. Philadelphia: JB Lippincott, 1984.)

shoulder dislocations are sufficiently uncommon that their occurrence creates a "diagnostic trap."

One of the largest series of posterior dislocations of the shoulder (37 cases) was recorded by Malgaigne[68] in 1855, 40 years before the discovery of x-rays. He and his

Subscapularis m.
Pectoralis major m.

Teres minor m.
Infraspinatus m.

Superior view

Latissimus dorsi m.
Teres major m.

FIGURE 16-82 Mechanism of posterior dislocation of the shoulder caused by an accidental electrical shock or a convulsive seizure. The strong internal rotators simply overpower the weak external rotators.

colleagues made the diagnosis by performing a proper physical examination! Cooper[67] stated that the physical findings are so classic that he called it "an accident which cannot be mistaken."

Posterior dislocation can result from axial loading of an adducted, internally rotated arm,[273] from violent muscle contraction, or from electrical shock or convulsive seizures[242,244,274-281] In the case of involuntary muscle contraction, the combined strength of the internal rotators (latissimus dorsi, pectoralis major, and subscapularis muscles) simply overwhelms the external rotators (infraspinatus and teres minor muscles) (Fig. 16-82). Heller and coworkers proposed a classification of posterior shoulder dislocations.[282]

Most traumatic "posterior dislocations" are actually impaction fractures of the anterior humeral articular surface from a fall, electroshock, or seizure. Because of the anterior impaction nature of the fracture, the posterior articular surface is left out the back of the glenohumeral joint. The nature of this injury indicates that it should be treated more like a fracture than a dislocation, with reduction and fixation or replacement of the injured fragments (Fig. 16-83).

Inferior Dislocations

Inferior dislocation of the glenohumeral joint was first described by Middeldorpf and Scharm[283] in 1859. Lynn[284] in 1921 carefully reviewed 34 cases, and Roca and Ramos-Vertiz[285] in 1962 reviewed 50 cases from the world literature. Laskin and Sedlin[286] reported a case in an infant. Three bilateral cases have been described by Murrard,[287] Langfritz,[288] and Peiro and coworkers.[289] Nobel[290] reported a case of subglenoid dislocation in which the acromion–olecranon distance was shortened by 1.5 inches.

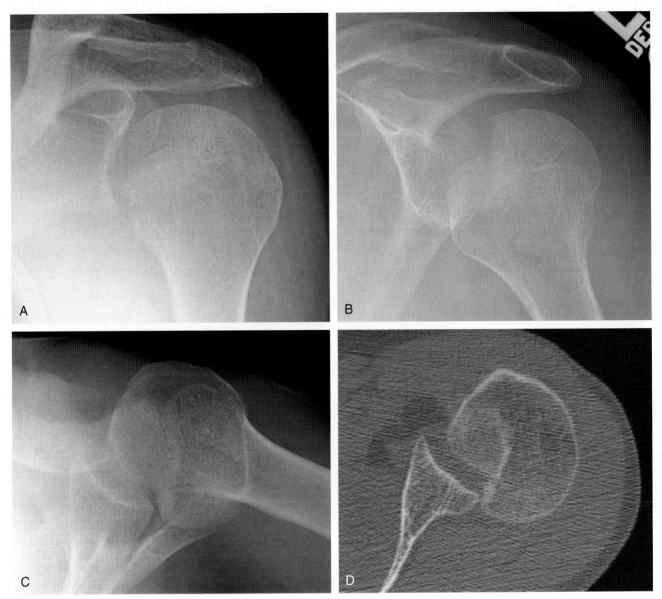

FIGURE 16-83 Images from a 40-year old cyclist who fell on the shoulder. Physical examination revealed an increased prominence of the coracoid anteriorly and inability to externally rotate the arm. **A,** AP view showing reduced radiographic joint space and impaction fracture. **B,** AP view showing discontinuity of articular surface. **C,** Axillary view showing impaction fracture with intact articular surface posterior to the glenoid. **D,** CT scan showing impaction of anterior articular surface with intact articular surface posterior to the glenoid.

Continued

Inferior dislocation can be produced by a hyperabduction force that causes abutment of the neck of the humerus against the acromion process and subsequent leverage of the head out of the glenoid inferiorly (see Figs. 16-84 to 16-87). The humerus is then locked with the head below the glenoid fossa and the humeral shaft pointing overhead, a condition called *luxatio erecta* (Fig. 16-88; see Figs. 16-84 to 16-87). The clinical picture of a patient with luxatio erecta is so clear that it can hardly be mistaken for any other condition. The humerus is locked in a position somewhere between 110 and 160 degrees of adduction (see Figs. 16-85 and 16-86). Severe soft tissue injury or fractures about the proximal end of the humerus occur with this dislocation (see Figs. 16-85 to 16-88). At the time of surgery or autopsy, various authors have found avulsion of the supraspinatus, pectoralis major, or teres minor muscles and fractures of the greater tuberosity.[283-287,291]

Neurovascular involvement is common.[284,292-294] Lev-El and Rubinstein[293] reported a patient with an injury to the axillary artery in whom a thrombus subsequently developed that required resection and a vein graft. Gardham

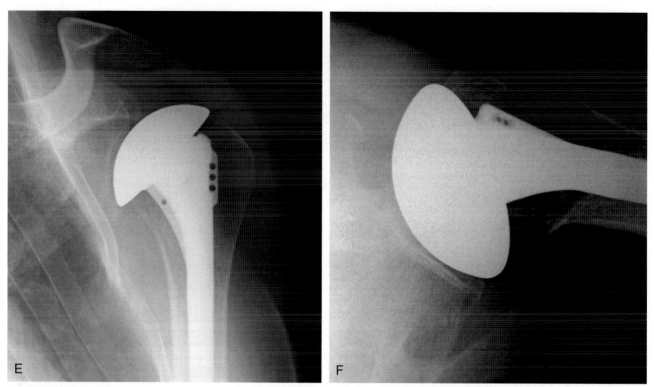

FIGURE 16-83, cont'd E, Postoperative AP view showing humeral head centered in the glenoid. **F,** Postoperative axillary view showing humeral prosthesis.

and Scott[292] reported a case in 1980 in which the axillary artery was damaged in its third part and was managed with a bypass graft using the saphenous vein. Rockwood and Wirth found that in 19 patients with this condition, all 19 had a brachial plexus injury and some vascular compromise before reduction.

The force may be so great that it forces the head out through the soft tissues and skin. Lucas and Peterson[295] reported the case of a 16-year-old boy who caught his arm in the power takeoff of a tractor and suffered an open luxatio erecta injury.

Reduction of an inferior dislocation can often be accomplished by traction and countertraction maneuvers (Fig. 16-89). When closed reduction cannot be achieved, the buttonhole rent in the inferior capsule must be surgically enlarged before reduction can occur.

Superior Dislocations

Speed[296] reported that Langier, in 1834, was the first to record a case of superior dislocation of the glenohumeral joint; Stimson[297] reviewed 14 cases that had been reported in the literature before 1912. In the current literature, little is mentioned about this type of dislocation, but undoubtedly occasional cases do occur. The usual cause is an extreme forward and upward force on an adducted arm. With displacement of the humerus upward, fractures can

occur in the acromion, acromioclavicular joint, clavicle, coracoid process, or humeral tuberosities (Fig. 16-90). Extreme soft tissue damage occurs to the capsule, rotator cuff, biceps tendon, and surrounding muscles. Clinically, the head rides above the level of the acromion. The arm is short and adducted to the side. Shoulder movement is restricted and quite painful, and neurovascular complications are usually present.

Bilateral Dislocations

Mynter[298] first described bilateral dislocation in 1902; according to Honner,[299] only 20 cases were reported before 1969. Bilateral dislocations have been reported by McFie,[278] Yadav,[300] Onabowale and Jaja,[280] Segal and colleagues,[281] and Carew-McColl.[244] Most of these cases were the result of convulsions or violent trauma. Peiro and coworkers[289] reported bilateral erect dislocation of the shoulders in a man caught in a cement mixer. Bilateral dislocation of the shoulder secondary to accidental electrical shock has been described by Carew-McColl[244] and by Fipp.[275] Nicola and coworkers[301] reported cases of bilateral posterior fracture-dislocation after a convulsive seizure. Ahlgren and associates[274] reported three cases of bilateral posterior fracture-dislocation associated with a convulsion. Lindholm and Elmstedt[277] presented a case of bilateral posterior fracture-dislocation after an epileptic seizure, which was treated by open reduction

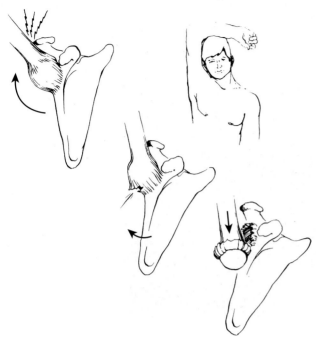

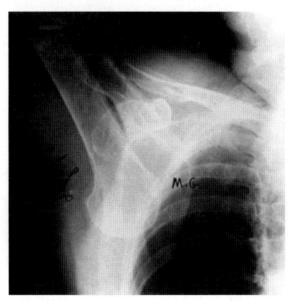

FIGURE 16-84 Mechanism of luxatio erecta. *Upper left,* With hyperabduction of the humerus, the shaft abuts the acromion process, which stresses and then tears the capsule inferiorly and levers the head out inferiorly. *Middle,* The head and neck may be buttonholed through a rent in the inferior capsule, or the entire capsule may be separated. *Lower right,* The rotator cuff muscles are always detached, and an associated fracture of the greater tuberosity may be present. (From Rockwood CA Jr, Green DP, Bucholz RW [eds]: Fractures in Adults. Philadelphia: JB Lippincott, 1991.)

FIGURE 16-85 An AP x-ray film of an inferior dislocation reveals that the entire humeral head and surgical neck of the humerus are inferior to the glenoid fossa. (From Rockwood CA Jr, Green DP, Bucholz RW [eds]: Fractures in Adults. Philadelphia: JB Lippincott, 1991.)

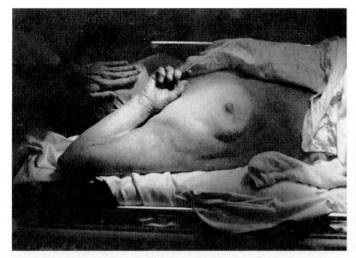

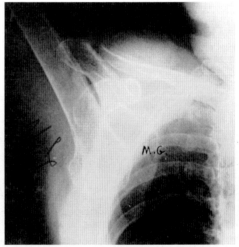

FIGURE 16-86 Inferior dislocation (*luxatio erecta*) of the right shoulder of a 75-year-old woman. Note that the arm is directed upward in relation to the trunk (*left*). The hand of the flexed elbow is lying on the anterior of the chest. An AP x-ray film of the inferior dislocation reveals that the entire humeral head and surgical neck of the humerus are inferior to the glenoid fossa (*right*). (From Rockwood CA Jr, Green DP, Bucholz RW [eds]: Fractures in Adults. Philadelphia: JB Lippincott, 1991.)

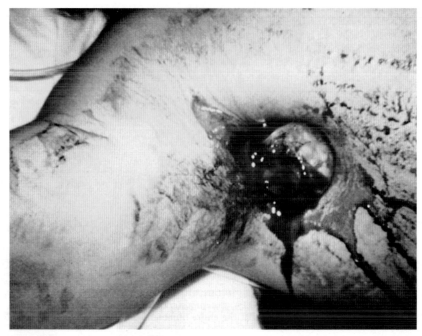

FIGURE 16-87 Photograph of the right shoulder and axilla of a patient who had an open inferior dislocation of the humeral head out through the axilla. (Courtesy of George Armstrong.)

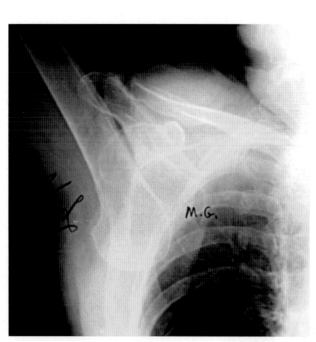

FIGURE 16-88 This AP radiograph of an inferior dislocation reveals that the entire humeral head and surgical neck of the humerus are inferior to the glenoid fossa.

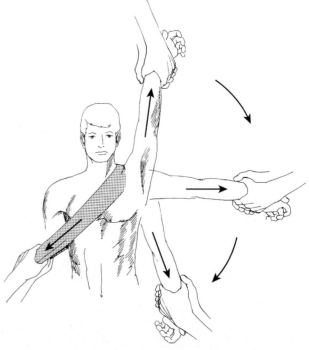

FIGURE 16-89 Technique of reduction of an inferior dislocation (*luxatio erecta*) of the glenohumeral joint. Countertraction is applied by an assistant using a folded sheet across the superior aspect of the shoulder and neck. Traction on the arm is first applied upward, and then gradually the arm is brought into less abduction and finally placed at the patient's side. (From Rockwood CA Jr, Green DP, Bucholz RW [eds]: Fractures in Adults. Philadelphia: JB Lippincott, 1991.)

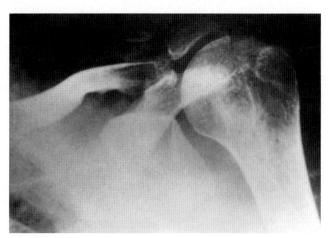

FIGURE 16-90 Superior dislocation of the left shoulder. Note that the head of the humerus is displaced superiorly from the glenoid fossa and that the fracture of the acromion process has also been displaced upward. (From Rockwood CA Jr, Green DP, Bucholz RW [eds]: Fractures in Adults. Philadelphia: JB Lippincott, 1991.)

and internal fixation with screws. Parrish and Skiendzielewski[302] reported a patient with bilateral posterior fracture-dislocation after status epilepticus. The diagnosis was missed for more than 12 hours. Pagden and associates[303] reported two cases of posterior shoulder dislocation after seizures related to regional anesthesia. Costigan and coworkers[304] reported a case of undiagnosed bilateral anterior dislocation of the shoulder in a 74-year-old patient admitted to the hospital for an unrelated problem. The patient had no complaints related to the shoulders and was able to place both hands on her head and behind her back.

DISLOCATION

CLINICAL FINDINGS

History

The history should define the mechanism of the injury, including the position of the arm, the amount of force applied, and the point of force application.[242,243,254] Injury with the arm in extension, abduction, and external rotation favors anterior dislocation. Electroshock, seizures, or a fall on the flexed and adducted arm are commonly associated with posterior dislocation. If the instability is recurrent, the history defines the initial injury, the position or action that results in instability, how long the shoulder stays out, whether radiographs are available with the shoulder out of joint, and what means have been necessary to reduce the shoulder. The history also solicits evidence of neurologic or rotator cuff problems after

previous episodes of shoulder instability. Previous treatment of the recurrent instability, as well as the effectiveness of this treatment, should be documented.

Physical Examination

Anterior Dislocation

An acutely dislocated shoulder is usually very painful, and muscles are in spasm in an attempt to stabilize the joint. The humeral head may be palpable anteriorly. The posterior and lateral aspect of the shoulder shows a hollow beneath the acromion. The arm is held in slight abduction. Passive and active motion are limited by pain. Because of the possible association of nerve injuries[305] and, to a lesser extent, vascular injuries,[306] an essential part of the physical examination of an anteriorly dislocated shoulder is assessment of the neurovascular status of the upper extremity and charting of the findings before reduction.

Posterior Dislocation

Because it is often more an impaction fracture than a dislocation, recognition of a posterior dislocation may be impaired by the lack of a striking deformity of the shoulder and by the fact that the shoulder is held in the traditional sling position of adduction and internal rotation. However, a directed physical examination will reveal the diagnosis. The classic features of a posterior dislocation include:

- Limited external rotation of the shoulder (often to <0 degrees)
- Limited elevation of the arm (often to <90 degrees)
- Posterior prominence and rounding of the shoulder in comparison to the normal side
- Flattening of the anterior aspect of the shoulder
- Prominence of the coracoid process on the dislocated side

Asymmetry of the shoulder contours can often best be visualized by viewing the shoulders from above while standing behind the patient (Fig. 16-91).

Motion is limited because the head of the humerus is fixed on the posterior glenoid rim by muscle forces, or the head might actually be impaled on the glenoid rim. With the passage of time, the posterior rim of the glenoid can further impact the fracture of the humeral head and produce a deep hatchet-like defect or a V-shaped compression fracture, which engages the head even more securely. Patients with old, unreduced posterior dislocations of the shoulder can have 30 to 40 degrees of glenohumeral abduction and some humeral rotation as a result of enlargement of the groove. With long-standing disuse of the muscles about the shoulder, atrophy will be present; such atrophy accentuates the flattening of the anterior portion of the shoulder, the prominence of the coracoid, and the fullness of the posterior portion of the shoulder.

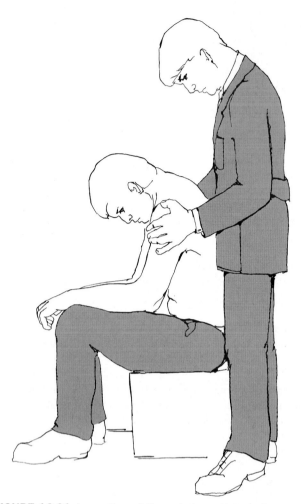

FIGURE 16-91 Inspection of the anterior and posterior aspects of the shoulders can best be accomplished by having the patient sit on a low stool with the examiner standing behind the patient. The injured shoulder can then be easily compared with the uninjured one. (From Rockwood CA, Green DP [eds]: Fractures, 3 vols, 2nd ed. Philadelphia: JB Lippincott, 1984.)

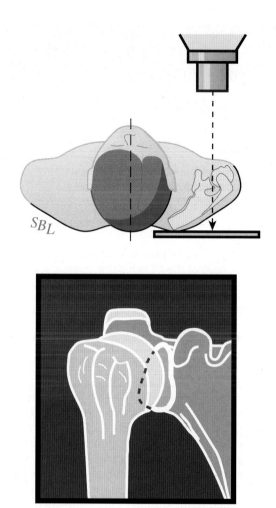

FIGURE 16-92 AP x-ray in the plane of the body. An AP view in the coronal plane of the body is of limited use in the evaluation of the glenohumeral joint, the joint space, or the relationship of the humeral head to the glenoid fossa. (From Matsen FA III, Lippitt SB: Shoulder Surgery: Principles and Procedures. Philadelphia: WB Saunders, 2004, p 7.)

Proper physical examination is essential. Rowe and Zarins[254] reported 23 cases of unreduced dislocation of the shoulder, 14 of which were posterior. Hill and McLaughlin[307] reported that in their series the average time from injury to diagnosis was 8 months. In the interval before the diagnosis of posterior dislocation of the shoulder is made, the injury may be misdiagnosed as a frozen shoulder[307,308] for which vigorous therapy may be mistakenly instituted in an attempt to restore range of motion.

Radiographic Evaluation

When a shoulder is dislocated, radiographs need to demonstrate the direction of the dislocation, the existence of associated fractures (displaced or not), and possible barriers to relocation. Dorgan[309] and McLaughlin[272] have

pointed out that reliance on anteroposterior (AP) and transthoracic radiographs will lead an unwary orthopaedist into a "diagnostic trap." The glenohumeral joint is most reliably imaged with four standardized views referred to the plane of the scapula. The complete series of four views oriented to the scapula provides much more information than does the commonly obtained view in the plane of the body (Fig. 16-92).

The first is an AP view in the plane of the scapula (Fig. 16-93). In 1923, Grashey[310] recognized that to take a true AP radiograph of the shoulder joint, the direction of the x-ray beam must be perpendicular to the plane of the scapula. This view is most easily accomplished by placing the scapula flat on the cassette (a position that the patient can help achieve) and passing the x-ray beam at right angles to this plane and centering it on the coracoid process (Fig. 16-94). This view can be taken with the arm

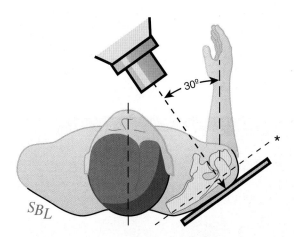

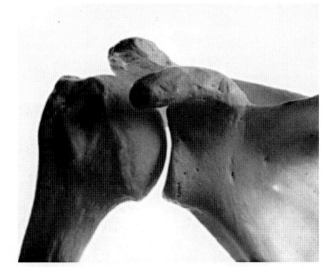

FIGURE 16-94 A simulated x-ray view of a scapular AP view using a backlighted skeletal model. This view reveals the radiographic glenohumeral joint space and provides a good opportunity to detect fractures of the humerus or glenoid lip.

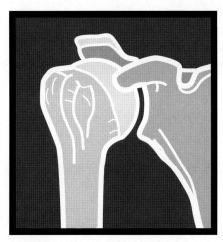

FIGURE 16-93 AP x-ray in the plane of the scapula. An AP view in the plane of the scapula reveals the glenohumeral joint space and demonstrates whether the humeral head has a normal relationship to the glenoid fossa. It is most easily taken by positioning the patient's scapula flat on the cassette and then passing the x-ray beam at right angles to the film, aiming at the coracoid process. (From Matsen FA III, Lippitt SB: Shoulder Surgery: Principles and Procedures. Philadelphia: WB Saunders, 2004, p 7.)

The downward stem of the Y is projected by the body of the scapula; the upper forks are projected by the coracoid process anteriorly and by the spine and acromion posteriorly (Figs. 16-100 and 16-101). The glenoid is located at the junction of the stem and the two arms of the Y. In a normal shoulder, the humeral head is at the center of the arms of the Y, that is, in the glenoid fossa. In posterior dislocations, the head is seen posterior to the glenoid (see Fig. 16-101); in anterior dislocations, the head is anterior to it (see Fig. 16-100).

in a sling and the body rotated to the desired position (Fig. 16-95). In a normal shoulder this view reveals clear separation of the humeral subchondral bone from that of the glenoid. In an injured shoulder, it often reveals the pathology (Fig. 16-96).

The second is a scapular lateral view (Fig. 16-97). This view is taken at right angles to the AP view in the plane of the scapula (Figs. 16-98 and 16-99).[272,308,311-313] Like the AP view, it can be obtained by positioning the body without moving the dislocated shoulder, which can remain in a sling. The radiographic beam is passed in a medial-to-lateral direction parallel to the body of the scapula while the cassette is held perpendicular to the beam at the anterolateral aspect of the shoulder.[313] In this view, the contour of the scapula projects as the letter Y.[314]

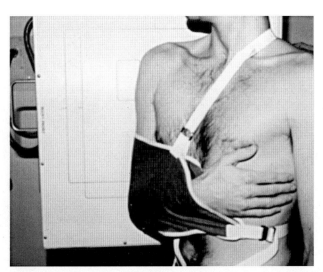

FIGURE 16-95 Positioning of the patient in a sling for an AP radiograph in the plane of the scapula. The scapula is placed flat on the cassette. The x-ray beam is positioned at right angles to the cassette and centered on the coracoid process.

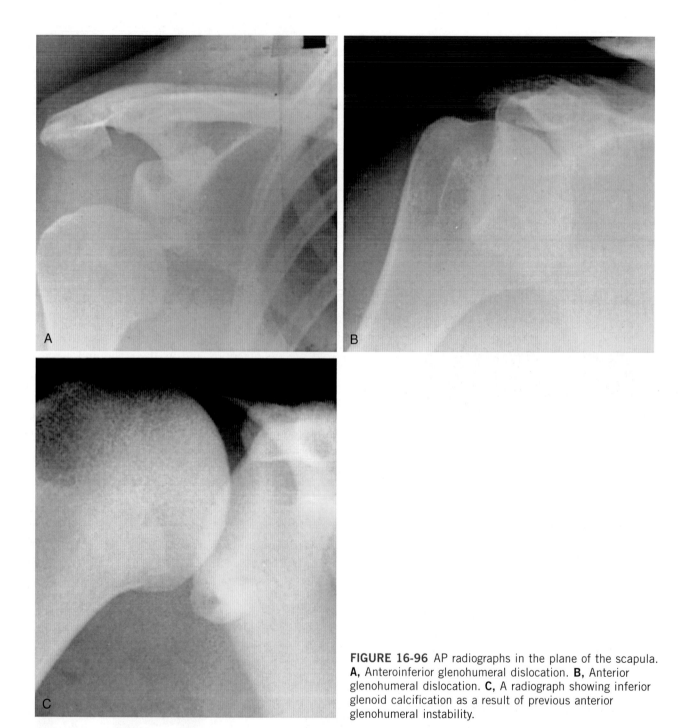

FIGURE 16-96 AP radiographs in the plane of the scapula.
A, Anteroinferior glenohumeral dislocation. **B,** Anterior
glenohumeral dislocation. **C,** A radiograph showing inferior
glenoid calcification as a result of previous anterior
glenohumeral instability.

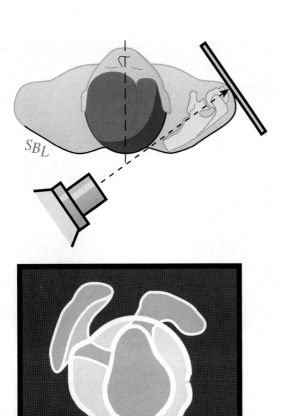

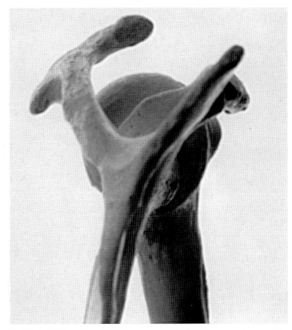

FIGURE 16-98 Simulated scapular lateral x-ray view with a backlighted skeletal model. The x-ray beam is passed parallel to the plane of the scapula and is centered on the scapular spine. The view reveals the AP relationship of the head of the humerus in the glenoid fossa. The glenoid fossa is identified as the intersection of the spine of the scapula, the coracoid process, and the body of the scapula.

FIGURE 16-97 Scapular lateral. The shoulder is placed against the radiographic cassette so that the scapular spine is perpendicular to it. The x-ray beam is passed parallel to the scapular spine and centered on the intersection of the coracoid process, the acromion process, and the plane of the scapular body. This intersection lies in the glenoid fossa. The humeral head should also lie centered at this intersection. (From Matsen FA III, Lippitt SB: Shoulder Surgery: Principles and Procedures. Philadelphia: WB Saunders, 2004, p 11.)

competence and version of the glenoid fossa, but the projection must be standardized to avoid misinterpretation (see Fig. 16-49).

In his text on radiographic positioning, Jordan demonstrated the various techniques for obtaining axillary

The third is an axillary view (Fig. 16-102). In this view, first described by Lawrence in 1915,[315,316] the cassette is placed on the superior aspect of the shoulder. This view requires that the humerus be abducted sufficiently to allow the radiographic beam to pass between it and the thorax. Fortunately, sufficient abduction can be achieved by gentle positioning of the dislocated shoulder or by modifications of the technique (Figs. 16-103 to 16-106). The axillary radiograph is critical in evaluation of a dislocated shoulder: It unambiguously reveals not only the direction and magnitude of head displacement relative to the glenoid but also the presence and size of head compression fractures, fractures of the glenoid, and fractures of the humeral tuberosities (Figs. 16-107 to 16-111). The axillary view might also be helpful in judging the bony

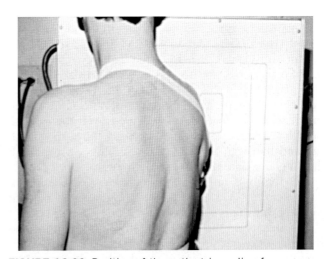

FIGURE 16-99 Position of the patient in a sling for a scapular lateral radiograph. The scapula is positioned perpendicular to the cassette. The beam should be placed parallel to the spine of the scapula and perpendicular to the cassette.

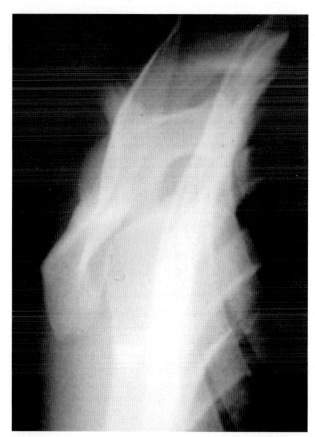

FIGURE 16-100 Scapular lateral view showing an anterior glenohumeral dislocation. Note that the humerus is no longer centered at the base of the Y.

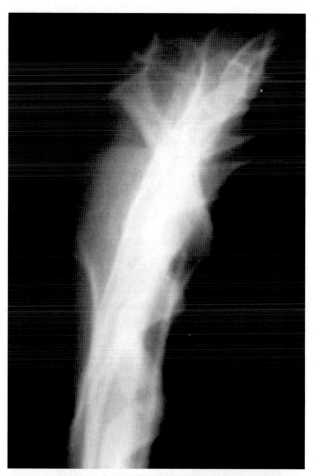

FIGURE 16-101 A scapular lateral view showing a posterior glenohumeral dislocation. The head of the humerus is dislocated posterior to the glenoid fossa and in this view appears to be sitting directly below the spine of the scapula.

lateral views.[317] Variations on this view have been described (see Fig. 16-104). Rockwood has pointed out that in a situation in which the patient cannot abduct the arm sufficiently, a curved cassette or a rolled cardboard cassette can be placed in the axilla and the radiographic beam passed from a superior position (see Fig. 16-103). Bloom and Obata[320] modified the axillary technique so that the arm does not have to be abducted (see Fig. 16-104). They called this modification the *Velpeau axillary lateral view.* While wearing a sling or Velpeau dressing, the patient leans backward 30 degrees over the cassette on the table. The x-ray tube is placed above the shoulder and the beam is projected vertically down through the shoulder onto the cassette.

The fourth is an apical oblique view of Garth and coworkers[241,321] (Fig. 16-112), introduced to us by our late friend, Doug Harryman.

In summary, in the evaluation of a possibly dislocated shoulder or a fractured-dislocated shoulder, we recommend the four projections of the shoulder that provide a sensitive assessment of shoulder anatomy. The use of fewer views or other less-interpretable projections can obscure significant pathologic processes. If these views cannot be taken, if a question has arisen regarding the diagnosis, or if the anatomy needs to be defined in greater detail, a CT scan may be of great assistance (Figs. 16-113 to 16-116; see Fig. 16-22).[322-324] By using modern methods of three-dimensional (3D) reconstruction, anterior-inferior glenoid lesions and posterior-lateral humeral head lesions can be shown in striking detail (Figs. 16-117 to 16-119). The patient whose shoulder is shown in these figures obtained an excellent result after nonoperative treatment in spite of the damage shown on the radiographic reconstructions.

INJURIES ASSOCIATED WITH ANTERIOR DISLOCATIONS

Ligaments and Capsule

A common feature of traumatic anterior dislocations is avulsion of the anteroinferior glenohumeral ligaments

Text continued on p. 671

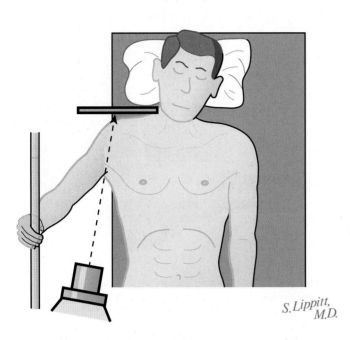

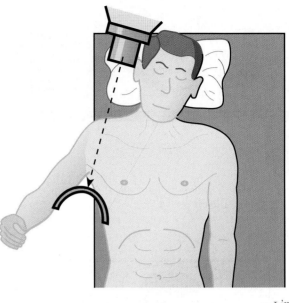

FIGURE 16-103 The axillary view with a curved cassette, a method that is useful if the arm cannot be adequately abducted for a routine axillary view.

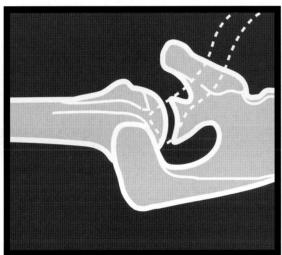

FIGURE 16-102 An axillary x-ray reveals the glenohumeral joint space and the AP position of the humeral head and glenoid fossa. It is obtained by having the patient's arm in abduction (e.g., holding onto an IV pole), the cassette on the superior aspect of the shoulder, and the x-ray beam passing up the axilla, aiming at the coracoid. (From Matsen FA III, Lippitt SB: Shoulder Surgery: Principles and Procedures. Philadelphia: WB Saunders, 2004, p 9.)

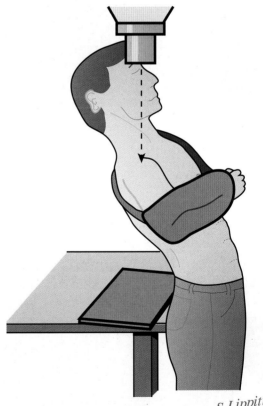

FIGURE 16-104 The Velpeau axillary lateral x-ray technique. With the arm in a sling, the patient leans backward until the shoulder is over the cassette. (Modified from Bloom MH, Obata WG: Diagnosis of posterior dislocation of the shoulder with use of the Velpeau axillary and angle-up roentgenographic views. J Bone Joint Surg Am 49:943-949, 1967.)

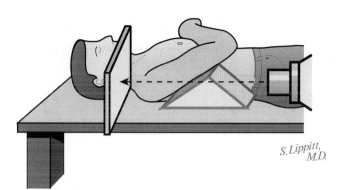

FIGURE 16-105 A trauma axillary lateral radiograph. This arm is flexed on a foam wedge.

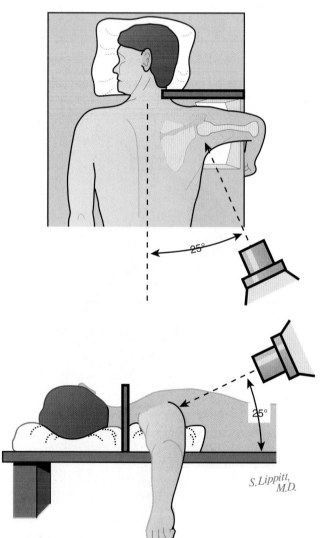

25°

25°

S. Lippitt, M.D.

FIGURE 16-106 The West Point axillary lateral view. The patient is prone with the beam inclined 25 degrees down and 25 degrees medially. (Modified from Rokous JR, Feagin JA, Abbott HG: Modified axillary roentgenogram. Clin Orthop Relat Res 82:84-86, 1972.)

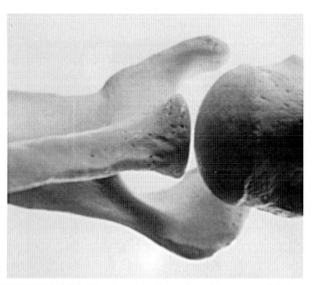

FIGURE 16-107 Simulated axillary view using a backlighted skeletal model. An x-ray beam is passed up the axilla to project the glenoid fossa between the coracoid process anteriorly and the scapular spine posteriorly. This projection reveals the radiographic glenohumeral joint space, the AP position of the head of the humerus relative to the glenoid, and a view of fractures of the glenoid lip and humerus.

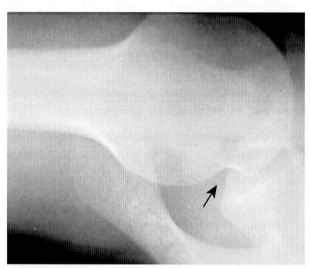

FIGURE 16-108 Axillary view. Note the posterior humeral head defect (Hill–Sachs lesion) secondary to a previous anterior glenohumeral dislocation.

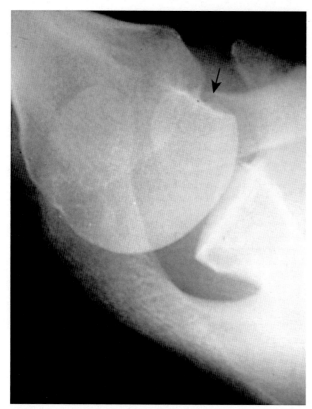

FIGURE 16-109 Axillary view. This patient has an anterior humeral head defect (*arrow*) that occurred as a result of a posterior glenohumeral dislocation.

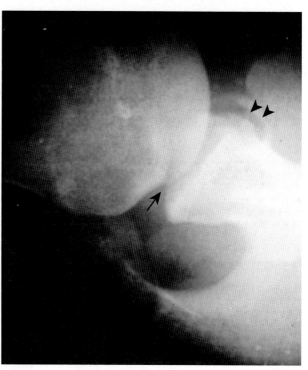

FIGURE 16-110 Axillary view showing an anterior glenoid defect and calcification (*arrowheads*) as a result of an anterior glenohumeral dislocation. A posterolateral humeral head defect is also seen (*arrow*).

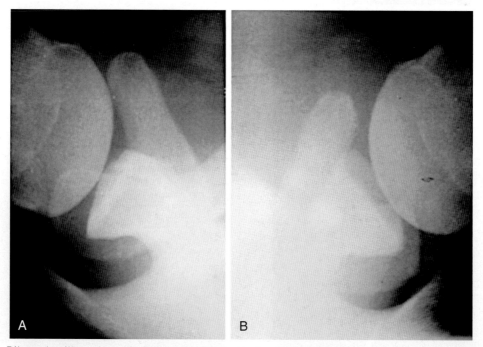

FIGURE 16-111 Bilateral axillary views. **A,** Rounding of the anterior glenoid rim as a result of recurrent anterior glenohumeral dislocation is evident on this axillary view. **B,** The normal side is shown for comparison.

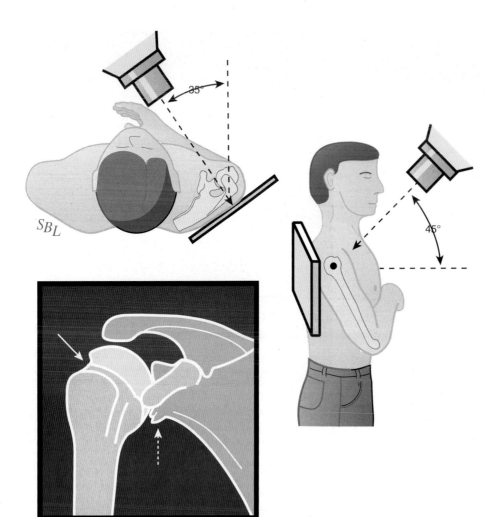

FIGURE 16-112 Apical oblique. The shoulder is positioned as for an anteroposterior view in the plane of the scapula except that the x-ray beam is angled inferiorly at an angle of 45 degrees. This reveals the contour of the posterolateral humeral head and the anteroinferior glenoid. *Solid arrow* indicates Hill–Sachs defect. *Dashed arrow* indicates anteroinferior glenoid defect. (From Matsen FA III, Lippitt SB: Shoulder Surgery: Principles and Procedures. Philadelphia: WB Saunders, 2004, p 12.)

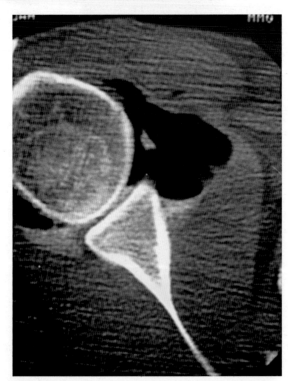

FIGURE 16-113 CT scan of the glenohumeral joint with air contrast. This study demonstrates a bony avulsion from the anterior glenoid rim.

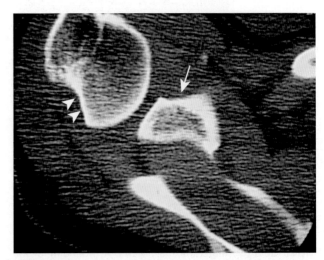

FIGURE 16-114 CT scan of the glenohumeral joint. The posterior humeral head defect (*arrowheads*) and the anterior glenoid defect (*arrow*) are well demonstrated.

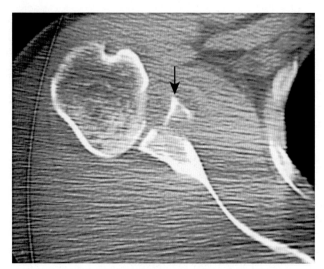

FIGURE 16-115 CT scan of the glenohumeral joint showing a fracture of the anterior glenoid rim (*arrow*) secondary to anterior glenohumeral dislocation.

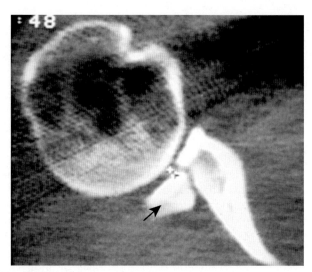

FIGURE 16-116 CT scan of the glenohumeral joint demonstrating a fracture of the posterior glenoid rim (*arrow*) as a result of posterior dislocation of the glenohumeral joint.

and capsule from the glenoid lip, especially in younger persons (Fig. 16-120). Nonhealing of this avulsion is a major factor in recurrent traumatic instability. The capsule might also be avulsed from the anteroinferior portion of the glenoid, sometimes with a fleck of bone (see Fig. 16-118).

Fractures

Fractures of the glenoid (Fig. 16-121; see also Figs. 16-6 and 16-116), humeral head (see Figs. 16-108 and 16-109),

and tuberosities (Figs. 16-122 to 16-124; see also Fig. 16-5) can accompany traumatic dislocations. A CT scan may be helpful in determining the degree of displacement of fractures (Figs. 16-125 and 16-126; see also Figs. 16-114 to 16-116).

It is important to seek evidence of a nondisplaced humeral neck fracture on the prereduction radiographs lest this fracture be displaced during attempted closed reduction (see Fig. 16-124).[325]

Other fractures, such as those of the coracoid process, may be associated with glenohumeral dislocations.[326,327]

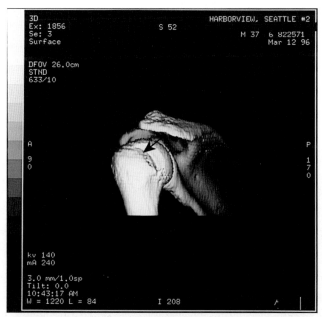

FIGURE 16-117 3D CT reconstruction after reduction of a first-time dislocation showing a posterolateral humeral head defect (*arrow*).

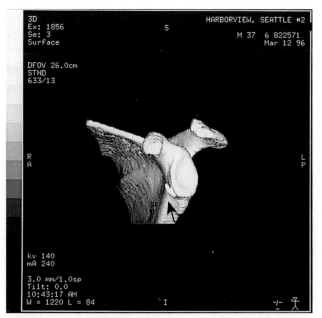

FIGURE 16-118 3D CT reconstruction after reduction of a first-time dislocation showing anterior glenoid avulsion (*arrow*).

Cuff Tears

Rotator cuff tears can accompany anterior and inferior glenohumeral dislocations (see Fig. 16-4). The frequency of this complication increases with age: In patients older than 40 years, the incidence exceeds 30%; in those older than 60 years, it exceeds 80%.[30,31,252,328-331]

Rotator cuff tears may be manifested as pain or weakness on external rotation and abduction.[47,119,330,332,333] Sonnabend reported a series of primary shoulder dislocations in patients older than 40 years.[262] Of the 13 patients who had complaints of weakness or pain after 3 weeks, 11 had rotator cuff tears. However, the presence of a rotator cuff tear may be masked by a coexisting axillary nerve palsy.[334,335]

Shoulder ultrasonography,[336] arthrography, or MRI is considered for evaluation of the possibility of an associated cuff tear when shoulder dislocations occur in patients older than 40 years, when initial displacement of the humeral head has been substantial (such as in a subglenoid dislocation), and when pain or loss of rotator cuff strength has persisted for 3 weeks after a glenohumeral dislocation. Toolanen found sonographic evidence of rotator cuff lesions in 24 of 63 patients older than 40 years at the time of anterior glenohumeral dislocation.[337]

Prompt operative repair of these acute cuff tears is usually indicated. Itoi and Tabata[328] reported 16 rotator cuff tears in 109 shoulders with a traumatic anterior dislocation. The cuff was surgically repaired in 11 shoulders, and the results were graded satisfactory in 73% of cases.

Neviaser and coauthors[338] reported on 37 patients older than 40 years in whom the diagnosis of cuff rupture was initially missed after an anterior dislocation of the shoulder. The weakness from the cuff rupture was often erroneously attributed to axillary neuropathy. Recurrent anterior instability caused by rupture of the subscapularis and anterior capsule from the lesser tuberosity developed in 11 of these patients. None of these shoulders had a Bankart lesion. Repair of the capsule and subscapularis restored stability in all of the patients. This study nicely points out that although younger patients with traumatic anterior instability often have anterior lesions (Bankart lesions or anterior rim fractures), older patients with traumatic anterior instability often have posterior lesions (cuff tears or tuberosity fractures).

Vascular Injuries

Several reports of arterial and neurologic injury with shoulder dislocation reinforce the importance of a thorough neurovascular evaluation.[339-341]

Vascular damage most often occurs in elderly patients with stiffer, more fragile vessels. The injury may be to the axillary artery or vein or to branches of the axillary

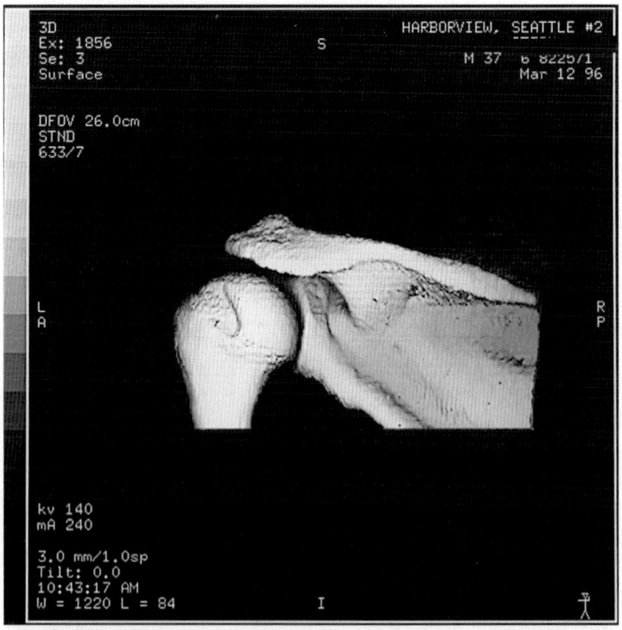

FIGURE 16-119 3D CT reconstruction of the left shoulder of a 37-year-old man 3 days after his first traumatic glenohumeral dislocation. The patient recovered normal shoulder function with nonoperative management.

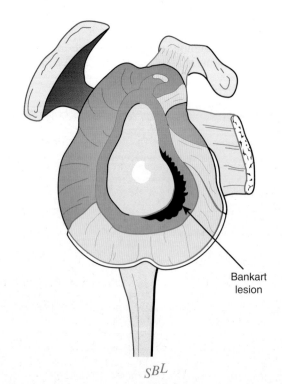

FIGURE 16-120 The capsulolabral detachment typical of traumatic instability. (Modified from Matsen FA III, Lippitt SB, Sidles JA, Harryman DT II: Practical Evaluation and Management of the Shoulder. Philadelphia: WB Saunders, 1994.)

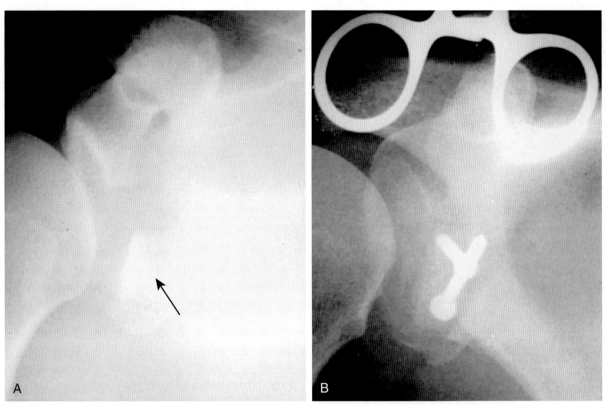

FIGURE 16-121 Anterior glenoid rim fracture. **A,** An AP radiograph demonstrates an anterior glenoid rim fracture secondary to traumatic anterior dislocation (*arrow*). **B,** An intraoperative AP radiograph shows reduction and screw fixation of an anterior glenoid rim fracture.

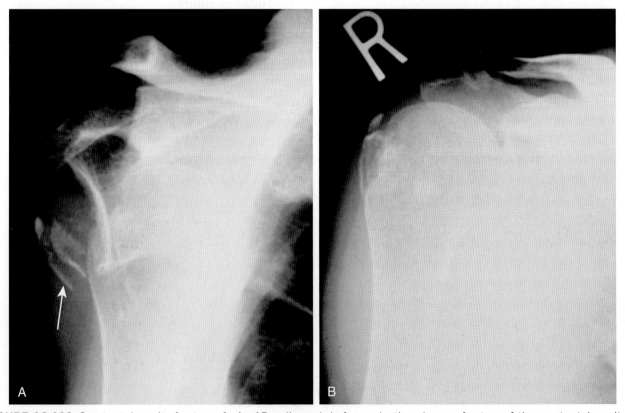

FIGURE 16-122 Greater tuberosity fracture. **A,** An AP radiograph before reduction shows a fracture of the greater tuberosity (*arrow*). **B,** Postreduction AP radiograph of a greater tuberosity fracture.

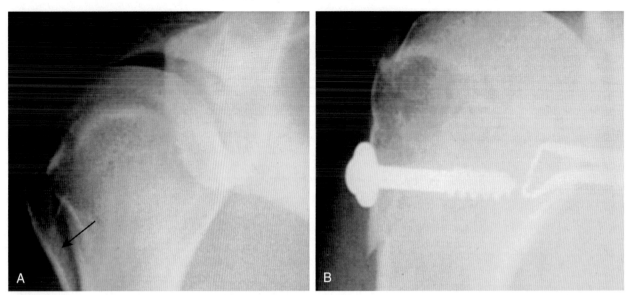

FIGURE 16-123 A, Radiograph showing a displaced greater tuberosity fracture (*arrow*). **B,** Intraoperative radiograph showing screw fixation of a greater tuberosity fracture.

artery: the thoracoacromial, subscapular, circumflex, and, rarely, the long thoracic. Sometimes these injuries can be combined, as pointed out by Kirker, who described a case of rupture of the axillary artery and axillary vein along with a brachial plexus palsy.[342] Injury can occur at the time of either dislocation or reduction.[343-346]

Anatomy

The axillary artery is divided into three parts that lie medial to, behind, and lateral to the pectoralis minor muscle (Fig. 16-127). Injuries most commonly involve the

second part, where the thoracoacromial trunk may be avulsed, and the third part, where the subscapular and circumflex branches may be avulsed or the axillary artery may be totally ruptured.

Mechanism of Injury

Damage to the axillary artery can take the form of a complete transection, a linear tear of the artery caused by avulsion of one of its branches, or an intravascular thrombus, perhaps related to an initial tear. The artery is relatively fixed at the lateral margin of the pectoralis

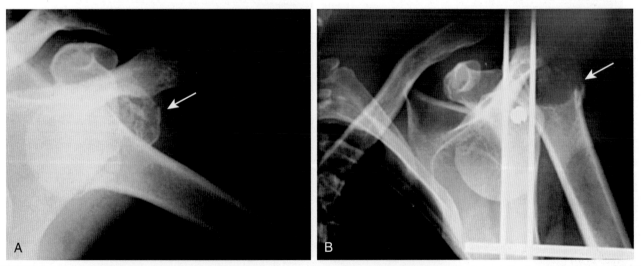

FIGURE 16-124 A, AP view showing an anteroinferior dislocation with an associated greater tuberosity fracture (*arrow*). **B,** AP view after a reduction attempt showing displacement of a humeral neck fracture (*arrow*).

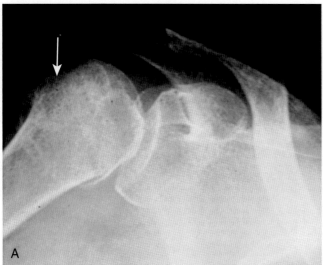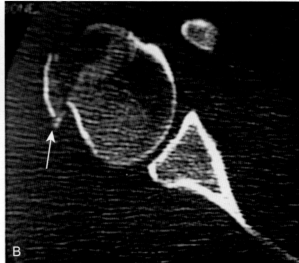

FIGURE 16-125 Minimally displaced greater tuberosity fracture. **A,** An AP radiograph shows a minimally displaced greater tuberosity fracture (*arrow*). **B,** A CT scan shows the position of the greater tuberosity (*arrow*).

minor muscle. With abduction and external rotation, the artery is taut; when the head dislocates, it forces the axillary artery forward, and the pectoralis minor acts as a fulcrum over which the artery is deformed and ruptured.[346-348]

Watson-Jones[349] reported the case of a man who had multiple anterior dislocations that he reduced himself. Finally, when the man was older, the axillary artery ruptured during one of the dislocations and he died. Vascular injuries can occur either at the time of dislocation or during attempted reduction. Sometimes it is unclear which is the case.[342,350,351]

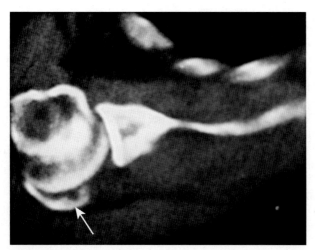

FIGURE 16-126 CT scan of a significantly displaced greater tuberosity fracture (*arrow*).

Injury at the Time of Dislocation

Vascular injuries are commonly associated with inferior dislocation.[284,292-294] Gardham and Scott[292] reported occlusion of the axillary artery with an erect dislocation of the shoulder in a 40-year-old patient who had fallen headfirst down an escalator. Although vascular injuries are most common in older persons, they can occur at any age.[352-357] Baratta and coworkers[358] reported the case of a 13-year-old boy who ruptured his axillary artery after a subcoracoid dislocation sustained while wrestling.

Injury at the Time of Reduction

Vascular damage at the time of reduction occurs primarily in the elderly, particularly when a chronic old anterior dislocation is mistaken for an acute injury and closed reduction is attempted. The largest series of vascular complications associated with closed reduction of the shoulder has been reported by Calvet and coworkers,[359] who in 1941 collected 90 cases. This paper, which revealed the tragic end results, must have accomplished its purpose because very few reports have appeared in the literature since then dealing with the complications that occur during reduction. In their series, in which 64 of 91 reductions were performed many weeks after the initial dislocation, the mortality rate was 50%. The other patients lost either the arm or function of the arm. Besides the long delay from dislocation to reduction, these injuries might also be due to the use of excessive force. Delpeche observed a case in which the force of 10 men was used to accomplish the shoulder reduction; such force damaged the axillary vessel.[360]

Signs and Symptoms

Vascular damage may be obvious or subtle. Findings can include pain, expanding hematoma, pulse deficit, periph-

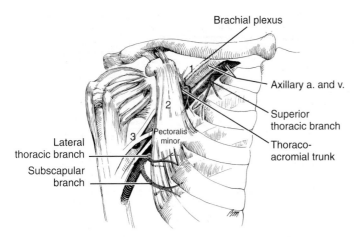

Brachial plexus

Axillary a. and v.

Superior thoracic branch

Thoraco-acromial trunk

Pectoralis minor

Lateral thoracic branch

Subscapular branch

FIGURE 16-127 The axillary artery is divided into three parts by the pectoralis minor muscle. The first part (*1*) is medial to the pectoralis minor, the second part (*2*) is behind it, and the third part (*3*) is lateral to it. (From Rockwood CA, Green DP [eds]: Fractures, 3 vols, 2nd ed. Philadelphia: JB Lippincott, 1984.)

eral cyanosis, peripheral coolness and pallor, neurologic dysfunction, and shock. Doppler or an arteriogram should confirm the diagnosis and locate the site of injury.

Treatment and Prognosis

A suspected major arterial injury is managed as a surgical emergency, including establishing a major intravenous (IV) line and obtaining blood for transfusion. Jardon and coworkers[346] pointed out that bleeding can be temporarily controlled by digital pressure on the axillary artery over the first rib. These authors also recommend that the axillary artery be explored through the subclavicular operative approach, as described by Steenburg and Ravitch.[361]

The treatment of choice for a damaged axillary artery is either direct repair or a bypass graft after resection of the injury. Excellent results have been reported with prompt management of these vascular injuries.[292,293,346,347,362-368] The results of simple ligation of the vessels in elderly patients have been disappointing, probably because of poor collateral circulation and the presence of arteriosclerotic vascular disease in these typically older persons.[342,369,370] Even when ligation has been performed in younger patients with good collateral circulation, approximately two thirds of these patients have lost function of the upper extremity, for example, because of the development of upper extremity claudication.

Nerve Injuries

The brachial plexus and the axillary artery lie immediately anterior, inferior, and medial to the glenohumeral joint.[111] It is not surprising, therefore, that neurovascular injuries often accompany traumatic anterior glenohumeral dislocations (Fig. 16-128).

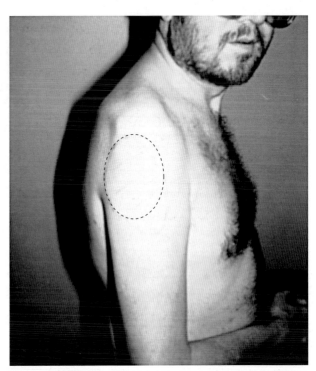

FIGURE 16-128 This patient sustained an axillary nerve palsy secondary to glenohumeral dislocation. Note the area of decreased sensation diagrammed on the lateral aspect of the proximal end of the humerus. Also note the significant wasting.

Anatomy

The axillary nerve originates off the posterior cord of the brachial plexus. It crosses the anterior surface of the subscapularis muscle and angulates sharply posteriorly to travel along the inferior shoulder joint capsule. It then leaves the axilla to exit through the quadrangular space below the lower border of the teres minor muscle, where it hooks around the posterior and lateral aspect of the humerus on the deep surface of the deltoid muscle.

Mechanism of Injury

The dislocated humeral head displaces the subscapularis and the overlying axillary nerve anteroinferiorly and creates traction and direct pressure on the nerve.[348,362,371] The injury to the nerve may be a neurapraxia (no structural damage, recovery in approximately 6 weeks), an axonotmesis (disruption of the axons, preservation of the nerve sheath, axonal regrowth at 1 inch per month), or a neurotmesis (complete nerve disruption, guarded prognosis for recovery).

Incidence

The reported incidence of nerve injuries in series of acute dislocations is substantial, often as high as 33%.[37,232,372-380] If careful electrodiagnostic studies are carried out prospectively, the incidence of nerve injury may be as high as 45%.[305]

The axillary nerve is most commonly involved; up to a third of first-time anterior dislocations are associated with axillary nerve involvement.[306,345,372,381,382] The likelihood of an axillary nerve injury increases with the age of the patient, the duration of the dislocation, and the amount of trauma that initiated the dislocation.[306,329] Other nerves injured are the radial, musculocutaneous, median, ulnar, and the entire brachial plexus.

Diagnosis

The diagnosis of nerve injury is considered in any patient with neurologic symptoms or signs such as weakness or numbness after a dislocation. A nerve injury can also be manifested as delayed recovery of active shoulder motion after glenohumeral dislocation. Blom and Dahlback[306] demonstrated that axillary neuropathy can exist without numbness in the usual sensory distribution of the axillary nerve. Electromyography provides objective evaluation of neurologic function, provided that 3 or 4 weeks has intervened between the injury and the evaluation.[306]

Treatment and Prognosis

Most axillary nerve injuries resulting from anterior dislocation are traction neurapraxias and will recover completely. However, if recovery has not occurred in 3 months, the prognosis is not as good.[305,306,373,383]

Recurrence of Instability After Anterior Dislocations

Effect of Age

The age of the patient at the time of the initial dislocation has a major influence on the incidence of redislocation.[232,384] Several authors have reported that patients younger than 20 years at the time of the initial dislocation have up to a 90% chance of recurrent instability.[7,232,374,384-392] In patients older than 40 years, the incidence drops sharply to 10% to 15%.[374,385] Hovelius and colleagues[393] reported a careful prospective study with a somewhat lower incidence of recurrence in each age group: 33% in those younger than 20 years, 25% between 20 and 30 years of age, and 10% between 30 and 40 years of age. The majority of all recurrences occur within the first 2 years after the first traumatic dislocation.[2,24,37,112,232,260,382,386,394,395]

Effect of Trauma, Sports, Sex, and Dominance

Rowe[232,385] has pointed out that the recurrence rate varies inversely with the severity of the original trauma; in other words, the more easily the dislocation occurred initially, the more easily it recurs. The recurrence rate in athletes may be higher than in nonathletes[384] and higher in men than women.[7] Dominance of the affected shoulder does not seem to have a major effect on the recurrence rate.[385]

Effect of Postdislocation Treatment

In many reports, the incidence of recurrence appears to be relatively insensitive to the type (sling versus plaster Velpeau) and duration of immobilization (0 versus 4 weeks) of the shoulder after the initial dislocation.[385,386,396,397] By contrast, others have reported that longer periods of immobilization (over 3 weeks) are associated with a reduced incidence of recurrence.[257,398]

In a definitive 10-year prospective study, Hovelius and coworkers studied the effect of immobilization on the incidence of recurrence.[393] After reduction, 247 primary anterior dislocations were partially randomized to either a 3- to 4-week period of immobilization or to a sling to be discarded after comfort was achieved. The authors concluded that the immobilization did not affect the rate of recurrence. The results provide useful general rules: Overall, half of these shoulders had recurrent dislocations, half the recurrences were treated surgically, and half of the recurrences treated nonoperatively were stable without surgery at 10 years. One of six patients had dislocation of the opposite shoulder. Eleven percent of the shoulders had at least mild evidence of secondary degenerative joint disease. Interestingly, this secondary disease was observed in both surgical and nonsurgical cases.

Aronen and Regan[399] reported a 3-year average follow-up study of 20 primary dislocations in Navy midshipmen treated with a 3-month aggressive postdislocation program. The program consisted of 3 weeks of sling immobilization followed by progressive strengthening. The patients were not allowed to return to activity until they had no evidence of weakness or atrophy and no apprehension on abduction and external rotation. In this series, there were no recurrent dislocations and two recurrent subluxations. Similarly, Yoneda[400] reported good results in 83% of patients in a program emphasizing postimmobilization exercises. Itoi and colleagues[401] has advocated immobilization in external rotation to hold the labrum in a reduced position to the glenoid during healing.

Effect of Fractures

The incidence of recurrence is lower when a first-time shoulder dislocation is associated with a greater tuberosity fracture.[226,232,245,374,387,393,402] Hovelius[387] reported that these fractures were three times as common in patients older than 30 years: 23% versus 8% in patients younger than 30 years. Other fractures, such as substantial posterolateral humeral head lesions and fractures of the glenoid lip, are likely to be associated with an increased incidence of recurrent instability.

In conclusion, it appears that the injuries sustained by young patients in association with traumatic dislocations are relatively unlikely to heal in a manner yielding a stable shoulder. Probably the most important of these nonhealing injuries are avulsion of the glenohumeral capsular ligaments from the anterior glenoid lip and defects of the posterolateral humeral head. Older patients tend to injure the posterior capsule or fracture the greater tuberosity, either of which is likely to heal and result in a stable shoulder unless the rotator cuff is substantially torn. In atraumatic instability, there is no traumatic lesion and thus a high chance of recurrence. The degree of trauma and the age of the patient seem to be the most important factors in determining the recurrence rate.

INJURIES ASSOCIATED WITH POSTERIOR DISLOCATIONS

Fractures

Fractures of the posterior glenoid rim and proximal part of the humerus (upper shaft, tuberosities, and head) are quite common in traumatic posterior dislocations of the shoulder.[266,403-405] The commonly associated compression fracture of the anteromedial portion of the humeral head is produced by the posterior cortical rim of the glenoid. It is best seen on an axillary view or a CT scan (Fig. 16-129; see also Fig. 16-109).

This lesion, sometimes called a *reverse Hill–Sachs lesion,* often occurs at the time of the original posterior dislocation. It becomes larger with multiple posterior dislocations of the shoulder. Large humeral head defects are also seen in old unreduced posterior dislocations.

The posterior rim of the glenoid may be fractured and displaced in posterior dislocations (see Fig. 16-116). Such injury occurs not only with direct forces from an anterior direction that push the humeral head out posteriorly but also with indirect types of dislocations such as occur during seizures or accidental electrical shock.

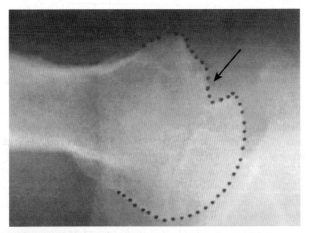

FIGURE 16-129 Axillary lateral x-ray film demonstrating an anteromedial compression fracture (*arrow*) of the humeral head (*dotted outline*) (reverse Hill–Sachs lesion) after a traumatic posterior shoulder dislocation. (From Rockwood CA Jr, Green DP, Bucholz RW [eds]: Fractures in Adults. Philadelphia: JB Lippincott, 1991.)

Fracture of the lesser tuberosity of the humerus can accompany posterior dislocations. The subscapularis muscle comes under considerable tension in this dislocation and can avulse the lesser tuberosity onto which it inserts. Although the fracture may be seen on AP and lateral radiographs of the glenohumeral joint, it is best seen on the axillary view and on CT scan.

Posterior dislocations of the humerus may be overlooked in the presence of a comminuted fracture of the proximal end of the humerus or humeral shaft fractures. In the series of 16 cases of posterior dislocation of the shoulder reported by O'Conner and Jacknow,[404] 12 had comminuted fractures of the proximal part of the humerus. In 8 of the 12 cases of fracture, the diagnosis of posterior dislocation was initially missed.

Other Associated Injuries

Injuries to the rotator cuff and neurovascular structures are less common with posterior than with anterior dislocations. However, they do occur. Moeller[273] reported a patient who had an open acute posterior dislocation of the left shoulder. The shoulder was totally unstable after reduction because of tears of the rotator cuff, biceps tendon, and subscapularis tendons. The patient had associated injury to the axillary and suprascapular nerves.

TREATMENT

Anterior Dislocations

Acute Traumatic Anterior Dislocations
Timing of Reduction and Analgesia

Acute dislocations of the glenohumeral joint should be reduced as gently and expeditiously as possible, ideally after a complete set of radiographs is obtained to rule out associated bone injuries. Early relocation promptly eliminates the stretch and compression of neurovascular structures, minimizes the amount of muscle spasm that must be overcome to effect reduction, and prevents progressive enlargement of the humeral head defect in locked dislocations.

The extent of anesthesia required to accomplish a gentle reduction depends on many factors, including the amount of trauma that produced the dislocation, the duration of the dislocation, the number of previous dislocations, whether the dislocation is locked, and to what extent the patient can voluntarily relax the shoulder musculature. When seen acutely, some dislocations can be reduced without the use of medication. At the other extreme, reduction of a long-standing, locked dislocation can require a brachial plexus block or general anesthesia with muscle relaxation. Many practitioners use narcotics and muscle relaxants to aid in the reduction of shoulder dislocations. A potential trap exists: the dosages required

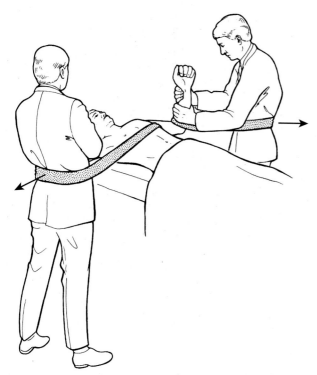

FIGURE 16-130 Reduction technique for an anterior glenohumeral dislocation. The patient lies supine with a sheet placed around the thorax and then around the assistant's waist to provide countertraction (*left arrow*). The surgeon stands on the side of the dislocated shoulder near the patient's waist with the elbow of the dislocated shoulder flexed to 90 degrees. A second sheet is tied loosely around the waist of the surgeon and looped over the patient's forearm, thus providing traction while the surgeon leans back against the sheet (*right arrow*) and grasps the forearm. Steady traction along the axis of the arm usually achieves reduction. The surgeon's hands are free to gently rock the humerus from internal to external rotation or provide gentle outward pressure on the proximal part of the humerus from the axilla.

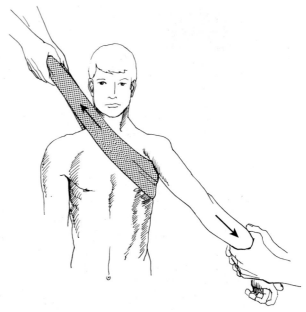

FIGURE 16-131 Closed reduction of the left shoulder with traction (*right arrow*) against countertraction (*left arrow*). (From Rockwood CA, Green DP [eds]: Fractures, 3 vols, 2nd ed. Philadelphia: JB Lippincott, 1984.)

to produce muscle relaxation while the shoulder is dislocated may be sufficient to produce respiratory depression once the shoulder is reduced. Our recommendation is that if these medications are to be used, they should be administered through an established IV line. Such practice produces a more rapid onset, a short duration of action, and the opportunity to adjust the required dose more appropriately. Furthermore, resuscitation (if necessary) is facilitated by the prospective presence of such a route of access. Airway management tools should be readily available.

Lippitt and colleagues[406,407] compared two methods of analgesia for the reduction of anterior dislocations: IV analgesia plus muscle relaxation and intra-articular lidocaine. With respect to the first, they found a 75% success rate and a 37% complication rate in a retrospective series of 52 reductions in which IV narcotics were used for analgesia. IV narcotics consisted of morphine 3 to 24 mg, or meperidine 12.5 to 100 mg, with or without diazepam 1.5 to 15 mg or midazolam 1 to 10 mg. They remarked on the difficulty of determining the appropriate IV dose of narcotics. The level of pain, age, smoking history, alcohol consumption, cardiac disease, and regional perfusion are just a few of the factors that can influence the narcotic requirement.[408] Older patients and intoxicated patients are more sensitive to the respiratory depressant effects of narcotics. Because pain counteracts the respiratory depressant effect, patients sedated by narcotics are at increased risk for respiratory depression after the painful stimulus is removed when the shoulder is reduced. Complications from IV analgesia included respiratory depression, hypotension, hyperemesis, and oversedation.

With respect to the second method, the use of 20 mL of 1% plain intra-articular lidocaine, Lippitt and associates found a 100% success rate in the reduction of 40 dislocations with no complications. One patient inadvertently received 400 mg instead of 200 mg of lidocaine, and transient tinnitus, perioral numbness, and mild dysarthria developed. A survey revealed that both patients and physicians were satisfied with this method. The authors speculated that the success of intra-articular injection may be due to a combination of pain relief allowing reduction, relief from muscle spasm, and venting of the joint. Intra-articular lidocaine has been shown to be effective in reducing dislocations in other studies as well.[409,410] This technique may be particularly useful in patients with

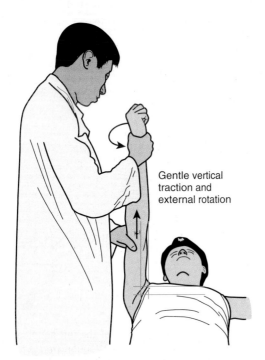

FIGURE 16-132 The Spaso technique for reducing anterior glenohumeral dislocations.

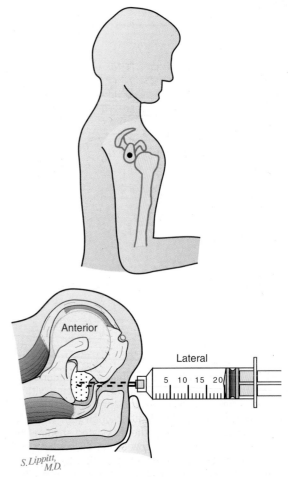

S. Lippitt,
M.D.

FIGURE 16-133 Intra-articular lidocaine injection for anesthesia during reduction of an anterior dislocation. The needle is inserted just posterior to the dislocated humeral head.

complicating factors such as medical problems or facial trauma and in whom respiratory depression with IV analgesia is not desired.

There is no need to put the patient through discomfort or potential risk by forcing a reduction in the emergency department. If a gentle, comfortable reduction cannot be obtained, we recommend reduction under formal anesthesia with muscle relaxation as needed. Once muscle relaxation is complete, reduction can usually be accomplished gently.

Method of Reduction
Once the shoulder is relaxed, a variety of gentle methods can be used to achieve reduction. Gentle traction on the arm is common to most (Figs. 16-130 and 16-131). One such method is known as the *Stimson technique*. Though the technique is named for Lewis A. Stimson,[297,411] Stimson credited Dr. Cole, a house staff physician of the Chambers Street Hospital. In the Stimson method, the patient is placed prone on the edge of the examining table while downward traction is gently applied.[411] The traction force may be applied by the weight of the arm, by weights taped to the wrist, or by the surgeon. It can take several minutes for the traction to produce muscle relaxation. It is important that patients not be left unattended in this position, particularly if narcotics and muscle relaxants have been administered.

A new method of reducing shoulder dislocations has been described as the *Spaso technique*. This method places the patient in the supine position with the arm at the side. Longitudinal traction is applied as the arm is brought into forward flexion to produce an external rotational moment (Fig. 16-132).[412]

Authors' Preferred Method of Anterior Reduction
Although analgesia might not be necessary to achieve reduction, we are impressed with the safety and effectiveness of intra-articular lidocaine as described by Lippitt and coworkers (Fig. 16-133).[406,407] In this method, a maximum of 20 mL of 1% plain lidocaine is injected with an 18-gauge needle placed 2 cm below the lateral edge of the acromion just posterior to the dislocated humeral head and directed toward the glenoid fossa. The amount of lidocaine is limited to 200 mg.[413] Placement of the needle in the joint is confirmed by a combination of feeling the needle penetrate the glenohumeral capsule, aspirating joint fluid or hemarthrosis and ensuring that the injection is not intravascular, gently palpating the glenoid fossa with the needle, and verifying easy flow on injection and return of the injected lidocaine solution. Fifteen minutes is allowed to maximize the analgesic effect of the lidocaine before manipulation.

Reduction of either anterior or posterior glenohumeral dislocations can usually be effected by traction on the abducted and flexed arm with countertraction on the body (see Figs. 16-130 and 16-131). The patient is placed supine with a sheet around the thorax and the loose ends on the side opposite the shoulder dislocation, where they are held by an assistant. The surgeon stands on the side of the dislocated shoulder near the patient's waist. The elbow of the dislocated shoulder is flexed to 90 degrees (to relax the neurovascular structures), and traction is applied through a sheet looped over the patient's forearm, or traction can be applied directly. Steady traction along the axis of the arm usually effects reduction.

To this basic maneuver, one may add gentle rocking of the humerus from internal to external rotation or outward pressure on the proximal end of the humerus from the axilla. These additions are particularly useful if prereduction axillary x-rays show the humeral head to be impaled on the glenoid rim. Postreduction x-rays are used to confirm reduction and detect fractures. A postreduction neurovascular examination and set of radiographs is routine.

Chronic Anterior Traumatic Dislocations
Reduction and Analgesia

A glenohumeral joint that has been dislocated for several days is a chronic dislocation. The principles and methods for reducing a chronic dislocation are similar to those relating to an acute dislocation, except that the patient and the shoulder are usually more fragile and the relocation is more difficult. As the chronicity of the dislocation increases, so do the difficulties and complications of reduction. When one encounters an elderly patient with pain in the shoulder whose radiographs reveal an anterior dislocation, a very careful history is needed to determine whether the initial injury occurred recently or quite a while earlier.

Chronic dislocations are seen most commonly in elderly people and in those whose general health or mental status might prevent them from seeking help for the injury. The event causing the injury may be relatively trivial.[43,414] Old age, chronicity of dislocation, and soft bone make closed reduction difficult and dangerous.[415] If closed reduction is to be performed, it should be done with minimal traction, without leverage, and with total muscle relaxation under controlled general anesthesia. If the dislocation is more than a week old, the humeral head is likely to be firmly impaled on the anterior glenoid with such soft tissue contraction that gentle closed reduction is impossible. When the risks of attempting reduction appear to outweigh the advantages, the dislocated position may be accepted.

Open Reduction

If a gentle attempt at closed reduction fails, open reduction may be considered. Open reduction can be a complex procedure because of the altered position of the axillary artery and branches of the brachial plexus and because the structures are tight and scarred. Sometimes the symptoms of chronic dislocation are surprisingly minimal.[416]

To perform an open reduction, the subscapularis and anterior portion of the capsule are incised near their insertion onto the lesser tuberosity to allow substantial external rotation of the dislocated shoulder. External rotation and lateral traction usually disimpact the humerus from the glenoid. While lateral traction is maintained, the humerus is gently internally rotated under direct vision to ensure that the articular surface of the humerus passes safely by the anterior glenoid lip and into the glenoid fossa. Leverage is avoided because the head is usually very soft. If the posterolateral head defect is greater than 40% or if the head collapses during reduction, a humeral head prosthesis may be necessary to restore a functional joint surface. The subscapularis and capsule are then repaired. The shoulder is carefully inspected for evidence of cuff tear or vascular damage.

Results of Treatment of Chronic Dislocations

Schulz and associates[417] reported a series of 17 posterior and 44 anterior chronic dislocations. These dislocations occurred primarily in elderly people, and more than half the dislocations were associated with fracture of the tuberosities, humeral head, humeral neck, glenoid, or coracoid process. More than a third involved neurologic deficits. Closed reduction was attempted in 40 shoulders and was successful in 20. Of the 20 shoulders successfully reduced (3 posterior and 17 anterior), the duration of dislocation exceeded 4 weeks in only 1 instance. Open reduction was performed in 20, humeral head excision was performed in 6, 8 patients were not treated, and 5 shoulders were not reducible.

Perniceni and Augereau[418] described reinforcement of the anterior shoulder complex in three patients after reduction of neglected anterior dislocations of the shoulder. They used the Gosset[419] technique, which places a rib graft between the coracoid and the glenoid rim. Rowe and Zarins[254] reported on 24 patients with unreduced dislocations of the shoulder and operated on 14 of them.

Management After Reduction of an Anterior Dislocation
Evaluation

After reducing the dislocation, AP and lateral x-ray views are obtained in the plane of the scapula to verify the adequacy of the reduction and provide an additional opportunity to detect fractures of the glenoid and proximal end of the humerus. The patient's neurologic status is again checked, including the sensory and motor function of all five major nerves in the upper extremity. The strength of the pulse is verified, and evidence of bruits or an expanding hematoma is sought.[345] The integrity of the rotator cuff is initially evaluated by observing the strength of isometric external rotation and abduction.

Trimmings[420] demonstrated that aspiration of hemarthrosis from the shoulder can be an effective means of decreasing discomfort after the shoulder is reduced.

Protection

Because recurrent glenohumeral instability is the most common complication of a glenohumeral dislocation, postreduction treatment focuses on optimizing shoulder stability. Thus, two potentially important elements in postreduction treatment are protection and muscle rehabilitation. Reeves demonstrated that after repair of the subscapularis in primates, 3 months was necessary before normal capsular patterns of collagen bundles were observed, 5 months before the tendon was histologically normal, and 4 to 5 months before tensile strength was regained.[23] It is unknown whether labral tears or ligamentous avulsions from the glenoid heal or how long it might take. In any event, it is apparent that the shoulder cannot be immobilized for the full length of time required for complete healing. Immobilization in external rotation rather than the standard internally rotated position is suggested by Itoi and colleagues, who used MRI to examine shoulders after dislocation and found the anterior labrum to have 1.9 mm of separation from the glenoid while the shoulder is in internal rotation but only 0.1 mm when the arm is externally rotated.[401] No clinical follow-up information was given.

We treat first-time dislocations in a manner similar to the postoperative management of dislocation repairs. Thus, younger patients are placed on the "90-0 program," in which flexion is limited to 90 degrees and external rotation is limited to 0 degrees for the first 3 weeks while strength is maintained with cuff and deltoid isometrics. The elbow is fully extended at least several times a day to prevent sling soreness. Because stiffness of the shoulder, elbow, and hand is more likely to develop in persons older than 30 years, the duration of immobilization is progressively reduced for persons of increasing age.[232,374,386,388,400] Patients are checked 3 weeks after relocation and examined for stiffness; if external rotation to 0 degrees is difficult, formal stretching exercises are started. Otherwise, the patient is allowed to increase use of the shoulder as comfort permits.

Strengthening

At 3 weeks, the patient institutes more-vigorous rotator cuff–strengthening exercises with rubber tubing or weights. The patient is informed that strong subscapularis and infraspinatus muscles are ideally situated to increase glenohumeral stability.[131]

Burkhead and Rockwood,[421] Glousman and coworkers,[189] and Tibone and Bradley[422] emphasized the importance of strengthening not only the rotator cuff but also the scapular stabilizing muscles because of their vital importance in providing a stable platform for shoulder function. Even in the case of recurrent instability, Burkhead and Rockwood[421] found that a complete exercise program was effective in the management of 12% of patients with traumatic subluxation, 80% with anterior atraumatic subluxation, and 90% with posterior instability.

Swimming is recommended at 6 weeks to enhance endurance and coordination. By 3 months after the dislocation, most patients should have almost full flexion and rotation of the shoulder. Patients are not allowed to use the injured arm in sports or for overhead labor until they have achieved normal rotator strength, comfortable and nearly full forward elevation, and confidence in their shoulder with it in the necessary positions. Any deviation from the expected course of recovery requires careful re-evaluation for occult fractures, loose bodies, rotator cuff tears, peripheral nerve injuries, and glenohumeral arthritis.

Early Surgery in Anterior Dislocations

Conventional wisdom has stated that nonoperative treatment is the conservative choice after an initial shoulder dislocation and that, in general, surgery is reserved for recurrent instability. However, in a study of functional outcome and risk of recurrent instability after primary anterior shoulder dislocation in young patients (15-35 years old), Robinson and coworkers[423] found that within 2 years instability was present in more than half. In young male patients, the risk of instability was the highest. The authors suggested clinical trials to examine the effects of interventions to reduce the prevalence of recurrent instability.

Soft Tissue Interposition

Tietjen[424] reported a case in which surgery was required to retrieve the avulsed supraspinatus, infraspinatus, and teres minor from their interposition between the humeral head and the glenoid.

Bridle and Ferris[425] reported a case of apparent successful closed reduction of an anterior shoulder dislocation that appeared to be confirmed on an AP radiograph. However, the patient continued to experience severe pain, and a subsequent axillary lateral view demonstrated persistent anterior subluxation of the glenohumeral joint. At the time of open reduction, the ruptured muscle belly of the subscapularis was found interposed between the humeral head and glenoid. Inao and associates[426] reported a case of an acute anterior shoulder dislocation that was irreducible by closed treatment because of interposition of the posteriorly displaced tendon of the long head of the biceps.

Displaced Fracture of the Greater Tuberosity

Although fractures of the greater tuberosity are not uncommonly associated with anterior shoulder dislocation, the tuberosity usually reduces into an acceptable position when the shoulder is reduced (see Figs. 16-5 and 16-122). Occasionally, the greater tuberosity fragment displaces up under the acromion process or is pulled posteriorly by the cuff muscles. If the greater tuberosity remains displaced after reduction of the shoulder joint (see Fig. 16-126), consideration should be given to anatomic reduction and internal fixation of the fragment and repair of the attendant split in the tendons of the rotator cuff (see Fig. 16-123).

It is relatively easy to determine the amount of superior displacement of the tuberosity fragment on an AP radiograph in the plane of the scapula. Posterior displacement can be more difficult to discern. It is important to look for the vacant tuberosity sign, wherein the normal contour of the greater tuberosity is lacking. If one is concerned about the AP position of the tuberosity on plain films, a CT scan should be considered. If the tuberosity is allowed to heal with posterior displacement, it can produce the functional equivalent of both a rotator cuff tear and a bony block to external rotation.

Glenoid Rim Fracture

Aston and Gregory[427] reported three cases in which a large anterior fracture of the glenoid occurred as a result of a fall on the lateral aspect of the abducted shoulder. A fracture of the glenoid lip can require open reduction and internal fixation if an intra-articular incongruity or an inadequate effective glenoid arc is present (see Fig. 16-116).

Special Problems

Occasionally, early surgical reconstruction may be considered in a patient who requires complete shoulder stability before being able to return to work or sports. Hertz and coauthors[428] reported a 2.4-year follow-up of 31 patients with an initial dislocation treated by primary repair of an arthroscopically demonstrated Bankart lesion: None had recurrent instability. Arciero and coworkers[389,429] initiated a study at West Point in which the Bankart lesion was repaired arthroscopically after the initial dislocation. Their initial data indicated a decrease in recurrent instability from 80% with nonoperative management to 14% with early repair.[389,429,430]

Posterior Dislocations

Reduction

Reduction of acute traumatic posterior dislocations may be much more difficult than reduction of acute traumatic anterior dislocations. Hawkins and coworkers[265] reviewed 41 cases of locked posterior shoulder dislocations. The average interval between injury and diagnosis was 1 year! In 7 shoulders the deformity was accepted. Closed reduction was successful in only 6 of the 12 cases in which it was attempted.

IV narcotics combined with muscle relaxants or tranquilizers can provide insufficient analgesia and muscle relaxation; general anesthesia with muscle paralysis may be required. Atraumatic closed reduction can usually be accomplished once the muscle spasm has been eliminated. With the patient in the supine position, longitudinal and lateral traction is applied to the arm while it is gently rocked in internal and external rotation. Once the head is disimpacted, it is lifted anteriorly

back into the glenoid fossa. In locked posterior dislocations, it may be necessary to gently stretch out the posterior cuff and capsule by maximally internally rotating the humerus before reduction is attempted. Care should be taken to not force the arm into external rotation before reduction is achieved; if the head is locked posteriorly on the glenoid rim, forced external rotation could produce a fracture of the head or shaft of the humerus.

If gentle closed reduction of a locked posterior glenohumeral dislocation is not possible, open reduction may be accomplished through an anterior deltopectoral approach.[265,311,431-436] Because local anatomy is significantly distorted, the tendon of the long head of the biceps is used as a guide to the lesser tuberosity. The subscapularis is released either by osteotomy of the lesser tuberosity or by direct incision. With the glenoid thus exposed, open reduction is carried out by gently pulling the humeral head laterally and then lifting its articular surface up on the face of the glenoid.

If after closed reduction the shoulder is stable in the sling position, this type of postreduction management is most convenient for the patient. However, if recurrent instability is a concern, the shoulder is immobilized in a shoulder spica or brace with the amount of external rotation necessary to provide stability.[437,438] Scougall[439] has shown experimentally in monkeys that a surgically detached posterior glenoid labrum and capsule heal soundly without repair. He concluded that the best position of immobilization, to allow healing of all the posterior structures, was in abduction, external rotation, and extension and that the position should be maintained for 4 weeks.

Although some have recommended pin fixation for 3 weeks after reduction,[405] this method carries a risk of pin breakage and infection.

Surgery

Indications for surgery include a displaced lesser tuberosity fracture, a significant posterior glenoid fracture, an irreducible dislocation, an open dislocation, or an unstable reduction. If the shoulder cannot be maintained in a reduced position, reconstructive surgery to reduce the impaction fracture, a tendon or bone transfer, an allograft, or replacement of the humeral head can be considered.

A major cause of recurrent instability after reduction of a posterior dislocation is the presence of a large anteromedial humeral head defect. If at the time of reduction stability cannot be obtained because of such a defect, it may be rendered extra-articular by filling it with the subscapularis tendon as described by McLaughlin[272,293,311,440,441] or the lesser tuberosity as described by Neer.[62,313] If the humeral head defect involves more than 30% of the articular surface, replacement with a prosthesis may be indicated; otherwise, instability can recur with internal rotation. Hawkins and coworkers demonstrated the use of each of these techniques in a series of locked posterior dislocations.[265]

After surgery, the arm may be immobilized in a sling and swathe for 2 weeks as recommended by McLaughlin, the arm may be positioned at the side posterior to the coronal plane with a strip of tape or canvas restraint as recommended by Rowe and Zarins,[254] or a modified spica in neutral rotation may be used for 6 weeks, followed by an additional 3 to 6 months of rehabilitative exercises as recommended by Rockwood.[313]

Keppler and colleagues suggested using rotational osteotomy of the humerus for the postreduction management of locked posterior dislocations.[442]

Authors' Preferred Method of Treatment

Our management of acute traumatic posterior dislocations begins with a thorough exploration of the cause of the dislocation, looking for evidence of seizures, substance abuse, and recurrent trauma. We then seek to define the extent and chronicity of the injury. A complete radiographic evaluation that includes AP and lateral views in the plane of the scapula and an axillary view is necessary. Careful note is made of associated fractures, including the extent of the impression fracture of the anteromedial humeral head. Under anesthesia and muscle relaxation, gentle closed reduction is attempted with the application of axial traction on the arm. If the head is locked on the glenoid rim, gentle internal rotation can stretch out the posterior capsule to facilitate reduction. Lateral traction on the proximal part of the humerus can unlock the humeral head. Once it is unlocked, the humerus is gently externally rotated. After reduction is achieved and confirmed by postreduction radiographs, a determination is made of the stability of the reduced shoulder and its bony anatomy.

If the shoulder appears to have a good chance of stability, the reduction is maintained for 3 weeks in a cummerbund handshake cast (Fig. 16-134) or orthotic (Fig. 16-135) in neutral rotation and slight extension. External rotation and deltoid isometrics are carried out during this period of immobilization. After removal of the cast, a vigorous *strengthening* program for the internal and external rotators is initiated. Range of motion is allowed to return with active use, beginning with elevation in the plane of the scapula. Vigorous physical activities are not resumed until the shoulder is strong and 3 months has elapsed since reduction. Swimming is encouraged because it helps to develop endurance and muscle coordination.

When a humeral head defect involves 20% to 40% of the humeral head, a subscapularis transfer into the defect can provide increased stability. When the humeral head defect is greater than 40%, a proximal humeral prosthesis to replace the lost articular surface is often necessary to prevent the glenoid from falling into the humeral defect (see Fig. 16-83). When the dislocation is obviously chronic, consideration may be given to accepting the dislocation and focusing on enhancing the patient's ability to carry out activities of daily living.

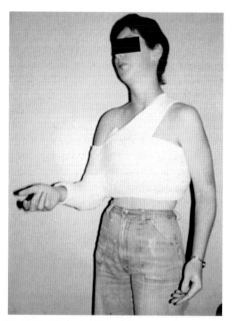

FIGURE 16-134 A handshake cast. After closed reduction of an acute traumatic posterior dislocation is confirmed by radiographs, a cast is applied in neutral rotation and slight extension for 3 weeks.

Chronic Posterior Dislocation

If a patient, especially an older patient, has had a chronic posterior dislocation for months or years with minimal pain and a functional range of motion, surgery might not be indicated. However, if disability exists and the glenohumeral joint has good bone stock, open reduction with a subscapularis or lesser tuberosity transfer or shoulder arthroplasty may be considered.[254]

RECURRENT DISLOCATION

EVALUATION

After an initial dislocation, the shoulder might return to functional stability, or it might fall victim to recurrent glenohumeral instability. Although intermediate forms of recurrent instability do occur, the great majority of recurrently unstable shoulders may be thought of as being either atraumatic or traumatic in origin.

Atraumatic Recurrent Instability

Atraumatic instability is instability that arises without the type of trauma necessary to tear the stabilizing soft tissues or create a humeral head defect, tuberosity fracture, or

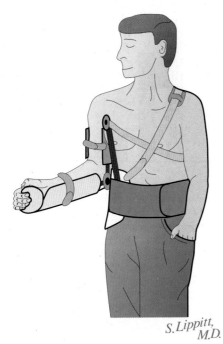

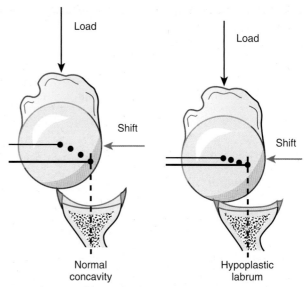

FIGURE 16-135 An orthosis is used to immobilize the arm after reduction of a posterior dislocation or a global capsular repair. (Modified from Matsen FA III, Lippitt SB, Sidles JA, Harryman DT II: Practical Evaluation and Management of the Shoulder. Philadelphia: WB Saunders, 1994.)

FIGURE 16-136 Compromised humeral head centering. When the labrum is excessively compliant, there is diminished resistance to the load and shift test. (From Matsen FA III, Lippitt SB: Shoulder Surgery: Principles and Procedures. Philadelphia: WB Saunders, 2004, p 195.)

glenoid lip fracture. Certain shoulders may be more susceptible to atraumatic instability. A small or functionally flat glenoid fossa can jeopardize the concavity compression, adhesion and cohesion, and glenoid suction-cup stability mechanisms (Fig. 16-136). Thin, excessively compliant capsular tissue can invaginate into the joint when traction is applied and thus limit the effectiveness of stabilization from limited joint volume. A large, potentially capacious capsule can allow humeroscapular positions outside the range of balance stability. Weak rotator cuff muscles can provide insufficient compression for the concavity compression–stabilizing mechanism. Poor neuromuscular control can fail to position the scapula to balance the net humeral joint reaction force. Voluntary or inadvertent malpositioning of the humerus in excessive anterior or posterior scapular planes can cause the net humeral joint reaction force to lie outside the balance stability angles. Once initiated, the instability may be perpetuated by compression of the glenoid rim as a result of chronically poor humeral head centering. Excessive labral compliance can predispose to this loss of effective glenoid depth.

Any of these factors, individually or in combination, could contribute to instability of the glenohumeral joint. For example, posterior glenohumeral subluxation may be caused by the combination of a relatively flat posterior glenoid and the tendency to retract the scapula during anterior elevation of the arm; such a combination results

in use of the elevated humerus in excessively anterior scapular planes. Excessively compliant capsular tissue in conjunction with relatively weak rotator cuff muscles could contribute to inferior subluxation on attempted lifting of objects with the arm at the side. If the lateral aspect of the scapula is allowed to droop (whether voluntarily or involuntarily), the superior capsular structures are relaxed and permit inferior translation of the humerus with respect to the glenoid (see Fig. 16-20).[443]

Because it usually results from loss of midrange stability, atraumatic instability is more likely to be multidirectional. Pathogenic factors such as a flat glenoid, weak muscles, and a compliant capsule can produce instability anteriorly, inferiorly, posteriorly, or in a combination of directions. Although the onset of atraumatic instability may be provoked by a period of disuse or a minor injury, many of the underlying contributing factors may be developmental. As a result, the tendency for atraumatic instability is likely to be bilateral and familial as well.

It is apparent that atraumatic instability is not a simple diagnosis, but rather a syndrome that can arise from a multiplicity of factors. To help recall the various aspects of this syndrome, we use the acronym AMBRII. The instability is *a*traumatic, usually associated with *m*ultidirectional laxity and with *b*ilateral findings. Treatment is predominantly by *r*ehabilitation directed at restoring optimal neuromuscular control. If surgery is necessary, it might need to include reconstruction of the rotator *i*nterval capsule–coracohumeral ligament mechanism and tightening of the *i*nferior capsule. The diagnosis and management of this condition have been presented in detail.[89,444-446]

TABLE 16-2 Characteristics of Patients With Traumatic Instability, Atraumatic Instability, and Failed Instability Repairs

Characteristic	TUBS	AMBRII	Failed Repairs
Patients			
Number	101	70	76
Female	26%	38%	28%
Right side	55%	68%	51%
Age (y)	29 ± 11	27 ± 10	31 ± 8
Able to Perform Function (%)			
Place coin on shelf	93	77	73
Place 1 lb on shelf	91	75	65
Tuck in shirt	89	81	54
Comfort by side	87	71	56
Toss underhand	83	70	44
Hand behind head	77	75	48
Carry 20 lb	73	61	46
Wash opposite shoulder	69	64	39
Do usual work	69	46	42
Place 8 lb on shelf	53	35	28
Sleep on side	43	19	11
Toss overhand	31	35	15
Health Status			
Emotional role	86	72	70
Physical function	85	78	71
Social function	84	73	66
General health	81	78	68
Mental health	78	74	68
Vitality	67	58	55
Comfort	60	43	43
Physical role	52	35	28

AMBRI, atraumatic instability; TUBS, traumatic instability.

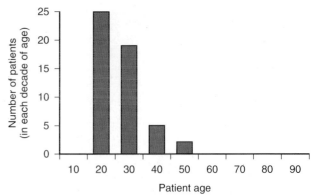

FIGURE 16-137 Age distribution of 51 patients with atraumatic instability. (From Matsen FA III, Lippitt SB, Sidles JA, Harryman DT II: Practical Evaluation and Management of the Shoulder. Philadelphia: WB Saunders, 1994.)

History

Most patients with AMBRII are younger than 30 years (Fig. 16-137). Because the instability occurs in the mid-range positions of the shoulder, atraumatic instability typically causes discomfort and dysfunction in ordinary activities of daily living. Commonly, such patients have the greatest difficulty sleeping, lifting overhead, and throwing (Table 16-2 and Fig. 16-138). Their general health status as revealed by the SF-36 health survey is not as good on average as that of a comparable group of patients with traumatic instability (Fig. 16-139).

The onset is usually insidious, but it can occur after a minor injury or period of disuse. The unwanted translations can range from a sensation of a minor slip in the joint to complete dislocation of the humeral head from the glenoid. The displacement characteristically reduces spontaneously, after which the patient is usually able to return to previous activities without much pain or problem. As the condition progresses, the patient notices that the shoulder has become looser and might feel it slip out and clunk back in with increasing ease and in an increasing number of activities. The shoulder can become uncomfortable, even with the arm at rest. Patients might volunteer that they can make the shoulder pop out and that at times the shoulder feels as though it needs to be popped out on purpose.

It is important to document from the history the circumstances surrounding the onset of the problem, as well as each and every position of the shoulder in which the patient experiences instability. It is also important to note whether the opposite shoulder is symptomatic as well. A family history might reveal other family members similarly affected, in addition to conditions known to predispose to atraumatic instability, such as Ehlers–Danlos syndrome.

Many patients admit that they had a habit of dislocating the joint but that they can now no longer control the stability of the joint. The surgeon must determine whether habitual dislocation remains a feature of the patient's problem. It is obvious that it is difficult for surgery to cure habitual instability.

Finally, it is important to document the patient's expectations for the shoulder to ensure that the goals are within reach before treatment is started. In this particular condition, shoulder pain may be a prominent component of the clinical picture and this pain might not be responsive to surgical management.

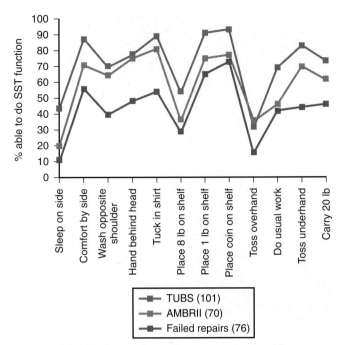

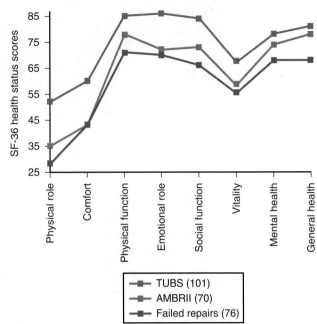

FIGURE 16-138 Comparison of responses to the 12 questions of the Simple Shoulder Test (SST) for groups of patients with traumatic instability (TUBS), atraumatic instability (AMBRII), and failed instability repairs.

FIGURE 16-139 Comparison of scores on the SF-36 general health status questionnaire for groups of patients with traumatic instability (TUBS), atraumatic instability (AMBRII), and failed instability repairs.

Physical Examination
Demonstration of Instability: The No-Touch Examination

Because glenohumeral instability is defined as a condition wherein the patient cannot maintain the humeral head in a centered position in the glenoid, it is critical to allow the patient to demonstrate his or her functional problem to the examiner. We invite the patient to "show me what your shoulder does that you don't like." In our experience, patients who respond "it just hurts" or "I don't know" are rarely good candidates for surgical reconstruction. On the other hand, patients who say "every time I put my arm in this position [e.g., abduction, extension, external rotation], it feels like it's going to slip out" define a mechanical problem that might be addressable with surgery. Patients who demonstrate a positive jerk test with posterior subluxation on cross-body adduction and reduction on abduction (Fig. 16-140; see Fig. 16-46) define the posterior direction of their problem and help the surgeon consider appropriate rehabilitative and surgical solutions. Patients who have instability with their arm at their side (see Figs. 16-20, 16-75, and 16-76) are usually not candidates for surgical reconstruction.

This no-touch examination coupled with a good history often gives most of the information needed to plan the management of the problem and has proved to be a much better predictor of outcome than tests of laxity, imaging, or arthroscopic evaluation.

Testing the Glenoid Concavity

In planning treatment for an unstable shoulder, it is important to know if the socket is sufficiently concave to center the humeral head. The adequacy of the concavity is assessed by the load and shift test, in which the humeral head is pressed into the glenoid and then displacing loads are applied in the directions of interest (Fig. 16-141). If the glenoid lip is insufficient and cannot be reconstructed with soft tissue methods, bony procedures need to be considered.

Laxity Tests. Laxity tests seek to define the amount of translation or rotation that an examiner can elicit in the relaxed shoulder. This translation is determined both by the position of the shoulder and by the properties of the ligaments and capsule. Translational and rotational laxity are closely related (see Figs. 16-52 to 16-55). When interpreting the significance of the degree of translation on laxity tests, it is important to use the contralateral shoulder as an example of what is "normal" for the patient.

In the past, laxity was confused with instability; treatments were directed at managing laxity rather than at enabling the head to stay centered in the glenoid. Shoulders without clear evidence of instability were tightened because they were lax and painful; the results were not good. For this reason, it is important to recognize that normal shoulders are lax and that laxity is often not increased in unstable shoulders (see Fig. 16-57).[105] Many

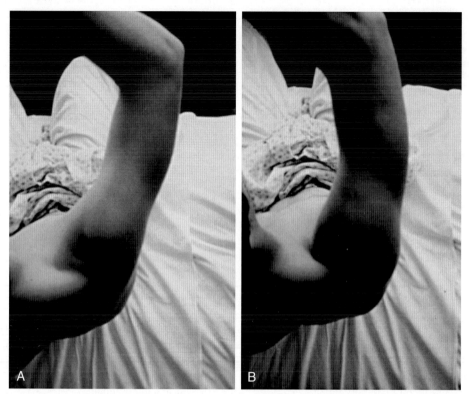

FIGURE 16-140 Voluntary jerk test. **A,** Normal appearance of the shoulder before the patient performs a jerk test. **B,** With movement of the arm horizontally across the body, the humeral head slides off the back of the glenoid with a jerk of dislocation and a prominence in the posterior aspect of the patient's shoulder. When the arm is moved back to the position shown in **A,** a jerk of reduction occurs.

normally stable shoulders, such as those of gymnasts, demonstrate substantial translation on laxity tests even though they are asymptomatic.

In performing the tests described next, it is important for examiner to note not only the amount of laxity but also any findings associated with the translation or rotation as well as the patient's subjective response to the test.

In the *drawer test* (Fig. 16-142), the patient is seated with the forearm resting on the lap and the shoulder relaxed. The examiner stands behind the patient. One of the examiner's hands stabilizes the shoulder girdle (scapula and clavicle) while the other grasps the proximal end of the humerus. These tests are performed with a minimal compressive load (just enough to center the head in the glenoid) and a substantial compressive load (to gain a feeling for the effectiveness of the glenoid concavity). Starting from the centered position with a minimal compressive load, the humerus is first pushed forward to determine the amount of anterior displacement relative to the scapula. The anterior translation of a normal shoulder reaches a firm end point with no clunking, no pain, and no apprehension. A clunk or snap on anterior subluxation or reduction can suggest a labral tear or Bankart lesion.[174]

In the *sulcus test* (Figs. 16-143 and 16-144), the patient sits with the arm relaxed at the side. The examiner centers the head with a mild compressive load and then pulls

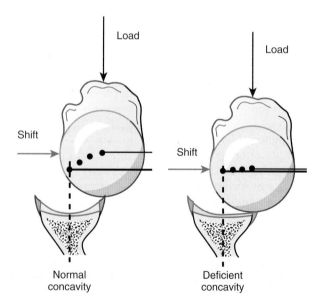

FIGURE 16-141 Load and shift test. The adequacy of the glenoid concavity in a given direction can be assessed by compressing the humeral head into the glenoid concavity and noting the amount of displacing force necessary to translate the head. The figure on the *left* shows a normal concavity and that on the *right* shows a diminished concavity in the direction of testing. (From Matsen FA III, Lippitt SB: Shoulder Surgery: Principles and Procedures. Philadelphia: WB Saunders, 2004, p 113.)

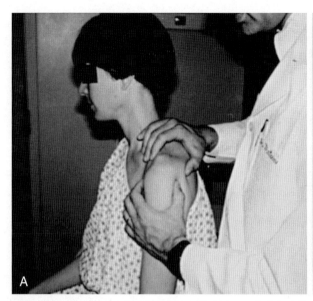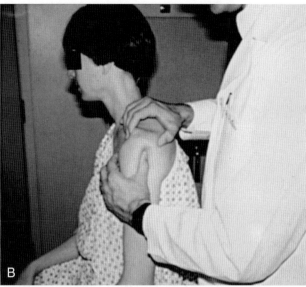

FIGURE 16-142 Drawer test. **A,** The patient is seated and the forearm is resting in the lap. The examiner stands behind the patient and stabilizes the shoulder girdle with one hand while grasping the proximal end of the humerus with the other and pressing the humeral head gently toward the scapula to center it in the glenoid. **B,** The head is then pushed forward to determine the amount of anterior displacement relative to the scapula. The head can then be returned to the neutral position, and a posterior force is applied to determine the amount of posterior translation relative to the scapula.

the arm downward. Inferior laxity is demonstrated if a sulcus or hollow appears inferior to the acromion.

In the *push–pull test* (Fig. 16-145), the patient lies supine with the shoulder off the edge of the table. The arm is in 90 degrees of abduction and 30 degrees of flexion. Standing next to the patient's hip, the examiner pulls up on the wrist with one hand while pushing down on the proximal part of the humerus with the other. Normal shoulders of relaxed patients often allow 50% posterior translation on this test.

Provocative Stability Tests. Stability tests examine the ability of the shoulder to resist challenges to stability in positions in which the ligaments are normally under tension. A key element of these tests is noting if the maneuver reproduces the symptoms of concern to the patient.

In the *fulcrum test* (Fig. 16-146), the patient lies supine at the edge of the examination table with the arm abducted to 90 degrees. The examiner places one hand on the table under the glenohumeral joint to act as a fulcrum. The patient's arm is gently and progressively extended and externally rotated over this fulcrum. Maintaining gentle passive external rotation for a minute fatigues the sub-scapularis and thereby challenges the capsular contribution to anterior stability of the shoulder. Normally no apprehension or translation occurs because the anterior ligaments are intact. A patient with anterior instability usually becomes apprehensive as this maneuver is carried out (watch the eyebrows for a clue that the shoulder is getting ready to dislocate); this finding suggests deficiency in the anterior stabilizing structures.

In the *crank* or *apprehension test* (Fig. 16-147), the patient sits with his or her back toward the examiner. The patient's arm is held in 90 degrees of abduction and external rotation. The examiner pulls back on the patient's wrist with one hand while stabilizing the back of the shoulder with the other. A patient with anterior instability usually becomes apprehensive with this maneuver.

In the *jerk test* (Fig. 16-148; see Fig. 16-140), the patient sits with the arm internally rotated and flexed forward to 90 degrees. The examiner grasps the elbow and axially loads the humerus in a proximal direction. While axial loading of the humerus is maintained, the arm is moved horizontally across the body. A positive test is indicated by a sudden jerk as the humeral head slides off the back of the glenoid. When the arm is returned to the original position of 90-degree abduction, a second jerk may be observed, that of the humeral head returning to the glenoid.

Strength Tests. The strength of abduction and rotation are tested to gauge the power of the muscles contributing to stability through concavity compression (Figs. 16-149 to 16-152). The strength of the scapular protractors and elevators is also tested to determine their ability to position the scapula securely (Fig. 16-153 and see Fig. 16-51).

Radiographs

In atraumatic instability, shoulder radiographs characteristically show no bony pathology, specifically, no postero-lateral humeral head defect, no glenoid rim fracture or new bone formation, and no evidence of tuberosity

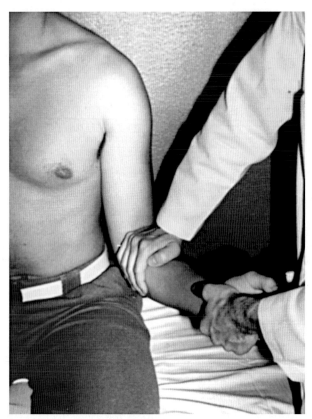

FIGURE 16-143 Sulcus test. The patient is seated with the arm relaxed and at the side. The examiner pulls downward on the arm. Inferior instability is demonstrated if a sulcus (or hollow) appears inferior to the acromion. The result of the sulcus test in this patient is negative.

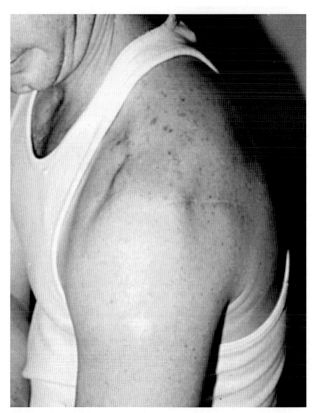

FIGURE 16-144 Sulcus sign. This patient had a posterior repair for glenohumeral instability. However, he continues to have inferior instability and demonstrates the sulcus (or hollow) just inferior to the anterior acromion during this sulcus test.

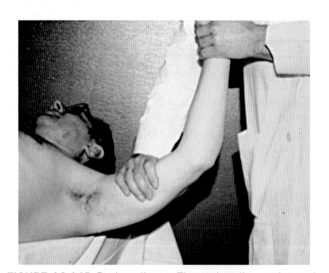

FIGURE 16-145 Push–pull test. The patient lies supine and relaxed with the shoulder at the edge of the examination table. The examiner pulls up on the wrist with one hand while pushing down on the proximal part of the humerus with the other. Approximately 50% posterior translation of the humerus on the glenoid is normal in relaxed patients.

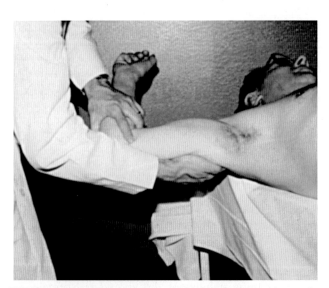

FIGURE 16-146 Fulcrum test. With the patient supine and the shoulder at the edge of the examination table, the arm is abducted to 90 degrees. The examiner's right hand is used as a fulcrum while the arm is gently and progressively extended and externally rotated. In the presence of anterior instability, the patient becomes apprehensive or the shoulder translates with this maneuver.

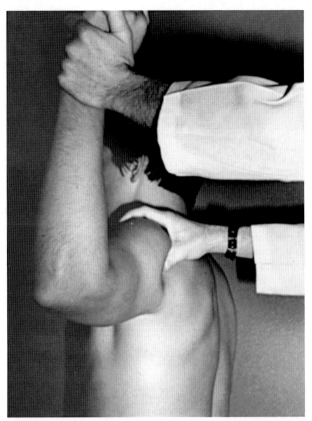

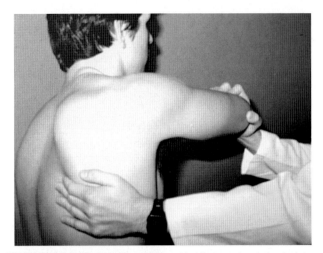

FIGURE 16-148 Jerk test. The patient's arm is abducted to 90 degrees and internally rotated. The examiner axially loads the humerus while the arm is moved horizontally across the body. The left hand stabilizes the scapula. A patient with a recurrent posterior instability might demonstrate a sudden jerk as the humeral head slides off the back of the glenoid or when it is reduced by moving the arm back to the starting position.

FIGURE 16-147 Crank test. The arm is held in 90 degrees of abduction and external rotation. The examiner's left hand is pulling back on the patient's wrist while the right hand stabilizes the back of the shoulder. A patient with anterior instability becomes apprehensive with this maneuver.

fracture. Because these patients typically demonstrate midrange instability, radiographs can show translation of the humeral head with respect to the glenoid; for example, the axillary view can show posterior subluxation. Occasionally, radiographs can suggest factors underlying the atraumatic instability, such as a relatively small or hypoplastic glenoid or a posteriorly inclined or otherwise dysplastic glenoid. The bony glenoid fossa can appear quite flat; however, it is difficult to relate the apparent depth of the bony socket to the effective depth of the fossa formed by cartilage and labrum covering the bone.

Arthroscopy

Using arthroscopy, Burkhart and colleagues have shown the bare spot of the glenoid to be a consistent reference point for the center of the glenoid.[447] Adequacy of the glenoid may be assessed by determining the amount of glenoid surrounding the bare area. The drive-through sign has been used as an indicator of laxity. In a study of 339 patients undergoing shoulder arthroscopy for any reason, the drive-through sign was found to have a sensitivity of 92% for the diagnosis of instability but only 37.6% specificity. The positive and negative predictive values were 29.9% and 94.2%, respectively.[448]

We do not use stress radiography, arthrography, MRI, or arthroscopy routinely in diagnosing atraumatic instability.

Traumatic Recurrent Instability

Traumatic instability is instability that arises from an injury of sufficient magnitude to tear the glenohumeral capsule, ligaments, labrum, or rotator cuff or produce a fracture of the humerus or glenoid. A typical patient is a 17-year-old skier whose recurrent anterior instability began with a fall on an abducted, externally rotated arm (although the condition has been reported in patients as young as 3 years).[449] To injure these strong structures, substantial force must be applied to them. The most common pathology associated with traumatic instability is avulsion of the anteroinferior capsule and ligaments from the glenoid rim. Considerable force is required to produce this avulsion in a healthy shoulder.

Although this load may be applied directly (for example, by having the proximal end of the humerus hit from behind), an indirect loading mechanism is more common. Indirect loading is most easily understood in terms of a simple model of the torques involved. When the upper extremity is abducted and externally rotated by a force applied to the hand, the following equation for torque equilibrium is a useful approximation, *if* we attribute the major stabilizing role to the ligament (see Fig. 16-61):

$$\text{IGHL tension} = \text{external load} \times \frac{\text{External load lever arm}}{\text{Humeral head radius}}$$

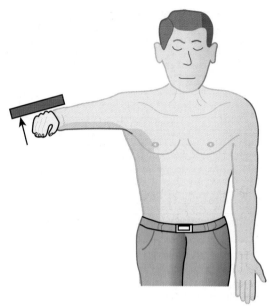

FIGURE 16-149 Supraspinatus test. The supraspinatus is tested by positioning the arm in 90 degrees of abduction in the plane of the scapula and in slight internal rotation. This puts the supraspinatus tendon on top of the humeral head. The patient holds this position while the examiner attempts to adduct the arm. (From Matsen FA III, Lippitt SB: Shoulder Surgery: Principles and Procedures. Philadelphia: WB Saunders, 2004, p 286.)

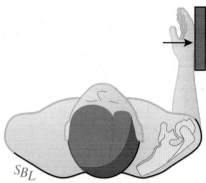

FIGURE 16-150 Infraspinatus test. The infraspinatus is tested by positioning the humerus with the elbow at the side and the forearm pointing straight ahead. The patient holds this position while the examiner attempts to push the arm into internal rotation. (From Matsen FA III, Lippitt SB: Shoulder Surgery: Principles and Procedures. Philadelphia: WB Saunders, 2004, p 287.)

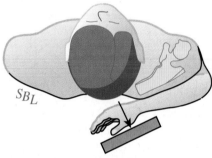

FIGURE 16-152 Lift-off test. The subscapularis may also be tested by having the patient push the hand away from the lumbar area posteriorly. (From Matsen FA III, Lippitt SB: Shoulder Surgery: Principles and Procedures. Philadelphia: WB Saunders, 2004, p 287.)

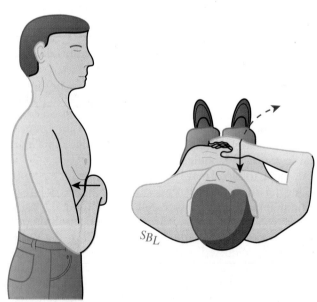

FIGURE 16-151 Subscapularis test. The subscapularis is tested by having the patient press the hand in toward the stomach. (From Matsen FA III, Lippitt SB: Shoulder Surgery: Principles and Procedures. Philadelphia: WB Saunders, 2004, p 287.)

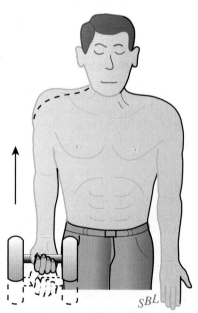

FIGURE 16-153 Trapezius shrug. The trapezius is strengthened by shrugging the shoulder upward while a weight is held in the hand. (From Matsen FA III, Lippitt SB: Shoulder Surgery: Principles and Procedures. Philadelphia: WB Saunders, 2004, p 345.)

If the radius of the humeral head is 1 in and the distance from the center of the head to the hand is 30 in, this formula suggests that the inferior glenohumeral ligament would experience a load 30 times greater than that applied to the hand. From this example we can see that a relatively small load is sufficient to produce the characteristic lesion of traumatic instability if this load is applied indirectly through the lever arm of the upper extremity.

Avulsion of the anterior glenohumeral ligament mechanism (see Figs. 16-3 and 16-120) deprives the joint of stability in positions in which this structure is a checkrein, such as in maximal external rotation and extension of the arm elevated near the coronal plane. Thus, it is evident that in recurrent traumatic instability, problems are most likely to occur when the arm is placed in a position approximating that in which the original injury occurred (see Figs. 16-146 and 16-147). Midrange instability can also result from a traumatic injury because the glenoid concavity may be compromised by avulsion of the labrum or fracture of the bony lip of the glenoid (see Fig. 16-31). Lessening of the effective glenoid arc compromises the effectiveness of concavity compression, reduces the balance stability angles, decreases the surface available for adhesion and cohesion, and compromises the ability of the glenoid suction cup to conform to the head of the humerus.

The corner of the glenoid abuts against the insertion of the cuff to the tuberosity when the humerus is extended, abducted, and externally rotated (Fig. 16-154).[98,450-452] Thus, the same forces that challenge the inferior glenohumeral ligament are also applied to the greater tuberosity–cuff insertion area. It is not surprising, therefore, that posterolateral humeral head defects, tuberosity fractures, and cuff injuries may be a part of the clinical picture of traumatic instability. The exact location and type of traumatic injury depend on the age of the patient and the magnitude, rate, and direction of force applied. Avulsions of the glenoid labrum, glenoid rim fractures, and posterolateral humeral head defects are more commonly seen in young persons. In patients older than 35 years, traumatic instability tends to be associated with fractures of the greater tuberosity and rotator cuff tears. This tendency increases with increasing age at the time of the initial traumatic dislocation. Thus, as a rule, younger patients require management of anterior lesions and older patients require management of posterior lesions.

Posterolateral humeral head defects are common features of traumatic instability. These lesions are often noted after the first traumatic dislocation and tend to increase in size with recurrent episodes. This impaction injury usually occurs when the anterior corner of the glenoid is driven into the posterolateral humeral articular surface. It is evident that this injury is close to the cuff insertion. Large head defects compromise stability by diminishing the articular congruity of the humerus.

To help recall the common aspects of traumatic instability, we use the acronym TUBS. The instability arises from a significant episode of *t*rauma, characteristically from abduction and extension of the arm elevated in the

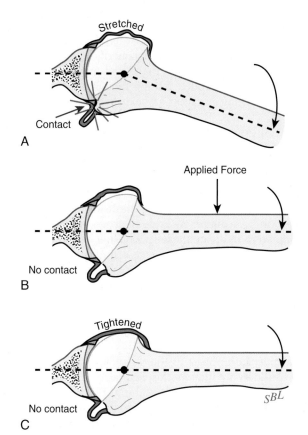

FIGURE 16-154 Posterior contact between the glenoid lip and the insertion of the cuff onto the tuberosity occurs in the apprehension, or fulcrum, position, especially if the anteroinferior aspect of the capsule has been stretched and is allowing the humerus to extend to an unusually posterior scapular plane. This contact can challenge the integrity of the posterior cuff insertion and the tuberosity (**A**). Application of a posteriorly directed force on the front of the shoulder can change the humeroscapular position enough to relieve this posterior abutment. This maneuver is similar to that described as the relocation test; however, this diagram suggests that the mechanism for relief of discomfort is avoidance of posterior abutment rather than elimination of subluxation (**B**). A similar protection from posterior abutment may be achieved by tightening the anterior part of the capsule, thus preventing extension of the humerus to a substantially posterior scapular plane (**C**). (From Matsen FA III, Lippitt SB, Sidles JA, Harryman DT II: Practical Evaluation and Management of the Shoulder. Philadelphia: WB Saunders, 1994.)

coronal plane. The resulting instability is usually *u*nidirectional in the anteroinferior direction. The pathology is generally an avulsion of the labrum and capsuloligamentous complex from the anterior inferior lip of the glenoid, commonly referred to as a *B*ankart lesion. With functionally significant recurrent traumatic instability, *s*urgical reconstruction of this labral and ligament avulsion is often required to restore stability.

The reader is referred to a review of the pathology and pathogenesis of traumatic instability by Wirth and Rockwood.[453]

History

Most patients with TUBS are between the ages of 14 and 34 years (Fig. 16-155). These patients characteristically have difficulty throwing overhand, but many patients also have problems sleeping, putting their hand behind their head, and lifting a gallon to head level (see Table 16-2 and Fig. 16-138). Their general health status as revealed by the SF-36 self-assessment questionnaire is better on average than that of a comparable group of patients with atraumatic instability (see Fig. 16-139).

The Initial Dislocation

The most important element in the history is a definition of the original injury. As is evident to anyone who has attempted to re-create these lesions in a cadaver, substantial force is required to produce a traumatic dislocation, and in most cadaver specimens, it is impossible to duplicate the Bankart injury mechanism because the humerus fractures first. In characteristic anterior traumatic instability, the structure that is avulsed is the strongest part of the shoulder's capsular mechanism: the anterior-inferior glenohumeral ligament. To tear this ligament, substantial force must be applied to the shoulder when the arm is in a position to tighten this ligament. Thus, the usual mechanism of injury involves the application of a large extension–external rotation force to the arm elevated near the coronal plane. Such a mechanism can occur in a fall while snow skiing, while executing a high-speed cut in water skiing, in an arm tackle during football, with a block of a volleyball or basketball shot, or in relatively violent industrial accidents in which a posteriorly directed force is applied to the hand while the arm is abducted and externally rotated. Awkward lifting on the job and rear-end automobile accidents would not be expected to provide the conditions or mechanism needed for this injury. Direct questioning and persistence are often necessary to elicit a full description of the mechanism of the initial injury, including the position of the shoulder and the direction and magnitude of the applied force, and this information is critical to establishing the diagnosis.

An initial traumatic dislocation often requires assistance in reduction rather than reducing spontaneously as is usually the case in atraumatic instability. Radiographs from previous emergency department visits may be available to show the shoulder in its dislocated position. Axillary or other neuropathy may have accompanied the glenohumeral dislocation. Any of these findings individually or in combination support the diagnosis of traumatic as opposed to atraumatic instability.

Traumatic instability can occur without a complete dislocation. In this situation, the injury produces a traumatic lesion, but the lesion is insufficient to allow the humeral head to completely escape from the glenoid. The shoulder may be unstable because as a result of the injury, it manifests apprehension or subluxation when the arm is placed near the position of injury. Such patients have no history of the need for reduction and have no

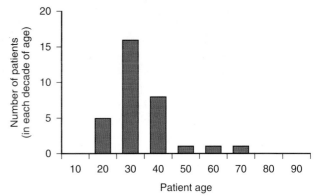

FIGURE 16-155 Age distribution of 32 patients with traumatic instability. (From Matsen FA III, Lippitt SB, Sidles JA, Harryman DT II: Practical Evaluation and Management of the Shoulder. Philadelphia: WB Saunders, 1994.)

radiographs with the shoulder in the dislocated position. Thus, the diagnosis rests to an even greater extent on a careful history that focuses on the position and forces involved in the initial episode.

Subsequent Episodes of Instability

Characteristically, a shoulder with traumatic instability is comfortable when troublesome positions are avoided. However, the apprehension or fear of instability can prevent the patient from returning to work or sports. Recurrent subluxation or dislocation can occur when the shoulder is unexpectedly forced into the abducted, externally rotated position or during sleep when the patient's active guard is less effective. The patient might have a history of increasing ease of dislocation as the remaining stabilizing factors are progressively compromised.

Physical Examination

We use the same approach to the physical examination of the recurrent traumatic unstable shoulder as we have described previously in this section for atraumatic instability: the no-touch examination, testing the glenoid concavity, laxity tests, and provocative tests.

The goal of physical examination is largely to confirm the impression obtained from the history: that a certain combination of arm position and application of force produces the actual or threatened glenohumeral instability that is of functional concern to the patient. If the diagnosis has been rigorously established from the history—for example, by documented recurrent anterior dislocations—it is not necessary to risk redislocation on the physical examination. If such rigorous documentation is not available, however, the examiner must challenge the ligamentous stability of the shoulder in the suspected position of vulnerability and be prepared to reduce the shoulder should a dislocation result.

The most common direction of recurrent traumatic instability is anteroinferior. Stability in this position is challenged by externally rotating and extending the arm

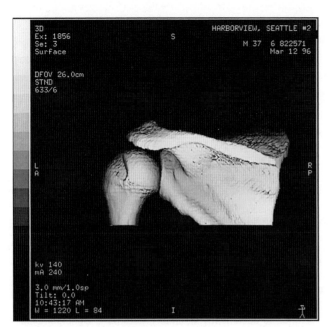

FIGURE 16-156 3D CT reconstruction of the left shoulder of a 37-year-old man 3 days after his first traumatic glenohumeral dislocation. The bony defect in the posterolateral aspect of the humeral head is clearly shown. The patient recovered normal shoulder function with nonoperative management.

elevated to various degrees in the coronal plane (see Figs. 16-146 and 16-147). It may be necessary to hold the arm in the challenging position for 1 to 2 minutes to fatigue the stabilizing musculature. When the muscle stabilizers tire, the capsuloligamentous mechanism is all that is holding the humeral head in the glenoid. At this moment a patient with traumatic anterior instability becomes apprehensive because of recognition that the shoulder is about to come out of joint. This recognition strongly supports the diagnosis of traumatic anterior instability.

The magnitude of translation on standard tests of glenohumeral laxity (see Figs. 16-142 to 16-145) does not necessarily distinguish stable from unstable shoulders (see Fig. 16-57). However, an experienced examiner can detect diminished resistance to anterior translation on the drawer test when the humeral head is compressed into the glenoid fossa; the diminished resistance in this case indicates loss of the anterior glenoid lip. This maneuver can also elicit grinding as the humeral head slides over the bony edge of the glenoid from which the labrum has been avulsed or elicit catching as the head passes over a torn glenoid labrum.

Pain on abduction, external rotation, and extension is not specific for instability. Such pain can relate to shoulder stiffness or alternatively to abutment of the glenoid against the cuff insertion to the head posteriorly.[98,451,452,454] Relief of this pain by anterior pressure on the humeral head can result from diminished stretch on the anterior capsule or from relief of the abutment posteriorly (see Fig. 16-154).

In all patients with traumatic instability, particularly those older than 35 years, the strength of internal and external rotation must be examined to explore the possibility of cuff weakness or tear. Finally, a neurologic examination is performed to determine the integrity of the axillary nerve and other branches of the brachial plexus.

Radiographs and Other Tests

Radiographs often help provide confirmation of traumatic glenohumeral instability.

Humeral Head Changes

One of the most common findings is indentation or impaction in the posterior aspect of the humeral head from contact with the anteroinferior corner of the glenoid when the joint was dislocated (Fig. 16-156; see Figs. 16-3 and 16-109). In their classic article,[11] Hill and Sachs evaluated the relationship of humeral head defects to shoulder instability. They concluded that more than two thirds of anterior shoulder dislocations are complicated by a bony injury of the humerus or scapula.

> Compression fractures as a result of impingement of the weakest portion of the humeral head, that is, the posterior lateral aspect of the articular surface against the anterior rim of the glenoid fossa, are found so frequently in cases of habitual dislocation that they have been described as a typical defect. These defects are sustained at the time of the original dislocation. A special sign is the sharp, vertical, dense medial border of the groove known as the line of condensation, the length of which is correlated with the size of the defect.[11]

They reported the defect in only 27% of 119 acute anterior dislocations but in 74% of 15 recurrent anterior dislocations. However, they stated that the incidence of the groove defect was low, undoubtedly because it was only in the last 6 months of their 10-year study (1930 to 1940) that they used special radiographic views. The size of the defect varied in length (cephalocaudal) from 5 mm to 3 cm, in width from 3 mm to 2 cm, and in depth from 10 mm to 22 mm.[455]

A number of special projections have been used to enhance visualization of the Hill–Sachs defect.[7,19,31,270,456-459] Two of these views bear special mention.

Stryker Notch View. The patient is supine on the table with the cassette placed under the shoulder.[458] The palm of the hand of the affected shoulder is placed on top of the head, with the fingers directed toward the back of the head. The elbow of the affected shoulder should point straight upward. The x-ray beam tilts 10 degrees toward the head and is centered over the coracoid process (Fig. 16-157). This technique was developed by William S. Stryker and reported by Hall and coworkers.[458] They stated that they could demonstrate the humeral head defect in 90% of 20 patients with a history of recurring anterior dislocation of the shoulder.

Apical Oblique View. Garth and coworkers[241,321] described the apical oblique projection of the shoulder (see Fig. 16-112). In this technique, the patient sits with the scapula flat against the cassette (as for the AP view in the plane of the scapula). The arm may be in a sling. The x-ray beam is centered on the coracoid and directed perpendicular to the cassette (45 degrees to the coronal plane), except that it is angled 45 degrees caudally. The beam passes tangential to the articular surface of the glenohumeral joint and the posterolateral aspect of the humeral head. This view is likely to reveal both anterior glenoid lip defects and posterolateral impression fractures of the humeral head.

The incidence of the Hill–Sachs defect reported depends on both the radiographic technique and the patient population. Symeonides[31] reported the humeral head defect in 23 of 45 patients who had recurrent anterior dislocations of the shoulder. However, at the time of surgery he could confirm only 18 of 45.

Eyre-Brook[460] reported a 64% incidence of the Hill–Sachs defect in 17 recurrent anterior dislocations, and Brav[461] recorded a rate of 67% in 69 recurrent dislocations. Rowe and colleagues[462] noted the defect in 38% of 125 acute dislocations and in 57% of 63 recurrent dislocations. Adams[394] reported that the defect was found at the time of surgery in 82% of 68 patients. Palmer and Widen[463] found the defect at surgery in all 60 patients.

Calandra and coworkers[464] used diagnostic arthroscopy to prospectively study the incidence of Hill–Sach lesions. In a young population of 32 patients with a mean age of 28 years, the frequency of this lesion was 47% for initial anterior shoulder dislocations.

Danzig and colleagues[465] reported that in cadaveric and clinical studies, no single view always reveals the humeral head compression fracture. Pavlov and coworkers[270] and Rozing and associates[466] found that the Stryker notch view taken in internal rotation best revealed the posterolateral humeral head defect (see Fig. 16-157).

The demonstration of a posterolateral humeral head defect strongly indicates that the shoulder has been subjected to a traumatic anterior dislocation. When these factors are already known—for example, in a 17-year-old whose recurrent anterior dislocations began with a well-documented abduction–external rotation injury in football—it is not necessary to spend a great deal of effort demonstrating the humeral head defect because it is very likely to be present even if not seen on radiographs and the existence of such a lesion does not in itself alter our management of the patient.

Glenoid Changes

Standard radiographs can reveal a periosteal reaction to the ligamentous avulsion at the glenoid lip or a fracture (see Figs. 16-6 and 16-115), erosion (see Fig. 16-111), or new bone formation (see Figs. 16-96 and 16-110) at the glenoid rim. Modifications of the axillary view can help in identifying glenoid rim changes. Rokous and colleagues[467] described the West Point axillary view.[313] In this technique, the patient is placed prone on the x-ray

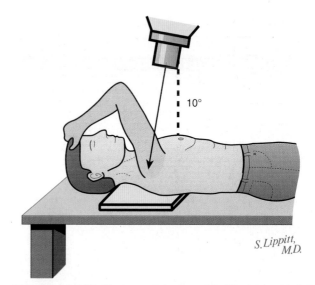

FIGURE 16-157 Stryker notch view. (Modified from Hall RH, Isaac F, Booth CR: Dislocations of the shoulder with special reference to accompanying small fractures. J Bone Joint Surg Am 41:489-494, 1959.)

table with the involved shoulder on a pad raised 7.5 cm from the top of the table. The head and neck are turned away from the involved side. With the cassette held against the superior aspect of the shoulder, the x-ray beam is centered on the axilla, 25 degrees downward from the horizontal and 25 degrees medial. The resulting radiograph is a tangential view of the anteroinferior rim of the glenoid (see Fig. 16-106). Using this view, Rokous and associates demonstrated bony abnormalities of the anterior glenoid rim in 53 of 63 patients whose histories indicated traumatic instability of the shoulder. Cyprien and coworkers[138] demonstrated lessening of the glenoid diameter and shortening of the anterior glenoid rim in shoulders with recurrent anterior dislocation. Blazina and Satzman[468] also reported anteroinferior glenoid rim fractures seen on the axillary view in nine of their cases. We have found that high-quality AP and axillary radiographs can give substantial information about the condition of the anterior glenoid lip (Figs. 16-158 and 16-159).

Special Radiographic Techniques

Most often the diagnosis of recurrent traumatic instability is clear from a careful history, physical examination, and plain radiographs. Although related pathology can be seen with additional radiographic views,[46,119,469,470] CT arthrography,[471-480] fluoroscopy,[481] or MRI, these additional tests are rarely cost-effective in the clinical evaluation and management of shoulders with characteristic traumatic instability.[482,483] Although CT evidence of labral or capsular pathology is unlikely to change management of the shoulder, contrast CT scans can help document flattening of the anteroinferior glenoid concavity caused by loss of articular cartilage (see Fig. 16-113). CT scans can also be useful in defining the magnitude of bone loss when sizable humeral head or glenoid defects are suggested on

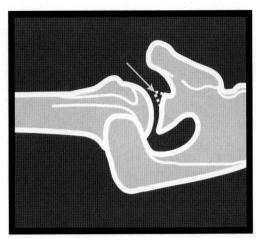

FIGURE 16-158 Axillary view showing anterior glenoid deficiency. This axillary view shows a bony defect (*arrow*) of the anterior glenoid lip. (From Matsen FA III, Lippitt SB: Shoulder Surgery: Principles and Procedures. Philadelphia: WB Saunders, 2004, p 117.)

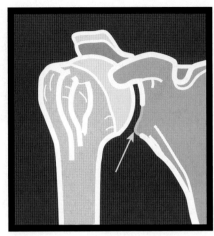

FIGURE 16-159 AP view showing loss of the anterior inferior cortical line. The normally sclerotic border of the anterior inferior glenoid lip has been worn away (*arrow*). (From Matsen FA III, Lippitt SB: Shoulder Surgery: Principles and Procedures. Philadelphia: WB Saunders, 2004, p 117.)

plain radiographs (see Figs. 16-114 and 16-115).[484,485] When previous glenoid bone blocks have been carried out or hardware inserted, CT scans are useful for examining the possibility of their encroachment on the humeral head.[13,471,486]

Although many articles have been written on the use of MRI for imaging the labrum and capsule of an unstable shoulder[463,487-489] (Fig. 16-160), the clinical cost-effectiveness of this examination awaits definition. Iannotti and colleagues[489] reported that the sensitivity and specificity of MRI in the diagnosis of labral tears associated with glenohumeral instability were 88% and 93%, respectively (Fig. 16-161). However, in a blinded study, Garneau and associates[490] found that it was insensitive and nonspecific for labral pathology. Even if MRI reliably yielded this information, it is unclear how it would be cost-effective in management because patients with refractory instability would be considered for surgery with or without such data.

MRI after postoperative recurrence of instability is less accurate than on unoperated shoulders. For imaging of recurrent labral lesions, MR arthrography has a higher sensitivity for detecting recurrent labral lesions than MRI does, 100% versus 71%, respectively.[491] The specificity of MR arthrography in this study was 60% versus 80% for standard MRI. Indirect MR arthrography in this study had 100% sensitivity and specificity in six shoulders, two of which had recurrent labral tears.

Rotator Cuff Imaging. Patients whose onset of traumatic instability occurred after the age of 35 years might have evidence of rotator cuff pathology on the history and physical examination. Particular concern arises if weakness of external rotation or elevation persists longer than a week or so. In these situations, preoperative imaging of cuff integrity can play an important role in surgical planning; for example, the approach for rotator cuff

repair is quite different from the approach for repair of an anteroinferior capsular lesion. Arthrography, ultrasound, or MRI can be useful in this situation.

Electromyography. Electromyography may be helpful in evaluating a patient with recurrent traumatic instability if the history and physical examination suggest residual brachial plexus lesions such as an axillary or suprascapular nerve palsy.

Arthroscopy. Because of the information gained from the history, physical examination, and plain films, diagnostic arthroscopy is not a necessary prelude to surgical repair of documented recurrent traumatic instability. Although it rarely changes the surgical approach, shoulder arthroscopy has helped define some of the pathology associated

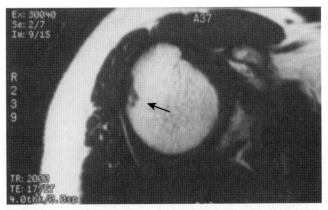

FIGURE 16-160 MRI demonstrating a focal abnormality in the posterolateral aspect of the humeral head (*arrow*) that is consistent with a recent episode of anterior glenohumeral instability. The plain x-ray films were interpreted as normal. (From Rockwood CA Jr, Green DP, Bucholz RW [eds]: Fractures in Adults. Philadelphia: JB Lippincott, 1991.)

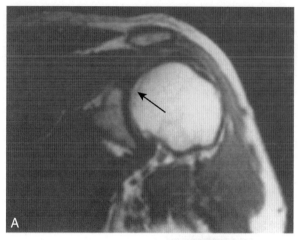

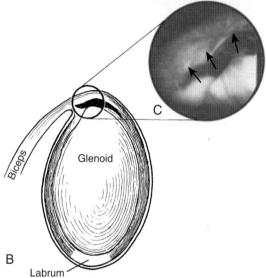

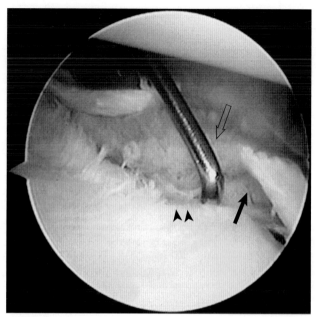

FIGURE 16-162 A Bankart lesion in a patient with recurrent anteroinferior instability. Note the traumatic disruption of the glenoid labrum (*solid arrow*), fraying of articular cartilage at the glenoid rim (*arrowheads*), and anterior capsular scarring with synovitis along the inferior glenohumeral ligament (*open arrow*). (Courtesy of Douglas T. Harryman II, MD, Department of Orthopaedics, University of Washington.)

FIGURE 16-161 Lesion of the long head of the biceps tendon origin and superior glenoid labrum. **A,** Lesion (*arrow*) as seen on MRI. **B,** Diagram of anatomy. **C,** Lesion (*arrows*) as seen on arthroscopic examination. (From Rockwood CA Jr, Green DP, Bucholz RW [eds]: Fractures in Adults. Philadelphia: JB Lippincott, 1991.)

with recurrent instability. Such lesions include labral tears, capsular rents, humeral head defects, and rotator cuff defects (see Fig. 16-161).[241,244,478,492-503]

An arthroscopic classification of anterior labral Bankart lesions was proposed by Green and Christensen.[504] In 37 cases, they described the arthroscopic appearance common to five separate groups:

Type I is the normal intact labrum.
Type II is a simple detachment of the labrum from the glenoid.
Type III is an intrasubstance tear of the glenoid labrum.
Type IV is a detachment of the labrum with significant fraying or degeneration.
Type V is complete degeneration or absence of the glenoid labrum.

Neviaser found that occasionally, the anterior labroligamentous periosteal sleeve is avulsed from the glenoid.[505] This injury has become known as the ALPSA lesion. The posterior labral periosteal sleeve avulsion (POLPSA lesion) described by Simons and colleagues has been shown to be associated with posterior instability,[506] tends to occur in younger patients, and is similar to the anterior version, the ALPSA lesion. The labrum is intact, but separated from the glenoid by an avulsion of its periosteum. The POLPSA lesion has been seen on MRI evaluation.[507]

Gleyze and Habermeyer noted that shoulders with more than five recurrent dislocations had erosion of the anterior articular cartilage.[508] Harryman detected labral damage in all patients treated for recurrent anterior traumatic instability (Fig. 16-162) and in 20% of patients treated for significant articular erosion to subchondral bone (Fig. 16-163).[509]

Other lesions may be associated with Bankart lesions. Snyder and associates[510] and Warner and coworkers[511] found an association of superior labral detachment and Bankart lesions.

Wolf and colleagues reported that 6 of 64 patients with anterior instability had avulsion of the glenohumeral ligaments from the humerus, whereas 47 had true Bankart lesions (73.5%).[512]

Arthroscopy has revealed defects in the articular cartilage of the posterolateral humeral head that would not be detected on radiographs (Figs. 16-164 to 16-166).

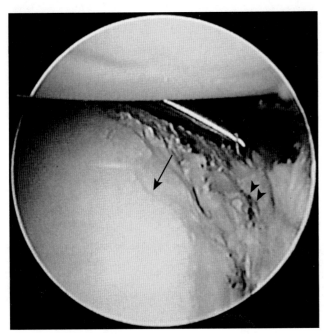

FIGURE 16-163 Chronic anteroinferior instability with evidence of erosion of articular cartilage to subchondral bone (*arrow*) and degenerative erosion of the labrum (*arrowheads*). (Courtesy of Douglas T. Harryman II, MD, Department of Orthopaedics, University of Washington.)

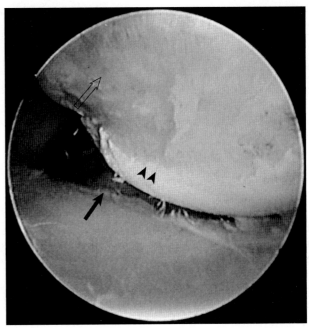

FIGURE 16-164 Visualizing the anterior rim of the glenoid (*solid arrow*) and the posterior edge of the humeral articular surface (*arrowheads*) adjacent to a large Hill–Sachs defect (*open arrow*) with the humerus in abduction and external rotation. (Courtesy of Douglas T. Harryman II, MD, Department of Orthopaedics, University of Washington.)

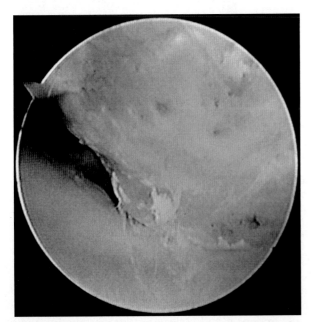

FIGURE 16-165 External rotation is increased until the humeral head suddenly dislocates over the edge of the anterior glenoid rim. After repair, external rotation of the glenohumeral joint must be checked adequately to maintain articular contact. (Courtesy of Douglas T. Harryman II, MD, Department of Orthopaedics, University of Washington.)

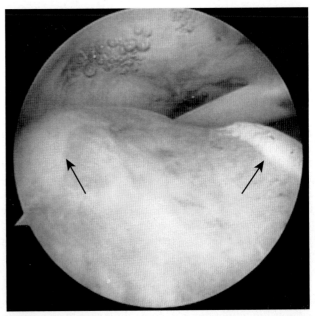

FIGURE 16-166 An extensive Hill–Sachs defect that crosses the superior humeral articular surface (*arrows*). Even with this degree of articular surface loss, an arthroscopic Bankart repair was performed with use of the Seattle Bankart guide and has been entirely successful. (Courtesy of Douglas T. Harryman II, MD, Department of Orthopaedics, University of Washington.)

TREATMENT

Nonoperative Management

As we emphasized in the section "Mechanisms of Glenohumeral Stability," coordinated, strong muscle contraction is a key element in stabilization of the humeral head in the glenoid. Patients with traumatic instability were found to have statistically significant humeral translation toward their direction of instability in abduction and external rotation. Patients with atraumatic instability also had decentralization of the humeral head, but in nonuniform directions. Those with traumatic instability were able to recenter the head with muscular action, whereas atraumatic patients were not.[513] This inability suggests that patients with atraumatic instability can have an insufficient glenoid concavity. Under these conditions, optimal neuromuscular control is required of the rotator cuff muscles, deltoid and pectoralis major, and the scapular musculature. These dynamic stabilizing mechanisms require muscle strength, coordination, and training. Such a program is likely to be of particular benefit in patients with atraumatic (AMBRII) instability[179,514] because optimizing neuromuscular control can help balance the humeral head in the glenoid. Nonoperative management is also an especially attractive option for children, for patients with voluntary instability,[514] for those with posterior glenohumeral instability, and for those requiring a supranormal range of motion (such as baseball pitchers and gymnasts, in whom surgical management often does not permit return to a competitive level of function).[245,514-516]

Strengthening of the rotator cuff, deltoid, and scapular motors can be accomplished with a simple series of exercises (Figs. 16-167 and 16-168; see also Figs. 16-51 and 16-153). During the early phases of the program, the patient is taught to use the shoulder only in the most stable positions, that is, those in which the humerus is elevated in the plane of the scapula (avoiding, for example, elevation in the sagittal plane with the arm in internal rotation if the patient has a tendency to posterior instability). As coordination and confidence improve, progressively less intrinsically stable positions are attempted. Taping can provide a useful reminder to avoid unstable positions (Fig. 16-169). The shoulder is then progressed to smooth repetitive activities such as swimming or rowing, which can play an essential role in retraining the neuromuscular patterns required for stability.

Finally, it is important to avoid all activities and habits that promote glenohumeral subluxation or dislocation; patients are taught that each time their shoulder goes out, it gets easier for it to go out the next time.

Rockwood and colleagues[517] and Burkhead and Rockwood[421] found that 16% of patients with traumatic subluxation, 80% of those with anterior atraumatic subluxation, and 90% of those with posterior instability responded to a rehabilitation program (Fig. 16-170). Brostrom and asso-

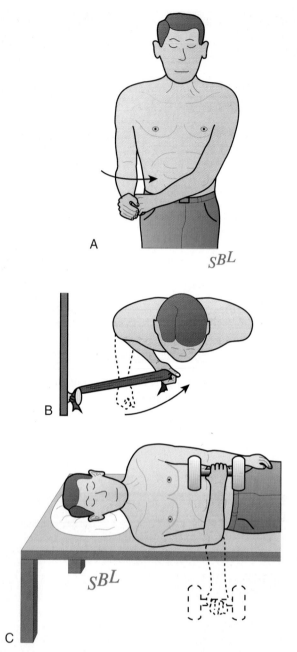

FIGURE 16-167 Internal rotation can be strengthened with isometrics (**A**), rubber tubing (**B**), or free weights (**C**). (From Matsen FA III, Lippitt SB, Sidles JA, Harryman DT II: Practical Evaluation and Management of the Shoulder. Philadelphia: WB Saunders, 1994.)

ciates[518] found that exercises improved all but 5 of 33 unstable shoulders, including traumatic and atraumatic types. Anderson and colleagues demonstrated the effectiveness of an exercise program that used rubber bands to improve internal rotator strength.[519]

Wirth and coworkers demonstrated that nonoperative management can be successful even in patients with a congenital factor in their instability. They reported 16 patients with hypoplasia of the glenoid.[231] A subset of this

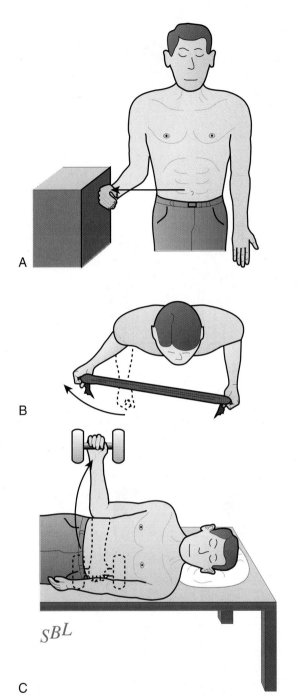

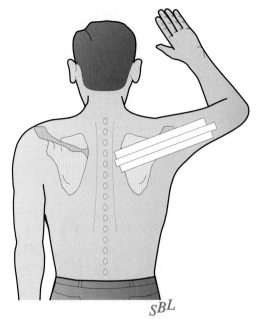

FIGURE 16-169 Training tape is applied across the back of the shoulder as a reminder to avoid unbalanced positions. (Modified from Matsen FA III, Lippitt SB, Sidles JA, Harryman DT II: Practical Evaluation and Management of the Shoulder. Philadelphia: WB Saunders, 1994.)

FIGURE 16-168 External rotation strengthening with isometrics (**A**), rubber tubing (**B**), or free weights (**C**). (From Matsen FA III, Lippitt SB, Sidles JA, Harryman DT II: Practical Evaluation and Management of the Shoulder. Philadelphia: WB Saunders, 1994.)

group consisted of 5 patients with bilateral glenoid hypoplasia and multidirectional instability as indicated by symptomatic increased translation of the humeral head during anterior, inferior, and posterior drawer testing. Generalized ligamentous laxity of the metacarpophalangeal joints, elbows, or knees was noted in all 5 patients in the subset. Four of the patients had been involved in

occupational or recreational activities, or both, that had placed heavy demands on the shoulders. All 4 had considerable improvement in ratings for pain and the ability to carry out work and sports activities at an average of 3 months after they had begun a strengthening program designed by Rockwood. None of the patients needed vocational rehabilitation despite the heavy demands on their shoulders associated with their occupational or recreational activities.

These results again support the concept of concavity compression and point out that when the concavity is compromised, stability can often be restored by optimizing balance of the compression mechanism.

Surgical Management of Traumatic Anterior Instability

Lenters and colleagues conducted a formal meta-analysis of the literature comparing open and arthroscopic repairs for anterior shoulder instability.[520] They concluded that the available evidence indicated that arthroscopic approaches are not as effective as open approaches in preventing recurrent instability or enabling patients to return to work. However, arthroscopic approaches resulted in better function as reflected by the Rowe scores in the randomized clinical trials. Arthroscopic repairs are discussed in other chapters in this text.

Open Operative Management

Surgical stabilization of the glenohumeral joint is considered for patients with traumatic instability if the condition

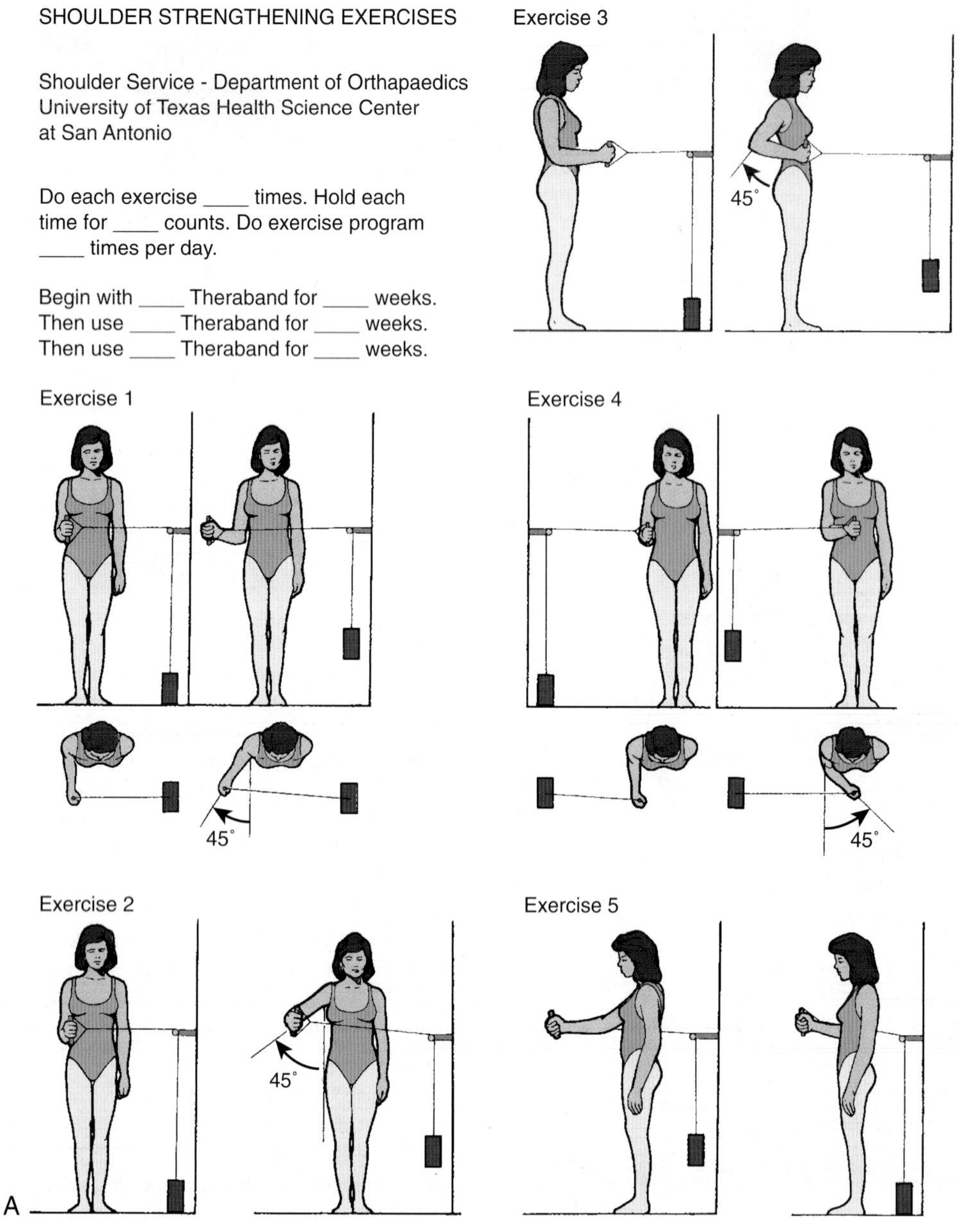

SHOULDER STRENGTHENING EXERCISES

Shoulder Service - Department of Orthapaedics
University of Texas Health Science Center
at San Antonio

Do each exercise _____ times. Hold each
time for _____ counts. Do exercise program
_____ times per day.

Begin with _____ Theraband for _____ weeks.
Then use _____ Theraband for _____ weeks.
Then use _____ Theraband for _____ weeks.

Exercise 1

Exercise 2

Exercise 3

Exercise 4

Exercise 5

FIGURE 16-170 Shoulder-strengthening exercises. **A,** Initially, the patient is given rubber exercise bands to strengthen the rotator cuff muscles and the three parts of the deltoid. After achieving proficiency in rubber resistance with exercises 1 to 5, the patient is given an exercise kit that consists of a pulley, hook, rope, and handle. The pulley is attached to the hook, which is fixed to the wall, and the five exercises are performed. Initially, the patient is instructed to use 5 or 10 lb of weight; the weight is gradually increased over a period of several months to as much as 25 lb. The purpose of the five exercises is to strengthen the three parts of the deltoid muscles, the internal rotators, and the external rotators.

Continued

repeatedly compromises shoulder comfort or function in spite of a reasonable trial of internal and external rotator strengthening and coordination exercises. When contemplating a surgical approach to anterior traumatic glenohumeral instability, it is essential to preoperatively identify any factors that can compromise the surgical result, such as a tendency for voluntary dislocation, generalized ligamentous laxity, multidirectional instability, seizures, alcoholism, occupational hazards, chemical dependency, smoking, or significant bony defects of the humeral head

or glenoid. If these conditions exist, it is necessary to modify the management approach. These factors can and should be identified preoperatively.

In the past, many surgical procedures have been described for treating recurrent anterior glenohumeral instability. Tightening and to some degree realigning the subscapularis tendon and partially eliminating external rotation were the goals of the Magnuson–Stack and the Putti–Platt procedures. The Putti–Platt operation also tightened and reinforced the anterior capsule. Reattach-

SHOULDER STRENGTHENING AND STRETCHING EXERCISES

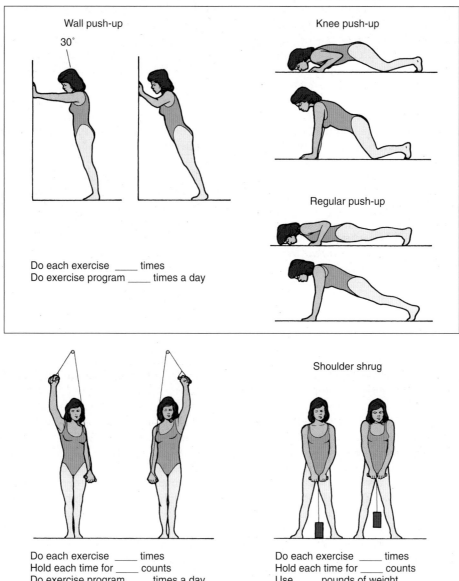

Wall push-up

30°

Knee push-up

Regular push-up

Do each exercise _____ times
Do exercise program _____ times a day

Shoulder shrug

Do each exercise _____ times
Hold each time for _____ counts
Do exercise program _____ times a day

Do each exercise _____ times
Hold each time for _____ counts
Use _____ pounds of weight
Do exercise program _____ times a day

B

FIGURE 16-170, cont'd B, In addition, the patient is instructed in exercises to strengthen the scapular stabilizer muscles. To strengthen the serratus anterior and the rhomboids, the patient is instructed to first do wall pushups, then gradually do knee pushups, and later do regular pushups. The shoulder-shrug exercise is used to strengthen the trapezius and levator scapulae muscles.

ment of the capsule and glenoid labrum to the glenoid lip was the goal of the DuToit staple capsulorrhaphy and the Eyre-Brook capsulorrhaphy.[395,521] The Bristow procedure transferred the tip of the coracoid process with its muscle attachments to create a musculotendinous sling across the anteroinferior glenohumeral joint. An anterior glenoid bone buttress was the objective of the Oudard and Trillat procedures. Augmentation of the bony anterior glenoid lip was the goal of anterior bone block procedures such as the Eden–Hybbinette procedure. Haaker

and coworkers[522] added an autogenous bone graft to the glenoid rim for recurrent instability. In their series of recurrent instabilities in 24 young soldiers, they used screws to fix an anterior iliac crest graft to the anterior glenoid rim. At the conclusion of graft placement, the glenoid labrum is replaced over the graft.

Large posterolateral humeral head defects have been approached by limiting external rotation, by filling the defect with the infraspinatus tendon, or by performing a rotational osteotomy of the humerus.[437,438,523,524]

As will be seen later, most of the reported series on the various types of reconstruction have yielded "excellent" results. However, it is very difficult to determine how each author graded the results. For example, if the patient has no recurrence after repair but has loss of 45 degrees of external rotation and cannot throw, is that a fair, good, or excellent result? The simple fact that the shoulder no longer dislocates cannot be equated with an excellent result. Although the older literature suggested that the goal of surgery for anterior dislocation of the shoulder was to limit external rotation, more modern literature suggests that a reconstruction can both prevent recurrent dislocation and allow nearly normal range of motion and comfortable function.

Capsulolabral Reconstruction

The objective of anatomic repair for traumatic instability is reconstruction of the avulsed capsule and labrum at the glenoid lip, often referred to as a *Bankart repair*. This type of repair was apparently first performed in 1906 by Perthes,[1] who recommended repair of the anterior capsule to the anterior glenoid rim. He was not in doubt about the pathology of traumatic instability: "In every case the anterior margin of the glenoid cavity will be found to be smooth, rounded, and free of any attachments, and a blunt instrument can be passed freely inwards over the bare bone on the front of the neck of the scapula." He reattached the capsule to the glenoid rim by placing drill holes through the bone.

Credit for this type of repair should go to Perthes, but the popularity of the technique is due to the work of Bankart,[2,21] who first performed the operation in 1923 on one of his former house surgeons. The procedure commonly used today is based on Bankart's 1939 article, in which he discusses repair of the capsule to the bone of the anterior glenoid through the use of drill holes and suture. The subscapularis muscle, which is carefully divided to expose the capsule, is reapproximated without any overlap or shortening. Bankart reported 27 consecutive cases with "full movements of the joint and in no case has there been any recurrence of the dislocation."[243,382,467,468]

There are several significant differences between Bankart's original method and the capsulolabral reconstruction currently recommended. Today we do not osteotomize the coracoid, we do not shave off bone from the anterior glenoid, and we strive to reattach the capsule and any residual labrum up on the surface of the glenoid lip rather than on the anterior aspect of the glenoid, as shown by Bankart.[139]

Hovelius and coworkers[525] found a 2% redislocation rate after the Bankart procedure versus a 19% rate after the Putti–Platt procedure. More than one third of the patients younger than 25 years were dissatisfied with the results of the Putti–Platt procedure. Rowe and Zarins[243] reported a series of 50 subluxating shoulders in which good or excellent results were achieved in 94% after a Bankart repair. A Bankart lesion was found in 64% of

these shoulders. Rowe and coworkers[462] reported on 51 shoulders with a fracture of the anterior rim of the glenoid; 18 shoulders had a fracture involving one sixth or less of the glenoid, 26 involved one fourth of the glenoid, and 7 had one third of the anterior glenoid fractured off. In this group of patients who were treated with a Bankart repair without particular attention paid to the fracture, the overall incidence of failure was 2%. Prozorovskii and colleagues[526] reported no recurrences in the long-term follow-up of 41 Bankart repairs. Martin and coworkers[527] reported excellent results and minimal degenerative change in a 10-year follow-up of 53 patients managed with a Bankart repair.

Although many variations on the method of attaching the capsule to the glenoid have been described, no method has been demonstrated to be safer or more secure than suture passed through drill holes in the lip of the glenoid.[528-530] Modifications of the technique do not seem to result in substantial improvement in the efficacy, cost, or safety of the procedure; for example, suture anchors do not have strength equal to that of sutures passed through holes in the glenoid lip.[531-533] Furthermore, when suture anchors are placed in the ideal location for capsulolabral reattachment, they have a substantial risk of rubbing on the articular surface of the humerus. In addition, it is difficult to restore the effective glenoid depth when suture anchors are used (see Fig. 16-32D).

Although some have advocated the addition of a capsular shift or capsulorrhaphy to the Bankart repair,[534] it does not seem necessary or advisable in the usual case of traumatic instability. Some believe that stretching of the capsular ligaments occurs at the time of injury as well and contend that these ligaments should be plicated, along with repair of the labrum. In a series of cadaveric simian shoulder dislocations, capsular microtears were seen in addition to a Bankart lesion in all shoulders.[535] The extent of the histologic findings was not quantified. In another series, the glenohumeral ligaments of cadaveric shoulders were placed in an anterior apprehension position until the ligament failed. Examination of the anterior band of these shoulders revealed a deformation of 0.04 to 0.53 mm, depending on the site of failure.[536] This finding implies that most of this deformation may be recovered with repair of the labrum to the glenoid alone in the majority of cases.

In fact, one of the outstanding features of Bankart's results was that "All these cases recovered full movement of the joint, and in no case has there been any recurrence of dislocation." Excessive tightening of the anterior capsule and subscapularis can lead to limited comfort and function, as well as to the form of secondary degenerative joint disease known as *capsulorrhaphy arthropathy*.[208,537-539] Rosenberg and colleagues[540] found that 18 of 52 patients had at least minimal degenerative changes at an average follow-up of 15 years; as a cautionary note against unnecessary capsular tightening, these authors found a correlation between loss of external rotation and the incidence

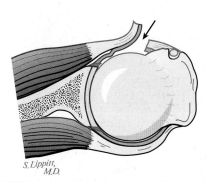

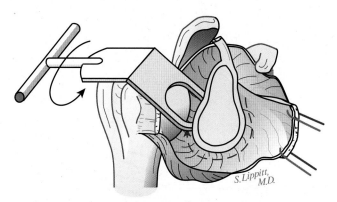

FIGURE 16-171 Subscapularis and capsular incision. The subscapularis and subjacent capsule are incised *(arrow)* so that strong tendinous tissue remains on either side of the incision. Sufficient tissue is left attached to the lesser tuberosity so that repair at the end of the case is facilitated. The subscapularis and capsule are not separated. (From Matsen FA III, Lippitt SB: Shoulder Surgery: Principles and Procedures. Philadelphia: WB Saunders, 2004, p 199.)

FIGURE 16-172 Capsular exposure. Twisting the inferior part of the humeral head retractor away from the glenoid exposes the inferior capsule. (From Matsen FA III, Lippitt SB: Shoulder Surgery: Principles and Procedures. Philadelphia: WB Saunders, 2004, p 201.)

of degenerative changes. To help guard against postoperative loss of motion, Rowe and associates[126] limit immobilization to just 2 to 3 days, after which the patient is instructed to gradually increase the motion and function of the extremity.

A clinical comparison has been made of the orientation of the capsulotomy performed in patients during an open Bankart repair. The group treated by horizontal capsulotomy recovered significantly more external rotation in abduction than did those treated by vertical capsulotomy, 112.9 versus 105 degrees, respectively.[541]

Thomas and Matsen described a simplified method of anatomically repairing avulsions of the glenohumeral ligaments directly to the glenoid lip without coracoid osteotomy, without splitting the capsule and the subscapularis, without metal or other anchors, and without tightening the capsule.[98,139] This method (described in detail in the section "Authors' Preferred Method") offers excellent range of motion and stability. Subsequently, Berg and Ellison[107] again recommended this simplified approach to capsulolabral repair.

When pathologically increased anterior laxity is combined with a Bankart lesion, the addition of capsular plication to reattachment of the capsulolabral avulsion has been recommended. Jobe and colleagues[542] and Montgomery and Jobe[543] achieved good or excellent results in athletes with shoulder pain secondary to anterior glenohumeral subluxation or dislocation. Two years after surgery, more than 80% had returned to their preinjury sport and level of competition.

Wirth and colleagues reported their results in 108 patients (142 shoulders) with recurrent anterior shoulder instability.[544] All patients were managed by repair of the capsulolabral injury, when present, and reinforcement of the anteroinferior capsular ligaments by an imbrication technique that decreases the overall capsular volume.

According to the grading system of Rowe and associates, 93% of the results were rated good or excellent at an average follow-up of 5 years (range, 2-12 years). The incidence of recurrent instability was approximately 1%.

Athletes in collision sports who were treated with open Bankart repair and capsulorrhaphy had a 3% redislocation rate. Eight percent had recurrent subluxation and 12% had rare subluxation, thus indicating the difficulty in treating instability in contact athletes.[545]

When the labrum is flattened or excessively compliant, a method of labrum augmentation using autologous blood has been described (Figs. 16-171 to 16-178).[146]

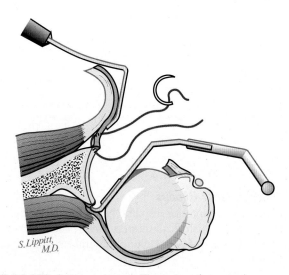

FIGURE 16-173 Suture passage. The suture is passed through the margin of the articular cartilage, around the labrum, and around 1 cm of capsule. (From Matsen FA III, Lippitt SB: Shoulder Surgery: Principles and Procedures. Philadelphia: WB Saunders, 2004, p 201.)

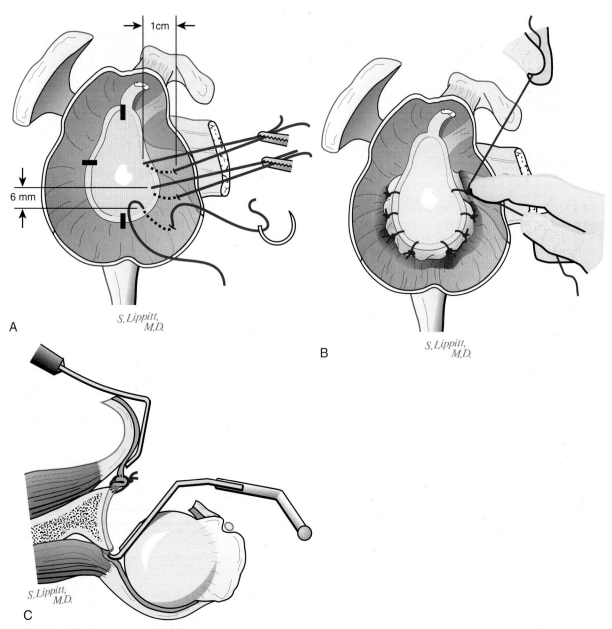

FIGURE 16-174 Suture placement and tying. **A,** Sutures are placed around the perimeter of the glenoid from 3 o'clock to 9 o'clock. **B,** These sutures are tied so that the knots overlie the capsule. **C,** Tying these sutures creates a substantial bumper, augmenting the glenoid concavity. (From Matsen FA III, Lippitt SB: Shoulder Surgery: Principles and Procedures. Philadelphia: WB Saunders, 2004, pp 202-204.)

Other Anterior Repairs

Many other anterior repairs have been described, but most are of historical interest only. The reader is also referred to a review of glenohumeral capsulorrhaphy by Friedman.[546]

Staple Capsulorrhaphy

In the DuToit staple capsulorrhaphy, the detached capsule is secured back to the glenoid with staples.[547,548] Actually, the staple repair had been described 50 years earlier by

Perthes. Rao and associates[549] reported the follow-up of 65 patients who underwent DuToit staple repair for avulsion of the capsule from the glenoid rim; 2 patients showed radiographic evidence of loose staples. Ward and colleagues[550] reviewed 33 staple capsulorrhaphies at an average of 50 months postoperatively; 50% continued to have apprehension and 12 had staple malposition.

O'Driscoll and Evans[238,551] reviewed 269 consecutive DuToit capsulorrhaphies in 257 patients at a median follow-up of 8.8 years; 53% had postoperative pain, and

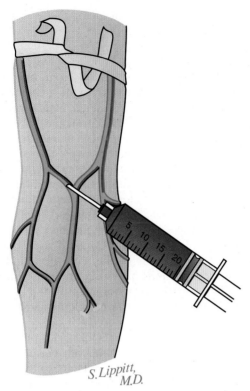

FIGURE 16-175 Blood harvest. From the ipsilateral antecubital fossa, 20 mL of blood is withdrawn. (From Matsen FA III, Lippitt SB: Shoulder Surgery: Principles and Procedures. Philadelphia: WB Saunders, 2004, p 205.)

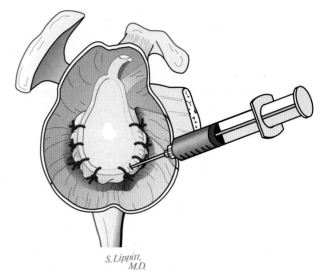

FIGURE 16-176 Labral inflation. The harvested blood is immediately injected into the rolled up capsule and labrum before it clots. A flat beveled needle is helpful here. (From Matsen FA III, Lippitt SB: Shoulder Surgery: Principles and Procedures. Philadelphia: WB Saunders, 2004, p 206.)

internal and external rotation was limited. Recurrence was reported in 28% if stapling alone was performed and in 8% if a Putti–Platt procedure was added; staple loosening, migration, or penetration of cartilage occurred in 11%. Staple complications contributed to pain, physical restriction, and osteoarthritis. Zuckerman and Matsen pointed out that the use of staples for surgical repair may be associated with major complications (Figs. 16-179 and 16-180).[552]

Subscapularis Muscle Procedures
Putti–Platt Procedure
In 1948, Osmond-Clarke[553] described this procedure, which was used by Sir Harry Platt of England and Vittorio

Putti of Italy. Platt first used this technique in November 1925. Some years later, Osmond-Clarke saw Putti perform essentially the same operation, which had been his standard practice since 1923. Scaglietta, one of Putti's pupils, revealed that the operation may well have been performed first by Codivilla, Putti's teacher and predecessor. Neither Putti nor Platt ever described the technique in the literature.

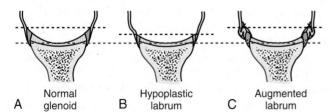

FIGURE 16-177 Augmented glenoid depth. The functional depth of the glenoid is increased by this labral augmentation. (From Matsen FA III, Lippitt SB: Shoulder Surgery: Principles and Procedures. Philadelphia: WB Saunders, 2004, p 207.)

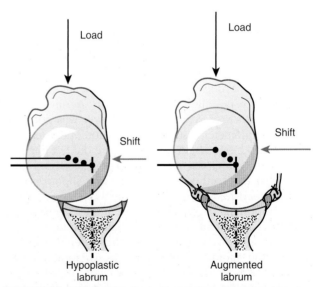

FIGURE 16-178 Restoration of centering. The augmented labrum restores the centering effect of the concavity, as demonstrated on the load and shift test. (From Matsen FA III, Lippitt SB: Shoulder Surgery: Principles and Procedures. Philadelphia: WB Saunders, 2004, p 207.)

In the Putti–Platt procedure, the subscapularis tendon is divided 2.5 cm from its insertion. The lateral stump of the tendon is attached to the "most convenient soft-tissue structure along the anterior rim of the glenoid cavity." If the capsule and labrum have been stripped from the anterior glenoid and neck of the scapula, the tendon is sutured to the deep surface of the capsule, and "it is advisable to raw the anterior surface of the neck of the scapula, so that the sutured tendo-capsule will adhere to it." After the lateral tendon stump is secured, the medial muscle stump is lapped over the lateral stump to produce substantial shortening of the capsule and subscapularis muscle. The exact placement of the lateral stump into the anterior soft tissues and the medial stump into the greater tuberosity is determined so that after conclusion of the procedure, the arm should externally rotate to the neutral position. Variations on the Putti–Platt procedure have been described by Blazina and Satzman,[468] Watson-Jones,[554] Müller,[211] and Symeonides.[31]

Quigley and Freedman[555] reported the results of 92 Putti–Platt operations; of these patients, 11 had more than 30% loss of motion and 7 had recurrent instability after their surgery. Leach and coworkers[556] in 1982 reported a series of 78 patients who had been treated with a modified Putti–Platt procedure. Loss of external rotation averaged between 12 and 19 degrees. Collins and associates[557] reviewed a series of 58 Putti–Platt procedures and 48 Putti–Platt–Bankart procedures. The redislocation rate was 11% (some because of significant trauma), 20% had residual pain, and the average restriction of external rotation was 20 degrees. Hovelius and colleagues,[525] in a follow-up of 114 patients who underwent either a Bankart or Putti–Platt reconstruction, found a recurrence rate of 2% in 46 patients treated with the Bankart procedure and 19% in 68 patients treated with a Putti–Platt procedure. Follow-up was between 1.5 and 10 years.

Fredriksson and Tegner[558] reviewed 101 patients who had had a Putti–Platt procedure with a mean follow-up of approximately 8 years (range, 5-14 years). Recurrent instability occurred in 20% of cases, and all patients demonstrated a decrease in the range of all measured movements, especially external rotation. Additionally, a significant decrease in strength and power was noted by Cybex dynamometer assessment. The authors stated that the restricted motion after this procedure did not improve with time as previous reports had suggested and concluded that this method of reconstruction should not be recommended for young active patients.

It is important to recognize that if this operation is carried out as described, a 2.5-cm lateral stump of subscapularis tendon is attached to the anterior glenoid. Because the radius of the humerus is approximately 2.5 cm, a 2.5-cm stump of subscapularis fused to the anterior glenoid would limit total humeral rotation to 1 radian, or 57 degrees. Angelo and Hawkins[208,559] presented a series of patients in whom osteoarthritis developed an average of 15 years after a Putti–Platt repair. It is now recognized that limitation of external rotation after repair for anterior instability is a factor predisposing to capsulorrhaphy arthropathy.[538,539]

Magnuson–Stack Procedure

Transfer of the subscapularis tendon from the lesser tuberosity across the bicipital groove to the greater tuberosity was originally described by Paul Magnuson and James Stack in 1940.[549,560-564] In 1955, Magnuson recommended that in some cases the tendon should be transferred not only across the bicipital groove but also distally into an area between the greater tuberosity and the upper shaft. DePalma[37] recommended that the tendon be transferred to the upper shaft below the greater tuberosity. Karadimas and colleagues,[560] in the largest single series of Magnuson–Stack procedures (154 patients), reported a 2% recurrence rate. Badgley and O'Connor[565] and Bailey[566] reported on a combination of the Putti–Platt and the Magnuson–Stack operations; they used the upper half of the subscapularis muscle to perform the Putti–Platt procedure and the lower half of the muscle to perform the Magnuson–Stack procedure.

Complications of the Magnuson–Stack procedure include excessive anterior tightening with posterior subluxation or dislocation (Fig. 16-181), damage to the biceps (Fig. 16-182), and recurrent instability.

Bone Block

Bone blocks are not the procedure of choice for routine cases of recurrent anterior glenohumeral instability. One must be concerned about procedures that can bring the humeral head into contact with bone that is not covered by articular cartilage because of the high risk of degenerative joint disease. Soft tissue repairs and reconstructions are safer and more effective for dealing with the usual case of recurrent traumatic instability. However, when a major anterior glenoid deficiency reduces the anterior or anteroinferior balance stability angle to an unacceptably small value, reconstruction of the anterior glenoid lip may be necessary. Matsen and Thomas[125] described a technique for using a contoured bone graft covered with joint capsule or other soft tissue to replace the missing glenoid bone in order to offer a smooth surface to articulate with the humeral head.

Eden–Hybbinette Procedure

The Eden–Hybbinette procedure was performed independently by Eden[567] in 1918 and by Hybbinette[568] in 1932. Eden first used tibial grafts, but both authors finally recommended the use of iliac grafts. This procedure is supposed to extend the anterior glenoid. It has been used by Palmer and Widen,[463] Lavik,[569] and Hovelius and colleagues[397] to treat shoulder subluxation and dislocation. Lavik modified the procedure by inserting the graft into the substance of the anterior glenoid rim. Lange[570] inserted the bone graft into an osteotomy on the anterior glenoid. Hehne and Hubner[268] reported a comparison of the Eden–Hybbinette–Lange and the Putti–Platt procedures in 170 patients; their results seemed to favor the latter.

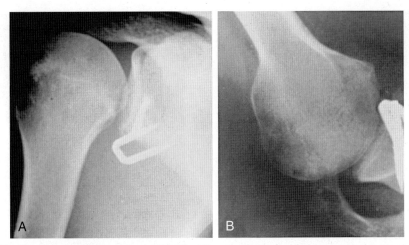

FIGURE 16-179 Complications of staple capsulorrhaphy. **A,** AP radiograph showing a prominent staple on the inferior glenoid rim. **B,** Axillary view showing impingement of a staple on the head of the humerus.

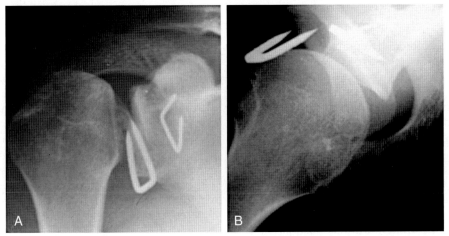

FIGURE 16-180 A loose staple after staple capsulorrhaphy. **A,** AP radiograph showing a loose staple in the glenohumeral joint. **B,** Axillary view.

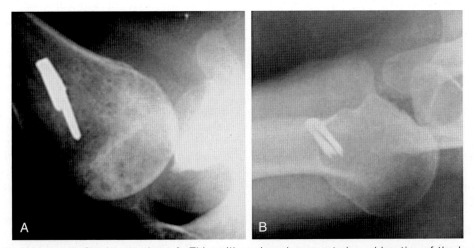

FIGURE 16-181 The Magnuson–Stack procedure. **A,** This axillary view shows posterior subluxation of the humeral head on the glenoid as a result of excessive anterior tightening with the Magnuson–Stack procedure. **B,** Another patient's axillary view shows excessive anterior tightening from the Magnuson–Stack procedure that resulted in posterior glenohumeral displacement of the humeral head.

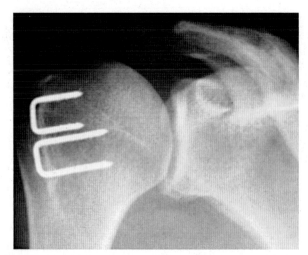

FIGURE 16-182 Impingement of a staple on the long head of the biceps tendon. This AP radiograph shows the position of the staple resulting in tendon impingement. The patient's anterior shoulder pain resolved when the staple was removed.

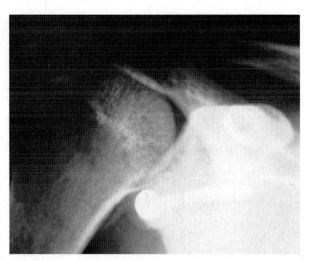

FIGURE 16-183 This AP radiograph shows impingement of a screw on the humeral head after the Bristow procedure.

Paavolainen and coworkers[571] reported on 41 patients treated with the Eden–Hybbinette procedure; 3 had recurrent instability, and external rotation was diminished an average of 10%. They found the results to be similar to those in their series of Putti–Platt operations. Degenerative joint disease developed in 10% in each group!

Niskanen and coworkers[572] reported a series of 52 shoulders, with a mean follow-up of 6 years, that had been treated with a modification of the Eden–Hybbinette procedure. The operation involved creating a trough through the capsule and into the anteroinferior aspects of the scapula neck. A tricortical iliac crest bone graft was then wedged into the trough without fixation. A 21% recurrence rate was attributed to one spontaneous dislocation and 10 traumatic redislocations. Postoperative arthrosis was noted in 9 shoulders and early degenerative changes in an additional 18 shoulders.

Oudard Procedure

In 1924, Oudard[573] described a method in which the coracoid process was prolonged with a bone graft from the tibia. The graft (4 × 3 × 1 cm) was inserted between the sawed-off tip and the remainder of the coracoid and was directed laterally and inferiorly. The graft acted as an anterior buttress that served to prevent recurrent dislocations. Oudard also shortened the subscapular tendon. Later, he published another method of achieving elongation of the coracoid: oblique osteotomy of the coracoid with displacement of the posterolateral portion to serve as a bone block.

Coracoid Transfer

In transfer of the coracoid process to the anterior glenoid, an attempt is made to create an anteroinferior musculotendinous sling. Some authors also refer to a bone block effect and intentional tethering of the subscapularis in front of the glenohumeral joint. Thus, it is apparent that these procedures do not address the usual pathology of traumatic instability. Redislocation rates after coracoid transfer for the usual case of traumatic instability are no lower than those for soft tissue reconstructions, but the rate of serious complications is substantially higher (Figs. 16-183 to 16-188). Furthermore, in contrast to soft tissue procedures, coracoid transfer procedures are extremely difficult and hazardous to revise: The subscapularis, musculocutaneous, and axillary nerves are scarred in abnormal positions; the subscapularis muscle is scarred and tethered; and the axillary artery may be displaced in scar tissue.

Trillat Procedure

Trillat and Leclerc-Chalvet[114,574-576] performed an osteotomy at the base of the coracoid process and then displaced the coracoid downward and laterally. The displaced coracoid is held in position by a special nail-pin or screw. The pin is passed into the scapula above the inferiorly displaced subscapularis muscle, which effectively shortens the muscle.

Bristow–Helfet Procedure

This procedure was developed, used, and reported by Arthur Helfet[577] in 1958 and was named the *Bristow operation* after his former chief at St. Thomas Hospital, W. Rowley Bristow of South Africa. Helfet originally described detaching the tip of the coracoid process from the scapula just distal to the insertion of the pectoralis minor muscle and leaving the conjoined tendons (the short head of the biceps and the coracobrachialis) attached. Through a vertical slit in the subscapularis tendon, the joint is exposed and the anterior surface of the neck of the scapula is "rawed up." The coracoid process with its attached tendons is then passed through

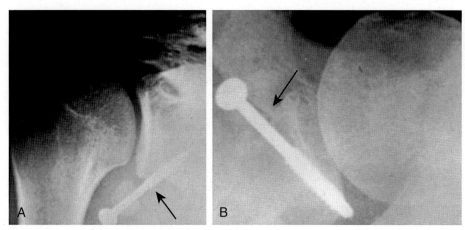

FIGURE 16-184 Nonunion of the coracoid process after the Bristow procedure. **A,** An AP radiograph shows nonunion of the coracoid process (*arrow*). **B,** An axillary view in a different patient shows nonunion of the coracoid process after the Bristow procedure (*arrow*).

the slit in the subscapularis and kept in contact with the raw area on the scapula by suturing the conjoined tendon to the cut edges of the subscapularis tendon. In effect, a subscapularis tenodesis is performed.

In 1958, T. B. McMurray (son of T. P. McMurray of hip osteotomy fame) visited Dr. Newton Mead[578] of Chicago and described modifications of the Bristow operation that were being used in Capetown, Johannesburg, and Pretoria. Mead and Sweeney[578] reported use of the modifications in over 100 cases. The modifications consist of splitting the subscapularis muscle and tendon unit in line with its fibers to open the joint and firmly securing the coracoid process to the anterior glenoid rim with a screw. May[579] modified the Bristow procedure further by vertically dividing the entire subscapularis tendon from the lesser tuberosity; after exploring the joint, he attached the tip of the coracoid process with the conjoined tendon to the anterior glenoid with a screw. The subscapularis tendon was then split horizontally and reattached—half the tendon above and half below the transferred conjoined tendon—to the site of its original insertion. Again, the net effect is a tenodesis of the subscapularis.

Helfet[577] reported that the procedure not only "reinforced" the defective part of the joint but also had a "bone block" effect. Mead and Sweeney,[578] however, do not regard the bone block as being a very important part of the procedure and believe that the transfer adds a muscle reinforcement at the lower anterior aspect of the shoulder joint that prevents the lower portion of the subscapularis muscle from displacing upward as the humerus is abducted.

Bonnin[580,581] modified the Bristow procedure in the following way: He did not shorten or split the subscapularis muscle tendon unit, but for exposure, he divided the subscapularis muscle at its muscle–tendon junction, and after attachment of the coracoid process to the glenoid with a screw, he reattached the subscapularis on top

of the conjoined tendon. The results of this modification in 81 patients have been reported by Hummel and associates.[582]

Torg and coworkers[583] reported their experience with 212 Bristow procedures. In their modification the coracoid was passed over the superior border rather than through the subscapularis. Their postoperative instability rate was 8.5% (3.8% redislocation and 4.7% subluxation rate). Ten patients required reoperation for screw-related problems; 34% had residual shoulder pain, and 8% were unable to do overhead work. Only 16% of athletes were able to return to their preinjury level of throwing.

Carol and associates[584] reported on the results of the Bristow procedure performed for 32 recurrently dislocating shoulders and 15 "spontaneous" shoulder instabilities. At an average follow-up of 3.7 years, only one patient had recurrent instability, and the average limitation of external rotation was 12 degrees.

Banas and coworkers[585] reported a 4% recurrence rate with an 8.6-year follow-up; however, additional surgery was required in 14%. Wredmark and colleagues[586] found only 2 of 44 recurrent dislocations at an average follow-up of 6 years, but 28% of patients complained of pain.

Hovelius and coworkers[397] reported follow-up on 111 shoulders treated with the Bristow procedure. At 2.5 years their postoperative instability rate was 13% (6% dislocation and 7% subluxation rate). External rotation was limited an average of 20 degrees, and 6% required a reoperation because of screw-related complications. Muscle strength was 10% less in the operated shoulder.

Chen and colleagues[587] found that after the Bristow procedure, the reduced strength of the short head of the biceps was compensated for by increased activity in the long head. Other series of Bristow procedures have been reported, each of which emphasizes the potential risks.[588]

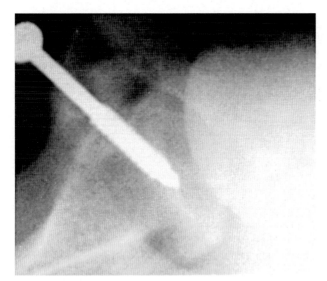

FIGURE 16-185 This axillary view shows the screw backing out of the glenoid after the Bristow procedure.

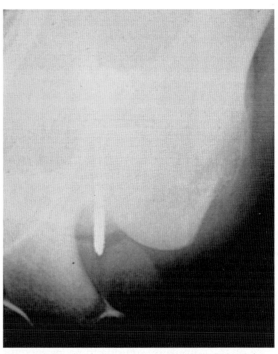

FIGURE 16-186 Axillary view showing an excessively long screw used during the Bristow procedure. The patient had an infraspinatus palsy as a result of injury to the nerve to this muscle.

Lamm and coworkers[589] and Lemmens and de Waal Malefijt[590] described four special x-ray projections to evaluate the position of the transplanted coracoid process: AP, lateral, oblique lateral, and modified axial. Lower and coworkers[591] used CT scans to demonstrate impingement of a Bristow screw on the head of the humerus. Collins and Wilde[235] and Nielsen and Nielsen[592] reported that although they had minimal problems with recurrence of dislocation, they did encounter problems with screw breakage, migration, and nonunion of the coracoid to the scapula. Hovelius and colleagues[593,594] reported only a 50% union rate of the coracoid to the scapula.

Norris and associates[595] evaluated 24 patients with failed Bristow repairs; only 2 had union of the transferred coracoid. Causes of failure included residual subluxation and osteoarthritis from screw or bone impingement or an overtight repair. They pointed to the difficulty of reconstructing a shoulder after a failed Bristow procedure. Singer and colleagues[596] conducted a 20-year follow-up study of the Bristow–Latarjet procedure; in spite of an average Constant–Murley score of 80 points, radiographic evidence of degenerative joint disease was detected in 71%.

Ferlic and DiGiovine[597] reported on 51 patients treated with the Bristow procedure. They had a 10% incidence

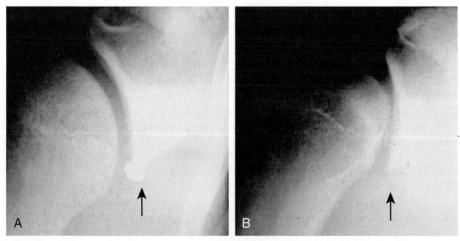

FIGURE 16-187 AP radiographs showing broken screws with the humerus in external rotation (**A**) and internal rotation (**B**).

of redislocation or subluxation and a 14% incidence of complications related to the screw. An additional surgical procedure was required in 14% of the patients. In a long-term follow-up study of 79 shoulders, Banas and colleagues[585] also reported complications necessitating reoperation in 14% of patients; 73% of reoperations were for hardware removal secondary to persistent shoulder pain.

Recurrent subluxation after the Bristow procedure also appears to be a significant problem.[278,594,595,597,598] Hill and coworkers[455] and MacKenzie[599] noted failure to manage subluxation with this procedure. Schauder and Tullos[600] reported 85% good or excellent results with a modified Bristow procedure in 20 shoulders at a minimum of 3 years of follow-up. Interestingly, the authors attributed the success to healing of the Bankart lesion because in many instances, the position of the transferred coracoid precluded it from containing the humeral head. The authors suggested that the 15% fair or poor results were secondary to persistent or recurrent subluxation.

In 1989, Rockwood and Young[601,602] reported on 40 patients who had previously been treated with the Bristow procedure. They commented on the danger and the technical difficulty of these repairs. Of the 40, 31 underwent subsequent reconstructive procedures: 10 had a capsular shift reconstruction, 4 required capsular release, 4 had total shoulder arthroplasty, 1 had an arthrodesis, and the rest had various combined procedures. The authors concluded the Bristow procedure was nonphysiologic and associated with too many serious complications and recommended that it not be performed for routine anterior reconstruction of the shoulder.

Latarjet Procedure

The Latarjet procedure,[603-605] described in 1954, involves the transfer of a larger portion of the coracoid process than used with the Bristow procedure, with the biceps and coracobrachialis tendons transferred to the anteroinferior aspect of the neck of the scapula. Instead of the raw cut surface of the tip of the coracoid process being attached to the scapula, as is done in the Bristow–Helfet procedure, the coracoid is laid flat on the neck of the scapula and held in place with one or two screws.

Tagliabue and Esposito[606] reported on the Latarjet procedure in 94 athletes. Wredmark and colleagues[586] analyzed 44 patients at an average follow-up of 6 years after a Bristow–Latarjet procedure for recurrent shoulder dislocation; 72% had no discomfort, but the remaining 28% complained of moderate exertional pain. Vittori has modified the procedure by turning the subscapularis tendon downward and holding it displaced downward with the transferred coracoid. Pascoet and associates[605] reported on use of the Vittori modification in 36 patients and noted 1 recurrence. Several reviews of the results of this procedure have been published.[607,608]

Other Open Repairs
Gallie Procedure

Gallie and LeMesurier[65,609] originally described the use of autogenous fascia lata to create new ligaments between the anteroinferior aspect of the capsule and the anterior neck of the humerus in 1927. Bateman[610] of Toronto has also used this procedure. Although fascia lata might not be the ideal graft material, exogenous autograft or allograft may be necessary for reconstructing deficient capsulolabral structures in the management of failed previous surgical repairs.

Nicola Procedure

Toufick Nicola's name is usually associated with this operation, but the procedure was first described by

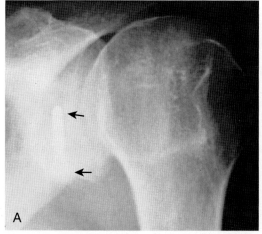
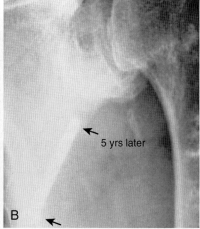

FIGURE 16-188 Late screw loosening after the Bristow procedure. **A,** An AP radiograph shows the position of the screw (*arrows*) in the transferred coracoid process. **B,** An AP radiograph taken 5 years later shows the screw backed out (*arrow*) and significant glenohumeral arthropathy.

Rupp[611] in 1926 and Heymanowitsch[612] in 1927. In 1929, Nicola[58] published his first article in which he described the use of the long head of the biceps tendon as a check-rein ligament. The procedure has been modified several times.[59-61,301] Recurrence rates have been reported to be between 30% and 50%.[524,613,614]

Saha Procedure

A. K. Saha[131,516,615-617] has described transfer of the latissimus dorsi posteriorly into the site of the infraspinatus insertion on the greater tuberosity. He reported that during abduction, the transferred latissimus reinforces the subscapularis muscle and the short posterior steering and depressor muscles by pulling the humeral head backward. He has used the procedure for traumatic and atraumatic dislocations, and in 1969 he reported 45 cases with no recurrence.

Boytchev Procedure

Boytchev first described this procedure in 1951 in the Italian literature,[618,619] and later modifications were developed by Conforty.[620] The muscles that attach to the coracoid process along with the tip of the coracoid are rerouted deep to the subscapularis muscle between it and the capsule. The tip of the coracoid with its muscles is then reattached to its base in the anatomic position. Conforty[620] reported on 17 patients, none of whom had a recurrence of dislocation. Ha'eri and Maitland[492] reported 26 cases with a minimum of 2 years' follow-up.

Osteotomy of the Proximal Humerus

Debevoise and associates[538,621] stated that humeral torsion is abnormal in a repeatedly dislocating shoulder. B. G. Weber[524,549,564,622,623] of Switzerland reported a rotational osteotomy whereby he increased the retroversion of the humeral head and simultaneously performed an anterior capsulorrhaphy. The indications were a moderate to severe posterolateral humeral head defect, which he found in 65% of his patients with recurrent anterior instability. By increasing the retroversion, the posterolateral defect is delivered more posteriorly and the anterior undisturbed portion of the articular surface of the humeral head then articulates against the glenoid. It is recognized that the effective articular surface of the humerus is reduced by the posterolateral head defect and that the osteotomy realigns the remaining articular surface in a position more compatible with activities of daily living. Weber and colleagues[623] reported a redislocation rate of 5.7%, with good to excellent results in 90%. Most patients required a reoperation for plate removal.

Osteotomy of the Neck of the Glenoid

In 1933, Meyer-Burgdorff reported on decreasing the anterior tilt of the glenoid with a posterior closing wedge osteotomy.[615] Saha has written[615] about an anterior opening wedge osteotomy with a bone graft placed into the neck of the glenoid to decrease the tilt.

Complications of Anterior Repairs

Complications of surgical repairs for anterior glenohumeral instability may be grouped into several categories.[624]

The first includes complications that can follow any surgical procedure. Of primary importance in this category is postoperative infection. Thorough skin preparation, adhesive plastic drapes, and prophylactic antibiotics are useful in reducing contamination by axillary bacterial flora. It is also important to prevent the accumulation of significant hematoma by achieving good hemostasis, obliterating any dead space, and using a suction drain if significant bleeding persists. It is important to keep the axilla clean and dry postoperatively by using a gauze sponge as long as the arm is held at the side.

The second category of complications consists of postoperative recurrent instability. The published incidence of recurrent dislocation after anterior repairs ranges from 0% to 30%. It is noteworthy that many of the reports in their tally included only recurrent dislocation rather than recurrent subluxation or recurrent apprehension. A 1975 review of 1634 reconstructions compiled from the literature revealed that the incidence of redislocation averaged 3%.[313] In a 1983 review of 3076 procedures, the incidence was unchanged.[285] This review included 432 Putti–Platt operations, 571 Magnuson–Stack operations or modifications, 513 Bankart operations or modifications, 45 Saha operations, 203 Bankart–Putti–Platt combinations, 639 Bristow operations, 115 Badgley combined procedures, 254 Eden–Hybbinette operations, 277 Gallie operations or modifications, and 27 Weber operations.

The incidence of recurrence is underestimated by studies with only 2 years of follow-up. Morrey and Janes,[240] in a long-term follow-up study of 176 patients that averaged 10.2 years, found a redislocation rate of 11%. The operative reconstructions were of the Bankart and Putti–Platt types. In 7 of the 20 patients, redislocation occurred 2 or more years after surgery. The need for long-term follow-up was further emphasized in a study by O'Driscoll and Evans,[551] who monitored 269 consecutive patients undergoing staple capsulorrhaphy for a minimum of 8.8 years. Twenty-one percent of 204 shoulders demonstrated redislocation; this incidence increased progressively with the length of follow-up.

Factors that have been shown to be significantly associated with a poor outcome after open surgical anterior stabilization are workers' compensation, voluntary instability, previous instability surgery, age of the patient, and shorter periods of postoperative immobilization.[625] Immobilization for less than 6 weeks and age 32 years or older were associated with significantly lower Rowe scores. The sex of the patient, Hill–Sachs lesions, the type of instability, labral tears, and the surgeon's experience were not statistically significant. The majority of these patients had Bankart repairs or capsular shifts.

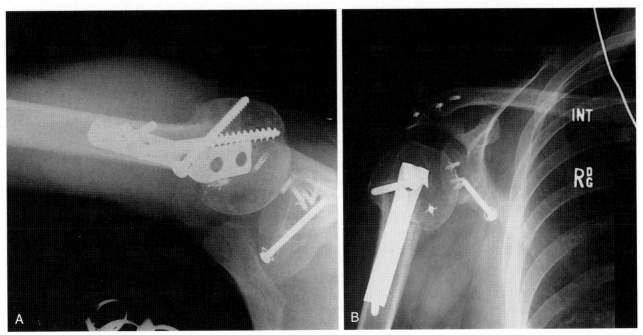

FIGURE 16-189 Axillary (**A**) and AP (**B**) radiographs of the shoulder of a young woman. The shoulder remained unstable after six surgeries for glenohumeral instability, including Bankart repairs, capsular shifts, and a Bristow and derotational osteotomy.

Rowe and colleagues[626] reported on the management of 39 patients with recurrence of instability after various surgical repairs. Of 32 who underwent reoperation, 84% did not have an effective repair of the Bankart lesion at the initial surgery. When the previously unrepaired Bankart lesion was repaired at revision surgery, almost all (22 of 24) the shoulders became stable and remained so for at least 2 years. Excessive laxity was thought to be the primary cause of instability in only 4 shoulders. Ungersböck and associates[127] also found that rounded or deficient glenoid rims and large unhealed Bankart lesions were associated with failure of surgical repair for anterior instability. Zabinski and coauthors reported similar findings: over half of their failed instability repairs were associated with unhealed Bankart lesions; most regained stability after revision repair.[627] By contrast, only 9 of the 21 shoulders with recurrent multidirectional instability obtained a good or excellent result from revision surgeries.

All 17 patients who had a significant traumatic event subsequent to instability surgery had excellent results after revision open stabilization. Of 33 patients with recurrent instability and no significant trauma after initial surgery, only 67% had good or excellent results.[628]

Refractory instability can be a major problem, whether caused by bone deficiency, poor-quality soft tissue, musculotendinous failure, or decompensation of neuromuscular control (Fig. 16-189). Richards and colleagues[629] described the challenges associated with trying to manage such cases of refractory or terminal instability by glenohumeral arthrodesis.

The third major category of complications arises from failure of diagnosis. It is essential to differentiate traumatic unidirectional instability (TUBS syndrome) from atraumatic multidirectional instability (AMBRII syndrome) before carrying out any surgical repair. The consequences of mistaking multidirectional instability for pure anterior instability are substantial. In this situation, if only the anterior structures are tightened, limited external rotation along with the resulting obligate posterior subluxation can lead to rapid loss of glenohumeral articular cartilage and capsulorrhaphy arthropathy.[208,538,539] This complication can be prevented only by accurate preoperative diagnosis and appropriate surgery that avoids unnecessary capsular tightening.

The importance of an accurate diagnosis and subsequent treatment cannot be overemphasized: 20 shoulders (53%) in the study of Cooper and Brems[140] and 22 shoulders (15%) in the report of Wirth and Rockwood[630] had previously been operated on for a mistaken diagnosis. In the latter report, diagnostic errors included (in order of decreasing frequency) rotator cuff disease, biceps tendinitis, thoracic outlet syndrome, and cervical disk herniation.

The fourth category of operative complications consists of neurovascular injuries. The musculocutaneous nerve runs as a single or multipartite structure obliquely through the coracobrachialis, a variable distance distal to the coracoid process. In this location it may be injured by dissection to free up the coracoid process, by retraction, or by inclusion in sutures.[472] Helfet[577] described one case in which the nerve had high penetration into the coraco-

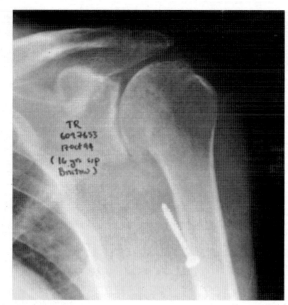

FIGURE 16-190 This patient experienced a pop while externally rotating the shoulder 5 months after a Bristow procedure. Shortly after this episode, he palpated a bump in his axilla while applying deodorant. (From Rockwood CA Jr, Green DP, Bucholz RW [eds] : Fractures in Adults. Philadelphia: JB Lippincott, 1991.)

brachialis and became injured where the conjoined tendon entered the slit made in the subscapularis tendon for a Bristow procedure. The axillary nerve may be injured during dissection and suture of the inferior capsule and subscapularis.[631]

Richards and associates[632] presented nine patients sustaining nerve injuries during anterior shoulder repair (three Bristow and six Putti–Platt procedures). Seven involved the musculocutaneous nerve and two involved the axillary nerve. Two of the nerves were lacerated, five were injured by suture, and two were injured

by traction. These nerve injuries are relatively more common during reoperation after a previous repair; in this situation, the nerves are tethered by scar tissue and are thus more difficult to mobilize out of harm's way. Neurovascular complications can best be avoided by good knowledge of local anatomy (including the possible normal variations), good surgical technique, and a healthy respect for the change in position and mobility of the neurovascular structures after a previous surgical procedure in the area. We recommend that the axillary nerve be routinely palpated and protected during all anterior reconstructions.[95,313]

The fifth category of complications includes those related to hardware inserted about the glenohumeral joint.[633,634] The screw used to fix the coracoid fragment in Bristow procedures has a particular potential for being problematic.[555,592] Loosening of the screw can result from rotation of the coracoid fragment as the arm is raised and lowered (Fig. 16-190). Artz and Huffer[635] and Fee and coauthors[636] reported a devastating complication in which the screw became loose and caused a false aneurysm of the axillary artery with subsequent compression of the brachial plexus and paralysis of the upper extremity. Similar complications have been reported as late as 3 years after surgery.[637] In other instances, the Bristow screw has damaged the articular surface of the glenoid and humeral head when placed too close to the glenoid lip, irritated the infraspinatus or its nerve when too long, or affected the brachial plexus when it became loose (see Figs. 16-183 to 16-188).

Staples used to attach the capsule to the glenoid can miss their target and damage the humeral or glenoid articular cartilage (Fig. 16-191; see also Figs. 16-179 to 16-181). Staples also can become loose from repeated pull of the muscles and capsule during shoulder use, particularly if they were not well seated in the first place. O'Driscoll and Evans[551] reported an 11% incidence of staple complications after the DuToit procedure. If screws

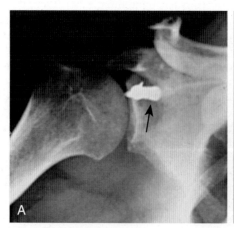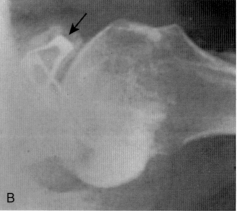

FIGURE 16-191 A, An AP radiograph shows the position of an arthroscopically placed staple (*arrow*). Contact of the staple with the humeral head is suggested by this view. **B,** An axillary view with contrast material demonstrates impingement of the staple on the humeral head (*arrow*).

and staples migrate into the intra-articular region, significant damage to the joint surfaces can result (Fig. 16-192). Metal fixation can injure the biceps tendon in a Magnuson–Stack procedure (see Fig. 16-182).

Zuckerman and Matsen[552] reported a series of patients with problems related to the use of screws and staples about the glenohumeral joint; 21 had problems related to the Bristow procedure and 14 to the use of staples (either for capsulorrhaphy or subscapularis advancement). The time between placement and symptom onset ranged from 4 weeks to 10 years. Screws and staples had been incorrectly placed in 10 patients, had migrated or loosened in 24, and had fractured in 3. Almost all patients required reoperation, at which time 41% had a significant injury to one or both of the joint surfaces.

Recent attempts to soften the potential complications of hardware by using bioabsorbable implants have been described. However, Edwards and colleagues[637] reported the adverse effects of a polyglyconate polymer in six shoulders after repair of the glenoid labrum. All patients had increasing pain and loss of motion requiring arthroscopic débridement. Dual-contrast arthrotomography revealed bony cystic changes around the implant, and histologic evaluation was consistent with a granulomatous reaction.

Taken together, these data suggest that primary repairs with hardware are more risky, yet no more effective than anatomic soft tissue repairs to bone with suture alone; the recurrence rates of techniques using screws and staples are no better than those with hardware-free repairs. With hardware, risks are incurred that simply do not exist with other repair techniques. The depth and variable orientation of the glenoid at surgery provide substantial opportunity for hardware misplacement (into the joint, under the articular cartilage, subperiosteally, out the back, too high, too low, too medial, too prominent anteriorly, and too insecurely). The large range of motion of the shoulder with frequent vigorous challenge to its stability creates an opportunity for loosening of hardware and for irreversible surface and neurovascular damage.

The sixth category of complications is limited motion. Limited range of motion, especially external rotation, has been reported after the Magnuson–Stack and the Putti–Platt procedures. It has also been noted after the Bristow procedure, which was supposed to be free of this problem.[50,638,639] Hovelius and colleagues[525] reported an average loss of external rotation of 21 degrees with the arm in abduction. In their series of 46 patients with continuing problems after shoulder reconstruction, Hawkins and Hawkins[276] found that 10 had stiffness related to limited external rotation.

MacDonald and colleagues[639] described release of the subscapularis muscle in 10 patients who had an internal rotation contracture after shoulder reconstruction for recurrent instability. At an average follow-up of 3 years, all patients reported less pain and demonstrated an average increase of 27 degrees of external rotation.

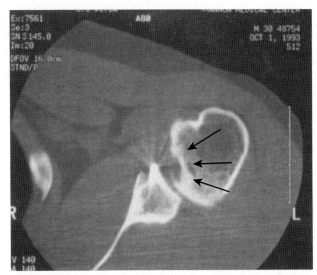

FIGURE 16-192 Significant humeral head erosion (*arrows*) secondary to intra-articular placement of an anterior capsular staple.

Lazarus and Harryman[624] pointed out that each centimeter of surgical lengthening of excessively tightened capsule regains approximately 20 degrees of rotation.

Lusardi and associates reported on 19 patients (20 shoulders) who had been treated for severe loss of external rotation of the glenohumeral joint after a previous anterior capsulorrhaphy for recurrent instability.[539] All 20 shoulders were managed by release of the anterior soft tissue. The average increase in external rotation was 45 degrees (range, 25-65 degrees).

The seventh complication is that of capsulorrhaphy arthropathy, or secondary degenerative joint disease resulting from surgery for recurrent instability.[98,538,539,559,624] This condition most commonly arises from excessive surgical tightening of the anterior capsule, causing obligate posterior translation with secondary degenerative joint disease (see Figs. 16-62 and 16-63). The condition can be prevented by ensuring that the shoulder has a functional range of motion after repair for instability and by performing a surgical release of shoulders with major limitations in external rotation. Severe capsulorrhaphy can require shoulder arthroplasty with normalization of the posteriorly inclined glenoid version.[284,538,539,624]

Angelo and Hawkins[559] reported eight patients with disabling degenerative arthritis seen an average of 15.1 years after a Putti–Platt procedure. None of the patients had ever gained external rotation beyond 0 degrees after their repair. Lusardi and colleagues[539] described 20 shoulders with severe loss of external rotation after anterior capsulorrhaphy and spoke about the risk of posterior subluxation and secondary degenerative joint disease in these circumstances.

Lusardi and coworkers[539] also reported on 7 shoulders in which the humeral head had been subluxated or dislocated posteriorly and 16 shoulders that had been affected by mild to severe degenerative joint disease after surgical repair for recurrent anterior dislocation. Nine required shoulder arthroplasty because of severe joint surface destruction. At a mean follow-up of 48 months, all shoulders had an improvement in ratings for pain and range of motion.

The eighth complication after surgical repair is failure of the subscapularis. As pointed out by Lazarus and Harryman,[624] the clinical manifestations of subscapularis failure can include pain, weakness of abdominal press and lumbar pushoff, apprehension, and frank instability. A failed subscapularis can sometimes be repaired directly and on other occasions might require a hamstring autograft, allograft, or transfer of the pectoralis major tendon (Figs. 16-193 to 16-200).

Wirth and coauthors[640] reported a series of failed repairs in which the subscapularis was completely disrupted and contracted medially into a dense connective tissue scar that precluded mobilization. Most of the shoulders had undergone multiple previous procedures. The subscapularis deficiency was reconstructed by transfer of either the upper portion of the pectoralis major or the pectoralis minor in five shoulders.

Matsen and Lippitt's Preferred Method of Management of Recurrent Traumatic Shoulder Instability

A patient with traumatic anterior glenohumeral instability usually has symptoms primarily when the arm is elevated near the coronal plane, extended, and externally rotated. Characteristically, the shoulder is relatively asymptomatic in other extreme positions or in midrange positions. Thus, appropriate management for some patients consists solely of education about the nature of the lesion and identification of the positions and activities that need to be avoided.

Strengthening the shoulder musculature can help prevent the shoulder from being forced into positions of instability. The exercise program previously described for atraumatic instability may be considered as an option for traumatic instability as well.

The option of surgical repair is discussed when careful clinical evaluation has documented the diagnosis of refractory anterior instability after an initial episode that was sufficiently traumatic to tear the anterior-inferior glenohumeral ligament and produce significant functional deficits (recurrent apprehension, subluxation, or dislocation) when the arm is in abduction, external rotation, and extension.

A patient desiring surgical stabilization is presented with a frank discussion of the alternatives and the risks of infection, neurovascular injury, stiffness, recurrent instability, pain, and the need for revision surgery.

Preoperative radiographs are obtained, including an AP view in the plane of the scapula (see Fig. 16-93), an apical oblique (Garth) view (see Fig. 16-112), and an axillary view (see Fig. 16-102). A preoperative rotator cuff ultrasound is obtained if cuff disease is suspected, for example, in a patient older than 40 years with pain between episodes of dislocation or with weakness of internal rotation, external rotation, or elevation. An electromyogram is performed if clinical evaluation suggests the possibility of nerve injury.

Surgical Technique

The goal of surgical management of traumatic anterior-inferior glenohumeral instability is safe, secure, and anatomic repair of the traumatic lesion and restoration of the attachment of the glenohumeral ligaments, capsule, and labrum to the rim of the glenoid from which they were avulsed. By ensuring that reattachment to the rim occurs, the effective depth of the glenoid is restored (Fig. 16-201 and see Fig. 16-32). This anatomic reattachment should re-establish not only the capsuloligamentous checkrein but also the fossa-deepening effect of the glenoid labrum. Unnecessary steps are avoided, such as coracoid osteotomy and splitting the subscapularis from the capsule. No attempt is made to modify the normal laxity of the anterior capsule in the usual case of traumatic instability. The repair must be secure from the time of surgery so that it will allow the patient to resume activities of daily living while the repair is healing. Such a secure repair allows controlled mobilization, thereby minimizing the possibility of unwanted stiffness. The tools needed for this repair are simple and commonly available (Fig. 16-202).

The procedure is performed with a brachial plexus block or general anesthetic. The glenohumeral joint is examined under anesthesia. Although this examination rarely changes the procedure performed, it provides helpful confirmation of the diagnosis.

The patient is positioned in a slight head-up position (~20 degrees) with the shoulder off the edge of the operating table (Fig. 16-203). This position provides a full range of humeral and scapular mobility and, if necessary, access to the posterior aspect of the shoulder. The neck, chest, axilla, and entire arm are prepared with iodine solution.

The shoulder is approached through the dominant anterior axillary crease (Fig. 16-204), which is marked before the application of an adherent, transparent plastic drape to facilitate a cosmetically acceptable scar.[641] If the incision is confined to the axillary crease, it is less noticeable than the scars from arthroscopic portals.

The skin is incised and the subcutaneous tissue is undermined up to the level of the coracoid process, which is then used as a guide to the cephalic vein and the deltopectoral groove (Fig. 16-205). The groove is opened by spreading with the two index fingers medial to the cephalic vein. A neurovascular bundle (a branch of the thoracoacromial artery and the lateral pectoral nerve) is commonly identified in the upper third of the groove[111]; this bundle is cauterized and transected. It is not necessary to release the upper pectoralis major unless

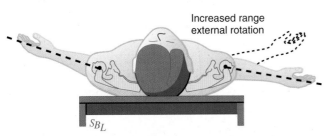

FIGURE 16-193 Loss of checkrein. When the anterior capsule is disrupted, the glenohumeral joint lacks its normal limitation of external rotation. (From Matsen FA III, Lippitt SB: Shoulder Surgery: Principles and Procedures. Philadelphia: WB Saunders, 2004, p 225.)

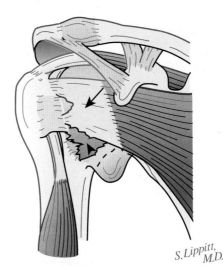

FIGURE 16-194 Compromised tissue quality. The quality of the subscapularis tendon (*arrow*) and anterior capsule (*arrowhead*) is insufficient for repair. (From Matsen FA III, Lippitt SB: Shoulder Surgery: Principles and Procedures. Philadelphia: WB Saunders, 2004, p 227.)

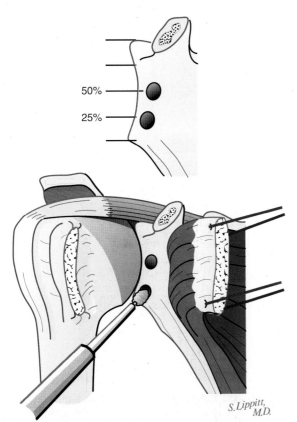

FIGURE 16-195 Glenoid drill holes. Using a pinecone bur, drill holes are placed in the middle and inferior aspects of the anterior glenoid, near the lip. (From Matsen FA III, Lippitt SB: Shoulder Surgery: Principles and Procedures. Philadelphia: WB Saunders, 2004, p 229.)

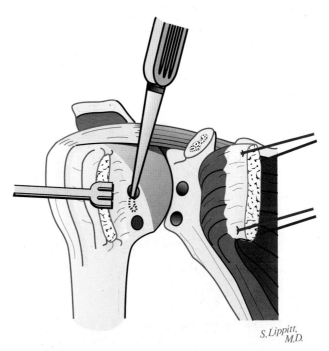

FIGURE 16-196 Humeral drill holes. Similarly, holes are made in the middle and inferior aspects of the proximal humerus, near the articular surface. (From Matsen FA III, Lippitt SB: Shoulder Surgery: Principles and Procedures. Philadelphia: WB Saunders, 2004, p 229.)

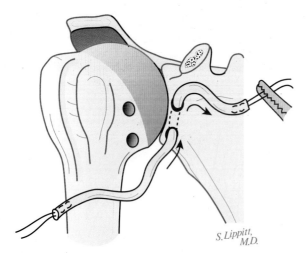

FIGURE 16-197 Passing the graft through the glenoid holes. The hamstring tendon graft is passed through the glenoid holes. (From Matsen FA III, Lippitt SB: Shoulder Surgery: Principles and Procedures. Philadelphia: WB Saunders, 2004, p 230.)

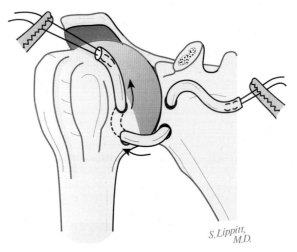

FIGURE 16-198 Passing the graft through the humeral holes. The hamstring tendon graft is then passed through the humeral holes. (From Matsen FA III, Lippitt SB: Shoulder Surgery: Principles and Procedures. Philadelphia: WB Saunders, 2004, p 231.)

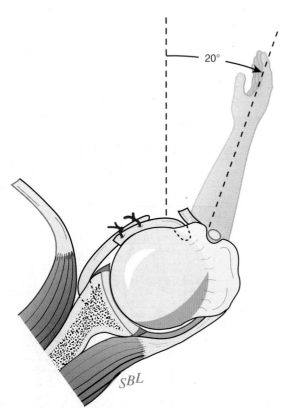

FIGURE 16-199 Tying the graft. The graft is tied so that external rotation is checked at 20 degrees. (From Matsen FA III, Lippitt SB: Shoulder Surgery: Principles and Procedures. Philadelphia: WB Saunders, 2004, p 231.)

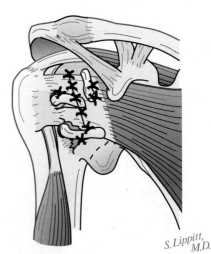

FIGURE 16-200 Reinforcing the graft. Any available capsular or tendon tissue is anchored to the graft. (From Matsen FA III, Lippitt SB: Shoulder Surgery: Principles and Procedures. Philadelphia: WB Saunders, 2004, p 231.)

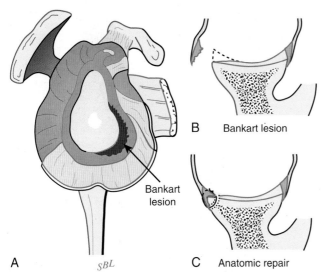

A   SBL   B   Bankart lesion   C   Anatomic repair

Bankart lesion

FIGURE 16-201 Anatomic repair of labral avulsion. If the labrum is avulsed from the glenoid (**A** and **B**), anatomic repair of the attachment of the labrum to the glenoid lip restores normal rotational laxity (**C**). (From Matsen FA III, Lippitt SB: Shoulder Surgery: Principles and Procedures. Philadelphia: WB Saunders, 2004, p 125.)

the humeroscapular motion interface (see Fig. 16-15) and exposes the subjacent subscapularis tendon and lesser tuberosity. The axillary nerve is routinely palpated as it crosses the anteroinferior border of the subscapularis. At this point it is useful to insert a self-retaining retractor, with one blade on the deltoid muscle and the other on the coracoid muscles. Care must be taken to ensure that the medial limb of this retractor does not compress the brachial plexus. Rotating the arm from internal to external rotation reveals, in succession, the greater tuberosity, the bicipital groove, the lesser tuberosity, and the subscapularis.

The anterior humeral circumflex vessels can usually be protected by bluntly dissecting them off the subscapularis muscle at its inferior border. The interval between the supraspinatus and subscapularis tendons is identified by palpation, and a blunt elevator is inserted through this interval into the joint. This elevator brings the upper subscapularis into the incision (Fig. 16-207). With care taken to protect the tendon of the biceps, the subscapularis tendon and subjacent capsule are then incised together approximately 1 cm medial to the lesser tuberosity (Fig. 16-208), beginning at the superior rounded edge of the tendon. A tag suture is placed in the upper rolled border of the subscapularis to mark it for subsequent repair. The incision is then extended inferiorly to the level of the anterior circumflex humeral vessels, which are not transected, cauterized, or ligated. It is important that the incision through the subscapularis tendon leaves strong tendinous material on both sides of the incision to facilitate a secure repair at the conclusion of the procedure (Fig. 16-209).

a prominent falciform border extends up to the superior extent of the bicipital groove.

The clavipectoral fascia is incised just lateral to the short head of the biceps, up to but not through the coracoacromial ligament (Fig. 16-206); the incision then enters

FIGURE 16-202 Instruments for surgical repair of recurrent glenohumeral instability. *Top,* A high-speed drill is used for drilling holes in the glenoid rim. *Left to right,* 000 angled curette and reaming tenaculum for connecting the holes drilled in the glenoid rim, curved-nosed needle holder for passing a No. 5 Mayo needle through these holes, self-retaining retractor, humeral head retractor, and sharp-tipped levering retractor.

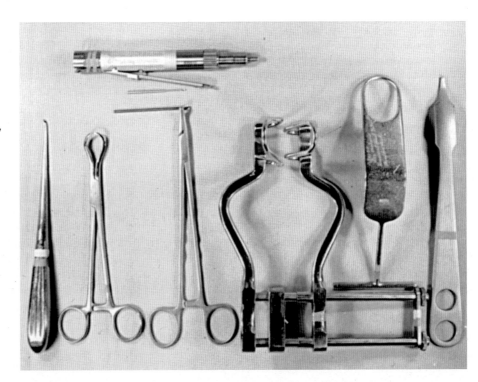

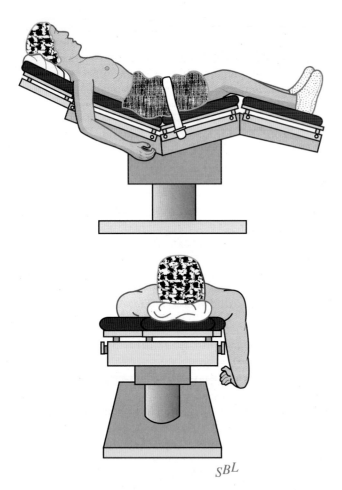

SBL

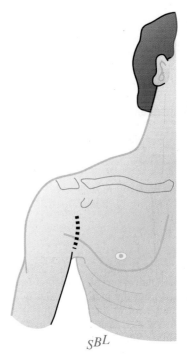

SBL

FIGURE 16-204 Skin incision for Bankart repair. If the incision is made in the major axillary crease, it usually heals with an excellent cosmetic result. (From Matsen FA III, Lippitt SB: Shoulder Surgery: Principles and Procedures. Philadelphia: WB Saunders, 2004, p 131.)

FIGURE 16-203 The beach chair position for surgery. The patient is placed in a comfortable position as in a beach chair with the thorax angled 30 degrees above the horizontal. The neck is in a neutral position. The glenohumeral joint is at the edge of the table, and the arm is completely free. Compressive stockings (not shown here) are applied to the legs. This position allows the skin preparation to be applied to the entire shoulder girdle and arm. (From Matsen FA III, Lippitt SB: Shoulder Surgery: Principles and Procedures. Philadelphia: WB Saunders, 2004, p 66.)

Without being separated, the subscapularis tendon and anterior shoulder capsule are retracted medially to provide an excellent view of the joint. If necessary for greater exposure, the joint capsule may be further divided parallel to the upper rolled border of the subscapularis. The biceps tendon is inspected and note taken of the integrity of the transverse humeral ligament. Particularly in patients older than 40 years, the shoulder is inspected for evidence of rotator cuff tears. In traumatic anterior instability, a posterolateral humeral head defect is usually palpable by passing an index finger over the top of the humeral head (see Fig. 16-3). If the humeral head defect is so large that it contributes to instability in functional positions, anterior capsular tightening may be necessary to keep the defect from entering the joint on external rotation.

The capsule and subscapularis are retracted together medially, and a humeral head retractor is placed so that it leans on the posterior glenoid lip and pushes the humeral head posterolaterally. This technique reveals the anterior inferior glenoid lip from which the labrum and capsule are avulsed in the great majority of patients with anterior traumatic instability (see Fig. 16-120). The labrum usually remains attached to the capsular ligaments, but it can remain on the glenoid side of the rupture, can be a separate (bucket handle) fragment, or can be absent. Occasionally, flimsy attempts to heal the lesion temporarily obliterate the defect. However, in these cases a blunt elevator easily separates the capsule from the glenoid lip and reveals the typical lesion in the anteroinferior quadrant of the glenoid. A spiked retractor is then placed through the capsular avulsion to expose the glenoid lip. The glenohumeral joint is inspected thoroughly for loose bodies, defects of the bony glenoid, and loss of cartilage from the remaining anterior glenoid.

Reconstruction of the capsulolabral detachment from the glenoid is necessary and sufficient for the surgical management of most cases of traumatic instability. Additional tightening jeopardizes the shoulder's range of motion. This repair is carried out from inside the joint, without separating the capsule from the subscapularis muscle and tendon. The glenoid is well exposed by a humeral head retractor laterally and a sharp-tipped lever-

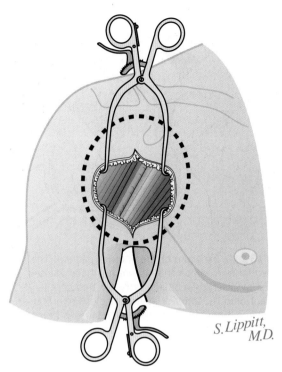

FIGURE 16-205 The deltopectoral interval. Subcutaneous dissection up to the level of the coracoid process exposes the cephalic vein in the deltopectoral groove. (From Matsen FA III, Lippitt SB: Shoulder Surgery: Principles and Procedures. Philadelphia: WB Saunders, 2004, p 131.)

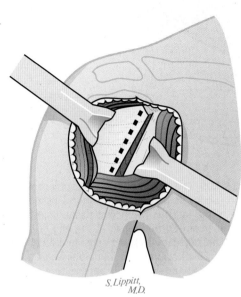

FIGURE 16-206 Clavipectoral fascia. Retraction of the deltoid and cephalic vein laterally and the pectoralis major medially exposes the clavipectoral fascia. This fascia is incised just lateral to the coracoid muscles and tendons (*dotted line*). (From Matsen FA III, Lippitt SB: Shoulder Surgery: Principles and Procedures. Philadelphia: WB Saunders, 2004, p 131.)

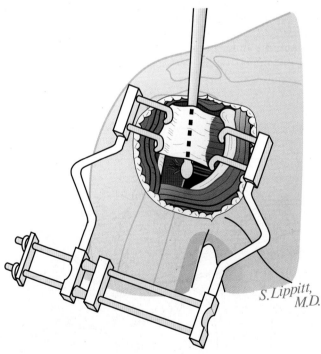

FIGURE 16-207 Subscapularis incision. The subscapularis is incised through its tendon, leaving good tissue on either side for later repair. The anterior humeral circumflex vessels are protected inferiorly. (From Matsen FA III, Lippitt SB: Shoulder Surgery: Principles and Procedures. Philadelphia: WB Saunders, 2004, p 133.)

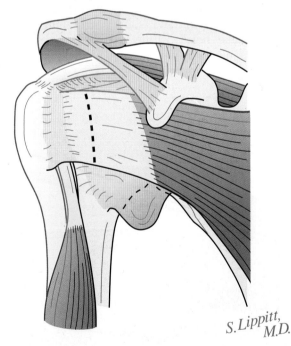

FIGURE 16-208 The subscapularis is incised medial to the lesser tuberosity (*heavy dashed line*), taking care to avoid the tendon of the long head of the biceps at the upper edge of the tendon. (From Matsen FA III, Lippitt SB: Shoulder Surgery: Principles and Procedures. Philadelphia: WB Saunders, 2004, p 134.)

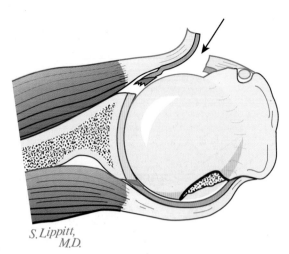

S. Lippitt, M.D.

FIGURE 16-209 The subscapularis and subjacent capsule are incised (*arrow*) so that strong tendinous tissue remains on either side of the incision. Sufficient tissue is left attached to the lesser tuberosity so that repair at the end of the case is facilitated. The subscapularis and capsule are not separated. (From Matsen FA III, Lippitt SB: Shoulder Surgery: Principles and Procedures. Philadelphia: WB Saunders, 2004, p 134.)

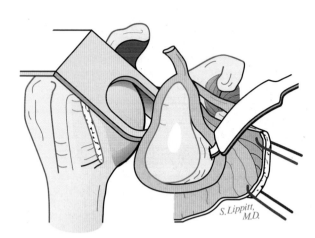

S. Lippitt, M.D.

FIGURE 16-210 Exposure of the anterior glenoid. The lip of the glenoid from which the labrum has been avulsed is exposed by inserting a spiked retractor through the detachment onto the anterior glenoid neck. (From Matsen FA III, Lippitt SB: Shoulder Surgery: Principles and Procedures. Philadelphia: WB Saunders, 2004, p 135.)

ing retractor inserted through the capsular defect onto the neck of the glenoid (Fig. 16-210). Bucket handle or flap tears of the glenoid labrum[641,643] are preserved for incorporation into the reconstruction of the glenoid lip.

The anterior, nonarticular aspect of the glenoid lip is roughened with a curette or a motorized bur, and care is taken to not compromise the bony strength of the glenoid lip (Figs. 16-211 and 16-212). A 1.8-mm drill bit is used to make holes on the articular aspect of the glenoid 3 to 4 mm back from the edge of the lip to ensure

a sufficiently strong bony bridge (Fig. 16-213). We place these holes 5 to 6 mm apart; thus the size of the defect dictates the number of holes used for the reconstruction (Fig. 16-214). Corresponding slots are placed on the anterior nonarticular aspect of the glenoid (Fig. 16-215). A 000 angled curette is used to establish continuity between the corresponding slots and holes (Fig. 16-216).

A strong No. 2 absorbable braided suture is passed through the holes in the glenoid lip with a trocar needle and an angled needle holder (Fig. 16-217). After each

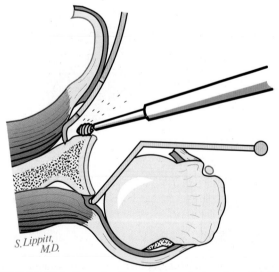

S. Lippitt, M.D.

FIGURE 16-211 Decortication of the anterior glenoid. With a pinecone bur, the cortex of the anterior, nonarticular aspect of the glenoid is roughened. (From Matsen FA III, Lippitt SB: Shoulder Surgery: Principles and Procedures. Philadelphia: WB Saunders, 2004, pp 136-137.)

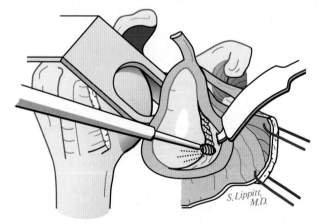

S. Lippitt, M.D.

FIGURE 16-212 The decortication of the anterior glenoid continues for the full length of the detachment to facilitate healing of the detached labrum. (From Matsen FA III, Lippitt SB: Shoulder Surgery: Principles and Procedures. Philadelphia: WB Saunders, 2004, pp 136-137.)

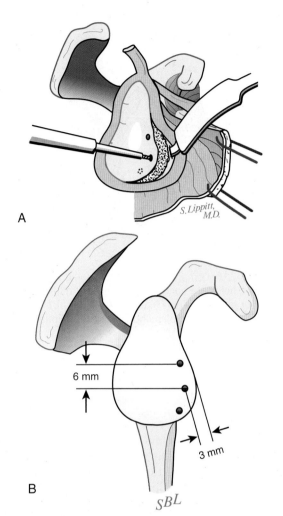

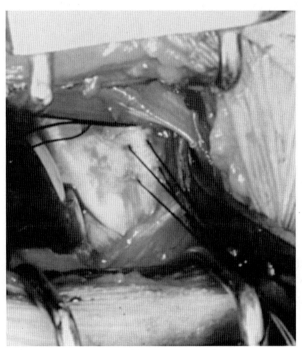

FIGURE 16-214 Intraoperative photograph of the Bankart procedure showing the placement of sutures through holes in the glenoid rim.

FIGURE 16-213 Holes in the glenoid lip. **A,** Holes are drilled through the cartilage and subchondral bone using a 1.8-mm drill. **B,** The holes are placed 6 mm apart for the length of the defect and 3 mm back from the edge of the glenoid lip. (From Matsen FA III, Lippitt SB: Shoulder Surgery: Principles and Procedures. Philadelphia: WB Saunders, 2004, p 138.)

suture is placed through the glenoid lip, the integrity of the bony bridge is checked by a firm pull on the suture.

When sufficient sutures have been placed to span the capsular defect, the spiked retractor is removed and replaced with a right-angled retractor positioned to reveal the trailing medial edge of the avulsed capsule and labrum. This edge is most easily identified by tracing the intact labrum around the glenoid to its point of detachment at the Bankart defect.

Next, by using the trocar needle, the anterior end of the suture (the limb exiting the anterior nonarticular aspect of the glenoid lip) is passed through the trailing medial edge of the capsule, with care taken to incorporate the glenoid labrum, if present, and the strong medial edge of the capsule (Figs. 16-218 and 16-219). To prevent unwanted tightening of the anteroinferior capsule, no

more capsule is taken than necessary to obtain firm purchase. In larger glenohumeral ligament avulsions, the detached medial edge of the capsule tends to sag inferiorly; in this situation, an effort is made to pass each suture through the capsule slightly inferior to the corresponding bone hole in the glenoid lip. Thus, when the sutures are tied, the inferiorly sagging medial capsule is repositioned anatomically (Fig. 16-220).

Once the sutures have been passed through the capsule, they are tied so that the labrum and medial edge of the capsule are brought up on the glenoid lip to restore the fossa-deepening effect of the labrum.[122] The knots are tied so that they come to rest over the capsule rather than on the articular surface of the glenoid. Because they lie over soft tissue, these sutures do not present a mechanical problem, even though they lie within the joint.

Once these sutures are tied, the smooth continuity between the articular surface of the glenoid fossa and the capsule should be re-established along with a reconstructed labrum-like structure (Figs. 16-221 and 16-222). No stepoff or discontinuity in the capsule should be present when the concavity is palpated. If a substantial anterior capsular defect exists anywhere but at the normal subcoracoid recess, it is closed.

Approximately 10% of TUBS patients have fractures or deficiencies of the anterior bony lip of the glenoid. It is reasonable to attempt to attach the avulsed anterior capsule to the lip of the remaining glenoid articular surface. Major anterior glenoid deficiencies or those associated with previous surgical failure might not be recon-

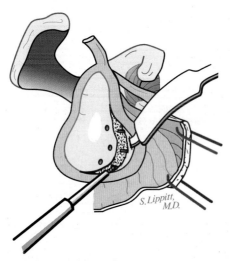

FIGURE 16-215 Slots in the anterior glenoid. If the anterior glenoid bone is dense, the 1.8-mm drill can be used to make slots to facilitate passage of the needle. (From Matsen FA III, Lippitt SB: Shoulder Surgery: Principles and Procedures. Philadelphia: WB Saunders, 2004, p 139.)

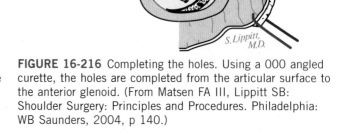

FIGURE 16-216 Completing the holes. Using a 000 angled curette, the holes are completed from the articular surface to the anterior glenoid. (From Matsen FA III, Lippitt SB: Shoulder Surgery: Principles and Procedures. Philadelphia: WB Saunders, 2004, p 140.)

structable with soft tissue methods alone (Figs. 16-223 and 16-224). In such cases we consider an extracapsular iliac crest graft. The bone at the glenoid defect is flattened (Fig. 16-225). Drill holes are placed for the capsular repair (Figs. 16-226 and 16-227). An iliac crest graft is harvested and contoured (Figs. 16-228 and 16-229) and docked on the host site (Figs. 16-230 and 16-231). The graft is then fixed into position (Figs. 16-232 to 16-235) and contoured (Figs. 16-236 and 16-237). The capsule is repaired to the glenoid lip (Fig. 16-238) and cancellous graft is added (Figs. 16-239 and 16-240).

A graft placed outside the repaired capsule becomes covered with periosteum or joint capsule, thereby preventing direct contact with the humeral head (Fig. 16-241). This technique is described in detail by Churchill and colleagues.[186] Its effectiveness in restoring glenoid stability has been demonstrated by Montgomery and colleagues.[147]

At the conclusion of the surgical repair, the capsule and subscapularis tendon are anatomically repaired to their mates at the lesser tuberosity (Figs. 16-242 and 16-243) and by using the upper rolled border of the subscapularis as a reference. At least six sutures of No. 2 braided nonabsorbable suture are used in this repair to ensure a good bite in both the medial and lateral aspects of the repair. If the tissue on the lateral side is insufficient, the tendon and capsule are repaired via drill holes at the base of the lesser tuberosity. A strong subscapularis

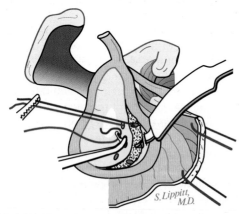

FIGURE 16-217 Passing the needle. Using an angled needle holder, a No. 5 trocar needle carrying No. 2 braided nonabsorbable suture is passed through each hole. (From Matsen FA III, Lippitt SB: Shoulder Surgery: Principles and Procedures. Philadelphia: WB Saunders, 2004, p 141.)

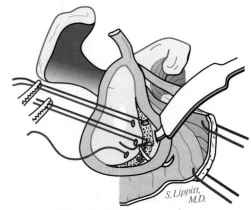

FIGURE 16-218 Suturing the labrum and capsule. Each suture is passed through the labrum, or if there is no residual labrum, through the trailing medial edge of the capsule. (From Matsen FA III, Lippitt SB: Shoulder Surgery: Principles and Procedures. Philadelphia: WB Saunders, 2004, p 142-143.)

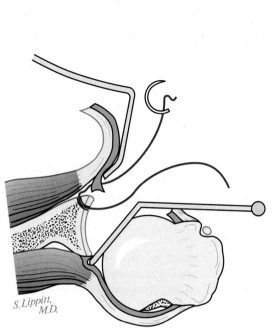

FIGURE 16-219 Cross-section view of the suture passing through the trailing medial edge of the labrum and capsule. (From Matsen FA III, Lippitt SB: Shoulder Surgery: Principles and Procedures. Philadelphia: WB Saunders, 2004, p 142-143.)

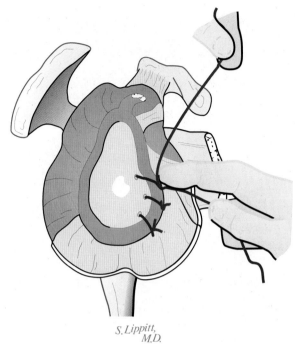

FIGURE 16-220 Tying the suture. Tying the suture over the capsule, rather than over the cartilage, keeps the knot from being interposed between the glenoid and humeral joint surfaces. The labrum is restored anatomically to the glenoid lip. (From Matsen FA III, Lippitt SB: Shoulder Surgery: Principles and Procedures. Philadelphia: WB Saunders, 2004, p 144.)

and capsule repair is essential to early rehabilitation. The shoulder should have at least 30 degrees of external rotation at the side after the subscapularis and capsule repair. Once this repair has been completed, shoulder stability is examined. If excessive anterior laxity remains— for example, external rotation in excess of 45 degrees

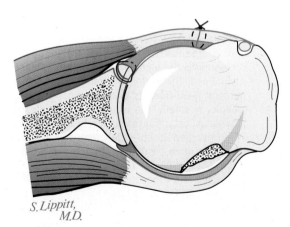

FIGURE 16-221 Final repair. Once the labrum has been reattached to the glenoid lip, the subscapularis and capsule are repaired anatomically. No capsular shift or capsular tightening is performed so that range of motion is not limited needlessly. (From Matsen FA III, Lippitt SB: Shoulder Surgery: Principles and Procedures. Philadelphia: WB Saunders, 2004, p 147.)

(which is rarely the case)—the lateral capsular and subscapularis reattachment may be advanced laterally or superolaterally as desired.

In the highly unusual situation in which a shoulder with the TUBS syndrome is found to not have capsular detachment, the shoulder should be inspected carefully for midsubstance capsular defects. If none are found, the anterior instability may be treated by reefing the anterior capsule and the subscapularis tendon (Fig. 16-244). Shortening these structures by 1 cm limits external rotation of the humerus by approximately 20 degrees. The goal of this restriction is to limit positions of the arm to those in which the net humeral joint reaction force will lie within the balance stability angle. Generally, restricting external rotation to 30 degrees at the operating table permits a very functional shoulder after rehabilitation is complete. If the patient has marked anterior ligamentous laxity, proportionately greater anterior tightening may be necessary, although the surgeon must be certain that the patient does not have multidirectional laxity before unidirectional tightening is carried out.

Standard wound closure is performed with a subcuticular suture, which is removed in 3 days.

After surgery, most patients are started on a self-conducted 90–0 rehabilitation program with instructions from a physical therapist or physician (Figs. 16-245 and

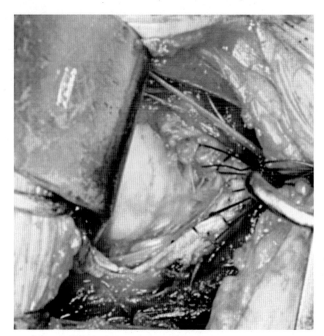

FIGURE 16-222 Intraoperative photograph during re-exploration of a Bankart repair. This patient ruptured the subscapularis tendon repair in a fall 2 months after a Bankart procedure. At the time of reoperation for repair of the subscapularis tendon, the anterior glenoid rim was explored and the Bankart repair was intact. The repair sutures were covered by synovium. The reconstructed labrum is strong.

16-246). We move the shoulder soon after surgery because the repair is strong enough that motion is safe for reliable patients and early motion can increase the ultimate strength of a ligament repair.[194] On the day after surgery, exercises five times daily are started, including assisted flexion to 90 degrees and external rotation to 0 degrees.

The contralateral arm is used as the assistant until the operated arm can conduct the exercises alone.

Patients are allowed to perform many activities of daily living as comfort permits within the 90-degree/0-degree range, as long as they avoid lifting anything heavier than a glass of water. Allowed activities include eating and personal hygiene, as well as certain vocational activities such as writing and keyboarding. Gripping, isometric external rotation, and isometric abduction exercises are started immediately after surgery to minimize the effects of disuse.

If a patient does not appear to be able to comply with this restricted-use program, the arm is kept in a sling for 3 weeks; otherwise, a sling is used only for comfort between exercise sessions and to protect the arm when the patient is out in public and at night while sleeping.

Driving is allowed as early as 2 weeks after surgery if the arm can be used actively and comfortably, particularly if the patient's car has an automatic transmission and the operated arm is not used to set the emergency brake. This rapid return to functional activities is made possible because of the strength of the repair and is encouraged to maintain the shoulder's strength and neuromuscular control. It minimizes the immediate postoperative disability and discomfort without jeopardizing the healing process.

At 2 weeks after surgery, the patient should return for an examination and should have at least 90 degrees of elevation and external rotation to 0 degrees. From 2 weeks to 6 weeks postoperatively, the patient is instructed to increase the range of motion to 140 degrees of elevation and 40 degrees of external rotation. At 6 weeks after surgery, if there is good evidence of active control of the shoulder, controlled repetitive activities such as swimming and using a rowing machine are instituted to help

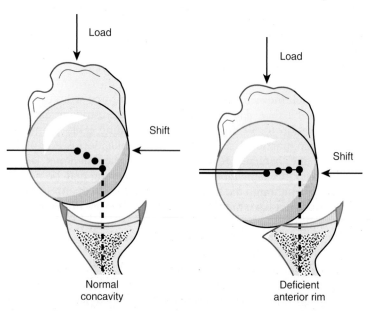

Normal
concavity

Deficient
anterior rim

FIGURE 16-223 Normal and pathologic load and shift. In the load and shift test, the humeral head is pressed into the glenoid, and while this loading is maintained, the examiner attempts to translate the humeral head from its position centered on the glenoid. Normally, the concavity of the glenoid provides substantial resistance to any translation. When the glenoid lip is deficient, the humeral head translates more easily from the centered position. (From Matsen FA III, Lippitt SB: Shoulder Surgery: Principles and Procedures. Philadelphia: WB Saunders, 2004, p 151.)

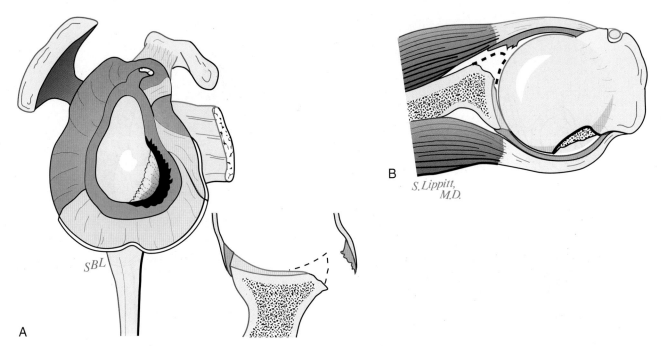

FIGURE 16-224 Eroded anterior glenoid lip. **A,** Deficient anterior glenoid lip. Loss of the glenoid labrum, the anterior glenoid cartilage, and anterior glenoid bone can each contribute to diminished resistance to translation from the centered position. **B,** Loss of the anterior bony lip. Deficiency of the bony lip of the glenoid compromises the potential for reattaching the residual capsule and labrum at their physiologic length. (From Matsen FA III, Lippitt SB: Shoulder Surgery: Principles and Procedures. Philadelphia: WB Saunders, 2004, p 153.)

rebuild coordination, strength, and endurance of the shoulder. More-vigorous activities such as basketball, volleyball, throwing, and serving in tennis should not be started until 3 months, and then only if the patient has excellent strength, endurance, range of motion, and coordination of the shoulder.

Vigilance must be exercised in patients older than 35 years to be sure that unwanted postoperative stiffness does not develop. Thus, particularly for these patients, the 2-week and 6-week checkups are very important to make sure that the range of elevation and external rotation are 90 and 0 degrees at 3 weeks and 140 and 40 degrees at 6 weeks.

In a 5.5-year follow-up of the first group of these repairs, we found 97% good to excellent results based on Rowe's[382] grading system. One of 39 shoulders had a single redislocation 4 years after repair while the patient was practicing karate. He became asymptomatic after completing a strengthening program and is back to full activities, including karate. The average range of motion at follow-up was 171 degrees of elevation, 68 degrees of external rotation with the arm at the side, and 85 degrees of external rotation at 90 degrees of abduction. Ninety-five percent of these patients reported that their shoulder felt stable with all activities; 80% had no shoulder pain, and 20% had occasional pain with activity. None had complications of posterior subluxation as a result of excessive anterior tightness, nor did any patient have complications related to hardware!

Rockwood and Wirth's Preferred Method for Management of Traumatic Shoulder Instability

Before surgery, all our patients are instructed in a series of exercises designed to strengthen the rotator cuff, deltoid, and scapular stabilizers (see Fig. 16-170). Our preferred method of surgical repair has been an anatomic reconstruction—that is, repair of the Perthes–Bankart lesion or double-breasting of the capsule. We rarely have to overlap, and thus shorten, the subscapularis tendon.

Surgical Incision

The standard anterior axillary incision begins in the anterior axillary crease and extends up toward and usually stops at the coracoid process (Fig. 16-247A). In large muscular men, the incision may extend proximally as far as the clavicle. In women, we use the modified axillary incision described by Leslie and Ryan.[69]

The skin is undermined subcutaneously in the proximal medial and distal lateral corners to expose the deltopectoral interval (see Fig. 16-247B). Usually, this interval is identified by the presence of the cephalic vein (see Fig. 16-247C), which may be absent or lying deep in the interval out of sight. When the vein is not present, we

Text continued on p. 734

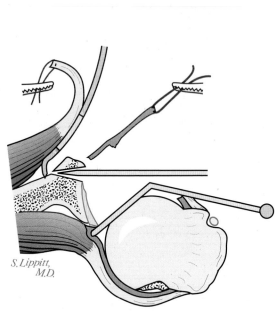

FIGURE 16-225 Flattening the host site. The selected host site is flattened with an osteotome, preserving the intact portion of the glenoid concavity. Ideally the host site should measure 25 × 25 mm. (From Matsen FA III, Lippitt SB: Shoulder Surgery: Principles and Procedures. Philadelphia: WB Saunders, 2004, p 159.)

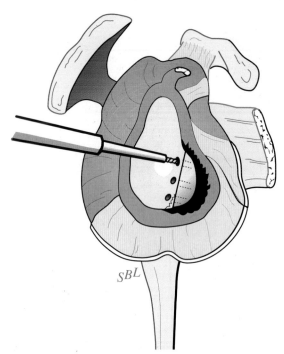

FIGURE 16-226 Capsular fixation holes. Drill holes are made at the margin of the intact glenoid for attachment of the capsule. (From Matsen FA III, Lippitt SB: Shoulder Surgery: Principles and Procedures. Philadelphia: WB Saunders, 2004, p 160.)

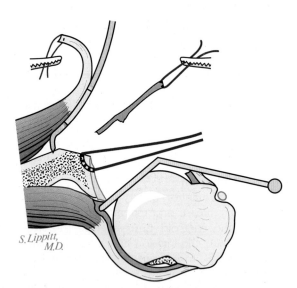

FIGURE 16-227 Suture passage. Strands of No. 2 braided nonabsorbable suture are passed through each hole in the glenoid lip. (From Matsen FA III, Lippitt SB: Shoulder Surgery: Principles and Procedures. Philadelphia: WB Saunders, 2004, p 161.)

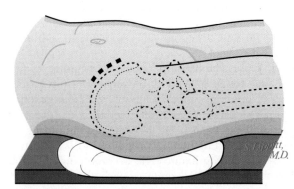

FIGURE 16-228 Graft incision. A skin incision (*heavy dotted line*) is made over the anterior iliac crest. (From Matsen FA III, Lippitt SB: Shoulder Surgery: Principles and Procedures. Philadelphia: WB Saunders, 2004, p 162.)

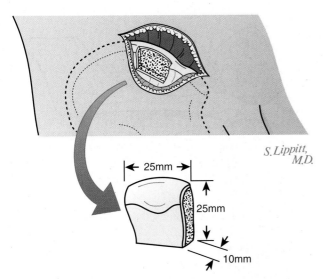

FIGURE 16-229 The graft. A 25 × 25 × 10 mm graft is harvested from the superolateral iliac crest. (From Matsen FA III, Lippitt SB: Shoulder Surgery: Principles and Procedures. Philadelphia: WB Saunders, 2004, p 163.)

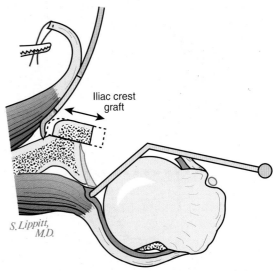

FIGURE 16-230 Docking the graft. The flat surface of the graft is placed on the flat surface of the host site. The graft is positioned so that it extends a few millimeters more laterally than the joint surface. (From Matsen FA III, Lippitt SB: Shoulder Surgery: Principles and Procedures. Philadelphia: WB Saunders, 2004, p 163.)

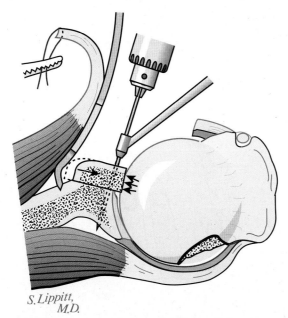

FIGURE 16-231 Pinning the graft. The graft is advanced laterally (*arrow*) until it just contacts the humeral head (*arrows*). Once the desired position of the graft is identified, it is temporarily fixed in position using two Kirschner wires. (From Matsen FA III, Lippitt SB: Shoulder Surgery: Principles and Procedures. Philadelphia: WB Saunders, 2004, p 165.)

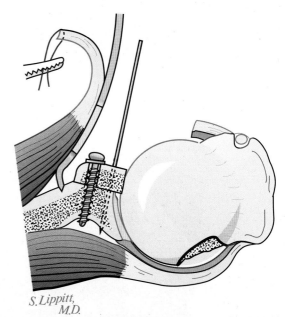

FIGURE 16-232 The first screw. A 3.5-mm self-tapping cortical screw with a washer is placed as far medially as the graft will allow. (From Matsen FA III, Lippitt SB: Shoulder Surgery: Principles and Procedures. Philadelphia: WB Saunders, 2004, p 166.)

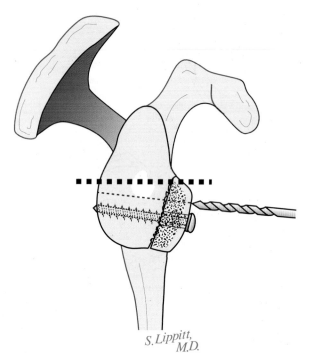

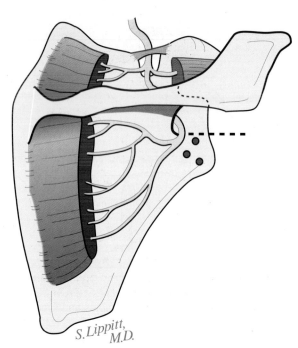

FIGURE 16-233 Second and third screws. Two additional self-tapping cortical screws are placed farther laterally in the graft. These screws are directed below the mid glenoid (*dotted line*) and clear of the joint surface. (From Matsen FA III, Lippitt SB: Shoulder Surgery: Principles and Procedures. Philadelphia: WB Saunders, 2004, p 167.)

FIGURE 16-234 Screw safety. Placing the screws below the mid glenoid (*dotted line*) reduces the risk to the nerve to the infraspinatus posteriorly. (From Matsen FA III, Lippitt SB: Shoulder Surgery: Principles and Procedures. Philadelphia: WB Saunders, 2004, p 167.)

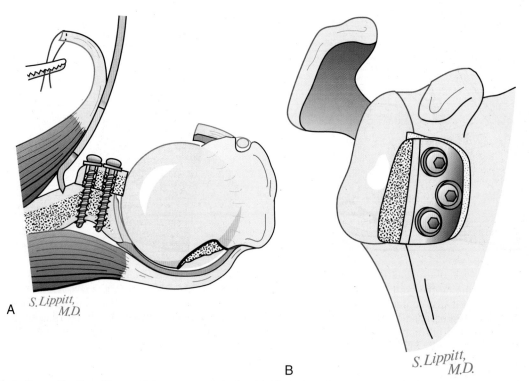

FIGURE 16-235 A, Screw fixation. The graft is now securely fixed with its flat side against the flat side of the host site. **B,** Triangulation. Arrangement of the three screws in a triangular configuration minimizes the risk of loosening. (From Matsen FA III, Lippitt SB: Shoulder Surgery: Principles and Procedures. Philadelphia: WB Saunders, 2004, p 168.)

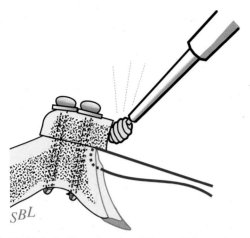

FIGURE 16-236 Graft contouring. The graft is contoured in situ using a pinecone bur. (From Matsen FA III, Lippitt SB: Shoulder Surgery: Principles and Procedures. Philadelphia: WB Saunders, 2004, p 169.)

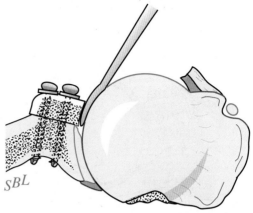

FIGURE 16-237 Fine-tuning. Shaping of the graft is continued until a thin elevator just passes between the graft and the humeral head centered in the glenoid. It is important that the graft not press the humeral head posteriorly. (From Matsen FA III, Lippitt SB: Shoulder Surgery: Principles and Procedures. Philadelphia: WB Saunders, 2004, p 169.)

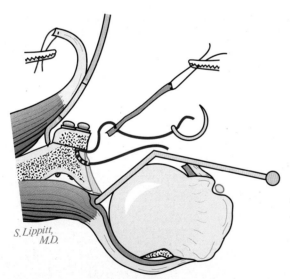

FIGURE 16-238 Capsule suturing. The capsule is closed to the margin of the glenoid using the previously placed sutures. (From Matsen FA III, Lippitt SB: Shoulder Surgery: Principles and Procedures. Philadelphia: WB Saunders, 2004, p 170.)

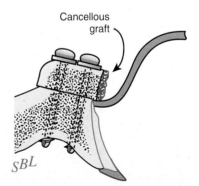

FIGURE 16-239 Cancellous grafting. Cancellous bone graft is added between the fixed graft and the capsule. (From Matsen FA III, Lippitt SB: Shoulder Surgery: Principles and Procedures. Philadelphia: WB Saunders, 2004, p 171.)

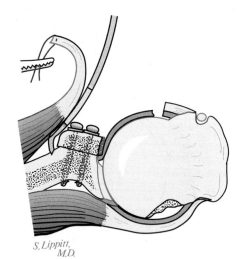

FIGURE 16-240 Extra-articular graft. The cancellous graft on top of the fixed graft provides moldable extracapsular support for the anterior capsule. (From Matsen FA III, Lippitt SB: Shoulder Surgery: Principles and Procedures. Philadelphia: WB Saunders, 2004, p 171.)

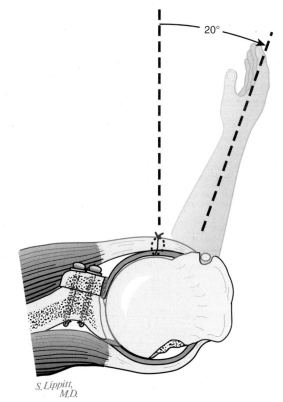

FIGURE 16-242 Subscapularis and capsular repair. If the capsule is sufficiently long, it is repaired back to its counterpart at the lesser tuberosity along with the subscapularis. (From Matsen FA III, Lippitt SB: Shoulder Surgery: Principles and Procedures. Philadelphia: WB Saunders, 2004, p 175.)

can define the deltopectoral interval proximally because in this area, it is easier to see the difference in angles of the muscle fibers between the pectoralis major and the deltoid.

The interval should be very carefully opened, with the vein taken laterally with the deltoid muscle. Routine ligation of the vein produces venous congestion in the area and in the upper extremity and increases postop-

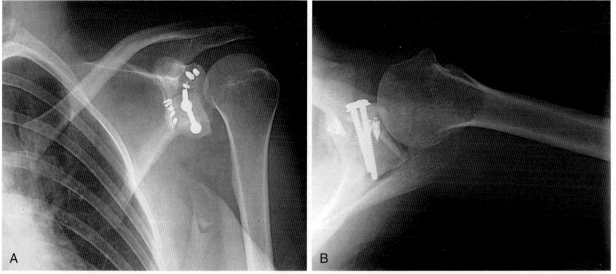

FIGURE 16-241 AP (**A**) and axillary (**B**) radiographs show a bone-reinforced Bankart repair performed for recurrent instability and anterior glenoid lip deficiency after multiple previous anterior repairs that used the suture anchors seen. In this procedure, the capsule is repaired to the lip of the remaining glenoid articular cartilage. The contoured iliac crest graft is then secured to the anterior glenoid outside the capsule, which provides a smooth covering for articulation with the humeral head. Final smoothing of the graft is carried out after it is in position to ensure that it presents the optimal congruent extension of the bony glenoid.

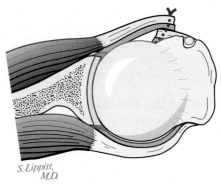

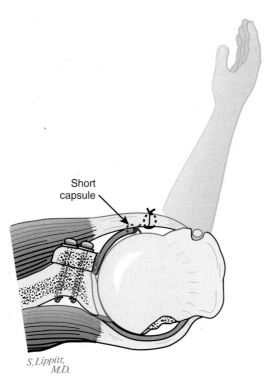

FIGURE 16-244 Transverse plane section showing reefing of the subscapularis tendon and capsule in a situation in which no Bankart lesion or other capsular defect is found with isolated anterior instability. Note the intact anterior glenoid rim and the strong repair of the subscapularis tendon. (From Matsen FA, Thomas SC: Glenohumeral instability. In Evarts CM [ed]: Surgery of the Musculoskeletal System, 2nd ed. New York: Churchill Livingstone, 1989.)

FIGURE 16-243 Subscapularis and capsular repair. If the capsule is too short to repair to itself, the lateral edge of the capsular flap is sewn to the deep surface of the subscapularis. (From Matsen FA III, Lippitt SB: Shoulder Surgery: Principles and Procedures. Philadelphia: WB Saunders, 2004, p 175.)

erative discomfort. Preservation of the vein contributes to an easier postoperative course (less pain and swelling). We use 8-0 nylon suture to repair any inadvertent nicks in the vein. The deltopectoral interval is developed all the way up to the clavicle without any need to detach any of the deltoid from the clavicle. We usually detach the upper 2 cm of the pectoralis major tendon to allow better visualization of the inferior capsule and make it easier to locate and protect the axillary nerve, which passes just inferior to the capsule. We do not find it necessary to detach the coracoid process or the conjoined tendon (see Fig. 16-247D).

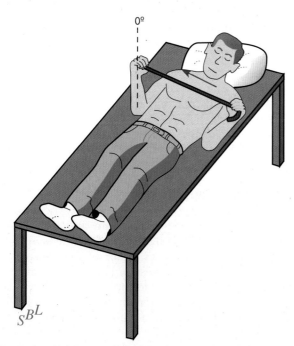

FIGURE 16-245 Immediate postoperative rehabilitation. Using the opposite hand and a cane or yardstick, the operated arm is passively externally rotated to 0 degrees. (From Matsen FA III, Lippitt SB: Shoulder Surgery: Principles and Procedures. Philadelphia: WB Saunders, 2004, p 148.)

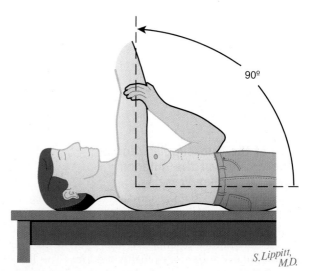

FIGURE 16-246 Immediate postoperative rehabilitation. Using the opposite hand, the operated arm is passively elevated to 90 degrees. (From Matsen FA III, Lippitt SB: Shoulder Surgery: Principles and Procedures. Philadelphia: WB Saunders, 2004, p 149.)

With the deltopectoral muscles retracted out of the way, the clavipectoral fascia is seen covering the conjoined tendon. This fascia is divided vertically along the lateral border of the conjoined tendon. Proximally, the clavipectoral fascia blends into the coracoacromial ligament.

Identification of the Musculocutaneous Nerve

Before a Richardson retractor is placed in the medial side of the incision to retract the conjoined muscles and pectoralis major muscle, we palpate for the musculocutaneous nerve as it enters the conjoined tendon. Ordinarily, the nerve enters the coracobrachialis and biceps muscles from the medial aspect approximately 5 cm distal to the tip of the coracoid process. However, it must be remembered that it might penetrate immediately below the tip of the coracoid. We have even seen the nerve visible on the lateral aspect of the conjoined tendon (Fig. 16-248). Usually, by palpating just medial to the conjoined tendon and muscles, one can feel the entrance of the musculocutaneous nerve.

Identification and Protection of the Axillary Nerve

Next, we locate the axillary nerve—an especially important step when performing the capsular shift procedure—by passing the finger down and along the lower and intact subscapularis muscle–tendon unit (see Fig. 16-247E). The right index finger should be used to locate the nerve in the left shoulder, and the left index finger should be used to locate the nerve in the right shoulder. When the finger is as deep as it will go, the volar surface of the finger should be on the anterior surface of the muscle. Then the distal phalanx is flexed and rotated anteriorly, which hooks under the axillary nerve before it dives back posteriorly under the inferior capsule. With the arm in external rotation, the nerve is displaced medially and IS difficult to locate. This large nerve can easily be located with the arm in adduction and neutral rotation. With the upper 2 cm of the pectoralis major tendon taken down, not only can the nerve be palpated, it can also be visualized. The nerve is at least 5/32 inch in size.

Division of the Subscapular Tendon and Preservation of the Anterior Humeral Circumflex Vessels

The arm is positioned in external rotation so that the upper and lower borders of the subscapularis tendon can be visualized and palpated. The soft spot at the superior border of subscapularis tendon is the interval between the subscapularis and supraspinatus tendons. The lower border of the tendon is identified by the presence of the anterior humeral circumflex artery and veins (see Fig. 16-247F). The upper three fourths of the subscapularis tendon will be vertically transected, usually 0.75 to 1 inch medial to its insertion into the lesser tuberosity. We cut only the upper two thirds of the subscapularis tendon and prefer to do so with the electric cautery (see Fig. 16-247F and G). We are very careful to divide only the tendon and usually try to leave a little of the subscapularis tendon on the capsule to add to its strength (see Fig. 16-247H). We avoid transecting the lower third of the subscapularis tendon and leave it in place to prevent injury to the anterior humeral circumflex artery and veins, to preserve a portion of the tendon's proprioceptive capability, and to protect the axillary nerve. The anterior humeral circumflex artery is the primary blood supply to the head of the humerus, and we believe that it should be preserved.

Once the vertical cut in the tendon has been completed, we very carefully reflect the medial part of the tendon off the capsule with curved Mayo scissors until there are no further connections between the tendon and the capsule. The tendon should have a rubbery bounce to it when lateral traction is applied to it. Three or four stay sutures of No. 2 Cottony Dacron are placed in the medial edge of the tendon; these sutures are used initially for retraction and later at the time of tendon repair.

The lateral stump of the subscapularis tendon is reflected off the capsule with a small sharp knife. This step is easy with the capsule intact when the arm is in external rotation and difficult when the capsule has been divided. Failure to perform this step will make the two-layer closure of the capsule and the subscapularis tendon more difficult.

With the divided portions of the subscapularis tendon reflected medially and laterally and with the arm in mild external rotation, we use an elevator to gently strip the intact lower fourth of the subscapularis muscle–tendon unit off the anteroinferior capsule. A narrow deep retractor (e.g., Scofield) should be used to retract the lower part of the subscapularis muscle anteriorly and distally, which allows easy visualization of the inferior capsule. The retractor holds not only the lower part of the subscapularis muscle but also the axillary nerve anteriorly and distally out of the way to prevent injury when the inferior capsule is opened, divided, and repaired (see Fig. 16-247L).

Division of the Capsule

The capsule is divided vertically midway between its usual attachment on the glenoid rim and the humeral head (see Fig. 16-247I-K). Division of the capsule at this location is easier and allows repair of the capsule if a Perthes–Bankart lesion is present. Furthermore, after the medial capsule is reattached to the glenoid rim, we have plenty of room to add strength to the anteroinferior capsule by double-breasting it with the planned capsular reconstruction.

This vertical incision begins at the superior glenohumeral ligament and extends all the way down to the most inferior aspect of the capsule. Occasionally, the superior capsular region is deficient, but such deficiency does not alter the vertical capsular incision (see Fig. 16-247L). We prefer to insert horizontal mattress sutures in the medial capsule just as we complete the division of the most inferior portion of the capsule. We explore the joint carefully and remove loose bodies and repair glenoid labrum tears. Close attention should be paid to stripping of the labrum, capsule, and periosteum from their normal attachments on the glenoid rim and neck of the scapula (i.e., the Perthes–Bankart lesion).

Capsular Shift and Reconstruction

If the capsule has secure fixation on the glenoid rim, capsular reconstruction can then be performed. However, if the capsule and periosteum have been stripped from the glenoid rim and neck of the scapula, the capsule must first be reattached before proceeding to capsular reconstruction. Formerly, we believed that if the capsule was stripped from the neck of the scapula, all that was needed was to roughen this area up with a curette or osteotome to create bleeding and then the capsule would spontaneously reattach or heal itself back to the glenoid rim. However, because of failures that required reoperation, it was obvious that this area had not healed and the capsule was still stripped off the glenoid neck. Most likely, synovial fluid within this area inhibits the usual healing process and prevents consistent firm reattachment of the capsule and periosteum to the bony glenoid rim.

In some situations, it may be necessary to horizontally split the medial part of the capsule in its midportion to better visualize and decorticate the anterior rim and neck of the scapula with an osteotome or an air bur. A special retractor developed by Dr. Carter Rowe, which we call the dinner fork because of its shape and three sharp teeth, is used to retract the capsule and muscles out of the way while the anterior glenoid rim and neck of the scapula are abraded. With the Bowen, Rowe, or Fukuda retractor holding the humeral head out of the way and the dinner fork retracting the medial capsule and subscapularis, an osteotome or bur is used to abrade the anterior surface of the neck of the scapula (see Fig. 16-247M). Absorbable anchors are placed into the anterior glenoid rim to ensure an anatomic repair of the capsulolabral structures. The anchors are evenly spaced from one another by 8 to 10 mm, and each is loaded with two No. 2 braided, nonabsorbable sutures (see Fig. 16-247N). The sutures are passed through the capsule and labrum in a horizontal mattress fashion and securely tied.

Before closure of the capsule, the joint is thoroughly irrigated with saline. Next, the rotator interval closure is performed with the arm in an adducted and externally rotated position (see Fig. 16-247O). This is followed by shifting the medial capsular flap under the lateral capsular flap, progressing in an inferior to superior direction. The arm is initially positioned in 90 degrees of abduction and the desired degree of external rotation during placement of the inferior capsular sutures and is progressively moved into adduction during each subsequent suture placement. External rotation is constantly reassessed during the cap-

sular shift procedure. This ensures that the capsule is adequately tensioned without compromising the laxity required for normal joint rotation.

Next, the lateral capsule is double-breasted by taking it medially and superiorly and suturing it down to the anterior surface of the medial capsule (see Fig. 16-247P and Q). These sutures are also placed with the arm in the desired rotation. Not only does this type of capsular reconstruction eliminate all laxity in the anterior and inferior capsular ligaments, but because of the double-breasting, the capsule is much stronger. The wound is again carefully irrigated with several liters of saline.

With the arm held in 25 degrees of external rotation, the medial subscapularis tendon is brought into view by pulling on the previously placed sutures. The two borders of the tendon are easily approximated with gentle traction, and the tendon is repaired without any overlapping. If the tendon is loose with the arm in 25 degrees of external rotation, double-breasting or overlapping of the tendon can be performed by using a two-layer closure with No. 2 Dacron horizontal mattress sutures.

Wound Closure

Before closure of the wound, we carefully irrigate with antibiotic solution and then infiltrate the joint, muscles, and subcutaneous tissue with 25 to 30 mL of 0.5% bupivacaine (Marcaine). This agent aids in decreasing the immediate postoperative pain. We are convinced that the use of bupivacaine before wound closure gives the patient an easier postoperative recovery period. The effect of the bupivacaine lasts 6 to 8 hours, which allows the patient to have relatively little pain on awakening; later in the day, as the anesthesia begins to wear off, the patient can request pain medications. Care should be taken to not overuse the bupivacaine or inject it directly into vessels. It is usually unnecessary to put any sutures in the deltopectoral interval. The deep subcutaneous layer is closed with 2-0 nonabsorbable suture, which helps prevent widening of the scar. Subcutaneous fat is closed with absorbable sutures, and a running subcuticular nylon suture is used in the skin.

Surgical Technique Summary

In contrast to a number of previously reported reconstructions for anterior shoulder instability, the procedure that we advocate is an anatomic method of reconstruction that affords great latitude in correcting any pathology encountered at the time of surgery. The anatomic capsular shift procedure is a physiologic repair that includes repair of capsulolabral injury, when present, and reinforcement of the anteroinferior capsular ligaments by a double-breasting technique that decreases overall capsule volume. This reconstruction is a modification of the published reports of the Putti–Platt, Bankart, and Neer capsular shift procedures, and several points deserve emphasis.

First, only the upper two thirds of the subscapularis tendon is detached and the inferior third of the tendon

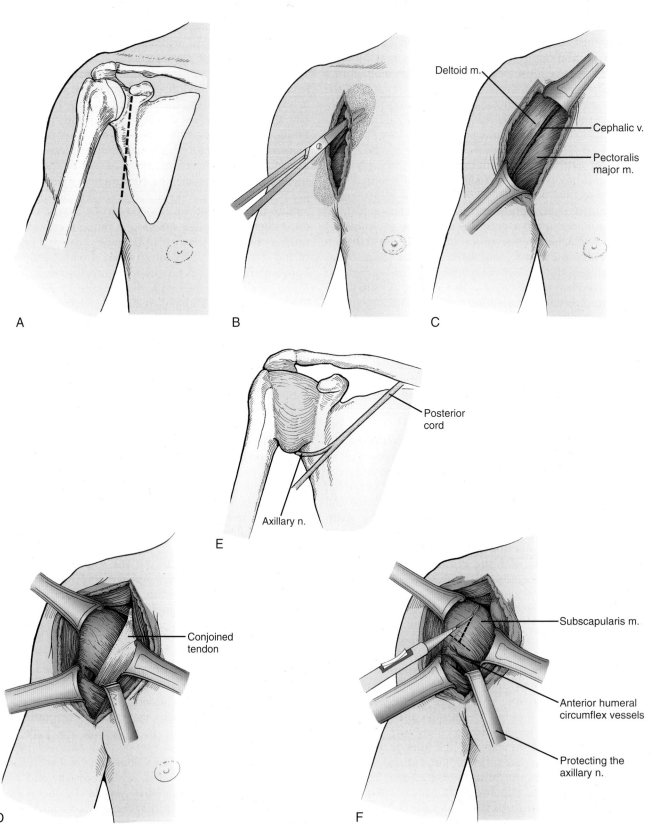

FIGURE 16-247 The precise details of the operative procedure can be followed in the detailed description of the author's preferred method of operative treatment in the text. **A** to **Q,** The procedure used if the anterior capsule is not stripped off the scapula. (**A** to **M, P, Q** from Wirth MA, Blatter G, Rockwood CA Jr: The capsular imbrication procedure for recurrent anterior instability of the shoulder. J Bone Joint Surg Am 78:246-259, 1996.)

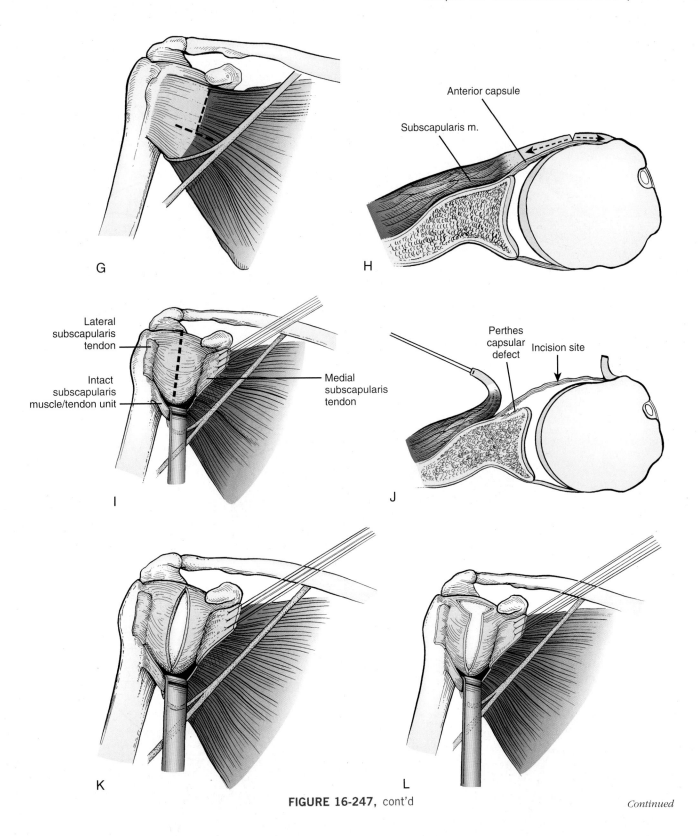

G

H

Anterior capsule

Subscapularis m.

Lateral subscapularis tendon

Intact subscapularis muscle/tendon unit

Medial subscapularis tendon

I

Perthes capsular defect

Incision site

J

K

L

FIGURE 16-247, cont'd

Continued

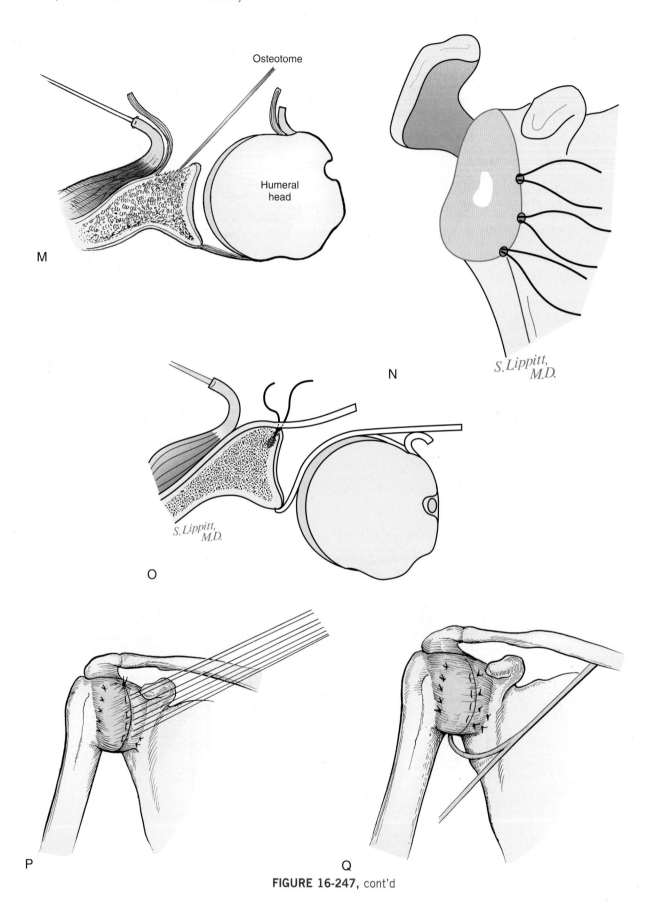

FIGURE 16-247, cont'd

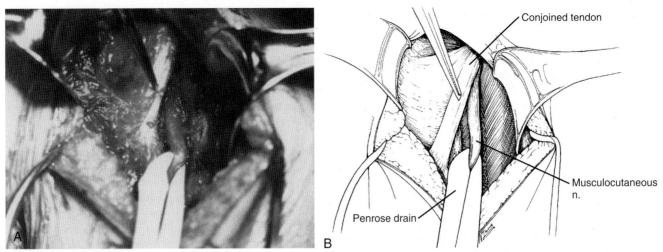

FIGURE 16-248 Intraoperative photograph (**A**) and correlative diagram (**B**) demonstrating the path of the musculocutaneous nerve as it courses lateral to the conjoined tendons. (From Rockwood CA Jr, Green DP, Bucholz RW [eds]: Fractures in Adults. Philadelphia: JB Lippincott, 1991.)

is left intact because of the theoretical advantages of preserving a portion of the tendon's proprioceptive capability and protecting the anterior humeral circumflex vessels, which are the primary blood supply to the humeral head. The intact portion of the tendon is also gently stripped and retracted from the underlying capsule to allow visualization of the inferior-most part of the capsule while protecting the axillary nerve and vessels.

Second, the deltopectoral interval should be carefully developed and the cephalic vein taken laterally with the deltoid because the majority of tributaries in this region arise from this muscle. In our experience, preservation of the vein contributes to an easier postoperative course, whereas routine ligation produces venous congestion in the upper extremity and increases postoperative discomfort.

Third, it is unnecessary to detach the coracoid or conjoined tendons to gain adequate exposure, but occasionally we release the upper 1 cm of the pectoralis major tendon to allow better visualization of the inferior capsule. Such release also facilitates identification of the axillary nerve, which passes just inferior to the capsule as it exits the quadrilateral space.

Fourth, proper identification of the musculocutaneous and axillary nerves cannot be overemphasized. Identification of the axillary nerve is especially critical so that it can be protected when opening and repairing the inferior capsule.

Fifth, the capsule is divided in a vertical fashion midway between its glenoid and humeral site of attachment. Division in this location provides excellent intra-articular exposure to repair a Perthes–Bankart lesion, and it is easy to perform and facilitates subsequent imbrication, which reinforces the capsular reconstruction.

Sixth, the upper two thirds of the subscapularis tendon is repaired anatomically to itself to help minimize the development of undesirable internal rotation contractures of the glenohumeral joint.

Postoperative Management

Postoperatively we prefer to use a commercial shoulder immobilizer because it is comfortable, quick, and simple to apply and it prevents abduction, flexion, and external rotation. Regardless of the type of immobilization, it is very important to temporarily remove the device when the patient is seen on the afternoon or evening of the day of surgery. For some reason, a patient who awakens from surgery with the arm in the device does not want to wiggle any part of the arm—almost as though it were frozen in the sling-and-swathe position. The commercial immobilizer can easily be removed to allow the patient to move the hand and wrist and then gradually extend the elbow down to the side and lay it on the bed. Such movement almost always relieves the aching pain in the arm and the muscle tension pain. We then tell the patient to flex and extend the elbow several times, which also relieves the generalized arm and shoulder discomfort. In many instances, a patient has related that the vague ache in the shoulder and elbow is more of a problem than pain at the operative site and that this simple release of the immobilizer to allow movement of the elbow and wrist eliminates the discomfort. We allow the patient to remove the immobilizer three to four times a day to exercise the elbow, but otherwise we instruct the patient to always keep the immobilizer in place. Specific instructions are given to the patient to avoid abduction, flexion, and external rotation when the device is removed.

Patients are usually discharged on the second or third postoperative day, and we allow them to remove the immobilizer two or three times a day while at home when sitting, reading, or watching television. The patient may return to school or work any time after discharge from the hospital. Five days after surgery, the patient may remove the small dressing, take a shower, and reapply the new bandage. We usually delay removing the running subcuticular nylon stitch for 2 weeks because such delay seems to help prevent a wide scar.

As a general rule, the older the patient, the shorter the postoperative immobilization; the younger the patient, the longer the immobilization. In patients younger than 20 years or in a competitive, aggressive athlete, we immobilize the shoulder for 3 to 4 weeks; in young, semiathletic people younger than 30 years, shoulders are immobilized for 3 weeks; the shoulders of patients 30 to 50 years are immobilized for 2 weeks; and the shoulders of patients older than 50 years are immobilized for 1 to 2 weeks. After removal of the shoulder immobilizer, we allow the patient to gently use the arm for everyday living activities but do not allow any rough use (e.g., lifting, moving furniture, pushing, pulling). At the end of the immobilization period, we start the patient on a stretching exercise program using an overhead pulley and rope set. After the return of motion, we institute a resisted-weight exercise and shoulder-strengthening program to strengthen the deltoid, internal rotators, external rotators, and scapular stabilizers (see Fig. 16-170). Athletes are not permitted to return to competitive sports until they have reached a full and functional range of motion and have regained normal muscle strength, which usually requires 4 to 6 months.

Results

In our series,[544] 93% of the results were rated good or excellent at an average follow-up of 5 years, with a high degree of patient satisfaction and marked improvement in ratings for pain, strength, stability, and function. The average loss of external rotation was 7 degrees, and the average loss of elevation was 6 degrees, which represents physiologic preservation of motion and compares favorably with other reports. The results after revision surgery were encouraging, with 45 (87%) good to excellent results and 7 (13%) fair to poor results. Despite this success, revision anterior shoulder surgery is a formidable challenge with a less-predictable outcome inasmuch as 7 of 10 patients graded fair or poor had failed previous reconstructive efforts. Although progressive symptoms of discomfort were noted in the subset of patients with previous surgery and degenerative changes in the glenohumeral joint, no relationship was found between symptomatic instability after the index procedure and the length of follow-up.

Operative Management of Posterior Instability

Considerations in the Decision for Surgery

In a current concepts review, Robinson and associates[644] concluded that recurrent posterior instability is a relatively uncommon debilitating condition that requires careful evaluation, vigorous nonoperative management, and carefully selected surgical approaches. In an important study, Kim and colleagues[645] performed magnetic reso-

nance arthrography on posteriorly unstable shoulders. They found that posterior glenoid depth was significantly reduced in the inferior and middle aspects of posteriorly unstable shoulders. The loss of depth was due to diminished osseous and chondrolabral height. Their findings might help explain recurrent instability after repairs that do not address the lack of what they refer to as *chondrolabral containment.*

The choice of management for recurrent posterior instability is complicated by several aspects. Most often, recurrent posterior instability is atraumatic, in contrast to the situation with anterior instability, in which only a small percentage of cases are obviously traumatic in etiology. The pathogenesis of recurrent posterior instability is multifactorial, complex, and less well understood than for anterior instability, and the results of the methods for posterior repair are at least 10 times worse than the average for anterior repair. As an example, Hawkins and coworkers[276,646,647] presented 50 shoulders in 35 patients treated for recurrent posterior instability. Only 11 of the 50 followed a traumatic event, and 41 demonstrated voluntary and involuntary instability. Of those operated on, 17 patients had a glenoid osteotomy, 6 had a reverse Putti–Platt procedure, and 3 had biceps tendon transfers. The dislocation rate after surgery was 50%, with complications occurring in 20% of the operated cases. Substantial degenerative osteoarthritis developed in two patients after glenoid osteotomy.

Many shoulders with posterior instability can be well managed by education, muscle strengthening, and neuromuscular retraining. Surgical stabilization of posterior glenohumeral instability may be considered when recurrent involuntary posterior subluxation or dislocation occurs in spite of a concerted effort at a well-structured rehabilitation program.[135] Before surgery, it is essential to identify all directions of instability and any anatomic factors that can predispose the joint to recurrent instability, such as humeral head or glenoid defect, abnormal glenoid version, rotator cuff tears, neurologic injuries, or generalized ligamentous laxity.[453,630] It is important for the patient to understand the high recurrence and complication rates associated with attempted surgical correction of posterior instability. Because the functional limitations and pain with recurrent posterior instability can be minimal, they suggested that some of these patients might do better without reconstructive procedures. Tibone and coworkers[648] stated that recurrent posterior dislocation of the shoulder is not a definite indication for surgery and stressed the need for careful patient selection before surgical reconstruction.

Posterior Surgical Approaches

Several surgical approaches have been described for treating recurrent posterior glenohumeral instability, including the posterior deltoid-splitting approach (see Fig. 16-254).[649] Shaffer and colleagues[650] described a surgical approach to the posterior glenohumeral joint through an infraspinatus-splitting incision that they found to offer safe and excellent exposure of the posterior capsule, labrum, and glenoid without requiring tendon detachment or causing neurologic compromise. Most surgeons prefer to split the deltoid at the posterior corner of the acromion and incise the infraspinatus tendon near its attachment to the greater tuberosity.

Posterior Soft Tissue Repairs

The goal of these procedures is to tighten the posterior capsule (the infraspinatus and posterior capsule) to restrict the range of positions attainable by the humerus in relation to the scapula.[626,651-655] In some cases, the infraspinatus and teres minor tendons may be used together in the plication. Boyd and Sisk[656] described transplanting the long head of the biceps tendon posteriorly around the humerus to the posterior glenoid rim.

One of the difficulties with these procedures is that the repair tends to stretch out as the shoulder resumes normal use. Hurley and associates[179] retrospectively reviewed 50 patients with recurrent posterior shoulder instability. Of the 25 patients treated surgically, 72% experienced recurrent instability. Tibone and Bradley[422] reported a failure rate of 30% after posterior staple capsulorrhaphy. Bayley and Kessel[657] stated that failure to distinguish between traumatic and habitual (atraumatic) types of instability led to inappropriate surgery and was a major cause of recurrence after operative repair. Bigliani and colleagues[658] reported a 20% failure rate for management of recurrent posteroinferior instability with a posterior capsular shift; most of the failures were in patients who had undergone previous attempts at surgical stabilization.

Tibone and Bradley[422] reviewed their experience with the management of posterior subluxation in athletes. They pointed out the difficulty in diagnosis, the unclear pathology, the importance of nonoperative management with exercises, and a 40% failure rate of surgical management with a posterior capsular shift. Of the failures, 11 were secondary to instability; 8 were a recurrence of posterior instability and 3 demonstrated anterior subluxation. These cases of conversion of posterior instability to anterior instability emphasize the importance of recognition and the challenge of management of multidirectional instability.

Arthroscopic capsular shift to the posterior and inferior labrum with closure of the rotator interval resulted in conversion of a positive to a negative jerk test in 85% of patients at a minimum of 12 months' follow-up.

Rotation Osteotomy of the Humerus[31,242,659]

Surin and colleagues[660] evaluated 12 shoulders that had recurrent posterior shoulder instability treated by external rotation osteotomy of the humerus. Recurrent instability developed in one shoulder with multidirectional instability.

Glenoid Osteotomy and Bone Blocks

Kretzler and Blue,[247,647] Scott,[661] English and Macnab,[662] Bestard,[663] Vegter and Marti,[664] Ahlgren and associates,[665]

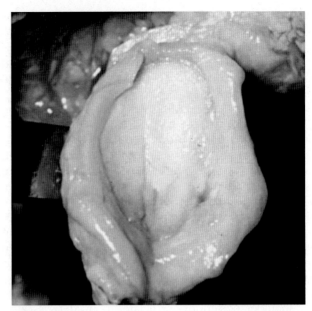

FIGURE 16-249 The articular surface of the glenoid after a posterior opening wedge osteotomy in a cadaver specimen.

and others[249,624,666-668] have reported using a posterior opening wedge glenoid osteotomy for recurrent posterior dislocations of the shoulder. In 1966, Kretzler and Blue[247] reported the use of this procedure in six patients with cerebral palsy. They used the acromion as the source of the graft to hold the wedge open. Kretzler[647] reported on 31 cases of posterior glenoid osteotomy in patients with voluntary (15 cases) and involuntary (16 cases) posterior dislocations, with recurrence in 4 patients, 2 from each category.

Extreme care must be taken during this procedure to prevent the osteotome from entering the glenoid, although cracks in subchondral bone are often experienced as the osteotomy is opened (Fig. 16-249). The suprascapular nerve above and the axillary nerve below are also at risk. English and Macnab[662] pointed out that the humeral head might have a tendency to subluxate anteriorly after osteotomy of the glenoid. Gerber and associates[669] demonstrated that with major angular changes, posterior glenoid osteotomy can thrust the humeral head forward and potentially cause abutment of the humeral head against the coracoid and produce pain and dysfunction. Their cadaver studies demonstrated that glenoplasty consistently resulted in squeezing of the subscapularis between the coracoid tip and the humeral head. In cadaveric shoulders, posteroinferior glenoplasty increased the posteroinferior glenoid depth from 3.8 to 7.0 mm and shifted the center of the humeral head anteriorly and superiorly by an average of 2.2 and 1.8 mm, respectively. This, along with an increase in the posterior slope, resulted in an increase in the stability ratio in the posteroinferior direction from 0.47 to 0.81.[177]

The posterior bone block, or glenoid osteotomy, has been combined with various soft tissue reconstructions.[670]

Mowery and associates[671] reported a series of five patients treated with a bone block for recurrent posterior dislocation. One patient had a subsequent anterior dislocation.

Wirth and colleagues[176] reported the use of glenoid osteotomy to manage recurrent posterior glenohumeral instability (Fig. 16-250).

Complications of Posterior Repairs

The principal cause of failure after a posterior soft tissue repair is recurrent instability.[646,672] Unless excellent dynamic stabilization is regained so that concavity compression rather than capsular restraint is the dominant mechanism of stability, the tightened posterior soft tissues are likely to stretch out as motion is regained. Even in its normal state, the posterior capsule is thin and often translucent. Its stretching out after surgical tightening is hastened if the posterior soft tissues are of poor quality, if the patient voluntarily or habitually tries to translate the shoulder posteriorly, or if large bony defects cause unphysiologic dependency on soft tissues for stability.

Occasionally, the opposite outcome can occur: Posterior repair can produce a shoulder that is too tight, which can push the shoulder out anteriorly. Insufficient posterior laxity can limit flexion, cross-body adduction, and internal rotation.

Complications can also result from bony procedures for posterior instability. Attempted posterior opening wedge osteotomy of the glenoid can result in an intraarticular fracture, in avascular necrosis of the osteotomized fragment, or in excessive anterior inclination and anterior instability. Posterior bone blocks placed in an excessively prominent position can cause severe degenerative joint disease.

Neurovascular injuries can also complicate posterior instability surgery. The axillary nerve may be injured as it exits the quadrangular space, or the nerve to the infraspinatus may be injured in the spinoglenoid notch.[190,654]

Matsen's Preferred Method for Treating Recurrent Posterior Glenohumeral Instability

Preoperative Considerations

Care is taken to identify the circumstances and directions of instability, the presence of generalized ligamentous laxity, and any anatomic factors that might potentially compromise the surgical result. We evaluate the possibilities of multidirectional and voluntary instability in each patient with posterior instability. All patients with posterior instability are started on the rehabilitation program described previously for atraumatic instability. A substantial number of patients with recurrent posterior instability respond to this program, particularly those with relatively atraumatic initiation of their condition. Straightforward patients who continue to have major symptomatic posterior instability after a reasonable rehabilitation effort may be considered for surgery. The type of posterior repair is influenced by the degree of trauma that initiated the repair and the quality of the posterior glenoid lip on the load and shift test and on imaging.

Shoulders with traumatic posterior instability might have pathology very similar to that of traumatic anterior instability (avulsion of the capsule and labrum from the glenoid rim or a capsular tear), which is amenable to primary repair. This condition must be diagnosed primarily from a history of an initial forcible posterior displacement of the humeral head on the glenoid, but it may be corroborated by a painful snap on the posterior drawer test.

Shoulders with lax posterior capsules may be managed with posterior capsulorrhaphy, but this capsular tightening is subject to stretching out again postoperatively, with resultant recurrent instability. This condition is suggested if the shoulder has an excessive range of cross-body adduction or internal rotation in abduction. If atraumatic multidirectional laxity is present, an inferior capsular shift may be performed from an anterior approach so that the rotator interval can be closed at the same procedure.

Shoulders without an effective posterior glenoid lip can require augmentation of the posterior lip with a labral reconstruction or posterior glenoid osteotomy. This situation is suggested if little resistance to posterior translation occurs when the humeral head is pressed into the glenoid when performing the posterior load and shift test (Fig. 16-251). The basis for this approach is presented by Metcalf and coworkers.[177]

Shoulders with major anteromedial humeral head defects (for example, more than one third of the humeral articular surface), might require insertion of a proximal humeral prosthesis. This situation needs to be identified preoperatively because the preferred surgical approach for this procedure is anterior.

Preoperatively, patients are informed of the alternatives and the risks of recurrent instability, excessive tightness with limited flexion and internal rotation, pain, neurovascular injury, infection, and the need for revision surgery.

Procedure

Before the patient is placed prone, the shoulder is examined under anesthesia, with particular attention paid to resistance to posterior translation with the humeral head pressed into the glenoid; such resistance indicates the degree of competence of the posterior glenoid lip.

The patient is placed prone with the shoulder off the operating table to allow a full range of humeral and scapular motion. After routine preparation of the arm, shoulder, neck, and back, a 10-cm incision is made in the extended line of the posterior axillary crease (Fig. 16-252). The deltoid muscle is split for a distance of 4 cm between its middle and posterior thirds. If necessary, additional exposure may be obtained by carefully dissecting the muscle for a short distance from the scapular spine and posterior acromion (Fig. 16-253). Retraction of the deltoid muscle inferiorly and laterally reveals the

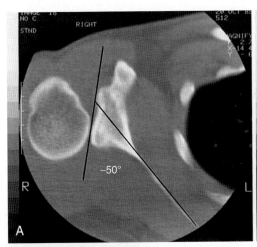
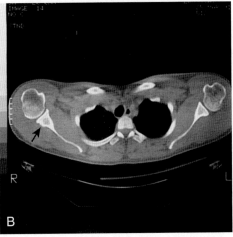

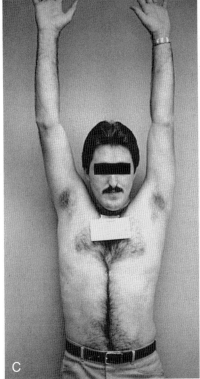
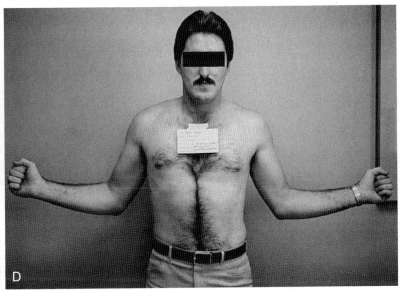

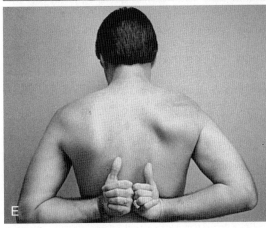

FIGURE 16-250 A, Preoperative CT scan demonstrating moderate glenoid retrotilt. **B,** Postoperative CT scan revealing a significant degree of correction of the glenoid version and incorporation of the tricortical bone graft after a posterior opening wedge osteotomy of the glenoid. **C** to **E,** Clinic photographs demonstrating full and symmetric motion. (From Wirth MA, Seltzer DG, and Rockwood CA Jr: Recurrent posterior glenohumeral dislocation associated with increased retroversion of the glenoid. Clin Orthop Relat Res 308:98-101, 1994.)

infraspinatus muscle, the teres minor muscle, and the axillary nerve emerging from the quadrangular space (Fig. 16-254). The spinoglenoid notch is palpated to determine the location of the important nerve to the infraspinatus.

The interval between the infraspinatus and teres minor and the attached capsule is split (Fig. 16-255) to expose the posterior capsule (Fig. 16-256), which is then split (Fig. 16-257). The joint is inspected for humeral head defects, wear of the anterior or posterior glenoid, tears in the glenoid labrum, loose bodies, and tears of the rotator cuff. Traumatic posterior capsular avulsions are repaired to the lip of the glenoid by a technique similar to that described for anterior repair.

Anteromedial humeral head defects of moderate size are managed by tightening the posterior capsule so that internal rotation is limited to 30 degrees. A shoulder with an anterior humeral head defect constituting more than a third of the articular surface often cannot be stabilized by soft tissue surgery. In these instances, insertion of a prosthetic head through the anterior approach is required to restore stability and function to the glenohumeral joint. Because it changes the surgical approach, a lesion of this size needs to be identified preoperatively.

In patients with deficiency of the posterior glenoid lip, increased glenoid retroversion, or undependable posterior soft tissues, a posteroinferior glenoid osteoplasty is considered. This osteotomy increases the effective glenoid arc and balances the stability angles posteriorly and inferiorly. It is most safely performed by exposing the posterior inferior glenoid neck and joint surface (Fig. 16-258) and measuring the thickness of the glenoid at the point of the planned osteotomy (Fig. 16-259). The osteotomy is carefully carried out to preserve an anterior bony hinge and to *avoid* entering the joint surface (Figs. 16-260 to 16-262). A graft is harvested from the scapular spine and contoured (Fig. 16-263; see also Fig. 16-262). The graft is then inserted into the opened osteotomy (Figs. 16-264 and 16-265) to construct the posterior glenoid rim (Fig. 16-266). The deltoid is carefully reconstructed (Fig. 16-267).

After surgery, rotator strengthening is started immediately. The arm is kept at the side for 6 weeks, after which active elevation is started in the plane of the thorax. Forward elevation is started at 3 months when optimal muscle control has been regained.

Rockwood and Wirth's Technique of Posterior Reconstruction for Traumatic Instability[649]

Standard Posterior Repair

The patient is placed in the lateral decubitus position with the operative shoulder upward. The best way to support the patient in this position is to use kidney supports and the bean bag.

The incision begins 2.5 cm medial to the posterolateral corner of the acromion and extends downward 7.5 cm toward the posterior axillary creases (Fig. 16-268A).[673] If a bone graft is to be taken from the acromion, the incision extends a little farther superiorly so that the acromion can be exposed. Next, the subcutaneous tissues are dissected medially and laterally so that the skin can be retracted to visualize the fibers of the deltoid.

A point 2.5 cm medial to the posterior corner of the acromion is selected, and the deltoid is then split distally for 10 cm in the line of its fibers. The deltoid can be easily retracted medially and laterally to expose the underlying infraspinatus and teres minor muscles. This deltoid split can be made down to the midportion of the teres minor muscle. Remember that the axillary nerve exits the quadrangular space at the lower border of the teres minor muscle.

When performing a posterior reconstruction, the teres minor tendon should be reflected inferiorly down to the level of the inferior joint capsule. If the infraspinatus tendon is divided and reflected medially and laterally, care should be taken to not injure the suprascapular nerve. When the infraspinatus tendon is very lax, it can be reflected off the capsule and retracted superiorly without having to divide the tendon.

With the infraspinatus and teres minor muscles retracted out of the way, a vertical incision can be made in the posterior capsule to expose and explore the joint. We prefer to make the incision midway between the humeral and glenoid attachment so that at closure we can double-breast it and make it stronger. When performing the posterior capsular shift procedure, it is essential to have the teres minor muscle reflected sufficiently inferior so that the vertical cut in the capsule goes all the way down to the most inferior recess of the capsule. If the capsule is thin and friable and it appears that a capsular shift alone will be insufficient, the infraspinatus tendon can be divided so that it can be double-breasted to shorten it.

With the capsule divided all the way down inferiorly, horizontal mattress sutures of No. 2 Cottony Dacron are inserted in the edge of the medial capsule. The arm should be held in neutral rotation and the medial capsule sutured laterally and superiorly under the lateral capsule. Next, the lateral capsule is reflected and sutured medially and superiorly over the medial capsule and again held in place with horizontal mattress sutures. This capsular shift procedure has effectively eliminated any of the posterior and inferior capsular redundancy.

The infraspinatus tendon is repaired next; this repair should also be performed with the arm in neutral rotation. If laxity exists, the tendon can be double-breasted. The wound is thoroughly irrigated, and the muscle and subcutaneous tissues are infiltrated with 25 to 30 mL of 0.5% bupivacaine. Care must be taken to not overuse the bupivacaine or inject it directly into vascular channels.

When the retractors are withdrawn, the deltoid falls nicely together and subcutaneous closure is performed. Care must be taken throughout closure of the capsule, infraspinatus tendon, and skin to maintain the arm in neutral rotation. The patient is then gently rolled into the

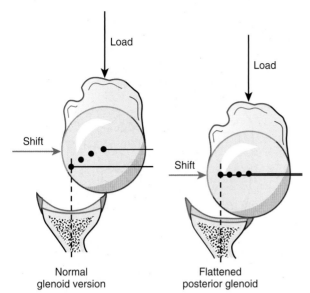

FIGURE 16-251 Diminished resistance to load and shift. A flat posterior glenoid diminishes the centering of the humeral head as reflected by the load and shift test. (From Matsen FA III, Lippitt SB: Shoulder Surgery: Principles and Procedures. Philadelphia: WB Saunders, 2004, p 209.)

supine position while making sure that the arm is in neutral rotation. When the anesthesia is completed, the patient is transferred to a bed, where the arm is maintained in neutral position and supported by skin traction. Usually within 24 hours after surgery the patient can stand, and a modified shoulder immobilizer cast is applied.

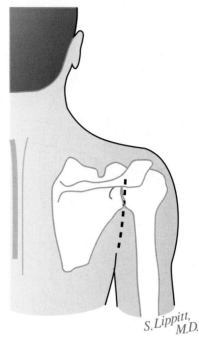

FIGURE 16-252 Skin incision. The posterior skin incision (*dashed line*) is made in the posterior axillary crease. (From Matsen FA III, Lippitt SB: Shoulder Surgery: Principles and Procedures. Philadelphia: WB Saunders, 2004, p 211.)

Posterior Glenoid Osteotomy

We do not use this procedure as a routine part of posterior reconstruction. Occasionally, when posterior glenoid deficiency is present or in patients with congenital retrotilt of the glenoid (i.e., >30 degrees), posterior

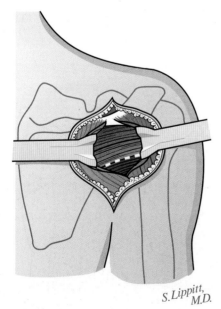

FIGURE 16-253 Opening the deltoid. Retracting the deltoid reveals the infraspinatus muscle. (From Matsen FA III, Lippitt SB: Shoulder Surgery: Principles and Procedures. Philadelphia: WB Saunders, 2004, p 211.)

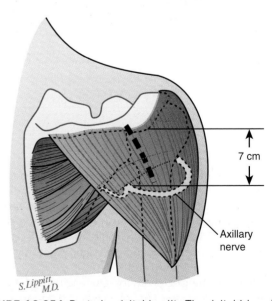

FIGURE 16-254 Posterior deltoid split. The deltoid is split (*heavy dashed line*) between the anterior two thirds and the posterior third of the muscle, being mindful of the axillary nerve inferiorly. (From Matsen FA III, Lippitt SB: Shoulder Surgery: Principles and Procedures. Philadelphia: WB Saunders, 2004, p 211.)

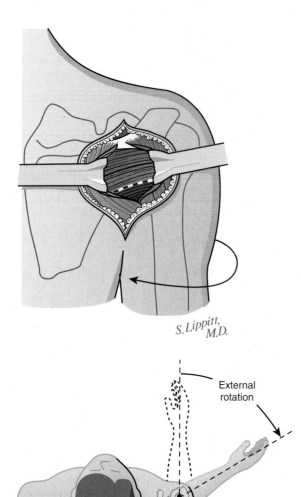

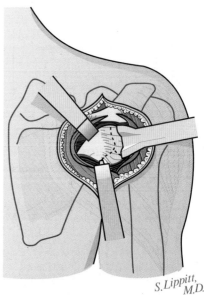

FIGURE 16-256 Exposure of the inferior glenoid neck. With the teres minor and axillary nerve retracted inferiorly, a spiked retractor is placed below the glenoid neck. The infraspinatus is retracted superiorly (toward its nerve supply) with a second spiked retractor. The *dotted lines* outline the glenoid (*left*) and the humeral head (*right*). This provides an excellent exposure of the capsule. (From Matsen FA III, Lippitt SB: Shoulder Surgery: Principles and Procedures. Philadelphia: WB Saunders, 2004, p 213.)

FIGURE 16-255 Splitting the external rotators. *Top,* The external rotators are split between the infraspinatus and the teres minor (*dashed line*). *Bottom,* These muscles are relaxed by external rotation of the humerus. (From Matsen FA III, Lippitt SB: Shoulder Surgery: Principles and Procedures. Philadelphia: WB Saunders, 2004, p 212.)

osteotomy should be considered. We have reported a patient who had failed two previous attempts at posterior capsulorrhaphy for recurrent posterior shoulder instability.[176] The patient had a previously unrecognized unilateral increase in glenoid fossa retrotilt and was successfully treated with a posterior opening wedge osteotomy of the scapular neck (see Fig. 16-250).

When performing a posterior glenoid osteotomy, the surgeon must take care to not overcorrect the retroversion because overcorrection can force the head out anteriorly. If a posterior osteotomy is to be performed, it is absolutely essential to know the anatomy and angle of the slope of the glenoid, which can best be determined by placing a straight, blunt instrument into the joint so that

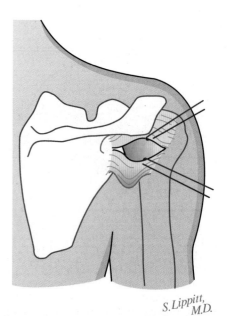

FIGURE 16-257 Capsulotomy. The posterior capsule is opened horizontally, making the incision through the weakest part of the capsule. (From Matsen FA III, Lippitt SB: Shoulder Surgery: Principles and Procedures. Philadelphia: WB Saunders, 2004, p 213.)

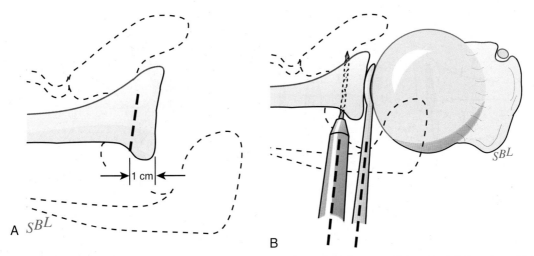

FIGURE 16-258 Marking the osteotomy. **A,** The intended osteotomy is marked 1 cm medial to the joint surface. **B,** With a smooth elevator on the joint surface, a 2-mm hole is drilled parallel to the joint in the plane of the osteotomy. (From Matsen FA III, Lippitt SB: Shoulder Surgery: Principles and Procedures. Philadelphia: WB Saunders, 2004, p 214.)

it lies on the anterior and posterior glenoid rim (see Fig. 16-268G). Next, the osteotome is placed intracapsularly and directed parallel to the blunt instrument. If one is unsure of the angle and does not have a guide instrument in place, the osteotomy can enter the joint (see Fig. 16-268). The osteotomy site is not more than 6.5 mm medial to the articular surface of the glenoid. If the osteotomy is more medial than 6.5 mm, the suprascapular nerve may be injured as it passes around the base of the spine of the scapula to supply the infraspinatus muscle.

Each time that the osteotome is advanced, the osteotomy site is pried open (see Fig. 16-268G-J) to help create a lateral plastic deformation of the posterior glenoid. The osteotomy should not exit anteriorly but should stop just at the anterior cortex of the scapula (see Fig. 16-268I). The intact anterior cortex periosteum and soft tissue act as a hinge and allow the graft to be secure in the oste-

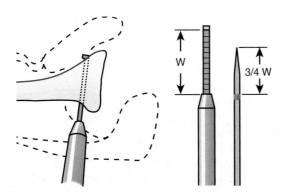

FIGURE 16-259 The depth of the osteotomy. The depth of the drill hole is measured with a depth gauge. A sterile paper tape is placed on the osteotome at a distance from the tip equal to three fourths of the depth of the hole. (From Matsen FA III, Lippitt SB: Shoulder Surgery: Principles and Procedures. Philadelphia: WB Saunders, 2004, p 215.)

otomy without any need for internal fixation. We generally use an osteotome that is 2.5 cm wide to make the original cut and then use smaller 1.25-cm osteotomes superiorly and inferiorly to complete the posterior division of bone.

Osteotomes are used to open up the osteotomy site, and the bone graft is placed into position (see Fig. 16-268M). If the anterior cortex is partially intact, internal fixation of the graft is not necessary because it is held securely in place by the osteotomy. We prefer to take the bone graft from the acromion (see Fig. 16-268). Either a small piece (8 × 30 mm) for the osteotomy or a large piece (15 × 30 mm) for a posteroinferior bone block can be taken from the top or the posterior edge of the acromion. If a larger piece of graft is required, it should be taken from the ilium. After completion of the osteotomy, a capsular shift, as described earlier, is performed.

After surgery, the patient lies supine with the forearm supported by the overhead bed frame and the arm held in neutral rotation. We usually let the patient sit up on the bed the evening of surgery while maintaining the arm in neutral rotation. We let the patient sit up in a chair the next day, again holding the arm in neutral rotation. Either 24 or 48 hours after surgery, when the patient can stand comfortably, we apply a lightweight long arm cast. Next, a well-padded iliac crest band that sits around the abdomen and iliac crest is applied. The arm is then connected to the iliac crest band with a broom handle support to maintain the arm in 10 to 15 degrees of abduction and neutral rotation. The cast is left in place for 6 to 8 weeks.

After the plaster is removed, the patient is allowed to use the arm for 4 to 6 weeks for everyday living activities. A rehabilitation program is begun that includes pendulum exercises, isometric exercises, and stretching of the shoulder with the use of an overhead pulley, after which resistive exercises are gradually increased.

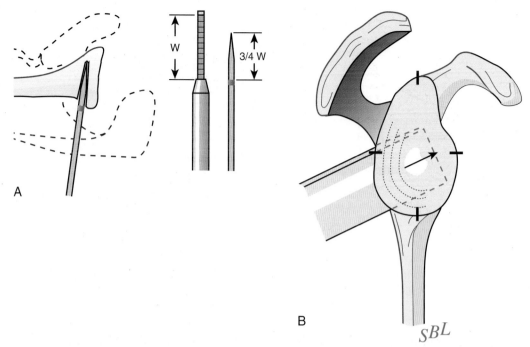

FIGURE 16-260 The cut. **A,** The osteotome is inserted parallel to the joint surface to the depth marked with the sterile tape. This should be three quarters of the AP thickness of the glenoid at the site of the osteotomy. **B,** The osteotome (*dotted outline*) is inserted from posterior inferior to anterosuperior (*arrow*). (From Matsen FA III, Lippitt SB: Shoulder Surgery: Principles and Procedures. Philadelphia: WB Saunders, 2004, p 216.)

Anterior Capsular Shift Reconstruction

We have used a capsular shift reconstruction in patients whose primary pathology is posterior shoulder instability if a recognizable component of multidirectional shoulder laxity is present (Fig. 16-269).[674] This procedure is indi-

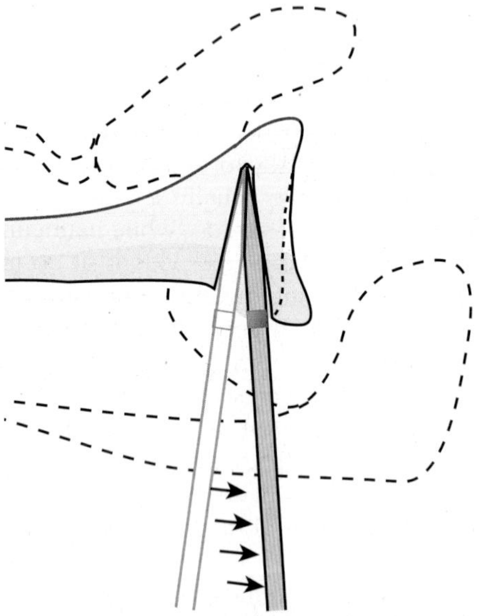

FIGURE 16-261 Opening the osteotomy. The osteotomy is opened with progressive gentle levering motions, attempting to bend, rather than fracture, the glenoid. (From Matsen FA III, Lippitt SB: Shoulder Surgery: Principles and Procedures. Philadelphia: WB Saunders, 2004, p 217.)

cated when instability or apprehension repeatedly compromises shoulder comfort or function in spite of an adequate trial of rotator cuff strengthening and coordination exercises.

The mainstay of the capsular shift procedure is reduction of excessive joint volume through symmetrical and anatomic plication of the redundant capsule. We have found it unnecessary to perform a combined anterior and posterior approach; instead, we reserve posterior capsular reconstruction for patients with recurrent traumatic posterior shoulder instability who do not have concomitant generalized ligamentous laxity and multidirectional laxity of the shoulder. Open anterior capsular shift procedures for posterior instability resulted in 10 of 11 patients having a stable shoulder at a minimum of 2 years of follow-up.[675] The patients lost motion in internal as well as external rotation.[676]

One explanation for the difficulties encountered with traditional posterior reconstructions has been the poor quality and unsubstantial nature of the posterior capsule, which precludes a strong surgical reconstruction. Additionally, surgically addressable lesions known to contribute to recurrent instability, such as associated fractures involving the posterior glenoid rim or anteromedial humeral head, are less common. In contrast to the capsulolabral injuries seen with traumatic anterior shoulder instability, posterior glenoid lateral pathology is often limited to degenerative changes rather than capsulolabral avulsions, which lend themselves to stable surgical repair. Finally and perhaps the most subtle reason for poor surgi-

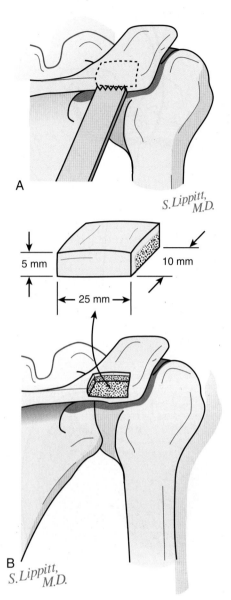

FIGURE 16-262 Graft harvest. **A,** The bone graft is harvested from the posterosuperior scapular spine. **B,** The graft should be approximately 25 mm wide, 5 mm thick, and 10 mm deep. (From Matsen FA III, Lippitt SB: Shoulder Surgery: Principles and Procedures. Philadelphia: WB Saunders, 2004, p 218.)

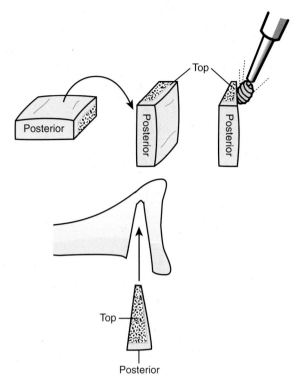

FIGURE 16-263 Shaping the graft. The graft is shaped to form a wedge with a base of 5 mm. (From Matsen FA III, Lippitt SB: Shoulder Surgery: Principles and Procedures. Philadelphia: WB Saunders, 2004, p 219.)

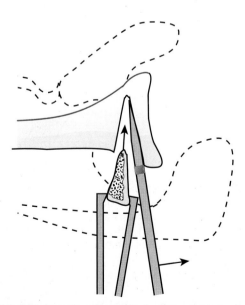

FIGURE 16-264 Inserting the graft. As the osteotomy is pried open, the graft is inserted with its cortical side toward the articular surface. (From Matsen FA III, Lippitt SB: Shoulder Surgery: Principles and Procedures. Philadelphia: WB Saunders, 2004, p 219.)

cal results is failure to recognize that some shoulders demonstrate multidirectional laxity even though the patient has a history, physical examination, and radiographs consistent with symptomatic posterior shoulder instability.

The basis for this seemingly unorthodox approach is supported by several reports in the literature. In 1988, Schwartz and colleagues[677] performed arthroscopically assisted selective sectioning of the shoulder capsule to quantitate the relative contribution of specific structures to glenohumeral stability. The superior glenohumeral

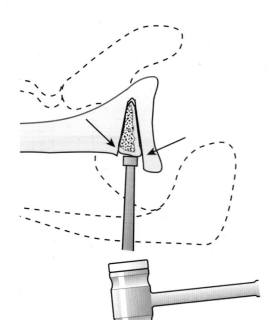

FIGURE 16-265 Recessing the graft. The graft is impacted until its base is within the cortex of the posterior glenoid. (From Matsen FA III, Lippitt SB: Shoulder Surgery: Principles and Procedures. Philadelphia: WB Saunders, 2004, p 219.)

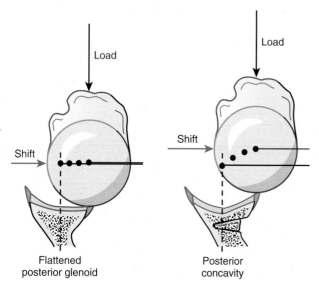

FIGURE 16-266 Re-establishment of centering. After the graft is in position, the restoration of humeral head centering is indicated by increased resistance to the posterior load and shift test. (From Matsen FA III, Lippitt SB: Shoulder Surgery: Principles and Procedures. Philadelphia: WB Saunders, 2004, p 220.)

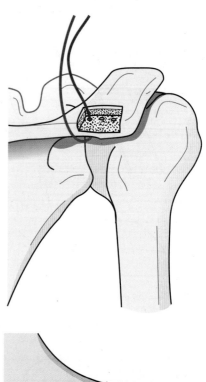

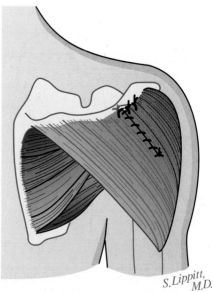

FIGURE 16-267 Deltoid repair. *Top,* The deltoid is repaired to drill holes at the osteotomy harvest site. *Bottom,* The deltoid is then closed side-to-side. (From Matsen FA III, Lippitt SB: Shoulder Surgery: Principles and Procedures. Philadelphia: WB Saunders, 2004, p 221.)

ligament was found to provide secondary restraint to posterior shoulder instability. In addition, posterior glenohumeral dislocation did not occur after incision of the posterior capsule until the anterosuperior capsular structures were also sectioned. In 1992, Harryman and associ-ates[89] investigated the role of selective capsular sectioning and imbrication of the rotator interval capsule. Surgical modifications were found to alter several different param-eters of shoulder motion, including rotation and transla-tion, which ultimately affected the stability of the shoulder joint. Specifically, the intrarotator interval was found to be a major component of stability against posterior and inferior glenohumeral displacement. Posterior and infe-rior glenohumeral dislocations usually occurred after sec-tioning of the rotator interval capsule, whereas imbrication

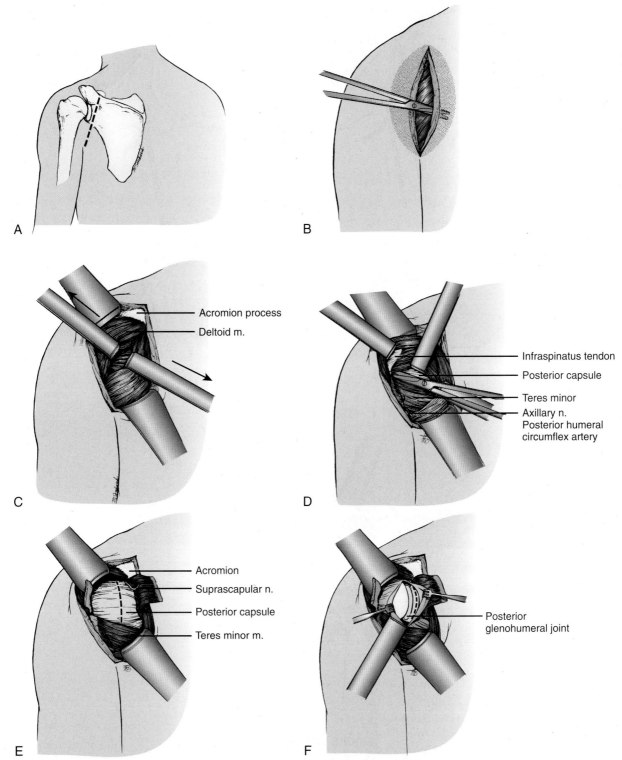

FIGURE 16-268 A-R, Rockwood's preferred posterior shoulder reconstruction. (See text for a detailed description of each step of the procedure.) (Modified from Rockwood CA, Green DP [eds]: Fractures, 3 vols, 2nd ed. Philadelphia: JB Lippincott, 1984.)

Continued

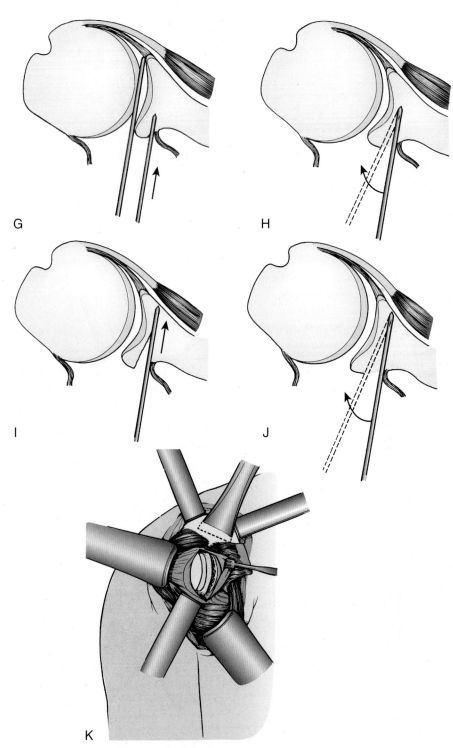

FIGURE 16-268, cont'd

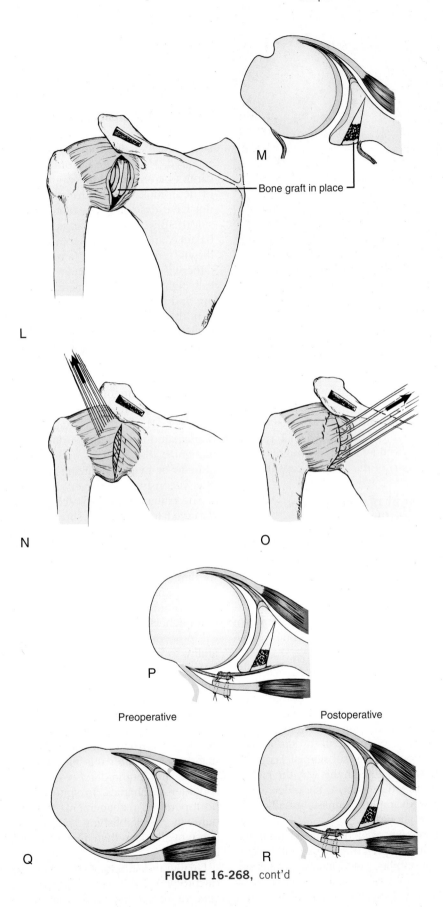

Bone graft in place

M

L

N

O

Preoperative

Postoperative

P

Q

R

FIGURE 16-268, cont'd

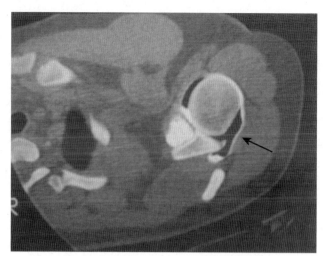

FIGURE 16-269 CT arthrogram in a patient with symptomatic posterior shoulder instability and multidirectional glenohumeral laxity. Note the overall capsular volume and the posterior capsular redundancy (*arrow*). (From Rockwood CA Jr, Green DP, and Bucholz RW [eds]: Fractures in Adults. Philadelphia: JB Lippincott, 1991.)

of this structure increased the resistance to translation in these directions. These authors concluded that patients with inferior or posterior shoulder instability might benefit from anterior reconstruction of the interval capsule.

Nonoperative Treatment of Recurrent Multidirectional Instability

The goal of treatment of patients with atraumatic instability is restoration of shoulder function by increasing the effectiveness of concavity compression. Many patients with AMBRII have simply become deconditioned from their normal state of dynamic glenohumeral stability. They have lost the proper neuromuscular control of humeroscapular positioning, and concavity compression has become dysfunctional.

Neuromuscular control cannot be restored surgically; rather, it requires prolonged adherence to a well-constructed reconditioning program. The patient may need to be convinced that training and exercises constitute a reasonable therapeutic approach. Many would prefer a surgical "cure." It is often useful to demonstrate that the contralateral shoulder has substantial laxity on examination, yet is clinically stable. In this way the patient and family can appreciate that a loose shoulder is not necessarily unstable; for example, gymnasts usually have very lax but very stable shoulders.

Nonoperative management of glenohumeral instability is discussed earlier in this chapter. In general, but particularly in atraumatic instability, glenohumeral stability depends on dynamic compression of the humeral head into the glenoid concavity (concavity compression) and excellence of neuromuscular control. Thus, the nonop-

erative and postoperative programs for an AMBRII shoulder need to optimize both.

Operative Treatment of Atraumatic Instability

Presurgical Considerations

The ability of surgery alone to *cure* atraumatic instability is limited. Usually, there is no single lesion that can be repaired. Most of the factors providing midrange stability cannot be enhanced by surgical reconstruction. Problems of neuromuscular control or relative glenoid flatness do not have easy surgical solutions. Even after a snug capsulorrhaphy, the midrange stabilizing mechanisms of balance and concavity compression must be optimized through muscle strengthening and kinematic training. Otherwise, excessive loads will be applied to the surgically tightened glenohumeral capsule and result in stretching and failure of the surgical reconstruction.

In this light, indications for surgical treatment of atraumatic instability need to be carefully considered. First, the patient must have major functional problems that are clearly related to atraumatic glenohumeral instability. Second, the patient must clearly understand that good strength and kinematic technique—rather than capsular tightness—are the primary stabilizing factors for the shoulder. Third, the patient must have conscientiously participated in a strengthening and training program and recognize that strength and proper technique will continue to be major stabilizing factors for the shoulder even after reconstructive surgery is performed.

The patient must also recognize that capsulorrhaphy is designed to stiffen the shoulder: The surgery will compromise range of motion in the hope of gaining stability. If attempts to regain totally normal range are made in the first postoperative year, instability is likely to recur. Thus, the limitations imposed by surgical capsulorrhaphy may be incompatible with the goals of normal or supernormal range of motion. Therefore, gymnasts, dancers, and baseball pitchers might not be good candidates for this surgical procedure. Similarly, this procedure has a limited ability to hold up under the demands of heavy physical labor unless it is accompanied by a superb strength and kinematic rehabilitation program.

The patient must understand that rehabilitation after a capsular shift procedure is protracted. It is important that the shoulder be immobilized in a brace for a month, during which time muscles get weak and normal kinematics is lost. After this month of immobilization, many months are required to re-establish good strength and shoulder kinematics. In spite of the best operative and postoperative management, the success of this procedure in re-establishing normal shoulder function is substantially less than that of procedures for traumatic instability.

Finally, the shoulder must have an identified mechanical problem for which surgery is the answer. The presence of shoulder pain and laxity does not indicate that the patient will be better after a surgical procedure.

The foregoing is a large amount of very important information about the surgical procedure that must be understood by the patient. The situation is further complicated by the fact that many patients with atraumatic midrange instability are young and may have difficulty understanding and accepting the ramifications of this information. Thus, during preoperative discussions with young patients, it may be important that parents participate actively. We find that many families who request that the shoulder be "fixed" are prepared to work more diligently on the nonoperative program after this discussion.

When the history and physical examination indicate that the shoulder is loose in all directions and when the patient has failed to respond to vigorous exercises for internal and external rotator strengthening, endurance, and coordination, an inferior capsular shift procedure may be considered as originally described by Neer and Foster.[141] The principle of the procedure is to symmetrically tighten the anterior, inferior, and posterior aspects of the capsule by advancing its humeral attachment.

However, it is now recognized that capsular laxity might not be the essential lesion in atraumatic instability. Procedures designed to improve the quality of the glenoid concavity might provide a more physiologic solution. In one study, capsulolabral augmentation of the posteroinferior labrum without capsular shift significantly increased glenoid depth (1.9 mm inferiorly, 2 mm posteroinferiorly, and 0.9 mm posteriorly) and the stability ratios posteroinferiorly and inferiorly (0.24 increase in both directions).[141a]

Results of Reconstructions for Atraumatic Instability

A capsular shift procedure is often considered in the surgical management of atraumatic instability. However, most of the existing reports of inferior capsular shift surgery include patients with both traumatic and atraumatic forms of instability.[140,141,534] Therefore, the results are substantially better than would be expected in the treatment of atraumatic instability.

Cooper and Brems[140] reported a 2-year follow-up of inferior capsular shift procedures and found that 9% continued to have significant instability. Altchek and colleagues[534] used a T-plasty modification of the Bankart procedure for multidirectional instability on 42 shoulders injured during athletics. Four patients experienced episodes of instability after the procedure, and throwing velocity decreased in the throwing athletes. Despite these shortcomings, patient satisfaction was noted to be excellent in 95% of shoulders.

Bigliani and associates[658] used an inferior capsular shift procedure to manage 68 shoulders in 63 athletes with anterior and inferior instability. Fifty-eight patients returned to their major sports, 75% at the same competitive level, but only 50% of elite throwing athletes returned to their previous level of competition. In contact-sport athletes, 92% had no further dislocations after an anterior-based capsular shift, and 88% of patients who underwent a posterior-based capsular shift had no further dislocations.

In the series of Choi and Olgivie-Harris, after an anterior procedure, 82% of athletes returned to their sport; 75% of athletes were able to return to their sport after a posterior procedure. Only 17% of patients with bilateral procedures were able to return to their sport, however.[678]

In a report by Pagnani and Dome, American football players were able to return to their sport 89% of the time after open anterior capsulorrhaphy along with repair of a Bankart lesion, if present.[679]

At an average 61-month follow-up by Pollack and colleagues, 94% of patients with primarily anterior multidirectional instability remained stable after the anterior capsular shift procedure, and all 15 patients with primarily posterior instability remained stable after posterior capsular shift.[680]

In general, better results are obtained with surgery whenever trauma is a contributing factor. In an attempt to evaluate the effectiveness of a homogeneous series of primary capsular shift surgery for purely atraumatic instability, Obremskey and coworkers[681] reviewed 26 patients with no history or radiographic or surgical evidence of a traumatic etiology. The patients in this series had failed an average of 17 months of vigorous physical rehabilitation before proceeding with surgery. Fifty-seven percent of the patients had bilateral symptoms. The average age was 22 ± 6 years (range, 13-34 years). Twenty-nine percent had generalized ligamentous laxity, and 15% had an industrial claim. At an average of 27 months after a standard capsular shift was performed,[141] 74% of the patients were satisfied with the condition of their shoulder; 46% were able to return to recreation, and 69% returned to their previous job. Thirty-nine percent had persistent pain and 57% had night pain that interfered with sleeping. Sixty-eight percent had at least occasional symptoms of instability and 10% required further surgery. By regression analysis, the most important correlate of patient dissatisfaction was not recurrent instability but rather persistent pain and stiffness. These results suggest that a key in the management of patients with atraumatic multidirectional instability is not the degree of surgical tightness achieved but rather restoration of comfort and motion.

Rockwood's Approach to Treatment of Atraumatic and Multidirectional Glenohumeral Instability

Treatment of patients with atraumatic instability requires that the physician differentiate between the voluntary and the involuntary types. Certainly, a patient with voluntary instability who has psychiatric problems should never be treated surgically. Rowe and Yee[682] reported on disasters in patients with psychiatric problems who had been treated with surgical reconstruction. Patients with emotional disturbances and psychiatric problems should be referred for psychiatric help. Rowe and Yee also pointed out that there are patients with voluntary instability who do not have psychiatric problems and can be significantly improved with a rehabilitation program.

Consistent with this recommendation, we place all patients with atraumatic instability problems on a very specific rehabilitation program to strengthen the three parts of the deltoid, the rotator cuff, and the scapular stabilizers. If the patient has an obvious psychiatric or emotional problem, we do our best to explain the problem to the patient and family and help them seek psychiatric help. Under no circumstances do we ever tell the patient or family that surgery is a possibility for an emotionally disturbed patient.

When we have ruled out congenital or developmental causes of the instability problem, we personally teach the patient how to perform the shoulder-strengthening exercises and give the patient a copy of the exercise diagrams (see Fig. 16-170).

We give the patient a set of TheraBands—yellow, red, green, blue, and black bands—and diagrams of the exercises to be performed. Each TheraBand is a strip 7.5-cm wide and 1.5-m long that is tied into a loop. The loop can be fastened over a doorknob or any fixed object to offer resistance to pull. The patient does five basic exercises to strengthen the deltoid and the rotator cuff. Each band offers a different amount of resistance to pull:

Yellow band: 1 lb
Red band: 2 lb
Green band: 3 lb
Blue band: 4 lb
Black band: 5 lb

The patient is instructed to perform the five exercises two or three times a day. Each exercise should be performed 5 to 10 times and each held for a count of 5 to 10. The patient is instructed to gradually increase the resistance (i.e., yellow to red and green, and so on) every 2 to 4 weeks.

After the black TheraBand becomes easy to use, the patient is given a pulley kit and is instructed to do the same five basic exercises, but now lifting weights, as shown in Figure 16-170. The pulley kit consists of a pulley, an open-eye screw hook, a handle, and a piece of rope, all in a plastic bag. The patient begins by attaching 7 to 10 lb of weight to the end of the rope and proceeds to the five basic exercises. Gradually over several months, the patient increases the weight of resistance, up to 15 lb for women and 20 to 25 lb for men.

When we start the basic strengthening of the rotator cuff and the deltoid, we also instruct the patient how to perform the exercises to strengthen the scapular stabilizer muscles. Pushups (wall pushups, knee pushups, and regular pushups) are used to strengthen the serratus anterior, rhomboids, and other muscles, and shoulder-shrugging exercises are performed to strengthen the trapezius muscles.

We have learned that the rehabilitation program is 80% successful in managing anterior instability problems and 90% successful in managing atraumatic posterior instability problems.[467] Regardless of any previous rehabilitation program that the patient has participated in, we always start the patient on our strengthening routine.

If the patient still has signs and symptoms of instability after 6 months of exercises, a very specific capsular shift procedure is performed. One must always remember that it is possible for a patient with laxity of the major joints to have a superimposed traumatic episode, which ordinarily does not respond to a rehabilitation program. A patient with atraumatic instability who has a history of significant trauma, pain, swelling, and so forth will probably require surgical reconstruction, but only after a trial with the rehabilitation program.

The details of the incision, surgical approach, protection of the axillary nerve, and preservation of the anterior humeral circumflex vessels are essentially the same as we use for management of a recurrent traumatic anterior instability problem (Fig. 16-270). The main difference is noted after the capsule is opened and the surgeon does not find a Perthes–Bankart lesion. The deficiency is simply a very redundant capsule anteriorly, inferiorly, or posteroinferiorly. The principle of the capsular shift is to divide the capsule all the way down inferiorly, midway between its attachment on the humerus and the glenoid rim. The joint is carefully inspected and then the shift is performed. As demonstrated in Figure 16-247P and Q, we prefer to take the medial capsule superiorly and laterally under the lateral capsule and then take the lateral capsule superiorly and medially over the medial capsule. We are careful that placement and tying of the sutures are done with the arm in approximately 15 to 20 degrees of external rotation for an anterior reconstruction and in neutral rotation for a posterior reconstruction. Ordinarily, the subscapularis is simply repaired to itself, but when there is laxity of the subscapularis with the arm in 15 to 20 degrees of external rotation, the subscapularis can be double-breasted. Normally, when performing a posterior capsular shift, the infraspinatus tendon can be reflected superiorly and the teres minor reflected inferiorly off the posterior capsule. As with the anterior shift, the posterior capsule is divided midway between its attachments, thus allowing a double-breasting or strengthening of the midportion of the capsule. The reader must remember, however, that posterior shifts are rarely required because most patients do so well with the rehabilitation program.

Surgical management of patients with atraumatic instability demands that the shoulder not be put up too tight, as can occur with the Magnuson–Stack, Putti–Platt, or Bristow procedure. If the surgeon fails to recognize that the patient has an atraumatic instability problem and if a routine muscle-tightening procedure is performed, the result may be that the humeral head will be pushed out in the opposite direction. The surgeon must also be careful, even in patients with atraumatic instability, to not perform a capsular shift that is so tight that it forces the head out in the opposite direction. As mentioned, we prefer to place and tie the sutures in the anterior capsular shift procedure with the arm in 15 to 20 degrees of external rotation and held in neutral rotation during the posterior capsular shift reconstruction. It is essential to isolate and protect the axillary nerve when performing an anterior or posterior capsular shift.

Treatment of Other Types of Recurrent Instability

The AMBRII and TUBS syndromes represent clearly defined clinical pathologic entities, each of which has specific diagnostic features and treatment strategies. Together, they account for the great majority of patients with glenohumeral instability. Patients who do not fit into one of these two categories have highly individualized problems and cannot be grouped together effectively. In evaluating these patients, a meticulous history and physical examination take on even greater importance.

When an initiating injury has occurred, it is essential to determine the position of the arm and the direction and magnitude of the force producing the injury so that the likelihood of a capsular tear can be determined. Unless this is clearly the case, the default assumption is that the shoulder has become dysfunctional without a substantial anatomic lesion and therefore needs to be managed with a rehabilitative approach that emphasizes strength, balance, endurance, and good technique. Unless a functionally significant instability can be determined by the history and physical examination, the emphasis on rehabilitation must continue.

When the history and physical examination do not indicate the nature of the shoulder problem, studies such as contrast CT, MRI, examination under anesthesia, and arthroscopy are unlikely to be helpful in determining the treatment. Findings on these tests, such as increased translation, "increased laxity," a large axillary pouch, or labral fraying, may be identified even in functionally normal shoulders and might have no relationship to the patient's functional problem. The risk, therefore, is that findings on these tests can distract the clinician from findings on the history and physical examination. Unless functional instability can be rigorously characterized by the history and physical examination, it is unlikely that surgical attempts to increase stability will be curative.

Summary

The history and physical examination constitute the most efficient and cost-effective methods for identifying treatable problems of glenohumeral instability. When these clinical tools do not clearly define the nature of the patient's functional problem, surgical management is unlikely to be effective. Expensive diagnostic approaches

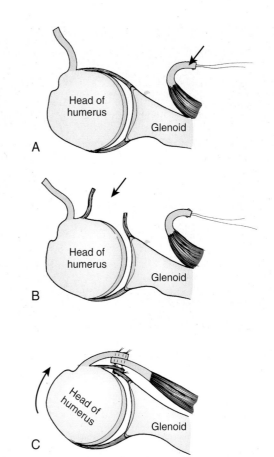

Procedure if anterior capsule is not stripped off scapula.

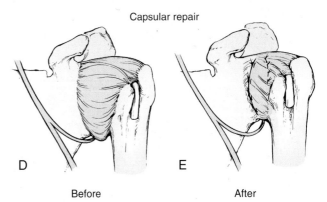

Capsular repair

Before   After

FIGURE 16-270 Capsular shift reconstruction for atraumatic anterior subluxation or dislocation. The Bankart–Perthes lesion is not present, and the capsule is shifted to eliminate the anterior inferior laxity. **A,** Reflection of the subscapularis (*arrow*). **B,** Incision of capsule (*arrow*). **C,** Imbrication of capsule and subscapularis.

can be reduced to a minimum. Surgery is reserved for those with clearly defined mechanical instability. This highly selective approach improves the overall results of surgical treatment of instability by helping minimize situations in which an operation fails to restore the patient's function (Fig. 16-271).

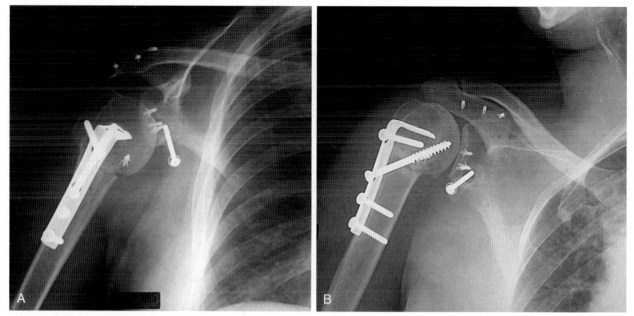

FIGURE 16-271 Radiographs of a shoulder with continued instability after five operations, including a capsular shift, a Bristow procedure, and a rotational osteotomy. **A,** Internal rotation. **B,** External rotation.

REFERENCES

1. Perthes G: Über Operationen bei habitueller Schulterluxation. Dtsch Z Chir 85:199-222, 1906.
2. Bankart ASB: The pathology and treatment of recurrent dislocation of the shoulder joint. Br J Surg 26:23-29, 1939.
3. Zimmerman LM, Veith I: Great Ideas in the History of Surgery: Clavicle, Shoulder, Shoulder Amputations. Baltimore: Williams & Wilkins, 1961.
4. Hussein MK: Kocher's method is 3,000 years old. J Bone Joint Surg Br 50:669-671, 1968.
5. Adams FL: The Genuine Works of Hippocrates. New York: William Wood, 1886.
6. Brockbank W, Griffiths DL: Orthopaedic surgery in the 16th and 17th centuries. J Bone Joint Surg Br 30:365-375, 1948.
7. Moseley HF: Recurrent Dislocations of the Shoulder. Montreal: McGill University Press, 1961.
8. Flower WH: On pathologic changes produced in the shoulder joint by traumatic dislocation. Trans Path Soc London 12:179-200, 1861.
9. Eve FS: A case of subcoracoid dislocation of the humerus with the formation of an indentation on the posterior surface of the head. Medico-Chirurg Trans Soc London 63:317-321, 1880.
10. Joessel D: Über die Recidine der Humerus-luxationen. Dtsch Z Chir 13:167-184, 1880.
11. Hill HA, Sachs MD: The grooved defect of the humeral head. A frequently unrecognized complication of dislocations of the shoulder joint. Radiology 35:690-700, 1940.
12. Kuster E: Über habituelle Schulter Luxation. Verh Deutsch Ges Chir 11:112-114, 1882.
13. Cramer F: Resection des Oberamkopfes wegen Habitueller Luxation (Nach einem im Arzlichen Verein zu Wiesbaden Gehaltenen Vortrage). Berliner Klin Wochenschr 19:21-25, 1882.
14. Löbker K: Einige Präparate von habitueller Schulterluxation. Arch Klin Chir 34:658-667, 1887.
15. Schüller M: Berlin Klin Wochenschr. 33:760, 1896.
16. Staffel F: Verh Dtsch Ges Chir 24(2):651-656, 1895.
17. Francke GH: Dislocations of shoulder. Dtsch Z Chir 48:399, 1898.
18. Caird FM: The shoulder joint in relation to certain dislocations and fractures. Edinb Med J 32:708-714, 1887.
19. Hermodsson I: Röntgenologische Studien über die Traumatischen und Habituellen Schultergelenk-Verrenkungen nach Vorn und nach Unten. Acta Radiol (Suppl) 20:1-173, 1934.
20. Pilz W: Zur Röntgenuntersuchung der habituellen Schulterverrenkung. Arch Klin Chir 135:1-22, 1925.
21. Bankart ASB: Recurrent or habitual dislocation of the shoulder joint. Br Med J 2:1132-1133, 1923.
22. Broca A, Hartman H: Contribution a l' étude des luxations de l' épaule. Bull Soc Anat Paris 4:312-336, 1890.
23. Reeves B: Experiments on the tensile strength of the anterior capsular structures of the shoulder in man. J Bone Joint Surg Br 50:858-865, 1968.
24. Townley CO: The capsular mechanism in recurrent dislocation of the shoulder. J Bone Joint Surg Am 32:370-380, 1950.
25. Moseley HF, Overgaard B: The anterior capsular mechanism in recurrent anterior dislocation of the shoulder: Morphological and clinical studies with special reference to the glenoid labrum and glenohumeral ligaments. J Bone Joint Surg Br 44:913-927, 1962.
26. DePalma AF, Cooke AJ, Prabhakar M: The role of the subscapularis in recurrent anterior dislocations of the shoulder. Clin Orthop Relat Res 54:35-49, 1967.
27. Hauser EDW: Avulsion of the tendon of the subscapularis muscle. J Bone Joint Surg Am 36:139-141, 1954.
28. McLaughlin HL: Recurrent anterior dislocation of the shoulder. I. Morbid anatomy. Am J Surg 99:628-632, 1960.
29. Jens J: The role of the subscapularis muscle in recurring dislocation of the shoulder [abstract]. J Bone Joint Surg Br 34:780, 1964.
30. Reeves B: Acute anterior dislocation of the shoulder. Clinical and experimental studies. Ann R Coll Surg Engl 43:255-273, 1969.
31. Symeonides PP: The significance of the subscapularis muscle in the pathogenesis of recurrent anterior dislocation of the shoulder. J Bone Joint Surg Br 54:476-483, 1972.
32. Hippocrates: Works of Hippocrates with an English Translation. London: William Heinemann, 1927.
33. Kocher T: Eine neue Reductionsmethode für Schulterverrenkung. Berlin Klin 7:101-105, 1870.
34. Milch H: Treatment of dislocation of the shoulder. Surgery 3:732-740, 1938.
35. Lacey T II: Reduction of anterior dislocation of the shoulder by means of the Milch abduction technique. J Bone Joint Surg Am 34:108-109, 1952.
36. Russell JA, Holmes EMI, Keller DJ: Reduction of acute anterior shoulder dislocations using the Milch technique: A study of ski injuries. J Trauma 21(9):802-804, 1981.
37. DePalma AF: Surgery of the Shoulder. Philadelphia: JB Lippincott, 1973.
38. Beattie TF, Steedman DJ, McGowan A, et al: A comparison of the Milch and Kochner techniques for acute anterior dislocation of the shoulder. Injury 17(5):349-352, 1986.
39. McMurray TB: Recurrent dislocation of the shoulder (proceedings). J Bone Joint Surg Br 43:402, 1961.
40. Janecki CJ, Shahcheragh GH: The forward elevation maneuver for reduction of anterior dislocations of the shoulder. Clin Orthop Relat Res (164):177-180, 1982.
41. Waldron VD: Dislocated shoulder reduction—a simple method that is done without assistants. Orthop Rev 11:105-106, 1982.
42. Liedelmeyer R: Letter to the editor: External rotation method of shoulder dislocation reduction. Ann Emerg Med 10:228, 1981.
43. Mirick MJ, Clinton JE, Ruiz E: External rotation method of shoulder dislocation reduction. J Am Coll Emerg Physicians 8:528-531, 1979.

44. Anderson D, Zvirbulis R, Ciullo J: Scapular manipulation for reduction of anterior shoulder dislocations. Clin Orthop Relat Res (164):181-183, 1982.

45. Lippert FG: A modification of the gravity method of reducing anterior shoulder dislocations. Clin Orthop Relat Res (165):259-260, 1982.

46. Parisien VM: Shoulder dislocation: An easier method of reduction. J Maine Med Assoc 70:102, 1979.

47. White ADN: Dislocated shoulder—a simple method of reduction. Med J Aust 2:726-727, 1976.

48. Clotteau JE, Premont M, Mercier V: A simple procedure for reducing dislocations of the shoulder without anesthesia. Nouv Presse Med 11:127-128, 1982.

49. Manes HR: A new method of shoulder reduction in the elderly. Clin Orthop Relat Res (147):200-202, 1980.

50. Bardenheuer BA: Die Verletzungen der oberen Extremitaten. Dtsch Chir 63:268-418, 1886.

51. Thomas TT: Habitual or recurrent anterior dislocation of the shoulder. Am J Med Sci 137:229-246, 1909.

52. Thomas TT: Habitual or recurrent dislocation of the shoulder: Forty-four shoulder operations in 42 patients. Surg Gynecol Obstet 32:291-299, 1921.

53. Albert E: Arthodese bei einer Habituellen Luxation der Schultergelenkes. Klin Rundschau 2:281-283, 1898.

54. Hildebrand: Zur operativen Behandlung der habituellen Schuterluxation. Arch Klin Chir 66:360-364, 1902.

55. Clairmont P, Ehrlich H: Ein neues Operations-Verfahren zur Behandlung der habituellen Schulterluxation mittels Muskelplastik. Verh Dtsch Ges Chir 38:79-103, 1909.

56. Finsterer H: Die operative Behandlung der habituellen Schulterluxation. Deutsch Ztschr Chir 141:354-497, 1917.

57. Clark KC: Positioning in Radiography. London: William Heinemann, 1941.

58. Nicola T: Recurrent anterior dislocation of the shoulder. J Bone Joint Surg 11:128-132, 1929.

59. Nicola T: Recurrent dislocation of the shoulder—its treatment by transplantation of the long head of the biceps. Am J Surg 6:815, 1929.

60. Nicola T: Anterior dislocation of the shoulder: The role of the articular capsule. J Bone Joint Surg 24:614-616, 1942.

61. Nicola T: Acute anterior dislocation of the shoulder. J Bone Joint Surg Am 31:153-159, 1949.

62. Nicola T: Recurrent dislocation of the shoulder. Am J Surg 86:85-91, 1953.

63. Henderson MS: Habitual or recurrent dislocation of the shoulder. Surg Gynecol Obstet 33:1-7, 1921.

64. Henderson MS: Tenosuspension operation for recurrent or habitual dislocation of the shoulder. Surg Clin North Am 5:997-1007, 1949.

65. Gallie WE, LeMesurier AB: An operation for the relief of recurring dislocations of the shoulder. Trans Am Surg Assoc 45:392-398, 1927.

66. Bateman JE: The shoulder and neck. Philadelphia: WB Saunders, 1972.

67. Cooper A: On the dislocation of the os humeri upon the dorsum scapula, and upon fractures near the shoulder joint. Guy's Hosp Rep 4:265-284, 1839.

68. Malgaigne JF: Traité des Fractures et des Luxations. Paris: JB Bailliere, 1855.

69. Leslie JT, Ryan TJ: The anterior axillary incision to approach the shoulder joint. J Bone Joint Surg Am 44:1193-1196, 1962.

70. Clark JM, Harryman DT II: Tendons, ligaments, and capsule of the rotator cuff. Gross and microscopic anatomy. J Bone Joint Surg Am 74(5):713-725, 1992.

71. Yung SW, Harryman DT II: The surgical anatomy of the subscapular nerves. Presented at the 62nd Annual meeting of the American Academy of Orthopaedic Surgeons, Orlando, Fla, March 1995.

72. Halder A, Zobitz ME, Schultz E, et al: Structural properties of the subscapularis tendon. J Orthop Res 18(5):829-834, 2000.

73. Ciccone WJ II, Hunt TJ, Lieber R, et al: Multiquadrant digital analysis of shoulder capsular thickness. Arthroscopy 16(5):457-461, 2000.

74. Schiffern SC, Rozencwaig R, Antoniou J, et al: Anteroposterior centering of the humeral head on the glenoid in vivo. Am J Sports Med 30(3):382-387, 2002.

75. Myers JB, Lephart SM: Sensorimotor deficits contributing to glenohumeral instability. Clin Orthop Relat Res (400):98-104, 2002.

76. Schlemm F: Über die Verstarkungsbander am Schultergelenk. Arch Anat Physiol Wissenschaft Med 22:45-48, 1853.

77. Delorme D: Die Hemmungsbander des Schultergelenks und ihre Bedeutung für die Schulterluxationen. Arch Klin Chir 92:79-101, 1910.

78. Ferrari DA: Capsular ligaments of the shoulder. Anatomical and functional study of the anterior superior capsule. Am J Sports Med 18(1):20-24, 1990.

79. DePalma AF: The management of fractures and dislocations, an Atlas. Philadelphia: WB Saunders, 1970.

80. Fick R: Handbuch der Anatomie und Mechanik der Gelenke unter Berucksichtigung der Bewegenden Muskeln. Jena: Fischer, 1904.

81. O'Connell PW, Nuber GW, Mileski RA, et al: The contribution of the glenohumeral ligaments to anterior stability of the shoulder joint. Am J Sports Med 18(6):579-584, 1990.

82. Codman EA: Rupture of the supraspinatus tendon and other lesions in or about the subacromial bursa. Boston: Thomas Todd & Co, 1934.

83. O'Brien SJ, Neves MC, Arnoczky SP, et al: The anatomy and histology of the inferior glenohumeral ligament complex of the shoulder. Am J Sports Med 18:449-456, 1990.

84. Williams MM, Snyder SJ, Buford D Jr: The Buford complex—the cord-like middle glenohumeral ligament and absent anterosuperior labrum complex: In a normal anatomic capsulolabral variant. Arthroscopy 10(3):241-247, 1994.

85. Uhthoff HK, Piscopo M: Anterior capsular redundancy of the shoulder: Congenital or traumatic? An embryological study. J Bone Joint Surg 67(3):363-366, 1985.

86. Eberly VC, McMahon PJ, Lee TQ: Variation in the glenoid origin of the anteroinferior glenohumeral capsulolabrum. Clin Orthop Relat Res (400):26-31, 2002.

87. DePalma AF, Callery G, Bennett GA: Variational anatomy and degenerative lesions of the shoulder joint. Instr Course Lect 255-281, 1949.

88. Clark JM, Sidles JA, Matsen FA III: The relationship of the glenohumeral joint capsule to the rotator cuff. Clin Orthop Relat Res (254):29-34, 1990.

89. Harryman DT II, Sidles JA, Harris S, et al: The role of the rotator interval capsule in passive motion and stability of the shoulder. J Bone Joint Surg Am 74(1):53-66, 1992.

90. Jerosch J, Moersler M, Castro WH: The function of passive stabilizers of the glenohumeral joint—a biomechanical study. Z Orthop Ihre Grenzgeb 128(2):206-212, 1990.

91. Kuboyama M: The role of soft tissues in downward stability of the glenohumeral joint—an experimental study with fresh cadavers. Igaku Kenkyu 61(1):20-33, 1991.

92. Ovesen J, Nielsen S: Experimental distal subluxation in the glenohumeral joint. Arch Orthop Trauma Surg 104(2):82-84, 1985.

93. Steiner D, Hermann B: Collagen fiber arrangement of the human shoulder joint capsule—an anatomical study. Acta Anat (Basel) 136(4):300-302, 1989.

94. Basmajian JV, Bazant FJ: Factors preventing downward dislocation of the adducted shoulder joint. J Bone Joint Surg Am 41:1182-1186, 1959.

95. Neer CS II, Satterlee CC, Dalsey RM, et al: On the value of the coracohumeral ligament release. Ortho Trans 13(2):235-236, 1989.

96. Nobuhara K, Ikeda H: Rotator interval lesion. Clin Orthop Relat Res (223):44-50, 1987.

97. Warner JJ, Deng XH, Warren RF, et al: Static capsuloligamentous restraints to superior–inferior translation of the glenohumeral joint. Am J Sports Med 20(6):675-685, 1992.

98. Matsen FA III, Lippitt SB, Sidles JA, et al: Practical Evaluation of Management of the Shoulder. Philadelphia: WB Saunders, 1994.

99. Itoi E, Motzkin NE, Morrey BP, et al: Scapular inclination and inferior stability of the shoulder. J Shoulder Elbow Surg 1:131-139, 1992.

100. Terry GC, Hammon D, France P: The stabilizing function of passive shoulder restraints. Am J Sports Med 19:26-34, 1991.

101. Turkel SJ, Panio MW, Marshall JL, et al: Stabilizing mechanisms preventing anterior dislocation of the glenohumeral joint. J Bone Joint Surg Am 63:1208-1217, 1981.

102. Morgan CD, Rames RD, Snyder SJ: Arthroscopic assessment of anatomic variants of the glenohumeral ligaments associated with recurrent anterior shoulder instability. Ortho Trans 15(3):727, 1992.

103. Warren RF, Kornblatt IB, Marchand R: Static factors affecting posterior shoulder stability. Orthop Trans 8:89, 1984.

104. Baeyens JP, Van Roy P, De Schepper A, et al: Glenohumeral joint kinematics related to minor anterior instability of the shoulder at the end of the late preparatory phase of throwing. Clin Biomech (Bristol, Avon) 16(9):752-757, 2001.

105. Harryman DT II, Sidles JA, Clark JM, et al: Translation of the humeral head on the glenoid with passive glenohumeral motion. J Bone Joint Surg Am 72(9):1334-1343, 1990.

107. Berg EE, Ellison AE: The inside-out Bankart procedure. Am J Sports Med 18(2):129-133, 1990.

108. Matsen FA III, Chebli C, Lippitt SB: Principles for the evaluation and management of shoulder instability. J Bone Joint Surg Am 88(3):648-659, 2006.

109. Weldon EJ III, Boorman RS, Smith KL, et al: Optimizing the glenoid contribution to the stability of a humeral hemiarthroplasty without a prosthetic glenoid. J Bone Joint Surg Am 86:2022-2029, 2004.

110. Gardner E: The prenatal development of the human shoulder joint. Surg Clin North Am 43:1465-1470, 1963.

111. Grant JCB: Grant's Atlas of Anatomy. Baltimore: Williams & Wilkins, 1972.

112. Moseley HF: Shoulder Lesions. Springfield Ill: Charles C Thomas, 1945.

113. Moseley HF: Shoulder Lesions. Edinburgh: Churchill Livingstone, 1972.

114. Trillat A, Leclerc-Chalvet F: Luxation Recidivante de L'Épaule. Paris: Masson, 1973.

115. Hertz H, Weinstabl R, Grundschober F, et al: Macroscopic and microscopic anatomy of the shoulder joint and the limbus glenoidalis. Acta Anat (Basel) 125(2):96-100, 1986.

116. Prodromos CC, Ferry JA, Schiller AL, et al: Histological studies of the glenoid labrum from fetal life to old age. J Bone Joint Surg Am 72(9):1344-1348, 1990.

117. Olsson O: Degenerative changes of the shoulder joint and their connection with shoulder pain. A morphological and clinical investigation with special attention to the cuff and biceps tendon. Acta Chir Scand Suppl 181:1-130, 1953.

118. Pagnani MJ, Deng XH, Warren RF, et al: Effect of lesions of the superior portion of the glenoid labrum on glenohumeral translation. J Bone Joint Surg Am 77(7):1003-1010, 1995.

119. Reeves B: Arthrography in acute dislocation of the shoulder. J Bone Joint Surg Br 48:182-187, 1968.

120. Fehringer EV, Kopjar B, Boorman RS, et al: Characterizing the functional improvement after total shoulder arthroplasty for osteoarthritis. J Bone Joint Surg Am 84(8):1349-1353, 2002.

121. Halder AM, Kuhl SG, Zobitz ME, et al: Effects of the glenoid labrum and glenohumeral abduction on stability of the shoulder joint through concavity-compression: An in vitro study. J Bone Joint Surg Am 83(7):1062-1069, 2001.

122. Lazarus MD, Sidles JA, Harryman DT II, et al: Effect of a chondral–labral defect on glenoid concavity and glenohumeral stability. A cadaveric model. J Bone Joint Surg Am 78(1):94-102, 1996.

123. D'Angelo D: Luxacaorecidivante anterior de ombro. Rio de Janeiro, Brazil University of Rio de Janeiro, 1970.

124. DePalma AF: Surgery of the Shoulder. Philadelphia: Lippincott, 1950.

125. Matsen FA III, Thomas SC: Glenohumeral instability. In Evart CMC (ed): Surgery of the Musculoskeletal System. New York: Churchill Livingstone, 1990, pp 1439-1469.

126. Rowe CR, Patel D, Southmayd WW: The Bankart procedure: Long-term end-result study. J Bone Joint Surg Am 60(1):1-16, 1978.

127. Ungersbock A, Michel M, Hertel R: Factors influencing the results of a modified Bankart procedure. J Shoulder Elbow Surg 4:365-369, 1995.

128. Matsen FA III, Fu FH, Hawkins RJ: The Shoulder: A Balance of Mobility and Stability. Rosemont, Ill: American Academy of Orthopaedic Surgeons, 1993.

129. Das SP, Roy GS, Saha AK: Observations on the tilt of the glenoid cavity of scapula. J Anat Soc India 15:114, 1966.

130. Maki S, Gruen T: Anthropomorphic studies of the glenohumeral joint. Trans Orthop Res Soc 1:173, 1976.

131. Saha AK: Dynamic instability of the glenohumeral joint. Acta Orthop Scand 42:491-505, 1971.

132. Howell SM, Galinat BJ: The glenoid-labral socket: A constrained articular surface. Clin Orthop Relat Res (243):122-125, 1989.

133. Howell SM, Galinat BJ, Renzi AJ, et al: Normal and abnormal mechanics of the glenohumeral joint in the horizontal plane. J Bone Joint Surg Am 70(2):227-232, 1988.

134. Poppen NK, Walker PS: Normal and abnormal motion of the shoulder. J Bone Joint Surg Am 58:195-201, 1976.

135. Poppen NK, Walker PS: Forces at the glenohumeral joint in abduction. Clin Orthop Relat Res (135):165-170, 1978.

136. Soslowsky LJ, Bigliani LU, Flatow EL, et al: Articular geometry of the glenohumeral joint. Clin Orthop Relat Res (285):181-190, 1992.

137. Lippitt SB, Vanderhooft JE, Harris SL, et al: Glenohumeral stability from concavity-compression: A quantitative analysis. J Shoulder Elbow Surg Am 2(1):27-35, 1993.

138. Cyprien JM, Vasey HM, Burdet A: Humeral retrotorsion and glenohumeral relationship in the normal shoulder and in recurrent anterior dislocation. Clin Orthop Relat Res (175):8-17, 1983.

139. Thomas SC, Matsen III FA: An approach to the repair of glenohumeral ligament avulsion in the management of traumatic anterior glenohumeral instability. J Bone Joint Surg 71:506-513, 1989.

140. Cooper RA, Brems JJ: The inferior capsular-shift procedure for multidirectional instability of the shoulder. J Bone Joint Surg Am 74(10):1516-1521, 1992.

141. Neer CS II, Foster CR: Inferior capsular shift for involuntary inferior and multidirectional instability of the shoulder. A preliminary report. J Bone Joint Surg Am 62(6):897-908, 1980.

141a. Metcalf MH, Pon JD, Harryman DT 2nd, et al: Capsulolabral augmentation increases glenohumeral stability in the cadaver shoulder. J Shoulder Elbow Surg 10(6):532-538, 2001.

142. Baker CL, Uribe JW, Whitman C: Arthroscopic evaluation of acute initial anterior shoulder dislocations. Am J Sports Med 18:25-28, 1990.

143. Bankart ASB: The pathology and treatment of recurrent dislocation of the shoulder joint. Brit J Surg 26:23-29, 1938.

144. Matsen FA III, Thomas SC, Rockwood CA Jr: Glenohumeral instability. In Rockwood CA Jr, Matsen FA III (eds): The Shoulder. Philadelphia: WB Saunders, 1990, pp 547-551.

145. Pappas AM, Goss TP, Kleinman PK: Symptomatic shoulder instability due to lesions of the glenoid labrum. Am J Sports Med 11:279-288, 1983.

146. Matsen LJ, Hettrich C, Tan A, et al: Direct injection of blood into the labrum enhances the stability provided by the glenoid labral socket. J Shoulder Elbow Surg 15(6):651-658, 2006.

147. Montgomery WH Jr, Wahl M, Hettrich C, et al: Anteroinferior bone-grafting can restore stability in osseous glenoid defects. J Bone Joint Surg Am 87(9):1972-1977, 2005.

148. Harryman DT II, Lazarus MD, Sidles JA, et al: Pathophysiology of shoulder instability. In McGinty JB, Caspari RB, Jackson RW et al (eds): Operative Arthroscopy. Philadelphia: Lippincott-Raven, 1996, pp 677-693.

149. Basmajian JV, DeLuca CJ: Muscles alive. Baltimore: Williams & Wilkins, 1985, pp 270-271.

150. Bassett RW, Browne AO, Morrey BF, et al: Glenohumeral muscle force and moment mechanics in a position of shoulder instability. J Biomech 23(5):405-415, 1990.

151. Blasier RB, Guldberg RE, Rothman ED: Anterior shoulder stability: Contributions of rotator cuff forces and the capsular ligaments in a cadaver model. J Shoulder Elbow Surg 1(3):140-150, 1992.

152. Cain PR, Mitschler T, Fu FH, et al: Anterior stability of the glenohumeral joint: A dynamic model. Am J Sports Med 15(2):144-148, 1987.

153. Itoi E, Kuechle DK, Newman SR, et al: Stabilizing function of the biceps in stable and unstable shoulders. J Bone Joint Surg Br 75(4):546-550, 1993.

154. Itoi E, Newman SR, Kuechle DK, et al: Dynamic anterior stabilizers of the shoulder with the arm in abduction. J Bone Joint Surg Br 76(5):834-836, 1994.

155. Karlsson D, Peterson B: Towards a model for force predictions in the human shoulder. J Biomech 25(2):189-199, 1992.

156. Perry J, Glousman RE: Biomechanics of throwing. In Nicholas JA, Hershman EB (eds): The Upper Extremity in Sports Medicine. St. Louis: CV Mosby, 1989, pp 727-751.

157. Rodosky MW, Harner CD, Fu FH: The role of the long head of the biceps muscle and superior glenoid labrum in anterior stability of the shoulder. Am J Sports Med 22(1):121-130, 1994.

158. Sarrafian AK: Gross and functional anatomy of the shoulder. Clin Orthop Relat Res (173):11-19, 1983.

159. Van der Helm FC: A finite element musculoskeletal model of the shoulder mechanics. J Biomech 27(5):551-569, 1994.

160. Van der Helm FC, Veeger HE, Pronk GM, et al: Geometry parameters for musculoskeletal modeling of the shoulder system. J Biomech 25(2):129-144, 1992.

161. Veeger HE, Van der Helm FC, Van der Woude LH, et al: Inertia and muscle contraction parameters for musculoskeletal modeling of the shoulder mechanism. J Biomech 24(7):615-629, 1991.

162. Wulker N, Rossig S, Korell M, et al: Dynamic stability of the glenohumeral joint. A biomechanical study. Sportverletz Sportschaden 9(1):1-8, 1995.

163. Lee SB, An KN: Dynamic glenohumeral stability provided by three heads of the deltoid muscle. Clin Orthop Relat Res (400):40-47, 2002.

164. Halder AM, Halder CG, Zhao KD, et al: Dynamic inferior stabilizers of the shoulder joint. Clin Biomech (Bristol, Avon) 16(2):138-143, 2001.

165. Kim SH, Ha KI, Kim HS, et al: Electromyographic activity of the biceps brachii muscle in shoulders with anterior instability. Arthroscopy 17(8):864-868, 2001.

166. Guanche C, Knatt T, Solomonow M, et al: The synergistic action of the capsule and the shoulder muscles. Am J Sports Med 23(3):301-306, 1995.

167. Hashimoto T, Hamada T, Sasaguri Y, et al: Immunohistochemical approach for the investigation of nerve distribution in the shoulder joint capsule. Clin Orthop Relat Res (305):273-282, 1994.

168. Jerosch J, Castro WH, Grosse-Hackman A, et al: Function of the glenohumeral ligaments in active protection of shoulder stability. Z Orthop Ihre Grenzgeb 133(1):67-71, 1995.

169. Vangsness CT Jr, Ennis M, Taylor JG, et al: Neural anatomy of the glenohumeral ligaments, labrum, and subacromial bursa. Arthroscopy 11(2):180-184, 1995.

170. Blasier RB, Carpenter JE, Huston LJ: Shoulder proprioception. Effect of joint laxity, joint position, and direction of motion. Orthop Rev 23(1):45-50, 1994.

171. Kronberg M, Brostrom LA, Nemeth G: Differences in shoulder muscle activity between patients with generalized joint laxity and normal controls. Clin Orthop Relat Res (269):181-192, 1991.

172. Zuckerman JD, Gallagher MA, Cuomo F, et al: Effect of instability and subsequent anterior shoulder repair on proprioceptive ability. Presented at the American Shoulder and Elbow Surgeons 12th Open Meeting, Atlanta, Ga, March 1996.

173. Itoi E, Lee SB, Berglund LJ, et al: The effect of a glenoid defect on anteroinferior stability of the shoulder after Bankart repair: A cadaveric study. J Bone Joint Surg Am 82(1):35-46, 2000.

174. Silliman JF, Hawkins RJ: Classification and physical diagnosis of instability of the shoulder. Clin Orthop Relat Res (291):7-19, 1993.

175. Lerat JL, Chotel F, Besse JL, et al: Dynamic anterior jerk of the shoulder. A new clinical test for shoulder instability. Preliminary study. Rev Chir Orthop Reparatrice Appar Mot 80(6):461-467, 1994.

176. Wirth MA, Seltzer DG, Rockwood CA Jr: Recurrent posterior glenohumeral dislocation associated with increased retroversion of the glenoid. Clin Orthop Relat Res (308):98-101, 1994.

177. Metcalf MH, Duckworth DG, Lee SB, et al: Posteroinferior glenoplasty can change glenoid shape and increase the mechanical stability of the shoulder. J Shoulder Elbow Surg 8(3):205-213, 1999.

178. Brewer BJ, Wubben RC, Carrera GF: Excessive retroversion of the glenoid cavity. A cause of non-traumatic posterior instability of the shoulder. J Bone Joint Surg Am 68(5):724-731, 1986.

179. Hurley JA, Anderson TE, Dear WA, et al: Posterior shoulder instability. Surgical versus conservative results with evaluation of glenoid version. Am J Sports Med 20(4):396-400, 1992.

180. Randelli M, Gambrioli PL: Glenohumeral osteometry by computed tomography in normal and unstable shoulders. Clin Orthop Relat Res (208):151-156, 1986.

181. Dias JJ, Mody BS, Finlay DB, et al: Recurrent anterior glenohumeral joint dislocation and torsion of the humerus. J Orthop Sports Phys Ther 18(1):379-385, 1993.
182. Dowdy PA, O'Driscoll SW: Recurrent anterior shoulder instability. Am J Sports Med 22(4):489-492, 1994.
183. Hirschfelder H, Kirsten U: Biometric analysis of the unstable shoulder. Z Orthop Ihre Grenzgeb 129(6):516-520, 1991.
184. Grasshoff H, Buhtz C, Gellerich I, et al: CT diagnosis in instability of the shoulder joint. Rofo 155(6):523-526, 1991.
185. Crockett HC, Gross LB, Wilk KE, et al: Osseous adaptation and range of motion at the glenohumeral joint in professional baseball pitchers. Am J Sports Med 30(1):20-26, 2002.
186. Churchill RS, Brems JJ, Kotschi H: Glenoid size, inclination, and version: An anatomic study. J Shoulder Elbow Surg 10(4):327-332, 2001.
187. Weishaupt D, Zanetti M, Nyffeler RW, et al: Posterior glenoid rim deficiency in recurrent (atraumatic) posterior shoulder instability. Skeletal Radiol 29(4):204-210, 2000.
188. Bradley JP, Tibone JE: Electromyographic analysis of muscle action about the shoulder. Clin Sports Med 10:789-805, 1991.
189. Glousman R, Jobe F, Tibone J: Dynamic electromyographic analysis of the throwing shoulder with glenohumeral instability. J Bone Joint Surg Am 70:220-226, 1988.
190. Inman VT, Saunders JB, Abbott LC: Observations on the function of the shoulder joint. J Bone Joint Surg 26:1-30, 1994.
191. Ozaki J: Glenohumeral movement of the involuntary inferior and multidirectional instability. Clin Orthop Relat Res (238):107-111, 1989.
192. Warner JJ, Micheli LJ, Arslanian LE, et al: Scapulothoracic motion in normal shoulders and shoulders with glenohumeral instability and impingement syndrome. A study using Moir'e topographic analysis. Clin Orthop Relat Res (285):191-199, 1992.
193. Atwater AE: Biomechanics of overarm throwing movements and of throwing injuries. Exerc Sports Sci Rev 8:43-85, 1980.
194. Frank CB: Ligament healing: Current knowledge and clinical applications. J Am Acad Orthop Surg 4(2):74-83, 1996.
195. Stefko JM, Tibone JE, McMahon PJ, et al: Strain of the anterior band of the glenohumeral ligament at the time of capsular failure. Paper presented at the American Shoulder and Elbow Surgeons Closed Meeting, LaQuinta, Calif, March 1995.
196. Emery RJ, Mullaji AB: Glenohumeral joint instability in normal adolescents. Incidence and significance. J Bone Joint Surg Br 73(3):406-408, 1991.
197. Cofield RH, Nessler JP, Weinstabl R: Diagnosis of shoulder instability by examination under anesthesia. Clin Orthop Relat Res (291):45-53, 1993.
198. Jerosch J, Goertzen M, Marquardt M: Possibilities of diagnostic sonography in assessment of instability of the shoulder joint. Unfallchirurg 94(2):88-94, 1991.
199. Jerosch J, Marquardt M, Winklemann W: Ultrasound documentation of translational movement of the shoulder joint. Normal values and pathologic findings. Ultraschall Med 12(1):31-35, 1991.
200. Jorgensen U, Bak K: Shoulder instability. Assessment of anterior-posterior translation with a knee laxity tester. Acta Orthop Scand 66(5):398-400, 1995.
201. Marquardt M, Jerosch J: Ultrasound evaluation of multidirectional instability of the shoulder. Unfallchirurg 94:295-301, 1991.
202. Harryman DT II, Sidles JA, Matsen FA III: Laxity of the normal glenohumeral joint: A quantitative in vivo assessment. J Shoulder Elbow Surg 1(2):66-76, 1992.
203. Lippitt SB, Harris SL, Harryman DT II, et al: In vivo quantification of the laxity of normal and unstable glenohumeral joints. J Shoulder Elbow Surg 3(4):215-223, 1994.
204. Sperber A, Wredmark T: Capsular elasticity and joint volume in recurrent anterior shoulder instability. Arthroscopy 10(6):598-601, 1994.
205. Lieber R: Skeletal Muscle Structure and Function. Baltimore: Williams & Wilkins, 1992, p 314.
206. Kaltsas DS: Comparative study of the properties of the shoulder joint capsule with those of other joint capsules. Clin Orthop Relat Res (173):20-26, 1983.
207. Bigliani LU, Pollock RG, Soslowsky LJ, et al: Tensile properties of the inferior glenohumeral ligament. J Orthop Res 10(2):187-197, 1992.
208. Hawkins RJ, Angelo RL: Glenohumeral osteoarthritis: A late complication of the Putti–Platt repair. J Bone Joint Surg Am 72(8):1193-1197, 1990.
209. Simkin PA: Structure and function of joints. In Schumacher HR, Klippel JH, Robinson DR (eds): Primer on the Rheumatic Diseases, 9th ed. Atlanta: Arthritis Foundation, 1988.
210. Levick JR: Joint pressure–volume studies: Their importance, design and interpretation. J Rheumatol 10:353-357, 1983.
211. Müller W: Über den negativen Luftdruck im Gelenkraum. Dtsch Z Chir 217:395-401, 1929.
212. Itoi EA, Motzkin NE, Browne AO, et al: Intraarticular pressure of the shoulder. Arthroscopy 9(4):406-413, 1993.
213. Humphry GM: A treatise on the human skeleton (including the joints). London: Macmillan, 1858, pp 73-74.
214. Kumar VP, Balasubramaniam P: The role of atmospheric pressure in stabilizing the shoulder. J Bone Joint Surg Br 67:719-721, 1985.
215. Neer CS II: Displaced proximal humeral fractures. I. Classification and evaluation. J Bone Joint Surg Am 52:1077-1089, 1970.
216. Cotton FJ: Subluxation of the shoulder downward. Boston Med Surg J 185:405-407, 1921.
217. Fairbank TJ: Fracture-subluxations of the shoulder. J Bone Joint Surg Br 30:454-460, 1948.
218. Ovesen J, Nielsen S: Stability of the shoulder joint: Cadaver study of stabilizing structures. Acta Orthop Scand 56:149-151, 1985.
219. Sidles JA, Harryman DT, Simkin PA: Passive and active stabilization of the glenohumeral joint. Submitted to J Bone Joint Surg, 1989.
220. Thompson FR, Winant WM: Unusual fracture-subluxations of the shoulder joint. J Bone Joint Surg Am 32:575-582, 1950.
221. Thompson FR, Winant WM: Comminuted fractures of the humeral head with subluxation. Clin Orthop 20:94-96, 1961.
222. Gibb TD, Harryman DT II, Sidles JA, et al: The effect of capsular venting on glenohumeral laxity. Clin Orthop Relat Res (268):120-127, 1991.
223. Wulker N, Sperveslage C, Brewe F: Passive stabilizers of the glenohumeral joint. A biomechanical study. Unfallchirurg 96(3):129-133, 1993.
224. Habermeyer P, Schuller U: Significance of the glenoid labrum for stability of the glenohumeral joint. An experimental study. Unfallchirurg 93(1):19-26, 1990.
225. Habermeyer P, Schuller U, Wiedemann E: The intra-articular pressure of the shoulder: An experimental study on the role of the glenoid labrum in stabilizing the joint. J Arthroscopy 8(2):166-172, 1992.
226. Roston JB, Haines RW: Cracking in the metacarpo-phalangeal joint. J Anat 81:165-173, 1947.
227. Unsworth A, Dowson D, Wright V: "Cracking joints": A bioengineering study of cavitation in the metacarpophalangeal joint. Ann Rheum Dis 30:348-358, 1971.
228. Ziegler DW, Harrington RM, Matsen FA III: The superior rotator cuff tendon and acromion provide passive superior stability to the shoulder. Unpublished.
229. Flatow EL, Raimondo RA, Kelkar R, et al: Active and passive restraints against superior humeral translation: The contributions of the rotator cuff, the biceps tendon, and the coracoacromial arch. Presented at the Annual American Academy of Orthopaedic Surgeons meeting, Atlanta, Ga, March 1996.
230. Largacha M, Parsons IM, Campbell B, et al: Deficits in shoulder function and general health associated with sixteen common shoulder diagnoses: A study of 2674 patients. J Shoulder Elbow Surg 15(1):30-39, 2006.
231. Wirth MA, Lyons FR, Rockwood CA Jr: Hypoplasia of the glenoid. A review of sixteen patients. J Bone Joint Surg Am 75(8):1175-1184, 1993.
232. Rowe CR: Prognosis in dislocations of the shoulder. J Bone Joint Surg Am 38:957-977, 1956.
233. DePalma AF: Surgery of the Shoulder. Philadelphia: JB Lippincott, 1983.
234. Rockwood CA Jr: Subluxation of the shoulder—the classification, diagnosis and treatment. Orthop Trans 4:306, 1979.
235. Collins HR, Wilde AH: Shoulder instability in athletes. Orthop Clin North Am 4:759-773, 1973.
236. Imazato Y: Etiological considerations of the loose shoulder from a biochemical point of view—biochemical studies on collagen from deltoid and pectoral muscles and skin. Nippon Seikeigeka Gakkai Zasshi 66(10):1006-1015, 1992.
237. Hirakawa M: On the etiology of the loose shoulder—biochemical studies on collagen from joint capsules. Nippon Seikeigeka Gakkai Zasshi 65(8):550-560, 1991.
238. O'Driscoll SW, Evans DC: Long-term results of staple capsulorrhaphy for anterior instability of the shoulder. J Bone Joint Surg Am 75:249-258, 1993.
239. Dowdy PA, O'Driscoll SW: Shoulder instability. An analysis of family history. J Bone Joint Surg Br 75(5):782-784, 1993.
240. Morrey BF, Janes JM: Recurrent anterior dislocation of the shoulder: Long-term follow-up of the Putti–Platt and Bankart procedures. J Bone Joint Surg Am 58:252-256, 1976.
241. Garth WP Jr, Allman FL, Armstrong WS: Occult anterior subluxations of the shoulder in noncontact sports. Am J Sports Med 15(6):579-585, 1987.
242. Protzman RR: Anterior instability of the shoulder. J Bone Joint Surg Am 62:909-918, 1980.
243. Rowe CR, Zarins B: Recurrent transient subluxation of the shoulder. J Bone Joint Surg Am 63:863-872, 1981.
244. Carew-McColl M: Bilateral shoulder dislocations caused by electrical shock. Br J Clin Prac 34:251-254, 1980.
245. Rowe CR, Pierce DS, Clark JG: Voluntary dislocation of the shoulder. A preliminary report on a clinical, electromyographic, and psychiatric study of 26 patients. J Bone Joint Surg Am 55:445-460, 1973.
246. Percy LR: Recurrent posterior dislocation of the shoulder. J Bone Joint Surg Br 42:863, 1960.
247. Kretzler HH, Blue AR: Recurrent posterior dislocation of the shoulder in cerebral palsy. J Bone Joint Surg Am 48:1221, 1966.
248. Sever JW: Obstetrical paralysis. Surg Gynecol Obstet 44:547-549, 1927.
249. Fairbank HAT: Birth palsy: Subluxation of the shoulder joint in infants and young children. Lancet 1:1217-1223, 1913.

250. L'Episcopo JB: Restoration of muscle balance in the treatment of obstetrical paralysis. N Y J Med 39:357-363, 1939.

251. Zachary RB: Transplantation of teres major and latissimus dorsi for loss of external rotation at the shoulder. Lancet 2:757-761, 1947.

252. Wickstrom J: Birth injuries of the brachial plexus: Treatment of defects in the shoulder. Clin Orthop 23:187-196, 1962.

253. Zorowitz RD, Idank D, Ikai T, et al: Shoulder subluxation after stroke: A comparison of four supports. Arch Phys Med Rehabil 76(8):763-771, 1995.

254. Rowe CR, Zarins B: Chronic unreduced dislocations of the shoulder. J Bone Joint Surg Am 64:494-505, 1982.

255. Lee AJ, Garraway WM, Hepburn W, et al: Influence of rugby injuries on players' subsequent health and lifestyle: Beginning a long term follow up. Br J Sports Med 35(1):38-42, 2001.

256. Marx RG, McCarty EC, Montemurno TD, et al: Development of arthrosis following dislocation of the shoulder: A case-control study. J Shoulder Elbow Surg 11(1):1-5, 2002.

257. Kazar B, Relovszky E: Prognosis of primary dislocation of the shoulder. Acta Orthop Scand 40:216-224, 1969.

258. Cave EF, Burke JF, Boyd RJ: Trauma Management. Chicago: Year Book Medical Publishers, 1974, p 437.

259. Glessner JR: Intrathoracic dislocation of the humeral head. J Bone Joint Surg Am 42:428-430, 1961.

260. Moseley HF: The basic lesions of recurrent anterior dislocation. Surg Clin North Am 43:1631-1634, 1963.

261. Patel MR, Pardee ML, Singerman RC: Intrathoracic dislocation of the head of the humerus. J Bone Joint Surg Am 45:1712-1714, 1963.

262. Sonnabend DH: Treatment of primary anterior shoulder dislocation in patients older than 40 years of age. Clin Orthop Relat Res (304):74-77, 1994.

263. West EF: Intrathoracic dislocation of the humerus. J Bone Joint Surg Br 31:61-62, 1949.

264. Wirth MA, Jensen KL, Agarwal A, et al: Fracture-dislocation of the proximal humerus with retroperitoneal humeral head displacement. J Bone Joint Surg Am 79:763-766, 1997.

265. Hawkins RJ, Neer CS 2nd, Pianta RM, Mendoza FX: Locked posterior dislocation of the shoulder. J Bone Joint Surg Am 69:9-18, 1987.

266. Thomas MA: Posterior subacromial dislocation of the head of the humerus. AJR Am J Roentgenol 37:767-773, 1937.

267. Engelhardt MB: Posterior dislocation of the shoulder: Report of six cases. South Med J 71:425-427, 1978.

268. Hehne HJ, Hubner H: Die Behandlung der Rezidivieremden Schulterluxation nach Putti-Platt-Bankart und Eden-Hybinette-Lange. Orthop Prax 16:331-335, 1980.

269. Mestdagh H, Maynou C, Delobelle JM, et al: Traumatic posterior dislocation of the shoulder in adults. A propos of 25 cases. Ann Chir 48(4):355-363, 1994.

270. Pavlov H, Warren RF, Weiss CBJ, et al: The roentgenographic evaluation of anterior shoulder instability. Clin Orthop Relat Res (194):153-158, 1985.

271. Verrina F: Para-articular ossification following simple dislocation of the shoulder. Minerva Orthop 210:480-486, 1975.

272. McLaughlin HL: Posterior dislocation of the shoulder. J Bone Joint Surg Am 3:584-590, 1952.

273. Moeller JC: Compound posterior dislocation of the shoulder. J Bone Joint Surg Am 57:1006-1007, 1975.

274. Ahlgren O, Lorentzon R, Larsson SE: Posterior dislocation of the shoulder associated with general seizures. Acta Orthop Scand 52:694-695, 1981.

275. Fipp GJ: Simultaneous posterior dislocation of both shoulders. Clin Orthop Relat Res 44:191-195, 1966.

276. Hawkins RH, Hawkins RJ: Failed anterior reconstruction for shoulder instability. J Bone Joint Surg Br 67(5):709-714, 1985.

277. Lindholm TS, Elmstedt E: Bilateral posterior dislocation of the shoulder combined with fracture of the proximal humerus. Acta Orthop Scand 51:485-488, 1980.

278. McFie J: Bilateral anterior dislocation of the shoulders: A case report. Injury 8:67-69, 1976.

279. Mills KLG: Simultaneous bilateral posterior fracture dislocation of the shoulder. Injury 6:39-41, 1974-1975.

280. Onabowale BO, Jaja MOA: Unreduced bilateral synchronous shoulder dislocations. Niger Med J 9:267-271, 1979.

281. Segal D, Yablon IG, Lynch JJ, Jones RP: Acute bilateral anterior dislocation of the shoulders. Clin Orthop Relat Res (140):21-22, 1979.

282. Heller KD, Forst J, Forst R, et al: Posterior dislocation of the shoulder. Arch Orthop Trauma Surg 113:228-231, 1994.

283. Middeldorpf M, Scharm B: De Nova Humeri Luxationis Specie. Clinique Europenne 2:12-16, 1859.

284. Lynn FS: Erect dislocation of the shoulder. Surg Gynecol Obstet 39:51-55, 1921.

285. Roca LA, Ramos-Vertiz JR: Luxacion erecta de hombro. Rev San Milit Argent 61:135-142, 1962.

286. Laskin RS, Sedlin ED: Luxatio erecta in infancy. Clin Orthop 80:126-129, 1971.

287. Murrard J: Un cas de luxatio erecta de l'épaule double et symétrique. Rev Orthop 7:423-429, 1920.

288. Langfritz HV: Die doppelseitige traumatische Luxatio Humeri Erecta eine seltene Verletzungsform. Monatschr Unfallheilkunde 59(367), 1956.

289. Peiro A, Ferrandis R, Correa F: Bilateral erect dislocation of the shoulders. Injury 6:294-295, 1975.

290. Nobel W: Posterior traumatic dislocation of the shoulder. J Bone Joint Surg Am 44:523-538, 1962.

291. Kubin Z: Luxatio humeri erecta: Kasuisticke sdeleni. Acta Chir Orthop Traumatol Cech 31:565-567, 1964.

292. Gardham JRC, Scott JE: Axillary artery occlusion with erect dislocation of the shoulder. Injury 11(2):155-158, 1980.

293. Lev-El A, Rubinstein Z: Axillary artery injury in erect dislocation of the shoulder. J Trauma 21:323-325, 1981.

294. Meadowcroft JA, Kain TM: Luxatio erecta shoulder dislocation: Report of two cases. Jefferson Orthop J 6:20-24, 1977.

295. Lucas GL, Peterson MD: Open anterior dislocation of the shoulder. J Trauma 17:883-884, 1977.

296. Speed K: Fractures and Dislocation. Philadelphia: Lea & Febiger, 1942.

297. Stimson LA: A Practical Treatise on Fractures and Dislocations. Philadelphia: Lea & Febiger, 1912.

298. Mynter H: Subacromial dislocation from muscular spasm. Ann Surg 36:117-119, 1902.

299. Honner R: Bilateral posterior dislocation of the shoulder. Aust N Z J Surg 38:269-272, 1969.

300. Yadav SS: Bilateral simultaneous fracture-dislocation of the shoulder due to muscular violence. J Postgrad Med 23:137-139, 1977.

301. Nicola FG, Ellman H, Eckardt J, et al: Bilateral posterior fracture-dislocation of the shoulder treated with a modification of the McLaughlin procedure. J Bone Joint Surg Am 63:1175-1177, 1981.

302. Parrish GA, Skiendzielewski JJ: Bilateral posterior fracture-dislocations of the shoulder after convulsive status epilepticus. Ann Emerg Med 14(3):264-266, 1985.

303. Pagden D, Halaburt AS, Wiroszo R, et al: Posterior dislocation of the shoulder complicating regional anesthesia. Anesth Analg 65(10):1063-1065, 1986.

304. Costigan PS, Binns MS, Wallace WA: Undiagnosed bilateral anterior dislocation of the shoulder. Injury 21:409, 1990.

305. de Laat EA, Visser CP, Coene LN, et al: Nerve lesions in primary shoulder dislocations and humeral neck fractures. A prospective clinical and EMG study. J Bone Joint Surg Br 76(3):381-383, 1994.

306. Blom S, Dahlback LO: Nerve injuries in dislocations of the shoulder joint and fractures of the neck of the humerus. Acta Chir Scand 136:461-466, 1970.

307. Hill NA, McLaughlin HL: Locked posterior dislocation simulating a "frozen shoulder." J Trauma 3:225-234, 1963.

308. McLaughlin HL: Dislocation of the shoulder with tuberosity fractures. Surg Clin North Am 43:1615-1620, 1963.

309. Dorgan JA: Posterior dislocation of the shoulder. Am J Surg 89:890-900, 1955.

310. Grashey R: Atlas Typischer Rontgenfilder. Munich: Lehman, 1923.

311. McLaughlin HL: Locked posterior subluxation of the shoulder: Diagnosis and treatment. Surg Clin North Am 43:1621-1622, 1963.

312. Neer CS II: Fractures of the distal third of the clavicle. Clin Orthop Relat Res 58:43-50, 1968.

314. Rubin SA, Gray RL, Green WR: Scapular Y—a diagnostic aid in shoulder trauma. Radiology 110:725-726, 1974.

315. Lawrence WS: New position in radiographing the shoulder joint. Am J Roentgenol 2:728-730, 1915.

316. Merrill V: Atlas of Roentgenographic Positions and Standard Radiologic Procedures. St Louis: CV Mosby, 1975.

317. Jordan H: New technique for the roentgen examination of the shoulder joint. Radiology 25:480-484, 1935.

318. Cleaves EN: A new film holder for roentgen examination of the shoulder. Am J Roentgenol Rad Ther Nucl Med 45:288-290, 1941.

319. Post M: The Shoulder. Surgical and Non-surgical Management. Philadelphia: Lea & Febiger, 1978.

320. Bloom MH, Obata WG: Diagnosis of posterior dislocation of the shoulder with use of Velpeau axillary and angle-up roentgenographic views. J Bone Joint Surg Am 49:943-949, 1967.

321. Garth WP Jr, Slappey CE, Ochs CW: Roentgenographic demonstration of instability of the shoulder: The apical oblique projection. A technical note. J Bone Joint Surg Am 66(9):1450-1453, 1984.

322. Kinnard P, Gordon D, Levesque RY, et al: Computerized arthrotomography in recurring shoulder dislocations and subluxations. Can J Surg 27:487-488, 1984.

323. Ribbans WJ, Mitchell R, Taylor GJ: Computerized arthrotomography of primary anterior dislocation of the shoulder. J Bone Joint Surg Br 72:181-185, 1990.

324. Shuman WP, Kilcoyne RF, Matsen FA III, et al: Double-contrast computed tomography of the glenoid labrum. AJR Am J Roentgenol 141:581-584, 1983.

325. Ferkel RD, Hedley AK, Eckardt JJ: Anterior fracture-dislocations of the shoulder: Pitfalls in treatment. J Trauma 24(4):363-367, 1984.

326. Benechetrit E, Friedman B: Fracture of the coracoid process associated with subglenoid dislocation of the shoulder. J Bone Joint Surg Am 61:295-296, 1979.

327. Wong-Pack WK, Bobechko PE, Becker EJ: Fractured coracoid with anterior shoulder dislocation. J Can Assoc Radiol 31:278-279, 1980.

328. Itoi E, Tabata S: Rotator cuff tears in anterior dislocation of the shoulder. Int Orthop 16:240-244, 1992.

329. Pasila M, Jaroma H, Kiviluoto O: Early complications of primary shoulder dislocations. Acta Orthop Scand 49:260-263, 1978.

330. Pettersson G: Rupture of the tendon aponeurosis of the shoulder joint in anterior inferior dislocation. Acta Chir Scand (Suppl) 77:1-187, 1942.

331. Tijmes J, Loyd HM, Tullos HS: Arthrography in acute shoulder dislocations. South Med J 72:564-567, 1979.

332. Hawkins RJ, Koppert G, Johnston G: Recurrent posterior instability (subluxation) of the shoulder. J Bone Joint Surg Am 66:169-174, 1984.

333. Neviaser RJ, Neviaser TJ, Neviaser JS: Concurrent rupture of the rotator cuff and anterior dislocation of the shoulder in the older patient. J Bone Joint Surg Am 70:1308-1311, 1988.

334. Gonzalez D, Lopez R: Concurrent rotator-cuff tear and brachial plexus palsy associated with anterior dislocation of the shoulder. A report of two cases. J Bone Joint Surg Am 73(4):620-621, 1991.

335. Johnson JR, Bayley JIL: Loss of shoulder function following acute anterior dislocation. J Bone Joint Surg Br 63:633, 1981.

336. Mack LA, Matsen FA III, Kilcoyne RF: US evaluation of the rotator cuff. Radiology 157:205-209, 1985.

337. Toolanen G, Hildingsson C, Hedlund T, et al: Early complications after anterior dislocation of the shoulder in patients over 40 years. An ultrasonographic and electromyographic study. Acta Orthop Scand 64(5):549-552, 1993.

338. Neviaser RJ, Neviaser TJ, Neviaser JS: Anterior dislocation of the shoulder and rotator cuff rupture. Clin Orthop Relat Res (291):103-106, 1993.

339. Helm AT, Watson JS: Compression of the brachial plexus in a patient with false aneurysm of the axillary artery as a result of anterior shoulder dislocation. J Shoulder Elbow Surg 11(3):278-279, 2002.

340. Martin SS, Limbird TJ: The terrible triad of the shoulder. J South Orthop Assoc 8(1):57-60, 1999.

341. Onyeka W: Anterior shoulder dislocation: An unusual complication. Emerg Med J 19(4):367-368, 2002.

342. Kirker JR: Dislocation of the shoulder complicated by rupture of the axillary vessels. J Bone Joint Surg Br 34:72-73, 1952.

343. Antal CS, Conforty B, Engelberg M: Injuries to the axillary due to anterior dislocation of the shoulder. J Trauma 13:564-566, 1973.

344. Curr JF: Rupture of the axillary artery complicating dislocation of the shoulder. Report of a case. J Bone Joint Surg Br 52:313-317, 1970.

345. Gugenheim S, Sanders RJ: Axillary artery rupture caused by shoulder dislocation. Surgery 95:55-58, 1984.

346. Jardon OM, Hood LT, Lynch RD: Complete avulsion of the axillary artery as a complication of shoulder dislocation. J Bone Joint Surg Am 55:189-192, 1973.

347. Brown FW, Navigato WJ: Rupture of the axillary artery and brachial plexus palsy associated with anterior dislocation of the shoulder—report of a case with successful vascular repair. Clin Orthop 60:195-199, 1968.

348. Milton GW: The mechanism of circumflex and other nerve injuries in dislocation of the shoulder and the possible mechanism of nerve injuries during reduction of dislocation. Aust N Z J Surg 23:24-30, 1953-1955.

349. Watson-Jones R: Fractures and Joint Injuries. Baltimore: Williams & Wilkins, 1957.

350. Ng KC, Singh S, Low YP: Axillary artery damage from shoulder trauma—a report of 2 cases. Chirurgie 116(2):190-193, 1990.

351. Stener B: Dislocation of the shoulder complicated by complete rupture of the axillary artery. J Bone Joint Surg Br 39:714-717, 1957.

352. Bertrand JC, Maestro M, Pequignot JP, et al: Les complications vasculaires des luxations anterieures fermes de l'épaule. Ann Chir 36:329-333, 1981.

353. Drury JK, Scullion JE: Vascular complications of anterior dislocation of the shoulder. Br J Surg 67:579-581, 1980.

354. Fitzgerald JF, Keates J: False aneurysm as a late complication of anterior dislocation of the shoulder. Ann Surg 181:785-786, 1975.

355. Lescher TJ, Andersen OS: Occlusion of the axillary artery complicating shoulder dislocation: Case report. Milit Med 144:621-622, 1979.

356. Sarma A, Savanchak H, Levinson ED, et al: Thrombosis of the axillary artery and brachial plexus injury secondary to shoulder dislocation. Conn Med 45:513-514, 1981.

357. Stein E: Case report 374: Posttraumatic pseudoaneurysm of axillary artery. Skeletal Radiol 15(5):391-393, 1986.

358. Baratta JB, Lim V, Mastromonaco E, et al: Axillary artery disruption secondary to anterior dislocation of the shoulder. J Trauma 23(11):1009-1011, 1983.

359. Calvet J, Leroy M, Lacroix L: Luxations de l'épaule et lesions vasculaires. J Chir 58:337-346, 1942.

360. Guibe M: Des lesions des vaisseaux de l'aiselle qui compliquent les luxations de l'épaule. Rev Chir 4:580-583, 1911.

361. Steenburg RW, Ravitch MM: Cervicothoracic approach for subclavian vessel injury from compound fracture of the clavicle: Considerations of subclavian axillary exposures. Ann Surg 157:839-846, 1963.

363. Cranley JJ, Krause RF: Injury to the axillary artery following anterior dislocation of the shoulder. Am J Surg 95:524-526, 1958.

364. Dolk T, Stenberg B: Arterial injury in fracture dislocation of the shoulder. Acta Orthop Scand 62(Suppl 246):17, 1991.

365. Gibson JMC: Rupture of the axillary artery following anterior dislocation of the shoulder. J Bone Joint Surg Br 44:114-115, 1962.

366. Henson GF: Vascular complications of shoulder injuries: A report of two cases. J Bone Joint Surg Br 38:528-531, 1956.

367. McKenzie AD, Sinclair AM: Axillary artery occlusion complicating shoulder dislocation. Am Surg 148:139-141, 1958.

368. Rob CG, Standeven A: Closed traumatic lesions of the axillary and brachial arteries. Lancet 1:597-599, 1956.

369. Johnston GW, Lowry JH: Rupture of the axillary artery complicating anterior dislocation of the shoulder. J Bone Joint Surg Br 44:116-118, 1962.

370. Van der Spek K: Rupture of the axillary artery as a complication of dislocation of the shoulder. Arch Chir Neerl 16:113-118, 1964.

371. Milton GW: The circumflex nerve and dislocation of the shoulder. Br J Phys Med 17:136-138, 1954.

372. Pasila M, Kiviluoto O, Jaroma H, et al: Recovery from primary shoulder dislocation and its complications. Acta Orthop Scand 51:257-262, 1980.

373. Brown JT: Nerve injuries complicating dislocation of the shoulder. J Bone Joint Surg Br 34:526, 1952.

374. McLaughlin HL, MacLellan DI: Recurrent anterior dislocation of the shoulder: II. A comparative study. J Trauma 7:191-201, 1967.

375. Gariepy R, Derome A, Laurin CA: Brachial plexus paralysis following shoulder dislocation. Can J Surg 5:418-421, 1962.

376. Mumenthaler M, Schliack H: Läsionen Peripherer Nerven. Stuttgart: Georg Thieme Verlag, 1965.

377. Parsons SW, Rowley DI: Brachial plexus lesions in dislocations and fracture dislocation of the shoulder. J R Coll Surg Edinb 31(2):85-87, 1986.

378. Tuszyński W: Anterior dislocation of the shoulder complicated by temporary brachial paresis. Chir Narzadow Ruchu Ortop Pol 46(2):129-131, 1981.

379. Volpin G, Langer R, Stein H: Complete infraclavicular brachial plexus palsy with occlusion of axillary vessels following anterior dislocation of the shoulder joint. J Orthop Trauma 4(2):121-123, 1990.

380. Watson-Jones R: Dislocation of the shoulder joint. Proc R Soc Med 29:1060-1062, 1936.

381. Leffert RD, Seddon H: Infraclavicular brachial plexus injuries. J Bone Joint Surg Br 47:9-22, 1965.

382. Rowe CR: Instabilities of the glenohumeral joint. Bull Hosp Joint Dis 39:180-186, 1978.

383. Assmus H, Meinel A: Schulterverletzung und Axillarparese. Hefte Unfallheilkd 79:183-187, 1976.

384. Simonet WT, Cofield RH: Prognosis in anterior shoulder dislocation. Presented at the American Orthopaedic Society for Sports Medicine, Homestead, Va, 1983.

385. Rowe CR, Sakellarides HT: Factors related to recurrences of anterior dislocations of the shoulder. Clin Orthop 20:40-48, 1961.

386. McLaughlin HL, Cavallaro WU: Primary anterior dislocation of the shoulder. Am J Surg 80:615-621, 1950.

387. Hovelius L: Anterior dislocation of the shoulder in teen-agers and young adults. Five-year prognosis. J Bone Joint Surg Am 69:393-399, 1987.

388. Kiviluoto O, Pasila M, Jaroma H, et al: Immobilization after primary dislocation of the shoulder. Acta Orthop Scand 51:915-919, 1980.

389. Arciero RA, Wheeler JH, Ryan JB, et al: Arthroscopic Bankart repair vs. nonoperative treatment for acute, initial, anterior shoulder dislocations. Am J Sports Med 22:589-594, 1994.

390. Henry JH, Genung JA: Natural history of glenohumeral dislocation—revisited. Am J Sports Med 10:135-137, 1982.

391. Hovelius L, Malmqvist B, Augustaini BG: Ten year prognosis of primary anterior dislocation of the shoulder in young (abstract 7). Presented at the 10th open meeting of the American Shoulder and Elbow Surgeons, New Orleans, March 1994.

392. Wheeler JH, Ryan JB, Arciero RA, et al: Arthroscopic versus nonoperative treatment of acute shoulder dislocations in young athletes. Arthroscopy 5(3):213-217, 1989.

393. Hovelius L, Augustini BG, Fredin H, et al: Primary anterior dislocation of the shoulder in young patients. J Bone Joint Surg Am 78(11):1677-1684, 1996.

394. Adams JC: Recurrent dislocation of the shoulder. J Bone Joint Surg Br 30:26-38, 1948.

395. Eyre-Brook AL: The morbid anatomy of a case of recurrent dislocation of the shoulder. Br J Surg 29:32-37, 1943.

396. Ehgartner K: Has the duration of cast fixation after shoulder dislocations had an influence on the frequency of recurrent dislocation? Arch Orthop Unfallchir 89:187-190, 1977.

397. Hovelius L, Akermark C, Albrektsson B: Bristow–Latarjet procedure for recurrent anterior dislocation of the shoulder. Acta Orthop Scand 54:284-290, 1983.

398. Stromsoe K, Senn E, Simmen B, et al: Rezidivhaufigkeit nach erstmaliger traumatischer Schulterluxation. Helv Chir Acta 47:85-88, 1980.

399. Aronen JG, Regan K: Decreasing the incidence of recurrence of first time anterior shoulder dislocations with rehabilitation. Am J Sports Med 12(4):283-291, 1984.

400. Yoneda B, Welsh RP, and MacIntosh DL: Conservative treatment of shoulder dislocation in young males (proceedings). J Bone Joint Surg Br 64:254-255, 1982.

401. Itoi E, Sashi R, Minagawa H, et al: Position of immobilization after dislocation of the glenohumeral joint. A study with use of magnetic resonance imaging. J Bone Joint Surg Am 83(5):661-667, 2001.

402. DePalma AF: Recurrent dislocation of the shoulder joint. Ann Surg 132:1052-1065, 1950.

403. O'Connor SJ: Posterior dislocation of the shoulder. Arch Surg 72:479-491, 1956.

404. O'Connor SJ, Jacknow AS: Posterior dislocation of the shoulder. J Bone Joint Surg Am 37:1122, 1955.

405. Wilson JC, McKeever FM: Traumatic posterior (retroglenoid) dislocation of the humerus. J Bone Joint Surg Am 31:160-172, 1949.

406. Lippitt SB, Kennedy JP, Thompson TR: Intraarticular lidocaine versus intravenous analgesia in the reduction of dislocated shoulders. Orthop Trans 15(3):804, 1991.

407. Lippitt SB, Kennedy JP, Thompson TR: Intraarticular lidocaine versus intravenous analgesia in the reduction of dislocated shoulders. Orthop Trans 16(1):230, 1992.

408. Bailey PL, Stanley TH: Pharmacology of the intravenous narcotic anesthetics. In Miller R (ed): Anesthesia. New York: Churchill Livingstone, 1986, pp 745-797.

409. Dhinakharan SR, Ghosh A: Towards evidence-based emergency medicine: Best BETs from the Manchester Royal Infirmary. Intra-articular lidocaine for acute anterior shoulder dislocation reduction. Emerg Med J 19(2):142-143, 2002.

410. Orlinsky M, Shon S, Chiang C, et al: Comparative study of intra-articular lidocaine and intravenous meperidine/diazepam for shoulder dislocations. J Emerg Med 22(3):241-245, 2002.

411. Stimson LA: Fractures and Dislocations. Philadelphia: Lea Brothers, 1900.

412. Yuen MC, Yap PG, Chan YT, et al: An easy method to reduce anterior shoulder dislocation: The Spaso technique. Emerg Med J 18(5):370-372, 2001.

413. Savarsee JJ, Covino BG: Basic and clinical pharmacology of local anesthetic drugs. In Miller RD (ed): Anesthesia. New York: Churchill Livingstone, 1986.

414. Bennett GE: Old dislocations of the shoulder. J Bone Joint Surg 18:594-606, 1936.

415. McLaughlin HL: Discussion of acute anterior dislocation of the shoulder by Toufick Nicola. J Bone Joint Surg Am 31:172, 1949.

416. Ganel A, Horoszowski H, Heim M: Persistent dislocation of the shoulder in elderly patients. J Am Geriatr Soc 28:282-284, 1980.

417. Schulz TJ, Jacobs B, Patterson RL: Unrecognized dislocations of the shoulder. J Trauma 9:1009-1023, 1969.

418. Perniceni B, Augereau A: Treatment of old unreduced anterior dislocations of the shoulder by open reduction and reinforced rib graft: Discussion of three cases. Ann Chir 36:235-239, 1983.

419. Gosset J: Une technique de greffe coraco-glenordienne dans le traitement des luxations recidivantes de l'époule. Mem Acad Chir 86:445-447, 1960.

420. Trimmings NP: Hemarthrosis aspiration in treatment of anterior dislocation of the shoulder. J R Soc Med 78(12):1023-1027, 1985.

421. Burkhead WZ, Rockwood CA Jr: Treatment of instability of the shoulder with an exercise program. J Bone Joint Surg Am 74(6):890-896, 1992.

422. Tibone JE, Bradley JP: The treatment of posterior subluxation in athletes. Clin Orthop Relat Res (291):124-137, 1993.

423. Robinson CM, Howes J, Murdoch H, et al: Functional outcome and risk of recurrent instability after primary traumatic anterior shoulder dislocation in young patients. J Bone Joint Surg Am 88(11):2326-2336, 2006.

424. Tietjen R: Occult glenohumeral interposition of a torn rotator cuff. J Bone Joint Surg Am 64:458-459, 1982.

425. Bridle SH, Ferris BD: Irreducible acute anterior dislocations of the shoulder: Interposed scapularis. J Bone Joint Surg Br 72:1078-1079, 1990.

426. Inao S, Hirayama T, Takemitsu Y: Irreducible acute anterior dislocation of the shoulder: Interposed bicipital tendon. J Bone Joint Surg Br 72:1079-1080, 1990.

427. Aston JW, Gregory CF: Dislocation of the shoulder with significant fracture of the glenoid. J Bone Joint Surg Am 55:1531-1533, 1973.

428. Hertz H, Kwasny O, Wohry G: Therapeutic procedure in initial traumatic shoulder dislocation (arthroscopy—limbus refixation). Unfallchirurgie 17(2):76-79, 1991.

429. Arciero RA, Taylor DC, Snyder RJ, et al: Arthroscopic bioabsorbable tack stabilization of initial anterior shoulder dislocations: A preliminary report. Arthroscopy 11(4):410-417, 1995.

430. Arciero RA: Arthroscopic stabilization of acute, initial anterior shoulder dislocation in current techniques in arthroscopy. Parisien S (ed): Techniques in Therapeutic Arthroscopy. Churchill Livingstone, 1996, pp 117-124.

431. Doege KW: Irreducible shoulder joint dislocations. Lancet 49:191-195, 1929.

432. Johnson HF: Unreduced dislocation of the shoulder. Nebr State Med J 16:220-224, 1931.

433. Kuhnen W, Groves RJ: Irreducible acute anterior dislocation of the shoulder: Case report. Clin Orthop Relat Res (139):167-168, 1979.

434. Lam SJS: Irreducible anterior dislocation of the shoulder. J Bone Joint Surg Br 48:132-133, 1966.

435. Romanes GJ: Cunningham's Textbook of Anatomy. London, Oxford University Press, 1972.

436. Saxena K, Stavas J: Inferior glenohumeral dislocation. Ann Emerg Med 12(11):718-720, 1983.

437. Cautilli RA, Joyce MF, Mackell JV Jr: Posterior dislocation of the glenohumeral joint. Jefferson Orthop J 7:15-20, 1978.

438. Cautilli RA, Joyce MF, Mackell JV Jr: Posterior dislocations of the shoulder: A method of postreduction management. Am J Sports Med 6:397-399, 1978.

439. Scougall S: Posterior dislocation of the shoulder. J Bone Joint Surg Br 39:726-732, 1957.

440. McLaughlin HL: On the "frozen" shoulder. Bull Hosp Joint Dis 12:383-393, 1951.

441. McLaughlin HL: Trauma. Philadelphia: WB Saunders, 1959.

442. Keppler P, Holz U, Thieleman FW, et al: Locked posterior dislocation of the shoulder. J Orthop Trauma 8(4):286-292, 1994.

443. Itoi E, Motzkin NE, Morrey BF, et al: Bulk effect of rotator cuff on inferior glenohumeral stability as function of scapular inclination angle: A cadaver study. Tohoku J Exp Med 171(4):267-276, 1993.

444. Cofield RH: Physical examination of the shoulder: Effectiveness in assessing shoulder stability. In Matsen III F, Fu F, Hawkins R (eds): The Shoulder: A Balance of Mobility and Stability. Rosemont, Ill: American Academy of Orthopaedic Surgeons, 1993, pp 331-344.

445. Lippitt SB, Harryman DT II, Sidles JA, et al: Diagnosis and management of AMBRI syndrome. Tech Orthop 6(1):61-73, 1991.

446. O'Driscoll SW: Atraumatic instability: Pathology and pathogenesis. In Matsen III F, Fu F, Hawkins R (eds): The Shoulder: A Balance of Mobility and Stability. Rosemont, Ill: American Academy of Orthopaedic Surgeons, 1993, pp 305-318.

447. Burkhart SS, Debeer JF, Tehrany AM, et al: Quantifying glenoid bone loss arthroscopically in shoulder instability. Arthroscopy 18(5):488-491, 2002.

448. McFarland EG, Neira CA, Gutierrez MI, et al: Clinical significance of the arthroscopic drive-through sign in shoulder surgery. Arthroscopy 17(1):38-43, 2001.

449. Endo S, Kasai T, Fujii N, et al: Traumatic anterior dislocation of the shoulder in a child. Arch Orthop Trauma Surg 112(4):201-202, 1993.

450. Liu SH, Boynton E: Posterior superior impingement of the rotator cuff on the glenoid rim as a cause of shoulder pain in the overhead athlete. Arthroscopy 9(6):697-699, 1993.

451. Walch G, Liotard JP, Boileau P, et al: Postero-superior glenoid impingement. Another impingement of the shoulder. J Radiol 74(1):47-50, 1993.

452. Walch G, Liotard JP, Boileau P, et al: Postero-superior glenoid impingement. Another shoulder impingement. Rev Chir Orthop Reparatrice Appar Mot 77(8):571-574, 1991.

453. Wirth MA, Rockwood CA Jr: Traumatic glenohumeral instability. In Matsen III F, Fu F, Hawkins R (eds): The Shoulder: A Balance of Mobility and Stability. Rosemont, Ill: American Academy of Orthopaedic Surgeons, 1993, pp 279-304.

454. Rossi F, Ternamian PJ, Cerciello G, et al: Posterosuperior glenoid rim impingement in athletes: The diagnostic value of traditional radiology and magnetic resonance. Radiol Med (Torino) 87(1-2):22-27, 1994.

455. Hill JA, Lombardo SJ, Kerlan RK, et al: The modified Bristow–Helfet procedure for recurrent anterior shoulder subluxations and dislocations. Am J Sports Med 9:283-287, 1981.

456. Adams JC: The humeral head defect in recurrent anterior dislocations of the shoulder. Br J Radiol 23:151-156, 1950.

457. Didiee J: Le radiodiagnostic dans la luxation recidivante de l'épaule. J Radiol Electrol 14:209-218, 1930.

458. Hall RH, Isaac F, Booth CR: Dislocations of the shoulder with special reference to accompanying small fractures. J Bone Joint Surg Am 41:489-494, 1959.

459. Oppenheim WL, Dawson EG, Quinlan C, et al: The cephaloscapular projection. A special diagnostic aid. Clin Orthop Relat Res (195):191-193, 1985.

460. Eyre-Brook AL: Recurrent dislocation of the shoulder. Physiotherapy 57:7-13, 1971.

461. Brav EA: Ten years' experience with Putti–Platt reconstruction procedure. Am J Surg 100:423-430, 1960.

462. Rowe CR, Patel D, Southmayd WW: The Bankart procedure—a study of late results (proceedings). J Bone Joint Surg 59:122, 1977.

463. Palmer I, Widen A: The bone block method for recurrent dislocation of the shoulder joint. J Bone Joint Surg Br 30:53-58, 1948.

464. Calandra JJ, Baker CL, Uribe J: The incidence of Hill–Sachs lesions in initial anterior shoulder dislocations. Arthroscopy 5:254-257, 1989.

465. Danzig LA, Greenway G, Resnick D: The Hill–Sachs lesion: An experimental study. Am J Sports Med 8:328-332, 1980.

466. Rozing PM, De Bakker HM, Obermann WR: Radiographic views in recurrent anterior shoulder dislocation. Comparison of six methods for identification of typical lesions. Acta Orthop Scand 57(4):328-330, 1986.

467. Rokous JR, Feagin JA, Abbott HG: Modified axillary roentgenogram. A useful adjunct in the diagnosis of recurrent instability of the shoulder. Clin Orthop Relat Res 82:84-86, 1972.

468. Blazina ME, Satzman JS: Recurrent anterior subluxation of the shoulder in athletes—a distinct entity. J Bone Joint Surg Am 51:1037-1038, 1969.

469. Green MR, Christensen KP: Magnetic resonance imaging of the glenoid labrum in anterior shoulder instability. Am J Sports Med 22(4):493-498, 1994.

470. Mishra DK, Fanton GS: Two-year outcome of arthroscopic Bankart repair and electrothermal-assisted capsulorrhaphy for recurrent traumatic anterior shoulder instability. Arthroscopy 17(8):844-849, 2001.

471. Cramer F, Von BM, Kramps HA: CT diagnosis of recurrent subluxation of the shoulder. Fortschr Rontgenstr 136(4):440-443, 1982.

472. Shively J, Johnson J: Results of modified Bristow procedure. Clin Orthop Relat Res (187):150-153, 1984.

473. Braunstein EM, O'Conner G: Double-contrast arthrotomography and the shoulder. J Bone Joint Surg Am 64:192-195, 1982.

474. El-Khoury GY, Kathol MH, Chandler JB, et al: Shoulder instability: Impact of glenohumeral arthrotomography on treatment. Radiology 160(3):669-673, 1986.

475. Kelley JP: Fractures complicating electroconvulsive therapy and chronic epilepsy. J Bone Joint Surg Br 36:70-79, 1954.

476. Kleinman PD, Kanzaria PK, Goss TP, et al: Axillary arthrotomography of the glenoid labrum. AJR Am J Roentgenol 142:993-999, 1984.

477. McGlynn FJ, El-Khoury G, Albright JP: Arthrotomography of the glenoid labrum in shoulder instability. J Bone Joint Surg Am 64:506-518, 1982.

478. McMaster WC: Anterior glenoid labrum damage: A painful lesion in swimmers. Am J Sports Med 14(5):383-387, 1986.

479. Rafii M, Firooznia H, Bonamo JJ: Athlete shoulder injuries: CT arthrographic findings. Radiology 162(2):559-564, 1987.

480. Rafii M, Firooznia H, Bonamo JJ: CT arthrography of capsular structures of the shoulder. AJR Am J Roentgenol 146(2): 361-367, 1986.

481. Norris TR: C-arm fluoroscopic evaluation under anesthesia for glenohumeral subluxations. In Bateman JE, Welsh RP (eds): Surgery of the Shoulder. Philadelphia: B.C. Decker, 1984, pp 22-25.

482. Engebretsen L, Craig EV: Radiologic features of shoulder instability. Clin Orthop Relat Res (291):29-44, 1993.

483. Liu SH, Henry MH: Anterior shoulder instability. Clin Orthop Relat Res (323):327-337, 1996.

484. Gould R, Rosenfield AT, Friedlaender GE: Loose body within the glenohumeral joint in recurrent anterior dislocation: CT demonstration. J Comput Assist Tomogr 9(2):404-405, 1985.

485. Seltzer SE, Weissman BN: CT findings in normal and dislocating shoulders. J Can Assoc Radiol 36(1):41-46, 1985.

486. Danzig LA, Resnick D, Greenway G: Evaluation of unstable shoulders by computed tomography. Am J Sports Med 10:138-141, 1982.

487. Chandnani VP, Yeager TD, DeBerardino T, et al: Glenoid labral tears: Prospective evaluation with MRI imaging, MR arthrography, and CT arthrography. Am J Roentgenol 161(6):1229-1235, 1993.

488. Gross ML, Seeger LL, Smith JB, et al: Magnetic resonance imaging of the glenoid labrum. Am J Sports Med 18:229-234, 1990.

489. Iannotti JP, Zlatkin MB, Esterhai JL, et al: Magnetic resonance imaging of the shoulder. Sensitivity, specificity, and predictive value. J Bone Joint Surg Am 73(1):17-29, 1991.

490. Garneau RA, Renfrew DL, Moore TE, et al: Glenoid labrum: Evaluation with MR imaging. Radiology 179(2):519-522, 1991.

491. Wagner SC, Schweitzer ME, Morrison WB, et al: Shoulder instability: Accuracy of MR imaging performed after surgery in depicting recurrent injury—initial findings. Radiology 222(1):196-203, 2002.

492. Ha'eri GB, Maitland A: Arthroscopy findings in the frozen shoulder. J Rheumatol 8:149-152, 1981.

493. Hintermann B, Gachter A: Theo van Rens Prize. Arthroscopic assessment of the unstable shoulder. Knee Surg Sports Traumatol Arthrosc 2(2):64-69, 1994.

494. Andrews J, Carson WCM, Hughston JC: Operative shoulder arthroscopy. Presented at the American Orthopaedics Association, Homestead, Va, 1983.

495. Frizziero L, Zizzi F, Facchini A: Arthroscopy of the shoulder joint: A review of 23 cases. Rheumatologie 11:267-276, 1981.

496. Johnson LL: Arthroscopy of the shoulder. Orthop Clin North Am 11:197-204, 1980.

497. Lilleby H: Arthroscopy of the shoulder joint. Acta Orthop Scand 53:708-709, 1982.

498. Mital MA, Karlin LI: Diagnostic arthroscopy in sports injuries. Orthop Clin North Am 11:771-785, 1980.

499. Older MWJ: Arthroscopy of the shoulder joint. J Bone Joint Surg Br 58:253, 1976.

500. Parisien JS: Shoulder arthroscopy technique and indications. Bull Hosp Joint Dis 43:56-69, 1983.

501. Wiley AM, Austwick DH: Shoulder Surgery Through the Arthroscope. Toronto: Department of Surgery, University of Toronto and Toronto Western Hospital. 1982.

502. Wiley AM, Older MWJ: Shoulder arthroscopy. J Sports Med 8:31-38, 1980.

503. Zizzi F, Frizziero L, Facchini A, et al: Artroscopia della spalla: Indicazioni e limiti. Reumatismo 33:429-432, 1981.

504. Green MR, Christensen KP: Arthroscopic Bankart procedure: Two- to five-year follow-up with clinical correlation to severity of glenoid labral lesion. Am J Sports Med 23(3):276-281, 1995.

505. Neviaser TJ: The anterior labroligamentous periosteal sleeve avulsion lesion: A cause of anterior instability of the shoulder. Arthroscopy 9(1):17-21, 1993.

506. Simons P, Joekes E, Nelissen RG, et al: Posterior labrocapsular periosteal sleeve avulsion complicating locked posterior shoulder dislocation. Skeletal Radiol 27(10):588-590, 1998.

507. Yu JS, Ashman CJ, Jones G: The POLPSA lesion: MR imaging findings with arthroscopic correlation in patients with posterior instability. Skeletal Radiol 31(7):396-399, 2002.

508. Gleyze P, Habermeyer P: [Arthroscopic aspects and chronologic outcome of lesions of the labro-ligament complex in post-traumatic antero-inferior instability of the shoulder. A prospective study of 91 cases]. Rev Chir Orthop Reparatrice Appar Mot 82(4):288-298, 1996.

509. Harryman DT II: Arthroscopic management of shoulder instability. Univ Research Washington Report 1:24-26, 1996. www.orthop.washington.edu/usersfiles/file/research/1966.pdf

510. Snyder SJ, Strafford BB: Arthroscopic management of instability of the shoulder. Orthopedics 16(9):993-1002, 1993.

511. Warner JJ, Miller MD, Marks P: Arthroscopic Barkart repair with the Suretac device. Part II. Experimental observations. Arthroscopy 11(1):14-20, 1995.

512. Wolf EM, Cheng JC, Dickson K: Humeral avulsion of glenohumeral ligaments as a cause of anterior shoulder instability. Arthroscopy 11(5):600-607, 1995.

513. von Eisenhart-Rothe RM, Jager A, Englmeier KH, et al: Relevance of arm position and muscle activity on three-dimensional glenohumeral translation in patients with traumatic and atraumatic shoulder instability. Am J Sports Med 30(4):514-522, 2002.

514. Neer CS II: Displaced proximal humeral fractures. I. Classification and evaluation. J Bone Joint Surg Am 52:1077-1089, 1970.

515. Huber H, Gerber C: Voluntary subluxation of the shoulder in children. J Bone Joint Surg Br 76(11): 118-122, 1994.

516. Saha AK: Anterior recurrent dislocation of the shoulder. Acta Orthop Scand 39:479-493, 1967.

517. Rockwood CA Jr, Burkhead WZ Jr, Brna J: Subluxation for the glenohumeral joint; response to rehabilitative exercise in traumatic vs. atraumatic instability. Presented at the American Shoulder and Elbow Surgeons Second Open Meeting, New Orleans, La, March 1986.

518. Brostrom LA, Kronberg M, Nemeth G, et al: The effect of shoulder muscle training in patients with recurrent shoulder dislocations. Scand J Rehab Med 24(1):11-15, 1992.

519. Anderson L, Rush R, Sherer L, et al: The effects of a Theraband exercise program on shoulder internal rotation strength. Phys Ther 72(Suppl 6):S40, 1992.

520. Lenters TR, Franta AK, Wolf FM, et al: Arthroscopic compared with open repairs for recurrent anterior shoulder instability. A systematic review and meta-analysis of the literature. J Bone Joint Surg Am 89(2):244-254, 2007.

521. Eyre-Brook AL: Recurrent dislocation of the shoulder. Lesions discovered in seventeen cases. Surgery employed, and intermediate report on results. J Bone Joint Surg Br 30:39-46, 1948.

522. Haaker RG, Eickhoff U, Klammer HL: Intraarticular autogenous bone grafting in recurrent shoulder dislocations. Mil Med 158(3):164-169, 1993.

523. Stufflesser H, Dexel M: The treatment of recurrent dislocation of the shoulder by rotation osteotomy with internal fixation. Technique and results. Ital J Orthop Traumatol 39(2):191-197, 1977.

524. Weber BG: Operative treatment for recurrent dislocation of the shoulder. Injury 1:107-109, 1969.

525. Hovelius L, Thorling J, Fredin H: Recurrent anterior dislocation of the shoulder. Results after the Bankart and Putti–Platt operations. J Bone Joint Surg Am 61:566-569, 1979.

526. Prozorovskii VF, Khvisiuk NI, Gevorkian AD: Surgical treatment of anterior instability of the shoulder joint. Ortop Traumatol Protez 4:14-18, 1991.

527. Martin B, Javelot T, Vidal J: Long-term results obtained with the Bankart method for the treatment of recurring anterior instability of the shoulder. Chir Organi Mov 76(3):199-207, 1991.

528. Levine WN, Richmond JC, Donaldson WR: Use of the suture anchor in open Bankart reconstruction: A follow-up report. Am J Sports Med 22(5):723-726, 1994.

529. McEleney ET, Donovan MJ, Shea KP, et al: Initial failure strength of open and arthroscopic Barkart repairs. Arthroscopy 11(4):426-431, 1995.

530. Richmond JC, Donaldson WR, Fu F, et al: Modification of the Barkart reconstruction with a suture anchor: Report of a new technique. Am J Sports Med 19:343-346, 1991.

531. Gohlke F, Schneider P, Siegel K, et al: Tensile strength of various anchor systems in surgical correction of instability of the shoulder joint. Unfallchirurg 96(10):546-550, 1993.

532. Harner CD, Fu FH: The Bankart lesion of the shoulder: A biochemical analysis following repair. Knee Surg Sports Traumatol Arthrosc 3(2):117-120, 1995.

533. Hecker AT, Shea M, Hayhurst JO, et al: Pull-out strength of suture anchors for rotator cuff and Bankart lesion repairs. Am J Sports Med 21(6):874-879, 1993.

534. Altchek DW, Warren RF, Skyhar MJ, et al: T-plasty modification of the Bankart procedure for multidirectional instability of the anterior and inferior types. J Bone Joint Surg Am 73(1):105-112, 1991.

535. Cooper ME, Hutchinson MR: The microscopic pathoanatomy of acute anterior shoulder dislocations in a simian model. Arthroscopy 18(6):618-623, 2002.

536. McMahon PJ, Dettling JR, Sandusky MD, et al: Deformation and strain characteristics along the length of the anterior band of the inferior glenohumeral ligament. J Shoulder Elbow Surg 10(5):482-488, 2001.

537. Bigliani LU, Weinstein DM, Glasgow MT, et al: Glenohumeral arthroplasty for arthritis after instability surgery. J Shoulder Elbow Surg 4(2):87-94, 1995.

538. Kronberg M, Brostrom LA: Humeral head retroversion in patients with unstable humeroscapular joints. Clin Orthop Relat Res (260):207-211, 1990.

539. Lusardi DA, Wirth MA, Wurtz D, et al: Loss of external rotation following anterior capsulorrhaphy of the shoulder. J Bone Joint Surg Am 75:1185-1192, 1993.

540. Rosenberg BN, Richmond JC, Levine WN: Long-term follow up of Bankart reconstruction. Amer J Sports Med 23(5):538-544, 1995.

541. Itoi E, Watanabe W, Yamada S, et al: Range of motion after Bankart repair. Vertical compared with horizontal capsulotomy. Am J Sports Med 29(4):441-445, 2001.

542. Jobe FW, Giangarra CE, Kvitne RS, et al: Anterior capsulolabral reconstruction of the shoulder in athletes in overhand sports. Am J Sports Med 19:428-434, 1991.

543. Montgomery WH, Jobe FW: Functional outcomes in athletes after modified anterior capsulolabral reconstruction. Am J Sports Med 22(3):352-357, 1994.

544. Wirth MA, Blatter G, Rockwood CAJ: The capsular imbrication procedure for recurrent anterior instability of the shoulder. J Bone Joint Surg Am 78:246-259, 1996.

545. Weber S: The gold standard revisited: Recent experience with the open Bankart repair for recurrent anterior glenohumeral dislocation. Presented at the American Academy of Orthopaedic Surgeons Specialty Day, American Shoulder and Elbow Surgeons, Orlando, Fla, February 19,1995.

546. Friedman RJ: Glenohumeral capsulorrhaphy. In Matsen III F, Fu F, Hawkins R (eds): The Shoulder: A Balance of Mobility and Stability. Rosemont, Ill: American Academy of Orthopaedic Surgeons, 1993, pp 445-458.

547. DuToit GT, Roux D: Recurrent dislocation of the shoulder. A 24 year study of the Johannesburg stapling operation. J Bone Joint Surg Am 38:1-12, 1956.

548. Sisk TD, Boyd HB: Management of recurrent anterior dislocation of the shoulder. DuToit-type or staple capsulorrhaphy. Clin Orthop Relat Res (103): 150-156, 1974.

549. Rao JP, Francis AM, Hurley J, et al: Treatment of recurrent anterior dislocation of the shoulder by duToit staple capsulorrhaphy. Results of long-term follow-up study. Clin Orthop Relat Res (204):169-176, 1986.

550. Ward WG, Bassett FHI, Garrett WEJ: Anterior staple capsulorrhaphy for recurrent dislocation of the shoulder: A clinical and biomechanical study. South Med J 83(5):510-518, 1990.

551. O'Driscoll SW, Evans DC: The DuToit staple capsulorrhaphy for recurrent anterior dislocation of the shoulder: Twenty years of experience in six Toronto hospital. Presented at the American Shoulder and Elbow Surgeons Fourth Open Meeting, Atlanta, March 1988.

552. Zuckerman JD, Matsen FA III: Complications about the glenohumeral joint related to the use of screws and staples. J Bone Joint Surg Am 66:175-180, 1984.

553. Osmond-Clarke H: Habitual dislocation of the shoulder. The Putti–Platt operation. J Bone Joint Surg Br 30:19-25, 1948.

554. Watson-Jones R: Recurrent dislocation of the shoulder. J Bone Joint Surg Br 30:6-8, 1948.

555. Quigley TB, Freedman PA: Recurrent dislocation of the shoulder. Am J Surg 128:595-599, 1974.

556. Leach RE, Corbett M, Schepsis A, et al: Results of a modified Putti–Platt operation for recurrent shoulder dislocation and subluxation. Clin Orthop Relat Res (164):20-25, 1982.

557. Collins KA, Capito C, Cross M: The use of the Putti–Platt procedure in the treatment of recurrent anterior dislocation, with special reference to the young athlete. Am J Sports Med 14(5):380-382, 1986.

558. Fredriksson AS, Tegner Y: Results of the Putti–Platt operation for recurrent anterior dislocation of the shoulder. Int Orthop 15:185-188, 1991.

559. Angelo RN, Hawkins RJ: Osteoarthritis following an excessively tight Putti–Platt repair. Presented at the American Shoulder and Elbow Surgeons Fourth Open Meeting, Atlanta, March 1988.

560. Karadimas J, Rentis G, Varouchas G: Repair of recurrent anterior dislocation of the shoulder using transfer of the subscapularis tendon. J Bone Joint Surg Am 62:1147-1149, 1980.

561. Magnuson PB: Treatment of recurrent dislocation of the shoulder. Surg Clin North Am 25:14-20, 1945.

562. Magnuson PB, Stack JK: Bilateral habitual dislocation of the shoulder in twins, a familial tendency. JAMA 144:2103, 1940.

563. Magnuson PB, Stack JK: Recurrent dislocation of the shoulder. JAMA 123:889-892, 1943.

564. Miller LS, Donahue JR, Good RP, Staerk AJ: The Magnuson–Stack procedure for treatment of recurrent glenohumeral dislocation. Am J Sports Med 12:133-137, 1984.

565. Badgley CE, O'Connor GA: Combined procedure for the repair of recurrent anterior dislocation of the shoulder. J Bone Joint Surg Am 47:1283, 1965.

566. Bailey RW: Acute and recurrent dislocation of the shoulder. J Bone Joint Surg Am 49(4):767-773, 1967.

567. Eden R: Zur Operation der habituellen Schulterluxation, unter Mitteilung eines neuen Verfahrens bei Abri β am inneren Pfannenrand. Dtsch Z Chir 144:269-280, 1918.

568. Hybbinette S: De la transplantation d'un fragment osseux pour remedier aux luxations recidivantes de l'épaule; constations et resultats operatoires. Acta Chir Scand 71:411-445, 1932.

569. Lavik K: Habitual shoulder luxation. Acta Orthop Scand 30:251-264, 1961.

570. Lange M: Die Operative Behandlung der Gewohnheitsmabigen Verrenkung an Schulter, Knie und Fuß. Z Orthop 75:162, 1944.

571. Paavolainen P, Bjorkenheim JM, Ahovuo J, et al: Recurrent anterior dislocation of the shoulder. Results of Eden–Hybinette and Putti–Platt operations. Acta Orthop Scand 55(5):556-560, 1984.

572. Niskanen RO, Lehtonen JY, Kaukonen JP: Alvik's glenoplasty for humeroscapular dislocation. Acta Orthop Scand 62:279-283, 1991.

573. Oudard P: La luxation récidivante de l'épaule (variété antéro-interne) procede operatoire. J Chir 23:13, 1924.

574. Bodey WN, Denham RA: A free bone block operation for recurrent anterior dislocation of the shoulder joint. Injury 15:184-188, 1983.

575. Noesberger B, Mader G: Die Modifizierte Operation nach Trillat bei Habitueller Schulterluxation. Z Unf Med Berufskr 69:34-36, 1976.

576. Trillat A: Traitement de la luxation récidivante de l'épaule: Considerations, techniques. Lyon Chir 49:986-993, 1954.

577. Helfet AJ: Coracoid transplantation for recurring dislocation of the shoulder. J Bone Joint Surg Br 40:198-202, 1958.

578. Mead NC, Sweeney HJ: Bristow procedure [letter]. Spectator July 9, 1964.

579. May VR: A modified Bristow operation for anterior recurrent dislocation of the shoulder. J Bone Joint Surg Am 52:1010-1016, 1970.

580. Bonnin JG: Transplantation of the coracoid tip: A definitive operation for recurrent anterior dislocation of the shoulder. R Soc Med 66:755-758, 1973.

581. Bonnin JG: Transplantation of the tip of the coracoid process for recurrent anterior dislocation of the shoulder. J Bone Joint Surg Br 51:579, 1969.

582. Hummel A, Bethke RO, Kempf L: Die Behandlung der habituellen Schulterluxation nach dem Bristow-Verfahren. Unfallheikunde 85:482-484, 1982.

583. Torg JS, Balduini FC, Bonci C, et al: A modified Bristow–Helfet–May procedure for recurrent dislocations and subluxation of the shoulder: Report of 212 cases. J Bone Joint Surg Am 69(6):904-913, 1987.

584. Carol EJ, Falke LM, Kortmann JH, et al: Bristow–Latarjet repair for recurrent anterior shoulder instability; an 8 year study. Neth J Surg 37(4):109-113, 1985.

585. Banas MP, Dalldorf PG, Sebastianelli WJ, et al: Long-term followup of the modified Bristow procedure. Am J Sports Med 21(5):666-671, 1993.

586. Wredmark T, Tornkvist H, Johansson C, et al: Long-term functional results of the modified Bristow procedure for recurrent dislocations of the shoulder. Am J Sports Med 20(2):157-161, 1992.

587. Chen SK, Perry J, Jobe FW, et al: Elbow flexion analysis in Bristow patients. A preliminary report. Am J Sports Med 12(5):347-350, 1984.

588. Weaver JK, Derkash RS: Don't forget the Bristow Latarjet procedure. Clin Orthop Relat Res (308):102-110, 1994.

589. Lamm CR, Zaehrisson BE, Korner L: Radiography of the shoulder after Bristow repair. Acta Radiol Diagn 23:523-528, 1982.

590. Lemmens JA, de Waal Malefitj J: Radiographic evaluation of the modified Bristow procedure for recurrent anterior dislocation of the shoulder. Diagn Imaging Clin Med 53(5):221-225, 1984.

591. Lower RF, McNiesh LM, Callaghan JJ: Computed tomographic documentation of intra-articular penetration of a screw after operations on the shoulder. A report of two cases. J Bone Joint Surg Am 67(7):1120-1122, 1985.

592. Nielsen AB, Nielsen K: The modified Bristow procedure for recurrent anterior dislocation of the shoulder. Acta Orthop Scand 53:229-232, 1982.

593. Hovelius L: Incidence of shoulder dislocation in Sweden. Clin Orthop Relat Res (166):127-131, 1982.

594. Hovelius L, Eriksson K, Fredin H, et al: Recurrences after initial dislocation of the shoulder. Results of a prospective study of treatment. J Bone Joint Surg Am 65:343-349, 1983.

595. Norris TR, Bigliani LU, Harris E: Complications following the modified Bristow repair for shoulder instability. Presented at the American Shoulder and Elbow Surgeons Third Open Meeting, San Francisco, March 1987.

596. Singer GC, Kirkland PM, Emery RJH: Coracoid transposition for recurrent anterior instability of the shoulder. J Bone Joint Surg Br 77:73-76, 1995.

597. Ferlic DC, DeGiovine NM: A long-term retrospective study of the modified Bristow procedure. Am J Sports Med 16:469-474, 1988.

598. Mackenzie DB: The treatment of recurrent anterior shoulder dislocation by the modified Bristow–Helfet procedure. S Afr Med J 65:325-330, 1984.

599. Mackenzie DB: The Bristow–Helfet operation for recurrent anterior dislocation of the shoulder. J Bone Joint Surg Br 62:273-274, 1980.

600. Schauder KS, Tullos HS: Role of the coracoid bone block in the modified Bristow procedure. Am J Sports Med 20:31-34, 1992.

601. Rockwood CA Jr, Young DC: Complications and management of the failed Bristow shoulder reconstructions. Orthop Trans 13(2):232, 1989.

602. Young DC, Rockwood CA Jr: Complications of a failed Bristow procedure and their management. J Bone Joint Surg Am 73:969-981, 1991.

603. Latarjet M, Vittori P. Résultat die traitement des luxations recidivantes de l'épaule pars le procédure de Latarjet, a propos de 42 cas. Lyon Clin 64:964-968,1968.

604. Latarjet M: Technique de la butée coracoïdienne preplenoidienne dans le traitement des luxations récidivantes de l'épaule. Lyon Chir 54:604-607, 1958.

605. Pascoet G, Jung F, Foucher G, et al: Treatment of recurrent dislocation of the shoulder by preglenoid artificial ridge using the Latarjet–Vittori technique. J Med Strasbourg 6:501-504, 1975.

606. Tagliabue D, Esposito A: L'intervento di Latarjet nella lussazione recidivante di spalla-dello sportivo. Ital J Orthop Traumatol 2:91-100, 1980.

607. Burkhart SS, De Beer JF: Traumatic glenohumeral bone defects and their relationship to failure of arthroscopic Bankart repairs: Significance of the inverted-pear glenoid and the humeral engaging Hill–Sachs lesion. Arthroscopy 16(7):677-694, 2000.

608. Hovelius L, Sandstrom B, Saebo M: One hundred eighteen Bristow-Latarjet repairs for recurrent anterior dislocation of the shoulder prospectively followed for fifteen years: Study II—the evolution of dislocation arthropathy. J Shoulder Elbow Surg 15(3):279-289, 2006.

609. Gallie WE, LeMesurier AB: Recurring dislocation of the shoulder. J Bone Joint Surg Br 30:9-18, 1948.

610. Bateman JE: Gallie technique for repair of recurrent dislocation of the shoulder. Surg Clin North Am 43:1655-1662, 1963.

611. Rupp F: Über ein vereinfachtes Operationverfahren bei habitueller Schulterluxatuion. Deutsch Z Chir 198:70-75, 1926.

612. Heymanowitsch Z: Ein Beitrag zur operativen Behandlung der habituellen Schulterluxationen. Zbl Chir 54:648-651, 1927.

613. Carpenter GI, Millard PH: Shoulder subluxation in elderly inpatients. J Am Geriatr Soc 30(7):441-446, 1982.

614. Jones FW: Attainment of upright position of man. Nature 146:26-27, 1940.

615. Saha AK: Theory of Shoulder Mechanism. Springfield, Ill: Charles C Thomas, 1961.

616. Saha AK: Mechanics of elevation of glenohumeral joint: Its application in rehabilitation of flail shoulder in upper brachial plexus injuries and poliomyelitis and in replacement of the upper humerus by prosthesis. Acta Orthop Scand 44:668-678, 1973.

617. Saha AK, Das NN, Chakravarty BF: Treatment of recurrent dislocation of shoulder: Past, present, and future: Studies on electromyographic changes of muscles acting on the shoulder joint complex. Calcutta Med J 53:409-413, 1956.

618. Boytchev B: Treatment of recurrent shoulder instability. Minerva Orthopedica 2:377-379, 1951.

619. Boytchev B, Conforty B, Tchokanov K: Operatiunaya Ortopediya y Travatologiya. Sofia: Meditsina y Fizkultura, 1962.

620. Conforty B: The results of the Boytchev procedure for treatment of recurrent dislocation of the shoulder. Int Orthop 4:127-132, 1980.

621. Debevoise NT, Hyatt GW, Townsend GB: Humeral torsion in recurrent shoulder dislocation. Clin Orthop Relat Res 76:87-93, 1971.

622. Kavanaugh JH: Posterior shoulder dislocation with ipsilateral humeral shaft fracture. A case report. Clin Orthop Relat Res (131):168-172, 1978.

623. Weber BG, Simpson LA, Hardegger F: Rotational humeral osteotomy for recurrent anterior dislocation of the shoulder associated with a large Hill–Sachs lesion. J Bone Joint Surg Am 66:1443-1450, 1984.

624. Lazarus MD, Harryman DT II: Complications of open anterior repairs for instability and their solutions. In Warner J, Iannotti J, Gerber R (eds): Complex and Revision Problems in Shoulder Surgery. Philadelphia: Lippincott–Raven, 1996.

625. Hattrup SJ, Cofield RH, Weaver AL: Anterior shoulder reconstruction: Prognostic variables. J Shoulder Elbow Surg 10(6):508-513, 2001.

626. Rowe CR, Zarins B, Ciullo JV: Recurrent anterior dislocation of the shoulder after surgical repair. Apparent causes of failure and treatment. J Bone Joint Surg Am 66:159-168, 1984.

627. Zabinski SJ, Callaway GH, Cohen S, et al: Long term results of revision shoulder stabilization. Presented at the American Shoulder and Elbow Surgeons Meeting, La Quinta, Calif, March 1995.

628. Levine WN, Arroyo JS, Pollock RG, et al: Open revision stabilization surgery for recurrent anterior glenohumeral instability. Am J Sports Med 28(2):156-160, 2000.

629. Richards RR, Beaton D, Hudson AR: Shoulder arthrodesis with plate fixation: Functional outcome analysis. J Shoulder Elbow Surg 2(5):225-239, 1993.

630. Wirth MA, Rockwood CA Jr: Complications of treatment of injuries to the shoulder. In Epps CH (ed): Complications in Orthopaedic Surgery. Philadelphia: JB Lippincott, 1994, pp 229-255.

631. Loomer R, Graham B: Anatomy of the axillary nerve and its relation to inferior capsular shift. Clin Orthop Relat Res (243):100-105, 1989.

632. Richards RR, Waddell JP, Hudson MB: Shoulder arthrodesis for the treatment of brachial plexus palsy: A review of twenty-two patients. Presented at the American Shoulder and Elbow Surgeons 3rd Open Meeting, San Francisco, March 1987.

633. Cayford EH, Tees FJ: Traumatic aneurysm of the subclavicular artery as a late complication of fractured clavicle. Can Med Assoc J 25:450-452, 1931.

634. Hawkins RJ, Neer CS II, Pianta R, et al: Missed posterior dislocations of the shoulder. Presented at the American Academy of Orthopaedic Surgery Annual Meeting, New Orleans, La, March 1982.

635. Artz T, Huffer JM: A major complication of the modified Bristow procedure for recurrent dislocation of the shoulder. A case report. J Bone Joint Surg Am 54:1293-1296, 1972.

636. Fee HJ, McAvoy JM, Dainko EA: Pseudoaneurysm of the axillary artery following a modified Bristow operation: Report of a case and review. J Cardiovasc Surg 19:65-68, 1978.

637. Edwards DJ, Hoy G, Saies AD, et al: Adverse reactions to an absorbable shoulder fixation device. J Shoulder Elbow Surg 3:230-233, 1994.

638. Braly WG, Tullos HS: A modification of the Bristow procedure for recurrent anterior shoulder dislocation and subluxation. Am J Sports Med 13:81-86, 1985.

639. MacDonald PB, Hawkins RJ, Fowler PJ, et al: Release of the subscapularis for internal rotation contracture and pain after anterior repair for recurrent dislocation of the shoulder. J Bone Joint Surg Am 74(5):734-737, 1992.

640. Wirth MA, Seltzer DG, Rockwood CA Jr: Replacement of the subscapularis with pectoralis muscle in anterior shoulder instability. Presented at the 62nd Annual Meeting of the American Academy of Orthopaedics Surgeons, Orlando, Fla, March 1995.

641. Harryman DT II: Common surgical approaches to the shoulder. Instr Course Lect 41:3-11, 1992.

642. Adams F: The Genuine Works of Hippocrates. New York: William Woods, 1891.

643. Barrett J: The clavicular joints. Physiotherapy 57:268-269, 1971.

644. Robinson CM, Aderinto J: Recurrent posterior shoulder instability. J Bone Joint Surg Am 87(4):883-892, 2005.

645. Kim SH, Noh KC, Park JS, et al: Loss of chondrolabral containment of the glenohumeral joint in atraumatic posteroinferior multidirectional instability. J Bone Joint Surg Am 87(1):92-98, 2005.

646. Hawkins RJ, Mohtadi NGH: Controversy in anterior shoulder instability. Clin Orthop Relat Res (272):152-161, 1991.

647. Kretzler HH: Posterior glenoid osteotomy. Presented at the American Academy of Orthopaedic Surgeons Meeting, Dallas, March 1944.

648. Tibone JE, Prietto C, Jobe FW, et al: Staple capsulorrhaphy for recurrent posterior shoulder dislocation. Am J Sports Med 9:135-139, 1981.

649. Wirth MA, Butters KP, and Rockwood CA Jr: The posterior deltoid-splitting approach to the shoulder. Clin Orthop Relat Res (296):92-98, 1993.

650. Shaffer BS, Conway J, Jobe FW, et al: Infraspinatus muscle-splitting incision in posterior shoulder surgery. An anatomic and electromyographic study. Am J Sports Med 22(1):113-120, 1994.

651. Gold AM: Fractured neck of the humerus with separation and dislocation of the humeral head (fracture-dislocation of the shoulder, severe type). Bull Hosp Joint Dis 32(1):87-99, 1971.

652. Howard FM, Shafer SJ: Injuries to the clavicle with neurovascular complications. J Bone Joint Surg Am 47:1335-1346, 1965.

653. Leyder P, Augereau B, Apoil A: Traitement des luxations postérieures invétérées de l'épaule par double abord et butée osseuse rétro-glénoïdienne. Ann Chir 34:806-809, 1980.

654. Neer CS II, Horwitz BS: Fracture of the proximal humeral epiphyseal plate. Clin Orthop Relat Res 41:24-31, 1965.

655. Valls J: Acrylic prosthesis in a case with fracture of the head of the humerus. Bal Soc Orthop Trauma 17:61, 1952.

656. Boyd HB, Sisk TD: Recurrent posterior dislocation of the shoulder. J Bone Joint Surg Am 54:779-786, 1972.

657. Bayley JIL, Kessel L: Posterior dislocation of the shoulder: The clinical spectrum. J Bone Joint Surg Br 60:440, 1978.

658. Bigliani LU, Pollock RG, McIlveen SJ, et al: Shift of the posteroinferior aspect of the capsule for recurrent posterior glenohumeral instability. J Bone Joint Surg Am 77(7):1011-1020, 1995.

659. Weber SC: Open versus arthroscopic repair of traumatic anterior glenohumeral instability. Presented at the American Academy Meeting of Orthopaedic Surgeons Specialty Day, Arthroscopy Assoc of North America, Orlando, Fla, March 1995.

660. Surin V, Blader S, Markhede G, et al: Rotational osteotomy of the humerus for posterior instability of the shoulder. J Bone Joint Surg Am 72:181-186, 1990.

661. Scott DJJ: Treatment of recurrent posterior dislocations of the shoulder by glenoplasty. Report of three cases. J Bone Joint Surg Am 49:471-476, 1967.

662. English E, Macnab I: Recurrent posterior dislocation of the shoulder. Can J Surg 17:147-151, 1974.

663. Bestard EA: Glenoplasty: A simple reliable method of correcting recurrent posterior dislocation of the shoulder. Orthop Rev 5:29-34, 1976.

664. Vegter J, Marti RK: Treatment of posterior dislocation of the shoulder by osteotomy of the neck of the scapula. J Bone Joint Surg 63:288, 1981.

665. Ahlgren SA, Hedlund T, Nistor L: Idiopathic posterior instability of the shoulder joint. Acta Orthop Scand 49:600-603, 1978.
666. Ghormley RK, Black JR, Cherry JH: Ununited fractures of the clavicle. Am J Surg 51:343-349, 1941.
667. Guilfoil PH, Christiansen T: An unusual vascular complication of fractured clavicle. JAMA 200:72-73, 1967.
668. Neer CS II: Degenerative lesions of the proximal humeral articular surface. Clin Orthop 20:116-124, 1961.
669. Gerber A, Warner JJ: Thermal capsulorrhaphy to treat shoulder instability. Clin Orthop Relat Res (400):105-116, 2002.
670. Dick W, Baumgartner R: Hypermobilität und wilkurliche hintere Schulter-luxation. Orthop Prax 16:328-330, 1980.
671. Mowery CA, Garfin SR, Booth RE, et al: Recurrent posterior dislocation of the shoulder: Treatment using a bone block. J Bone Joint Surg Am 67(5):777-781, 1985.
672. Neumann CH, Petersen SA, Jahnke AH: MR Imaging of the labral capsular complex: Normal variation. AJR Am J Roentgenol 157:1015-1021, 1991.
673. Butters KP, Curtis RJ, Rockwood CA Jr: Posterior deltoid splitting shoulder approach. J Bone Joint Transactions 11:233, 1987.
674. Wirth MA, Groh GI, Rockwood CA Jr: The treatment of symptomatic posterior glenohumeral instability with an anterior capsular shift. Presented at the Western Orthopaedic Association 58th Annual Meeting, 1994.
675. Wirth MA, Groh GI, Rockwood CA Jr: Capsulorrhaphy through an anterior approach for the treatment of atraumatic posterior glenohumeral instability with multidirectional laxity of the shoulder. J Bone Joint Surg Am 80(11):1570-1578, 1998.
676. Antoniou J, Duckworth DT, Harryman DT II: Capsulolabral augmentation for the management of posteroinferior instability of the shoulder. J Bone Joint Surg Am 82(9):1220-1230, 2000.
677. Schwartz RE, O'Brien SJ, Warren RF, et al: Capsular restraints to anterior–posterior motion in the shoulder. Orthop Trans 12(3):727, 1988.
678. Choi CH, Ogilvie-Harris DJ: Inferior capsular shift operation for multidirectional instability of the shoulder in players of contact sports. Br J Sports Med 36(4):290-294, 2002.
679. Pagnani MJ, Dome DC: Surgical treatment of traumatic anterior shoulder instability in American football players. J Bone Joint Surg Am 84(5):711-715, 2002.
680. Pollock RG, Owens JM, Flatow EL, et al: Operative results of the inferior capsular shift procedure for multidirectional instability of the shoulder. J Bone Joint Surg Am 82(7):919-928, 2000.
681. Obremskey WT, Lippitt SB, Harryman DT, et al: Follow-up of the inferior capsular shift procedure for atraumatic multidirectional instability. Unpublished data.
682. Rowe CR, Yee LBK: A posterior approach to the shoulder joint. J Bone Joint Surg Am 26:580-584, 1944.

BIBLIOGRAPHY

Arciero RA: Arthroscopic stabilization of initial anterior shoulder dislocations. Presented at the American Academy of Orthopaedic Surgeons Specialty Day, Arthroscopy Association of North America, New Orleans, La, 1994.
Cotton FJ: Subluxation of the shoulder downward. Boston Med Surg J 185:405-407, 1921.
Coughlin L, Rubinovich M, Johansson J, et al: Arthroscopic staple capsulorrhaphy for anterior shoulder instability. Am J Sports Med 20(3):253-256, 1992.
Cuckler JM, Bearcroft J, Asgian CM: Femoral head technologies to reduce polyethylene wear in total hip arthroplasty. Clin Orthop Relat Res (317):57-63, 1995.
Fairbank TJ: Fracture-subluxations of the shoulder. J Bone Joint Surg Br 30:454-460, 1948.
Geiger DF, Hurley JA, Tovey JA, et al: Results of arthroscopic versus open Bankart suture repair. Presented at the American Academy of Orthopaedic Surgeons Specialty Day, San Francisco, CA, 1993.
Green MR, Christensen KP: Arthroscopic versus open Bankart procedures: A comparison of early morbidity and complications. Arthroplasty 9(4):371-374, 1993.
Gross RM: Arthroscopic shoulder capsulorrhaphy: Does it work? Am J Sports Med 17(4):495-500, 1989.
Hawkins RB: Arthroscopic stapling repair for shoulder instability: A retrospective study of 50 cases. Arthroscopy 5(2):122-128, 1989.
Henderson WD: Arthroscopic stabilization of the anterior shoulder. Clin Sports Med 6(3):581-586, 1987.
Johnson LL: Symposium: The controversy of arthroscopic versus open approaches to shoulder instability and rotator cuff disease: A new perspective, a new opportunity, a new challenge. Presented at the American Shoulder and Elbow Surgeons 4th Open Meeting, Atlanta, March 1988.
Landsiedl F: Arthroscopic therapy of recurrent anterior luxation of the shoulder by capsular repair. Arthroscopy 8(3):296-304, 1992.
Luetzow WF, Atkin DM, Sachs RA: Arthroscopic versus open Bankart repair of the shoulder for recurrent anterior dislocations. Presented at the American Academy of Orthopaedic Surgeons Specialty Day, American Shoulder and Elbow Surgeons, Orlando, Fla, February 19,1995.
Matthews L, Vetter W, Oweida S, et al: Arthroscopic staple capsulorrhaphy for recurrent anterior shoulder instability. Arthroscopy 4(2):106-111, 1988.
McIntyre LF, Caspari RB: The rationale and technique for arthroscopic reconstruction of anterior shoulder instability using multiple sutures. Orthop Clin North Am 24(1):55-58, 1993.
Mologne TS, Lapoint JM, Morin WD, et al: Arthroscopic anterior labral reconstruction using a transglenoid suture technique: Results in the active duty military patient. Presented at the American Academy of Orthopaedic Surgeons Specialty Day, American Shoulder and Elbow Surgeons, Orlando, Fla, February 19,1995.
Moran MC, Warren RF: Development of a synovial cyst after arthroscopy of the shoulder. J Bone Joint Surg Am 71(1):127-129, 1989.
Morgan CD: Arthroscopic transglenoid Bankart suture repair. Oper Tech Orthop 1(2):171-179, 1991.
Morgan CD, Bordenstab AB: Arthroscopic Bankart suture repair: Technique and early results. Arthroscopy 3(2):111-122, 1987.
Ovesen J, Nielsen S: Stability of the shoulder joint: Cadaver study of stabilizing structures. Acta Orthop Scand 56:149-151, 1985.
Resch H: Current aspects in the arthroscopic treatment of shoulder instability. Orthopade 20(4):273-281, 1991.
Rockwood CA Jr: Shoulder arthroscopy. J Bone Joint Surg Am 70:639-640, 1988.
Rose DJ: Arthroscopic suture capsulorrhaphy for recurrent anterior and anteroinferior shoulder instability: 2-6 year followup. Presented at the American Academy of Orthopaedic Surgeons Specialty Day, Arthroscopy Assoc of North America, 1994.
Savoie FH III: Arthroscopic reconstruction of recurrent traumatic anterior instability. Presented at the American Academy of Orthopaedic Surgeons Specialty Day, American Shoulder and Elbow Surgeons, Orlando, Fla, February 19,1995.
Sidles JA, Harryman DT, Simkin PA: Passive and active stabilization of the glenohumeral joint. J Bone Joint Surg 72:1334-1343, 1990.
Small NC: Complications in arthroscopic surgery performed by experienced arthroscopists. Arthroscopy 4(3):215-221, 1988.
Small NC: Complications in arthroscopic surgery of the knee and shoulder. Orthopedics 16(9): 985-988, 1993.
Speer KP, Deng X, Borrero S, et al: A biomechanical evaluation of the Bankart lesion. Presented at the American Academy of Orthopaedic Surgeons Specialty Day, American Shoulder and Elbow Surgeons, Orlando, Fla, February 19,1995.
Speer KP, Pagnani M, Warren RF: Arthroscopic anterior shoulder stabilization: 2-5 year follow-up using a bioabsorbable tac. Presented at the American Shoulder and Elbow Surgeons 10th Open Meeting, New Orleans, La, March 1994.
Thompson FR, Winant WM: Unusual fracture-subluxations of the shoulder joint. J Bone Joint Surg Am 32:575-582, 1950.
Thompson FR, Winant WM: Comminuted fractures of the humeral head with subluxation. Clin Orthop 20:94-96, 1961.
Tibone J, Ting A: Capsulorrhaphy with a staple for recurrent posterior subluxation of the shoulder. J Bone Joint Surg Am 72(7):999-1002, 1990.
Uhorchak JM, Arciero RA, Taylor DC: Recurrent instability after open shoulder stabilization in athletes. Presented at the American Academy of Orthopaedic Surgeons Specialty Day, American Shoulder and Elbow Surgeons, Orlando, Fla, February 19,1995.
Uribe JW, Hechtman KS: Arthroscopically assisted repair of acute Bankart lesion. Orthopedics 16(9): 1019-1023, 1993.
Walch G, Boileau P, Levigne C, et al: Arthroscopic stabilization for recurrent anterior shoulder dislocation: Results of 59 cases. J Arthroscopy 11(2):173-179, 1995.
Wolf EM: Arthroscopic capsulolabral reconstruction using suture anchors. Presented at the American Academy of Orthopaedic Surgeons Specialty Day, American Shoulder and Elbow Surgeons, New Orleans, February 1994.
Wolf EM: Arthroscopic capsulolabral repair using suture anchors. Orthop Clin North Am 24(1):59-69, 1993.
Yahiro MA, Matthews LS: Arthroscopic stabilization procedures for recurrent anterior shoulder instability. Orthop Rev 18(11):1161-1168, 1989.
Youssef JA, Carr CF, Walther CE, et al: Arthroscopic Bankart suture repair for recurrent traumatic unidirectional anterior shoulder dislocations. Arthroscopy 11(5):561-563, 1995.

Index

Note: Page numbers followed by f refer to figures; page numbers followed by t refer to tables; page numbers followed by b refer to boxes.

A

Abrasion test, 807, 807f
Abscess. *See also* Sepsis
  scapular, 567, 567f
  sternoclavicular, 551
  subacromial, 563
  subdeltoid, 563
Acromial artery, 41, 82f, 83
Acromial process. *See* Acromion
Acromial traction spur, 780f, 781–782, 781f, 1123f
Acromioclavicular joint, 453–517. *See also* Acromion; Clavicle
  active compression test of, 468, 469f
  age-related changes in, 466, 515
  anatomy of, 41–43, 42f, 453–458, 454f, 455f, 456f, 457f, 984
    variational, 103–104, 103f
  anesthetic injection of, 469–470, 469f
  anteroposterior stress test of, 478, 478f
  arthritis of, 515, 516f
    crystal, 515
    degenerative, 466, 509, 511f, 515, 516f
    distal clavicle excision in, 984–985
    post-traumatic, 411–412, 490
    rheumatoid, 515
    vs. rotator cuff tear, 818
  biomechanics of, 214–217, 215f, 216f, 230–231, 463–466, 463f
    with arm elevation, 216, 217f, 463–466, 464f–466f
  blood supply to, 41, 453
  Buchberger test of, 468
  capsule of, 41, 455
    stability and, 215–216
  computed tomography of, 197, 457f, 471
  cross-body adduction stress test of, 467, 468f
  cyst of, 515–516, 516f, 517f
  development of, 9, 10f, 453
  disorders of, 466. *See also* Acromioclavicular joint injury
  evaluation of, 467–474
    active compression test in, 468, 469, 469f
    anesthetic injection in, 469–470, 469f
    anteroposterior stress test in, 478, 478f
    Buchberger test in, 468
    computed tomography in, 471
    cross-body adduction test in, 165–166, 166f, 467, 468f
    hug test in, 160, 161f, 468–469, 469f
    magnetic resonance imaging in, 472–474, 474f

Acromioclavicular joint *(Continued)*
  pain in, 467
  palpation in, 154, 155f, 467, 467f, 469
  patient history in, 467
  Paxinos test in, 468, 468f
  physical examination in, 467–470, 467f, 468f, 469f
  radiography in, 194–199, 194f–197f, 470–471, 470f–473f
  resisted extension test in, 468, 468f
  scintigraphy in, 472, 473f
  ultrasonography in, 474
  gout of, 515
  hug test of, 160, 161f, 468–469, 469f
  infection of, 517. *See also* Sepsis
  injury to. *See* Acromioclavicular joint injury
  innervation of, 453–454
  intra-articular disk of, 455
  ligaments of, 41–42, 42f, 455–456, 455f
  loose body in, 509, 511f
  magnetic resonance imaging of, 197, 472–474, 474f
  osteoarthritis of, 509, 511f, 515, 516f
  osteolysis of, 514–515, 514f
  osteophytes of, 783–784, 784f
  pain in, 467
  palpation of, 154, 155f, 467, 467f, 469
  Paxinos test of, 468, 468f
  physical examination of, 467–470, 467f, 468f, 469f
  pseudodislocation of, 389t, 391, 391f
  radiography of, 194–197, 194f, 470–471
    Alexander view for, 196–197, 197f
    anteroposterior view for, 195–196, 196f, 470, 470f, 471, 471f, 472f
    axillary lateral view for, 196, 470–471, 471f
    lateral view for, 470–471, 471f
    stress views for, 195–196, 196f, 471, 472f, 473f
    Zanca view for, 194–195, 195f, 470, 470f, 471f
  radionuclide imaging of, 197, 472, 473f
  reduction of, 484, 485f
  resisted extension test of, 468, 468f
  sagittal plane orientation of, 455, 455f
  separation of, 398, 398f. *See also* Acromioclavicular joint injury
    vs. clavicular fracture, 406
    distal clavicle resection after, 985
  ultrasonography of, 474
Acromioclavicular joint injury, 466, 474–514
  acute, 476–498
    type I, 476–478, 476f

Acromioclavicular joint injury *(Continued)*
    complications of, 478
    treatment of, 477
    type II, 476f, 478–480, 478f, 480f
      complications of, 479–480
      degenerative changes with, 480, 480f
      imaging of, 478, 479f
      treatment of, 479, 480
    type III, 476f, 480–497
      acromial fracture and, 361
      arthritis after, 490
      arthroscopic treatment of, 487–488, 990–992, 991f, 992f
      clinical manifestations of, 480–481, 481f
      complications of, 482, 485f, 489–491, 490f, 491f, 492f, 493f
      coracoid process fracture and, 359–360, 364f, 498–499, 499f, 500f, 501f, 502f
      deformity with, 482
      experimental investigations for, 488–489
      failed stabilization of, 490
      graft erosion in, 490, 490f, 491f–492f
      hook plate loosening in, 490, 493f
      imaging of, 481, 481f, 482f
      nonoperative treatment of, 482–483, 483f, 484f, 485f
      open operative treatment of, 483–497, 485f
        arthroscopic, 487–488, 990–992, 991f, 992f
        Bosworth screw for, 486, 486f, 488, 489, 493f
        complications of, 489–490, 490f, 491f, 492f, 493f
        coracoclavicular ligament reconstruction in, 487, 487f, 488–489, 488f
        experimental investigations in, 488–489
        failure of, 490
        hook plate for, 484, 486f, 489, 493–497, 493f, 494f–497f
        muscle transfer for, 487, 489
        reduction in, 484, 485f
        results of, 489
        revision, 490
        sutures for, 487, 487f, 493, 493f, 494f, 495f
      outcomes of, 489
      pathoanatomy of, 481
      physeal injury with, 497–498, 498f, 499f
      pin breakage in, 489–490, 490f
      screw loosening in, 490, 493f
      suture failure in, 490, 493f

Acromioclavicular joint injury *(Continued)*
  Thurston-Holland fragment with, 497, 498f
  variants of, 497–498, 498f, 499f
  type IV, 476f, 499–500, 502–504, 504f, 505f
    clinical manifestations of, 499–500, 504f
    imaging of, 500, 502, 504f, 505f
    nonoperative treatment of, 502
    operative treatment of, 502–505
  type V, 476f, 504–507
    clinical manifestations of, 504–505, 506f
    imaging of, 506, 507f
    treatment of, 506–507
  type VI, 476f, 507–509
    clinical manifestations of, 507, 508f
    imaging of, 507–508, 508f
    treatment of, 509, 510f
  chronic, 507–509, 508f
    complete (types III and V), 511–514
      clinical manifestations of, 511–512, 511f
      nonoperative treatment of, 512
      operative treatment of, 512–514, 513f
    incomplete (types I and II), 509, 511, 511f
  classification of, 475, 476f
  claviculectomy in. *See* Claviculectomy
  evaluation of. *See* Acromioclavicular joint, evaluation of
  in golfer, 1446
  mechanisms of, 475–476, 477f
  pain with, 148
Acromioclavicular ligaments, 41–43, 384, 384f, 455–456, 455f. *See also specific ligaments*
  stabilizing properties of, 456, 457f
  strain of, 391–392, 392f
Acromion
  absence of, 130
  age-related changes in, 779–780
  anatomy of, 44, 44f, 45f, 296, 454, 775–776, 776f
    comparative, 1–2, 2f
    variational, 112, 112f
  classification of, 44, 44f, 961, 961f
  development of, 10, 11f, 12, 12f, 453
  double, 126, 127f
  elongated, 127
  fracture of, 335, 335f, 353, 354f, 360–361.
    See also Scapular fracture
    after acromioplasty, 903
    with arthroscopy, 916
    in children, 611
    coracoid fracture and, 360–361, 360f
    grade III acromioclavicular joint disruption and, 361
    segmental, 361, 363f
    stress, 903
    treatment of, 369, 370f
  functions of, 353
  lateral extension of, rotator cuff tear and, 247–248
  ossification centers of, 122, 122f
  resection of. *See also* Acromioplasty
    in Apert's syndrome, 132
    instability after, 779, 779f, 833
    in rotator cuff disease, 779–781, 780f, 781f
  sclerosis of, 810f, 811, 811f
  traction spur of, 780f, 781–782, 781f, 1123f
  type I, 112, 112f, 780, 961
  type II, 112, 112f, 780, 781, 961
  type III, 112, 112f, 779–780, 781, 961, 961f
  unfused, 44, 44f
Acromionectomy
  in Apert's syndrome, 132
  instability after, 779, 779f, 833

Acromioplasty
  in Apert's syndrome, 132
  arthroscopic
    in impingement syndrome, 961–964, 963f, 965f
    with rotator cuff repair, 976–977, 979
    in subacromial abrasion, 825–828, 832–834
  in calcifying tendinitis, 1302
  deltoid detachment in, 774f, 775
  deltoid split for, 774f, 775, 827f, 829, 831, 831f
  failed, 808, 808t, 891–906
    acromial stress fracture and, 903
    deltoid insufficiency and, 903–905, 904f
    evaluation of, 891–893, 894f
    heterotopic ossification and, 902–903
    patient self-assessment in, 809–810, 809f
    persistent subacromial impingement and, 897–899
    stiffness and, 899–902, 901f
    after subacromial abrasion treatment, 832–834
    treatment of, 894–897, 895f
  kinematic effects of, 231
  open, in subacromial abrasion, 824–825, 832–835
  revision, in failed rotator cuff tear surgery, 898–899
  rotator cuff tear after, 781
Active compression test, 468, 469f, 1455
Acupuncture, in stiff shoulder, 1418
Adhesions, in rotator cuff evaluation, 805f, 807
Adhesive capsulitis. *See also* Stiff shoulder
  vs. biceps tendinitis, 1341
  biceps tendinitis with, 1339
  diagnosis of, 899–900, 994–995, 996f
  gender and, 146
  movement with, 228–229, 230f
  pain in, 148
  refractory, arthroscopic arthrolysis for, 1085–1087, 1086f, 1087f
  secondary, 998
  stages of, 994, 994b
  treatment of
    arthroscopic, 995–998, 997f, 998f
    arthroscopic arthrolysis for, 1085–1087, 1086f, 1087f
    arthroscopic capsular release for, 997f, 998f
    biceps tenodesis in, 1342, 1342f
    closed manipulation in, 995
    corticosteroid injections in, 995
    nonoperative, 995
Adipose tissue, 89–92, 92f
Adson test/maneuver, 175–176, 175f, 1376, 1483
Age/aging
  acromial changes with, 779–780
  acromioclavicular joint changes with, 466, 515
  calcifying tendinitis and, 1285, 1288–1289
  glenohumeral joint dislocation and, 677
  glenoid labrum changes with, 232, 232f
  osteoarthritis and, 146
  in patient history, 146
  recurrent atraumatic glenohumeral joint instability and, 686, 686f
  rotator cuff changes with, 791–793, 791f
  stiff shoulder and, 1410
  tumors and, 1531, 1532f
Air, arthroscopy-related extravasation of, 911
Air embolism, 289, 911
Airway
  arthroscopy-related obstruction of, 911
  surgical management of, 288

AMBRII acronym, 685, 952. *See also* Glenohumeral joint instability, recurrent, atraumatic (multidirectional)
American Shoulder and Elbow Surgeons (ASES) Standardized Assessment Form Shoulder Score Index, 272
American With Disabilities Act, 1503–1504
Amputation (congenital), 1558
Amputation (surgical), 1557–1574
  in arterial injury, 84–85
  in brachial plexus injury, 1381–1382, 1574
  disarticulation, 1557, 1560–1561, 1560f, 1562f
  in Ewing's sarcoma, 1549–1550
  indications for, 1558
  intercalary resection, 1557–1558, 1565–1566, 1566f
  pain after, 290, 1574
  prosthetic rehabilitation after, 1568–1574
    body-powered functional prostheses for, 1569–1570, 1570f, 1571f, 1572f
    externally powered prostheses for, 1570, 1572
    lightweight passive prostheses for, 1569, 1569f
    postural abnormalities and, 1572–1573
    targeted nerve transfers for, 1572, 1573f
  scapulothoracic (forequarter), 1557, 1561, 1563f, 1564–1565
    anterior approach to, 1561, 1563f, 1564
    posterior approach to, 1564–1565, 1565f
  through surgical neck, 1558–1560, 1559f
  types of, 1557–1558
Amputation (traumatic), 1558
Anesthesia, 279–285
  airway management for, 288
  in arthroscopic procedures, 288–289, 910–911, 929–930
  examination under, 929–930
  general, 279–280
    interscalene block with, 287
  interscalene brachial plexus block for, 280–285, 281f–284f, 284t, 287. *See also* Interscalene brachial plexus block
  manipulation under, in stiff shoulder, 1418–1420, 1423–1424
  monitoring of, 287–289
  nerve injury and, 286–287, 286b
  in pain treatment, 289–291
  postarthroscopy complications from, 910–911
  postoperative considerations with, 280, 289
  preoperative evaluation for, 287
  regional, 279–280
    axillary sheath for, 87–88, 88f, 89f
  selection of, 279–280
Anesthetics, local, 283, 284t
  acromioclavicular joint injection of, 469–470, 469f
  arterial injection of, 285
  intraneuronal injection of, 287
  in pain treatment, 289–291
Aneurysm, clavicular fracture and, 410, 411f
Angiography
  in brachial plexus injury, 1379
  in clavicular fracture, 400f, 401
  in osteosarcoma, 1518
Angiosomes, 53–54, 80
Angle phenomenon, at deltoid, 1074
Ankylosing spondylitis, coracoclavicular joint in, 456, 458f
Antebrachial cutaneous nerve, 71
Anterior drawer test, 158
Anterior interosseous nerve injury, clavicular fracture and, 411
Anterior slide test, 167t, 168, 168f

Anteroposterior stress test, of acromioclavicular joint, 478, 478f
Antibiotics
  in arthroplasty, 579
  in glenoid component reimplantation, 1281–1282, 1281f
  in infected arthroplasty, 1279
  perioperative, 288
  in sepsis, 575–578, 576f, 577t
Apert's syndrome, 132, 132f, 133f
Apprehension tests, 158–159, 158f, 159f
  in athlete, 1454–1455
  in atraumatic recurrent glenohumeral instability, 689, 691f
Arcuate artery, 83
Aristotle, 37
Arm elevation. See also Glenohumeral joint, biomechanics of
  acromioclavicular joint motion with, 216, 217f, 463–466, 464f–466f
  biceps in, 254
  center of rotation for, 226–228, 227f
  clavicle in, 386–388, 386f, 387f, 389
  deltoid in, 252–255, 254f, 255f, 258, 260
  external humerus rotation with, 225–226, 227f
  glenohumeral joint forces in, 254–258, 257f, 258f
  glenohumeral joint motion with, 224, 225f, 226f
  infraspinatus in, 253
  scapulothoracic joint motion with, 224, 225f, 226f, 229f, 230
  serratus anterior in, 254
  sternoclavicular joint motion with, 216, 217f
  supraspinatus in, 252–255, 254f, 255f, 257–258, 260
  teres minor in, 253
  torque generation in, 259–260, 259f, 259t
  trapezius in, 254
Arteriography. See Angiography
Artery (arteries), 80–85. See also specific arteries
  absence of, 84
  collateral, 84–85, 85f
  evaluation of, 175–176
  glenohumeral capsule, 28
  glenohumeral ligament, 28
  glenoid labrum, 27–28, 29f
  nonpathologic anomalies of, 84
  oblique course of, 80, 81f, 84
  rotator cuff, 26–27, 26f, 27f
Arthritis
  acromioclavicular joint. See Acromioclavicular joint, arthritis of
  degenerative. See Osteoarthritis
  glenohumeral. See Glenohumeral joint arthritis
  rheumatoid. See Rheumatoid arthritis
  septic, 566–567, 567t, 571. See also Sepsis
    synovial fluid examination in, 572, 572t
    treatment of, 575–579, 576f, 577t
  sternoclavicular joint. See Sternoclavicular joint, arthritis of
Arthrodesis, 1135–1143, 1139f, 1140f
  in brachial plexus injury, 1382, 1382f
  extra-articular, 1136–1137, 1138t
  function after, 1136, 1137f, 1138f
  indications for, 1135, 1137t
  in infected arthroplasty, 1280
  intra-articular, 1136–1137, 1138f, 1138t
  Matsen's technique for, 1137–1143, 1141f, 1142f, 1145f
    bone graft in, 1142, 1143f, 1144f, 1145f
    neutralization plate in, 1142–1143, 1145f
  position for, 229, 229f

Arthrodesis (Continued)
  postresection, 1545–1547
  pseudarthrosis after, 1140t
  Rockwood's technique for, 1143
  in rotator cuff tear arthropathy, 1255f, 1256
  in septic arthritis, 579
Arthrography
  in biceps tendon lesions, 1335–1336, 1336f
  distention, in stiff shoulder, 1417
  geyser sign on, 813, 814f
  of normal shoulder, 812f, 813
  of rotator cuff, 200–201, 203f, 813–814, 813f, 814f
  in shoulder instability, 189
  in stiff shoulder, 921, 1414, 1417
  in throwing-related SLAP lesion, 1459, 1460f
Arthrolysis, arthroscopic, 1085–1087, 1086f, 1087f
Arthroplasty, 1144–1191. See also Hemiarthroplasty
  arthroscopy after, 1008–1009
  balance stability angle in, 1101–1104, 1102f
  biomechanics of, 1089–1107, 1155–1159
    articular concentricity in, 1097–1098, 1097f, 1098f
    capsular, 1089–1096, 1090f–1095f
    coracoacromial concavity in, 1097–1098, 1097f
    distributed load transfer in, 1107, 1107f, 1108f
    glenoid articular surface in, 1096–1097, 1097f
    glenoid concavity in, 1101–1104, 1102f, 1103f, 1104f
    glenoid orientation in, 1099f, 1100–1101, 1100f, 1101f, 1102f
    humeral articular surface in, 1096, 1096f, 1097f, 1099–1100
    humeroscapular motion interface in, 1098–1099, 1098f, 1099f, 1107
    joint stuffing in, 1089–1096, 1091f–1095f, 1106–1107, 1106f
    muscle strength in, 1106–1107
    net humeral joint reaction force in, 1104–1106, 1104f, 1105f, 1106f
    smoothness in, 1107, 1107f, 1108f
  complications of, 1222–1229
    deltoid, 1229
    fracture, 1228
    glenoid component, 1223–1225, 1224f, 1225f, 1226f
    humeral component, 1223, 1224f, 1225–1226, 1225f
    infectious, 1222–1223, 1228–1229, 1277–1282
    instability, 1227–1228, 1227f
    neurologic, 1228
    rotator cuff, 1228
    scapular notching, 1323, 1324f
  computed tomography in, 192, 193, 1110–1111
  computer-assisted, 1579–1580
  coracoacromial concavity in, 1097–1098, 1097f
  cost of, 1167, 1172
  distributed load transfer in, 1107, 1107f, 1108f
  glenoid articular surface in, 1096–1097, 1097f
  glenoid centerline in, 1099f, 1100–1101, 1100f, 1101f, 1102f
  glenoid concavity in, 1101–1104, 1102f, 1103f, 1104f
  glenoid deficiency in, management of, 1580–1581, 1580f, 1581f
  in glenoid hypoplasia, 125

Arthroplasty (Continued)
  glenoid prosthesis for, 1161–1165, 1162f, 1163f, 1164f
    alternative bearing surfaces for, 1581–1583, 1582f
    arthroscopic removal of, 1009
    arthroscopic revision of, 1083–1085, 1083f, 1084f, 1085f
    bearing surfaces of, 1581–1583, 1582f
    bone support for, 1162–1163, 1163f
    fixation of, 1161–1162, 1162f, 1163f
    glenoid concavity and, 1163–1164, 1164f
    glenoidogram for, 1164, 1164f
    loosening of, 260, 260f, 1009, 1223, 1225, 1237f, 1238, 1581–1583, 1582f
    reimplantation of, 1280–1282, 1280f, 1281f
    removal of, 1009, 1237f, 1238
    wear of, 1225, 1226f
  glenoid version in, 1110, 1111f
  goals of, 1155–1159
  hemi-, 1159–1160, 1160f, 1161. See also Hemiarthroplasty
  historical perspective on, 1144–1151, 1145f–1158f, 1146t, 1155t, 1158t
  humeral articular surface in, 1096, 1096f, 1097f
  humeral convexity in, 1097–1098, 1098f
  humeral prosthesis for, 1165–1172, 1165f–1171f, 1167t
    fixation of, 1166, 1169f, 1170f, 1171f
    humeral version and, 1166, 1167f, 1168f
    loosening of, 1224f, 1225–1226, 1234, 1236f
    orthopaedic axis and, 1165–1166, 1165f, 1166f, 1167f
    procrustean grafting and, 1166, 1171f
    reaming for, 1165, 1165f
    register and, 1166, 1168f
    removal of, 1236f, 1238
    varus-valgus adaptability and, 1166, 1169f
  humeral version in, 1099–1100, 1166, 1167f, 1168f
  humeroscapular motion interface in, 1098–1099, 1098f, 1099f, 1107
  impingement syndrome after, 1009
  indications for, 1151–1155, 1158t
  infection after, 561, 562f, 570, 571, 910f, 911–912, 1222–1223, 1228–1229, 1277–1282
    aspiration in, 1278
    catheter-related, 290
    classification of, 1277
    diagnosis of, 1278–1279, 1278f
    pain with, 1277
    perineural interscalene catheter and, 290
    physical examination in, 1277–1278
    treatment of, 1279–1282, 1280f, 1281f
      antibiotics in, 1279
      débridement in, 1279
      reimplantation in, 1280–1282, 1280f, 1281f
      resection arthroplasty in, 1279–1280, 1280f
  interposition, resection, 1134–1135
  joint stuffing in, 1089–1096, 1106–1107, 1106f, 1159, 1159f
    capsular release for, 1089–1090, 1091f
    glenoid component in, 1092, 1093f
    humeral component in, 1092–1093, 1093f, 1094f
    range of motion effects of, 1090, 1091f, 1092f
    revision surgery and, 1231, 1232f
    translation and rotation effects of, 1090–1091, 1092f, 1093–1096, 1095f, 1095t

Arthroplasty (Continued)
  Matsen's technique of, 1172–1197
    in capsulorrhaphy arthropathy, 1192
    in degenerative disease, 1191, 1192
    glenoid preparation for, 1175, 1180–1186,
      1182f–1190f
    humeral insertion in, 1186–1187, 1190f,
      1191, 1191f
    humeral preparation for, 1172, 1174–1175,
      1176f–1181f
    incisions for, 1172, 1173f, 1174f, 1175f
    position for, 1172, 1173f
    ream and run in, 1180, 1182f, 1183f, 1184,
      1184f, 1185f, 1186f
    rehabilitation after, 1192–1197, 1193f–1196f
    in rheumatoid disease, 1191–1192
    in rotator cuff tear arthropathy, 1192
  methylmethacrylate in, 289
  minimally invasive, 1579–1580
  motion goals of, 1156
  net humeral joint reaction force in,
    1104–1106, 1104f, 1105f, 1106f
  nonconstrained, 1202–1222
    Anchor Peg Glenoid prosthesis in, 1205f,
      1206–1209, 1206f–1209f
    in degenerative disease, 1216–1218,
      1217f, 1221f
    humeral head resection in, 1202–1206,
      1202f–1205f
    humeral head size in, 1211, 1211f
    keeled glenoid prosthesis in, 1210–1211,
      1210f
    outcome assessment after, 1218–1219, 1220t
    patient self-assessment after, 1221–1222,
      1221f
    results of, 1213–1216, 1214t, 1215t, 1216f,
      1216t, 1217t
    in rheumatoid disease, 1218
    subscapularis tendon repair in, 1211–1213,
      1211f, 1212f, 1213f
    survivorship analysis after, 1219, 1221
  nonprosthetic, 1159
  optimal prosthetic design for, 230
  osteophyte resection in, 1098, 1098f
  in postinfectious glenohumeral arthritis, 579
  postresection, 1545–1547, 1546f
  prophylactic antibiotics in, 579
  in proximal humeral fracture, 318–327. See
    also Humeral fracture (proximal),
    arthroplasty for
  radiography of, 192–193, 193f
  rehabilitation after, 1192–1197, 1193f, 1194f,
    1195f, 1196f
  resection, 1133–1135, 1136f
    in infected arthroplasty, 1133, 1136f,
      1279–1280, 1280f
    in septic arthritis, 579, 1133
  revision, 1229–1238
    glenoid bone loss and, 1580–1581, 1581f
    for glenoid component failure, 1083–1085,
      1083f, 1084f, 1085f
    infection and, 1279
    Matsen's technique of, 1229–1238
      bone abutment and, 1229, 1231f
      component removal for, 1236f, 1237f,
        1238, 1238f
      glenoid defect in, 1237f, 1238, 1238f
      humeral component loosening and, 1234,
        1236f
      instability and, 1232f, 1233f, 1234, 1234f,
        1235f
      overstuffing and, 1231, 1231f, 1232f
      periprosthetic fracture and, 1229, 1229f,
        1230f

Arthroplasty (Continued)
    in rotator cuff tear arthropathy, 1269–1270,
      1272f
  rocking horse effect in, 1105–1106, 1105f
  Rockwood's technique of, 1197–1202
    anatomic landmarks in, 1197
    axillary nerve in, 1197, 1200, 1200f
    capsule release for, 1201–1202, 1202f
    incision for, 1199, 1199f, 1200f
    musculocutaneous nerve in, 1197–1198,
      1200, 1200f
    position in, 1198, 1198f
    subscapularis tendon release for, 1201,
      1201f
  in rotator cuff tear arthropathy. See Rotator
    cuff tear arthropathy
  sepsis after, 561, 562f, 570, 571
  smoothness goals of, 1159
  stability in, 1099–1106
    glenoid arc in, 1004f, 1101–1104, 1102f,
      1103f
    glenoid orientation in, 1099f, 1100–1101,
      1100f
    goals for, 1156–1159
    humeral articular surface area and,
      1099–1100
    net humeral joint reaction force in,
      1104–1106, 1104f, 1105f
  stability ratio in, 232, 233f
  types of, 1159–1161
Arthroscopy, 921–1043
  anatomy on, 922–928, 1045–1046, 1047–1048,
    1047f. See also specific structures
    anterior, 1047f, 1048, 1048f
    extra-articular, 927–928
    interior, 1047f, 1066–1067
    intra-articular, 922–927, 922f, 923f, 924f,
      925f, 926f
    superoposterior, 1047f, 1072–1073
  complications of, 909–918
    anesthesia-related, 910–911
    fluid extravasation, 914–915
    historical perspective on, 909–910
    implant-related, 916–917, 917f
    infectious, 910f, 911–912
    muscular, 915–916
    neurovascular, 912–914, 913f
    osseous, 916
    stiffness, 914
    thermal, 917–918
  diagnostic, 921–939
    anatomy on, 922–928, 922f, 923f, 924f, 925f,
      926f
    anesthesia for, 929–930
    in biceps tendon lesions, 922–923, 922f,
      1011–1012, 1011f, 1013f, 1338–1339,
      1338f, 1339f
    biceps tendon on, 922–923, 922f, 935–936,
      935f
    blood pressure during, 915
    capsular ligaments on, 924–926, 924f, 925f,
      926f
    drive-through test on, 936–937
    equipment for, 929
    examination under anesthesia with, 929–930
    in glenohumeral joint instability, 697–698,
      698f, 699f, 941–942, 941b
    glenohumeral ligaments on, 924–926, 924f,
      925f, 926f, 936, 936f, 938
    glenoid labrum on, 922f, 923–924, 923f, 937
    glenoid on, 924
    humeral head on, 926–927, 926f, 937–938
    in overhead throwing disorders, 1033–1034,
      1459–1460

Arthroscopy (Continued)
    portals for, 931–939
      acromioclavicular, 934–935
      anterior acromioclavicular, 934
      anterior subacromial, 934
      anteroinferior, 932
      anteromedial, 932
      anterosuperior, 931–932, 931f, 932f
      lateral subacromial, 933–934
      posterior, 289, 931, 931f
      posterior subacromial, 933
      posteroinferior, 933
      scapulothoracic, 935
      subacromial, 933–934
      superior acromioclavicular, 934–935
      superolateral, 933
      supraspinatus, 933
    positioning for, 928f, 929, 930–931, 930f
    primary examination in, 934f, 935–939,
      935f, 936f, 937f, 938f
    rotator cuff on, 927, 937–938, 937f, 938f,
      1034
    scapulothoracic articulation on, 927–928,
      928f
    subacromial space on, 927, 938–939
    subscapularis tendon on, 924–926, 924f
    in throwing-related SLAP lesion, 1459–1460
  historical perspective on, 921–922
  portals for. See Arthroscopy, diagnostic,
    portals for
  surgical, 1045–1087
    acromial fracture after, 916
    in acromioclavicular joint stabilization,
      990–992, 991f, 992f
    in adhesive capsulitis, 995–998, 997f, 998f,
      1085–1087, 1086f, 1087f
    air embolism with, 289, 911
    air extravasation with, 911
    airway compromise with, 911
    anatomy for, 1045–1046, 1047–1048, 1047f
      anterior, 1047f, 1048, 1048f
      interior, 1047f, 1066–1067
      superoposterior, 1047f, 1072–1073
    anesthesia for, 288–289
    complications of, 910–911
    in anterior HAGL lesion, 1054–1055, 1054f,
      1055f, 1056f
    in anterior iliac crest bone block procedure,
      1065–1066, 1065f, 1066f
    in arthrolysis, 1085–1087, 1086f, 1087f
    after arthroplasty, 1008–1009
    in axillary nerve pathology, 1068–1070,
      1069f, 1070f
    in Bennett's lesion, 1043
    in biceps tendon transfer, 1017–1018,
      1018f
    in biceps tendotomy, 1016–1017, 1017f
    in biceps tenodesis, 1013–1016, 1345–1348,
      1347f, 1348f, 1349f, 1350f, 1351f
    bioabsorbable tack–related complications
      of, 916–917
    blood pressure during, 915
    bupivacaine-induced chondrolysis after, 918
    in calcifying tendinitis, 1000–1001,
      1300–1303, 1301f, 1304
    in capsulolabral double row fixation,
      1050–1053, 1051f, 1052f, 1053f
    in cartilage lesions, 1048–1050, 1049f, 1050f,
      1051f
    chondrolysis after, 918
    in clavicular excision, 984–990. See also
      Claviculectomy, arthroscopic
    in coracoclavicular ligament reconstruction,
      1076–1079, 1078f, 1079f

Arthroscopy *(Continued)*
in coracoid fracture, 1060–1061, 1061f,
1062f
in coracoplasty, 981, 981f
epinephrine in, 915
in failed rotator cuff tear surgery, 896–897,
897f
fluid extravasation with, 914–915
in full-thickness rotator cuff tear, 865–868
in glenohumeral arthritis, 1003–1008. *See
also* Glenohumeral joint arthritis,
arthroscopic treatment of
in glenohumeral joint instability (anterior),
942–949, 946f–949f
in glenohumeral joint instability (atraumatic/
multidirectional), 691, 917–918, 952–956,
955f
in glenohumeral joint instability (posterior),
950–952, 951f, 952f
in glenoid component revision, 1083–1085,
1083f, 1084f, 1085f
in glenoid resurfacing, 1007–1008
in glenoid rim fracture, 1053–1054, 1054f
in glenoidplasty, 1007
after hemiarthroplasty, 1008–1009
heterotopic ossification after, 916
hypotension during, 288
in impingement syndrome, 961–964, 963f,
965f, 1009
implant-related complications in, 916–917,
917f
infectious complications of, 564–565, 910f,
911–912
in inferior HAGL lesion, 1067–1068, 1067f,
1068f
in interposition capsuloplasty, 1048–1050,
1049f, 1050f, 1051f
in Latarjet procedure, 1061–1065, 1063f,
1064f, 1065f
in latissimus dorsi transfer, 1070–1071
in lesser tuberosity fracture, 1058–1059,
1058f, 1059f
muscle injury with, 915–916
neurovascular complications of, 912–914
in os acromiale, 1075–1076, 1076f, 1077f
in osteonecrosis, 1008
in partial-thickness rotator cuff tear,
835–836
in PASTA lesion, 975–976, 1465–1470,
1466f, 1467f
in pectoralis minor transfer, 1059–1060,
1059f, 1060f, 1061f
pneumothorax after, 911
portals for, 931–939, 1046–1047, 1046f,
1048, 1048f, 1066–1067, 1073
positioning-related complications of,
912–913, 913f
in posterosuperior retracted cuff tear,
1073–1075, 1074f, 1075f
in proximal humeral rotational osteotomy,
1071–1072, 1071f, 1072f, 1073f
in renal arthropathy, 1008
in rotator cuff tear, 835–836, 865–868,
964–980. *See also* Rotator cuff tear(s),
arthroscopic treatment of
in rotator cuff tear arthropathy, 1256
rotator cuff tears with, 915–916
safe zone in, 1047, 1047f
sepsis after, 564–565
in SLAP lesion, 1024–1026, 1037–1038,
1460–1462, 1461f, 1463f, 1464f, 1465f
in spinoglenoid notch cyst, 1027–1028
in stiff shoulder capsule release, 1414,
1422–1423, 1424–1425, 1427f, 1428f

Arthroscopy *(Continued)*
stiffness after, 914, 999–1000
in subacromial abrasion, 825–828, 832–834
in subscapularis tendon tears, 980–982,
981f, 982f, 1055–1058, 1057f, 1058f,
1059–1060, 1059f, 1060f
in suprascapular nerve procedures,
1079–1083, 1079f, 1080f, 1081f, 1082f
in synovectomy, 1008
tendon injury with, 915–916
thromboembolism after, 914
in throwing-related dislocation, 1474–1477,
1475f, 1476f, 1478f–1479f
in throwing-related exostosis, 1042–1043
in throwing-related internal impingement,
1034–1035, 1036f–1037f
in throwing-related rotator cuff tears,
1038–1042, 1040f, 1041f
in throwing-related SLAP lesion, 1035,
1037–1038, 1460–1462, 1461f, 1463f,
1464f, 1465f
in throwing-related subacromial
impingement, 1042
topographic anatomy for, 1047–1048,
1047f
traction-related complications of, 912–913
in type III acromioclavicular joint injury,
487–488, 990–992, 991f, 992f
Aspiration (needle), in infected arthroplasty,
1278
Assessment. *See* Clinical evaluation; Outcome
assessment
Atherosclerosis, stiff shoulder and, 1411
Athlete, 1437–1483
acromioclavicular pain evaluation in, 1455
active compression test in, 1455
apprehension relocation test in, 1454–1455
baseball. *See* Overhead throwing
burner (stinger) syndrome in, 1479–1480
cervical radiculitis in, 1480–1481
dead arm in, 1450
effort thrombosis in, 1483
evaluation of, 1454–1455, 1455f
golf
acromioclavicular joint disease in, 1446
arthritis in, 1446
biomechanics in, 1445
glenohumeral instability in, 1446
rotator cuff injury in, 1445–1446
SLAP lesion in, 1446
subacromial impingement in, 1445–1446
Hawkins impingement sign in, 1455
inspection of, 1454
kinetic chain in, 1437–1438
Neer impingement sign in, 1455
overhead throwing in. *See* Overhead throwing
palpation examination in, 1454
physical examination of, 1454–1455, 1455f
quadrilateral space syndrome in, 1481
range of motion in, 1454
scapular assistance test in, 1455
scapular retraction test in, 1455
spinal accessory nerve injury in, 1481
strength testing in, 1454
suprascapular nerve entrapment in, 1482,
1482f
swimming
biomechanics in, 1442–1445, 1444f
impingement in, 1445
instability in, 1444–1445
symptom history in, 1454
tennis, 1442, 1443f
thoracic outlet syndrome in, 1483
trauma in, 1472–1479

Athlete *(Continued)*
anterior instability with, 1472–1478, 1473f,
1474f
arthroscopic treatment of, 1474–1477,
1475f, 1476f
nonoperative treatment of, 1473–1474
burner syndrome with, 1479–1480
cervical radiculitis with, 1480–1481
neurovascular injury with, 1479–1483
posterior instability with, 1477–1479,
1478f–1479f
quadrilateral space syndrome with, 1481
spinal accessory nerve injury with, 1481
suprascapular nerve entrapment with,
1482
thoracic outlet syndrome with, 1483
venous thrombosis with, 1483
Atlantoaxial rotatory subluxation, with clavicular
fracture, 596–597, 596f
Atraumatic recurrent glenohumeral joint
instability. *See* Glenohumeral joint
instability, recurrent, atraumatic
(multidirectional)
Avascular necrosis
distal clavicle, 517
humeral head, 1112b, 1126t
arthroplasty for, 1128–1129. *See also*
Arthroplasty
arthroscopic decompression in, 1008
degenerative joint disease with, 1128, 1128f,
1129f
fracture and, 328, 594, 1127f, 1128
steroid-related, 1128f, 1129, 1129f
Avulsion fracture, scapular, 361–364, 369
imaging of, 362, 365f
inferior angle, 364, 365f
nonoperative treatment of, 362–363, 364f
operative treatment of, 363–364, 364f
Axilla
anterior wall of, 385
lymph nodes of, 86, 86f
Axillary artery
anatomy of, 80, 81–83, 82f, 85f, 86–87, 106,
296f, 674, 676f
anomalies of, 84
injury to
amputation in, 84–85
collateral circulation and, 84–85
glenohumeral joint dislocation and, 672,
674–676, 676f
inferior glenohumeral dislocation and,
657–658
proximal humeral fracture and, 297
Axillary nerve
anatomy of, 29, 29f, 51, 53f, 73, 74f, 296f,
622–623, 623f, 624–625, 625f, 676,
1363–1364
variational, 110
in arthroplasty, 1197, 1200, 1200f
deltoid course of, 59, 622–623, 623f
in humeroscapular motion interface, 624–625,
625f
injury to. *See* Axillary nerve injury
in tumor treatment, 1512
Axillary nerve injury, 1363–1366
arthroscopy of, 1068–1070, 1069f, 1070f
clinical manifestations of, 1364, 1364f
electrophysiologic evaluation of, 1069
etiology of, 1364, 1364f
glenohumeral joint dislocation and, 676–677,
676f
interscalene block and, 286
nonoperative treatment of, 1069, 1364–1365
operative treatment of, 1069, 1365–1366

Axillary nerve injury (*Continued*)
  recurrent glenohumeral joint instability
    treatment and, 716
  rotator cuff tear treatment and, 903–905, 904f
  thermal, 1364
Axillary pouch, of inferior glenohumeral
    ligament complex, 17, 20, 21f, 22f, 24f
Axillary sheath, 87–88, 88f, 89f
Axillary space, 90, 92f
Axillary vein, 85–86
Axillopectoral muscle, 137, 137f
Axiohumeral muscles. *See* Latissimus dorsi;
    Pectoralis major; Pectoralis minor
Axioscapular muscles. *See* Levator scapulae;
    Rhomboid(s); Serratus anterior; Trapezius
Axon, 67

B

Balance stability angle, 630, 631f, 632f, 633–634,
    634f
Bankart lesion, 666, 671, 672f, 697–698, 698f,
    940, 942. *See also* Glenohumeral
    instability, recurrent, traumatic (anterior)
  arthroscopy of, 698, 698f
  classification of, 698
  historical perspective on, 618, 619f
  magnetic resonance imaging of, 947f
  reverse, 950–952, 951f, 952f. *See also*
    Glenohumeral instability, recurrent,
    traumatic (posterior)
Bankart repair, 249, 249f, 704–705, 705f, 706f,
    707f
  arthroscopic, 946–949, 947f, 948f, 949f
  capsulorrhaphy arthropathy after, 704–705,
    1127
  Matsen and Lippitt's preferred method of, 718,
    721–737
    anterior glenoid decortication for, 724,
      724f
    anterior glenoid exposure for, 722, 724,
      724f
    clavipectoral fascia exposure for, 721, 723f
    glenoid holes for, 724, 725f
    goals of, 718, 721f
    graft for, 726, 730f, 731f, 732f, 733f, 734f
    incision for, 718, 721, 722f
    instruments for, 718, 721f
    position for, 718, 722f
    rehabilitation after, 727–729, 735f
    subcutaneous dissection for, 721, 723f
    subscapularis incision for, 721, 723f, 724f
    subscapularis repair for, 726–727, 734f, 735f
    subscapularis tendon reefing for, 727, 735f
    sutures for, 724–725, 725f, 726f, 727f
  motion loss after, 250
Barrier effect, in active motion, 245
Baseball pitching. *See* Overhead throwing
Basilia, 1, 2f
Beach chair position, 288, 928f, 929, 930
Bear hug test, 160, 161f, 468–469, 469f
Belly-press test, 160, 161f
Bennett's lesion, in throwing athlete, 1042–1043,
    1470–1472
Bezold-Jarisch reflex, 285, 910
Biceps brachii
  anatomy of, 5, 65–66, 454
  in arm elevation, 254
  blood supply of, 66
  cross-sectional area of, 252t
  distal head of, 1314
  electromyography of, 1324–1325
  function of, 66
  innervation of, 66

Biceps brachii (*Continued*)
  long head of. *See* Biceps tendon
  rupture of, 1397–1399, 1398f
    in athlete, 1397–1398, 1398f
    clinical findings in, 1397–1398, 1398f
    complications of, 1398
    mechanism of, 1397
    treatment of, 1398–1399
  short head of, 1314
  Speed's test of, 1332, 1332f
  stabilizing function of, 246–247
  strength testing of, 173–174
Biceps instability test, 1332, 1333f
Biceps load test, 167t, 168–169, 169f, 170f
Biceps reflex, 175
Biceps resistance test (Speed's test), 166, 167t,
    1332, 1332f
Biceps tendinitis, 1326. *See also* Biceps tendon,
    lesions of
  vs. adhesive capsulitis, 1341
  adhesive capsulitis with, 1339
  attrition, 1326–1327, 1327f
  bicipital groove in, 1320–1321, 1320f
  calcific, 1296, 1329–1330, 1330, 1331
  classification of, 1326–1327, 1326b, 1328,
    1328b
  clinical presentation of, 1331
  vs. coracoid impingement syndrome, 1341
  differential diagnosis of, 1339–1341
  etiology of, 1330–1331
  vs. glenohumeral arthritis, 1341
  vs. glenohumeral instability, 1340
  vs. glenoid labrum tears, 1340–1341
  in golfer, 1446
  historical perspective on, 1311–1312
  impingement, 1326, 1327f
    treatment of, 1350–1352, 1353f
    vs. impingement syndrome, 1340
  magnetic resonance imaging in, 1336, 1338
  pathogenesis of, 47–48, 1319–1321
  physical examination in, 1331–1335, 1332f,
    1333f, 1334f
  prevention of, 1331
  with rotator cuff tear, 1328–1329, 1330, 1339
  supratubercular ridge in, 1321, 1322f
  treatment of, 1341–1355
    arthroscopic, 1345–1348, 1347f–1351f
    nonoperative, 1341–1342
    open, 1342–1345, 1343f, 1344f, 1348,
      1350–1353
Biceps tendon, 1309–1355
  anatomy of, 14–15, 115–116, 116f, 1312–1321
    arthroscopic, 922–923, 922f, 935–936, 935f
    attachment, 1312–1313, 1312f
    comparative, 1318, 1318f
    cross-sectional, 1313, 1313f
    developmental, 1318–1319, 1319f
    extracapsular, 1313, 1313f, 1321, 1323f
    intra-articular, 922–923, 922f, 1314, 1321,
      1323f
    pathologic, 1319–1321, 1320f, 1322f, 1323f
    variant, 115–116, 116f, 922–923
    vascular, 1313
    zonal, 1314
  arthroscopic tenodesis of, 1013–1016,
    1345–1348, 1347f–1351f
  arthroscopic tenotomy of, 1016–1017, 1017f
  arthroscopic transfer of, 1017–1018, 1018f
  arthroscopy of, 922–923, 922f, 935f, 1011–
    1013, 1013f, 1338–1339, 1338f, 1339f
    in active compression test, 1011, 1011f
  biomechanics of, 1311f, 1312, 1321,
    1323–1325, 1323f
  blood supply to, 1313

Biceps tendon (*Continued*)
  developmental anomalies of, 115
  dislocation of, 47–48, 1018–1019, 1326, 1327f
    bicipital groove in, 1320, 1320f
    clinical presentation of, 1331
    etiology of, 1330
    historical perspective on, 1309–1310
    magnetic resonance imaging of, 207, 207f,
      1336, 1337f
    operative treatment of, 1345, 1346f
    pathogenesis of, 1319
    pathologic anatomy of, 1319
    physical examination in, 1331–1335, 1332f,
      1333f, 1334f
    prevention of, 1331
    pulley lesion and, 1311f, 1312
    with rotator cuff tear, 1329, 1352–1354,
      1353f, 1354f
    traumatic, 1330
    treatment of, 1018–1019, 1342, 1345, 1346f,
      1352–1353
  electromyography of, 1324–1325
  entrapment of, 1019, 1019f, 1326, 1327f,
    1350–1352, 1353f
  extracapsular, 1313, 1313f, 1321, 1323f
  function of, 1321, 1323–1326, 1323f
  historical perspective on, 1309–1312, 1310f,
    1311f
  hourglass, 1019, 1019f, 1339
  hypertrophy of, in rotator cuff tear, 796, 796f
  imaging of, 206f, 207, 1334–1339, 1335f,
    1336f, 1337f, 1338f
  inflammation of. *See* Biceps tendinitis
  innervation of, 29
  intra-articular, 922–923, 922f, 1314, 1321,
    1323f
  lesions of. *See also* Biceps tendinitis
    vs. adhesive capsulitis, 1341
    arthrography in, 1335–1336, 1336f
    associated disorders with, 1018–1019
    bony pathoanatomy and, 1320–1321, 1322f
    classification of, 1326–1329, 1326b, 1327f,
      1328b, 1329b
    complications of, 1339
    vs. coracoid impingement syndrome, 1341
    dialysis-related, 1331
    differential diagnosis of, 1339–1341
    etiology of, 1330–1331
    evaluation of, 166, 167f
      arthrography in, 1335
      arthroscopy in, 922–923, 922f, 1011–1020,
        1011f, 1013f, 1338–1339, 1338f, 1339f
      biceps instability test in, 1332, 1333f
      deAnquin's test in, 1333, 1334f
      Hueter's sign in, 1334
      Lippmann's test in, 1333
      Ludington's test in, 1332–1333
      magnetic resonance imaging in,
        1336–1338, 1337f, 1338f
      palpation in, 1331, 1332f
      physical examination in, 1331–1335,
        1332f, 1333f, 1334f
      Popeye sign in, 1013, 1013f, 1334, 1334f
      radiography in, 207, 1334–1335, 1335f
      Speed's test in, 1332, 1332f
      ultrasonography in, 1012–1013, 1012f,
        1336, 1337f
      Yergason's sign in, 1332, 1333f
    vs. glenohumeral arthritis, 1341
    vs. glenohumeral instability, 1340
    vs. glenoid labrum tears, 1340–1341
    in golfer, 1446
    historical perspective on, 1309–1312, 1310f,
      1311f

Biceps tendon (*Continued*)
　vs. impingement syndrome, 1340
　incidence of, 1329–1330
　interval, 1328, 1328b
　isolated, 1353–1354, 1354f
　origin, 1327–1328, 1328b
　at origin, 1327–1328
　prevention of, 1331
　supratubercular ridge and, 1321, 1322f
　TLC classification of, 1329, 1329b
　treatment of, 1013–1018, 1341–1355
　　arthroscopic tenodesis in, 431, 1013–1016,
　　　1345–1348, 1347f–1351f
　　arthroscopic tenotomy in, 1016–1017,
　　　1017f
　　arthroscopic transfer in, 1017–1018, 1018f
　　care after, 1354
　　conservative, 1341–1342, 1348
　　failure of, 1355
　　operative, 1342–1345, 1342f, 1343f, 1344f,
　　　1348, 1350
　pulley lesion of, 1311f, 1312, 1336
　in rotator cuff tears, 1324–1325
　rupture of, 1326
　　acute, 1354, 1354f
　　after arthroscopic thermal capsulorrhaphy,
　　　918
　　chronic, 1352
　　clinical presentation of, 1331
　　isolated, 1328, 1353–1354, 1354f
　　magnetic resonance imaging of, 1336, 1338f
　　nonoperative treatment of, 1341–1342
　　in older patient, 1342, 1354, 1354f
　　with rotator cuff tear, 1319, 1329
　　treatment of, 1354, 1354f
　　in young patient, 1353–1354
　in SLAP lesion, 246–247
　sliding zone of, 1314
　stabilization of, 1314–1316, 1315f, 1316f
　stabilizing function of, 246–247, 1324
　subluxation of, 1326, 1327f, 1328, 1328b
　　prevention of, 1331
　　treatment of, 1345, 1346f, 1352–1353
　tenderness in, 1331, 1332f
　tenotomy of, 1016–1017, 1017f
　tensile properties of, 1313
　in throwing, 1325
　traction zone of, 1314
Biceps tendotomy, 1016–1017, 1017f
Biceps tenodesis
　in adhesive capsulitis, 1342, 1342f
　arthroscopic, 1013–1016, 1345–1348,
　　1347f–1351f
　failure of, 1355
　Hitchcock's, 1342, 1343f, 1344–1345
　keystone, 1343, 1344, 1344f
Biceps tenosynovitis, 1319, 1320, 1329
　treatment of, 1341, 1342–1343, 1343f
Biceps tension test, 167–168
Biceps transfer
　arthroscopic, 1017–1018, 1018f
　in type III acromioclavicular joint injury,
　　487
Bicipital groove
　anatomy of, 13, 14f, 47–48, 48f, 295,
　　1316–1317, 1317f, 1320–1321, 1320f
　variant, 115–116, 116f, 1317, 1317f
　injection of, 1340
　lips of, 48
　narrow, 1320, 1320f, 1322f
　palpation of, 154
　point tenderness in, 1331, 1332f
　radiography of, 206f, 207, 1334–1335, 1335f
　in rotator cuff evaluation, 805f, 806

Bicipital groove (*Continued*)
　shallow, 1320, 1320f
　spurs of, 1321, 1323f
Bicipital sheath, loose bodies in, 1320
Bioabsorbable tacks, complications of, 916–917
Biomechanics
　acromioclavicular joint, 214–217, 215f, 216f,
　　230–231, 463–466, 463f, 464f–466f
　arthroplasty-related. *See* Arthroplasty,
　　biomechanics of
　biceps tendon, 246–247, 1311f, 1312, 1321,
　　1323–1325, 1323f
　clavicle, 213–217, 215f, 216f, 217f
　glenohumeral joint. *See* Glenohumeral joint,
　　biomechanics of
　overhead throwing, 1029–1030, 1030f,
　　1437–1442, 1438f
　rotator cuff. *See* Rotator cuff, biomechanics
　　of
　sternoclavicular joint, 214f
　swimming, 1442–1445, 1444f
Biopsy, tumor, 1538–1540, 1539f, 1550
Bipolar (floating) anterior-inferior glenohumeral
　ligament, 945
Birth
　clavicular fracture with, 394, 595
　　clinical manifestations of, 396, 596
　　treatment of, 413, 419–420
　　ultrasonography of, 403
　humeral fracture with, 584, 586
Blastema, 6, 7f
Blood, operative loss of, 289
Blood pressure, during arthroscopy, 915
Blood vessels, 79–86. *See also specific arteries
　and veins*
Bone. *See also specific bones*
　chondrosarcoma of, 1520–1522, 1521f, 1533f,
　　1548–1549, 1551
　cyst of
　　aneurysmal, 1523, 1523f
　　simple, 1522f, 1523, 1533f
　Ewing's sarcoma of, 1525–1526, 1527f,
　　1549–1550, 1551–1552
　fibrous dysplasia of, 1524, 1524f, 1537
　giant cell tumor of, 1525, 1551
　metastatic disease of, 1530, 1536, 1536f,
　　1550
　multiple myeloma of, 1525, 1526f
　myositis ossificans of, 1517
　nonossifying fibroma of, 1524, 1525f
　osteoblastoma of, 1517
　osteoid osteoma of, 1515–1516
　Paget's disease of, 1526–1528, 1528f, 1529f,
　　1537
　sarcoma of, 1516f, 1517–1518, 1517b, 1518f.
　　See also Osteosarcoma
　tumors of, 1533f
　　benign, 1515–1517
　　　treatment of, 1547–1548
　　malignant, 1517–1518, 1518f
　　　staging of, 1512t, 1513–1515
　　　treatment of, 1548–1550
　　reticuloendothelial, 1525–1526, 1526f
Bone block
　for failed Latarjet procedure, 1065–1066,
　　1065f, 1066f
　in recurrent anterior glenohumeral instability,
　　708, 710
　in recurrent posterior glenohumeral instability,
　　743–744
Bone graft
　in arthrodesis, 1142, 1143f, 1144f, 1145f
　in humeral fracture–related arthroplasty, 324,
　　324f

Bone scan. *See* Radionuclide imaging
Bosworth screw, in type III acromioclavicular
　joint injury, 486, 486f, 488
Boutonnière deformity, 781f, 797, 1104f, 1105
Boytchev procedure, 714
Brachial artery, 82f, 85f
Brachial cutaneous nerve
　lateral, 73
　medial, 71
Brachial plexitis, idiopathic (Parsonage-Turner
　syndrome), 287, 1376–1377, 1377f, 1412
　diagnosis of, 1377, 1377f
　long thoracic nerve palsy in, 1369, 1370f
　prognosis for, 1377, 1377f
　suprascapular nerve injury in, 1372, 1373
　treatment of, 1377, 1377f
Brachial plexus, 68–77
　anatomy of, 280, 1378f
　anomalous, 107, 109f, 110f
　autonomic fibers of, 74–75
　blood supply of, 72, 72f
　at clavicle, 41, 384, 384f
　cords of, 69–70, 70f
　cutaneous representation of, 95
　divisions of, 69–70, 70f
　injury to. *See* Brachial plexus injury
　nonpathologic variants of, 75–77, 76f, 78f
　postfixed, 69, 76
　prefixed, 69, 76
　roots of, 69, 70f
　terminal branches of, 70–74. *See also specific
　　nerves*
　trunks of, 69–70, 70f
　tumors of, 1511, 1535
Brachial plexus block. *See* Interscalene brachial
　plexus block
Brachial plexus injury, 1377–1385
　clavicular fracture and, 399–401, 400f, 411,
　　412f, 603
　closed, 1378, 1380
　diagnosis of, 1378–1380, 1379f, 1380f
　Horner's syndrome with, 175
　humeral fracture and, 297, 593
　imaging in, 1379–1380, 1380f
　mechanisms of, 1378, 1378f, 1379f
　nonoperative treatment of, 1380
　operative treatment of, 1380–1385
　　amputation in, 1381–1382, 1574
　　fusion in, 1382, 1382f
　　indications for, 1380–1381
　　muscle transfer in, 1384
　　nerve reimplantation in, 1384
　　nerve repair in, 1382
　　nerve transfer in, 1382–1384, 1383f
　　outcomes of, 1384
　　planning of, 1381
　　technique of, 1381
　postganglionic, 69, 75
　preganglionic, 69, 75
　scapular fracture and, 612
　scapulothoracic dissociation and, 365
　in Sprengel's deformity treatment, 122
　types of, 1378
Brachialis, strength testing of, 173–174
Brachiocephalic veins, 106
Brachioradialis reflex, 175
Breast cancer
　radiation therapy in, glenohumeral joint injury
　　and, 1129–1130, 1130f
　surgery for, stiff shoulder and, 1411
Brisement, in stiff shoulder, 1417
Bristow-Helfet procedure, 710–713, 710f, 711f,
　　713f
　complications of, 716, 716f

Bronchitis, stiff shoulder and, 1411
Buchberger test, 468
Buford complex, 114, 115f, 936, 936f, 1457, 1457f
Bupivacaine, 283, 284t
    chondrolysis with, 918
Burner (stinger) syndrome, 1479–1480
Bursa (bursae)
    abscess of, 563
    anatomy of, 22, 25–26, 25f, 26f, 92–93, 93f
        sepsis and, 563
    coracobrachial, 92–93
    subacromial, 92, 93f, 112
    subdeltoid, 92
    subscapular, 22, 25, 25f, 26f, 92
    thickness of, in rotator cuff evaluation, 805f, 807
    unintentional injection of, 563
Bursectomy, subacromial, 938–939, 938f
Bursography
    in rotator cuff disorders, 814
    subacromial, 201, 814
Bursoscopy, 927
    subacromial, 927, 938, 938f

C

Calcification. See also Calcifying tendinitis
    in chondroblastoma, 1519
    coracoacromial ligament, 777, 777f
    diffuse, 1296
    dystrophic, vs. calcifying tendinitis, 1286, 1289, 1295, 1296
    in enchondroma, 1520
Calcifying tendinitis, 1283–1305
    age and, 1285, 1288–1289
    anatomy of, 1283–1284
    bursitis in, 1292–1293
    calcific stage of, 1287f, 1288f, 1289f, 1290, 1290f, 1291t, 1292, 1292f
    chondrocytes in, 1286–1287, 1287f
    classification of, 1285–1286
    clinical features of, 1291–1293, 1292f
    complications of, 1296
    differential diagnosis of, 1296
    vs. dystrophic calcification, 1286, 1289, 1295, 1296
    historical perspective on, 1283
    HLA-A1 in, 1295
    hyperemia in, 1292, 1292f
    incidence of, 1284–1285
    laboratory evaluation in, 1295–1296
    magnetic resonance imaging in, 206f, 207, 1001, 1001f
    microspheroliths in, 1288
    occupation and, 1285, 1293
    pain in, 1291, 1291t, 1292–1293
    pathogenesis of, 1288–1291, 1289f, 1290f, 1291t
    pathology of, 1283–1284, 1284f, 1286–1288, 1286f, 1287f, 1288f
    postcalcific stage of, 1289f, 1290–1291, 1291t, 1292–1293, 1292f, 1293f, 1304
    precalcific stage of, 1286f, 1289–1290, 1289f, 1291–1292, 1291t
    psammomas in, 1287, 1288f
    radiography in, 205f, 207, 811, 811f, 1001, 1001f, 1286, 1293–1295, 1293f, 1294f
    rotator cuff tear and, 1303
    stiffness and, 1293, 1296
    treatment of, 1296–1304, 1303t
        acromioplasty in, 1302
        arthroscopic, 1000–1001, 1300–1303, 1301f, 1304

Calcifying tendinitis (Continued)
        extracorporeal shock wave therapy in, 1297–1299, 1298t, 1302–1303
        lavage in, 1299, 1303t
        needling in, 1299, 1303t
        nonoperative, 1000, 1296–1300, 1298t, 1303–1304, 1303t, 1304
        open procedures in, 1301, 1304
        radiation therapy in, 1299–1300
    ultrasonography in, 1295, 1295f
Calcitonin, in stiff shoulder, 1418
Calcium, rotator cuff tendon, 1283–1305. See also Calcifying tendinitis
    dystrophic, 1286, 1289, 1295, 1296
    pain with, 147
    radiography of, 205f, 207
Cancer. See Tumor(s) and specific tumors
Capsular distention, in stiff shoulder, 1417
Capsular ligament, 529, 530f, 531f
Capsular plication, in atraumatic glenohumeral joint instability, 953–954, 955–956, 955f
Capsular shift procedure
    in atraumatic glenohumeral joint instability, 758–759, 759f, 953
    in traumatic anterior glenohumeral joint instability, 737, 740f
    in traumatic posterior glenohumeral joint instability, 750–752, 756, 756f
Capsule
    acromioclavicular joint, 41, 455
        stability and, 215–216
    glenohumeral joint
        anatomy of, 15–16, 15f, 16f
        blood supply of, 28
        collagen of, 235
        development of, 10–11
        innervation of, 28–29
        laxity of, 1089–1090, 1090f
        mechanoreceptors of, 248
        redundancy of, 235
        stability contribution of, 235, 237, 237f, 238f
        synovial lining of, 20, 22, 22f, 23f, 115
        tensile strength of, 235, 237f, 238f
        thickness of, 22, 22f, 23f
    sternoclavicular joint, 105
Capsulolabral double row fixation, arthroscopic, 1050–1053, 1051f, 1052f, 1053f
Capsulolabral reconstruction. See Bankart repair
Capsulorrhaphy
    DuToit staple, 706–707, 709f
        complications of, 716–717
    thermal, 954–955
        complications of, 917–918
Capsulorrhaphy arthropathy, 646, 647f, 704–705, 717, 1092f, 1100f, 1112b, 1126t
    arthroplasty for, 1126–1128, 1192. See also Arthroplasty
Carcinoma. See Tumor(s) and specific tumors
Cardiac arrest
    clavicular fracture and, 411
    interscalene block and, 285
Cardiac catheterization, stiff shoulder and, 1411
Carotid artery
    anesthetic injection into, 285
    clavicular fracture–related obstruction of, 410
Carotid bruit, interscalene block and, 285
Cartilage, hyaline (articular), 563–564, 564f
    arthroscopic surgery on, 1048–1050, 1049f, 1051f, 1059f
    bacterial colonization of, 565–566, 566f
Cartilaginous tumors
    benign, 1518–1520, 1519f, 1520f, 1521f
    malignant, 1520–1522, 1521f

Cassiopeia capsulolabral double row fixation, 1050–1053, 1051f, 1052f, 1053f
Cephalic vein, 86, 105f, 112
    arthroscopy-related laceration of, 912
Cervical plexus, 280
Cervical plexus block, 280, 281f
Cervical radiculitis, in athlete, 1480–1481
Cervical radiculopathy, 148
    vs. rotator cuff tear, 818
Cervical spine
    atlantoaxial rotatory subluxation of, clavicular fracture and, 596–597, 596f
    degenerative disease of, stiff shoulder and, 1411
    examination of, 152–153, 152f
Cervical spondylosis, vs. rotator cuff tear, 818
Charcot joint, 1129
Cheiroarthropathy, in diabetes mellitus, 1410
Chemotherapy, 1551–1552
    in osteosarcoma, 1551
    in soft tissue sarcoma, 1552
Chest wall
    clavicular fracture–related injury to, 596
    tumor involvement of, 1535
Chief complaint, 146–151. See also Clinical evaluation
Children
    clavicular fracture in, 394, 594–604
        anatomy of, 594–595, 595f
        atlantoaxial rotatory subluxation with, 596–597, 596f
        birth-related, 394, 595
            clinical manifestations of, 396, 596
            vs. congenital pseudarthrosis, 403, 404–406
            treatment of, 413, 419–420
            ultrasonography of, 403
        chest wall injury with, 596
        classification of, 391–392, 392f, 599–601, 599f
        clinical manifestations of, 397, 397f
        complications of, 603–604
        differential diagnosis of, 598–599
        distal (lateral), 391–392, 392f, 421–422, 421f, 599, 599f, 600f, 601f
            radiography of, 403–404
            treatment of, 601–602, 602f
        greenstick, 403, 403f, 413
        implant complications of, 603–604
        incidence of, 595
        malunion of, 603
        mechanism of, 595–596
        medial, 421–422, 599f, 600–601
            treatment of, 602–603, 603f
        neurovascular complications of, 603
        nonunion of, 603
        radiography of, 403, 403f, 597–598, 597f, 598f
        Rockwood's classification of, 391–392, 392f
        shaft, 599, 599f, 601, 602f
        signs and symptoms of, 596
        treatment of, 413, 420–422, 421f, 601–603
            nonoperative, 601, 601f
        vascular injury with, 596
    congenital amputation in, 1558
    congenital clavicular absence in, 41, 385–386
    congenital clavicular pseudarthrosis in, 118, 118f, 403, 404–406, 598–599
    floating shoulder in, 608, 609f
    greater tuberosity fracture in, 590
    lesser tuberosity fracture in, 590
    os acromiale in, 608, 608f
    postamputation scoliosis in, 1573
    proximal humeral fracture in, 583–594

Children (*Continued*)
anatomy of, 583–584
classification of, 585–586, 586f, 587f
complications of, 592–594, 594f
incidence of, 584
mechanism of, 584–585, 584f, 585f
nonaccidental, 585
pathologic, 584, 585f
radiography of, 587–588, 588f
rehabilitation after, 592
signs and symptoms of, 586–587
treatment of, 588–591, 589f
complications of, 593, 594
immobilization for, 589–590, 590f, 591
intramedullary nail fixation for, 590, 592f
operative, 590, 591f, 592, 592f, 594
percutaneous pin fixation for, 590, 591f, 593f
reduction for, 589–590, 590f, 590t
varus after, 593, 594f
scapular fracture in, 604–612
anatomy of, 604, 604f, 605f
associated injury with, 605
classification of, 608–610, 609f, 610f
clinical manifestations of, 605
complications of, 612
coracoid process, 608, 611
differential diagnosis of, 608
glenoid, 608, 610, 610f, 612
incidence of, 605
mechanism of, 605
neck, 608, 609f
neurovascular complications of, 612
radiography of, 605–607, 606f, 607f, 608f
treatment of, 611–612, 611f
scapulothoracic dissociation in, 607, 608f, 610, 612
Chinese medicine, 33
Chondroblastoma, 1519, 1520f, 1533f
Chondroepitrochlear muscle, 133, 134f
Chondrolysis
bupivacaine-induced, 918
after thermal capsulorrhaphy, 918
Chondroma, periosteal, 1519, 1533f
Chondromatosis, synovial, 1008, 1522–1523
Chondrosarcoma, 1520–1522, 1521f, 1533f, 1551
resection of, 1548–1549, 1551
secondary, 1520–1521
Chromosome translocations, in neoplasms, 1515, 1516t
α-Chymotrypsin injection, in stiff shoulder, 1417
Circulus articuli vasculosus, 563
Circumflex humeral artery, 26, 26f, 27f, 29f
anterior, 82f, 83, 85f
posterior, 59, 82f, 83, 85f
compression of, 87
Circumflex scapular artery, 82f, 85f
Clavicle. *See also* Sternoclavicular joint
absence of, 41, 385–386
anatomy of, 40–41, 41f, 594–595, 595f
comparative, 4
surgical, 385
variational, 101–103, 102f, 103f
anterior torsion of, 102–103, 102f
in arm elevation, 216, 217f, 386–388, 386f, 387f, 389
bifurcated, 126
biomechanics of, 213–217, 215f, 216f, 217f, 386–388
blood supply of, 384–385
brachial plexus at, 384, 384f
congenital absence of, 41, 385–386
congenital pseudarthrosis of, 118, 118f, 403, 404–406, 598–599

Clavicle (*Continued*)
cosmetic function of, 389
curvature of, 102, 102f, 103
development of, 11–12, 12f, 382–383, 453, 594
dislocation of, 537–538. *See also* Sternoclavicular joint dislocation
distal (lateral), 40, 41f, 454, 454f
osteolysis of, 514–515, 514f, 985, 986f
osteonecrosis of, 517
duplication of, 126, 126f
epiphysis of, 11–12, 12f, 40
excision of. *See* Claviculectomy
fasciae about, 385
floating, 391, 398
fracture of. *See* Clavicular fracture
function of, 385–389, 386f
length of, 457
ligament attachment to, 40, 41f
medial, 40, 41f. *See also* Sternoclavicular joint
condensing osteitis of, 536
epiphysis of, 529, 531f
middle suprascapular nerve foramen of, 126, 126f
moment of inertia of, 383
morphology of, 383–385, 383f, 384f
muscle attachments of, 40–41, 41f, 388
neurovascular structures at, 384, 384f, 385f, 389
osteotomy of, in sternoclavicular joint dislocation, 547, 553, 554f, 555f
porosity of, 383
pseudoarthrosis of, 118, 118f, 403, 404–406, 598–599
pseudodislocation of, 599
radiography of, 193f, 194
resection of. *See* Claviculectomy
in respiration, 389
scapular osseous bridge from, 128
shape of, 383–384, 383f
stabilization of, 386f
stresses on, 383–384
subclavian vein relationship to, 41
surgical anatomy of, 385
tumors of. *See* Tumor(s) *and specific tumors*
type I, 102f, 103
type II, 102f, 103
type III, 102f, 103
Clavicle index, 102, 102f
Clavicular artery, 82f, 83
Clavicular fracture, 381–444
vs. acromioclavicular separation, 406
aneurysm and, 410, 411f
arthritis after, 411–412
associated injuries with, 398–401, 398f, 399f, 400f
birth-related, 394, 595
clinical manifestations of, 396, 596
vs. congenital pseudarthrosis, 403
treatment of, 413, 419–420
ultrasonography of, 403
brachial plexus injury with, 399–401, 400f, 411, 412f, 603
classification of, 389–394, 389b
Craig's, 389–391, 389b, 390f, 391f
Robinson's, 392–394, 393f
Rockwood's, 391–392, 392f
vs. cleidocranial dysostosis, 406
clinical manifestations of, 396–401
complications of, 406–413. *See also* Clavicular fracture, nonunion of
arthritic, 411–412
compressive, 410–411, 412f
malunion, 387–388, 387f, 388f, 409–410, 410f, 412f

Clavicular fracture (*Continued*)
neurologic, 411, 412f
neurovascular, 410–411, 411f, 419
computed tomography in, 198–199, 199f
vs. congenital pseudarthrosis, 404–406
Craig's classification of, 389–391, 389b, 390f, 391f
differential diagnosis of, 404–406
distal third (group II), 389b, 390–391, 390f, 391f
articular extension of, 404, 405f
computed tomography in, 404, 405f
conoid ligament in, 440, 441f
coracoclavicular screw for, 441–443, 442f, 443f, 444f
displaced, 440, 441f
hybrid fixation for, 443, 444f
Kirschner-wire fixation for, 441
nondisplaced, 439–440
nonunion of, 407. *See also* Clavicular fracture, nonunion of
plate fixation for, 440–441, 442f
radiography of, 403–404, 404f, 405f, 440, 441f
Rockwood's classification of, 391–392, 392f
in scapulothoracic dissociation, 365–366, 366f
treatment of, 439–444, 442f, 443f, 444f
care after, 443–444, 444f
coracoclavicular screw in, 441–443, 442f, 443f, 444f
Kirschner-wire fixation in, 441
plate fixation in, 440–441, 442f
sling in, 439
type I, 361, 362f, 389t, 390, 390f
type II, 389t, 390–391, 390f, 391f
coracoid fracture and, 361, 361b, 362f
radiography of, 403–404, 405f
type III, 389t, 391
type IV, 389t, 391, 391f
type V, 389t
exercises after, 419
historical perspective on, 381–382
incidence of, 394–395
infection after, 578–579
malunion of, 387–388, 387f, 388f, 409–410, 410f, 412f
thoracic outlet syndrome after, 1374–1376, 1375f
mechanisms of, 394–396, 395f
middle third (group I), 389–390, 389b
glenoid neck fracture and, 358–359, 358f
greenstick, 403, 403f
intramedullary fixation for, 426–436, 427f
care after, 435–436, 437f, 438f
closure for, 435, 436f
drilling and tapping for, 429–431, 430f, 431f, 432f, 433f
incision for, 428–429, 429f
pin fixation for, 431, 435, 435f
pin insertion for, 431, 434f
positioning for, 428, 429f
supraclavicular nerve in, 429, 430f
malunion of, 412f, 436, 438f, 439f, 440f
nonunion of, 395, 395f, 402f, 403f, 408, 408f, 410, 411f, 412f. *See also* Clavicular fracture, nonunion of
plate fixation for, 423f, 424–426, 424f, 425f
radiography of, 401–403, 401f, 402f, 403f
seat-belt, 395, 395f, 407
treatment of, 413–416, 414f, 423–436
intramedullary fixation for, 426–436, 427f
plate fixation for, 423f, 424–426, 424f, 425f

Clavicular fracture (Continued)
neurovascular complications of, 399–401, 400f, 410–411, 411f, 412f, 419
nontraumatic, 396, 396f
nonunion of, 387–388, 406–409, 412f
diagnosis of, 402, 402f, 403f, 408–409
displacement and, 407
fracture location and, 407
inadequate immobilization and, 406
open reduction and, 407–408, 408f
physical examination in, 409
radiography of, 402, 402f, 403f, 408–409
refracture and, 407
symptoms of, 409
tape-related, 396
trauma severity and, 407
treatment of, 416–418
vascular injury with, 410, 411f
pediatric. See Children, clavicular fracture in
physical examination in, 398
pneumothorax with, 399, 399f
proximal third (group III), 389b, 391
nonunion of, 418. See also Clavicular fracture, nonunion of
pulmonary complications of, 401
radiography of, 404
sternoclavicular joint injury with, 537–538, 539f
treatment of, 416, 422
radiography of, 193f, 194, 401–404, 401f, 402f, 403f
recurrent, 407
rehabilitation after, 418
return-to-play after, 418–419
rib fracture and, 398–399, 399f
Robinson's classification of, 392–394, 393f
Rockwood's classification of, 391–392, 392f
seat-belt, 395, 395f, 407
shaft. See Clavicular fracture, middle third (group I)
shock with, 401
vs. sternoclavicular dislocation, 406
stress, 396, 396f
subclavian artery injury with, 393, 399–401, 400f, 411f
thoracic outlet syndrome after, 1374–1376, 1374f, 1375f
treatment of, 413–419
care after, 419
in children, 413, 419–422, 421f
complications of, 416, 416f
in distal third fracture, 439–444, 441f, 442f, 443f, 444f
external fixation in, 415
figure-of-eight bandage in, 413–415, 414f, 415f
immobilization in, 406, 413
nonunion after. See Clavicular fracture, nonunion of
open reduction and internal fixation in, 407–408, 415–416, 416f
in proximal third fracture, 416, 422
Rahmanzadeh plate in, 416
reduction in, 414–416, 414f, 415f
in shaft fracture, 422, 423–426. See also Clavicular fracture, middle third (group I)
sling in, 413, 414f
supports in, 413, 414f
vascular injury with, 399–401, 400f, 410–411, 411f, 412f, 419
Clavicular reflex, 174
Claviculectomy, 457–463, 1558, 1567–1568, 1567f
arthroscopic, 460, 460f, 984–990
in acromioclavicular arthritis, 984–985

Claviculectomy (Continued)
contraindications to, 985
indications for, 984–985
instability after, 460, 460f
lateral subacromial (indirect) approach in, 985–989, 987f, 988f, 989f, 990
vs. open procedure, 460
in osteolysis, 985, 986f
superior (direct) approach in, 460, 989–990
complete, 457–459
in complete acromioclavicular joint injury, 512, 513f
complications of, 386, 386f, 460, 460f
heterotopic ossification after, 460, 462
kinematic effects of, 231
open, 460–462, 461f, 462f
partial, 459, 459f
in fracture nonunion, 417
in neurovascular lesions, 419
in refractory infection, 579
results of, 459–460, 460f
in type III acromioclavicular joint injury, 487, 985
Clavipectoral fascia, 91–92, 105f, 106
Cleidocranial dysostosis, 117–118, 117f, 385–386, 406
Cleitrum, 1, 2f
Clinical evaluation, 145–176. See also Outcome assessment
acromioclavicular joint examination in, 165–166, 166f
Adson's maneuver in, 175–176, 175f
age in, 146
anterior slide test in, 167t, 168, 168f
apprehension tests in, 158–159, 158f
bear hug test in, 160, 161f
belly-press test in, 160, 161f
biceps load test in, 167t, 168–169, 169f, 170f
biceps tendon examination in, 166, 167f, 167t
biceps tension test in, 167–168
cervical spine examination in, 152–153, 152f
crank test in, 167t, 168, 168f
crepitus in, 151, 171
cross-body adduction maneuver for, 157, 165–166, 166f
Halstead's test in, 176
Hawkins-Kennedy impingement test in, 163–164, 163f, 166t
hyperabduction syndrome test in, 176
impingement tests in, 162–165, 163f, 166t
inspection in, 153–154, 153f, 154f
instability in, 150–151, 151b
internal rotation resistance stress test in, 164–165, 164f, 166t
Jobe-Yocum test in, 164, 164f
joint translation in, 157–158, 158f
Kim test in, 169
lift-off test in, 160, 160f
Ludington's test in, 166
Napoleon test in, 160, 161f
Neer impingement test in, 162–163, 163f, 166t
neurologic testing in, 173–174, 173f, 174f
O'Brien test in, 166–167, 167t, 168f
pain in, 147–150, 149f, 150b
pain provocation test in, 167t, 168, 169f
painful arc test in, 165, 165f
palpation in, 154, 155f
paresthesias in, 151
patient history in, 145–151
posterior-inferior labrum examination in, 169
posterior instability test in, 159, 159f
presenting complaint in, 146–151
range of motion in, 154–157, 155f, 156f, 157f
reflex testing in, 174–175, 174t

Clinical evaluation (Continued)
relocation test in, 159, 159f, 165, 165f
resting scapular positional measurements in, 171
rotator cuff examination in, 159–162, 160f, 161f
scapular assistance test in, 171
scapular dyskinesis tests in, 170–171, 171f
scapular stabilization test in, 170–171, 171f
sensory testing in, 175, 175t
sex in, 146
shoulder examination in, 153–162
active elevation for, 156
active total elevation for, 156f, 157
apprehension tests for, 158–159, 158f, 159f
cross-body adduction for, 157, 165–166, 166f
Hawkins-Kennedy impingement test for, 163–164, 163f, 166t
impingement tests for, 162–165, 163f, 166t
inspection for, 153–154, 153f, 154f
internal rotation resistance test for, 164–165, 164f, 166t
Jobe-Yocum test for, 164, 164f, 166t
modified relocation test for, 165, 165f
Neer impingement sign in, 162–163, 163f, 166t
painful arch test for, 165, 165f
palpation for, 154, 155f
passive elevation for, 155, 155f
passive external rotation for, 155f, 156, 156f
passive internal rotation for, 156f, 157
posterior instability testing for, 159, 159f
range of motion for, 154–157, 155f, 156f, 157f
rotator cuff examination of, 159–162, 160f, 161f, 162f, 165
stability assessment for, 157–158, 157f, 158f
Speed's test in, 166, 167t
stability assessment in, 157–158, 157f, 158f
strength testing in, 171–173, 172f, 172t, 173f
subcoracoid impingement test in, 169–170, 170f
superior labrum examination in, 166–169, 167t, 168f, 169f, 170f
vascular examination in, 175–176
weakness in, 151
Wright test in, 176
Yergason's test in, 166, 167f
Codman's paradox, 218, 218f, 219f
Codman's tumor, 1519, 1520f
Collateral circulation, 84–85, 85f
Compartment(s)
anesthesia, 87–88, 89f
tumor, 87, 1514
Compartment syndrome, 87, 88f
triceps rupture and, 1396
Compression devices, perioperative, 288
Computed tomography (CT), 192b
of acromioclavicular joint, 197, 457f, 471
in acromioclavicular joint injury, 500, 502, 505f
in arthroplasty, 1110–1111
in brachial plexus injury, 1379
of clavicle, 197
in clavicular fracture, 404, 405f, 598, 598f
in fibrous dysplasia, 1524, 1524f
in glenohumeral arthritis, 192, 192f, 193f
in glenohumeral arthroplasty, 193
in glenohumeral fracture, 182
in glenohumeral joint evaluation, 670f, 671, 671f, 672f
in glenoid cavity fracture, 345, 346f, 347f
in glenoid neck fracture, 344, 344f
in Hill-Sachs lesion, 188, 188f

Computed tomography *(Continued)*
  in lesser tuberosity fracture, 1058, 1058f
  in osteosarcoma, 1518f
  in Paget's disease, 1528, 1528f, 1529f
  in pediatric scapular fracture, 605, 607, 607f
  in proximal humeral fracture, 298
  in recurrent glenohumeral joint instability,
    696–697
  of scapula, 205f, 207
  in scapular fracture, 336, 338f, 339f
  in sepsis, 573
  in shoulder instability, 189–190, 189f
  of sternoclavicular joint, 198–199, 199f, 200f,
    541, 542f, 543f
Computed tomography (CT) arthrography
  of biceps tendon, 1335, 1336f
  of rotator cuff, 200, 817
Concavity-compression effect, in humeral head
    positioning, 244–245, 244f
Congenital abnormalities, 8, 117–137. *See also*
    Children *and specific abnormalities*
Conoid ligament
  anatomy of, 40, 41f, 103f, 104, 455–456,
    455f
  assessment of, 440, 441f
  clavicular motion and, 215, 216f
Constant-Murley shoulder score, 272, 273
Contracture
  deltoid, 133–134
  Dupuytren's, 1409
  posterior capsular, 1451, 1455–1457, 1456f
Coracoacromial arch
  anatomy of, 623–624, 623f, 624f, 777
  bursoscopy of, 927
  development of, 9–10
  function of, 104, 777–778
Coracoacromial ligament
  acromial traction spur in, 780f, 781–782, 781f,
    1123f
  anatomy of, 42f, 44, 45f, 455f, 456, 456f,
    776–777
    variational, 104
  bursoscopy of, 927
  calcification of, 777, 777f
  development of, 10, 11f
  resection of, 628, 779, 779f
  stabilizing properties of, 237–238, 650, 651f
  tensile properties of, 238
Coracoacromial ligament transposition, in
    acromioclavicular joint injury, 487,
    488–489, 512, 513–514, 513f
Coracobrachial bursa, 92–93
Coracobrachialis
  anatomy of, 63, 454
  cross-sectional area of, 252t
  function of, 63
  innervation of, 63, 73
  multiple insertions of, 136, 136f
  rupture of, 1400
Coracoclavicular articulation, 41, 127, 127f,
    456–458, 457f, 458f
Coracoclavicular ligament
  anatomy of, 41–42, 42f, 104, 384, 384f, 457
  ossification of, shoulder motion and, 216,
    218f
  reconstruction of
    all-arthroscopic, 1076–1079, 1078f, 1079f
    in type III acromioclavicular joint injury,
      487, 487f, 488–489, 488f
  stabilizing properties of, 456, 457f
Coracoclavicular screw, in distal clavicular
    fracture, 441–443, 442f, 443f, 444f
Coracoclaviculosternal muscle, 133, 134f
Coracoglenoid ligament, 43

Coracohumeral ligament, 60. *See also* Conoid
    ligament; Trapezoid ligament
  anatomy of, 15–16, 15f, 47, 627
    variational, 113
  in biceps tendon stabilization, 1314–1315,
    1315f
  stabilizing properties of, 238–239
Coracoid
  anatomy of, 353, 354f, 454, 624, 624f, 776
    comparative, 1–2, 2f, 3–4, 4f
    variational, 105–107, 105f, 106f
  anomalies of, 43
  arthroscopic osteotomy of, 1063–1064, 1064f
  development of, 10f, 12, 12f, 453
  double, 126, 127f
  fracture of, 335, 335f, 353–355, 354f, 355f,
    359–361. *See also* Scapular fracture
    acromial fracture and, 360–361, 360f
    arthroscopic treatment of, 1060–1061, 1061f,
      1062f
    clavicular fracture and, 361, 361b, 362f, 398
    glenoid neck fracture and, 361
    mechanisms of, 353–354
    radiography of, 205, 205f, 354, 355f, 498,
      499f, 500f
    treatment of, 369, 369f, 370f
      arthroscopic, 1060–1061, 1061f, 1062f
    type II distal clavicular fracture and, 361,
      361b, 362f
    type III acromioclavicular joint injury and,
      359–360, 364f, 498–499, 499f, 500f, 501f,
      502f
  functions of, 353
  osteotomy of, 1063–1064, 1064f
  safe side/suicide side division by, 624, 624f
  triple, 126
Coracoid-to-humeral distance, 1341
Coracoid transfer, 710–713, 710f, 711f, 713f
Coracoplasty, arthroscopic, 981, 981f
Coracosternal bone, 128
Corticosteroid injection
  in adhesive capsulitis, 995
  in stiff shoulder, 1416–1417, 1419–1420
Costoclavicular ligaments, 39, 39f, 40, 41f, 105,
    527–529, 529f, 530f
Costoclavicular space, 384, 384f
  fracture-related narrowing of, 410–411
  surgical enlargement of, 419
Costoclavicular syndrome, in clavicular fracture,
    410
Costoclavicular test, in thoracic outlet syndrome,
    1483
Costoclavicular triangle, 107
Costocoracoid band, 128
Costocoracoid ligament, in clavicular fracture–
    related subclavian vein compression, 410
Costocoracoid membrane, 105f, 106, 385
Costosternal band, 128
Costosternal bone, 128
Costovertebral band, 128, 128f
Cranial nerve XI. *See* Spinal accessory nerve
Cranial sutures, metopic, 117
Crank test, 167t, 168, 168f, 689, 691f
Crepitus
  evaluation of, 151, 171, 807, 807f
  glenohumeral, 171
  palpation for, 807, 807f
  scapulothoracic, 171, 367–368, 367f, 368f, 376
Cross-body adduction maneuver/test, 157,
    165–166, 166f, 467, 468f
Cuff tear arthropathy, 1254. *See also* Rotator cuff
    tear arthropathy
Cyst(s)
  acromioclavicular, 515–516, 516f, 517f

Cyst(s) *(Continued)*
  bone
    aneurysmal, 1523, 1523f
    simple, 585f, 1522f, 1523, 1533f
  ganglion, 1528
    vs. rotator cuff tear, 819, 819f
    suprascapular nerve injury with, 1372,
      1372f, 1373f, 1374, 1482, 1482f
Cytokines, in idiopathic stiff shoulder, 1409

D

Da Vinci, Leonardo, 34f, 35–36
Dead arm, 1450
Dead man's angle, 967, 968f
DeAnguin's test, 1333, 1334f
Débridement
  in glenohumeral osteoarthritis, 1004–1006,
    1004f, 1005f
  in infected arthroplasty, 1279
  in throwing-related SLAP lesion, 1035, 1037
Degenerative joint disease. *See* Osteoarthritis
Deltoid
  activity of, 252–255, 254f, 255f
  anatomy of, 58–59, 58f, 59f, 87, 88f, 454,
    622–623, 774f, 775, 1394
    comparative, 4, 4f
    variational, 109–110, 110f, 111–112
  angle phenomenon at, 1074
  anterior head of, 112
  in arm elevation, 252–255, 254f, 255f, 258,
    260
  atrophy of, 1364–1365
  blood supply of, 59
  clavicular head of, 109
  contracture of, 133–134
  cross-sectional area of, 252t
  dissection of, 51, 53f, 73, 89
  function of, 58, 59f
  heterotopic ossification of, after arthroscopy,
    916
  injection-related contracture of, 133–134
  innervation of, 59, 73
  insertion of, 58
  inspection of, 153, 153f
  insufficiency of, after rotator cuff tear surgery,
    903–905, 904f
  internal structure of, 58, 58f
  lateral head of, 111–112
  origin of, 40, 41f, 58
  palpation of, 154
  postarthroplasty dysfunction of, 58
  posterior head of, 109–110
  rupture of, 1394–1395
    in elderly, 1394
  stabilizing function of, 247–248
  strength testing of, 173, 173f
Deltoid artery, 82–83, 82f, 85f
Deltoid splitting incision, 51, 53f, 89
  for acromioplasty, 774f, 775, 827f, 829, 831,
    831f
Deltoidplasty, 905
Desmoid, 1528–1530
Development, 5–11
  embryonic, 6–8, 6f, 7f, 8f, 9f
  fetal, 8–11, 10f, 11f
  postnatal, 11–12, 12f, 13f
Diabetes mellitus
  cheiroarthropathy in, 1410
  limited joint motion syndrome in, 1410–1411
  stiff shoulder and, 1410–1411
Diagnosis. *See* Clinical evaluation
Dialysis, 1008, 1331
Diaphysis, development of, 8–9

Disabilities of the Arm, Shoulder and Hand
(DASH) questionnaire, 268–269, 274
Disability. *See also* Occupational shoulder
disorders
compensation systems for, 1503–1505
evaluation of, 1501–1503
Disarticulation. *See also* Amputation (surgical)
shoulder, 1557, 1560–1561, 1560f, 1562f
Dislocation
biceps tendon. *See* Biceps tendon,
dislocation of
glenohumeral joint. *See* Glenohumeral
joint dislocation
scapular. *See* Scapula (scapulae),
dislocation of
sternoclavicular joint. *See* Sternoclavicular
joint dislocation
Dorsal epitrochlearis, 136–137, 136f
Dorsal scapular artery, 80, 85f
Dorsal scapular nerve, 70
Drawer test, 688, 689f
Drive-through sign, 955f
Drive-through test, 936–937
Drugs
overdose of, compression syndromes with, 87
stiff shoulder with, 1412
Duchenne, G.B., 36, 36f
Dupuytren's contracture, 1409
DuToit staple capsulorrhaphy, 706–707, 709f
complications of, 716–717
Dysostosis
cleidocranial, 117–118, 117f, 385–386, 406
mutational, 117
Dysplasia, fibrous, 1524, 1524f, 1533f, 1536,
1537

E

Ecchymosis, 154
Ectoderm, 5
Eden-Hybbinette procedure, 708, 710
Eden-Lange procedure, 1368–1369
Effort thrombosis, 1483
Effusion, subacromial, 154, 154f
Elbow dislocation, 235, 237f
Electric shock injury, posterior shoulder
instability and, 151
Electromyography
of biceps brachii, 1324–1325
in proximal humeral fracture, 297
in recurrent glenohumeral joint instability, 697
Embolism
air, 289, 911
pulmonary, 914
Embryology, 6–8, 6f, 7f, 8f, 9f
Emphysema, stiff shoulder and, 1411
Empty groove sign, 1336
Enchondroma, 1519–1520, 1520f, 1521f, 1533f
Ender rod fixation, in proximal humeral fracture,
317–318, 318f
Endoderm, 5
Endoneurium, 67
Eosinophilic granuloma, vs. tumor, 1538
Epidural block, with interscalene block, 285
Epilepsy, posterior shoulder instability and, 151
Epinephrine
in arthroscopy, 915
in local anesthetic solution, 287
Epineurium, 68
Epiphysis
clavicular, 11–12, 12f, 40
development of, 8–9
dysplasia of, 132, 133f
humeral tuberosity, 12

Epitrochlearis, dorsal, 136–137, 136f
Ergonomics, in occupational shoulder disorders,
1495, 1496–1498
Erythema, 154
Erythrocyte sedimentation rate (ESR), 1413
Eulerian angles, 218, 220–221, 221f
Evaluation. *See* Clinical evaluation
Ewing's sarcoma, 1525–1526, 1527f
chemotherapy in, 1551
fracture with, 1536
treatment of, 1549–1550
Exercise program
after arthroplasty, 1192–1197, 1193f, 1194f,
1195f, 1196f
after clavicular fracture, 419
in glenohumeral joint arthritis, 1131, 1132f,
1133f, 1134f, 1135f
after glenohumeral joint stabilization
procedures, 956
Jackins. *See* Jackins program
for rotator cuff tear in elderly, 851–865, 853f,
855f–865f
after subacromial abrasion treatment, 831–832,
832f, 833f
Exostoses, 1533f
osteochondroma and, 1518–1519
throwing-related, 1042–1043
Extracellular matrix graft, in rotator cuff tear
treatment, 1577–1579, 1578t
Extracorporeal shock wave therapy, in calcifying
tendinitis, 1297–1299, 1298t, 1302–1303
Eyebrow sign, 810f, 811

F

Facioscapulohumeral muscular dystrophy, 1377,
1377f
Fallen-leaf sign, 1523
Fascial planes, 89, 90f
hypovascular, 80, 89, 90f
Fascial spaces, 37f, 89, 90f
Fascicles, 68, 76–77, 78f
Federal Employer's Liability Act, 1505
Fetus, 8–11, 10f, 11f
Fibroblasts, in idiopathic stiff shoulder, 1409
Fibroma, nonossifying, 1524, 1525f
Fibromatosis, 1528–1530, 1548
Fibrosarcoma, congenital, 1530
Fibrous cortical defect, 1524
Fibrous dysplasia, 1524, 1524f, 1533f, 1537
fracture with, 1536
Figure-of-eight bandage, in clavicular fracture,
413, 414f, 415f, 420–421
Fish, fins of, 1, 2f
Flail shoulder, 1544–1545
Floating clavicle, 391
Floating shoulder, 358–359, 358f, 399
in children, 608, 609f
Fluid extravasation, arthroscopy-related, 914–915
Fluid-fluid level, in aneurysmal bone cyst, 1523,
1523f
Forelimb, comparative anatomy of, 1–5, 2f, 3f,
4f, 5f
Forequarter amputation, 1557, 1561, 1563f,
1564–1565
anterior approach to, 1561, 1563f, 1564
posterior approach to, 1564–1565, 1565f
Fossa axillaris, 6
Fracture. *See also specific fracture*
cyst-related, 584, 585f
periprosthetic, 1228, 1229, 1229f, 1230f
tumor-related, 1536, 1536f
Frozen shoulder. *See* Stiff shoulder, idiopathic
(frozen shoulder)

Fulcrum test, 689, 690f
Fungal infection, vs. tumor, 1537

G

Galen, 34–35
Gallie procedure, 713
Ganglion cyst, 1026–1028, 1528
arthroscopic treatment of, 1027–1028
diagnosis of, 1027, 1027f
nonoperative treatment of, 1027
vs. rotator cuff tear, 819, 819f
suprascapular nerve injury with, 1372, 1372f,
1373f, 1374, 1482, 1482f
Gaucher's disease, 1526
Gender, in patient history, 146
Germ layers, 5
Geyser sign, 813, 814f
Giant cell tumor, 1525, 1533f, 1551
Gilliatt-Sumner hand, 1374
Glenohumeral index, 231
Glenohumeral internal rotation deficit, throwing-
related, 1451–1452, 1451f
Glenohumeral joint. *See also* Glenoid; Humerus
anatomy of, 12–15, 13f, 14f, 15f
comparative, 1–5, 2f, 3f, 4f
historical perspective on, 33–38, 34f, 35f,
36f, 37f
arthritis of. *See* Glenohumeral joint arthritis
biomechanics of, 629–650, 1406–1407, 1406f
constraint (stability), 214t, 230–250, 230t,
629–650
acromial load transduction and, 650,
651f
adhesion-cohesion in, 646–647
articular contribution to, 231–235, 231f,
232f, 233f, 234f, 235f, 236f
balance stability angle in, 630, 631f, 632f,
633–634, 634f
barrier effect in, 245
biceps tendon in, 246–247, 1324, 1325
capsular contribution to, 235, 237,
237f, 238f
clinical applications of, 248–250,
249f, 251f
compressive forces in, 649–650,
649f, 650f
concavity-compression effect in,
243–245, 244f
coracoacromial ligament in, 237–238,
650, 651f
coracohumeral ligament in, 238–239
deltoid in, 247–248
at end range of motion, 231
in glenohumeral arthroplasty, 1099–1106.
See also Arthroplasty, biomechanics of
glenoidogram in, 634–637, 635f, 636f,
637t
inferior glenohumeral ligament in, 239f,
240–243, 240f, 241f, 243f, 644–646,
644f, 645f, 646f
ligaments in, 235, 237–245, 238f, 644–646,
644f, 645f, 646f
limited joint volume effect in, 647–648,
648f
at mid range of motion, 231
middle glenohumeral ligament in, 238f,
239f, 240, 644–646
net humeral joint reaction force in, 630,
631f, 632–633, 632f, 633f
passive muscle tension in, 243, 244f
resting, 648–649
rotator cuff in, 245–246, 246f
rotator interval in, 239

Glenohumeral joint (Continued)
    scapular positioning and, 234–235, 236f,
      639–640, 640f
    stability ratio in, 633–634, 634f, 636f, 637
    suction cup effect in, 647, 647f
    superior, 649–650, 649f, 650f, 651f
    superior glenohumeral ligament in,
      239–240, 239f, 240f, 644–646
  force transmission (strength), 214t, 250,
    252–258
    with arm elevation, 254–258, 256f,
      257f, 258f
    clinical applications of, 260, 260f
    in glenohumeral arthroplasty, 1106–1107,
      1106f
    joint contact pressure in, 258–259
    maximal torque in, 259–260, 259f, 259t
    muscle activity in, 252–254, 254f, 255f
    muscle orientation in, 250, 252f, 253f,
      254f
    muscle size in, 250
  glenoid arc in, 630, 631f, 632f
  glenoid version in, 637–639, 638f, 639f
  glenoidogram of, 634–637, 635f, 636f, 637t
  vs. hip joint, 630, 630f
  kinematic (motion), 214t, 217–230
    arm elevation, 224, 225f, 226f
    articular surface in, 222–224, 223f, 224f
    biceps brachii in, 1325
    center of rotation in, 226–228, 228f
    clinical applications of, 228–230, 228f,
      229f, 230f
    Codman's paradox in, 218, 218f
    description of, 218–220, 220f
    Eulerian angles in, 220–221, 221f
    external humerus rotation, 225–226, 227f
    in glenohumeral arthroplasty, 1089–1099.
      See also Arthroplasty
    glenoid in, 223–224, 224f
    humeroscapular motion interface in,
      624–626, 625f
    humerus in, 222–223, 223f
    measurement of, 218–219
    resting posture and, 222, 222f
    rolling, 220, 220f
    rotator cuff in, 1325
    in rotator cuff tear, 230, 230f
    screw axis in, 221, 222f, 228, 228f
    sliding, 220, 220f
    spinning, 220, 220f
    three-dimensional, 220–221, 221f, 222f
    two-dimensional, 219–220, 220f
    vs. knee joint, 630, 630f
  ligaments in, 626–628, 627f, 640–644, 641f,
    642f, 643f
  scapular positioning in, 639–640, 640f
  stability ratio in, 633–634, 635f
  capsule of
    anatomy of, 15–16, 15f, 16f
    blood supply of, 28
    collagen of, 235
    development of, 10–11
    innervation of, 28–29
    laxity of, 1089–1090, 1090f
    mechanoreceptors of, 248
    redundancy of, 235
    stability contribution of, 235, 237, 237f, 238f
    synovial lining of, 20, 22, 22f, 23f, 115
    tensile strength of, 235, 237f, 238f
    thickness of, 22, 22f, 23f
  center of rotation of, 226–228, 228f
  chondrolysis of, thermal capsulorrhaphy
    and, 918
  contact pressure of, 258–259

Glenohumeral joint (Continued)
  dislocation of. See Glenohumeral joint
    dislocation; Glenohumeral joint
    instability
  evaluation of. See Clinical evaluation
  forces at, 254–258, 256f, 257f, 258f
  fracture of. See Humeral fracture (proximal)
  vs. hip joint, 630, 630f
  infection of. See Sepsis
  instability of. See Glenohumeral joint
    instability
  intra-articular pressure of, 235, 236f
    loss of, 250, 251f
  vs. knee joint, 630, 630f
  osteoarthritis of. See Glenohumeral joint
    arthritis, dégénerative
  radiography of, 228, 228f. See also
    Radiography
  resection of, 1543f, 1544
  rheumatoid arthritis of. See Glenohumeral
    joint arthritis, rheumatoid
  subluxation of, 654. See also Glenohumeral
    joint dislocation; Glenohumeral joint
    instability
  type A, 13–14
  type B, 13–14
  type C, 13–14
Glenohumeral joint arthritis, 1089–1238. See also
  Capsulorrhaphy arthropathy;
  Osteonecrosis; Rotator cuff tear
  arthropathy
  arthrodesis for, 1135–1143
    indications for, 1137t
    in infected arthroplasty, 1280
    Matsen's technique for, 1137–1143, 1141f,
      1142f, 1143f, 1144f, 1145f
    position for, 229, 229f, 1137–1138
    postresection, 1545–1547
    Rockwood's technique for, 1143
    in septic disease, 579
  arthroplasty for, 1144–1191. See also
    Arthroplasty
  arthroscopic treatment of, 1002–1010
    capsular release in, 1006
    débridement in, 1004–1006, 1004f, 1005f
    distal clavicle excision in, 1006
    glenoid resurfacing in, 1007–1008
    glenoidplasty in, 1007
    imaging for, 1003–1004
    indications for, 1003
    loose body removal in, 1004–1005, 1004f
    microfracture technique in, 1007
    physical examination for, 1003
    setup for, 1004
    subacromial decompression in, 1006
  vs. biceps tendinitis, 1341
  computed tomography in, 192f, 193f
  degenerative, 1100f, 1115, 1115b
    after anterior instability treatment, 101–102
    after arthroscopic procedures, 957
    epidemiology of, 1003
    imaging in, 1003–1004
    occupational disorders and, 1495–1496
    physical examination in, 1003
    primary, 1112b, 1114f, 1115, 1115b, 1115f,
      1126t, 1191, 1254–1255
    secondary, 957, 1112b, 1116f, 1117–1118,
      1118b, 1118f, 1126t, 1192
  evaluation of, 1107–1115
    comorbidities in, 1108
    patient history in, 1107–1108
    physical examination in, 1109
    radiography in, 1109–1111, 1109f, 1110f,
      1111f, 1114f, 1115f

Glenohumeral joint arthritis (Continued)
    self-assessment in, 1108, 1111, 1113–1115,
      1113b, 1113t, 1114t
  in golfer, 1446
  neurotrophic, 1129, 1130f
  nonoperative treatment of, 1131, 1132f, 1133f,
    1134f, 1135f
  pain in, 148
  periarticular osteotomy for, 1144
  vs. radiation-related injury, 1129–1130
  radiography in, 191–192, 191f, 1109–1111
    anteroposterior view for, 1109–1110, 1109f
    axillary view for, 1109–1110, 1109f
    templating view for, 1110, 1110f, 1111f
  range of motion in, 1089, 1090f
  rheumatoid, 1102f, 1112b, 1118–1122, 1119f,
    1120f, 1121f, 1122b, 1122f, 1126t
  vs. rotator cuff tear, 818, 818f
  self-assessment in, 1108, 1111, 1113–1115,
    1113b, 1113t, 1114t
  septic, 566–567, 567t, 571, 1130. See also
    Sepsis
  synovial fluid examination in, 572, 572t
  treatment of, 575–579, 576f, 577t
  synovectomy for, 1131–1133
  vs. tumor-related pain, 1130, 1131f
Glenohumeral joint dislocation, 654, 661–678.
    See also Glenohumeral joint instability
  anterior, 654–655, 654f, 655f, 666, 671–678
    age and, 677
    axillary artery injury with, 672, 676–677,
      676f
    axillary nerve injury with, 676–677, 676f
    fracture with, 671, 673f, 674f, 675f, 677–678,
      682–683
    glenohumeral ligament injury with, 666,
      671, 672f
    historical perspective on, 619–620, 620f
    intrathoracic, 655, 655f
    joint volume and, 250
    nerve injury with, 676–677, 676f
    patient history in, 661
    physical examination in, 661
    proprioceptive function and, 248
    radiography of, 183, 185f, 186f, 662–666,
      664f, 666f, 668f, 669f
    recurrence of, 677–678. See also
      Glenohumeral joint instability, recurrent
    retroperitoneal, 655, 655f
    rotator cuff tears with, 672
    soft tissue interposition in, 682
    subclavicular, 655
    subcoracoid, 654, 654f
    subglenoid, 655
    in throwing athlete, 1472–1478, 1473f,
      1474f, 1475f, 1476f
    treatment of, 678–683, 680f
      for acute dislocation, 678–681, 680f
      analgesia in, 678–680, 680f
      arthroscopic, 945
      in athlete, 945
      capsulolabral double row fixation in,
        1050–1053, 1051f, 1052f, 1053f
      for chronic dislocation, 681
      displaced greater tuberosity fracture
        fragment and, 682–683
      early surgery in, 682–683
      evaluation of, 681
      glenoid rim fracture and, 683
      magnetic resonance arthrography of,
        190–191, 191f
      open reduction in, 681
      operative, 682–683
      recurrent instability after, 677

Glenohumeral joint dislocation (*Continued*)
    reduction technique for, 678–681, 679f,
        680f
        rehabilitation after, 682
        soft tissue interposition and, 682
        strengthening exercises after, 682
        vascular injury with, 675
    vascular injury with, 672, 674–676, 676f
    bilateral, 658, 661
    computed tomography in, 670f, 671, 671f,
        672f
    congenital, 133
    force required for, 235, 237f
    historical perspective on, 617–622, 618f, 620f
    inferior, 656–658, 659f, 660f
    patient history in, 661
    physical examination in, 661–662
    posterior, 655–656, 656f, 657f–658f, 678
        chronic, 684
        cuff injury with, 678
        fractures with, 678, 678f
        historical perspective on, 621–622
        mechanisms of, 151, 656f, 657
        nerve injury with, 678
        patient history in, 661
        physical examination in, 661–662, 662f
        radiography of, 188–189, 662–666, 666f,
            669f, 1898f
        subacromial, 655, 656f
        subglenoid, 655
        subspinous, 655
        in throwing athlete, 1477–1479
        treatment of, 683–684, 684f, 685f
            operative, 683–684
            reduction for, 683, 684, 684f
    radiography in, 183, 662–666
        anteroposterior view for, 662–663, 662f,
            663f, 664f
        apical oblique view for, 183, 186f, 666,
            669f, 670f
        axillary view for, 665–666, 667f, 668f, 669f
        scapular lateral view for, 663, 665f, 666f
        Velpeau axillary lateral view for, 666, 667f
        West Point axillary lateral view for, 183,
            185f, 666f, 668f
    recurrent. *See* Glenohumeral joint instability,
        recurrent
    superior, 658, 661f
Glenohumeral joint instability, 617–760. *See also*
        Glenohumeral joint dislocation
    acute, 651
    anatomy of, 622–629
        coracoacromial arch in, 623–624, 623f, 624f
        coracoid process in, 624, 624f
        cutaneous, 622, 622f
        glenoid concavity in, 628–629, 628f, 629f
        glenoid labrum in, 629, 629f
        humeroscapular motion interface in,
            624–626, 625f
        ligamentous, 626–628, 626f, 627f
        muscular, 622–623, 623f
        rotator cuff in, 626, 626f
    apprehension with, 654
    vs. biceps tendinitis, 1340
    biomechanics of, 629–650. *See also*
        Glenohumeral joint, biomechanics of
    as chief complaint, 147
    chronic, 651
    congenital, 651
    degree of, 654
    evaluation of, 150–151, 151b, 157–158, 157f
        arthroscopic, 941–942, 941b
        imaging in, 662–666, 662f–672f
        jerk test in, 637, 637f, 638f, 688f, 689, 691f

Glenohumeral joint instability (*Continued*)
    magnetic resonance imaging in, 189f, 190,
        190f
    patient history in, 661
    physical examination in, 661–662
    gender and, 146
    in golfer, 1446
    historical perspective on, 617–622, 618f, 619f,
        620f
    involuntary, 652
    jerk test in, 637, 637f, 638f, 688f, 689, 691f
    magnetic resonance imaging in, 189f, 190,
        190f
    neuromuscular, 652
    occupational consequences of, 654
    postarthroplasty, 1227–1228, 1227f
        revision arthroplasty for, 1232f, 1233f, 1234,
            1234f, 1235f
    recurrent, 651, 652, 654, 684–760. *See also*
        Glenohumeral joint dislocation
        atraumatic (multidirectional), 651, 652, 652f,
            940–941
            age and, 686, 686f
            apprehension test in, 689, 691f
            arthroscopic treatment of, 952–956
                capsular plication in, 953–954, 955–956,
                    955f
                capsular shift in, 953
                capsular volume reduction with,
                    953–954
                management after, 956
                rotator interval closure in, 955
                thermal capsulorrhaphy in, 917–918,
                    954–955
            capsular shift reconstruction for, 758–759,
                759f
            crank test in, 689, 691f
            drawer test in, 688, 689f
            evaluation of, 684–691, 686t, 687f–692f
            fulcrum test in, 689, 690f
            generalized laxity and, 652, 652f
            infraspinatus test in, 692f
            jerk test in, 688f, 689, 691f
            laxity tests in, 687–689, 689f
            lift-off test in, 689, 692f
            load and shift test in, 687, 688f
            no-touch examination in, 687, 688f
            nonoperative treatment of, 700–701, 701f,
                702f–703f, 757–758
            open operative treatment of, 756–759,
                759f, 953
                results of, 757
                Rockwood's approach to, 757–759,
                    759f
            patient history in, 686, 686t, 687f
            physical examination in, 687–689, 688f
            provocative stability tests in, 689, 690f,
                691f
            push-pull test in, 688–689, 690f
            radiography in, 689, 691
            rehabilitation program for, 757–758
            strength tests in, 689, 692f
            subscapularis test in, 692f
            sulcus test in, 688, 690f
            supraspinatus test in, 692f
            TheraBand rehabilitation program for,
                757–758
            trapezius shrug test in, 692f
            vs. traumatic, 715
        failed treatment of, 759, 759f
        nonoperative treatment of, 700–701, 701f,
            702f–703f
        traumatic (anterior), 652, 654, 691,
            693–742

Glenohumeral joint instability (*Continued*)
    arthroscopic evaluation of, 697–698, 698f,
        699f
    arthroscopic treatment of, 942–949
        complications of, 957
        contraindications to, 944
        HAGL lesion and, 944–945
        indications for, 945–946, 946f
        management after, 956
        vs. open treatment, 943–944
        results of, 942–943
        suture anchors in, 943, 948, 948f
        technique of, 946–949, 947f, 948f, 949f
    vs. atraumatic instability, 715
    computed tomography in, 696–697
    electromyography in, 697
    evaluation of, 691, 694–699, 694f, 695f,
        696f, 697f, 698f, 699f, 941–942, 941b
    failed repair of, 714–718, 715, 715f, 716f,
        719f, 720f
    historical perspective on, 619–621, 620f
    magnetic resonance imaging in, 697,
        697f, 698f
    mechanisms of, 691, 693, 693f, 940
    nonoperative treatment in, 700–701, 700f,
        701f, 702f–703f
    open operative treatment of, 701–742,
        942
        bone block in, 708, 710
        Boytchev procedure in, 714
        capsulolabral reconstruction in,
            704–705, 705f, 706f, 707f
        capsulorrhaphy arthropathy after, 101
        complications of, 714–718, 715f, 716f,
            717f, 719f, 720f
        coracoid transfer in, 710–713, 711f,
            712f, 713f
        degenerative arthritis after, 101–102
        degenerative disease after, 717–718
        Eden-Hybbinette procedure in, 708,
            710
        Gallie procedure in, 713
        glenoid neck osteotomy in, 714
        hardware-related complications of,
            716–717, 716f, 717f
        Helfet-Bristow procedure in, 710–713,
            711f, 712f, 713f, 716, 716f
        historical perspective on, 621
        humeral osteotomy in, 714
        infection after, 714
        Latarjet procedure in, 713
        limited motion after, 717
        Magnuson-Stack procedure in, 708,
            709f, 710f, 717
        Matsen and Lippitt's preferred method
            of, 718, 721–737
            anterior glenoid decortication for,
                724, 724f
            anterior glenoid exposure for, 722,
                724, 724f
            clavipectoral fascia exposure for,
                721, 723f
            glenoid holes for, 724, 725f
            goals of, 718, 721f
            graft for, 726, 730f, 731f, 732f, 733f,
                734f
            incision for, 718, 721, 722f
            instruments for, 718, 721f
            position for, 718, 722f
            rehabilitation after, 727–729, 735f
            subcutaneous dissection for, 721,
                723f
            subscapularis incision for, 721, 723f,
                724f

Glenohumeral joint instability *(Continued)*
  subscapularis repair for, 726–727,
    734f, 735f
  subscapularis tendon reefing for,
    727, 735f
  sutures for, 724–725, 725f, 726f, 727f
  misdiagnosis and, 715
  neurovascular complications of,
    715–716
  Nicola procedure in, 713–714
  Oudard procedure in, 710
  Putti-Platt procedure in, 707–708, 717
  recurrent instability after, 715, 715f
  Rockwood and Wirth's preferred
    method of, 729, 734–742
    axillary nerve in, 736, 738f
    capsule division for, 736–737,
      738f–739f
    capsule shift and reconstruction for,
      737, 740f
    care after, 741–742
    closure for, 737
    incision for, 729, 734–735, 738f–740f
    musculocutaneous nerve in, 736,
      741f
    results of, 742
    subscapular tendon division for, 736,
      738f–739f
    summary of, 737, 741
  Saha procedure in, 714
  staple capsulorrhaphy in, 706–707,
    709f, 716–717, 716f, 717f
  subscapularis failure after, 718, 719f,
    720f
  Trillat procedure in, 710
patient history in, 694, 694f
physical examination in, 694–695
radiography in, 695–699, 695f
  apical oblique view for, 696
  axillary view for, 696, 697f
  glenoid changes on, 696, 697f
  humeral head changes on, 695–696
  Stryker notch view for, 695, 696f
refractory, 715, 715f
rotator cuff imaging in, 697
strengthening exercises in, 700–701, 700f,
  701f, 702f–703f
taping in, 700, 701f
traumatic (posterior), 941
  arthroscopic treatment of, 950–952, 951f,
    952f
    complications of, 957
    management after, 956
  evaluation of, 159, 159f, 941–942, 941b
  historical perspective on, 621–622
  open operative treatment of, 742–756
    anterior capsular shift reconstruction in,
      750–752, 756, 756f
    bone block in, 743–744
    complications of, 744
    evaluation for, 744, 747f
    glenoid osteotomy in, 248–249, 249f,
      743–744, 743f, 745f, 747–749,
      754f–755f
    humeral osteotomy in, 743
    indications for, 742
    Matsen's preferred method of, 744, 746
      deltoid repair for, 746, 752f
      deltoid split for, 744, 747f
      external rotator split for, 746, 748f
      glenoid osteotomy for, 746, 749f,
        750f
      graft for, 746, 751f, 752f
      incision for, 744, 747f

Glenohumeral joint instability *(Continued)*
    posterior capsule exposure for, 746,
      748f
  Rockwood and Wirth's preferred
    method of, 746–756, 753f–755f
    capsular shift reconstruction for,
      750–752, 756, 756f
    glenoid osteotomy for, 747–749,
      754f–755f
    incision for, 746, 753f
    soft tissue repair in, 743
  in swimmer, 1444–1445
  voluntary, 652, 653f, 757–758
Glenohumeral ligament(s)
  anatomy of, 16–22, 18f, 19f, 626–628, 626f
    arthroscopic, 924–926, 924f, 925f, 926f, 936,
      936f, 938
    variational, 113–114, 113f, 114f, 115f
  anterior-inferior, 17f, 62
  bipolar (floating), 945
  arthroscopy of, 924–926, 924f, 925f, 926f
  avulsion of, 644–646, 645f
  blood supply of, 28
  checkrein effect of, 644, 644f, 645f
  countervailing force effect of, 644–645, 645f
  development of, 10–11
  elasticity of, 640–641, 641f, 643
  Hawkins' load-shift maneuver for, 929
  inferior. *See also* Inferior glenohumeral
    ligament complex
    anatomy of, 17–22, 17f, 18f, 19f, 113f, 114,
      240–242, 241f, 627–628, 924–925, 924f,
      925f
    anterior band of, 2f, 18–22, 20f, 21f, 25f,
      242, 924, 925–926, 925f, 926f, 936
    arthroscopy of, 17–22, 19f, 21f, 22f,
      924–925, 925f, 936
    avulsion of, 249–250, 644–646, 645f
    posterior band of, 18–22, 20f, 21f, 22f, 23f,
      24f, 241–242, 924–925, 926, 937–938,
      938f
    stabilizing properties of, 238f, 240–243,
      240f, 241f, 644–646, 644f, 645f
    superior band of, 17, 19f
  laxity of, 231, 641, 641f, 642f, 687–689
  middle, 17f
    absence of, 16–17
    anatomy of, 16–17, 18f, 62, 113–114, 113f,
      115f, 627, 924, 925f
    arthroscopy of, 924, 924f, 925, 925f, 936,
      936f
    cord-like, 114, 115f
    stabilizing properties of, 238f, 239f, 240,
      240f, 241f, 242, 644–646, 644f, 645f
    thickness of, 17, 18f
  plastic deformability of, 640–641, 641f
  resting length of, 640, 641f
  rotational laxity of, 641, 641f, 687–689
  strength of, 641
  stretchiness of, 643
  superior
    anatomy of, 16, 17f, 18f, 113f, 114, 627,
      924, 924f
    arthroscopy of, 924, 924f, 925, 936
    in biceps tendon stabilization, 1314–1315,
      1315f
    stabilizing properties of, 238f, 239–240,
      239f, 240f, 241f, 242, 644–646, 644f,
      645f
  throwing-related changes in, 1446–1447
  translational laxity of, 641, 641f, 642f, 643,
    643f, 687–689
Glenohumeral ratio, 223–224
Glenohumeral recesses, 113–114, 114f

Glenoid. *See also* Glenoid labrum
  anatomy of, 13–14, 14f, 44, 296, 924
    variational, 114–115
  anteversion of, 231, 638–639
  arthroscopic evaluation of, 924
  arthroscopic resurfacing of, 1007–1008
  articular surface of, 223–224, 224f
  balance stability angle of, 630, 631f, 632f,
    633–634, 634f
  bare area of, 13, 14f, 233
  cartilage lesions of, arthroscopic treatment of,
    1048–1050, 1049f, 1050f, 1051f
  center line of, 634–635, 635f
  center of rotation of, 623–624, 623f
  deficiency of
    in arthroplasty, 1580–1581, 1580f, 1581f
    hypoplastic, 124–125, 125f, 638, 639f
    in revision arthroplasty, 1237f, 1238, 1238f
    in rotator cuff tear arthropathy, 1251,
      1251b, 1251f
    in throwing athlete, 1473, 1473f
  dentated, 129, 129f
  depth of, 232
  development of, 11, 12
  dysplasia of, 234, 637–638, 638f
  fracture of. *See* Glenoid fracture
  humeral head centering in, 244–245, 244f,
    628–629, 628f
  hypoplasia of, 124–125, 125f, 638, 639f
  inclination of, 115
  joint reaction force effects on, 258
  loosening of
    after arthroplasty, 260, 260f
    in rotator cuff–deficient shoulder, 260
  motion of, 233–234, 234f. *See also*
    Glenohumeral joint, biomechanics of
  osteoarthritis of, arthroplasty and, 1580–1581,
    1580f, 1581f
  osteotomy of, in posterior glenohumeral joint
    instability, 248–249, 249f, 743–744, 743f,
    745f, 746, 749f, 750f
  retroversion of, 114–115, 231, 638–639, 639f
  rocking horse, 260, 1105, 1105f
  in rotator cuff tear, 797, 797f, 798f
  size of, 114
  superoinferior line of, 13, 14f
  upward tilt of, 234, 235f
  version of, 231, 231f, 637–639, 638f
Glenoid arc
  in arthroplasty, 1101–1104, 1102f, 1103f, 1104f
  effective, 630, 631f, 632f, 633–634, 634f
Glenoid center line, 634–635, 635f
Glenoid fracture
  cavity, 335, 335f, 344–352, 344f, 345b
    classification of, 344, 345f
    fossa, 345, 345f, 346f, 347f, 348–342
      treatment of, 374–375, 374f, 375f
      type II, 345f, 348, 349f
      type III, 345f, 348, 349f, 350
      type IV, 345f, 350, 350f
      type V, 345f, 350, 351f
      type VI, 345f, 350, 352
    imaging of, 345, 346f, 347f
    rim (type I), 345, 345f, 346f, 348, 373–374
      anterior glenohumeral dislocation and,
        620f, 671, 671f, 673f, 683
      arthroscopic treatment of, 1053–1054,
        1054f
      posterior glenohumeral joint dislocation
        and, 671f, 678, 678f
      treatment of, 369–375, 371b, 371f, 372f,
        373f, 374f, 375f
    neck, 335, 335f, 336–338, 340–344, 340b,
      340f, 361

Glenoid fracture *(Continued)*
    anatomy of, 337–338, 340f, 341f
    computed tomography of, 344, 344f
    coracoid fracture and, 361
    fragment angulation with, 341, 341f, 343f
    mechanisms of, 337–338, 340f, 341f
    midshaft clavicular fracture and, 358–359,
        358f
    radiography of, 344, 344f
    treatment of, 341–344, 369–373, 371b, 371f,
        372f, 373f, 374f, 375–376, 376f
    type I, 338, 341f
    type II, 338, 340–341, 341f, 342f, 343f
Glenoid labrum
    age-related changes in, 232, 232f
    anatomy of, 14, 15f, 628–629, 628f, 629f,
        1457, 1457f
        arthroscopic, 922f, 923–924, 923f, 937
        biceps tendon relationship to, 1020–1021
        variational, 115, 923–924, 923f, 1021,
            1457, 1457f
    arteries of, 27–28, 28f
    arthroscopy of, 923–924, 923f, 925, 934f,
        935–936, 935f
    Bankart repair of. *See* Bankart repair
    cadaveric studies of, 629
    Cassiopeia double row fixation of, 1050–1053,
        1051f, 1052f, 1053f
    collagen fibers of, 231–232
    development of, 7, 8f, 9
    double row fixation of, 1050–1053, 1051f,
        1052f, 1053f
    evaluation of, 166–169, 167t, 168f
        arthroscopic, 923–924, 923f, 934f, 935–936,
            935f
    function of, 923, 1457–1458
    sulcus of, 923, 923f
    tears of, 629. *See also* Bankart lesion; Bankart
        repair; SLAP (superior labrum anterior
        and posterior) lesion
    vs. biceps tendinitis, 1340–1341
    tensile strength of, 235, 237f
Glenoid osteotomy
    in anterior glenohumeral joint instability,
        714
    in posterior glenohumeral joint instability,
        248–249, 249f, 743–744, 743f, 745f, 746,
        749f, 750f
Glenoid prosthesis, 1161–1165, 1162f, 1163f,
        1164f. *See also* Arthroplasty
    alternative bearing surfaces for, 1581–1583,
        1582f
    arthroscopic revision of, 1083–1085, 1083f,
        1084f, 1085f
    bearing surfaces of, 1581–1583, 1582f
    loosening of, 260, 260f, 1009, 1223, 1225,
        1237f, 1238, 1581–1583, 1582f
    reimplantation of, 1280–1282, 1280f, 1281f
    removal of, 1009, 1237f, 1238
    wear of, 1225, 1226f
Glenoidogram, 634–637, 635f, 636f, 637t
Glenoidplasty. *See also* Arthroplasty
    in glenohumeral osteoarthritis, 1007
Glenopolar angle, 611, 611f
Golfer
    acromioclavicular joint disease in, 1446
    arthritis in, 1446
    glenohumeral instability in, 1446
    rotator cuff injury in, 1445–1446
    SLAP lesion in, 1446
    subacromial impingement in, 1445–1446
    swing biomechanics in, 1445, 1445f
Gout, acromioclavicular joint, 515
Gram stain, in septic arthritis, 572, 572t

Greater tuberosity. *See* Humeral tuberosity,
        greater
Greenstick fracture, 403, 403f, 413
Growth factors, in rotator cuff tear repair, 1578

H

HAGL (humeral avulsion of glenohumeral
        ligaments) lesion
    anterior, 1054–1055, 1054f, 1055f
    arthroscopic identification of, 944–945
    inferior, 1067–1068, 1067f, 1068f
Halstead's test, 176
Handshake cast, in posterior glenohumeral joint
        dislocation, 684, 684f
Hatchet head shoulder, 133f
Hawkins-Kennedy impingement test, 163–164,
        163f, 166t
    in athlete, 1455
Hawkins' load-shift maneuver, 929
Hemangioma, 1528
Hemiarthroplasty, 1159–1160, 1160f, 1161.
        See also Arthroplasty
    arthroscopy after, 1008–1009
    in humeral fracture, 318–327. *See also*
        Humeral fracture (proximal),
        arthroplasty for
    Matsen's technique of, 1172–1184
        glenoid preparation for, 1175, 1180–1186,
            1182f–1190f
        humeral insertion in, 1186–1187, 1190f,
            1191, 1191f
        humeral preparation for, 1172, 1174–1175,
            1176f–1181f
        incisions for, 1172, 1173f, 1174f, 1175f
        position for, 1172, 1173f
        ream and run in, 1180, 1182f, 1183f, 1184,
            1184f, 1185f, 1186f
        rehabilitation after, 1192–1197, 1193f–1196f
    nonconstrained, 1202–1206, 1202f–1205f
    results of, 1213, 1214t
    in rotator cuff tear arthropathy. *See* Rotator
        cuff tear arthropathy, hemiarthroplasty for
    vs. total arthroplasty, 1161, 1216–1218
Hemidiaphragmatic paresis, interscalene brachial
        plexus block and, 285
Hemiplegia, stiff shoulder in, 1411–1412
Hemodialysis, 1008, 1331
Herophilus, 34
Heterotopic ossification
    after arthroscopy, 916
    after claviculectomy, 460, 462
    after proximal humeral fracture, 328
    after rotator cuff tear surgery, 902–903
Hill-Sachs lesion
    arthroscopy of, 926–927, 926f, 937, 946f
    computed tomography in, 188, 188f
    historical perspective on, 618, 619f
    magnetic resonance imaging of, 947f
    radiography in, 186–188, 186f, 187f, 668f,
        695–696, 696f
    in recurrent glenohumeral joint instability,
        698, 699f
    reverse, 188–189, 189f, 671f, 678, 678f,
        951, 951f
    in throwing athlete, 1473, 1473f, 1474f
Hill-Sachs sign, 186, 186f
    reverse, 188–189, 189f
Hilton's law, 29
Hip joint, 630, 630f
Hippocrates, 34
Histiocytosis, vs. tumor, 1538
History, in clinical evaluation, 145–151
Holt-Oram syndrome, 130–131

Horner's syndrome, 175, 285
Hueter's sign, 1334
Hug test, 160, 161f, 468–469, 469f
Humeral artery, 296f
Humeral avulsion of glenohumeral ligament
        (HAGL) lesion
    anterior, 1054–1055, 1054f, 1055f
    arthroscopic identification of, 944–945
    inferior, 1067–1068, 1067f, 1068f
Humeral fracture (proximal), 295–328
    anatomic neck, 295–296
    anatomy of, 295–297, 296f
    anterior glenohumeral dislocation and, 668f,
        669f, 671, 673f, 674f, 675f, 678, 682–683
    AO classification of, 298–299
    arthroplasty for, 318–327
        biceps tendon identification in, 320f, 321
        bone graft in, 324, 324f
        cementation for, 324, 324f
        complications of, 325
        drill holes for, 322–324, 323f
        incision for, 319–321, 320f
        positioning for, 319, 319f
        radiography after, 326f
        rehabilitation after, 325
        results of, 326
        retroversion for, 321–322, 322f
        reverse, 326–327
        revision, 327
        sutures for, 321, 321f, 324–325, 325f
        template for, 321, 321f
        trial implant for, 321–324, 322f, 323f, 324f
    in children. *See* Children, proximal humeral
        fracture in
    classification of, 298–300, 299f, 300f
    clinical evaluation of, 297
    Codman classification of, 298, 299–300, 299f,
        300f
    complications of, 327–328
    four-part, 306–307, 307f, 311, 313, 313f, 314f
    greater tuberosity, 301–303, 301f, 302f, 303f,
        304f
        anterior glenohumeral dislocation and, 671,
            673f, 674f, 675f, 678, 682–683
        in children, 590
        inferior head subluxation after, 250, 251f
        malunion of, 810f, 811
    heterotopic bone formation after, 328
    humeral head ischemia with, 299–300, 300f
    inferior head subluxation after, 250f, 251f
    Kocher classification of, 298, 299f
    lesser tuberosity, 303, 305f, 678
        arthroscopic treatment of, 1058–1059,
            1059f
        in children, 590
        computed tomography of, 1058, 1058f
        posterior glenohumeral joint dislocation
            and, 678
    malunion of, 328, 810f, 811
    mechanism of, 297
    minimally displaced, 309
    neck, anterior glenohumeral dislocation and,
        671, 674f
    Neer classification of, 299, 300f
    nondisplaced, 309
    nonunion of, 328
        infection with, 578
    osteonecrosis after, 328
    pathologic, 584, 585f, 1536, 1536f
    pediatric. *See* Children, proximal humeral
        fracture in
    posterior glenohumeral joint dislocation and,
        671f, 678, 678f
    radiography of, 297–298

Humeral fracture (proximal) *(Continued)*
  anteroposterior view for, 177–178, 178f,
    179f, 297, 298f
  apical-oblique view for, 180–181, 184f
  axillary lateral view for, 178–179, 180f,
    181–182, 185f
  scapulolateral view for, 179–180, 180f, 181f,
    297–298, 298f
  Stripp axial lateral view for, 181
  Velpeau axillary lateral view for, 180, 183f
 stiffness after, 327–328, 999
 surgical neck, 303, 305–307, 306f, 307f, 308f
 three-part, 305–306, 307f, 311
 treatment of
  arthroscopic osteosynthesis for, 1071–1072,
    1071f, 1072f, 1073f
  nonoperative, 300–301, 305, 306, 309
  operative, 307, 309–325. *See also* Humeral
    fracture (proximal), arthroplasty for
    approaches for, 307, 309, 309f, 310f
    Ender rod and tension band fixation for,
     317–318, 318f
    in four-part fracture, 306–307, 308f, 311,
     313, 314f, 323f
    intramedullary fixation for, 315, 317–318,
     317f, 318f
    locking plate for, 314–315, 316f, 318
    nonlocking plate for, 314–315
    open reduction and internal fixation for,
     313–318, 314f, 316f, 317f, 318f
    percutaneous, 310–313, 311f, 312f, 313f,
     314f
    in three-part fracture, 306, 307f, 311
    in two-part fracture, 307, 308f, 310–311,
     312f
 two-part, 310–311, 312f, 313f
 vascular injury with, 295–296, 296f, 297
Humeral fracture-dislocation, 307, 308f
 in children, 591
Humeral head. *See also* Glenohumeral joint
 absence of, 130
 anatomy of, 45–49, 46f, 47f, 48f, 115, 295,
  296f
  arthroscopic, 926–927, 926f
 in Apert's syndrome, 132, 132f
 arthroscopy of, 926–927, 926f
 bare area of, 926–927, 926f
 blood supply of, 311f
 center of rotation of, 226–228, 227f
 contact points of, 233, 233f, 234f. *See also*
  Glenohumeral joint, biomechanics of
 glenoid centering of, 243–245, 244f, 628–629,
  628f
 glenoidogram of, 244–245, 244f, 634–637,
  635f, 636f, 637t
 intertubercular groove of. *See* Bicipital groove
 ischemia of, fracture-related, 299–300, 300f
 obligate translation of, 646, 646f
 osteonecrosis of, 1112b, 1126t, 1128–1129
  arthroplasty for, 1128–1129. *See also*
   Arthroplasty
  arthroscopic decompression in, 1008
  degenerative joint disease with, 1128, 1128f,
   1129f
  steroid-related, 1128f, 1129
 posterior superior compression fracture of.
  See Hill-Sachs lesion
 resting position of, 222
 resurfacing of, 1160
 retroversion of, 47, 115, 1313, 1313f
 supratubercular ridge of, 115–116, 116f
Humeral prosthesis, 1165–1172, 1165f–1171f,
  1167t. *See also* Arthroplasty
 fixation of, 1166, 1169f, 1170f, 1171f

Humeral prosthesis *(Continued)*
 humeral version and, 1166, 1167f, 1168f
 loosening of, 1224f, 1225–1226, 1234, 1236f
 orthopaedic axis and, 1165–1166, 1165f,
  1166f, 1167f
 procrustean grafting and, 1166, 1171f
 reaming for, 1165, 1165f
 register and, 1166, 1168f
 removal of, 1236f, 1238
 varus-valgus adaptability and, 1166, 1169f
Humeral tuberosity
 greater, 46f, 47f, 296
  development of, 12
  fracture of, 301–303, 301f, 302f, 303f, 304f
   anterior glenohumeral dislocation and,
    671, 673f, 674f, 675f, 678, 682–683
   in children, 590
   epidemiology of, 301
   inferior head subluxation after, 250, 251f
   malunion of, 810f, 811
   mechanisms of, 301
   nonoperative treatment of, 301–302
   operative treatment of, 302, 303, 303f,
    304f
   radiography of, 301f, 302f, 304f
   rehabilitation after, 302
  in hemiarthroplasty, 1261–1262, 1261f, 1262f
 lesser, 46f, 47, 47f
  development of, 12
  fracture-dislocation of, biceps tendon
   subluxation with, 1328
  fracture of, 303, 305f
   arthroscopic treatment of, 1058–1059,
    1059f
   in children, 590
   computed tomography of, 1058, 1058f
   posterior glenohumeral joint dislocation
    and, 678
  spurs of, 1321, 1322f
Humeroscapular motion interface, 624–626, 625f,
  775–776, 776f, 777, 778
 in arthroplasty, 1098–1099, 1098f, 1099f
 spheric model of, 782–783, 782f, 783f
Humerus. *See also* Glenohumeral joint
 amputation through, 1558–1560, 1559f
 anatomic neck of, 47, 47f, 295–296, 296f
 anatomy of, 12–14, 13f, 14f, 45–49, 46f, 47f,
  48f, 295–297, 296f
  in children, 583–584
  comparative, 4, 4f
  variational, 115
 articular surface of, 222–223, 223f
 blood supply of, 296, 296f, 562–563
 development of, 12, 13f, 583
 external rotation of, 225–226, 227f, 233,
  233f
 fracture of. *See* Humeral fracture (proximal)
 head of. *See* Humeral head
 innervation of, 296f, 297
 motion of. *See also* Glenohumeral joint,
  biomechanics of
  Codman's paradox of, 218, 218f, 219f
  contact points in, 233, 233f, 234f
 ossification of, 583
 osteotomy of, in recurrent glenohumeral joint
  instability, 714
 pectoralis minor insertion into, 136, 136f
 physis of, injury to, 584, 584f, 585, 586f, 588,
  589f, 593–594
 resection of
  long, 1543–1544, 1543f
  short, 1542–1543, 1543f
 retroversion of, 223, 583
 rotational center of, 623–624, 623f

Humerus *(Continued)*
 rotational osteotomy of
  arthroscopic, 1071–1072, 1071f, 1072f, 1073f
  in recurrent posterior glenohumeral joint
   instability, 743
 surgical neck of, 47, 295, 296f
  fracture of, 303, 305–307. *See also* Humeral
   fracture (proximal)
 throwing-related changes in, 1447
 tumors of. *See* Tumor(s) *and specific tumors*
Humerus varus, 125–126, 125f, 593, 594f
 idiopathic, 126
Hylase injection, in stiff shoulder, 1417
Hyperabduction syndrome test, 176
Hyperlaxity
 elbow, 157, 157f
 shoulder, 235
Hyperostosis, sternoclavicular joint, 536
Hyperthyroidism, stiff shoulder and, 1411
Hypotension
 after interscalene block, 285
 intraoperative, in arthroscopic surgery, 288
Hypothyroidism, stiff shoulder and, 1411

I

Imaging. *See* Computed tomography (CT);
  Magnetic resonance imaging (MRI);
  Radiography
Immobilization
 in clavicular fracture, 406, 413
 in proximal humeral fracture, 300–301, 309,
  589–590, 590f, 591
 stiff shoulder and, 1411
Immune system, in idiopathic stiff shoulder,
  1408–1409
Impairment. *See also* Occupational shoulder
  disorders
 evaluation of, 1501–1503
Impingement syndrome, 927. *See also* Rotator
  cuff tear(s)
 arthroscopic management of, 961–964, 964f,
  1009
  examination for, 963
  technique of, 962–964, 963f, 965f
 bicipital tendinitis and, 1326, 1327f
  treatment of, 1350–1352, 1353f
 stages of, 961
Impingement test, 162–165, 163f, 166t
 Hawkins-Kennedy, 163–164, 163f, 166t
 Neer, 162–163, 163f, 166t, 1455
 subcoracoid, 169–170, 170f
Indium scintigraphy, in sepsis, 573
Infant. *See* Neonate
Infection, 87. *See also* Osteomyelitis; Sepsis
 acromioclavicular, 517
 after arthroplasty. *See* Arthroplasty, infection
  after
 after recurrent anterior glenohumeral
  instability treatment, 714
 sternoclavicular joint, 536–537, 538f, 550–551
 vs. tumor, 1537
Inferior glenohumeral ligament complex, 18–19,
  25f. *See also* Glenohumeral ligament(s),
  inferior
 anterior band of, 18, 19, 20f, 25f
 attachments of, 18, 20f, 21f
 axillary pouch of, 19, 21f, 22f, 24f
 definition of, 18–19, 19f
 development of, 10–11
 fetal, 10–11
 histology of, 19–22, 22f, 23f, 24f
 motion-associated changes in, 18, 20f, 21f
 origin of, 18, 20f

Inferior glenohumeral ligament complex (Continued)
  posterior band of, 18, 19, 20f, 21f, 22f, 23f, 24f
  thickness of, 18–19, 21f
Infrascapular bone, 128–129, 129f
Infraspinatus
  anatomy of, 61, 62f, 784
    comparative, 4–5
  in arm elevation, 253
  cross-sectional area of, 252t
  function of, 61
  innervation of, 61, 73
  inspection of, 153, 154f
  rupture of, 1401
  stabilizing function of, 245–246, 246f
  strength testing of, 174
  tendinous portion of, 16, 16f
Infraspinatus fossa, suprascapular nerve injury at, 1081–1083
Infraspinatus tendon, 16, 16f, 1283. See also Rotator cuff tendon(s)
Infraspinatus test, 162, 162f
  in atraumatic recurrent glenohumeral instability, 692f
  in rotator cuff evaluation, 804f, 805
Injection, corticosteroid. See Corticosteroid injection
Innominate vein, 385
Inspection, in shoulder examination, 153–154, 153f, 154f
Intercalary shoulder resection, 1557–1558, 1565–1566, 1566f
Interclavicular ligament, 39, 39f, 105, 529, 530f
Intercostal brachial nerve, 77
Internal impingement, throwing-related, 1030–1031, 1030f, 1031f, 1450–1451, 1451f
  arthroscopic treatment of, 1034–1035, 1036f–1037f
Internal rotation resistance stress test, 164–165, 164f, 166t
Interposition capsuloplasty, arthroscopic, 1048–1050, 1049f, 1050f, 1051f
Interscalene brachial plexus block, 280–285, 284f, 284t
  anatomy for, 284, 284f
  for arthroscopic procedures, 288–289, 910
  care after, 289
  complications of, 283–285, 284f, 286–287, 910
  continuous, 283
  contraindications to, 280, 285
  under general anesthesia, 287
  monitoring of, 287
  nerve injury with, 286–287
  paresthesia technique of, 281–282
  peripheral nerve stimulation for, 282–283
  postarthroscopy complications from, 910
  postoperative, 289–290
  ultrasound for, 281, 282, 282f, 283, 283f
  Winnie approach to, 281, 281f, 282
Interscalene triangle, 107
Intersternal ligament, 105
Intertubercular groove (sulcus). See Bicipital groove
Intertubercular ligament, 47
Intra-articular disk ligament, 527, 528f
Intramedullary fixation
  in clavicular fracture, 426–436
  in proximal humeral fracture, 315, 317–318, 317f, 318f
Intrathecal block, with interscalene block, 285
Iron cross maneuver, 50–51
Isometric testing, in rotator cuff evaluation, 804–805, 804f

J
Jackins program
  step 1 (avoid repeated injury), 821–822
  step 2 (restore normal flexibility), 821f, 822, 822f
  step 3 (restore normal strength), 822–824, 823f, 824f, 825f
  step 4 (aerobic exercise), 824
  step 5 (modify work/sport), 824
  in stiff shoulder, 1423
  in subacromial abrasion, 820–824, 821f, 822f, 823f, 824f, 825f
Jahnke test, 159, 159f
Jerk test, 159, 159f
  negative, 637, 637f
  positive, 637, 637f, 638f
  in recurrent glenohumeral instability, 688f, 689, 691f
Jobe-Yocum test, 164, 164f
Jugular vein, 385
  injury to, clavicular fracture and, 401
  at sternoclavicular joint, 384, 384f

K
Kenny-Howard shoulder harness, 482, 484f, 485f
Kidney failure, 1008, 1331
Kim test, 169
Knee joint, 630, 630f
Kosenow's syndrome, 132–133

L
Labrum. See Glenoid labrum
Langer's armbogen/arm arch, 137, 137f
Laryngeal palsy, 285
Latarjet procedure
  arthroscopic, 1061–1065
    coracoid osteotomy for, 1063–1064, 1064f
    evaluation for, 1063, 1063f
    exposure for, 1063–1064
    graft fixation for, 1065, 1065f
    indications for, 1063, 1063f
    subscapularis split for, 1064–1065, 1065f
  failure of, 1065–1066, 1065f, 1066f
  open, 713, 1127
Lateral anterior thoracic nerve, 70–71
Lateral brachial cutaneous nerve, 73
Lateral decubitus position, 929, 930
Lateral pectoral nerve, 70–71
  variant, 76–77
Lateral thoracic artery, 56–57, 82f, 83
  absence of, 84
Latissimus dorsi
  anatomy of, 5, 64f, 65
  blood supply of, 65
  cross-sectional area of, 252t
  innervation of, 65
Latissimus dorsi tendon transfer
  arthroscopic, 1070–1071
  open, 895, 895f
Lavage, in calcifying tendinitis, 1299, 1303t
Lesser tuberosity. See Humeral tuberosity, lesser
Levator scapulae
  anatomy of, 4–5, 55–57, 56f
  strength testing of, 174
Levator scapulae transfer, in spinal accessory nerve injury, 1368–1369
Liang, artery of, 296
Lidocaine, 283, 284t
Lift-off test, 160, 160f
  in atraumatic recurrent glenohumeral instability, 689, 692f
  in rotator cuff evaluation, 804f, 805

Ligament. See specific ligaments
Limb buds, 6, 6f
  extension of, 8, 8f
  layers of, 7
  rotation of, 8, 8f
Limb-salvage surgery, 1541–1544, 1543f, 1552
Limited joint motion syndrome, in diabetes mellitus, 1410–1411
Lipoma, 1528, 1530f, 1533–1534
Liposarcoma, 1530
Lippmann's test, 1333, 1334f
Lipstick sign, 1326
Load-and-shift test, in atraumatic recurrent glenohumeral instability, 687, 688f
Long head of biceps brachii. See Biceps tendon
Long thoracic nerve, 56–57, 70, 1369
Long thoracic nerve injury, 1369–1371
  etiology of, 1369
  nonoperative treatment of, 1369
  operative treatment of, 1369–1371, 1370f, 1371f
Loose bodies
  acromioclavicular joint, 509, 511f
  bicipital sheath, 1320
  in glenohumeral osteoarthritis, 1004–1005, 1004f
  in osteochondromatosis, 1522–1523
Ludington's test, 166, 1332–1333, 1333f
Lung disease
  preoperative assessment of, 287
  stiff shoulder and, 1411
Luxatio erecta, 657, 659f, 660f
Lymphatic system, 86, 86f

M
Mac stitch, 969, 969f
Magnetic resonance arthrography (MRA), in shoulder instability, 190–191, 191f
Magnetic resonance imaging (MRI)
  of acromioclavicular joint, 197, 472–474, 474f
  in adhesive capsulitis, 995, 996f
  anatomy on, 1511f
  in aneurysmal bone cyst, 1523, 1523f
  in Bankart lesion, 947f
  in biceps tendon dislocation, 1336, 1337f
  in biceps tendon lesions, 1336–1338
  in biceps tendon rupture, 1336, 1338f
  in bicipital instability, 207, 207f
  in brachial plexus injury, 1379–1380
  in calcifying tendinitis, 1001, 1001f
  in chondroblastoma, 1519, 1520f
  in chondrosarcoma, 1521, 1521f
  in distal clavicle osteolysis, 986f
  in Ewing's sarcoma, 1526, 1527f
  in failed rotator cuff tear surgery, 893, 894f
  in fracture, 182–183
  in ganglion cyst, 819, 819f, 1027, 1027f
  in glenohumeral osteoarthritis, 1003–1004
  in Hill-Sachs lesion, 947f
  in lipoma, 1528, 1530f
  in osteosarcoma, 1518f
  in overhead throwing disorders, 1033, 1033f
  in Paget's disease, 1528, 1528f, 1529f
  in pectoralis major rupture, 1392, 1392f
  in proximal humeral fracture, 298
  in recurrent glenohumeral joint instability, 697, 697f, 698f
  of rotator cuff, 203–206, 203f, 204f, 814–815
  in sepsis, 573, 574
  in shoulder instability, 189f, 190, 190f
  in SLAP lesion, 1024, 1024f
  in spinoglenoid notch ganglion cyst, 819, 819f, 1027, 1027f

Magnetic resonance imaging (Continued)
  of sternoclavicular joint, 199, 200f, 541, 543f
  in stiff shoulder, 1413
  in supraspinatus atrophy, 815
Magnuson-Stack procedure, 708, 709f, 710f
  complications of, 717
Malignant fibrous histiocytoma, 1530
Malunion
  clavicular fracture, 387–388, 387f, 388f,
    409–410, 410f, 412f, 436, 438f, 439f, 440f,
    603
    thoracic outlet syndrome after, 1374–1376,
      1375f
  greater tuberosity fracture, 810f, 811
  humeral fracture, 328
  middle third clavicular fracture, 412f, 436,
    438f, 439f, 440f
  scapular fracture, 336
Manipulation under anesthesia, in stiff shoulder,
  1418–1420, 1423–1424
Margin-convergence repair, in rotator cuff tear,
  974, 974f
Maritime workers' compensation system, 1505
Matrix metalloproteinases, in idiopathic stiff
  shoulder, 1409
Matsen's technique
  for arthrodesis, 1137–1143, 1141f, 1142f,
    1145f
  for arthroplasty, 1172–1197. See also
    Arthroplasty, Matsen's technique of
  for Bankart repair, 718, 721–737. See also
    Bankart repair, Matsen and Lippitt's
    preferred method of
  for failed acromioplasty, 834–835
  for full-thickness rotator cuff tears, 869–876,
    871f–876f
  for hemiarthroplasty, 1172–1184. See also
    Hemiarthroplasty, Matsen's technique of
  for partial-thickness cuff tears, 836–839, 837f,
    838f, 839f
  for revision arthroplasty, 1229–1238. See also
    Arthroplasty, revision, Matsen's technique
    of
  for subacromial smoothing, 827f, 828f,
    829–830, 829f
Mechanoreceptors, 248
Medial antebrachial cutaneous nerve, 71
Median nerve, 71
Melbourne Instability Shoulder Scale, 269
Menopause, sternoclavicular osteoarthritis after,
  536, 537f, 549, 550f
Mepivacaine, 283, 284t
Mesoderm, 5, 6, 6f, 7f
Methylmethacrylate, 289
Microfracture, arthroscopic, 1007
Milwaukee shoulder syndrome, 1254. See also
  Rotator cuff tear arthropathy
Möbius syndrome, 136
Modified Adson's maneuver, 176
Moment arm, 250, 254f
Motion/movement. See Arm elevation;
  Biomechanics; Glenohumeral joint,
  biomechanics of
Multiple epiphyseal dysplasia, 132, 133f
Multiple myeloma, 1525, 1526f
Muscle(s), 48–67. See also specific muscles
  actions of, 49–51, 50f, 51f
  activity of, 252–254, 254f, 255f
  angiosomes of, 53–54, 80
  blood supply to, 51, 53–54, 53f, 79–80
  concavity-compression effect of, 243–244, 244f
  cross section of, 250, 252f, 252t
  dissection of, 51, 53f
  fibers of, 49, 49f

Muscle(s) (Continued)
  glenohumeral. See Coracobrachialis; Deltoid;
    Infraspinatus; Subscapularis;
    Supraspinatus; Teres major; Teres minor
  landmark, 66–67
  moment arm of, 250, 254f
  movements of, 49–51, 50f, 51f
  multiple joint. See Biceps brachii; Latissimus
    dorsi; Pectoralis major; Triceps brachii
  nerves to, 51, 53, 53f
  orientation of, 250, 252f, 253f, 254f
  parallel, 49, 49f
  passive tension of, 243, 244f
  pennate (multipennate), 49, 49f
  physiologic cross section of, 250
  rotator cuff. See Coracobrachialis;
    Infraspinatus; Subscapularis;
    Supraspinatus; Teres major; Teres minor
  rupture of, 1389–1402. See also specific
    muscles
  scapulothoracic. See Levator scapulae;
    Pectoralis minor; Rhomboid(s); Serratus
    anterior; Subclavius; Trapezius
  size of, 250
  stabilizing function of, 243–250
    barrier effect in, 245
    biceps, 246–247
    clinical relevance of, 248–250, 249f
    concavity-compression effect in, 243–245,
      244f
    deltoid, 247–248
    passive tension in, 243, 244f
    rotator cuff, 245–246, 246f
  strength testing of, 171–173, 172f, 172t, 173f
  torque data on, 259–260, 259t
Muscle transfer
  in axillary nerve injury, 1365–1366
  biceps, 487
  in brachial plexus injury, 1384
  latissimus dorsi, 1070–1071
  in musculocutaneous nerve injury, 1363
  pectoralis major, 1370–1371, 1370f
  pectoralis minor, 1059–1060, 1059f, 1060f, 1061f
  in spinal accessory nerve injury, 1368–1369
Musculocutaneous nerve
  anatomy of, 29, 63, 73, 75f, 296f, 625–626,
    1362
  in arthroplasty, 1197–1198, 1200, 1200f
Musculocutaneous nerve injury, 1362–1363
  arthroscopy and, 1362–1363
  biceps rupture and, 1398
  clavicular fracture and, 411
  interscalene block and, 286
  proximal humeral fracture and, 297
  recurrent glenohumeral joint instability
    treatment and, 715–716
  treatment of, 1363
Musculoskeletal tumors. See Tumor(s) and
  specific tumors
Muybridge, Eadweard, 37, 37f
Myalgia, 1492–1493. See also Occupational
  shoulder disorders
Myositis ossificans, 1517

N

Nail-patella syndrome, 131, 131f
Napoleon test, 160, 161f
Neck. See also Cervical spine
  examination of, 152–153, 152f
  extension of, 152, 152f
  flexion of, 152, 152f
  lateral bending of, 152, 152f
  Spurling test of, 152, 152f

Necrotizing fasciitis, amputation in, 1558
Needle biopsy, 1539–1540
Needling therapy, in calcifying tendinitis, 1299
Neer impingement test, 162–163, 163f, 166t,
  1455
Neonate. See also Children
  clavicular fracture in, 394, 595
    clinical manifestations of, 396, 596
    treatment of, 413, 419–420
  proximal humeral fracture in, 583–594, 584,
    586, 588f. See also Children, proximal
    humeral fracture in
Neoplasm. See Tumor(s) and specific tumors
Nerve(s), 28–29, 29f, 67–78. See also specific
  nerves
  blood supply to, 68, 69f
  duplication of, 77, 78f
  evaluation of, 173–175, 173f
  function of, 67–68
  microanatomy of, 67–68, 69f
Nerve action potentials, in brachial plexus
  injury, 1381
Nerve block. See also Anesthesia; Interscalene
  brachial plexus block
  postoperative, 289–290
  in stiff shoulder, 1418
Nerve graft
  in brachial plexus injury, 1382
  in spinal accessory nerve injury, 1368, 1368f
Nerve injury, 1361–1385. See also specific
  nerves
  evaluation of, 1361–1362
  perioperative, 285–287, 286b
    anesthetic causes of, 286–287, 286b
    mechanical causes of, 286, 286b
Nerve reimplantation, in brachial plexus injury,
  1384
Nerve transfer
  in axillary nerve injury, 1365
  in brachial plexus injury, 1382–1384, 1383f,
    1385
  in long thoracic nerve injury, 1369
  in musculocutaneous nerve injury, 1363
  in postamputation prosthetic rehabilitation,
    1572, 1573f
  in spinal accessory nerve injury, 1368
Net humeral joint reaction force, 630, 631f,
  632–633, 632f, 633f
  in arthroplasty, 1104–1106, 1104f, 1105f,
    1106f
Neurologic disorders. See also specific nerve
  injuries
  postarthroscopy, 912–914, 1228
  stiff shoulder and, 1411–1412
Neurologic examination, 173–175, 173f, 174f,
  174t, 175t
  in nerve injury, 1361–1362
  in rotator cuff lesion evaluation, 818
Neurolysis
  in axillary nerve injury, 1365
  in long thoracic nerve injury, 1369
Neuropathy. See Nerve injury and specific nerve
  injuries
Neurosarcoma, 1511
Neurotrophic arthropathy, 1129, 1130f
Neurotrophic neuropathy, 1129, 1130f
Newton, Sir Isaac, 37
Nicola procedure, 713–714
No-touch examination, in atraumatic recurrent
  glenohumeral instability, 687, 688f
Nonossifying fibroma, 1524, 1525f
Nonsteroidal anti-inflammatory drugs
  postoperative, 291
  in stiff shoulder, 1415

Nonunion
    clavicular fracture, 406–409, 603. *See also*
        Clavicular fracture, nonunion of
    proximal humeral fracture, 328, 578
    scapular fracture, 336
Nutraceuticals, in patient history, 150

O

Oberlin transfer, in musculocutaneous nerve
    injury, 1363
O'Brien test, 166–167, 167t, 168f
Observed repetitive forward elevation, 170
Occupational Safety and Health Administration,
    1497–1498
Occupational shoulder disorders, 1489–1506
    case studies of, 1498–1499, 1500b
    climatic factors and, 1492
    definition of, 1489, 1490, 1506
    degenerative joint disease and, 1495–1496
    disability compensation systems in, 1503–1505
    disability evaluation in, 1501–1503
    epidemiology of, 1490–1492, 1491t
    etiology of, 1491–1493, 1491t, 1493f
    Federal Employer's Liability Act and, 1505
    grading of, 1494, 1494b, 1495b
    impairment evaluation in, 1501–1503
    management of, 1493–1495, 1494b
    organic (physiologic) theory of, 1492–1493
    posture and, 1491–1492, 1491t
    prevention of, 1496–1499
    primary prevention of, 1497–1498
    private disability insurance in, 1505
    psychosocial theory of, 1493
    repetitive work and, 1491, 1491t
    secondary prevention of, 1498
        case studies of, 1498–1499, 1500f
    Social Security Disability Insurance program
        in, 1505
    sports activity and, 1492
    stress and, 1495
    treatment of, 1499–1501
        client matching in, 1498
        ergonomic changes in, 1495, 1496–1498
        job restructuring in, 1498
        multidisciplinary approach to, 1494–1495
        secondary gain and, 1500–1501
    workers' compensation system in, 1504–1505
Ollier's disease, 1519, 1520f
Omohyoid, 66–67, 105
Omovertebral bone, 118, 119f
Onycho-osteodysplasia, 131, 131f
Opioids, postoperative, 289, 290, 291
Orthotherapy, for rotator cuff tear in elderly,
    851–865, 853f, 855f–865f
Os acromiale, 122–124, 123f, 608, 608f, 775–776,
    776f
    rotator cuff tear and, 776
    treatment of, 123–124, 124f, 1075–1076
        arthroscopic, 1075–1076, 1076f, 1077f
        nonoperative, 123
Osteitis deformans (Paget's disease), 1526–1528,
    1528f, 1529f
Osteoarthritis
    acromioclavicular joint, 509, 511f, 515, 516f
    age and, 146
    glenohumeral joint, 1100f, 1115, 1115b. *See
        also* Glenohumeral joint arthritis
        after anterior instability treatment, 101–102
        after arthroscopic procedures, 957
        epidemiology of, 1003
        imaging in, 1003–1004
        occupational disorders and, 1495–1496
        physical examination in, 1003

Osteoarthritis *(Continued)*
        primary, 1112b, 1114f, 1115, 1115b, 1115f,
            1126t, 1191, 1254–1255
        secondary, 957, 1112b, 1116f, 1117–1118,
            1118b, 1118f, 1126t
        glenoid, arthroplasty and, 1580–1581, 1580f,
            1581f
        sternoclavicular joint, 535–536, 535f, 536f,
            549–550, 551f
            postmenopausal, 536, 537f, 549–550, 550f
        vs. tumor, 1537, 1537f
Osteoblastoma, 1517
Osteochondroma, 1518–1519, 1519f
Osteochondromatosis, 1522–1523
    loose bodies with, 1320
Osteoid osteoma, 1515–1516, 1533f
Osteolysis, acromioclavicular joint, 514–515, 514f
Osteoma, osteoid, 1515–1516
Osteomalacia, vs. tumor, 1538
Osteomyelitis, 565, 567–568, 567f, 567t, 576f. *See
    also* Sepsis
    hematogenous, 567–568, 567f
        vs. tumor, 1537
    treatment of, 575–578, 576f, 577t
Osteonecrosis
    distal clavicle, 517
    humeral head, 1112b, 1126t
        arthroplasty for, 1128–1129. *See also*
            Arthroplasty
        arthroscopic decompression in, 1008
        degenerative joint disease with, 1128, 1128f,
            1129f
        fracture and, 328, 594, 1127f, 1128
        steroid-related, 1128f, 1129, 1129f
Osteopenia, in stiff shoulder, 1413
Osteopontin, in calcifying tendinitis, 1296
Osteoporosis, vs. tumor, 1538
Osteoporosis circumscripta (Paget's disease),
    1526–1528, 1528f, 1529f
Osteosarcoma, 1516f, 1517–1518, 1517b, 1518f,
    1533f
    vs. aneurysmal bone cyst, 1523
    biopsy of, 1538–1540, 1539f, 1550
    chemotherapy in, 1551
    fracture with, 1536
    incidence of, 1530, 1531, 1532f
    limb-salvage surgery for, 1541–1544, 1543f,
        1552
    postresection reconstruction for, 1544–1547
    resection of, 1540–1547, 1541f, 1542t, 1549
Osteotomy
    clavicular, 547, 553, 554f, 555f
    coracoid, 1063–1064, 1064f
    glenoid, 248–249, 249f, 714, 743–744, 743f,
        745f, 746, 749f, 750f
    humeral, 714, 743, 1071–1072, 1071f, 1072f,
        1073f
    periarticular, 1144
Oto-onycho-peroneal syndrome, 132
Oudard procedure, 710
Outcome assessment, 267–277, 270b
    aggregate scores in, 269–270
    application of, 269–270, 275, 276f
    categorical rankings in, 269–270
    disease-specific instruments for, 269
    generic health instruments for, 268, 271–272
    historical perspective on, 267–268
    instrument reliability in, 271
    instrument responsiveness in, 271
    instrument validity in, 270–271
    joint-specific instruments for, 268, 272–274
    limb-specific instruments for, 268–269, 274
    medical comorbidities in, 274–275
    pain assessment in, 269

Overhead reach. *See* Arm elevation;
    Glenohumeral joint, biomechanics of
Overhead throwing, 1438f, 1439f, 1440f, 1441f
    asymptomatic adaptations to, 1446–1449,
        1448f, 1449f
    Bennett's lesion with, 1042–1043, 1470–1472
    biceps tendon in, 1325, 1330
    biomechanics of, 1029–1030, 1030f, 1437–
        1442, 1438f, 1439f, 1440f, 1441f, 1442f
    bone adaptations to, 1447
    capsuloligamentous changes with, 1447–1448,
        1448f, 1449f
    dislocation with, 1472–1479, 1475f, 1476f,
        1478f–1479f
    exostosis with, 1042–1043
    glenohumeral internal rotation deficit with,
        1451–1452, 1451f
    internal impingement with, 1030–1031, 1030f,
        1031f, 1450–1451, 1451f
        arthroscopic treatment of, 1034–1035,
            1036f–1037f
        evaluation of, 1454–1455
    kinetic chain in, 1437–1438
    muscle changes with, 1448
    PAINT lesion with, 1468f, 1469f, 1470, 1471f
    PASTA lesion with, 1462, 1464–1470, 1466f,
        1467f
        arthroscopic treatment of, 1465–1470, 1466f,
            1467f
        nonoperative treatment of, 1465
    pathologic changes with, 1449–1453, 1450f
        evaluation of, 1031–1033, 1033f, 1454–1455
            arthroscopy in, 1033–1034
            patient history in, 1454
            physical examination in, 1031–1033,
                1032f, 1454–1455, 1455f
        imaging in, 1033, 1033f
        treatment of, 1033–1043, 1455–1472
            anterior capsulolabral reconstruction in,
                1034–1035
            capsular plication in, 1035, 1036f–1037f
            diagnostic arthroscopy in, 1033–1034
            labral débridement in, 1035, 1037
            labral repair in, 1037–1038
            rehabilitation in, 1033
    peel back phenomenon with, 1030–1031,
        1031f, 1452, 1452f
    posterior capsular contracture with, 1451
        nonoperative treatment of, 1455–1456, 1456f
        operative treatment of, 1456–1457
    proprioceptive changes with, 1448
    rotator cuff tears with, 1470
        arthroscopic treatment of, 1038–1042, 1040f,
            1041f
    scapular changes with, 1448–1449, 1450f,
        1452–1453
    scapulothoracic motion with, 1448–1449,
        1450f
    SICK scapula with, 1452–1453, 1453f
    SLAP lesion with, 1457–1462
        arthroscopic treatment of, 1035, 1037–1038,
            1460–1462, 1461f, 1463f, 1464f, 1465f
        nonoperative treatment of, 1460
    subacromial impingement with, 1042
Oxford score, 273

P

Paget's disease, 1526–1528, 1528f, 1529f, 1537
Paget-Schroetter syndrome, 1483
Pain, 147–150, 150b
    acromioclavicular joint, 467
    aggravating factors in, 148
    alleviation of, 149, 149f

Pain (Continued)
  assessment of, 269
  in calcifying tendinitis, 1291, 1291t, 1292
  description of, 147
  hemodialysis-related, 1331
  localization of, 148
  night, 148
  onset of, 147–148
  patient-controlled analgesia for, 290, 291
  perception of, 147
  postamputation, 290, 1574
  postoperative, 289–291
  radicular, 148
  in tumor, 1532, 1533
Pain provocation test, 167t, 168, 169f
Painful arc test, 165, 165f
PAINT (partial articular tear with intratendinous
    extension), 975–976, 976f, 1468f, 1469f,
    1470, 1471f
Palpation, 154, 155f
  acromioclavicular joint, 154, 155f, 467, 467f,
    469
  in athlete, 1454
  bicipital groove, 154
  for crepitus, 807, 807f
  deltoid, 154
  in rotator cuff lesions, 804f, 806, 807, 807f
Panclavicular dislocation, 391, 398
Pancoast tumor, 1411
Paralysis. See specific nerve injuries
Paresthesias, 151
Parkinson's disease, stiff shoulder in, 1411
Parsonage-Turner syndrome, 287, 1376–1377,
    1377f
  diagnosis of, 1377, 1377f
  long thoracic nerve palsy in, 1369, 1370f
  prognosis for, 1377
  stiff shoulder in, 1412
  suprascapular nerve injury in, 1372, 1373
  treatment of, 1377
PASTA (partial articular-sided supraspinatus
    tendon avulsion) lesion, 975–976, 1462,
    1464–1470, 1466f, 1467f
Pathologic fracture
  clavicular, 396
  humeral, 584, 585f, 1536, 1536f
Patient-controlled analgesia, 290, 291
Patient history, 145–151. See also Clinical
    evaluation
Paxinos test, 468, 468f
Pectoral artery, 65, 82–83, 82f
Pectoral girdle, 1, 2f
Pectoral nerve, 64
  lateral, 70–71
    variant, 76–77
  medial, 71
Pectoralis major, 385
  absence of, 64
  anatomy of, 5, 64–65, 65f, 1390
  blood supply of, 65, 82–83
  clavicular insertion of, 388
  clavicular portion of, 109
  congenital absence of, 134–135, 135f
  cross-sectional area of, 252t
  function of, 64
  innervation of, 64
  origin of, 40, 41f, 64
  rupture of, 1390–1394
    in athlete, 1391, 1391f, 1392f
    classification of, 1390–1391
    clinical findings in, 1391–1392, 1391f, 1392f
    complications of, 1392
    in elderly, 1391
    incidence of, 1391

Pectoralis major (Continued)
    magnetic resonance imaging in, 1392, 1392f
    mechanisms of, 1391
    radiography in, 1392
    treatment of, 1392–1394
  transfer of, in long thoracic nerve injury,
    1370–1371, 1370f
Pectoralis minor, 385
  absence of, 57
  anatomy of, 5, 57, 57f
  blood supply of, 57
  humeral insertion of, 136, 136f
  rupture of, 1401
  transfer of, 1059–1060, 1060f, 1061f
Pectoralis minor tendon, in acromioclavicular
    joint injury treatment, 489
Pectoralis reflex, 174
Peel back phenomenon, in throwing athlete,
    1452, 1452f
Pelvis-shoulder dysplasia, 132–133
Periarthritis personality, 1412
Periarticular osteotomy, 1144
Perineurium, 67–68
Periosteal chondroma, 1519, 1533f
Peripheral nerve stimulator, in interscalene
    block, 282–283
Persistent subacromial impingement, in failed
    rotator cuff tear surgery, 893, 897–899
Personality disorders, stiff shoulder and, 1412
Phantom pain, postamputation, 1574
Phocomelia, 129–130, 129f, 130f, 131f
Phrenic nerve blockade, 285
Physeal injury
  acromioclavicular, 497–498, 498f, 499f
  sternoclavicular, 547, 549, 549f, 556–557
Physical examination. See Clinical evaluation
Physical therapy. See also Exercise program;
    Jackins program
  in calcifying tendinitis, 1296–1297
  in stiff shoulder, 1415–1416
Pigmented villonodular synovitis, 1008, 1522
Pitching, 1438–1442, 1438f, 1439f, 1440f, 1441f.
    See also Overhead throwing
Planes, surgical, 89, 90f, 91f
Plate fixation
  in distal third clavicular fracture, 440–441,
    442f
  in middle third clavicular fracture, 423f,
    424–426, 424f, 425f
  in proximal humeral fracture, 314–315, 316f,
    318
  in sternoclavicular joint dislocation, 547, 548f
Platelets, in rotator cuff tear repair, 1578
Pneumothorax
  arthroscopy and, 911
  clavicular fracture and, 399, 399f
  interscalene block and, 285
Poland's syndrome, 134–135, 135f
Popeye sign, 1013, 1013f, 1334, 1334f
Porcupine shoulder, 516
Positioning, surgical, 288. See also specific
    procedures
Positron emission tomography, in osteogenic
    sarcoma, 1515, 1516f
Posterior capsular contracture, throwing-related,
    1447, 1448f, 1449f, 1451
  nonoperative treatment of, 1455–1456, 1456f
  operative treatment of, 1456
Posterior capsular tightness, 808
  evaluation of, 800f, 801f, 802f, 803
  mechanism of, 782f, 783
  treatment of, 819
Posterior drawer test, 158
Posterior load test, 159, 159f

Postural deformity, postamputation, 1572–1573
Presenting complaint, 146–151
Profunda brachii artery, 82f, 85f
Proprioception, 248
  in throwing shoulder, 1448
Prostheses
  glenoid, 1161–1165, 1162f, 1163f, 1164f.
    See also Glenoid prosthesis
  humeral, 1165–1172, 1165f–1171f, 1167t.
    See also Humeral prosthesis
  postamputation, 1568–1574
    body-powered, 1569–1570, 1570f, 1571f,
      1572f
    externally powered, 1570, 1572
    lightweight passive, 1569, 1569f
    postural abnormalities and, 1572–1573
    targeted nerve transfers for, 1572, 1573f
Pseudarthrosis, clavicular, 118, 118f, 403,
    404–406
Pseudoaneurysm
  clavicular fracture and, 410
  venous, arthroscopy and, 912
Pseudomalignant myositis ossificans, 1517
Pseudoparalysis, 260
  in sepsis, 571
Pulmonary embolism, after arthroscopy, 914
Pulse oximetry, during arthroscopy, 912
Push-pull test, 688–689, 690f
Push-up test, 170
Putti-Platt procedure, 707–708
  capsulorrhaphy arthropathy after, 1126–1127
  complications of, 717
Pyarthrosis, glenohumeral, 565

Q

Quadrangular space, 109–110
Quadrilateral space syndrome, 87, 1365
  in athlete, 1481
QuickDASH (Quick Disabilities of the Arm,
    Shoulder and Hand) questionnaire, 274

R

Radial head fracture, triceps rupture with, 1396
Radial nerve, 71
Radials, 1, 2f
Radiation therapy
  in calcifying tendinitis, 1299–1300
  glenohumeral joint changes with, 1129–1130,
    1130f
  in soft tissue sarcoma, 1550, 1552
  in stiff shoulder, 1418
Radiography, 177–207. See also Computed
    tomography (CT); Magnetic resonance
    imaging (MRI)
  in acromial fracture, 353, 354f
  in acromioclavicular cyst, 516, 516f, 517f
  of acromioclavicular joint, 194–197, 194f, 195f,
    196f, 197f, 470–471, 470f, 471f, 472f, 473f
  in acromioclavicular joint injury type III, 478,
    479f, 481, 481f, 482f
  in acromioclavicular joint injury type IV,
    500–501, 503f, 504f
  in acromioclavicular joint injury type V, 506,
    507f
  in acromioclavicular joint injury type VI,
    507–508, 508f, 510f
  in acromioclavicular joint osteolysis, 514, 514f
  in anterior glenohumeral joint instability, 183,
    185f, 186f
  in arthroplasty, 192–193, 1278, 1278f
  in atraumatic recurrent glenohumeral
    instability, 689, 691

Radiography *(Continued)*
in biceps rupture, 1398
of biceps tendon, 206f, 207
of bicipital groove, 1334–1335, 1335f
in brachial plexus injury, 1379, 1380
in calcifying tendinitis, 205f, 207, 811, 811f, 1001, 1001f, 1286, 1293–1295, 1293f, 1294f
in chondroblastoma, 1519, 1520f
in chondrosarcoma, 1521, 1521f
of clavicle, 193f, 194
in clavicular fracture, 193f, 194, 401–404, 401f, 402f, 403f, 404f, 405f, 597–598, 597f, 598f
in clavicular fracture nonunion, 402, 402f, 403f
of coracoclavicular ligament, 457f, 458f
in coracoid fracture, 205, 205f, 354, 355f, 498, 499f, 500f
in distal clavicle osteolysis, 986f
in enchondroma, 1519, 1520f
in Ewing's sarcoma, 1526, 1527f
in failed rotator cuff tear surgery, 893, 894f
in fibrous dysplasia, 1524, 1524f
of glenohumeral joint, 228, 228f
in glenohumeral joint arthritis, 191–192, 191f, 193f, 1109–1111, 1109f, 1110f, 1111f
in glenohumeral joint dislocation, 183, 188–189, 662–666. *See also* Glenohumeral joint dislocation, radiography in
in glenoid cavity fracture, 345, 346f, 347f
in glenoid neck fracture, 344, 344f
in greater tuberosity fracture, 301f, 302f, 304f
in Hill-Sachs lesion, 186–188, 186f, 187f, 668f, 695–696, 696f
in infected arthroplasty, 1278, 1278f
in intrathoracic scapular dislocation, 367, 367f
in lesser tuberosity fracture, 303, 305f
in nonossifying fibroma, 1524, 1525f
in Ollier's disease, 1519, 1520f
in osteochondroma, 1518, 1519f
in osteogenic sarcoma, 1516f
in osteosarcoma, 1518f
in pectoralis major rupture, 1392
in pediatric proximal humerus fracture, 587–588, 588f
in pediatric scapular fracture, 605–607, 606f, 607f
in posterior glenohumeral joint instability, 188–189, 189f, 190f
in proximal humeral fracture, 177–183, 178f–183f, 297–298, 298f
in pseudomeningocele, 1380, 1380f
reduced voltage for, 194, 194f
of rotator cuff, 199–201, 201f, 202f, 203f, 810–817, 810f, 811f
of scapula, 206–207
in scapular fracture, 335, 335f, 336, 336b, 337f
in sepsis, 572–573, 573f, 574f
in simple bone cyst, 1522f, 1523
of sternoclavicular joint, 197–198, 198f, 199f, 200f, 539–542, 540f, 541f, 542f
in stiff shoulder, 1413
in thoracic outlet syndrome, 1374f, 1375f
trauma series, 177–182, 178f–185f
in triceps rupture, 1396
in tumor evaluation, 1515, 1516f, 1534–1535
views for
Alexander, 196–197, 197f
anteroposterior, 177–178, 178f, 179f, 195–196, 196f, 200
in glenohumeral joint arthritis, 1109–1110, 1109f
in glenohumeral joint dislocation, 662–663, 662f, 663f, 664f
in internal rotation, 188

Radiography *(Continued)*
anteroposterior stress, 195–196, 196f
apical oblique, 180–181, 183, 184f, 186f, 670f, 696
in glenohumeral joint dislocation, 183, 186f, 666, 669f, 670f
axillary lateral, 178–179, 180f, 181–182, 185f, 196, 196f, 200
in glenohumeral joint arthritis, 1109–1110, 1109f
in glenohumeral joint dislocation, 665–666, 667f, 668f, 669f
bicipital groove, 1334–1335, 1335f
Fisk's, 1334, 1335f
Heinig, 540, 541f
Hobbs, 540, 541f
scapular outlet, 200, 202f
scapulolateral, 179–180, 180f, 181f, 663, 665f, 666f
serendipity, 198, 198f, 199f, 540–541, 542f
Stripp axial lateral, 181
Stryker notch, 187f, 188, 204f, 207, 695, 696f
templating, in glenohumeral joint arthritis, 1110, 1110f, 1111f
thirty-degree caudal tilt, 200, 201f
Velpeau axillary lateral, 180, 183f, 666, 667f
West Point axillary lateral, 183, 185f, 666f, 668f, 696
Zanca, 194–195, 195f
Radionuclide imaging
acromioclavicular joint, 197
in Ewing's sarcoma, 1526, 1527f
in Paget's disease, 1528, 1529f
in sepsis, 573
sternoclavicular joint, 199
in stiff shoulder, 1413
Railroad workers' compensation system, 1505
Rami communicantes, 74–75
Range of motion, 154–162
active supine elevation for, 156
active total shoulder elevation for, 156f, 157
in athlete, 1454
cross-body adduction for, 157
passive external rotation for, 155f, 156, 156f
passive internal rotation for, 156f, 157
passive supine elevation for, 155, 155f
sternoclavicular joint, 529, 531f
in stiff shoulder, 1413
Reflexes
biceps, 175
brachioradialis, 175
clavicular, 174
evaluation of, 174–175
pectoralis, 174
scapular, 174
triceps, 175
Rehabilitation program (Orthotherapy). *See also* Exercise; Jackins program
for rotator cuff tears, 851–865, 853f, 855f–865f
Reliability, of outcome assessment instrument, 271
Relocation test, 159, 159f, 165, 165f
Resisted extension test, 468, 468f
Resisted forward elevation test, 170
Respiration, clavicle in, 389
Respiratory failure, interscalene block and, 285
Responsiveness, of outcome assessment instrument, 271
Reticuloendothelial tumors, 1525–1526, 1526f, 1527f
Rheumatoid arthritis
acromioclavicular joint, 515

Rheumatoid arthritis *(Continued)*
glenohumeral joint, 1008, 1112b, 1118–1122, 1122b, 1126t, 1191–1192, 1254. *See also* Glenohumeral joint arthritis; Rotator cuff tear arthropathy
arthroplasty for, 1121–1122, 1191–1192. *See also* Arthroplasty
erosion in, 1102f, 1118, 1121f
radiography in, 1119f, 1120f, 1121f, 1122f
rotator cuff defect in, 1118–1119, 1121f
synovectomy for, 1131–1133
sepsis with, 571
sternoclavicular joint, 536, 536f
Rhomboid(s)
absence of, 136
anatomy of, 4–5, 55, 56f
strength testing of, 174, 174f
Rhomboid ligament. *See* Costoclavicular ligaments
Rib fracture, 398–399, 399f
Rim rent, 792f, 793, 799–800, 799f
Rocking horse effect, 260, 1105–1106, 1105f, 1256
Rockwood's technique
for anterior glenohumeral joint instability, 729, 734–742, 738f–741f
for arthrodesis, 1143
for arthroplasty, 1197–1202. *See also* Arthroplasty, Rockwood's technique of
for posterior glenohumeral joint instability, 746–756, 753f–756f
Roos test, 1376
Ropivacaine, 283, 284t
Rotator cuff, 771–880
age-related changes in, 792–793
anatomy of, 16, 16f, 626, 626f, 784–786
arthroscopic, 927, 937, 937f, 1034
variational, 113
arteries of, 26–27, 26f, 27f, 778–779
arthrography of, 201, 203f, 813–814, 813f, 814f
arthroscopy of, 927, 937, 937f, 1034
asymptomatic failure of, 808
treatment of, 819
biomechanics of, 786–791
bending loads and, 788f, 789–790
compressive forces in, 786f, 787
compressive loads and, 790
concentric loads and, 789f, 790
coracoacromial arch in, 779–780, 779f
eccentric loads and, 788f, 790
humeral torque in, 784f, 786
humeroscapular motion interface in, 775–776, 776f, 777, 778
load transfer in, 778–779, 778f
muscle excursion and, 785f, 787
muscle force and, 786f, 787
muscular balance and, 787–788, 787f
rotational forces in, 787, 787f
shearing loads and, 789f, 790, 790f
spacer effect in, 779, 779f
Boutonnière deformity of, 781, 781f, 797
calcifying tendinitis of, 1283–1305. *See also* Calcifying tendinitis
clinical evaluation of, 159–162, 160f, 161f, 162f, 165–166
disruption of, 799. *See also* Rotator cuff tear(s)
evaluation of. *See also* Rotator cuff, lesions of, clinical evaluation of
arthroscopic, 937, 937f, 1034
physical, 159–162, 160f, 161f, 162f
in recurrent glenohumeral joint instability, 697
historical perspective on, 771–774
hypovascular critical zone of, 26–27, 27f

Rotator cuff (Continued)
lesions of, 799–817. See also Posterior capsular tightness; Rotator cuff tear(s); Rotator cuff tear arthropathy; Subacromial abrasion
acromial shape in, 779–781, 780f, 781f
acromioclavicular joint in, 783–784, 784f
arthrography of, 201, 203f, 813–814, 813f, 814f
clinical evaluation of, 802–807
bicipital groove in, 805f, 806
crepitance in, 807, 807f
instability in, 806–807
palpation in, 804f, 806, 807, 807f
physical tests in, 159–162, 160f, 161f, 162f
roughness in, 805f, 806f, 807, 807f, 808f
stiffness in, 800f, 801f, 802f, 803, 803f, 1000
suture knots in, 806f, 807
weakness in, 803–806, 803f, 804f, 805f
coracoacromial arch in, 777–778, 779f
historical perspective on, 771–774
incidence of, 800–802
magnetic resonance imaging of, 814–815
occupation and, 802
os acromiale and, 776, 776f
patient self-assessment in, 809–810, 809f, 810f
prevalence of, 808t
radiography of, 199–201, 810–817, 810f, 811f
anteroposterior view for, 200, 810f, 811, 811f
axillary lateral view for, 200
eyebrow sign on, 810f, 811
indications for, 812
scapular outlet view for, 200, 202f
thirty-degree caudal tilt view for, 200, 201f
ultrasonography of, 815–817, 815f, 816f
magnetic resonance imaging of, 203–206, 203f, 204f, 814–815
muscles of, 59–63, 784–786. See also Coracobrachialis; Infraspinatus; Subscapularis; Supraspinatus; Teres major; Teres minor
passive tension of, 245
stabilizing function of, 245–246
ultrasonography of, 201–203, 815–817, 815f, 816f
Rotator cuff tear(s). See also Rotator cuff tear arthropathy
acromioclavicular cyst in, 516, 516f, 517f
acromioclavicular joint osteophytes and, 783–784, 784f
after acromioplasty, 781
age and, 791–793, 791f
vs. arthritis, 818, 818f
arthrography of, 201, 203f, 812f, 813–814, 813f, 814f
arthroscopic evaluation of, 937, 937f
arthroscopic treatment of, 960–982
acromioplasty and, 976–977
cuff footprint restoration in, 970–972, 970f
development of, 964–966
double-row repair in, 970–971, 970f
knot typing in, 969–970
margin-convergence repair in, 974, 974f
in massive tears, 974–975, 974f
outcomes of, 972–974
in partial-thickness tears, 975–976, 976f
portals for, 967
Pushlock anchor in, 972, 972f
in retracted posterosuperior tear, 1073–1075, 1074f, 1075f

Rotator cuff tear(s) (Continued)
stiffness and, 977, 1000
suture anchors in, 967, 968f
suture placement in, 968–969, 969f
tear configuration in, 966–967, 966f
technique of, 977–980, 978f
tendon release in, 967
transosseous-equivalent repair in, 971, 971f, 978f
biceps dislocation with, 1329, 1352–1354, 1353f, 1354f
biceps rupture with, 1319, 1329
biceps tendinitis with, 1328–1329, 1330, 1339
biceps tendon in, 1324–1325
vs. bursitis, 817
calcifying tendinitis and, 1303–1304
vs. cervical radiculopathy, 818
vs. cervical spondylosis, 818
clinical evaluation of, 159–162, 160f, 161f, 162f, 802–807
instability in, 806–807
isometric testing in, 803f, 804–805, 804f
roughness in, 805f, 806f, 807, 807f, 808f
stiffness in, 800f, 801f, 802f, 803, 803f, 1000
weakness in, 803–806, 803f, 804f, 805f
computed tomography arthrography of, 817
coracoacromial ligament in, 237–238
differential diagnosis of, 817–819, 818f, 819f
edge of, 806f, 807
electromyography in, 1324–1325
failed surgery on, 808, 808t, 877, 879–880, 891–906
acromial stress fracture and, 903
arthroscopic evaluation of, 894
arthroscopic treatment of, 896–897, 897f
deltoid insufficiency and, 903–905, 904f
diagnosis of, 891–893, 892b, 893, 894f
etiology of, 892–893
heterotopic ossification and, 902–903
latissimus dorsi transfer in, 895, 895f
magnetic resonance imaging of, 893, 894f
patient self-assessment of, 809–810, 809f
persistent subacromial impingement and, 893, 897–899
physical examination in, 892, 893
radiography of, 893, 894f
stiffness and, 899–902, 901f
treatment of, 894–897, 895f, 897f
ultrasonography of, 892, 893
vs. frozen shoulder, 817
full-thickness, 808
arthrography of, 813–814, 814f
concentricity loss in, 783, 783f
evaluation of, 839–840
incidence of, 800–802
irreparable, 866–868
smooth and move procedure for, 876–877, 876f, 877f, 878f, 879f, 880f
nonoperative treatment of, 840–841, 840t, 841f
open operative treatment of, 841–851. See also Rotator cuff tear(s), arthroscopic treatment of
approaches to, 844
arthroscopically assisted, 865–866, 867–868
capsule release in, 843, 843f
cost-effectiveness of, 868–869, 869t, 870f
deltoid flap in, 845
failed, 877, 879–880, 879f, 880f
fascia lata graft in, 845
grafts in, 845
indications for, 842–843

Rotator cuff tear(s) (Continued)
in irreparable defects, 866–868, 876–877, 876f, 877f, 878f, 879f
laboratory studies on, 843–844, 843f
latissimus transfer in, 845
Matsen's method of, 869–876, 871f–876f
patient selection for, 869–870
position for, 870
pain control after, 846
patient selection for, 841–843, 842t
porcine small intestine submucosa implant in, 846
results of, 846–851, 848t, 849t, 850f, 850t, 851f, 851t
smooth and move procedure in, 876–877, 876f–880f
subscapular nerve in, 843–844
subscapularis transfer in, 845
synthetic prosthesis in, 845
techniques for, 844–846
ultrasonography after, 848, 850
in overhead throwing athlete, 1042, 1470
patient self-assessment in, 809–810, 809f
in throwing athlete, 1470
ultrasonography of, 815–817, 815f, 816f
vs. ganglion cyst, 819, 819f
gender and, 146
glenohumeral dislocation and, 620f, 672
glenohumeral joint kinematics in, 230, 230f
global fatty degeneration index in, 799
in golfer, 1445–1446
historical perspective on, 619, 620f
iatrogenic, 915–916
magnetic resonance imaging of, 814–815
muscle atrophy with, 1578–1579
occupation and, 802
occupation ratio in, 815
os acromiale and, 776, 903
pain in, 149, 149f
partial-thickness, 799–800, 799f, 808
arthrography of, 813–814, 813f
arthroscopic treatment of, 835–836, 975–976, 976f
evaluation of, 824f, 834f, 835
arthroscopic, 937, 937f
incidence of, 800–802
nonoperative treatment of, 836
operative treatment of, 836–839, 837f, 838f, 839f
in overhead throwing athlete, 1038–1042, 1040f, 1041f, 1450, 1462, 1464–1470, 1466f, 1467f, 1468f, 1469f, 1471f
patient self-assessment in, 809–810, 809f
stiffness in, 834f, 835
subacromial abrasion with, 835
treatment of. See also Rotator cuff tear(s), treatment of
arthroscopic, 835–836, 975–976, 976f
nonoperative, 836
ultrasonography of, 815–817, 815f, 816f
pathogenesis of, 791–799
aging-related changes in, 791–794, 791f, 792f, 793f
biceps tendon length in, 796, 796f
boutonnière deformity in, 797
canine model of, 798
circulatory compromise in, 795, 795f
fiber failure propagation in, 794–796, 794f, 795f, 796f, 797f
glenoid concavity in, 797, 797f, 798f
load concentration in, 793f, 794
muscle atrophy in, 796, 796f
notch phenomenon in, 795f, 796
sheep model of, 798

Rotator cuff tear(s) (*Continued*)
  superior rim loss in, 797, 798f
  synovial fluid exposure in, 795, 795f
  tendon insertion degeneration in, 793f, 794
  unified theory of, 793f–798f, 794–799
 postarthroplasty, 1228
 posterosuperior, retracted, arthroscopic
    treatment of, 1073–1075, 1074f, 1075f
 radiography in, 811–814, 811f, 812f, 813f, 814f
 rehabilitation program (Orthotherapy) for,
    851–865
  home-based, 863–864
  instruction for, 853, 853f
  patient evaluation for, 852–853
  phase I (pain control) of, 853
  phase II (stretching) of, 853–854, 855, 856f,
    857f, 858f
  phase III (strengthening) of, 854, 859f, 860f,
    861f, 862f, 863f, 864f, 865f
  phase IV (maintenance) of, 854
  results of, 854, 859–860
  summary of, 864–865
 vs. snapping scapula, 818
 subacromial effusion with, 154, 154f
 vs. suprascapular neuropathy, 818–819
 tangent sign in, 815
 vs. tendinitis, 817
 treatment of. *See also* Rotator cuff tear(s),
    full-thickness; Rotator cuff tear(s),
    partial-thickness
  acromial stress fracture after, 903
  arthroscopic. *See* Rotator cuff tear(s),
    arthroscopic treatment of
  biological enhancement for, 1577–1579,
    1578t
  crepitus after, 151
  deltoid insufficiency after, 903–905, 904f
  extracellular matrix graft for, 1577–1579,
    1578t
  growth factors in, 1578
  heterotopic ossification after, 902–903
  historical perspective on, 771–774
  infection after, 578
  open. *See* Rotator cuff tear(s), full-thickness,
    open operative treatment of
  outcomes of, 892–893. *See also* Rotator cuff
    tear(s), failed surgery on
  platelet gels in, 1578
  revision. *See* Rotator cuff tear(s), failed
    surgery on
  stiffness after, 899–902, 901f
  supraspinatus outlet narrowing after, 893,
    897–899
 ultrasonography of, 815–817, 815f, 816f
Rotator cuff tear arthropathy, 797, 798f, 808,
    808t, 1112b, 1122–1126, 1126t, 1247–1275.
    See also Rotator cuff tear(s)
 arthrodesis for, 1255f, 1256
 arthroscopic treatment for, 1256
 bipolar arthroplasty for, 1258, 1258f
 classification of, 1249–1254, 1250f, 1251b,
    1253t
  biomechanical, 1251–1252, 1253t
  Burkhart, 1253
  Favard, 1250f, 1252–1253
  Hamada-Fukuda, 1252
  Seebauer, 1253–1254, 1253f
 coracoacromial arch in, 781f, 782
 differential diagnosis of, 1254–1255
 evaluation of, 1102f, 1103, 1255, 1255f
 glenoid defects in, 1251, 1251b, 1251f
 hemiarthroplasty for, 1125–1126, 1160, 1256f,
    1256t, 1257–1258, 1257f
  anesthesia for, 1259

Rotator cuff tear arthropathy (*Continued*)
  bipolar, 1258, 1258f
  care after, 1263
  complications of, 1275
  exposure for, 1259–1261, 1259f
  failed, 1269–1270, 1272f
  greater tuberosity preparation for,
    1261–1262, 1261f, 1262f
  head resection for, 1260f, 1261
  head size for, 1262, 1262f
  implantation for, 1262–1263, 1263f
  indications for, 1259
  positioning for, 1259
  results of, 1269–1270, 1270f, 1271f, 1272f
  Seebauer's approach to, 1259–1263,
    1260f–1263f
  subscapularis reattachment for, 1262–1263,
    1263f
 mechanisms of, 807, 808f, 1122–1125, 1123f,
    1124f, 1125f
 nonoperative treatment of, 1255
 patient self-assessment in, 809–810, 809f
 radiography of, 812, 812f, 1123f, 1251f,
    1253–1254, 1253f, 1254f
 reverse arthroplasty for, 1126, 1258–1259,
    1263–1269
  closure for, 1267
  complications of, 1274–1275
  Ekelund's approach to, 1263–1269,
    1264f–1270f
  exposure for, 1263–1264, 1264f, 1265f
  glenoid component for, 1264–1265, 1265f,
    1266f, 1267f
  historical perspective on, 1247–1249, 1248f,
    1249f
  humerus preparation for, 1265, 1267f
  positioning for, 1263
  rehabilitation after, 1267, 1269
  results of, 1270, 1273–1274, 1273t, 1274
  trial reduction for, 1266–1267, 1268f, 1269f
 rocking horse effect in, 1256
 treatment of, 807–808, 1125–1126, 1255–1275
  arthrodesis in, 1255f, 1256
  arthroplasty in, 1192, 1256–1275. *See also*
    Rotator cuff tear arthropathy,
    hemiarthroplasty for; Rotator cuff tear
    arthropathy, reverse arthroplasty for
  bipolar, 1258, 1258f
  complications of, 1274–1275
  dislocation after, 1274
  historical perspective on, 1247–1249,
    1248f, 1249f
  infection after, 1275
  results of, 1125–1126, 1269–1274, 1270f,
    1271f, 1272f, 1273t
   glenoid notching and, 1273t, 1274
  total, 1126, 1256–1257
 arthroscopic, 1256
 nonoperative, 1255
Rotator cuff tendon(s)
 age-related changes in, 791–793, 791f
 anatomy of, 1283–1284, 1284f
 avulsion of, 799, 799f
 bending load on, 788f, 789–790
 calcium in, 1283–1305. *See also* Calcifying
    tendinitis
  incidence of, 1284–1285
  pain with, 147
  radiography of, 205f, 207
 compressive loads on, 790
 concentric loads on, 789f, 790
 degenerative changes in, 791–799. *See also*
    Rotator cuff tear(s)
 eccentric loads on, 788f, 790

Rotator cuff tendon(s) (*Continued*)
 insertion of, 791, 791f
  bone avulsion at, 799, 799f
  degeneration of, 793f, 794
 rim rents in, 792f, 793, 799–800, 799f
 shearing loads on, 789f, 790, 790f
 strength of, 791, 791f
 vascular anatomy of, 788–789, 1283–1284,
    1284f
Rotator cuff–deficient arthritic shoulder. *See*
    Rotator cuff tear arthropathy
Rotator interval, 26
 arthroscopy of, 927
 in biceps tendon stabilization, 1314–1315,
    1315f
 closure of, 955
 fetal, 11
 lesions of, 1328
 stabilizing properties of, 239
 type I, 1315
 type II, 1315
 variants of, 927
Russell-Silver syndrome, 134

S

Saha position, 149, 149f
Saha procedure, 714
Sarcoma. *See also* Osteosarcoma; Tumor(s)
 Ewing's, 1525–1526, 1527f
  treatment of, 1549–1550
 Paget's disease and, 1527–1528, 1528f
 soft tissue, 1530, 1533
  incidence of, 1530, 1531, 1532f
  staging of, 1513–1515, 1513t
  treatment of, 1550, 1552
Sayre bandage, in clavicular fracture, 413, 414f
Scalenus anterior, 66, 67f
Scalenus medius, 66, 67f
Scapula (scapulae)
 abduction of, 775, 775f
 adduction of, 775, 775f
 anatomy of, 42f, 43–45, 43f, 44f, 45f, 333–334,
    334f
  in children, 604, 605f, 606f
  comparative, 2, 3–4, 3f, 4f, 5f
 assistance test of, 171, 1455
 blood supply to, 45
 center of rotation of, 227f, 228
 clasp-like cranial margin of, 126, 127f
 clavicular osseous bridge to, 128
 computed tomography of, 205f, 207
 development of, 6, 7f, 12, 12f, 604, 604f
 dislocation of
  intrathoracic, 366–367, 367f, 376
  lateral, 364–366, 365b, 366f, 376
   pediatric, 607, 608f, 610, 612
   sternoclavicular dislocation and, 538
 duplication of, 127, 127f
 dyskinesis of, 170–171, 171f, 1452–1453, 1453f
 elevation of, 50, 51f
 evaluation of, 153–154, 170–171, 171f
 fracture of. *See* Scapular fracture
 in glenohumeral joint stability, 639–640, 640f
 in Holt-Oram syndrome, 130–131
 in humeral head motion, 234–235, 236f
 hypoplasia, 132–133
 inferior angle of, avulsion fracture of, 364,
    365f
 inspection of, 153–154
 lateral drooping of, 627, 627f
 notched inferior angle of, 129, 129f
 ossification centers of, 604, 604f
 osteomyelitis of, 567, 567f, 571f

Scapula (scapulae) (Continued)
in overhead throwing, 1448–1449, 1450f
positional measurements of, 171
protraction of, 775, 775f
pseudowinging of, 387f, 388, 409
push-up test of, 170
radiography of, 205f, 206–207
resection of, 1543f, 1544, 1558, 1566–1567, 1566f
reconstruction after, 1547, 1548f
resisted forward elevation test of, 170
resting measurements of, 171
resting position of, 222, 222f, 223f
SICK, 1452–1453, 1453f
snapping, 367–368, 367f, 368f
vs. rotator cuff tear, 818
in spinal accessory nerve injury, 1367
spine of, 43–44
Sprengel's deformity of, 118–122, 119f, 120f, 120t, 121f
stabilization test of, 170–171, 171f
tumors of. See Tumor(s) and specific tumors
winging of
evaluation of, 170–171, 171f, 1362
in facioscapulohumeral dystrophy, 1377, 1377f
after Sprengel's deformity treatment, 122
Scapular assistance test, 171
in athlete, 1455
Scapular dyskinesis, 170–171, 171f, 1452–1453, 1453f
Scapular fracture, 333–376
acromial process, 353, 354f, 360–361, 360f, 363f
treatment of, 369, 370f
anatomy of, 333–334, 334f
associated injuries with, 335–336
avulsion, 354, 361–364, 369
imaging of, 362, 365f
inferior angle, 364, 365f
nonoperative treatment of, 362–363, 364f, 369
operative treatment of, 363–364, 364f, 369
body, 352–353, 352f, 368
classification of, 334–335
clinical features of, 335, 335f
complications of, 335–336
computed tomography of, 336, 338f, 339f
coracoid process, 353–355, 354f, 355f, 359–361, 360f, 362f
treatment of, 369, 369f, 370f
glenoid cavity, 344–352, 344f, 345b
classification of, 344, 345f
fossa, 345, 345f, 346f, 347f, 348–342
treatment of, 374–375, 374f, 375f
type II, 345f, 348, 349f, 374, 374f
type III, 345f, 348, 349f, 350, 374–375
type IV, 345f, 350, 350f, 375
type V, 345f, 350, 351f, 375
type VI, 345f, 350, 352, 375
imaging of, 345, 346f, 347f
operative treatment of, 369–375, 371b, 374f, 375f
approaches to, 370–371, 371f, 372f
fixation techniques for, 372, 373f
management after, 372–373
rim (type I), 345, 345f, 346f, 348, 373–374, 375f
glenoid neck, 336–338, 340–344, 340b, 340f, 361
anatomy of, 337–338, 340f, 341f
computed tomography of, 344, 344f
fragment angulation with, 341, 341f, 343f
mechanisms of, 337–338, 340f, 341f

Scapular fracture (Continued)
nonoperative treatment of, 341–344
operative treatment of, 369–373, 371b, 373f, 375–376
approaches to, 370–371, 371f, 372f
fixation techniques for, 376, 376f
radiography of, 344, 344f
type I, 338, 341f
type II, 338, 340–341, 341f, 342f, 343f
incidence of, 333, 334, 334b, 335f
malunion of, 336
nonunion of, 336
pediatric. See Children, scapular fracture in
radiography of, 335, 335f, 336, 336b, 337f
treatment of, 368–376
for acromial process fracture, 369, 370f
for body fracture, 368
complications of, 336
for coracoid process fracture, 369, 369f, 370f
for glenoid cavity fracture, 373–375, 374f, 375f
for glenoid neck fracture, 369–373, 371b, 371f, 372f, 373f, 374f, 375–376, 376f
Scapular index, 3, 3f
Scapular nerve, 70
Scapular reflex, 174
Scapular retraction test, 1455
Scapular stabilization test, 170–171, 171f
Scapular winging
evaluation of, 170–171, 171f, 1362
in facioscapulohumeral dystrophy, 1377, 1377f
after Sprengel's deformity treatment, 122
Scapulectomy, 1543f, 1544, 1558, 1566–1567, 1566f
reconstruction after, 1547, 1548f
Scapulohumeral muscles. See Deltoid; Infraspinatus; Subscapularis; Supraspinatus; Teres major; Teres minor
Scapulohumeral resection, 1543f, 1544
Scapuloiliac dysostosis, 132–133
Scapulothoracic (forequarter) amputation, 1557, 1561, 1563f, 1564–1565
anterior approach to, 1561, 1563f, 1564
posterior approach to, 1564–1565, 1565f
Scapulothoracic articulation, 38. See also Acromioclavicular joint; Sternoclavicular joint
arthroscopy of, 927–928, 928f
dissociation of, 364–366, 365f, 366f, 376
clavicular fracture and, 399
pediatric, 607, 608f, 610, 612
sternoclavicular dislocation and, 538
motion of, 217–221. See also Glenohumeral joint, biomechanics of
with arm elevation, 224, 225f, 226f, 229f, 230
Scapulothoracic bursitis, 368
Scapulothoracic crepitus, 367–368, 367f, 368f, 376
Scapulothoracic fusion, in long thoracic nerve injury, 1369–1370
Scapulothoracic muscles. See Levator scapulae; Pectoralis minor; Rhomboid(s); Serratus anterior; Subclavius; Trapezius
Scoring systems, in outcome assessment, 269–270
Screw axis, 221, 222f, 228, 228f
Seat-belt fracture, 395, 395f, 407
Sensory testing, 175, 175t
Sepsis, 561–580, 562f, 565f, 1130
age-related aspects of, 562
anatomic aspects of, 562–563, 563f
breast cancer radiation therapy and, 571

Sepsis (Continued)
classification of, 564–565, 564b
clinical presentation of, 570–571, 570f
complications of, 574–575, 574f
differential diagnosis of, 571
foreign bodies and, 565, 566, 568
historical perspective on, 561–562
hyaline cartilage in, 563–564, 564f
imaging in, 572–574, 573f, 574f
immune system disorders and, 561
injection and, 565, 571, 571f
intra-articular, 566–567, 568–569, 568f
laboratory evaluation of, 571–574, 572t
microanatomic aspects of, 563–564, 564f
microbial adhesion and, 568–569, 568f, 569f
osteomyelitis and, 565, 567–568, 567f, 567t, 576f
pathogenesis of, 562, 563f, 565–568, 566f, 567f, 569f
pathogens in, 561, 569–570, 570t
surface attachment of, 568–569, 568f, 569f
surface substrate for, 565–566, 566f
in pectoralis major rupture, 1392
postarthroplasty, 561, 562f, 570, 571
postarthroscopy, 564–565
postoperative, 564, 565f
prevention of, 579
prognosis for, 578–579
pseudoparalysis with, 571
in rheumatoid arthritis, 571
synovial fluid analysis in, 572, 572t
treatment of, 574f, 575–578, 576f, 577t, 579
antibiotics in, 575, 577–578, 577t
drainage in, 579
results of, 578–579
Septic arthritis, 566–567, 567t, 571, 1130. See also Sepsis
synovial fluid examination in, 572, 572t
treatment of, 575–579, 576f, 577t
Serratus anterior
anatomy of, 4–5, 55–57, 56f, 57f
in arm elevation, 254
blood supply of, 56–57
innervation of, 56–57
paralysis of, 56–57
rupture of, 1399–1400
Serratus anterior space, anatomy of, 927–928, 928f
Shock, clavicular fracture and, 401
Short Form-36 questionnaire, 271–272, 274–275
in rotator cuff conditions, 809–810, 809f
Short thoracic arteries, 57
Shoulder. See also Glenohumeral joint
amputation at. See Amputation
anatomy of, 12–15, 13f, 14f, 15f. See also specific components
comparative, 1–5, 2f, 3f, 4f
historical perspective on, 33–38, 34f, 35f, 36f, 37f
arthrodesis of. See Arthrodesis
arthroplasty of. See Arthroplasty
arthroscopy of. See Arthroscopy
development of, 5–11
coracoacromial arch in, 9–10, 11f
embryonic, 6–8, 6f, 7f, 8f, 9f
fetal, 8–11, 10f, 11f
germ layers in, 5–6, 6, 6f, 7f
glenohumeral capsule in, 10–11
glenohumeral ligaments in, 10–11
glenoid in, 11
limb buds in, 6, 6f, 7–8, 8f
postnatal, 11–12, 12f, 13f
dislocation of. See Glenohumeral joint dislocation

Shoulder *(Continued)*
  examination of. *See* Clinical evaluation
  frozen. *See* Stiff shoulder, idiopathic (frozen
    shoulder)
  instability of. *See* Glenohumeral joint
    instability
  motion of. *See* Glenohumeral joint,
    biomechanics of
  replacement of. *See* Arthroplasty
  stability of. *See* Glenohumeral joint,
    biomechanics of
  stiffness of. *See* Stiff shoulder
Shoulder Disability Questionnaire, 273, 274
Shoulder Pain and Disability Index, 272, 274
Shoulder Rating Questionnaire, 273–274
Shoulder suspensory complex, 604, 605f,
  606f
Sibson's fascia, 69
SICK scapula, 1452–1453, 1453f
Simple Shoulder Test, 272–273, 809–810, 809f
Skin, 93–96
  circulation of, 93–94, 94f
  cleavability of, 95
  congenital fossa of, 134, 134f
  cosmetic incision of, 622, 622f
  innervation of, at clavicle, 453–454
  noncosmetic incision of, 622, 622f
  sensation of, 94–95, 95f
  tension lines of, 95–96, 96f
SLAP (superior labrum anterior and posterior)
    lesion
  anatomy of, 1020–1021
  arthroscopic treatment of, 1024–1026
  biomechanics of, 1021
  classification of, 1021–1022, 1021f, 1458–1459,
    1458f
  diagnosis of, 166–169, 167t, 168f, 169f,
    1022–1024, 1024f
  in golfer, 1446
  long head of the biceps in, 246–247
  magnetic resonance imaging in, 1024,
    1024f
  mechanism of, 1022–1023
  physical examination in, 1023
  provocative tests in, 1023
  radiography in, 1024
  throwing-related, 232, 1035, 1037–1038,
    1457–1462
    anatomy in, 1457, 1457f
    arthroscopic treatment of, 1037–1038
    arthroscopy in, 1459–1460
    classification of, 1458–1459, 1458f
    imaging in, 1459, 1460f
    labral débridement in, 1035, 1037
    nonoperative treatment of, 1460
    operative treatment of, 1460–1462, 1461f,
      1462f, 1463f, 1464f, 1465f
    patient history in, 1459
    physical examination in, 1459
  type I, 1021, 1021f, 1458, 1458f
  type II, 232, 1021f, 1022, 1022f, 1458, 1458f,
    1463f
  type III, 1021f, 1022, 1458, 1458f
  type IV, 1021f, 1022, 1458, 1458f
  type IX, 1022, 1023f
  type V, 1022, 1023f
  type VI, 1022, 1023f
  type VII, 1022, 1023f
  type VIII, 1022, 1023f
  type X, 1022, 1023f
Sling, in clavicular fracture, 413, 414f
Snapping scapula, 367–368, 367f, 368f, 818
Social Security Disability Insurance program,
  1505

Somatosensory evoked potentials
  after arthroscopy, 912
  in brachial plexus injury, 1381
Somites, 6, 7f
Sourcil sign, 810f, 811
Spaso reduction, in anterior glenohumeral joint
    dislocation, 680, 680f
Speed's test, 166, 167t, 1332, 1332f
Spinal accessory nerve
  anatomy of, 77, 79f, 1366–1367
  trapezius-related course of, 55, 55f
Spinal accessory nerve injury, 1366–1369
  in athlete, 1481
  diagnosis of, 1367–1368
  etiology of, 1366, 1366f, 1367f
  muscle transfer for, 1368
  nerve transfer for, 1368–1369
  treatment of, 1368–1369, 1368f
Spinal nerves, 69
Spinoglenoid notch, 43
  ganglion cyst of, 1026–1028
    arthroscopic treatment of, 1027–1028
    diagnosis of, 1027, 1027f
    nonoperative treatment of, 1027
    vs. rotator cuff tear, 819, 819f
    in suprascapular nerve entrapment, 1482,
      1482f
  suprascapular nerve injury at, 1081–1083,
    1082f
Sports-related injury. *See* Athlete; Overhead
    throwing
Sprain, sternoclavicular joint, 535, 551
Sprengel's deformity, 41, 118–122, 119f
  concurrent deformities with, 120, 120t
  treatment of, 120–122, 121f
    complications of, 122
    results of, 122
Spur(s)
  acromial, 777, 780f, 781–782, 781f, 1123f
  acromioclavicular, 783–784, 784f
  bicipital groove, 1321, 1323f
  lesser tuberosity, 1321, 1322f
Spurling test, 152, 152f
Stability ratio, 232, 233f, 633–634, 634f, 636f, 637
Standardized response mean, in outcome
    assessment, 271
Staple capsulorrhaphy, 706–707, 709f
  complications of, 716–717, 716f, 717f
Sternalis, 137, 137f
Sternoclavicular joint, 384, 527–559
  abscess of, 551
  anatomy of, 38–40, 39f, 40f
    in children, 595, 595f
    surgical, 527–533, 528f, 529f, 530f, 531f,
      532f, 533f
    variational, 104f, 105
    vascular, 40, 532–533, 532f, 533f
  arthritis of, 535–536, 535f, 536f, 537f
    clavicular fracture–related, 411–412
    postmenopausal, 536, 537f
    treatment of, 549–550, 550f
  arthrotomy of, 551
  biomechanics of, 39–40, 213–214, 214f, 529,
    530f, 531f
    with arm elevation, 216, 217f
  blood supply to, 40
  bone scan of, 199
  capsular ligament of, 529, 530f, 531f
  capsule of, 105
  computed tomography of, 40f, 198–199, 199f,
    541, 542f, 543f
  in congenital syphilis, 537
  costoclavicular ligaments of, 39, 39f, 40, 41f,
    105, 527–529, 529f, 530f

Sternoclavicular joint *(Continued)*
  cross section of, 532f
  depression of, 39–40
  dislocation of. *See* Sternoclavicular joint
    dislocation
  fibrocartilage disk of, 105
  hyperostosis of, 536
  infection of, 536–537, 538f. *See also* Sepsis
    treatment of, 550–551
  injury to, 527–559. *See also* Sternoclavicular
    joint dislocation
    anatomy of, 527–533, 528f–533f
    classification of, 534–537
    clinical manifestations of, 539
    complications of, 557–558, 558f, 559t
    computed tomography in, 541, 542f, 543f
    incidence of, 537–538
    magnetic resonance imaging in, 541, 543f
    mechanism of, 533–534, 534f
    physeal, 547, 549, 549f, 556–557, 557f
    radiography of. *See* Sternoclavicular joint,
      radiography of
    treatment of, 551–559. *See also specific
      injuries*
    type II. *See* Sternoclavicular joint,
      subluxation of
    type III. *See* Sternoclavicular joint
      dislocation
    ultrasonography in, 542
    vascular anatomy in, 532–533, 532f, 533f
  interclavicular ligament of, 39, 39f, 105, 529,
    530f
  ligaments of, 527–529, 529f, 530f
  magnetic resonance imaging of, 199, 200f,
    541, 543f
  motion of, 39–40, 213–214, 214f
  osteoarthritis of, 535–536, 535f, 536f
    treatment of, 549–550, 550f536f
    vs. tumor, 1537, 1537f
  physeal injury of, 547, 549, 549f, 556–557,
    557f
    treatment of, 549, 549f
  radiography of, 197–198, 198f, 539–542
    anteroposterior view for, 539, 540f
    Heinig view for, 540, 541f
    Hobbs view for, 540, 541f
    serendipity view for, 198, 198f, 199f,
      540–541, 542f
  range of motion of, 39–40, 529, 531f
  sprain of, 535, 551
  subluxation of, 551
    anterior, 542–543
    atraumatic, 539, 549
    clinical manifestations of, 539
    posterior, 543–544
    spontaneous, 535, 549, 550f
    treatment of, 542–544, 549
  tomography of, 198–199
  ultrasonography of, 542
  vascular anatomy of, 532–533, 532f, 533f
Sternoclavicular joint dislocation
  acute, 535
  anterior, 499, 534, 534f
    clinical manifestations of, 539
    complications of, 557–558, 558f
    mechanism of, 534, 534f
    spontaneous, 535, 535f, 549
    treatment of, 543, 551, 558, 559t
  atraumatic, 539
  classification of, 534–537, 534f, 535f
  clinical manifestations of, 539
  vs. epiphyseal clavicular fracture, 406
  mechanism of, 533–534, 534f
  posterior, 534, 534f, 542f

Sternoclavicular joint dislocation (*Continued*)
  clinical manifestations of, 539
  closed reduction for, 544, 545f, 546f, 552, 557, 557f
  complications of, 557–558, 558f
  computed tomography of, 528f, 544, 544f
  mechanism of, 534, 534f
  operative treatment of, 544–547, 552–554
    arthrodesis for, 547, 548f
    capsular ligament transfer for, 553, 556f
    care after, 554, 556, 557f
    clavicle exposure for, 552, 553f
    clavicular osteotomy for, 547, 553, 554f, 555f
    clavicular resection for, 547
    complications of, 558, 559t
    fascia lata for, 544
    incision for, 552, 552f
    intra-articular disk ligament in, 552, 553f
    plate fixation for, 547, 548f
    semitendinosus tendon for, 545, 547, 547f
    subclavius tendon for, 544–545
    sutures for, 553, 556f
    spontaneous, 549
  radiography of, 539–542, 540f, 541f, 542f
  recurrent, 535
  scapulothoracic dissociation and, 538
  spontaneous, 535, 535f, 549
Sternoclavicular ligament
  anterior, 39, 39f, 105
  posterior, 39, 105
Sternocleidomastoid muscle, 40–41, 41f, 66, 388
Sternohyoid muscle, 41, 41f, 105
Sternothyroid muscle, 105
Stiff shoulder, 1405–1429
  acquired, 998–1000, 1405, 1406f
    arthrography in, 1414
    after arthroplasty, 999–1000
    arthroscopic treatment of, 999–1000, 1414, 1422–1423
    clinical features of, 1412–1413
    diagnostic criteria for, 1409, 1410
    epidemiology of, 1410
    with failed rotator cuff tear surgery, 899–902, 901f
    after fracture, 327–328, 999
    immobilization and, 1411
    laboratory examination in, 1413
    magnetic resonance imaging in, 1413
    nonshoulder surgery and, 1411
    nuclear imaging in, 1413
    open operative release for, 1420–1421, 1425–1427
    pathomechanics of, 1406–1408, 1407f, 1408f
    physical examination in, 1413
    postarthroplasty, 999–1000
    postarthroscopy, 914
    postoperative, 999–1000, 999f
    after proximal humeral fracture, 327–328
    radiography in, 1413
    rotator cuff disease and, 1000
    after rotator cuff repair, 899–902, 901f
    ultrasonography in, 1414
  calcifying tendinitis and, 1293, 1296
  classification of, 1405, 1406f
  definition of, 1405
  diagnosis of, 1409–1410
  glenohumeral articulation in, 1406–1407, 1406f, 1407f
  humeroscapular motion interface in, 1407–1408, 1407f, 1408f
  idiopathic (frozen shoulder)
    age and, 1410
    arthrography in, 1414

Stiff shoulder (*Continued*)
    cardiac disease and, 1411
    cervical disk disease and, 1411
    clinical features of, 1412
    diabetes mellitus and, 1410–1411
    diagnostic criteria for, 1409–1410
    Dupuytren's contracture and, 1409
    epidemiology of, 1410
    fibroplasia and, 1409
    genetic factors in, 1412
    immobility and, 1411
    immune factors in, 1408–1409
    laboratory examination in, 1413
    magnetic resonance imaging in, 1413
    medication-related, 1412
    natural history of, 1414
    neoplasms and, 1412
    neurologic disorders and, 1411–1412
    nonshoulder surgery and, 1411
    nuclear imaging in, 1413
    personality disorders and, 1412
    physical examination in, 1413
    pulmonary disorders and, 1411
    radiography in, 1413
    vs. rotator cuff tear, 817
    stages of, 1412
    synovitis in, 1420
    thyroid disorders and, 1411
    treatment of, 1414–1423
      acupuncture in, 1418
      arthroscopic capsular release for, 1414, 1422–1423, 1424–1425, 1427f, 1428f
      calcitonin in, 1418
      capsular distention in, 1417
      intra-articular injections in, 1416–1417
      manipulation and arthroscopy in, 1420
      manipulation under anesthesia for, 1418–1420, 1423–1424
      medication in, 1415
      nerve blockade in, 1418
      nonoperative, 1414–1420, 1423
      open operative release for, 1420–1421, 1425–1427
      operative, 1418–1421
      periarticular trigger point injection in, 1417–1418
      physical therapy in, 1415–1416
      radiation therapy in, 1418
      subacromial decompression in, 1425
      subscapularis lengthening in, 1426–1427
    ultrasonography in, 1414
  pathomechanics of, 1406–1408, 1406f, 1407f
  pathophysiology of, 1408–1409
  post-traumatic. *See* Stiff shoulder, acquired
  scapulothoracic mechanics in, 1408
  secondary. *See* Stiff shoulder, acquired
Stimson reduction, in anterior glenohumeral joint dislocation, 680
Stinger (burner) syndrome, 1479–1480
Strength tests, 171–173, 172f, 172t
  in atraumatic recurrent glenohumeral instability, 689, 692f
Strengthening exercises
  in anterior glenohumeral joint dislocation, 682
  in Jackins program, 822–824, 823f, 824f, 825f
  in traumatic recurrent glenohumeral joint instability, 700–701, 700f, 701f, 702f–703f
Stress fracture
  acromion, 903
  clavicular, 396, 396f
Stretching exercises
  in Jackins program, 821f, 822, 822f
  in posterior capsular contracture, 1455–1456, 1456f

Subacromial abrasion, 808, 808t, 819–835
  evaluation of, 807, 807f, 808
  nonoperative treatment of, 820–824, 821f, 822f, 823f, 824f, 825f
  operative treatment of, 824–835
    arthroscopic acromioplasty in, 825–828
      failed, 832–835
      vs. open, 826–827
    care after, 831–832, 832f, 833f
    Matsen's subacromial smoothing procedure in, 827f, 828f, 829–830, 829f
    open acromioplasty in, 824–825
      vs. arthroscopic, 826–827
      failed, 832–835
    subacromial decompression without acromioplasty in, 828
  patient self-assessment in, 809–810, 809f
  radiography of, 811, 811f
Subacromial block, in postoperative pain, 290
Subacromial bursa, 92, 93f, 112
Subacromial bursectomy, 938–939, 938f
Subacromial bursography, 201, 927, 938, 939
Subacromial decompression, arthroscopic
  in glenohumeral joint arthritis, 1006
  in impingement syndrome, 962–964, 963f
  in osteoarthritis, 1006
  in stiff shoulder, 1425
  in subacromial abrasion, 828
  in throwing-related impingement, 1042
Subacromial impingement. *See also* Impingement syndrome; Rotator cuff tear(s)
  in golfer, 1445–1446
  persistent, 893, 897–899
  subacromial injection in, 149, 149f
  in throwing athlete, 1042
Subacromial injection, in subacromial impingement pain, 149, 149f
Subacromial space, bursoscopy of, 201, 927, 938–939
Subclavian artery
  anatomy of, 80–81, 82f, 85f, 86–87, 105f, 106
  aneurysm of, 410, 411f
  brachial plexus relationship to, 70
  clavicle relationship to, 41
  compression of, 410
  injury to
    amputation in, 84–85
    clavicular fracture and, 393, 399–401, 400f, 411f
Subclavian groove, 40, 41f
Subclavian vein
  clavicle relationship to, 41
  clavicular fracture–related injury to, 401, 410
Subclavius
  anatomy of, 57, 58f
  clavicular insertion of, 40, 41f, 57, 388
  innervation of, 70
Subcoracoid decompression, arthroscopic, 981–982, 981f, 982f
Subcoracoid impingement test, 169–170, 170f
Subdeltoid bursa, 92
Subdural block, with interscalene block, 285
Subscapular artery, 26, 82f, 83, 85f
  anomalies of, 84
Subscapular bursa, 22, 25, 25f, 26f
Subscapular nerves, 62, 72–73, 90
Subscapularis
  anatomy of, 4, 62, 63f, 784
  barrier effect of, 245
  blood supply of, 62
  cross-sectional area of, 252t
  evaluation of, 160, 160f, 161f
  excursion of, 785f, 787

Subscapularis (Continued)
  failure of, after recurrent glenohumeral joint
    instability treatment, 718, 719f, 720f
  functions of, 62
  innervation of, 62, 72–73
  lengthening of, in stiff shoulder surgical
    release, 1426–1427
  passive tension of, 245
  rupture of, 957, 1400–1401
  stabilizing function of, 245–246, 246f
  strength testing of, 174
Subscapularis bursa, 92
Subscapularis space, 927–928, 928f
Subscapularis tendon. See also Rotator cuff
    tendon(s)
  anatomy of, 16, 16f, 17f, 925, 926f, 1283,
    1315, 1316f
  arthroscopic evaluation of, 925, 926f, 936,
    936f, 981
  tears of
    arthroscopic treatment of, 980–982, 982f,
      1055–1058, 1057f, 1058f
      coracoplasty in, 981, 981f
      pectoralis minor transfer in, 1059–1060,
        1059f, 1060f
    classification of, 1056–1057, 1056f, 1056t
    pectoralis minor transfer for, 1059–1060,
      1059f, 1060f
Subscapularis-teres-latissimus muscle, 133, 134f
Subscapularis test
  in atraumatic recurrent glenohumeral
    instability, 692f
  in rotator cuff evaluation, 1105 33f
Sulcus
  glenoid, 923, 923f
  intertubercular. See Bicipital groove
Sulcus test, 157, 157f, 930
  in atraumatic recurrent glenohumeral
    instability, 688, 690f
Superior shoulder suspensory complex
  anatomy of, 355, 356f
  double disruption of, 335, 355–359, 356f,
    357b, 357f, 369
    acromial fracture and, 357–358
    coracoid fracture and, 357
    glenoid neck fracture and, 358–359, 358f
    imaging of, 336, 337f
  single disruption of, 357, 357f
Superior thoracic artery, 82f
Supraclavicular nerve
  anatomy of, 77, 79f
  clavicular fracture–related injury to, 411
  entrapment of, 383, 383f
Suprahumeral artery, 26
Suprascapular artery, 26, 26f, 60–61, 82f, 85f,
  296f
Suprascapular ligament
  congenital duplication of, 111, 111f
  ossification of, 111
Suprascapular nerve, 29, 29f, 62, 73–74, 111,
  296f, 1079, 1079f, 1372
Suprascapular nerve block, in stiff shoulder,
  1418
Suprascapular nerve injury, 1372–1374
  arthroscopic treatment of, 1079–1083
    at spinoglenoidal notch, 1081–1083, 1082f
    subacromial approach to, 1082–1083, 1082f
    at suprascapular notch, 1080–1081, 1080f,
      1081f
    transarticular, 1082
  in athlete, 1482, 1482f
  clinical manifestations of, 1373
  diagnosis of, 1373
  etiology of, 1372, 1372f, 1373f

Suprascapular nerve injury (Continued)
  ganglion cyst and, 1372, 1372f, 1373f, 1374
  with interscalene block, 286
  nonoperative treatment of, 1373
  open operative treatment of, 1080, 1373–1374
  with proximal humeral fracture, 297
  vs. rotator cuff tear, 818–819
  at spinoglenoidal notch, 1081–1083, 1082f
  at suprascapular notch, 1080–1081, 1080f
Suprascapular notch, 43
  nerve entrapment in, 74
  suprascapular nerve injury at, 1080–1081,
    1080f
  variational anatomy of, 111, 111f
Supraspinatus
  activity of, 252–254, 254f, 255f
  anatomy of, 59–61, 60f, 61f, 784
    comparative, 4, 5f
  in arm elevation, 252–254, 254f, 255f,
    257–258, 260
  atrophy of, 815
  blood supply of, 60–61, 788–789
  cross-sectional area of, 252t
  evaluation of, 162, 162f, 174
  function of, 60–61, 61f
  inspection of, 153
  magnetic resonance imaging of, 815
  rupture of, 1401
  stabilizing function of, 245–246, 246f
  strength testing of, 174
  tear of, 253
Supraspinatus fossa, suprascapular nerve injury
  at, 1081–1083
Supraspinatus outlet, 44, 60
  narrowing of, in failed rotator cuff tear
    surgery, 893, 897–899
Supraspinatus tendon. See also Rotator cuff
    tendon(s)
  anatomy of, 788–789, 1283–1284, 1284f, 1315,
    1316f
  bending loads on, 788f, 789–790
  calcific deposits in. See Calcifying tendinitis
  compressive loads on, 790–791
  concentric loads on, 789f, 790
  degeneration of, 793f, 794–795, 794f. See also
    Rotator cuff tear(s)
  eccentric loads on, 788f, 790
  insertion of, 788f, 789
  Jobe-Yocum test of, 164, 164f
  shearing loads on, 789f, 790, 790f
  vascular anatomy of, 788–789, 1283–1284,
    1284f
Supraspinatus test
  in atraumatic recurrent glenohumeral
    instability, 692f
  in rotator cuff evaluation, 803f, 805
Supratubercular ridge, 115–116, 116f
  in biceps tendon disorders, 1321, 1322f
Sural nerve graft
  in brachial plexus injury, 1382
  in spinal accessory nerve injury, 1368, 1368f
Surgery. See also specific disorders
  anesthesia for. See Anesthesia
  antibiotics for, 288
  arthroscopic. See Arthroscopy, surgical
  blood loss in, 289
  fusion. See Arthrodesis
  joint replacement. See Arthroplasty
  nonshoulder, stiff shoulder and, 1411
  pain after, 289–291
  positioning for, 288
Swimming. See also Athlete
  after anterior glenohumeral joint dislocation
    treatment, 682

Swimming (Continued)
  impingement in, 1445
  instability in, 1444–1445
  stroke biomechanics in, 1442–1445, 1444f
Synovectomy
  arthroscopic, 1008
  in glenohumeral joint rheumatoid arthritis,
    1131–1133
  in synovial dysplasias, 1522–1523
Synovial chondromatosis, 1008, 1522–1523
Synovial dysplasias, 1522–1523
Synovial fluid analysis, in sepsis, 571, 572, 572t
Synovial recesses, 22, 25–26, 26f
Synovitis
  in stiff shoulder, 1420
  villonodular, pigmented, 1008, 1522
Syphilis, congenital, sternoclavicular joint
    enlargement in, 537

T

Tendinitis
  biceps. See Biceps tendinitis
  calcifying. See Calcifying tendinitis
Tendon(s), 51, 52f. See also specific tendons
  direct insertion of, 51, 52f
  indirect insertion of, 51, 52f
Tendon transfer
  biceps tendon, 1017–1018, 1018f
  latissimus dorsi tendon, 1070–1071
  in long thoracic nerve injury, 1370
  teres major tendon, 1070–1071
Tennis, 1442, 1443f
TENS (transcutaneous nerve stimulation), in stiff
    shoulder, 1415
Tension band fixation, in proximal humeral
    fracture, 317–318, 318f
Tension lines, of skin, 95–96, 96f
Teres major
  anatomy of, 4, 62–63, 64f, 784
  cross-sectional area of, 252t
  function of, 63
  rupture of, 1402
Teres major tendon transfer, arthroscopic,
  1070–1071
Teres minor
  anatomy of, 4, 61–62, 62f
  in arm elevation, 253
  cross-sectional area of, 252t
  evaluation of, 162, 162f
  function of, 61–62
  innervation of, 73
  stabilizing function of, 245–246, 246f
  strength testing of, 174
  tendinous portion of, 16, 16f. See also Rotator
    cuff tendon(s)
Thermal capsulorrhaphy, 954–955
  complications of, 917–918
Thoracic artery
  lateral, 56–57, 82f, 83
  short, 57
  superior, 82f
Thoracic outlet syndrome, 1374–1376
  anomalous bands in, 106f, 107, 107f, 108f
  in athlete, 1483
  clinical manifestations of, 1374, 1374f, 1375f
  diagnosis of, 175–176, 175f, 1376, 1483
  stiff shoulder in, 1412
  treatment of, 1376
Thoracoacromial artery, 26, 27f, 59, 65, 82–83,
  82f
Thoracodorsal artery, 56–57, 82f, 83, 85f
Thoracodorsal nerve, 71, 77, 90
Thromboembolism, after arthroscopy, 914

Thrombosis, effort, 1483
Thrower's shoulder. *See* Overhead throwing, pathologic changes with
Throwing. *See* Overhead throwing
Thurston-Holland fragment, 497, 498f
Thyroid gland disorders, stiff shoulder and, 1411
Tikhoff-Linberg intercalary shoulder resection, 1557–1558, 1565–1566, 1566f
Torque, muscle, 259–260, 259f, 259t
Transcutaneous electrical nerve stimulation, in postamputation pain, 1574
Transmission electron microscopy, 37, 37f
Transverse cervical artery, 82f
Transverse humeral ligament, 16, 16f, 47
  in biceps tendon stabilization, 1315–1316, 1316f
Trapezius
  absence of, 136
  accessory spinal nerve and, 55, 55f
  anatomy of, 4–5, 54–55, 55f, 454
  in arm elevation, 254
  blood supply of, 55
  clavicular insertion of, 40, 41f, 54, 388
  congenital absence of, 54–55
  imbalance of, stiff shoulder and, 1415
  origin of, 54
  paralysis of, 54–55
    scapular depression with, 39
  strength testing of, 174, 174f
Trapezius shrug, in atraumatic recurrent glenohumeral instability, 692f
Trapezoid ligament, 455–456, 455f
  anatomy of, 40, 41f, 103f, 104
  clavicular motion and, 215, 216f
Triceps brachii
  anatomy of, 5, 66, 1395
  cross-sectional area of, 252t
  function of, 66
  rupture of, 1395–1397
    in athlete, 1396
    complications of, 1396
    treatment of, 1396–1397
  strength testing of, 174
Triceps reflex, 175
Trigger point injection, in stiff shoulder, 1417–1418
Trillat procedure, 710
Tuberculosis
  stiff shoulder and, 1411
  vs. tumor, 1537
TUBS acronym, 952. *See also* Glenohumeral joint instability, recurrent, traumatic
Tumor(s), 1509–1552. *See also specific tumors*
  age and, 1531, 1532f
  anatomic factors in, 1510–1512, 1511f
  benign
    cartilaginous, 1518–1520, 1519f, 1520f, 1521f
    osseous, 1515–1517, 1523–1525
      treatment of, 1547–1548
    soft tissue, 1528–1530, 1530f
    spread of, 1512
    staging of, 1512
  biopsy of, 1538–1540, 1539f, 1550

Tumor(s) *(Continued)*
  cartilaginous
    benign, 1518–1520, 1519f, 1520f, 1521f
    malignant, 1520–1523, 1521f
  clinical features of, 1532–1534, 1533f
  complications of, 1536, 1536f
  density of, 1535
  differential diagnosis of, 1536–1538, 1537f, 1537t
  evaluation of, 1534–1535
  historical perspective on, 1509–1510
  incidence of, 1530–1531, 1532f
  laboratory studies in, 1535
  location of, 1533f, 1534
  malignant
    biopsy of, 1538–1540, 1539f, 1550
    cartilaginous, 1520–1523, 1521f
    chemotherapy in, 1551–1552
    chromosomal translocations in, 1515, 1516t
    compartment classification of, 87, 1514
    complications of, 1536, 1536f
    computed tomography in, 1515
    laboratory studies in, 1535
    magnetic resonance imaging in, 1515
    molecular biology of, 1515, 1516t
    osseous, 1517–1518, 1518f
      staging of, 1512t, 1513–1515
      treatment of, 1548–1550
    positron emission tomography in, 1515, 1516f
    radiography in, 1515, 1516f
    resection of, 1540–1552
      axillary nerve in, 1512
      follow-up after, 1534
      glenohumeral, 1543f, 1544
      limb-salvage with, 1541–1544, 1543f, 1552
      long, 1543–1544, 1543f
      margin in, 1540–1551, 1540t, 1541f, 1542t
      reconstruction after, 1544–1547, 1545f, 1546f, 1548f
      scapular, 1543f, 1544
      scapulohumeral, 1543f, 1544
      short, 1542–1543, 1543f
    soft tissue, 1530, 1531f
      staging of, 1513–1515, 1513t
      treatment of, 1550
    staging of, 1512t, 1513–1515, 1513t, 1535
  metastatic, 1130, 1131f, 1530, 1536, 1536f
    treatment of, 1550
  molecular biology of, 1515, 1516t
  osseous
    benign, 1515–1517, 1523–1525
      treatment of, 1547–1548
    malignant, 1517–1518, 1518f
      staging of, 1512t, 1513–1515
      treatment of, 1548–1550
  pain with, 1532, 1533
  physical examination in, 1533, 1534
  radiography of, 1515, 1516f, 1534–1535
  reticuloendothelial, 1525–1526, 1526f, 1527f
  soft tissue
    benign, 1528–1530, 1530f
    malignant, 1530, 1531f
      staging of, 1513–1515, 1513t
      treatment of, 1550

U
UCLA Shoulder Scale, 273
Ulnar nerve, 72
  injury to, triceps rupture and, 1396
  transfer of, in musculocutaneous nerve injury, 1363
Ultrasonography
  of acromioclavicular joint, 474
  of biceps tendon, 1012–1013, 1012f, 1336, 1337f
  in birth-related clavicular fracture, 403
  in calcifying tendinitis, 1295, 1295f
  in interscalene block, 282, 282f, 283, 283f
  of rotator cuff, 201–203, 815–817, 815f, 816f
  in sepsis, 573–574
  of sternoclavicular joint, 542
  in stiff shoulder, 1414
University of Pennsylvania Shoulder Score, 273

V
Validity, of outcome assessment instrument, 270–271
Vanishing epiphysis sign, 587
Vascular examination, 175–176, 175f
Vasovagal episode, after interscalene block, 285
Veins, 85–86. *See also specific veins*
  oscillating, 54
Ventral bar, 1, 2f
Vertebral artery, 81
  anesthetic injection into, 285
Vesalius, A., 35f, 36, 36f
Vimentin, in Dupuytren's contracture, 1409
Viral infection, vs. bacterial sepsis, 571–572

W
Weakness
  as chief complaint, 147
  evaluation of, 151
  in rotator cuff tear evaluation, 803–806, 803f, 804f, 805f
Weaver-Dunn procedure, in type III acromioclavicular joint injury, 487, 488–489
Western Ontario Rotator Cuff Index, 269, 274
Western Ontario Shoulder Instability Index (WOSI), 269
Woodward procedure, 121, 121f
Worker's compensation, 1504–1505
Wright's test, 176
  in thoracic outlet syndrome, 1376, 1483

X
Xenograft, in failed rotator cuff tear surgery repair, 895

Y
Yergason's test, 166, 167f, 1332, 1333f